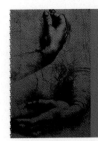

Rehabilitation of the Hand and Upper Extremity

Terri M. Skirven, OTR/L, CHT

Director, Hand Therapy, The Philadelphia and
South Jersey Hand Centers, P.C.
Director, Hand Rehabilitation Foundation
Philadelphia, PA

A. Lee Osterman, MD

Professor, Orthopaedic and Hand Surgery
Chairman, Division of Hand Surgery
Department of Orthopaedic Surgery
Jefferson Medical College
Thomas Jefferson University;
President, The Philadelphia and South Jersey Hand Centers, P.C.
and Hand Surgery Fellowship Program
Philadelphia, PA

Jane M. Fedorczyk, PT, PhD, CHT, ATC

Associate Clinical Professor
Director, Post-Professional Clinical Programs
Department of Physical Therapy and Rehabilitation Sciences
College of Nursing and Health Professions
Drexel University
Philadelphia, PA

Peter C. Amadio, MD

Lloyd A. and Barbara A. Amundson
Professor of Orthopedic Surgery
Mayo Clinic
Rochester, MN

Rehabilitation of the Hand and Upper Extremity

SIXTH EDITION

ELSEVIER
MOSBY

ELSEVIER
MOSBY

1600 John F. Kennedy Blvd.
Ste. 1800
Philadelphia, PA 19103-2899

REHABILITATION OF THE HAND AND UPPER EXTREMITY,
SIXTH EDITION

ISBN: 978-0-323-05602-1

Notices

Knowledge and best practice in this field are constantly changing. As new research and experience
broaden our understanding, changes in research methods, professional practices, or medical treatment
may become necessary.

Practitioners and researchers must always rely on their own experience and knowledge in evaluating
and using any information, methods, compounds, or experiments described herein. In using such
information or methods they should be mindful of their own safety and the safety of others, including
parties for whom they have a professional responsibility.

With respect to any drug or pharmaceutical products identified, readers are advised to check the
most current information provided (i) on procedures featured or (ii) by the manufacturer of each
product to be administered, to verify the recommended dose or formula, the method and duration of
administration, and contraindications. It is the responsibility of practitioners, relying on their own
experience and knowledge of their patients, to make diagnoses, to determine dosages and the best
treatment for each individual patient, and to take all appropriate safety precautions.

To the fullest extent of the law, neither the Publisher nor the authors, contributors, or editors,
assume any liability for any injury and/or damage to persons or property as a matter of products
liability, negligence or otherwise, or from any use or operation of any methods, products, instructions,
or ideas contained in the material herein.

Previous editions copyrighted 1978, 1984, 1990, 1995, 2002

Library of Congress Cataloging-in-Publication Data

Rehabilitation of the hand and upper extremity.—6th ed. / [edited by]
Terri M. Skirven ... [et al.].
    p. ; cm.
  Includes bibliographical references and index.
  ISBN 978-0-323-05602-1
 1. Hand–Wounds and injuries. 2. Hand–Surgery. 3. Hand–Surgery–Patients–
Rehabilitation. I. Skirven, Terri M.
  [DNLM: 1. Hand–Surgery. 2. Arm Injures–rehabilitation. 3. Hand Injuries–
rehabilitation. 4. Shoulder Joint–injuries. WE 830 R345 2010]
  RD559.R43 2010
  617.5'75059—dc22

                                        2009044037

Acquisitions Editor: Dan Pepper
Developmental Editor: Lucia Gunzel
Publishing Services Manager: Pat Joiner-Myers
Design Direction: Steven Stave

Printed in Canada

Last digit is the print number: 9 8 7 6 5

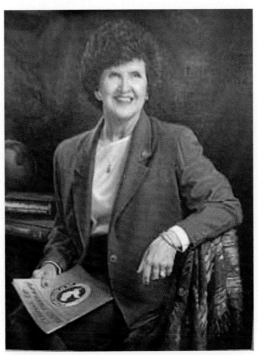

Evelyn J. Mackin, PT

LEADER   EDUCATOR   MENTOR   FRIEND

It is with great pride and gratitude that we dedicate this sixth edition of *Rehabilitation of the Hand and Upper Extremity* to Evelyn J. Mackin, PT. Evelyn's vision, commitment, and determination elevated Hand Rehabilitation to a specialty practice recognized for excellence. Countless therapists and surgeons have been inspired to emulate the team approach to the care of the hand-injured patient modeled by Evelyn and her Hand Surgery colleagues James Hunter, MD, and Lawrence Schneider, MD. This partnership gave rise to groundbreaking contributions, including the world-renown annual Philadelphia symposium *Surgery and Rehabilitation of the Hand*, which has been held annually for over 35 years. Evelyn was one of the founders and past presidents of the American Society of Hand Therapists; the first president of the International Federation of Societies for Hand Therapy; and founding editor of the *Journal of Hand Therapy*, a peer-reviewed scientific journal. With the first edition of this text in 1976, Evelyn, along with her co-editors, lit a flame that has burned brightly and steadily ever since. It is our intention with this sixth edition to honor Evelyn and to keep the flame burning.

SIXTH EDITION EDITORS

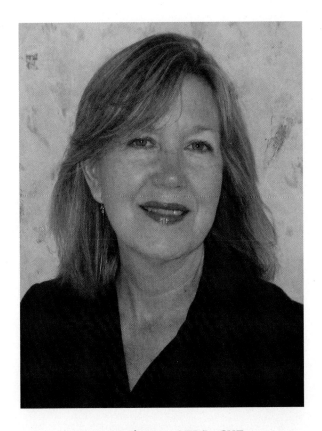

Terri M. Skirven, OTR/L, CHT
Editions 5, 6

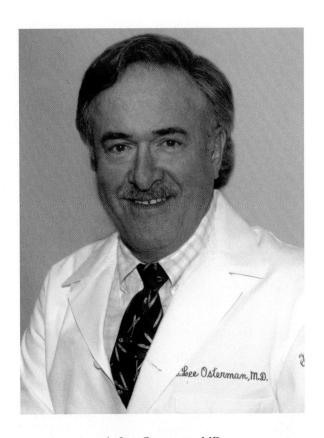

A. Lee Osterman, MD
Editions 5, 6

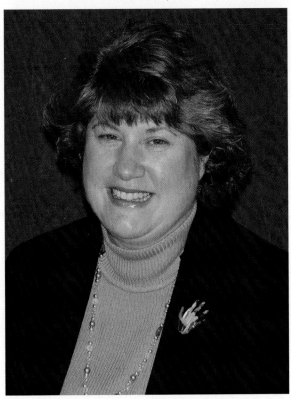

Jane M. Fedorczyk, PT, PhD, CHT, ATC
Edition 6

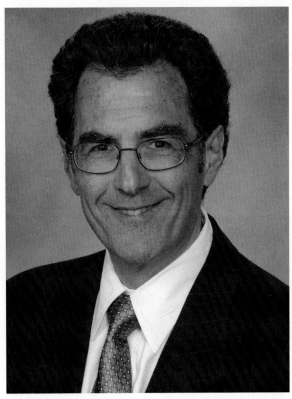

Peter C. Amadio, MD
Edition 6

CONTRIBUTORS

Joshua Abzug, MD
Fellow, Hand Surgery
Thomas Jefferson University Hospital
The Philadelphia and South Jersey Hand Centers, P.C.
Philadelphia, Pennsylvania

Julie E. Adams, MD
Assistant Professor
Orthopaedic Surgery
University of Minnesota
Minneapolis, Minnesota

Steven Alter, MD
Orthopedic Hand Surgeon
Orthopedic Surgical Associates
Lowell, Massachusetts

Emily Altman, PT, DPT, CHT
Senior Physical Therapist
Hand Therapy Center
Hospital for Special Surgery
New York, New York

Peter C. Amadio, MD
Lloyd A. and Barbara A. Amundson Professor of Orthopedic
    Surgery
Mayo Clinic
Rochester, Minnesota

Thomas J. Armstrong, BSE, MPH, PhD
Professor, Industrial and Operations Engineering and
    Biomedical Engineering
The University of Michigan
Ann Arbor, Michigan

Sandra M. Artzberger, MS, OTR, CHT
Certified Hand Therapist
Rocky Mountain Physical Therapy and Sports Injury Center
Pagosa Springs, Colorado

Sarah Ashworth, OTR/L
Shriners Hospital for Children
Philadelphia, Pennsylvania

Pat L. Aulicino, MD
Sentara Hand Surgery Specialists
Chesapeake, Virginia

Alejandro Badia, MD, FACS
Badia Hand to Shoulder Center
Doral, Florida

Mark E. Baratz, MD
Professor and Executive Vice Chairman
Director, Division of Upper Extremity Surgery
Program Director, Orthopedic Residency and Upper
    Extremity Fellowship
Department of Orthopedics
Drexel University for the Health Sciences
Allegheny General Hospital
Pittsburgh, Pennsylvania

Mary Barbe, PhD
Professor of Anatomy and Cell Biology
Temple University School of Medicine
Philadelphia, Pennsylvania

Ann E. Barr, DPT, PhD
Vice Provost and Executive Dean
College of Health Professionals
Pacific University
Hillsboro, Oregon

Mary Bathen, BS
Medical Student
University of California, San Diego, School of Medicine
La Jolla, California

Jeanine Beasley, EdD, OTR, CHT
Assistant Professor
Grand Valley State University;
Hand Therapist
Cherry Street Hand Therapy
Advent Health;
Hand Therapist
East Paris Hand Therapy
Mary Free Bed Rehabilitation Hospital
Grand Rapids, Michigan

John M. Bednar, MD
Clinical Associate Professor of Orthopaedic Surgery
Thomas Jefferson Medical College
The Philadelphia and South Jersey Hand Centers, P.C.
Philadelphia, Pennsylvania

Judith A. Bell Krotoski, MA, OTR/L, CHT, FAOTA
CAPTAIN, United States Public Health Service (retired);
Guest Lecturer/Instructor
Texas Women's University
Houston, Texas;
Private Research, Teaching, and Consulting
Hand Therapy Research
Baton Rouge, Louisiana

Mark R. Belsky, MD
Clinical Professor
Tufts University School of Medicine
Boston, Massachusetts;
Chief, Orthopaedic Surgery
Newton-Wellesley Hospital
Newton, Massachusetts

Pedro K. Beredjiklian, MD
Associate Professor of Orthopaedic Surgery
Thomas Jefferson School of Medicine;
Chief, Hand Surgery Division
The Rothman Institute
Philadelphia, Pennsylvania

Richard A. Berger, MD, PhD
Professor of Orthopaedic Surgery and Anatomy
Dean, Mayo School of Continuous Professional Development
College of Medicine
Mayo Clinic;
Consultant, Orthopedic Surgery;
Chair, Division of Hand Surgery
Mayo Clinic
Rochester, Minnesota

Thomas H. Bertini, Jr., DPT, ATC
Department of Physical Therapy & Rehabilitation Sciences
Drexel University
Philadelphia, Pennsylvania

Sam J. Biafora, MD
Fellow
Thomas Jefferson University
The Philadelphia Hand Center
Philadelphia, Pennsylvania

Teri M. Bielefeld, PT, CHT
PT Clinical Specialist
Outpatient Clinic
Zablocki Veterans Affairs Medical Center
Milwaukee, Wisconsin

Susan M. Blackmore, MS, OTR/L, CHT
Assistant Director of Hand Therapy
The Philadelphia Hand Center
King of Prussia, Pennsylvania

Salvador L. Bondoc, OTD, OTR/L, CHT
Associate Professor of Occupational Therapy
Quinnipiac University
Hamden, Connecticut

Michael J. Botte, MD
Clinical Professor
University of California, San Diego;
Attending Surgeon
VA San Diego Healthcare System
San Diego, California;
Co-Director, Hand and Microvascular Surgery
Scripps Clinic
La Jolla, California

David J. Bozentka, MD
Chief of Orthopedic Surgery
Penn Presbyterian Medical Center
University of Pennsylvania School of Medicine
Philadelphia, Pennsylvania

Zach Broyer, MD
Thomas Jefferson University Medical School
Philadelphia, Pennsylvania

Donna Breger-Stanton, MA, OTR/L, CHT, FAOTA
Associate Professor
Academic Fieldwork Coordinator
Samuel Merritt University
Oakland, California

Anne M. Bryden, OTR/L
The Cleveland FES Center
Cleveland, Ohio

**Katherine Butler, B Ap Sc (OT) AHT (BAHT)
  A Mus A (flute)**
Clinical Specialist in Hand Therapy
London Hand Therapy
London, Great Britain

Nancy N. Byl, MPH, PhD, PT, FAPTA
Professor Emeritus
University of California, San Francisco, School of
  Medicine
Department of Physical Therapy and Rehabilitation
  Science;
Clinical Professor
San Francisco State University
Physical Therapy Program;
Physical Therapist
Physical Therapy Health and Wellness Program
University of California, San Francisco, Faculty Practice
San Francisco, California

Nancy Cannon, OTR, CHT
Director
Indiana Hand to Shoulder Center
Indianapolis, Indiana

Roy Cardoso, MD
Assistant Professor of Clinical Orthopaedics
University of Miami Leonard Miller School Medicine;
Orthopaedic Surgeon
Bascom Palmer Eye Hospital
Miami, Florida

James Chang, MD
Professor and Chief of Plastic and Reconstructive Surgery
Stanford University
Stanford, California

Nancy Chee, OTR/L, CHT
Adjunct Assistant Professor
Samuel Merritt University
Oakland, California;
Hand Therapist
California Pacific Medical Center
San Francisco, California

Jill Clemente, MS
Research Coordinator
Department of Orthopaedics
Allegheny General Hospital
Pittsburgh, Pennsylvania

Mark S. Cohen, MD
Professor and Director, Hand and Elbow Section;
Director, Orthopaedic Education
Department of Orthopaedic Surgery
Rush University Medical Center
Chicago, Illinois

Judy C. Colditz, OTR/L, CHT, FAOTA
HandLab
Raleigh, North Carolina

Ruth A. Coopee, MOT, OTR/L, CHT, MLD, CDT, CMT
Hand Therapist
Lymphedema Therapist
Largo Medical Center
Largo, Florida

Cynthia Cooper, MFA, MA, OTR/L, CHT
Clinical Specialist in Hand Therapy
Faculty, Physical Therapy Orthopedic Residency Program
Scottsdale Healthcare
Scottsdale, Arizona

Randall W. Culp, MD, FACS
Professor of Orthopaedic, Hand and Microsurgery
Thomas Jefferson University Hospital
Philadelphia, Pennsylvania;
Physician
The Philadelphia and South Jersey Hand Centers, P.C.
King of Prussia, Pennsylvania

Leonard L. D'Addesi, MD
The Reading Hospital and Medical Center
Reading, Pennsylvania

Phani K. Dantuluri, MD
Assistant Clinical Professor
Department of Orthopaedics
Emory University Midtown Hospital
Atlanta Medical Center
Resurgens Orthopaedics
Atlanta, Georgia

Sylvia A. Dávila, PT, CHT
Hand Rehabilitation Associates of San Antonio, Inc.
San Antonio, Texas

Paul C. Dell, MD
Chief of the Hand Surgery Division
Department of Orthopaedics
University of Florida Orthopaedics and Sports Medicine
Gainesville, Florida

Ruth B. Dell, MHS, OTR, CHT
Chief of the Hand Therapy Division
Department of Orthopaedics
University of Florida Orthopaedics and Sports Medicine
Gainesville, Florida

Lauren M. DeTullio, MS, OTR/L, CHT
Assistant Director
The Philadelphia and South Jersey Hand Centers, P.C.
Philadelphia, Pennsylvania

Cecelia A. Devine, OTR, CHT
Adjunct Instructor
Department of Occupational Therapy
Mount Mary College;
Clinical Coordinator, Hand Therapy
Froedtert Hospital
Milwaukee, Wisconsin

Madhuri Dholakia, MD
Thomas Jefferson University Medical School
The Rothman Institute
Philadelphia, Pennsylvania

Edward Diao, MD
Professor Emeritus
Departments of Orthopaedic Surgery and Neurosurgery;
Former Chief
Division of Hand, Upper Extremity, and Microvascular Surgery
University of California, San Francisco
San Francisco, California

Annie Didierjean-Pillet, Psychoanalyst
Strasbourg, France

Susan V. Duff, EdD, PT, OTR/L, CHT
Associate Professor
Department of Physical and Occupational Therapy
Thomas Jefferson University;
Clinical Specialist, Occupational Therapy
Children's Hospital of Philadelphia
Philadelphia, Pennsylvania

Matthew D. Eichenbaum, MD
Chief Resident in Orthopaedic Surgery
Thomas Jefferson University Hospital
Philadelphia, Pennsylvania

Bassem T. Elhassan, MD
Assistant Professor of Orthopedics
Mayo Clinic
Rochester, Minnesota

Melanie Elliott, PhD
Instructor of Neurosurgery
Thomas Jefferson University
Philadelphia, Pennsylvania

Timothy Estilow, OTR/L
Occupational Therapist
Children's Hospital of Philadelphia
Philadelphia, Pennsylvania

Roslyn B. Evans, OTR/L, CHT
Director/Owner
Indian River Hand and Upper Extremity Rehabilitation
Vero Beach, Florida

Marybeth Ezaki, MD
Professor of Orthopaedic Surgery
University of Texas Southwestern Medical School;
Director of Hand Surgery
Texas Scottish Rite Hospital for Children
Dallas, Texas

Frank Fedorczyk, PT, DPT, OCS
Physical Therapist
Yardley, Pennsylvania

Jane M. Fedorczyk, PT, PhD, CHT, ATC
Associate Clinical Professor
Director, Post-Professional Clinical Programs
Department of Physical Therapy & Rehabilitation Sciences
College of Nursing and Health Professions
Drexel University
Philadelphia, Pennsylvania

Lynne M. Feehan, BScPT, MSc(PT), PhD, CHT
Postdoctoral Fellow
Michael Smith Foundation for Health Research
Department of Physical Therapy
University of British Columbia
Vancouver, British Columbia, Canada

Paul Feldon, MD
Associate Professor of Orthopaedic Surgery
Tufts University School of Medicine
Boston, Massachusetts

Sheri B. Feldscher, OTR/L, CHT
Senior Hand Therapist
The Philadelphia and South Jersey Hand Centers, P.C.
Philadelphia, Pennsylvania

Elaine Ewing Fess, MS, OTR, FAOTA, CHT
Adjunct Assistant Professor
School of Allied Health and Rehabilitation
Indiana University
Indianapolis, Indiana

Lynn Festa, OTR, CHT
Certified Hand Therapist
Crouse Hospital
Syracuse, New York

Mitchell K. Freedman, DO
Clinical Assistant Professor
Thomas Jefferson University Medical School;
Director of Physical Medicine and Rehabilitation
The Rothman Institute
Philadelphia, Pennsylvania

Alan E. Freeland, MD
Professor Emeritus
University of Mississippi Medical Center
Jackson, Mississippi

Mary Lou Galantino, PT, PhD, MSCE
Professor
Richard Stockton College of New Jersey
Pomona, New Jersey;
Adjunct Research Scholar
University of Pennsylvania
Philadelphia, Pennsylvania;
Clinician
PT Plus Christiana Care
Wilmington, Delaware

Kara Gaffney Gallagher, MS, OTR/L, CHT
Occupational Therapist/Hand Therapist
King of Prussia Physical Therapy and Sports Injury Center
King of Prussia, Pennsylvania

George D. Gantsoudes, MD
Assistant Professor
Riley Hospital for Children
Indianapolis, Indiana

Marc Garcia-Elias, MD, PhD
Consultant, Hand Surgery
Institut Kaplan
Barcelona, Spain

Bryce W. Gaunt, PT, SCS, CSCS
Director of Physical Therapy
HPRC at St. Francis Rehabilitation Center
Columbus, Georgia

Charles L. Getz, MD
Assistant Professor
Department of Orthopaedic Surgery
Thomas Jefferson Medical School;
The Rothman Institute
Philadelphia, Pennsylvania

Thomas J. Graham, MD
Chief, Cleveland Clinic Innovations
Vice Chair, Orthopaedic Surgery
Cleveland Clinic
Cleveland, Ohio

Rhett Griggs, MD
Alpine Orthopaedics, Sports Performance & Regional Hand
  Center
Gunnison, Colorado

Brad K. Grunert, PhD
Professor, Plastic Surgery;
Professor, Psychiatry and Behavioral Medicine
Medical College of Wisconsin
Milwaukee, Wisconsin

Ranjan Gupta, MD
Professor and Chair
Orthopaedic Surgery
University of California, Irvine;
Principal Investigator
University of California, Irvine;
Peripheral Nerve Research Laboratory
Irvine, California

Maureen A. Hardy, PT, MS, CHT
Director
Rehabilitation Services and Hand Management Center
St. Dominic Hospital
Jackson, Mississippi

Michael Hausman, MD
Robert K. Lippmann Professor of Orthopedic Surgery
Mount Sinai School of Medicine;
Vice Chairman
Department of Orthopedic Surgery;
Chief, Hand and Elbow Surgery
Mount Sinai Medical Center
New York, New York

David Hay, MD
Chief Resident
Stanford University Hospital and Clinics
Standford, California

Eduardo Hernandez-Gonzalez, MD
Private Practice
Miami, Florida

Heather Hettrick, PhD, PT, CWS, FACCWS, MLT
Assistant Clinical Professor
Drexel University
Philadelphia, Pennsylvania
Vice President, Academic Affairs and Education
American Medical Technologies
Irvine, California

Alan S. Hilibrand, MD
Professor of Orthopaedic Surgery
Professor of Neurology
Thomas Jefferson University Medical School;
The Rothman Institute
Philadelphia, Pennsylvania

Leslie K. Holcombe, MScOT, CHT
Consultant
Pillet Hand Prostheses, Ltd.
New York, New York

Harry Hoyen, MD
Assistant Professor
Department of Orthopaedic Surgery
Case Western Reserve University Medical School
Cleveland, Ohio

Deborah Humpl, OTR/L
Children's Hospital of Philadelphia
Philadelphia, Pennsylvania

Larry Hurst, MD
Professor and Chairman
Department of Orthopaedics
SUNY Stony Brook
Stony Brook, New York

Asif M. Ilyas, MD
Assistant Professor of Orthopaedic Surgery
Thomas Jefferson University;
The Rothman Institute
Philadelphia, Pennsylvania

Dennis W. Ivill, MD
Clinical Assistant Professor
Thomas Jefferson University Medical School;
Staff Psychiatrist
The Rothman Institute
Philadelphia, Pennsylvania

Sidney M. Jacoby, MD
Assistant Professor
Department of Orthopaedic Surgery
Jefferson Medical College
Thomas Jefferson University;
The Philadelphia and South Jersey Hand Centers, P.C.
Philadelphia, Pennsylvania

Neil F. Jones, MD, FRCS
Professor of Orthopedic Surgery
Professor of Plastic and Reconstructive Surgery
Chief of Hand Surgery
University of California, Irvine
Irvine, California;
Consulting Hand Surgeon
Shriners Hospital
Los Angeles, California;
Consulting Hand Surgeon
Children's Hospital of Orange County
Orange, California

Lana Kang, MD
Assistant Professor
Weil Cornell Medical College of Cornell University;
Attending Orthopaedic Surgeon
Hospital for Special Surgery;
Attending Orthopaedic Surgeon
New York–Presbyterian Hospital of Cornell University
New York, New York

Parivash Kashani, OTR/L
Hand Therapist
University of California, Los Angeles
Los Angeles, California

Leonid Katolik, MD
Attending Surgeon
The Philadelphia and South Jersey Hand Centers, P.C.
Assistant Professor
Thomas Jefferson University School of Medicine
Philadelphia, Pennsylvania

Michael W. Keith, MD
Professor
Case Western Reserve University;
Orthopedic Surgeon
MetroHealth Medical Center;
Principle Investigator
Case Western Reserve University
Cleveland, Ohio

Martin J. Kelley, PT, DPT, OCS
Good Shepherd Penn Partners
Penn Presbyterian Medical Center
Philadelphia, Pennsylvania

David M. Kietrys, PT, PhD, OCS
Associate Professor
University of Medicine and Dentistry of New Jersey
Stratford, New Jersey

Yasuko O. Kinoshita, ORT/L, CHT
La Jolla, California

Diana L. Kivirahk, OTR/L, CHT
Scripps Clinic Division of Orthopaedic Surgery
La Jolla, California

Zinon T. Kokkalis, MD
Consultant
First Department of Orthopaedic Surgery "Attikon" University
    General Hospital
University of Athens School of Medicine
Athens, Greece

L. Andrew Koman, MD
Professor and Chair
Department of Orthopaedic Surgery
Wake Forest University School of Medicine
Winston-Salem, North Carolina

Scott H. Kozin, MD
Professor
Department of Orthopeadic Surgery
Temple University;
Hand Surgeon
Shriners Hospital for Children
Philadelphia, Pennsylvania

Leo Kroonen, MD
Assistant Director of Hand Surgery
Naval Medical Center
San Diego, California

Tessa J. Laidig, DPT
Department of Physical Therapy & Rehabilitation Sciences
Drexel University
Philadelphia, Pennsylvania

Amy Lake, OTR, CHT
Texas Scottish Rite Hospital for Children
Dallas, Texas

Paul LaStayo, PhD, PT, CHT
Department of Physical Therapy
Department of Orthopaedics
Department of Exercise and Sport Science
University of Utah
Salt Lake City, Utah

Mark Lazarus, MD
Rothman Institute
Philadelphia, PA

Marilyn P. Lee, MS, OTR/L, CHT
Supervisor, Hand and Upper Extremity Rehabilitation
Crozer Keystone Health System, Springfield Division
Springfield, Pennsylvania

Michael Lee, PT, DPT, CHT
Clinical Director
Maximum Impact Physical Therapy
Tucson, Arizona

Brian G. Leggin, PT, DPT, OCS
Team Leader
Penn Presbyterian Medical Center
Philadelphia, Pennsylvania

Matthew Leibman, MD
Assistant Clinical Professor
Orthopaedic Surgery
Tufts University School of Medicine
Boston, Massachusetts;
Newton-Wellesley Hospital
Newton, Massachusetts

L. Scott Levin, MD, FACS
Professor and Chairman
Department of Orthopaedic Surgery
Professor, Plastic Surgery
Hospital of the University of Pennsylvania
Philadelphia, Pennsylvania

Zhongyu Li, MD, PhD
Assistant Professor
Department of Orthopaedic Surgery
Wake Forest University School of Medicine
Winston-Salem, North Carolina

Chris Lincoski, MD
Hand Surgery Fellow
Thomas Jefferson University Hospital
Philadelphia, Pennsylvania

Kevin J. Little, MD
Assistant Professor
Department of Orthopaedic Surgery
University of Cincinnati School of Medicine;
Cincinnati Children's Hospital Medical Center
Cincinnati, Ohio

Frank Lopez, MD, MPH
Assistant Professor
University of Pennsylvania
Philadelphia, Pennsylvania

John Lubahn, MD
Orthopaedic Residency Program Director
Hamot Medical Center
Erie, Pennsylvania

Göran Lundborg, MD, PhD
Professor
Lund University;
Senior Consultant
Department of Hand Surgery
Skåne University Hospital
Malmö, Sweden

Joy C. MacDermid, BScPT, PhD
Assistant Dean, Rehabilitation Science
Professor, Rehabilitation Science
McMaster University School of Rehabilitation Science
Hamilton, Ontario, Canada;
Co-Director of Clinical Research
Hand and Upper Limb Center
London, Ontario, Canada

Glenn A. Mackin, MD, FRAN, FACP
Associate Professor of Clinical Neurology
Pennsylvania State University/Milton S. Hershey Medical
    Center
Hershey, Pennsylvania;
Director and Staff Neurologist
Neuromuscular Diseases Center and ALS Clinic
Lehigh Valley Health Network
Allentown, Pennsylvania

Leonard C. Macrina, MSPT, SCS, CSCS
Sports Certified Physical Therapist
Certified Strength and Conditioning Specialist
Champion Sports Medicine
Birmingham, Alabama

Kevin J. Malone, MD
Assistant Professor
Department of Orthopaedic Surgery
Case Western Reserve University
MetroHealth Medical Center
Cleveland, Ohio

Gregg G. Martyak, MD
Orthopedic Surgery, Hand and Upper Extremity
San Antonio Military Medical Center
Fort Sam Houston, Texas

John A. McAuliffe, MD
Hand Surgeon
Broward Health Orthopaedics
Fort Lauderdale, Florida

Philip McClure, PT, PhD, FAPTA
Professor
Arcadia University
Glenside, Pennsylvania

Pat McKee, MSc, OT Reg (Ont), OT(C)
Associate Professor
Department of Occupational Science and Occupational
    Therapy
Faculty of Medicine
University of Toronto
Toronto, Ontario, Canada

Kenneth R. Means, Jr., MD
Attending Hand Surgeon
The Curtis National Hand Center
Union Memorial Hospital
Baltimore, Maryland

Robert J. Medoff, MD
Assistant Clinical Professor
University of Hawaii John A Burns School of Medicine
Honolulu, Hawaii

Jeanne L. Melvin, MS, OTR, FAOTA
Owner
Solutions for Wellness
Private Practice
Santa Monica, California

R. Scott Meyer, MD
Section Chief, Orthopaedic Surgery
VA San Diego Healthcare System;
Associate Clinical Professor
Department of Orthopaedic Surgery
University of California at San Diego
San Diego, California

Susan Michlovitz, PT, PhD, CHT
Adjunct Associate Professor
Rehabilitation Medicine
Columbia University
New York, New York;
Physical Therapist
Cayuga Hand Therapy
Ithaca, New York

Steven L. Moran, MD
Professor of Plastic Surgery
Associate Professor of Orthopedic Surgery
Chair of Plastic Surgery
The Mayo Clinic
Rochester, Minnesota;
Staff Surgeon
Shriners Hospital for Children
Twin Cities
Minneapolis, Minnesota

William B. Morrison, MD
Professor of Radiology
Thomas Jefferson University Hospital
Philadelphia, Pennsylvania

Edward A. Nalebuff, MD
Clinical Professor
Orthopaedic Surgery
Tufts University School of Medicine;
Hand Surgeon
New England Baptist Hospital
Boston, Massachusetts

Donald A. Neumann, PT, PhD, FAPTA
Professor, Physical Therapy
Marquette University
Milwaukee, Wisconsin

Richard Norris, MD
Director
Northampton Spine Medicine
Northampton, Massachusetts;
Board Certified, Physical Medicine and Rehabilitation
    Fellowship, Orthopedics;
Founder and Former Director
The National Arts Medicine Center
Washington, District of Columbia

Michael J. O'Brien, MD
Assistant Professor
Department of Orthopaedics
Tulane Institute for Sports Medicine
New Orleans, Louisiana

Scott N. Oishi, MD
Texas Scottish Rite Hospital for Children
Dallas, Texas

A. Lee Osterman, MD
Professor, Orthopaedic and Hand Surgery
Chairman, Division of Hand Surgery
Department of Orthopaedic Surgery
Jefferson Medical College
Thomas Jefferson University;
President, The Philadelphia and South Jersey Hand Centers, P.C.
    and Hand Surgery Fellowship Program
Philadelphia, Pennsylvania

Lorenzo L. Pacelli, MD
Consultant
Ascension Orthopedics
Austin, Texas

Allen E. Peljovich, MD, MPH
Attending Surgeon
The Hand and Upper Extremity Center of Georgia;
Clinical Instructor
Department of Orthopaedic Surgery
Atlanta Medical Center;
Attending Surgeon
Shepherd Center;
Medical Director
Hand and Upper Extremity Program
Children's Healthcare of Atlanta
Atlanta, Georgia

Karen Pettengill, MS, OTR/L, CHT
Clinical Coordinator
NovaCare Hand and Upper Extremity Rehabilitation
Springfield, Massachusetts

Nicole M. Pettit, DPT
Department of Physical Therapy & Rehabilitation Sciences
Drexel University
Philadelphia, Pennsylvania

Cynthia A. Philips, MA, OTR/L, CHT
Hand Therapist
Farmingham, Massachusetts

Jason Phillips, MD
Orthopaedic Resident
Albert Einstein Medical Center
Philadelphia, Pennsylvania

Jean Pillet, MD
Strasbourg, France

Marisa Pontillo, PT, DPT, SCS
Senior Physical Therapist
GSPP Penn Therapy and Fitness at Penn Sports Medicine
    Center
Philadelphia, Pennsylvania

Ann Porretto-Loehrke, PT, DPT, CHT, COMT
Therapy Manager
Hand and Upper Extremity Center of Northeast Wisconsin
Appleton, Wisconsin

Neal E. Pratt, PhD, PT
Emeritus Professor
Department of Physical Therapy and Rehabilitation Sciences
Drexel University
Philadelphia, Pennsylvania

Victoria W. Priganc, PhD, OTR, CHT, CLT
Owner, Hand Therapy Consultation Services
Richmond, Vermont

Joshua A. Ratner, MD
The Hand Treatment Center
Atlanta, Georgia

Christina M. Read, DPT
Department of Physical Therapy & Rehabilitation Sciences
Drexel University
Philadelphia, Pennsylvania

Mark S. Rekant, MD
Assistant Professor
Department of Orthopaedic Surgery
Thomas Jefferson University
Philadelphia, Pennsylvania

David Ring, MD, PhD
Associate Professor of Orthopaedic Surgery
Harvard Medical School;
Director of Research
MGH Orthopaedic Hand and Upper Extremity Service
Massachusetts General Hospital
Boston, Massachusetts

Annette Rivard, MScOT, PhD(Can)
Assistant Professor
Department of Occupational Therapy
University of Alberta
Edmonton, Alberta, Canada

Marco Rizzo, MD
Associate Professor
Department of Orthopedic Surgery
Mayo Graduate School of Medicine;
Associate Professor
Department of Orthopedic Surgery
Mayo Clinic
Rochester, Minnesota

Sergio Rodriguez, MD
McAllen Hand Center
Edinburg, Texas

Birgitta Rosén, OT, PhD
Associate Professor
Lund University;
Occupational Therapist
Department of Hand Surgery
Skåne University Hospital
Malmö, Sweden

Erik A. Rosenthal, MD
Retired Clinical Professor of Orthopaedic Surgery
Tufts University School of Medicine
Boston, Massachusetts;
Honorary Staff
Baystate Medical Center
Springfield, Massachusetts

Ralph Rynning, MD
Fellow
Thomas Jefferson University Hospital
Philadelphia, Pennsylvania

Douglas M. Sammer, MD
Assistant Professor of Surgery
Washington University School of Medicine
St. Louis, Missouri

Rebecca J. Saunders, PT, CHT
Clinical Specials
Curtis National Hand Center
Union Memorial Hospital
Baltimore, Maryland

Michael Scarneo, DPT
Department of Physical Therapy and Rehabilitation Sciences
Drexel University
Philadelphia, Pennsylvania

Christopher C. Schmidt, MD
Shoulder, Elbow, and Hand Surgery
Department of Orthopaedic Surgery
Allegheny General Hospital
Pittsburgh, Pennsylvania

Lawrence H. Schneider, MD
Retired Clinical Professor
Department of Orthopaedic Surgery
Jefferson Medical College
Thomas Jefferson University
Philadelphia, Pennsylvania

Karen Schultz-Johnson, MS, OTR, CHT, FAOTA
Director
Rocky Mountain Hand Therapy
Edwards, Colorado

Jodi L. Seftchick, MOT, OTR/L, CHT
Senior Occupational Therapist
Human Motion Rehabilitation
Allegheny General Hospital
Pittsburgh, Pennsylvania

Michael A. Shaffer, PT, ATC, OCS
Coordinator for Sports Rehabilitation
UI Sports Medicine;
Clinical Supervisor
University of Iowa Hospitals and Clinics;
Department of Rehabilitation Therapies
Institute for Orthopaedics, Sports Medicine and
  Rehabilitation
Iowa City, Iowa

Aaron Shaw, OTR/L, CHT
Clinical Specialist
Harborview Medical Center
Seattle, Washington

Eon K. Shin, MD
Assistant Professor in Orthopaedic Surgery
Department of Orthopaedic Surgery
Jefferson Medical College
Thomas Jefferson University;
The Philadelphia and South Jersey Hand Centers, P.C.
Philadelphia, Pennsylvania

**Conor P. Shortt, MB, BCh, BAO, MSc, MRCPI, FRCR,
    FFR RCSI**
Assistant Professor of Radiology
Thomas Jefferson University Hospital
Philadelphia, Pennsylvania

Roger L. Simpson, MD, FACS
Assistant Professor of Surgery
State University of New York, Stony Brook, New York;
Director of Plastic and Reconstructive Surgery and the Burn
    Center
Nassau University Medical Center
Long Island Plastic Surgical Group
Garden City, New York

Terri M. Skirven, OTR/L, CHT
Director of Hand Therapy
The Philadelphia and South Jersey Hand Centers, P.C.
Director
Hand Rehabilitation Foundation
Philadelphia, Pennsylvania

David J. Slutsky, MD, FRCS(C)
Assistant Clinical Professor of Orthopedics
Chief of Reconstructive Hand Surgery
Harbor-UCLA Medical Center
David Geffen UCLA School of Medicine
Los Angeles, California

Beth Paterson Smith, PhD
Associate Professor
Department of Orthopaedic Surgery
Wake Forest University School of Medicine
Winston-Salem, North Carolina

Kevin L. Smith, MD, MS
Private Practice
Charlotte Plastic Surgery
Charlotte, North Carolina;
Associate Clinical Professor of Plastic Surgery
University of North Carolina, Chapel Hill
Chapel Hill, North Carolina

Thomas L. Smith, PhD
Professor
Department of Orthopaedic Surgery
Wake Forest University School of Medicine
Winston-Salem, North Carolina

Elizabeth Soika, PT, DPT, CHT
Physical Therapist, Certified Hand Therapist
Results Physiotherapy
Clarksville, Tennessee

Dean G. Sotereanos, MD
Professor
Drexel University
Philadelphia, Pennsylvania
Vice Chairman
Department of Orthopaedic Surgery
Hand and Upper Extremity Surgery
Allegheny General Hospital
Pittsburgh, Pennsylvania

Alexander M. Spiess, MD
Clinical Instructor
Allegheny General Hospital
Pittsburgh, Pennsylvania

David Stanley, MBBS, BSc(Hons), FRCS
Honorary Senior Lecturer
University of Sheffield;
Consultant Elbow and Shoulder Surgeon
Northern General Hospital
Sheffield, South Yorkshire, United Kingdom

Pamela J. Steelman, CRNP, PT, CHT
Nurse Practitioner, Certified Hand Therapist
The Philadelphia and South Jersey Hand Centers, P.C.
Philadelphia, Pennsylvania

Scott P. Steinmann, MD
Professor of Orthopedic Surgery
Mayo Clinic
Rochester, Minnesota

Stephanie Sweet, MD
Clinical Assistant Professor
Department of Orthopaedic Surgery
Thomas Jefferson University;
Attending Hand Surgeon
The Philadelphia and South Jersey Hand Centers, P.C.
Philadelphia, Pennsylvania

Virak Tan, MD
Professor
Department of Orthopaedics
University of Medicine and Dentistry of New Jersey
The New Jersey Medical School;
Director
Hand and Upper Extremity Fellowship
University of Medicine and Dentistry of New Jersey
The New Jersey Medical School
Newark, New Jersey;
Attending Surgeon
Overlook Hospital
Summit, New Jersey

John S. Taras, MD
Associate Professor
Department of Orthopaedic Surgery
Drexel University and Thomas Jefferson University;
Chief
Division of Hand Surgery
Drexel University;
The Philadelphia Hand Center, PC
Philadelphia, Pennsylvania

Angela Tate, PT, PhD
Adjunct Faculty
Arcadia University
Glenside, Pennsylvania;
Clinical Director
H/S Therapy, Inc
Lower Gwynedd, Pennsylvania

Matthew J. Taylor, PT, PhD, RYT
Founder and Director
Dynamic Systems Rehabilitation Clinic
Scottsdale, Arizona

Andrew L. Terrono, MD
Clinical Professor
Orthopaedic Surgery
Tufts University School of Medicine;
Chief
Hand Surgery
New England Baptist Hospital
Boston, Massachusetts

Allen Tham, MD
Resident
Department of Orthopaedic Surgery
Temple University Hospital
Philadelphia, Pennsylvania

Michael A. Thompson, MD
Scripps Clinic Medical Group
La Jolla, California

Wendy Tomhave, OTR/L
Shriners Hospital for Children
Twin Cities
Minneapolis, Minnesota

Patricia A. Tufaro, OTR/L
Senior Occupational Therapist
William Randolph Hearst Burn Center at New York–
  Presbyterian Hospital Weill-Cornell Medical Center
New York, New York

Thomas H. Tung, MD
Associate Professor of Surgery
Division of Plastic and Reconstructive Surgery
Washington University School of Medicine
St. Louis, Missouri

Chris Tuohy, MD
Assistant Professor
Orthopaedic Surgery
Wake Forest University School of Medicine;
Orthopaedic Surgeon
North Carolina Baptist Hospital
Wake Forest University Health Sciences
Winston-Salem, North Carolina

Sheryl S. Ulin, MS, PhD
Research Program Officer
University of Michigan
Ann Arbor, Michigan

Gwendolyn van Strien, LPT, MSc
Director/Owner
Hand Rehabilitation Consultancy
Den Haag, the Netherlands;
Director
Hand Therapy Unit
Lange Land Hospital
Zoetermeer; the Netherlands;
Clinical Instructor
Department of Rehabilitation
Erasmus University Rotterdam
Rotterdam, the Netherlands;
Course Director and Instructor
Post Graduate Allied Health Education
National Institute for Allied Health
Amersfoort, the Netherlands

June P. Villeco, MBA, OTR/L, MLDC, CHT
Montgomery Hospital
Norristown, Pennsylvania

Rebecca L. von der Heyde, PhD, OTR/L, CHT
Associate Professor of Occupational Therapy
Maryville University;
Certified Hand Therapist
Milliken Hand Rehabilitation Center
Shriner's Hospital for Children
St. Louis, Missouri

Ana-Maria Vranceanu, PhD
Clinical Staff Psychologist
Massachusetts General Hospital
Boston, Massachusetts

Heather Walkowich, DPT
Physical Therapist
The New Jersey Center of Physical Therapy
Riverdale, New Jersey

Mark T. Walsh, PT, DPT, MS, CHT, ATC
Assistant Clinical Professor
Department of Physical Therapy and Rehabilitation Sciences
College of Nursing and Health Professions
Drexel University
Philadelphia, Pennsylvania;
President, Co-Founder/Owner
Hand and Orthopedic Physical Therapist Associates, PC
Levittown, Pennsylvania;
Consultant
Hand Therapy and Upper Extremity Rehabilitation
Department of Physical Therapy and Rehabilitation
Lower Bucks Hospital
Bristol, Pennsylvania

Jo M. Weis, PhD
Associate Professor, Psychiatry and Behavioral Medicine
Medical College of Wisconsin
Milwaukee, Wisconsin

Lawrence Weiss, MD
Assistant Professor of Orthopaedic Surgery
Pennsylvania State University School of Medicine;
Chief
Division of Hand Surgery
Lehigh Valley Hospital
Allentown, Pennsylvania

Kevin E. Wilk, PT, DPT
Associate Clinical Director
Champion Sports Medicine;
Director of Rehabilitative Research
American Sports Medicine
Birmingham, Alabama

Gerald R. Williams, Jr., MD
Professor, Orthopaedic Surgery;
Chief, Shoulder and Elbow Service
The Rothman Institute
Thomas Jefferson University
Philadelphia, Pennsylvania

Scott Wolfe, MD
Chief, Hand and Upper Extremity Surgery
Attending Orthopedic Surgeon
Hospital for Special Surgery;
Professor of Orthopedic Surgery
Weill Medical College of Cornell University
New York, New York

Terri L. Wolfe, OTR/L, CHT
Director
Hand and Upper Body Rehabilitation Center
Erie, Pennsylvania

Raymond K. Wurapa, MD
The Cardinal Orthopaedic Institute
Columbus, Ohio

Michael J. Wylykanowitz, Jr., DPT
Department of Physical Therapy & Rehabilitation Sciences
Drexel University
Philadelphia, Pennsylvania

Theresa Wyrick, MD
Assistant Professor
Department of Orthopaedic Surgery
Arkansas Children's Hospital
University of Arkansas for Medical Sciences
Little Rock, Arkansas

Kathleen E. Yancosek, PhD, OTR/L, CHT
MAJOR
United States Army

Jeffrey Yao, MD
Assistant Professor of Orthopaedic Surgery
Robert A. Chase Hand and Upper Limb Center
Stanford University Medical Center
Stanford, California

David S. Zelouf, MD
Clinical Instructor
Department of Orthopaedic Surgery
Jefferson Medical College
Thomas Jefferson University;
Assistant Chief of Trauma Surgery
Thomas Jefferson University Hospital;
The Philadelphia and South Jersey Hand Centers, P.C.
Philadelphia, Pennsylvania

FOREWORD

As was true in previous editions of *Rehabilitation of the Hand and Upper Extremity,* the editors' purpose in this sixth edition is to bring updated contributions from recognized experts in the field.

When I think of the sixth edition, for me it's not just a new volume with new authors and new information. I recognize in each chapter a fulfillment and tribute to what came before. The depth and quality of experience lived by pioneering hand surgeons and therapists, readily available to us in the literature, influences every facet of hand rehabilitation as we know it today. Those who had the vision to create our unique medical specialty put us in a position to see old problems with fresh eyes and invite us to use our creativity to find new ways to help our patients. We honor our predecessors through our passion for continuous improvement. We stand, truly, on the shoulders of giants. They would be proud, as am I, of this new edition.

It was not always so. In the War between the States (1861–1865), no special consideration was given to treatment of the injured hand and little was recorded. Despite the number of wrist and hand fractures due to gunshot and other injuries, only a few pages of the *Medical and Surgical History of the War of the Rebellion* dealt with hand wounds and surgery.

In World War I, somewhat less than three hundred lines covered hand injuries in the Medical Department of the United States Army's *World War, Volume XI, Surgery, Part I.*

Prior to World War II, surgery for hand injuries sustained by military personnel consisted essentially of drainage of infections, amputations, and wound closure, with only isolated efforts at repair. Physical and occupational therapy were used inadequately or ignored.

World War II stimulated significant interest in reparative hand surgery. Much of the early success in managing severe hand injuries was due to the wise leadership of the Surgeon General, Major General Norman T. Kirk. Rather than giving hand wounds routine treatment, he considered them a separate category worthy of specialized treatment. Nine "hand centers" in selected military hospitals were established across the country where officers trained in plastic, orthopedic, and neurological surgery were entrusted with the repair of wounded hands.

Under the guidance of Sterling Bunnell, MD, civilian consultant to the Surgeon General, a two-phase plan for managing hand injuries was implemented. Instructional courses and technical manuals outlined primary care for field surgeons. Soldiers receiving emergency wound closure in the Mediterranean and European Theaters of Operations were returned to the United States via advanced transport for definitive repair of tendons, nerves, and fractures.

Dr. Bunnell realized that postoperative therapy was as critical to recovery and socioeconomic well-being as the surgery itself. Patients with hand injuries who reached the desired stage of healing were placed in a single ward close to physical and occupational therapy departments. His seminal idea of therapists participating as part of a fully coordinated team to deliver optimal care gained momentum with hand injuries that occurred during the Vietnam War.

Dr. Bunnell's pioneering efforts attracted the interest of younger hand surgeons who recognized the advantages of a total care approach in civilian practice. One of these surgeons, James M. Hunter, MD, as civilian consultant in orthopedic surgery to the department of the Army at Valley Forge General Hospital (1964–1973), envisioned the team approach in his private hand practice. Along with his partner, Lawrence H. Schneider, MD, the Philadelphia Hand Center was founded in 1972 in a former Horn and Hardart bakery.

The remarkable progress in total care of the injured hand and upper extremity over the past half century is reflected in the founding of the American Society for Surgery of the Hand (ASSH) in 1946, the International Federation of Societies for Surgery of the Hand (IFSSH) in 1968, the American Society of Hand Therapists (ASHT) in 1978, and the International Federation of Societies of Hand Therapy (IFSHT) in 1986. Just as important, however, it is reflected in the rapid growth and high quality of peer-reviewed scientific literature on hand rehabilitation, most notably in the *Journal of Hand Surgery* and the *Journal of Hand Therapy.*

Although there were textbooks on the surgical management of hand injuries, in the 1960s there were few references for therapists who were eager to learn more about postoperative management. When I began working with Dr. Hunter in the 1960s, the only reference available was a text on hand rehabilitation by Wing Commander Wynn Parry, MD, who was Consultant in Physical Medicine to the Royal Air Force of England.

Six soft-covered manuals by Maude Malick, OTR (1967–1972) describing hand splinting, management of the quadriplegic upper extremity, and management of the burn patient took their place beside Wynn Parry's text in the early literature on postoperative management.

During this time, another book was published abroad— *The Hand: Principles and Techniques of Simple Splintmaking in Rehabilitation* by Nathalic Barr, MBE, FBAOT of Great Britain. It was intended to serve as a splinting guide in the management of hand conditions. Nathalie was a major contributor to hand rehabilitation in Europe, especially in the early years after World War II.

Four years after the founding of the Philadelphia Hand Center, an educational symposium was launched, chaired by Drs. Hunter and Schneider and Evelyn Mackin, PT. The meeting, "Rehabilitation of the Hand," set a pattern and high standard for future meetings. Together at the podium, surgeons and therapists discussed mutual problems before a rapt audience of 450 of their peers. The success of the 1976 meeting set the stage for increasingly sophisticated "Philadelphia Meetings" sponsored by the Philadelphia Hand Rehabilitation Foundation and held every year since the original meeting. Under the leadership of Terri Skirven, OTR/L, CHT, and Lee Osterman, MD, the symposium has continued to evolve, with a concurrent symposium directed to surgeons introduced in 1999. Both meetings are considered must-attend events by new and returning participants alike.

The papers presented at the first Philadelphia meeting were incorporated into the first edition of *Rehabilitation of the Hand,* edited by James Hunter, Lawrence Schneider, Evelyn Mackin, and Judith Bell, OTR, FAOTA, CHT, which brought surgeons and therapists together again as authors. Chapters addressed functional anatomy, processes of wound healing, surgical and postoperative care of hand injuries, and the development of hand centers, among other topics.

With each succeeding edition (1984, 1990, 1995) edited by James Hunter, Lawrence Schneider, Evelyn Mackin, and Anne Callahan, MS, OTR/L, CHT, the text has been recognized as the "bible" of an eager band of dedicated and enthusiastic therapists (JBJS) and as a "living classic" (JAMA).

It is impossible to reminisce without remembering the hundreds of surgeons and therapists, leaders in their respective fields, who have made the editions and the meetings possible, and to have known personally some of the giants of in our field: Dr. William Littler, who in 1945 as Maj. J. William Littler, MC, established a ward at the Cushing General Hospital designated specifically for the care of hand injuries, in accordance with Dr. Bunnell's plan. Dr. Paul Brand pioneered the surgical treatment of the hands of leprosy patients in India, and established centers where patients with reconstructed hands, under the care of physical and occupational therapists, could learn a trade that would make them self-reliant. Dr. Earl Peacock, having visited Dr. Brand in India, was influenced by Dr. Brand's advocating the team approach in the care of the hand patient. He brought this model of practice back to Chapel Hill, North Carolina, and formed the "Hand House," which was the first civilian hand center in the United States. Joining him in the effort were Irene Hollis, OTR; John Madden, MD; and Gloria DeVore, OTR. I was inspired by these people. I still am.

If anyone should be mentioned especially as having influenced my career, it is Dr. Hunter, my mentor and friend. His forward vision, enthusiasm, and unwavering support of the hand therapist in the early years was so important to the development of hand therapy and the recognition it now enjoys. He had the rare ability to lift those around him, hand surgery fellows and hand therapists alike, to the level of excellence that he always expected of them.

Almost a decade has passed since publication of the fifth edition of *Rehabilitation of the Hand and Upper Extremity* edited by Evelyn Mackin, Anne Callahan, Terri Skirven, Lawrence Schneider, and Lee Osterman. It remains an indispensible reference. However, with the continuing advances in hand surgery and hand therapy, it becomes more important than ever that new editions deliver the latest information to our growing professional community worldwide.

It is an honor and a very much appreciated privilege, for several reasons, to have been invited to write the foreword to the sixth edition edited by Terri Skirven, Lee Osterman, Jane Fedorczyk, PT, PhD, CHT, ATC, and Peter Amadio, MD. Foremost is the respect I have for the editors. Then there is the list of participating authors, who are recognized experts on their subjects. Perhaps most of all, I have no doubt that the hard work and dedicated efforts of the editors will ensure that this groundbreaking and ever-evolving book will remain for many years the most authoritative work on rehabilitation of the hand and the upper extremity.

The Chinese say, "May you live in interesting times." I have.

Evelyn J. Mackin

PREFACE

Synergy, in general, may be defined as two or more agents working together to produce a result not obtainable by any of the agents independently. Synergy is the ability of a group to outperform even its best individual member. The sixth edition of *Rehabilitation of the Hand and Upper Extremity* is the product of the synergy of editors, authors, publishers and many others involved in its publication.

The impetus for the first edition of *Rehabilitation of the Hand* grew out of a unique symposium that featured hand surgery correlated with hand therapy, sponsored by the Hand Rehabilitation Foundation in Philadelphia in 1976. The original editors of the book were also the chairpersons and faculty for the symposium: James M. Hunter, MD; Lawrence Schneider; Evelyn Mackin, PT; and Judith A. Bell Krotoski, OTR, FAOTA, CHT. Joining the effort with the second through fifth editions was Anne D. Callahan, MS, OTR/L, CHT. These extraordinary individuals introduced a working partnership of hand surgeons and hand therapists for the care of the hand patient that has endured and flourished over the years and is evidenced by the publication of the sixth edition of this book.

The expansion of this text and its readership is in keeping with the growth of the specialty of hand rehabilitation. This current two-volume edition features a total of 143 chapters, 37 of which are new, and more than 75 new authors. The authors of the text include physical and occupational therapists, certified hand therapists, orthopedic and plastic surgeons, physiatrists, neurologists, psychologists, psychiatrists, clinicians, researchers, and educators—all having expertise in the care of the hand and upper extremity patient.

Since the first edition, the table of contents has expanded with each edition to include separate sections on the shoulder, elbow, and wrist, as well as the hand. Many returning sections have been modified and expanded to reflect current practice. For example, the term *orthosis* is used to refer to the custom fabricated devices typically referred to as *splints*. Far from just a technical skill, the design and fabrication of hand and upper extremity orthoses require an in-depth knowledge of anatomy and pathology, as well as the healing and positioning requirements for the range of conditions and surgeries encountered. Hand, occupational, and physical therapists are uniquely qualified to design, apply, monitor, and modify orthotic devices as part of the rehabilitation treatment plan.

Taking advantage of the advances in information technology, this edition is complemented by a companion web site allowing supplemental information and video clips of therapy and surgery procedures to be included.

Given the emphasis on evidence-based practice in the current healthcare environment, special focus has been placed on providing peer-reviewed literature support for the information given in this text. However, published research in hand and upper extremity rehabilitation is limited in many areas. In some cases the best evidence is the clinical experience of the individual authors. Where it is stated that no evidence exists to support a particular approach or technique, the intention is not to suggest that it be abandoned; rather the goal is to stimulate the reader to adopt a critical attitude and to pursue clinical research, whether as a single case study or a multicenter randomized controlled trial.

We have dedicated this edition to Evelyn Mackin, who has been the driving force behind the book, as well as so many other groundbreaking achievements. Her leadership, dedication, determination, and inspiration have been instrumental in advancing the specialty of hand rehabilitation, as well as inspiring countless others (including the current editors) to follow her lead and further her initiatives. Available on the book's web site is a fascinating interview with Evelyn, recounting the early days of hand therapy, the formation of the American Society of Hand Therapists, the development of the *Journal of Hand Therapy*, and many other aspects of her extraordinary career.

The publication of the sixth edition of *Rehabilitation of the Hand and Upper Extremity* is the result of the efforts of many people over more than 3 years and acknowledgments are due. First and foremost, we would like to thank all of the authors who have contributed their clinical expertise and insights to this text.

Our special thanks is extended to Evelyn Mackin, who has written the foreword for this edition and who has provided guidance, support, and encouragement to the current editors.

We would like to acknowledge our editors at Elsevier for their ongoing support and persistence to see the text through to publication. In particular, Lucia Gunzel has been the perfect combination of coach, cheerleader, and disciplinarian. With Dan Pepper's diplomacy and wise counsel, rough patches were navigated and resolved. Ellen Sklar deserves recognition for her professional management of the final stages of the editing process, a daunting task.

Thanks to Leslie Ristine, Administrator of the Philadelphia Hand Rehabilitation Foundation, for providing administrative support, and to Andrew Cooney, Executive Director of the Philadelphia and South Jersey Hand Centers, who has provided encouragement and support during the work on the sixth edition, as well as for prior editions.

Finally, we thank our families, friends, and colleagues who have provided encouragement and patience during the 3 years that it has taken to complete the book.

We are proud to present this sixth edition of *Rehabilitation of the Hand and Upper Extremity.*

Terri M. Skirven
A. Lee Osterman
Jane M. Fedorczyk
Peter C. Amadio

CONTENTS

ONLINE SUPPLEMENTAL ELEMENTS

ONLINE VIDEO LIST

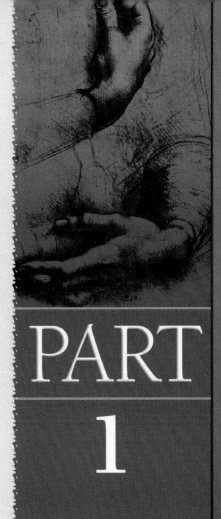

PART

1

Anatomy and Kinesiology

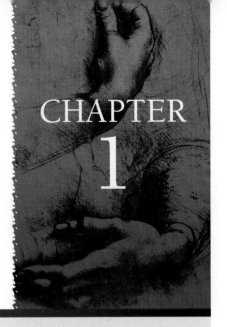

CHAPTER 1

Anatomy and Kinesiology of the Hand

NEAL E. PRATT, PhD, PT

OSTEOLOGY OF THE HAND
ARTICULATIONS OF THE HAND
SKIN, RETINACULAR SYSTEM, AND
   COMPARTMENTATION OF THE HAND
INTRINSIC MUSCLES OF THE HAND

TENDONS OF THE EXTRINSIC MUSCLES OF
   THE HAND
DIGITAL BALANCE
NERVE SUPPLY OF THE HAND
BLOOD SUPPLY OF THE HAND

CRITICAL POINTS

- The hand can assume almost countless positions and postures that allow it to perform numerous functions and manipulations.
- The muscles of the hand permit it to perform tasks that require both great strength and delicate precision.
- The skin of the hand, particularly that of the palm, is richly supplied with a large variety of sensory receptors that allow it to detect minute differences in texture and shape.
- The joints and muscles of the hand contain large numbers of proprioceptive receptors that enable it to detect miniscule differences in position and thus perform precise manipulations extremely smoothly.

Osteology of the Hand

The bones of the hand form its framework and are important in maintaining its shape and providing a stable base on which to anchor its various soft tissue structures. The bones are arranged to maximize the functional efficiency of the intrinsic muscles and the tendons of the extrinsic muscles of the hand. The 19 major bones are of only two types: the metacarpals and the phalanges (Fig. 1-1). All of these bones are classified as long bones and have central shafts and expanded proximal and distal ends (epiphyses). Additional small bones, sesamoids, are usually found in the tendons of certain intrinsic thumb muscles.

One *metacarpal* is associated with each digit, that of the thumb being considerably shorter than the others. These bones form the bony base of the hand, and their integrity is essential for both its natural form and function. Each bone has a *dorsally bowed shaft* with an *expanded base* (proximally) and *head* (distally) (Fig. 1-2). From closely positioned bases, the bones diverge distally to their heads. This arrangement determines the shape of the hand and separates the digits so they can function independently as well as manipulate large objects. The metacarpal of the thumb is anterior to the others and rotated approximately 90 degrees so it is ideally positioned to oppose (see Fig. 1-1).

The *shaft of each metacarpal* is triangular in cross section, with the apex of this triangle directed volarly and composed of more dense bone than the dorsal aspect of the shaft.[1] This concentration of dense bone reflects the significant compressile force on the flexor side of the bone. The overall shape of each metacarpal (along with that of the phalanges) contributes to the *longitudinal arch of the hand*. The dorsal convexities of the metacarpals along with their triangular cross sections provide significant room for the soft tissue of the palm, the bulk of which consists of the intrinsic interossei muscles and the more volarly positioned long digital flexor tendons and accompanying intrinsic lumbrical muscles. The mechanical advantage of these muscles is also enhanced by the metacarpal shape; their lines of pull are located volar to the flexion–extension axes of the metacarpophalangeal (MCP) joints.

The *bases of the four medial metacarpals* are irregular in shape and less wide volarly than dorsally, thus contributing to the *proximal transverse arch* (Fig. 1-3). Articular surface is found on the sides as well as the proximal aspect of the base. The *base of the thumb metacarpal* is significantly different. The somewhat flattened proximal surface is in the shape of a

3

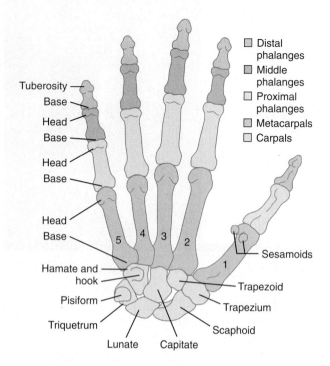

Bones of right wrist and hand (palmar view)

Figure 1-1 *Volar view of the bones of the hand and wrist. Note that the thumb is rotated approximately 90 degrees relative to the rest of the digits.*

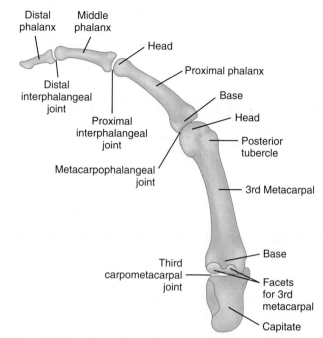

Figure 1-2 *Lateral view of the middle finger and the capitate. Note the dorsal convexities of the metacarpal and proximal and middle phalanges.*

shallow saddle, all of which is articular surface. The concave surface is oriented from medial to lateral; the convex from anterior to posterior. (Keep in mind that this bone is rotated about 90 degrees relative to the other metacarpals and this description is based on the anatomic position.) The most *medial aspect of the base* protrudes more proximally than the rest of the base and thus presents a triangular *beak*.

The *heads of all the metacarpals* are similar. The articular surface is rounded, both from side to side as well as dorsal to palmar. The side-to-side dimension is considerably shorter than the length from dorsal to palmar, but it is wider on the palmar aspect than it is dorsally. And importantly, the surface extends farther onto the volar aspect of the bone than dorsally. Prominent *dorsal tubercles* are found dorsally on each side of the head, just proximal to the articular surface.

The shapes of the metacarpals also contribute to the *proximal and distal transverse arches* of the hand (see Fig. 1-3). The proximal arch is at the level of the distal row of carpal bones and the bases of the metacarpals. The bases of the metacarpals as well as the distal row of carpals are wedge-shaped in cross section, and the apex of each wedge is directed volarly. Since the metacarpal bases and distal carpals are positioned very close to one another and are held tightly together, they collectively form a dorsal convexity and thus a side-to-side arch. The distal transverse arch is at the level of the metacarpal heads and is also a dorsal convexity. This arch is larger than the proximal arch and merely reflects the orientation of the metacarpals and the fact that the metacarpal heads are farther apart than their bases.

The hand contains 14 *phalanges*; the thumb has only 2, whereas each of the other digits has 3. The *proximal and middle phalanges*, like the metacarpals, are bowed dorsally along their long axis and thus contribute to the longitudinal arch of the hand. The *shafts of the phalanges* serve as anchors for the long digital flexor tendons. The volar aspect of the shaft is flat from side to side and rounded dorsally. The junctions of the rounded and flat surfaces are marked by longitudinal ridges that serve as the attachments for the fibrous part of the digital tendon sheath (see Fig. 1-1). Each bone has an expanded epiphysis on each end, with the *base* (proximally) being larger than the head (distally).

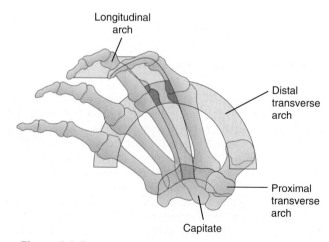

Figure 1-3 *The transverse and longitudinal arches of the hand.*

The *surface of the base of the proximal phalanx* is biconcave and consists entirely of articular surface. The *bases of both the middle and distal phalanges* are concave from dorsal to ventral, with a *central ridge* oriented in the same direction. This surface is entirely articular surface. The *heads of the proximal and middle phalanges* are cylindrical from side to side with a *central groove* oriented perpendicular to the cylinder. This surface is also articular surface. The *distal phalanx* is shorter than the others. It has no head but rather ends in an expanded and roughened palmar elevation, which supports the pulp of the fingertip as well as the fingernail.

Articulations of the Hand

The *carpometacarpal (CMC) joints* are the most proximal joints in the hand and connect it to the wrist. Even though they are all synovial joints, the thumb CMC joint is significantly different from those of the four medial digits. The CMC joint of the thumb allows significant and complex motion; those of the other digits allow a small amount to virtually none.

The *four medial joints* are between the bases of the four medial metacarpals and the distal row of carpal bones: the trapezium, trapezoid, capitate, and hamate. The articular surfaces of both sets of bones are irregular, continue on the medial and lateral aspects of the metacarpal bases and the carpals, but are quite congruent so the bones fit closely together. Each metacarpal base articulates with one, two, or even three carpal bones. Strong ligaments hold all of the bones tightly together, both side to side and across the CMC joint space. A single joint capsule encloses all of these joints so there is a single synovial cavity. This cavity extends not only across the span of the collective joints but also somewhat distally between the metacarpal bases and proximally between the distal carpal bones.

The *motion* available at these joints is variable and minimal. There is essentially no motion permitted at the CMC joints of the index and middle fingers. These two metacarpals along with the distal carpal row form the rigid and stable central base of the hand. A small amount of motion is permitted at the CMC joints of the ring and small fingers. This motion, primarily a bit of flexion, permits slight cupping of the medial side of the hand and is important in both manipulation and grip (Fig. 1-4).

The *first CMC (trapeziometacarpal) joint* is between the *base of the first metacarpal* and the *trapezium*. Since the thumb articulates with only the trapezium, its location and orientation is the basis for the position of the thumb. The trapezium is obliquely oriented, almost in the sagittal plane, and projects more volarly than the trapezoid or scaphoid with which it articulates.

The *articular surfaces* (Fig. 1-5) of both the base of the first metacarpal and the distal aspect of the trapezium are shaped like shallow saddles. As a result, each surface has a convex and a concave component, and these elements are perpendicular to one another. The shapes dictate that the major amount of motion occurs in two planes, which also are perpendicular to one another. *Motion in the coronal plane,* where the thumb moves across the palm, is flexion and extension. These motions occur as the concave surface of the

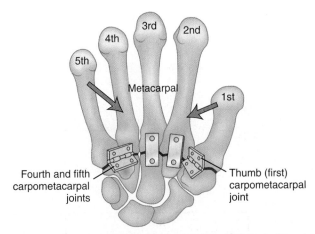

Figure 1-4 Volar view of the metacarpal and carpal bones of the right hand, showing the relative motion of the five carpometacarpal joints. Note that there is more motion at the thumb, ring, and little finger joints than at the index and middle fingers.

metacarpal base moves on the convex surface of the trapezium. *Motion in the sagittal plane,* where the thumb moves toward and away from the index finger, is adduction (toward) and abduction (away). This occurs as the convex surface of the metacarpal base moves on the concave surface of the trapezium. Since both saddles are shallow and the soft tissue restraints are somewhat lax, axial rotation is also permitted. This rotation, *opposition* (pronation), occurs primarily at this first CMC joint and represents an essential ingredient for the usefulness of the thumb. *Retroposition* (supination) is the opposite of opposition. In reality, certain motions are coupled. Abduction is accompanied by a bit of medial rotation (opposition). This is due to the slightly curved concave surface of the trapezium. Retroposition, then, is a combination of lateral rotation and adduction. Flexion and extension also involve some rotation, albeit less. Flexion is accompanied by a bit of opposition and extension by a bit of retroposition.[2] This is caused by the slightly curved convex surface of the

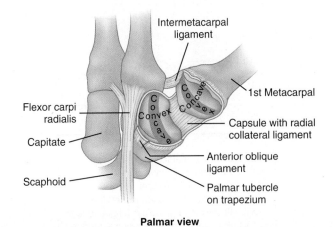

Palmar view

Figure 1-5 Palmar view of the carpometacarpal joint of the right thumb. The joint is open and the metacarpal reflected radially. Note the saddle-shaped articular surfaces of both bones and the concave and convex aspects of each.

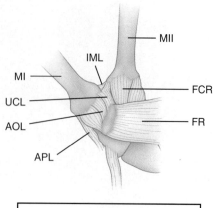

Key	
AOL,	Anterior oblique ligament
UCL,	Ulnar collateral ligament
IML,	First intermetacarpal ligament
APL,	Abductor pollicis longus tendon
FCR,	Flexor carpi radialis
FR,	Flexor retinaculum
MI,	First metacarpal
MII,	Second metacarpal

Figure 1-6 *Palmar view of the ligaments of the carpometacarpal joint of the left thumb.*

trapezium. Hanes[3] suggested the coupling was due to the tautness of certain of the ligaments of the joint; Zancolli and colleagues[4] considered the coupling was due both to the articular surfaces and the ligaments.

The *ligaments* (Figs. 1-6 and 1-7) of this joint are found on all sides of the joint. Their nomenclature can be confusing because several systems are used to name them and there are differences of opinion relative to how many ligaments there are. The *anterior oblique*, or beak, ligament is a strong liga-

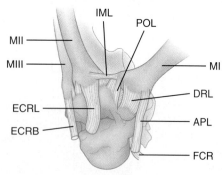

Key	
IML,	First intermetacarpal ligament
POL,	Posterior oblique ligament
DRL,	Dorsoradial ligament
APL,	Abductor pollicis longus tendon
ECRL,	Extensor carpi radialis longus tendon
ECRB,	Exensor carpi radialis brevis tendon
MIII,	Third metacarpal

Figure 1-7 *Dorsal view of the ligaments of the carpometacarpal joint of the left thumb.*

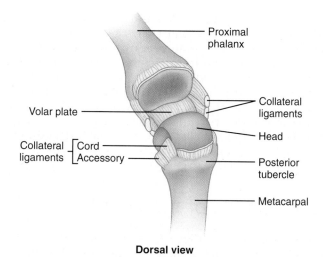

Dorsal view

Figure 1-8 *Dorsal view of the metacarpophalangeal joint that is opened dorsally to show the articular surfaces. Note the biconvex metacarpal head and the biconcave proximal phalangeal base.*

ment that interconnects the palmar tubercle (beak) of the metacarpal base and the distal part of a ridge on the tubercle of the trapezium. This ligament is generally considered a major stabilizing ligament of the joint and is taut in abduction, extension, and opposition.[5] Bettinger and coworkers[6] described a superficial anterior oblique ligament and a deep anterior oblique ligament, which they considered the beak ligament. The *ulnar collateral* ligament is on the volar and medial aspects of the joint and extends from the transverse carpal ligament to the palmar-medial aspect of the first metacarpal base. The *posterior oblique* ligament is on the dorsal aspect of the joint and interconnects the dorsal aspect of the trapezium and the ulnar (medial) base of the metacarpal. An *intermetacarpal* ligament (or pair of intermetacarpal [anterior and posterior] ligaments) interconnects the bases of the first and second metacarpals. The *dorsoradial* ligament extends from the dorsolateral aspect of the trapezium to the dorsal base of the first metacarpal. The joint capsule is complete and somewhat loose, which is necessary for axial rotation.

The *metacarpophalangeal (MCP) joints* (Fig. 1-8) of the four medial digits are formed by the bases of the proximal phalanges and the heads of the metacarpals. The articular surface of the *metacarpal head* is biconvex, cam-shaped so it extends farther volarly than dorsally, and it is wider volarly than dorsally. The articular surface of the *phalangeal base* is biconcave, shallow and smaller in area than the articular surface of the metacarpal head. These shapes would appear to permit the phalanx to move in virtually any plane on the metacarpal head. However, due to soft tissue restraints, *active motion* is limited to flexion and extension and adduction and abduction. Adduction is movement of the digits toward the middle finger; abduction is movement away from the middle finger. The middle finger can be deviated either radially (laterally) or ulnarly (medially). Axial rotation is available only passively.

The *joint capsule of the MCP* (Fig. 1-9) joint is highly specialized. Like any capsule it encloses the joint space and attaches to the edges of both articular surfaces. It is different in that its volar aspect is formed by a strong plate of

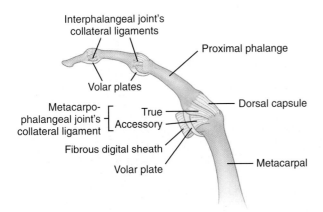

Figure 1-9 *Lateral view of the joint capsules of the metacarpophalangeal and interphalangeal joints of a finger.*

fibrocartilage—*palmar ligament*, or *volar plate*. The medial and lateral edges of the plate serve as attachments for the fibrous part of the digital tendon sheath, specifically the first annular ligament (A1 pulley). Thus, the plate is important in the stability and positioning of the long digital flexor tendons. The plate is thick and rigid distally and its volar aspect has a thin side-to-side attachment to the volar base of the proximal phalanx. This hingelike attachment allows the plate to move as a unit relative to the proximal phalanx. Proximally the plate thins, is a bit loose and flexible, and attaches to volar base of the metacarpal head. *With flexion the volar plate slides proximally* (Fig. 1-10); this is possible because the proximal part of the plate can fold.

The *collateral ligament* (see Fig. 1-10) is triangular in shape and consists of two distinct parts, both of which attach proximally to the dorsal tubercle of the metacarpal. From that attachment, the fibers of the ligament diverge as they pass distally. The *true*, or *band, part of the ligament* extends more distally and is the strongest part of the ligament. From the dorsal tubercle it passes obliquely volarly and attaches to the volar aspect of the side of the proximal phalangeal base. This true ligament is somewhat loose in extension and thus permits abduction and adduction. As the proximal phalanx is flexed, this part tightens because of the cam shape of the metacarpal head and because the metacarpal head is wider volarly. As a result of the tightness, abduction and adduction are very limited in flexion. The *accessory*, or *fan, part of the ligament* is more obliquely oriented and attaches to the volar plate. Since the fibrous tendon sheath also attaches to the volar plate, the accessory collateral ligament plays an important role in stabilizing the long digital flexor tendons. The accessory ligament loosens slightly as flexion occurs.

The MCP joints are reinforced dorsally and laterally by the *extensor hood* (see Fig. 1-20, online). This hood consists of a flat layer of fibers that is oriented perpendicular and oblique to the long axis of the digit and sweep around the joint from one edge of the volar plate to the other. The fibers on either side of the joint are in the sagittal plane and called the *sagittal bands*. The hood blends with the long digital extensor tendon, slides proximally and distally, respectively, with extension and flexion, and is the mechanism through which the proximal phalanx is extended. The hood is also important in centralizing the extensor tendons at the MCP joint.

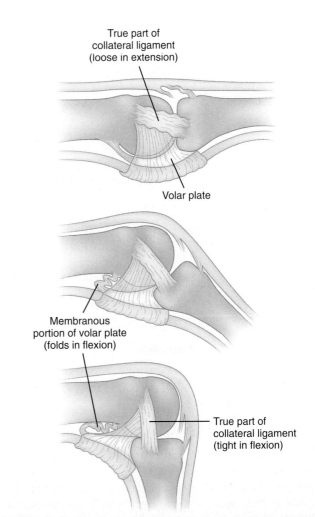

Figure 1-10 *Lateral view of the metacarpophalangeal joint of a finger. The band part of the collateral ligament and the volar plate are depicted in full extension, partial flexion, and flexion. Note how the tension of the band part of the ligament changes as the proximal phalanx is flexed. Note also how the proximal part of the volar plate folds as flexion occurs.*

The *MCP joint of the thumb* is both similar to and different from the other MCP joints. The articular surfaces and collateral ligaments are quite similar. In general, the joint capsule is similar but part of it, the volar plate, varies. The *volar plate* contains two sesamoids bones, which form a trough for the tendon of the flexor pollicis longus muscle. The sesamoids are also partial insertions for the adductor pollicis muscle on the ulnar side and the flexor pollicis brevis muscle on the radial side. The more superficial layer of fibrous support is a somewhat *modified extensor hood*. The ulnar side of the hood is stronger and heavier than the radial side and formed by the tendon and aponeurosis of the adductor pollicis muscle. It extends dorsally to blend with the tendons of the extensor pollicis brevis and extensor pollicis longus muscles. The radial side of the hood is formed by the tendons of the abductor pollicis brevis and flexor pollicis brevis, which also blend with the extensor pollicis brevis and extensor pollicis longus tendons dorsally. The aponeurosis on the ulnar side forms a strong restraint against abduction forces. However, since the thumb is in a different plane than the other digits it is more vulnerable to adduction and abduction forces.

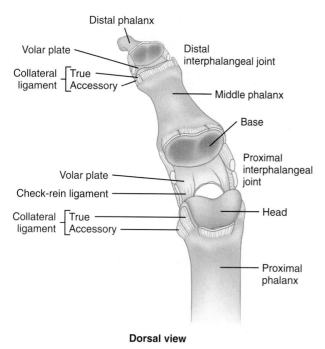

Dorsal view

Figure 1-11 *Dorsal view of the interphalangeal joints of a finger. The joints are opened dorsally to view the articular surfaces. Note the sagittal groove of the phalangeal heads and the sagittal ridge of the phalangeal bases.*

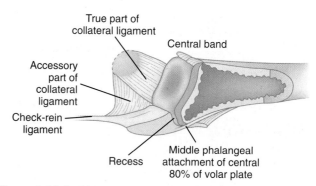

Figure 1-12 *Sagittal view of the proximal aspect of the middle phalanx and volar plate of the proximal interphalangeal joint. Note that only one half of the volar plate is depicted.*

The *motion* available at the thumb MCP is similar in direction to the other MCP joints but more limited because of the stability of the joint. Flexion and extension are less free, and adduction and abduction are significantly more limited. However, motion varies considerably from person to person so possible limitation should be compared with motion on the opposite side.

The *proximal interphalangeal (PIP) joint* (Fig. 1-11) is formed by the head of the proximal phalanx, which is shaped like a short transverse cylinder, and the base of the middle phalanx, which is concave from dorsal to ventral and thus conforms to the cylindrical head. In addition, the phalangeal head has a sagittally oriented groove and the phalangeal base has a sagittally oriented ridge. These surfaces enhance the stability of the joint and ensure that the motion is limited to one degree of freedom, which is in the sagittal plane (flexion and extension).

The *joint capsule* is similar to that of the MCP joint. It is reinforced by the volar plate palmarly, the collateral and retinacular ligaments and the lateral bands on both sides, and the triangular membrane and central band dorsally. These structures blend with the capsule to different degrees and thus move (glide) differently relative to the capsule and to each other.

The *volar plate* (Fig. 1-12) is similar to that of the MCP joint and moves in the same way during flexion and extension. The sides of the proximal attachment are longer than the central part and are referred to as the "*check-rein ligaments.*"[7] These ligaments tighten as the middle phalanx is extended and thus limit hyperextension at the PIP joint. The volar plate is also the attachment for the third annular liga-

ment (A3 pulley) of the fibrous flexor digital tendon sheath. This pulley attaches along the sides of the plate and ensures the flexor tendons stay in place as they cross the joint. The stability of this plate is therefore essential for proper flexor tendon position and function.

The *collateral ligaments* (see Figs. 1-11 and Fig. 1-12) are similar to those of the MCP joints, are triangular in shape, and consist of true (band) and accessory (fan) parts. From their attachment to the dorsal tubercle of the proximal phalanx, the two parts diverge as they cross the joint—the true part attaching to the side of the base of the middle phalanx and the accessory part attaching to the volar plate. The true part is taut throughout the range of motion and thus stabilizes the joint in all positions; the accessory part stabilizes the volar plate.

Like the MCP joints, the PIP joints are reinforced to some degree by components of the extensor mechanism. The central band and triangular membrane are positioned dorsally, and the lateral band and retinacular ligament located on the sides. The tendons of both the flexor digitorum profundus and flexor digitorum superficialis pass volar to the joint.

The *distal interphalangeal (DIP) joint* is quite similar to the PIP joint. The architecture of the articular surfaces is similar, so the motion is limited to only the sagittal plane and that is flexion and extension. The joint capsule, volar plate, and collateral ligaments are also similar, so the motion of each and the support they provide are very much the same as the PIP joints. The volar plate provides an attachment for the fibrous part of the flexor digital tendon sheath; in this case it is the fifth annular ligament (A5 pulley).

The extra-articular structures that cross the joint are quite different. Only the tendon of the flexor digitorum profundus crosses its volar aspect. Dorsally, only the central band blends with the joint capsule as it crosses the joint.

Skin, Retinacular System, and Compartmentation of the Hand

The skin on the dorsum of the hand is different from that on the palmar aspect. The *dorsal skin* is thin, loose, and quite mobile. This mobility is due to a very thin subcutaneous

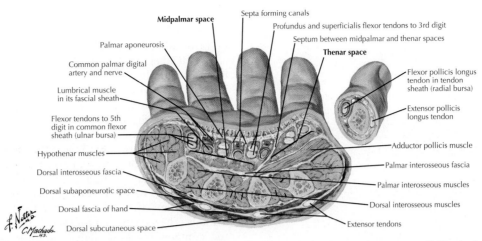

Figure 1-13 Transverse section through the palm of the hand. (Netter illustration from www.netterimages.com. © Elsevier Inc. All rights reserved.)

tissue (superficial fascia) that is loosely attached to the deep fascia. The *palmar skin* is thicker and less mobile. The subcutaneous tissue of the thenar and hypothenar eminences is thick and fatty and thus forms considerable pads. Centrally the palmar skin is firmly attached to the palmar aponeurosis by multiple septa and is thus almost immobile. This arrangement greatly enhances grasp.

The entire upper limb is enclosed in a sleeve of connective tissue called the *investing fascia*. In the arm and forearm this layer is connected medially and laterally to the bones by intermuscular septa with resulting anterior and posterior compartments. This same layer continues into the hand, where it becomes a complex system of fibrous layers and septa that form multiple compartments. Structures of similar function are isolated and confined to individual compartments. Since a retinaculum is a structure (usually composed of connective tissue) that retains other anatomic structures, this is called the *retinacular system*.

At the wrist the investing fascia is reinforced by circumferential bands of fibers both dorsally (extensor retinaculum) and volarly (flexor retinaculum). Both of these retinacula stabilize tendons that enter the hand from the forearm. The *flexor retinaculum* has a more proximal *superficial part*, the superficial part of the flexor retinaculum or the volar carpal ligament, and a deeper distal part called the *deep part* of the flexor retinaculum or the transverse carpal ligament. The deep part forms the volar boundary of the carpal tunnel and is significantly thicker and stronger.

In the hand the investing fascia attaches to both the first and fifth metacarpals (Fig. 1-13). Dorsally it is thin, attaches to the other metacarpals, and is called the *dorsal interosseous fascia*. In the palm it is thin over the thenar (*thenar fascia*) and hypothenar (*hypothenar fascia*) eminences. Centrally it is greatly thickened to form the *palmar aponeurosis*.

This *palmar aponeurosis* (palmar fascia) is a strong fibrous structure composed of fibers that are oriented from proximal to distal. It is narrow proximally where it is continuous with the tendon of the palmaris longus muscle and blends with the transverse carpal ligament. It widens as it is followed distally, and just proximal to the MCP joints it separates into four *digital slips,* which contribute to the formation of the fibrous digital tendon sheaths. The digital slips are interconnected by *transverse fasciculi* proximally and the transversely oriented *superficial transverse metacarpal ligament* at the level of the MCP joints. The palmar aponeurosis is firmly attached to the skin by multiple septa and to the metacarpals by several septa.

Additional fibrous layers separate various structures in the palm and define four definitive compartments. The *thenar septum* extends from the junction of the thenar fascia and the palmar aponeurosis to the first metacarpal and with the thenar fascia forms the *thenar compartment*. Similarly, on the ulnar side of the hand, the *hypothenar septum* extends from the junction of the hypothenar fascia and the palmar aponeurosis to the fifth metacarpal and with the hypothenar fascia forms the *hypothenar compartment*. A deep layer crosses the palm, attaching to the first, third, fourth, and fifth metacarpals. This *adductor–interosseous fascia*, together with a dorsal interosseous fascia that interconnects all of the metacarpals dorsally, forms the *adductor–interosseous compartment*, which more or less is between the metacarpals. The central area of the palm, the *central compartment*, is deep to the palmar aponeurosis, bounded medially and laterally by the hypothenar and thenar septa, respectively, and limited deeply by the adductor–interosseous fascia. Like the compartments in the arm and forearm, these compartments contain muscles that have similar function and are innervated by one or two nerves. The contents of the compartments are listed in Table 1-1 (online).

In addition to these literal compartments that contain muscles and other structures, some *potential spaces* are fascial planes, bursae, or synovial tendon sheaths. These structures normally enhance movement between adjacent structures. However, these potential spaces can become actual spaces when they accumulate blood or inflammatory material, which would, in each case, produce a characteristic swelling.

The *thenar* and *midpalmar clefts* (Figs. 1-13 and 1-14), or spaces, are in a fascial plane between the long digital flexor

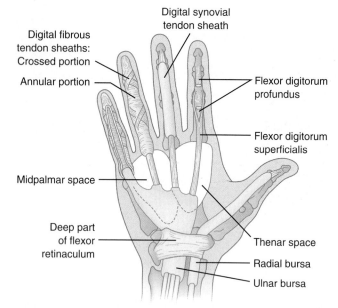

Figure 1-14 Volar view of the hand and wrist depicting the radial and ulnar bursae, digital tendon sheaths, and the thenar and midpalmar spaces.

tendons and the adductor–interosseous fascia. This plane is separated into ulnar midpalmar and radial thenar space by the midpalmar septum that extends between the palmar aponeurosis and the third metacarpal. The thenar space is located on the volar aspect of the adductor pollicis muscle; the midpalmar space on the volar aspects of the medial interossei muscles.

The *radial* and *ulnar bursae* (see Fig. 1-14) are parts of the synovial tendon sheaths of the long digital flexor muscles.

The radial bursa is associated with the flexor pollicis longus muscle and extends from just proximal to the carpal tunnel to the distal phalanx of the thumb. The ulnar bursa is associated with all eight tendons of the flexor digitorum superficialis and profundus muscles in the palm but continues distally into the digit with only those to the little finger. This bursa extends from proximal to the carpal tunnel into the palm and distally to the distal phalanx of the little finger. Digits two, three, and four have individual *synovial digital tendon sheaths* that extend from just proximal to the MCP joints to the distal phalanges. Each of these can also become enlarged.

On the dorsum of the hand there are *two potential planes* (see Fig. 1-13) where fluid can collect: one in the subcutaneous tissue and the other associated with the long extensor tendons. The subcutaneous tissue is dorsal to the metacarpals and contains the long digital extensor tendons, cutaneous nerves, dorsal venous network, and most of the afferent lymphatics from the hand. Since these lymphatics drain most of the hand, inflammation in virtually any part of the hand can lead to a general swelling on the dorsum of the hand. The long extensor tendons, aside from those to the thumb, are enclosed by *supratendinous* and *infratendinous layers of fascia*. These two layers unite on both sides of the group of tendons, thus forming a type of compartment around the tendons. Since the tendons do not occupy the entire side-to-side dimension of the dorsum of the hand, the subcutaneous plane is wider than the tendon plane.

Intrinsic Muscles of the Hand

The intrinsic muscles (Figs. 1-15 and 1-16) are those small muscles that both arise and insert within the hand and generally are involved in the finer movements of the digits. With the exception of the palmaris brevis, these muscles are found

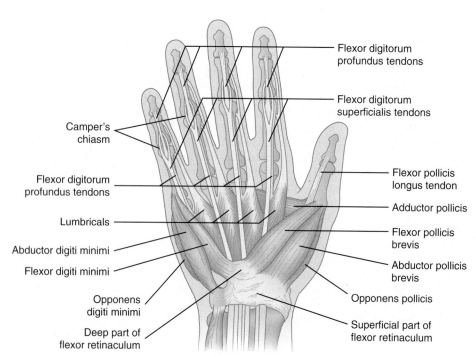

Figure 1-15 Volar view of the superficial muscles of the hand.

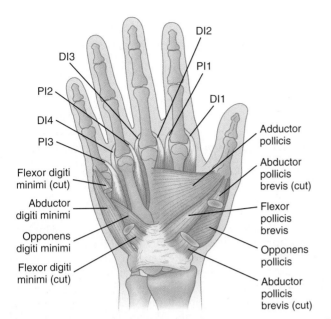

Figure 1-16 Volar view of the deep muscles of the hand. DI, dorsal interosseous; PI, palmar interosseous.

DI2
DI3
PI1
PI2
DI1
DI4
PI3
Adductor pollicis
Flexor digiti minimi (cut)
Abductor pollicis brevis (cut)
Abductor digiti minimi
Flexor pollicis brevis
Opponens digiti minimi
Opponens pollicis
Flexor digiti minimi (cut)
Abductor pollicis brevis (cut)

in the compartments of the hand, and those of each compartment have similar actions. The palmaris brevis is found in the subcutaneous tissue of the palm on the ulnar side at the base. This variable muscle extends from the ulnar side of the palmar aponeurosis to the skin of the medial hand. It is supplied by the superficial branch of the ulnar nerve and pulls the medial skin radially, which aids in grasp.

The *thenar compartment* contains three of the four intrinsic thumb muscles, and all three are supplied by the *recurrent (thenar, motor) branch of the median nerve.* The *abductor pollicis brevis* is superficial and volarly positioned, arising from the transverse carpal ligament and the trapezium and inserting on the ventral aspect of the base of the proximal phalanx of the thumb. It abducts the thumb; that is, moves it away from the index finger in the sagittal plane. The *flexor pollicis brevis* is in the same plane as the abductor and more medial in position. It arises from the transverse carpal ligament and trapezium and inserts on the ventromedial base of the thumb's proximal phalanx. It flexes (coronal plane) both the thumb metacarpal and proximal phalanx. The *opponens pollicis* is the deepest of the three muscles and covers a good part of the shaft of the first metacarpal. From an origin on the transverse carpal ligament and trapezium its fibers pass radially and insert on a line along the volar aspect of the metacarpal. Since its fibers are oblique and it has a linear attachment to the metacarpal, the muscle is ideally positioned to produce axial rotation (opposition) of the metacarpal.

The muscles in the *hypothenar compartment* are similar to those of the thenar compartment and produce similar motions. All three of these muscles are supplied by the *deep branch of the ulnar nerve.* The *abductor digiti minimi* is the most medial in position and extends from the pisiform to the medial aspect of the base of the fifth proximal phalanx. It abducts the little finger at the MCP joint (moves the digit away from the middle finger). The *flexor digiti minimi* is positioned volarly and laterally. From its origin on the hook

of the hamate and the transverse carpal ligament, it extends distally and a bit medially to insert on the medial base of the fifth proximal phalanx. This muscle flexes the little finger at the MCP joint. The *opponens digiti minimi* arises from the hook of the hamate. Its fibers diverge as they pass medially and distally, crossing the metacarpal obliquely, and insert along a line on the medial shaft of the fifth metacarpal. This muscle is in an ideal position to rotate the fifth metacarpal but due to the limited motion at the CMC joint it produces only a small amount of cupping of the medial aspect of the hand.

The *central compartment* contains the *four lumbrical muscles.* Each muscle arises from the flexor digitorum profundus tendon on its ulnar side or from both tendons between which it is positioned. The muscles pass distally, cross volar to the flexion–extension axes of the MCP joints, then insert into both the central and lateral bands of the extensor mechanism. Their actions are to produce flexion at the MCP joints and extension at both the PIP and DIP joints. The mechanism of these functions is more fully explained in the section on the extensor mechanism. The *innervation* of these muscles is similar to that of the flexor digitorum profundus muscle: the two ulnar muscles are supplied by the ulnar nerve; the two radial by the median.

The *adductor–interosseous* compartment contains all of the interossei muscles as well as an intrinsic thumb muscle, the adductor pollicis. All of these muscles are supplied by the *deep branch of the ulnar nerve.* The *adductor pollicis* is the largest of the intrinsic muscles and the only thumb intrinsic not in the thenar compartment. It has two heads: an oblique head, which arises from the lateral distal carpals and adjacent bases of the metacarpals and a transverse head, which arises from the shaft of the third metacarpal. The fibers from this wide origin converge and insert on the ventromedial base of the proximal phalanx of the thumb. This is the major muscle with the capability of adducting the thumb, that is, moving it toward the index finger.

The *palmar* and *dorsal interossei muscles* are found between the metacarpals and are responsible for adducting and abducting the four medial digits. Since the middle finger is the reference for this motion, the location and attachments relative to that finger determine their actions. The *palmar interossei* are the *adductors (PAD)* and the *dorsal* are the *abductors (DAB).* The interossei are also part of the extensor mechanism so they, like the lumbricals, produce *flexion at the MCP joints* and *extension at both the PIP and DIP joints.*

The three *palmar interossei* are positioned so they move the index, ring, and little fingers *toward the middle finger.* Hence, they arise from the lateral aspects of the fourth and fifth metacarpal shafts and the medial aspect of the second metacarpal shaft. They pass distally dorsal to the deep transverse metacarpal ligament but volar to the flexion–extension axis of the MCP joints and insert into both the central and lateral bands of the extensor mechanism. An insertion on the base of the proximal phalanx is variable.

Even though the four *dorsal interossei* are associated with the motion of only the index, middle, and ring fingers, they arise from all five metacarpals. Each of these muscles has two heads of origin so each muscle arises from the sides of adjacent metacarpal shafts. The muscles cross the MCP joints volar to the flexion–extension axes, insert into the sides of the bases of the proximal phalanges, and continue to insert into both the central and lateral bands of the extensor mechanism. The middle finger has two dorsal interossei, which deviate the finger medially and laterally; both of these motions are really abduction because they are moving the digit away from the central reference point.

Tendons of the Extrinsic Muscles of the Hand

The *extrinsic muscles* of the hand are those muscles that arise in the forearm and insert within the hand. These muscles, the long digital flexors and extensors, have muscle bellies located within the forearm and long tendons that cross the wrist and continue into the digits. These tendons have long courses through the hand, and their relationships and surrounding structures are constantly changing as they are followed from the wrist and into the digits. Since they are commonly injured, it is important to understand their relationships along their courses because different adjacent structures may be injured along with the tendons themselves and present different clinical issues. A general comparison of the long digital flexor and extensor tendons is presented in Table 1-2 (online).

The *long digital flexor tendons* (see Fig. 1-15) of the *flexor digitorum profundus (FDP)* and the *flexor digitorum superficialis (FDS)* muscles enter the hand by passing through the carpal tunnel. Just proximal to the tunnel the tendons are in three rows: the FDS tendons to the middle and ring fingers are volar, those to the index and little fingers are intermediate, and all four FDP tendons are dorsal. As the tendons continue into the tunnel, the FDS tendons are volar to those of the FDP. In the palm, they diverge toward their respective digits with the FDP tendons dorsal or deep to the FDS tendons. A lumbrical muscle is on the radial side of each pair of tendons. Each pair of tendons enters the digital tendon sheath just proximal to the volar plate of the MCP joint. The FDS tendon splits (Champer's chiasm) as it crosses the proximal phalanx; the two parts curve dorsally around the FDP tendon and insert on the volar base of the middle phalanx. The orientation of the fibers at this split minimizes the constrictive force transferred to the FDP tendon as it passes through the chiasm.[8] The FDP tendon continues across the middle phalanx and DIP joint and inserts on the volar base of the distal phalanx. The blood supply to these tendons is provided by vessels that enter the tendons in the palm and form longitudinal channels within the tendon itself and through the long and short vincula in the digits. Additionally, vessels enter both tendons through their boney insertions.[9]

The *zones of the flexor tendons* are described and summarized in Table 1-3 (online). These zones are numbered from distal to proximal, and in each zone both the number of structures and the biomechanical considerations change.

The *effectiveness of the extrinsic digital flexor muscles depends on the positions of the joints that they cross.* The FDP affects motion primarily at the DIP joints; the FDS, at the PIP joints. The force generated at all joints by muscle contraction is directly related to the position of the wrist because that

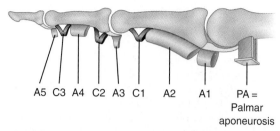

Figure 1-17 *Lateral view of the annular (A) and cruciate (C) ligaments (pulleys) of the fibrous part of the flexor digital tendon sheath as described by Doyle. (Doyle JR. Anatomy of the finger flexor tendon sheath and pulley system.* J Hand Surg. *1988;13A:473-484.)*

position determines the physiologic range in which the muscle operates. Thus, most activities of the hand occur with the wrist in some degree of extension. The tendons of these two muscles glide differently and that is determined by the positions of the joints of the digits (Table 1-4, online). The lumbricals produce flexion at the MCP joints and extension at the PIP and DIP joints. When the FDP shortens the proximal attachments of the lumbrical moves proximally, which increases the physiologic advantage of the lumbrical. Likewise, when flexion occurs at the MCP joint, the proximal movement of the FDP tendon compensates for the shortened lumbrical.

The *flexor tendon sheaths* have two distinct components: a *synovial sheath* that facilitates motion and a *fibrous sheath* that maintains tendon position. In most locations in the body, as in the digits, both components are present. In the palm, however, the synovial sheath is present by itself.

The *fibrous digital tendon sheath* (Fig. 1-17) is limited to each digit and extends from the proximal end of the MCP volar plate to the distal edge of the DIP volar plate. The sheath is considered to be anatomically continuous, but there are multiple points at which it is greatly reinforced by a *concentration of transversely oriented fibers (annular ligaments or annular [A] pulleys)* and points where less robust, *obliquely oriented fibers (cruciform ligaments or curiae [C] pulleys)* are found. The A pulleys are numbered from proximal to distal, so pulleys 1, 3, and 5 are attached to the MCP, PIP, and DIP volar plates, respectively, and pulleys 2 and 4 are associated with the proximal and middle phalanges, respectively.[10] These A pulleys are strong and important functionally because they hold the tendons exactly in position at the most critical places. *Pulleys A2 and A4* are the most important because they ensure the tendons follow the concave volar shafts of the proximal and middle phalanges. The reduction in motion caused by the loss of each A pulley is indicated in Table 1-5 (online). In addition to their importance in preventing bowstringing, the A2 and A4 pulleys, together with the head of the proximal phalanx, maintain a three-point force system that facilitates the onset of flexion at the PIP joint. In the extended digit, the flexor tendons are dorsal in position along the shafts of the proximal and middle phalanges and volar as they cross the PIP joint. As the flexor tendons tighten, they exert a dorsal force on the head of the proximal phalanx and volar forces on the A2 and A4 pulleys, which initiate flexion. This also occurs at the DIP joint but to a lesser degree.

The *cruciate, or C, pulleys* are also numbered from proximal to distal. The term *cruciate* implies that these pulleys are X-shaped, but in reality they may exist only in an oblique form.[11] The two most consistently present are C1 and C3, which are distal to the A2 and A4 pulleys, respectively. Pulley C1 extends from the proximal phalanx to the PIP volar plate; C3 interconnects the middle phalanx and the DIP volar plate. The presence of a C pulley proximal to either pulley A2 or A4 is highly variable.[12] These pulleys may aid in preventing bowstringing, but if so it appears to be minimal.

The *fibrous sheath of the thumb extends* from the proximal margin of the MCP volar plate to the distal margin of the IP volar plate. Annular pulleys are associated with both the MCP and IP volar plates. The pulley associated with the proximal phalanx is oblique, extending from the ulnar base of the proximal phalanx to its radial side near the IP joint. Loss of any single pulley does not appreciably reduce motion. Loss of the proximal annular and the oblique pulleys significantly reduces motion.[13]

The *synovial tendon sheath* (Figs. 1-14 and 1-18) is very much like a bursa in that it consists of two layers, which are continuous and thus form a closed space. Think of a balloon that has lost all its air, so although it is collapsed it still has a potential space if it were reinflated. A bursa is generally more or less flat; a synovial tendon sheath wraps around a tendon until the two sides meet so it doesn't entirely encircle the tendon. The *two layers of the synovial sheath attach to whatever is adjacent to them.* In the case of a digital tendon sheath, *the inner (visceral) layer attaches to the tendon,* and *the outer (parietal) layer attaches to the fibrous part of the tendon sheath.* When a tendon moves, the *gliding motion occurs between the two layers of the synovial tendon sheath* as opposed to between the tendon and the fibrous sheath. The inner surface of the sheath is lined by cells that are similar to those that line the synovial layer of a synovial joint capsule. These cells regulate a minuscule amount of lubricating fluid that is in the space, and they are sensitive to a variety of insults and react by initiating inflammation within the space. Inflammation within a synovial tendon sheath interferes with normal gliding of the tendon and forces the finger into flexion because the space can accommodate more fluid in that position.[14]

The *fibrous part of the digital tendon sheath* forms a very tight and rigid fibro-osseous canal, so there is very little room beyond that taken by the tendons and the synovial part of the sheath. Since the pulleys of the fibrous sheath are not continuous, the sheath is thinner, and thus weaker, between pulleys. Under normal circumstances the synovium bulges slightly, forming "cul-de-sacs," in the weaker areas, either between or next to pulleys; this is particularly true proximal to the A1 pulley because the synovial sheath extends proximal to the fibrous sheath and forms a pouch.[15] With flexion, the visceral layer of the synovial sheath slides proximally with the tendon so the pouch enlarges. With any inflammation in the sheath the bulges enlarge, particularly the pouch proximal to the A1 pulley.

There are *five different synovial tendon sheaths in the palmar hand:* the *ulnar and radial bursae* and *three separate digital tendon sheaths* (see Fig. 1-14). The *ulnar bursa* is associated with all of the tendons of the FDS and FDP muscles. It begins proximal to the carpal tunnel, extends through the tunnel into the palm, and follows the FDS and FDP tendons into the little finger, where it becomes its synovial digital tendon sheath. That part of the ulnar bursa associated with the tendons of the index, middle, and ring fingers ends in the midpalm so there is a *"bare area"* in the palm where there is no synovial sheath. The *radial bursa* is associated with the FPL tendon and extends from proximal to the carpal tunnel to the distal phalanx of the thumb. The three separate *digital synovial sheaths* are associated with the index, middle, and ring fingers and extend from just proximal to the MCP joints to the distal phalanges of those digits.

The *tendons of the extrinsic extensor muscles* enter the hand by passing deep to the extensor retinaculum; these muscles are *three wrist extensors,* the *abductor pollicis longus,* and *five digital extensors.* The *extensor retinaculum* extends from the radius laterally to the ulna medially and is connected to those bones by five septa that form *six separate compartments* deep to the retinaculum. These compartments are numbered from radial to ulnar and illustrated in Figure 1-19. The tendons of the extrinsic extensors pass through these compartments and thus are stabilized at the wrist. While in the compartments, the tendons have synovial sheaths that begin proximal to and extend distal to the retinaculum. Generally, a single synovial sheath is associated with all tendons in a compartment but there is variability, particularly in first compartment. The contents of these compartments, the synovial sheaths, and the terminations (insertions) of the tendons are summarized in Table 1-6 (online).

On the dorsolateral hand, in the region of the base of the thumb, the tendons of the APL, EPB, and EPL define the *anatomic "snuff box"* (see Fig. 1-19). The APL and EPB tendons form the anterior boundary. The EPL tendon forms the posterior boundary; it is positioned more posteriorly because it passes around the dorsal radial tubercle (of Lister) as it enters the hand. The floor of the snuff box is formed by the scaphoid. The radial artery passes diagonally across the scaphoid toward the first web space, and branches of the superficial radial nerve cross the tendons forming the boundaries.

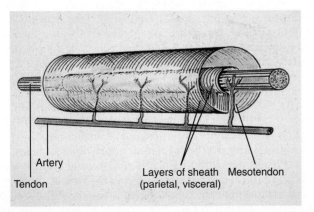

Figure 1-18 View of a synovial tendon sheath. Note that the sheath does not totally surround the tendon and that there is a space within the sheath in this illustration. In reality, that space is a potential space because the two layers of the sheath are separated only by a thin layer of fluid.

Artery

Tendon

Layers of sheath (parietal, visceral) Mesotendon

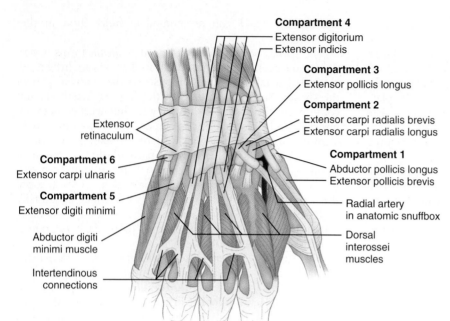

Compartment 4
Extensor digitorium
Extensor indicis

Compartment 3
Extensor pollicis longus

Compartment 2
Extensor carpi radialis brevis
Extensor carpi radialis longus

Compartment 1
Abductor pollicis longus
Extensor pollicis brevis

Radial artery
in anatomic snuffbox

Dorsal
interossei
muscles

Extensor
retinaculum

Compartment 6
Extensor carpi ulnaris

Compartment 5
Extensor digiti minimi

Abductor digiti
minimi muscle

Intertendinous
connections

Figure 1-19 View of the tendons of the extrinsic extensor muscles on the dorsum of the wrist and hand.

The *tendons to the four medial digits are the extensor digitorum (ED), extensor indicis proprius (EI), and the extensor digiti minimi (EDM)*. The tendons of the ED and EI muscles pass through extensor compartment four, and that of the EDM passes through compartment five. Distal to the wrist, the ED tendons diverge toward the MCP joints, with the EI and EDM tendons passing to the index and the little fingers, respectively. These tendons are thin and flat, and because there is minimal subcutaneous tissue, they are close to the metacarpals and dorsal interossei and the skin. Just proximal to the MCP joints, the ED tendons to all four digits may be interconnected by *intertendinous connections* (juncture tendinum) (see Fig. 1-19), but those of the middle, ring, and little fingers almost always are. These connections are oblique, passing distally from the ring finger tendon to those of the middle and little fingers. Because of this orientation, independent motion of the three fingers is limited, meaning that when the middle and little fingers are flexed at the MCP joints, it is difficult to actively extend the ring finger.[16]

The *extensor mechanism (retinaculum, aponeurosis)* (Fig. 1-20, online) is the system of fibrous bands on the dorsum and sides of the digits that extends from just proximal to the MCP joint to the distal phalanx on each digit. This structure is very important to both the motion and balance of the digit and has multiple components.

As the extensor tendon crosses the MCP joint, it is not functionally attached to the proximal phalanx but rather to the *extensor hood*. This hood is a circumferential band of fibers that sweeps around the joint. The sides of this hood are in the sagittal plane and attach volarly to the volar plate. They are known as the *sagittal bands*.[17] Distal to the sagittal bands the fibers of the hood are more obliquely oriented. The hood functions as a sling, sliding distally with flexion and proximally with extension, and is the mechanism through which the extensor tendon(s) extends the proximal phalanx

at the MCP joint. The hood also anchors and stabilizes the extensor tendon in its central position.

Just distal to the MCP joint the extensor tendon separates into a single *central band* (slip) and a pair of *lateral bands* (slips). The central band continues along the proximal phalanx, crosses the PIP joint, and attaches to the dorsal base of the middle phalanx. The lateral bands diverge as they pass distally, crossing the sides of the PIP joint just dorsal to its flexion–extension axis. They continue distally and converge dorsally to form a single band that crosses the dorsal aspect of the DIP joint and attaches to the dorsal base of the distal phalanx. Even though both the lateral and central bands are direct continuations of the extensor tendons, they are only minimally controlled by the extensor muscles because the excursion of the ED muscle is primarily utilized at the MP joint.[18] However, *since both the lumbrical and interossei muscles attach to the central and lateral bands, they effectively are the tendons of those muscles*. The lumbricals and interossei pass ventral to the flexion–extension axis of the MCP joint and thus flex the proximal phalanx, and by virtue of their attachments to the central and lateral bands, these muscles extend both the middle and distal phalanges.

The *maintenance of the position of the lateral bands* as they cross the PIP joint is critical to the normal position and motion of the digit. This position is maintained by two fibrous supports. The *triangular membrane* interconnects the lateral bands dorsal to the middle phalanx and the PIP joint and prevents them from migrating volarly. That is, the membrane ensures that the lateral bands cross the PIP dorsal to the flexion–extension axis. The *retinacular ligament* has two components, and both of these prevent dorsal migration of the lateral bands.[19] The transverse retinacular ligament originates from the volar capsule of the PIP joint and flexor pulleys and inserts at the conjoined lateral tendon at the proximal half of the middle plalanx. The oblique retinacular (Landsmeer's) ligament originates on the palmar plate and flexor sheath volar to the PIP joint and inserts in the terminal tendon.[20] The oblique retinacular ligament is likely the more important in stabilizing the lateral band. It passes volar to the flexion–extension axis of the PIP joint and it *links motion at the PIP and DIP joints*. As the distal phalanx is flexed, the lateral bands are pulled distally, which adds tension to the oblique ligaments. This increases the flexion force at the PIP joint and thus causes flexion of the middle phalanx. Conversely, as the middle phalanx is extended, the oblique ligaments are stretched, which adds tension to the lateral bands and causes extension of the distal phalanx. In other words, the distal phalanx cannot be flexed without the middle phalanx also being flexed, nor can the middle phalanx be extended without the distal phalanx also being extended. However, if Landsmeer's ligaments are a bit slack, the lateral bands can slide dorsally and the PIP joint can be "locked" in extension. Then, the distal phalanx can be flexed while the middle phalanx remains extended.

Even though the *thumb has a modified extensor hood*, extension of the middle and distal phalanges is rather straightforward and performed by the extensor pollicis brevis (EPB) and extensor pollicis longus (EPL), respectively. The modified hood is the superficial layer of fibrous support on the dorsum and sides of the thumb and is considerably stronger and heavier on the ulnar side. That side is formed by the tendon and aponeurosis of the AP; it is wide and extends dorsally to blend with the tendons of the EPB and EPL. The radial side is formed by the APB and FPB tendons, which also pass dorsally to blend with the EPB and EPL tendons.

Digital Balance

The position of a digit at rest, as well as during motion, is dependent on the forces on the flexor and extensor sides of the finger. These forces are both dynamic (muscular) and static (ligamentous). The relaxed posture of each digit— slight flexion at each joint with the amount of flexion increasing from the index to little fingers—reflects these forces and that the flexor forces exceed those on the extensor side. Loss of any force produces a predictable change in the natural posture (deformity) and typically an opposite dynamic loss. For example, loss of the central band as it crosses the DIP joint produces a flexed distal phalanx (mallet finger) and an inability to extend the distal phalanx.

The *normal dorsal and volar forces* at the MCP, PIP, and DIP joints are summarized in Table 1-7 (online) and illustrated in Figure 1-20 (online). On the volar aspect of the digit, the FDP muscle is the only force at the DIP joint, and it contributes to the flexor forces at both the PIP and MP joints. The FDS muscle is the primary force at the PIP joint, and it contributes to the volar force at the MP joint. Flexor force at the MP joint is provided by the lumbrical and interossei muscles as well as from the two long digital flexors. Although the flexor force at the MP joint is provided by multiple muscles, the specific source of that force varies considerably and is largely dependent on the position of the wrist. The force in a strong grasp occurs at the DIP and PIP joints, and, if the wrist is extended, at the MCP joints as well.

Flexion of the proximal phalanges by the lumbricals and interossei occurs when the hand is performing delicate maneuvers. The only *static force on the flexor side* of the digit is at the PIP joint, which is provided by the oblique part of the retinacular ligament.

The only *extensor force* across the MP joint is provided by the ED, EI, and EDM muscles; if they provide any force across the PIP and DIP joints it is minimal. At both the PIP and DIP joints, the major muscular force is supplied by the lumbrical and interossei muscles. The oblique portion of the retinacular ligament is a static support across the extensor aspect of the DIP joint, and the triangular membrane is a static support across the PIP joint.

Incompetence of the oblique retinacular ligament or the transverse retinacular ligament results in a dorsal displacement of the lateral bands, which increases the extensor force at the PIP joint. Loss of the oblique ligament also removes a flexor force at the PIP joint, so the net result is an imbalance of force in favor of the extensor side so there is hyperextension of the middle phalanx. This hyperextension causes an increase in the tension in the tendons of both the FDP and FDS muscles, which produces flexion of both the distal and proximal phalanges. The resulting position, hyperextension at the PIP joint and flexion at both the DIP and MP joints, is referred to as a *swan-neck deformity*.

Destruction of the soft structures dorsal to the PIP joint produces a different deformity. This is an example of a *deformity resulting from loss of both static and dynamic forces*. Loss of the *central band* removes the lumbrical and interossei force (and that of the ED if any exists) and loss of the *triangular membrane* allows the lateral bands to slide volarly. Force across the extensor side of the joint is reduced; if the volar displacement of the lateral bands is sufficient (volar to the flexion–extension axis), virtually all extensor force is lost, and force may be added to the flexor side. In either case the balance of power shifts toward the flexor side of the PIP joint and flexion results. The passive tension in the tendons of the FDP and FDS muscles is reduced, resulting in extension of the distal and proximal phalanges. This position, flexion of the PIP joint and extension at both the MP and DIP joints, is referred to as a *boutonnière (buttonhole) deformity*.

A deformity resulting from a *nerve injury results from loss of dynamic forces*. An injury of the ulnar nerve in Guyon's canal is considered a *"low" ulnar nerve injury*. This type of injury results in loss of the AP, all interossei, the two medial lumbricals, and the muscles in the hypothenar compartment. Of those muscles, the ones contributing to the flexion–extension balance of the digits are the interossei and lumbricals. The deformity resulting from such an injury is aptly called the *incomplete claw*. The loss of the interossei and lumbrical muscles reduces the dynamic force across the volar aspect of the MCP joint and most, if not all, of the dynamic force across the dorsal aspects of the PIP and DIP joints. This reduces the flexor force at the MCP joints and the extensor force at the PIP and DIP joints, which results in an increase in extensor force at the MCP joints and the flexor force at the PIP and DIP joints. The result is the clawlike posture when hyperextension occurs at the MCP joints and flexion occurs at the PIP and DIP joints. Since the lumbricals and interossei are both lost in the little and ring fingers and only the interossei are lost in the ring and middle fingers, the claw is more severe in the little and ring fingers.

Nerve Supply of the Hand

The muscular and cutaneous nerve supply to the hand is summarized in Table 1-8 (online).

Three *peripheral nerves*, the median, ulnar, and superficial radial, supply the hand (Figs. 1-21 and 1-22, online). The *median* nerve is the major cutaneous nerve of the hand. It has a small *palmar* branch in the distal forearm that passes superficially into the hand and supplies the skin of the base of the thumb. Just proximal to the wrist the median nerve is located between the tendons of the palmaris longus and flexor carpi radialis muscles. It enters the hand, passing through the carpal tunnel as the most volar structure. Just distal to the tunnel it branches into its terminal branches: the recurrent (motor, muscular) branch and several digital branches. The *recurrent branch* passes laterally and supplies the muscles in the thenar compartment. It is in a superficial position, about midway between the pisiform and the thumb MCP joint, and therefore vulnerable to laceration. The *digital branches* are of two types. A *common palmar digital nerve* supplies adjacent sides of two fingers; it passes toward a webspace, where it divides into two proper palmar digital nerves. Each *proper digital nerve* supplies the side of a single digit. It extends to the end of a digit and supplies the volar half of the skin to the PIP joint and the volar and dorsal aspects distal to that. A proper digital nerve also supplies the joints of the digit.

The *ulnar nerve* is the major muscular nerve of the hand. Just proximal to the wrist it is positioned deep to the tendon of the flexor carpi ulnaris muscle. It enters the hand in company with the ulnar artery by passing lateral to the pisiform, superficial to the pisohamate ligament, deep to the palmaris brevis muscle, and then medial to the hook of the hamate (Guyon's canal). This is a vulnerable part of its course because it is superficial and thus vulnerable to laceration, and it crosses the robust pisohamate ligament so it is vulnerable to external compression. In the canal or just distal, the nerve branches into superficial and deep branches. Aside from supplying the palmaris brevis muscle, the *superficial branch* is a cutaneous nerve and usually divides into one common palmar and one proper palmar digital nerve. The *deep branch* is muscular and has no cutaneous distribution. It passes through the hypothenar compartment and then accompanies the deep palmar arterial arch, passing laterally in a position deep to the long digital flexor tendons. The deep branch terminates laterally, where it enters the adductor pollicis muscle. The ulnar nerve has a *dorsal cutaneous branch*, which arises proximal to the wrist. This branch enters the hand by passing dorsally across the medial aspect of the wrist. On the dorsum of the hand it has common and proper dorsal digital branches. Its distribution is variable but typically it supplies the medial digit and a half as far distally as the PIP joint and the corresponding part of the dorsum of the hand.

The *superficial radial nerve* is purely cutaneous and supplies the dorsolateral aspect of the hand. It enters the hand by passing superficially across the anatomic snuff box and the tendon of the extensor pollicis longus. It branches into common and proper dorsal digital nerves and, although variable, typically supplies the lateral three and a half digits as far distally as the PIP joints and the corresponding part of the dorsal hand.

The *segmental innervation* is provided by four spinal cord segments. The skin of the lateral hand, thumb, and index finger is supplied by spinal cord segment C6; that of the middle finger by C7; and the medial hand, ring, and little fingers by C8. The intrinsic muscles of the hand are supplied by spinal cord segments C8 and T1, the lateral ones by C8 and the medial by T1.

Blood Supply of the Hand

The hand is supplied by the *radial* and *ulnar arteries* (see Figs. 1-21 and 1-22, online). These arteries form two arterial arches, and the branches of these arches have multiple interconnections so arterial collateralization in the hand is rich.

The *ulnar artery* enters the hand by passing lateral to the pisiform and medial to the hook of the hamulus, in Guyon's canal. It is accompanied by the ulnar nerve. While in the canal or just distally, the artery splits into its larger superficial branch and smaller deep branch. The *superficial branch* sweeps laterally across the palm and is the primary contributor to the *superficial palmar arterial arch*. This arch is at the level of the distal aspect of the fully extended thumb and positioned between the palmar aponeurosis and the long digital flexor tendons. The arch is typically completed by the *superficial palmar branch* of the radial artery although the connection may be very small or even absent. The branches of the arch are *common palmar digital arteries* to adjacent sides of two digits and *proper palmar digital arteries* to one side of a single digit. Typically, the branches are a proper digital to the medial aspect of the little finger and three common digitals to the little, ring, middle, and index fingers. The arteries to the thumb and lateral aspect of the index finger are usually branches of the radial artery but may branch from the superficial arch or both. The *deep branch* of the ulnar artery passes through the hypothenar compartment and then turns laterally to complete the deep palmar arterial arch.

Proximal to the wrist the *radial artery* is just lateral to the tendon of the flexor carpi radialis, where its superficial palmar branch arises. The radial artery then passes dorsally across the lateral aspect of the wrist and passes through the anatomic snuff box. Just distal to the tendon of the EPL it reaches the first webspace, where it turns volarly, passing between the two heads of the first dorsal interosseous to reach the palm. Once in the palm the radial artery becomes the *deep palmar arterial arch*; this arch is completed by the deep branch of the ulnar artery and positioned about a thumb's width proximal to the superficial arch between the long digital flexor tendons and the interossei and metacarpals. The deep arch is accompanied by the deep branch of the ulnar nerve. The most lateral branch of the deep arch is usually the *princeps pollicis artery* to the thumb. The next branch is the *radialis indicis artery*, which supplies the lateral aspect of the index finger. A variable number of *metacarpal arteries* branch from the deep arch and join the common digital branches of the superficial arch in the distal palm.

Both the radial and ulnar arteries have *palmar* and *dorsal carpal branches*. The branches unite off of their respective surfaces of the carpus to form *palmar* and *dorsal arches (rete)* that are somewhat variable.

REFERENCES

The complete reference list is available online at www.expertconsult.com.

Anatomy and Kinesiology of the Wrist 📹

RICHARD A. BERGER, MD, PhD

BONY ANATOMY	VASCULAR ANATOMY
JOINT ANATOMY	KINEMATICS
LIGAMENT ANATOMY	KINETICS
TENDONS	SUMMARY

CRITICAL POINTS

Anatomy
- Bones: Two rows
- Ligaments: Dorsal, palmar, intercarpal
- Membranes: Scapholunate and triquetrolunate
- Pedicles: Radioscapholunate

Normal Kinetics
- Proximal row moves as a unit
- Proximal row is intercalated segment—no tendons attach to it
- Ligaments provide stability
- Lunate is keystone

The wrist is a unique joint interposed between the distal aspect of the forearm and the proximal aspect of the hand. All three regions have common or shared elements, which integrate form and function to maximize the mechanical effectiveness of the upper extremity. The wrist enables the hand to be placed in an infinite number of positions relative to the forearm and also enables the hand to be essentially locked to the forearm in those positions to transfer the forces generated by the powerful forearm muscles.

Although the wrist is truly a mechanical marvel when it is intact and functioning, loss of mechanical integrity of the wrist inevitably causes substantial dysfunction of the hand and thus the entire upper extremity. It is vital that a thorough understanding of the wrist, including efforts at diagnosis, treatment, and rehabilitation, be acquired by all who treat the wrist. This chapter provides such a foundation by explor-

ing the general architecture of the wrist; the bones; and joints that comprise the wrists and the soft tissues that stabilize, innervate, and perfuse the wrist. In addition, an overview of the mechanics of the wrist, with a discussion of its motions and subparts and the force distribution across the wrist, is provided.

Bony Anatomy

There are eight carpal bones, although many consider the pisiform to be a sesamoid bone within the tendon of the flexor carpi ulnaris (FCU), and thus not behaving as a true carpal bone. The bones are arranged into two rows (proximal and distal carpal row), each containing four bones. All eight carpal bones are interposed between the forearm bones and the metacarpals to form the complex called the *wrist* joint.

Distal Radius and Ulna

The distal surface of the radius articulates with the proximal carpal row through two articular fossae separated by a fibro-cartilaginous prominence oriented in the sagittal plane called the *interfossal ridge* (Figs. 2-1 and 2-2). The scaphoid fossa is roughly triangular in shape and extends from the interfossal ridge to the tip of the radial styloid process. The lunate fossa is roughly quadrangular in shape and extends from the interfossal ridge to the sigmoid notch. On the dorsal cortex of the distal radius, immediately dorsal and proximal to the interfossal ridge, is a bony prominence called the *dorsal tubercle of the radius,* or *Lister's tubercle* (see Fig. 2-1). It serves as a divider between the second and third extensor compartments and functionally behaves as a trochlea for the

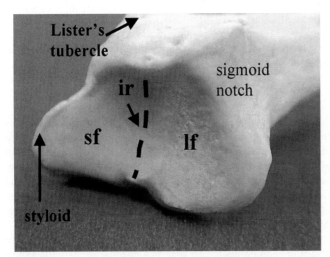

Figure 2-1 Distal radius from a distal and ulnar perspective. ir, Interfossal ridge; lf, lunate fossa; sf, scaphoid fossa.

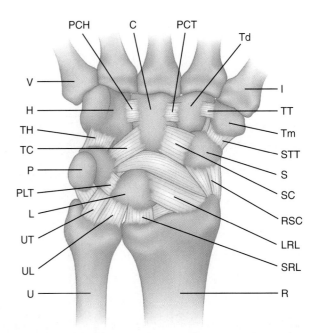

Figure 2-3 Wrist from palmar perspective. Bones: C, Capitate; H, hamate; I, first metacarpal; L, lunate; P, pisiform; R, radius; S, scaphoid; Td, trapezoid; Tm, trapezium; U, ulna; V, fifth metacarpal. *Ligaments:* LRL, Long radiolunate; PCH, palmar capitohamate; PCT, palmar trapezocapitate; PLT, palmar lunotriquetral; RSC, radioscaphocapitate; SC, scaphocapitate; SRL, short radiolunate; STT, scaphoid-trapezium-trapezoid; TC, triquetrocapitate; TH, triquetrohamate; TT, trapezium-trapezoid; UL, ulnolunate; UT, ulnotriquetral.

tendon of extensor pollicis longus. On the medial surface of the distal radius is the sigmoid notch. This concave surface articulates with the ulnar head to form the distal radioulnar joint (DRUJ). It has a variable geometry across a population, both in shape and orientation, but is largely felt to be symmetrical in any given individual.

Under normal circumstances, the ulna does not articulate directly with the carpus. Rather, a fibrocartilaginous wafer called the *triangular disk* is interposed between the ulnar head and the proximal carpal row (see Fig. 2-2). Even the ulnar styloid process is hidden from contact with the carpus by the ulnotriquetral (UT) ligament. The ulnar head is roughly cylindrical in shape, with a distal projection on its posterior border, called the *ulnar styloid process.* Approximately three fourths of the ulnar head is covered by articular carti-

lage, with the ulnar styloid process and the posterior one fourth as exposed bone or periosteum. A depression at the base of the ulnar styloid process, called the *fovea,* is typically not covered in articular cartilage.

Proximal Carpal Row Bones

The proximal row consists of, from radial to ulnar, the scaphoid (navicular), lunate, triquetrum, and pisiform (Figs. 2-3 and 2-4). The scaphoid is shaped somewhat like a kidney bean. The scaphoid anatomy is divided into three regions: the proximal pole, waist, and distal pole. The proximal pole has a convex articular surface that faces the scaphoid fossa and a flat articular surface that faces the lunate. The dorsal surface of the waist is marked by an oblique ridge that serves as an attachment plane for the dorsal joint capsule. The medial surface of the waist and distal surface of the proximal pole is concave and articulates with the capitate. The distal pole also articulates with the capitate medially, but distally it articulates with the trapezium and trapezoid. Otherwise, the distal pole is nearly completely covered with ligament attachments.

The lunate is crescent-shaped in the sagittal plane, such that the proximal surface is convex and the distal surface concave, and it is somewhat wedge-shaped in the transverse plane. With the exception of ligament attachment planes on its dorsal and palmar surfaces, the lunate is otherwise covered with articular cartilage. It articulates with the scaphoid laterally, the radius and triangular fibrocartilage proximally, the triquetrum medially, and the capitate distally. In some individuals, the lunate has a separate fossa for articulation with

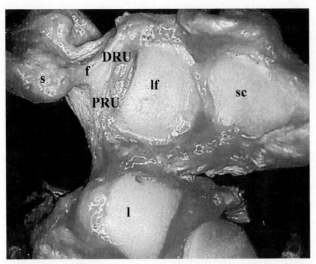

Figure 2-2 Radiocarpal joint from a distal perspective, prepared by palmar-flexing the proximal carpal row. The triangular disk is seen between the distal radioulnar (DRU) and palmar radioulnar (PRU) ligaments. The interfossal ridge is seen between the scaphoid and lunate fossae. f, Foveal attachment of triangular fibrocartilage complex (TFCC); l, lunate; lf, lunate fossa of the distal radius; s, styloid attachment of TFCC; sf, scaphoid fossa.

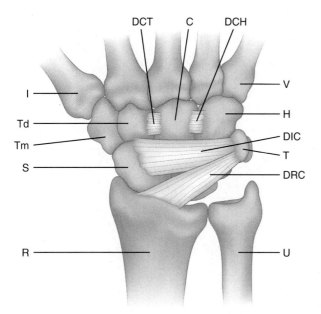

Figure 2-4 *Wrist from dorsal perspective. Bones:* C, Capitite; H, hamate; I, first metacarpal; R, radius; S, scaphoid; T, triquetrum; Td, trapezoid; Tm, trapezium; U, ulna; V, fifth metacarpal. *Ligaments:* DCH, Dorsal capitohamate; DCT, dorsal trapezocapitate; DIC, dorsal intercarpal; DRC, dorsal radiocarpal.

the hamate, separated from the fossa for capitate articulation by a prominent ridge.

The triquetrum has a complex shape, with a flat articular surface on the palmar surface for articulation with the pisiform; a concave distal articular surface for articulation with the hamate; a flat lateral surface for articulation with the lunate; and three tubercles on the proximal, medial, and dorsal surfaces, respectively. The proximal tubercle is covered in cartilage for contact with the triangular disk, and the medial and dorsal tubercles serve as ligament attachment surfaces.

The pisiform, which means "pea-shaped," is oval in profile with a flat articular facet covering the distal half of the dorsal surface for articulation with the triquetrum. Otherwise, it is entirely enveloped within the tendon of the FCU and serves as a proximal origin of the flexor digiti minimi muscle.

Distal Carpal Row Bones

The distal carpal row consists of, from radial to ulnar, the trapezium, trapezoid, capitate, and hamate (see Figs. 2-3 and 2-4). The trapezium, historically referred to as the *greater multangular*, has three articular surfaces. The proximal surface is slightly concave and articulates with the distal pole of the scaphoid. The medial articular surface is flat and articulates with the trapezoid. The distal surface is saddle-shaped and articulates with the base of the first metacarpal. The remaining surfaces are nonarticular and serve as attachment areas for ligaments. The anterolateral edge of the trapezium forms an overhang, referred to as the *beak*, which is part of the fibro-osseous tunnel for the tendon of flexor carpi radialis (FCR).

The trapezoid, referred to historically as the *lesser multangular*, is a small bone with articular surfaces on the proximal,

lateral, medial, and distal surfaces for articulation with the scaphoid, trapezium, capitate, and base of the second metacarpal, respectively. The palmar and dorsal surfaces serve as ligament insertion areas.

The capitate is the largest carpal bone and is divided into head, neck, and body regions. The head is almost entirely covered in articular cartilage and forms a proximally convex surface for articulation with the scaphoid and lunate. The neck is a narrowed region between the body and the head and is exposed to the midcarpal joint without ligament attachment. The body is nearly cuboid in shape with articular surfaces on its medial, lateral, and distal aspects for articulation with the trapezoid, hamate, and base of the third metacarpal, respectively. The large, flat palmar and dorsal surfaces serve as ligament attachment areas.

The hamate has a complex geometry, with a pole, body, and hamulus (hook). The pole is a conical proximally tapering projection that is nearly entirely covered in articular cartilage for articulation with the triquetrum, capitate, and variably the lunate. The body is relatively cuboid, with medial and distal articulations for the capitate and fourth and fifth metacarpal bases, respectively. The dorsal and palmar surfaces serve as ligament attachment areas, except the most medial aspect of the body, where the hamulus arises. The hamulus forms a palmarly directed projection that curves slightly lateral at the palmar margin. This also serves as a broad area for ligament attachment.

Joint Anatomy

Before a discussion of the anatomy of the wrist can be pursued, it is important that a consensus be reached on term definitions. The terms *proximal* and *distal* are universally understood, but some confusion may exist regarding terms defining relationships in other planes. Although the terms *medial* and *lateral* are anatomically correct, they require a virtual positioning of the upper extremity in the classic anatomic position to be interpretable. Therefore the terms *radial* and *ulnar* have been introduced by clinicians to enable an instant understanding of orientation independent of upper extremity positioning, because the reference to these terms (the orientation of the radius and ulna) does not change significantly relative to the wrist. Likewise, the terms *anterior, volar,* and *palmar* all describe the front surface of the wrist, whereas *dorsal* and *posterior* describe the back surface of the wrist. Some may object to using the term *palmar* in reference to the wrist, but they should be reminded that the palmar, glabrous skin covers the anterior surface of the carpus; therefore it seems to have an acceptable use in the wrist.

Composed of eight carpal bones as the wrist proper, the wrist should be functionally considered as having a total of 15 bones. This is because of the proximal articulations with the radius and ulna and the distal articulations with the bases of the first through fifth metacarpals. The geometry of the wrist is complex, demonstrating a transverse arch created by the scaphoid and triquetrum/pisiform column proximally and the trapezium and hamate distally. In addition, the proximal carpal row demonstrates a substantial arch in the frontal plane.

The distal radioulnar joint (DRUJ) is mechanically linked to the wrist and provides two additional degrees of motion to the wrist/forearm joint. The DRUJ is the distal of two components of the forearm joint (with the proximal radioulnar joint, or PRUJ). The motion exhibited through the DRUJ is a combination of translation and rotation, created as a pivot of the radius about the ulna through an obliquely oriented axis of rotation passing between the radial head proximally and the ulnar head distally.

From an anatomic standpoint, the carpal bones are divided into proximal and distal carpal rows, each consisting of four bones. This effectively divides the wrist joint spaces into radiocarpal and midcarpal spaces. Although mechanically linked to the distal radioulnar joint (DRUJ), the wrist is normally biologically separated from the DRUJ joint space by the triangular fibrocartilage complex (TFCC).

Radiocarpal Joint

The radiocarpal joint is formed by the articulation of confluent surfaces of the concave distal articular surface of the radius and the triangular fibrocartilage, with the convex proximal articular surfaces of the proximal carpal row bones.

Midcarpal Joint

The midcarpal joint is formed by the mutually articulating surfaces of the proximal and distal carpal rows. Communications are found between the midcarpal joint and the interosseous joint clefts of the proximal and distal row bones, as well as to the second through fifth carpometacarpal joints. Under normal circumstances, the midcarpal joint is isolated from the pisotriquetral, radiocarpal, and first carpometacarpal joints by intervening membranes and ligaments. The geometry of the midcarpal joint is complex. Radially, the scaphotrapezial trapezoidal (STT) joint is composed of the slightly convex distal pole of the scaphoid articulating with the reciprocally concave proximal surfaces of the trapezium and trapezoid. Forming an analog to a "ball-and-socket joint" are the convex head of the capitate and the combined concave contiguous distal articulating surfaces of the scaphoid and the lunate. In 65% of normal adults, it has been found that the hamate articulates with a medial articular facet at the distal ulnar margin of the lunate, which is associated with a higher rate of cartilage eburnation of the proximal surface of the hamate. The triquetrohamate region of the midcarpal joint is particularly complex, with the mutual articular surfaces having both concave and convex regions forming a helicoid-shaped articulation.

Interosseous Joints: Proximal Row

The interosseous joints of the proximal row are relatively small and planar, allowing motion primarily in the flexion–extension plane between mutually articulating bones. The scapholunate (SL) joint has a smaller surface area than the lunatotriquetral (LT) joint. Often, a fibrocartilaginous meniscus extending from the membranous region of the SL or LT interosseous ligaments is interposed into the respective joint clefts.

Interosseous Joints: Distal Row

The interosseous joints of the distal row are more complex geometrically and allow substantially less interosseous motion than those of the proximal row. The capitohamate joint is relatively planar, but the mutually articulating surfaces are only partially covered by articular cartilage. The distal and palmar region of the joint space is devoid of articular cartilage, being occupied by the deep capitohamate interosseous ligament. Similarly, the central region of the trapeziocapitate joint surface is interrupted by the deep trapeziocapitate interosseous ligament. The trapezium-trapezoid joint presents a small planar surface area with continuous articular surfaces.

Ligament Anatomy

Overview

The ligaments of the wrist have been described in a number of ways, leading to substantial confusion in the literature regarding various features of the carpal ligaments. Several general principles have been identified to help simplify the ligamentous architecture of the wrist. No ligaments of the wrist are truly extracapsular. Most can be anatomically classified as capsular ligaments with collagen fascicles clearly within the lamina of the joint capsule. The ligaments that are not entirely capsular, such as the interosseous ligaments between the bones within the carpal row, are intra-articular. This implies that they are not ensheathed in part by a fibrous capsular lamina. The wrist ligaments carry consistent histologic features, which are, to a degree, ligament-specific. The majority of capsular ligaments are made up of longitudinally oriented laminated collagen fascicles surrounded by loosely organized perifascicular tissue, which are in turn surrounded by the epiligamentous sheath. This sheath is generally composed of the fibrous and synovial capsular lamina. The perifascicular tissue has numerous blood vessels and nerves aligned longitudinally with the collagen fascicles. The function of these nerves is currently not well understood. It has been hypothesized that these nerves are an integral part of a proprioceptive network, following the principals of Hilton's law of segmental innervation. The palmar capsular ligaments are more numerous than the dorsal, forming almost the entire palmar joint capsules of the radiocarpal and midcarpal joints. The palmar ligaments tend to converge toward the midline as they travel distally and have been described as forming an apex-distal V. The interosseous ligaments between the individual bones within a carpal row are generally short and transversely oriented and, with specific exceptions, cover the dorsal and palmar joint margins. Specific ligament groups are briefly described in the following sections and are divided into capsular and interosseous groups.

Distal Radioulnar Ligaments

Although a description of the DRUJ is beyond the scope of this chapter, a brief description of the anatomy of the palmar and dorsal radioulnar ligaments is required to understand the origin of the ulnocarpal ligaments. The dorsal and palmar

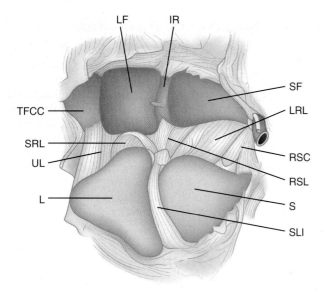

Figure 2-5 Radiocarpal joint from distal perspective after palmar-flexing the proximal carpal row. IR, Interfossal ridge; L, lunate; LF, lunate fossa of distal radius; LRL, long radiolunate ligament; RSC, radioscaphocapitate ligament; RSL, radioscapholunate ligament; S, scaphoid; SF, scaphoid fossa of distal radius; SLI, scapholunate interosseous; SRL, short radiolunate ligament; TFCC, triangular fibrocartilage complex; UL, ulnolunate ligament.

DRUJ ligaments are believed to be major stabilizers of the DRUJ. These ligaments are found deep (proximal) in the TFCC and form the dorsal and palmar margins of the TFCC in the region between the sigmoid notch of the radius and the styloid process of the ulna (see Fig. 2-2). Attaching radially at the dorsal and palmar corners of the sigmoid notch, the ligaments converge ulnarly and attach near the base of the styloid process, in the region called the *fovea*. The palmar ligament has substantial connections to the carpus through the ulnolunate (UL), UT, and ulnocapitate (UC) ligaments. The dorsal ligament integrates with the sheath of extensor carpi ulnaris (ECU). The concavity of the TFCC is deepened by more superficial fibers of the distal radioulnar ligament complex, which attaches to the styloid process.

Palmar Radiocarpal Ligaments

The palmar radiocarpal ligaments arise from the palmar margin of the distal radius and course distally and ulnarly toward the scaphoid, lunate, and capitate (Figs. 2-3 and 2-5). Although the course of the fibers can be defined from an anterior view, the separate divisions of the palmar radiocarpal ligament are best appreciated from a dorsal view through the radiocarpal joint (see Fig. 2-5). The palmar radiocarpal ligament can be divided into four distinct regions. Beginning radially, the radioscaphocapitate (RSC) ligament originates from the radial styloid process, forms the radial wall of the radiocarpal joint, attaches to the scaphoid waist and distal pole, and passes palmar to the head of the capitate to interdigitate with fibers from the UC ligament. Very few fibers from the RSC ligament attach to the capitate. Just ulnar to the RSC ligament, the long radiolunate (LRL) ligament arises to pass palmar to the proximal pole of the scaphoid and the SL interosseous ligament to attach to the radial margin of the palmar horn of the lunate. The interligamentous sulcus

separates the RSC and LRL ligaments throughout their courses. The LRL ligament has been called the *radiolunato-triquetral ligament* historically, but the paucity of fibers continuing toward the triquetrum across the palmar horn of the lunate renders this name misleading. Ulnar to the origin of the LRL ligament, the radioscapholunate (RSL) "ligament" emerges into the radiocarpal joint space through the palmar capsule and merges with the SL interosseous ligament and the interfossal ridge of the distal radius. This structure resembles more of a "mesocapsule" than a true ligament, because it is made up of small-caliber blood vessels and nerves from the radial artery and anterior interosseous neurovascular bundle. Very little organized collagen is identified within this structure. The mechanical stabilizing effects of this structure have recently been shown to be minimal. The final palmar radiocarpal ligament, the short radiolunate (SRL) ligament, arises as a flat sheet of fibers from the palmar rim of the lunate fossa, just ulnar to the RSL ligament. It courses immediately distally to attach to the proximal and palmar margin of the lunate.

Dorsal Radiocarpal Ligament

The dorsal radiocarpal (DRC) ligament arises from the dorsal rim of the radius, essentially equally distributed on either side of Lister's tubercle (see Fig. 2-4). It courses obliquely distally and ulnarly toward the triquetrum, to which it attaches on the dorsal cortex. There are some deep attachments of the DRC ligament to the dorsal horn of the lunate. Loose connective and synovial tissue forms the capsular margins proximal and distal to the DRC ligament.

Ulnocarpal Ligaments

The ulnocarpal ligament arises largely from the palmar margin of the TFCC, the palmar radioulnar ligament, and in a limited fashion, the head of the ulna. It courses obliquely distally toward the lunate, triquetrum, and capitate (Fig. 2-6). The ulnocarpal ligament has three divisions, designated by their distal bony insertions. The UL ligament is essentially continuous with the SRL ligament, forming a continuous palmar capsule between the TFCC and the lunate. Confluent with these fibers is the UT ligament, connecting the TFCC and the palmar rim of the triquetrum. In 60% to 70% of normal adults, a small orifice is found in the distal substance of the UT ligament, which leads to a communication between the radiocarpal and pisotriquetral joints. Just proximal and ulnar to the pisotriquetral orifice is the prestyloid recess, which is generally lined by synovial villi and variably communicates with the underlying ulnar styloid process. The UC ligament arises from the foveal and palmar region of the head of the ulna, where it courses distally, palmar to the UL and UT ligaments, and passes palmar to the head of the capitate, where it interdigitates with fibers from the RSC ligament to form an arcuate ligament to the head of the capitate. Few fibers from the UC ligament insert to the capitate.

Midcarpal Ligaments

The midcarpal ligaments on the palmar surface of the carpus are true capsular ligaments, and as a rule, they are short and

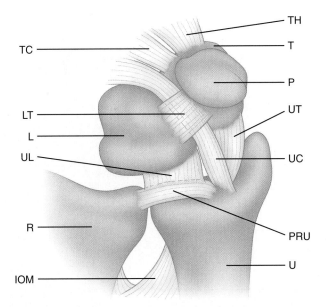

Figure 2-6 *Ulnocarpal and distal radioulnar joint complex from palmar perspective. Bones: L, Lunate; P, pisiform; R, radius; T, triquetrum; U, ulna. Ligaments: LT, Palmar lunotriquetral; PRU, palmar radioulnar; TC, triquetrocapitate; TH, triquetrohamate; UC, ulnocapitate; UL, ulnolunate; UT, ulnotriquetral. IOM, interosseous membrane.*

stout, connecting bones across a single joint space (see Figs. 2-3 and 2-6). Beginning radially, the STT ligament forms the palmar capsule of the STT joint, connecting the distal pole of the scaphoid with the palmar surfaces of the trapezium and trapezoid. Although no clear divisions are noted, it forms an apex-proximal V shape. The scaphocapitate (SC) ligament is a thick ligament interposed between the STT and RSC ligaments, coursing from the palmar surface of the waist of the scaphoid to the palmar surface of the body of the capitate. There are no formal connections between the lunate and capitate, although the arcuate ligament (formed by the RSC and UC ligaments) has weak attachments to the palmar horn of the lunate. The thick triquetrocapitate (TC) ligament, which is analogous to the SC ligament, passes from the palmar and distal margin of the triquetrum to the palmar surface of the body of the capitate. Immediately adjacent to the TC ligament, the triquetrohamate (TH) ligament forms the ulnar wall of the midcarpal joint and is augmented ulnarly by fibers from the TFCC. The dorsal intercarpal (DIC) ligament, originating from the dorsal cortex of the triquetrum, crosses the midcarpal joint obliquely to attach to the scaphoid, trapezoid, and capitate (see Fig. 2-4). The attachment of the DIC ligament to the triquetrum is confluent with the triquetral attachment of the DRC ligament. In addition, a proximal thickened region of the joint capsule, roughly parallel to the DRC ligament, extends from the waist of the scaphoid across the distal margin of the dorsal horn of the lunate to the triquetrum. This band, called the *dorsal scaphotriquetral ligament,* forms a "labrum," which encases the head of the capitate, analogous to the RSC and UC ligaments palmarly.

Proximal Row Interosseous Ligaments

The SL and LT interosseous ligaments form the interconnections between the bones of the proximal carpal row and share

several anatomic features. Each forms a barrier between the radiocarpal and midcarpal joints, connecting the dorsal, proximal, and palmar edges of the respective joint surfaces (see Fig. 2-5). This leaves the distal edges of the joints without ligamentous coverage. The dorsal and palmar regions of the SL and LT interosseous ligaments are typical of articular ligaments, composed of collagen fascicles with numerous blood vessels and nerves. However, the proximal regions are made up of fibrocartilage, devoid of vascularization and innervation and without identifiable collagen fascicles. The RSL ligament merges with the SL interosseous ligament near the junction of the palmar and proximal regions. The UC ligament passes directly palmar to the LT interosseous ligament with minimal interdigitation of fibers.

Distal Row Interosseous Ligaments

The bones of the distal carpal row are rigidly connected by a complex system of interosseous ligaments (see Figs. 2-3 and 2-4). As is discussed later, these ligaments are largely responsible for transforming the four distal row bones into a single kinematic unit. The trapezium-trapezoid, trapeziocapitate, and capitohamate joints are each bridged by palmar and dorsal interosseous ligaments. These ligaments consist of transversely oriented collagen fascicles and are covered superficially by the fibrous capsular lamina, also consisting of transversely oriented fibers. This lamina gives the appearance of a continuous sheet of fibers spanning the entire palmar and dorsal surface of the distal row. Unique to the trapeziocapitate and capitohamate joints are the "deep" interosseous ligaments (Fig. 2-7). These ligaments are entirely intra-articular, spanning the respective joint spaces between voids in the articular surfaces. Both are true ligaments with dense, colinear collagen fascicles, but they are also heavily invested with nerve fibers. The deep trapeziocapitate interosseous ligament is located midway between the palmar and dorsal limits of the joint, obliquely oriented from palmar-ulnar to dorsal-radial, and each measures approximately 3 mm in diameter. The respective attachment sites of the trapezoid and capitate are angulated in the transverse plane to accommodate the orthogonal insertion of the ligament. The deep capitohamate interosseous ligament is found

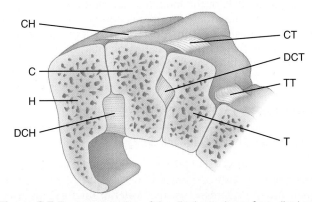

Figure 2-7 *Transverse section of the distal carpal row from distal and radial perspective. C, Capitate; CH, dorsal capitohamate ligament; CT, dorsal trapezocapitate ligament; DCH, deep capitohamate ligament; DCT, deep trapezocapitate ligament; H, hamate; T, trapezoid; TT, dorsal trapezium-trapezoid ligament.*

transversely oriented at the palmar and distal corner of the joint. It traverses the joint from quadrangular voids in the articular surfaces and measures approximately 5 × 5 mm in cross-sectional area.

Tendons

The tendons that cross the wrist can be divided into two major groups: those that are responsible primarily for moving the wrist and those that cross the wrist in their path to the digits. Both groups impart some moment to the wrist, but obviously those that are primary wrist motors have a more substantial influence on motion of the wrist. The five primary wrist motors can be grouped as either radial or ulnar deviators and as either flexors or extensors.

The extensor carpi radialis longus (ECRL) and extensor carpi radialis brevis (ECRB) muscles are bipennate and originate from the lateral epicondyle of the humerus from a common tendon. Over the distal radius epiphysis, they are found in the second extensor compartment, from which they emerge to insert into the radial cortices of the bases of the second and third metacarpals, respectively. The ECRL imparts a greater moment for radial deviation than the ECRB, whereas the opposite relationship is found for wrist extension. Both the ECRL and the ECRB muscles are innervated by the radial nerve.

The ECU muscle is bipennate and originates largely from the proximal ulna and passes through the sixth extensor compartment. Within the sixth extensor compartment, the ECU tendon is contained within a fibro-osseous tunnel between the ulnar head and the ulnar styloid process. Distal to the extensor retinaculum, the ECU tendon inserts into the ulnar aspect of the base of the fifth metacarpal. The ECU muscle is innervated by the radial nerve.

The FCR muscle is bipennate and originates from the proximal radius and the interosseous membrane. The tendon of FCR enters a fibro-osseous tunnel formed by the distal pole of the scaphoid and the beak of the trapezium; it then angles dorsally to insert into the base of the second metacarpal. This fibro-osseous tunnel is separate from the carpal tunnel. The FCR muscle is innervated by the median nerve.

The FCU muscle is unipennate and originates from the medial epicondyle of the humerus and the proximal ulna. It is not constrained by a fibro-osseous tunnel, in distinction to the other primary wrist motors. It inserts into the pisiform and ultimately continues as the pisohamate ligament. The FCU muscle is innervated by the ulnar nerve.

Vascular Anatomy

Extraosseous Blood Supply

The carpus receives its blood supply through branches from three dorsal and three palmar arches supplied by the radial, ulnar, anterior interosseous, and posterior interosseous arteries (Fig. 2-8). The three dorsal arches are named (proximal to distal) the *radiocarpal, intercarpal,* and *basal metacarpal transverse arches.* Anastomoses are often found between the arches, the radial and ulnar arteries, and the interosseous

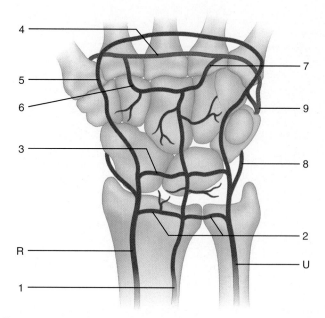

Figure 2-8 Palmar extraosseous blood supply of the wrist. *1,* Anterior interosseous artery; *2-4,* transverse anastomotic arches; *5,* deep branch of radial artery; *6-9,* longitudinal anastomotic network. *R,* Radial artery; *U,* ulnar artery.

artery system. The palmar arches are named (proximal to distal) the *radiocarpal, intercarpal,* and *deep palmar* arches.

Intraosseous Blood Supply

All carpal bones, with the exception of the pisiform, receive their blood supply through dorsal and palmar entry sites and usually from more than one nutrient artery. Generally, a number of small-caliber penetrating vessels are found in addition to the major nutrient vessels. Intraosseous anastomoses can be found in three basic patterns. First, a direct anastomosis can occur between two large-diameter vessels within the bone. Second, anastomotic arcades may form with similar-sized vessels, often entering the bone from different areas. A final pattern, although rare, has been identified in which a diffuse arterial network virtually fills the bone.

Although the intraosseous vascular patterns of each carpal bone have been defined in detail, studies of the lunate, capitate, and scaphoid are particularly germane because of their predilection to the development of clinically important vascular problems. The lunate has only two surfaces available for vascular penetration: the dorsal and palmar. From the dorsal and palmar vascular plexuses, two to four penetrating vessels enter the lunate through each surface. Three consistent patterns of intraosseous vascularization have been identified, based on the pattern of anastomosis. When viewed in the sagittal plane, the anastomoses form a Y, X, or an I pattern with arborization of small-caliber vessels stemming from the main branches. The proximal subchondral bone is consistently the least vascularized. The capitate is supplied by both the palmar and dorsal vascular plexuses; however, the palmar supply is more consistent and originates from larger caliber vessels. Just distal to the neck of the capitate, vessels largely from the ulnar artery penetrate the palmar-ulnar cortex, whereas dorsal penetration occurs just distal to the midwaist level. The intraosseous vascularization pattern consists of proximally directed retrograde flow, with minimal anastomoses between dorsal and palmar vessels. When present, the dorsal vessels principally supply the head of the capitate, whereas the palmar vessels supply both the body and the head of the capitate. The scaphoid typically receives its blood supply through three vessels originating from the radial artery: lateral-palmar, dorsal, and distal arterial branches. The lateral-palmar vessel is believed to be the principal blood supply of the scaphoid. All vessels penetrate the cortex of the scaphoid distal to the waist of the scaphoid, coursing in a retrograde fashion to supply the proximal pole. Although there have been reports of minor vascular penetrations directly into the proximal pole from the posterior interosseous artery, substantial risk for avascular necrosis of the proximal pole remains with displaced fractures through the waist of the scaphoid. Overall, it is thought that the remaining carpal bones generally have multiple nutrient vessels penetrating their cortices from more than one side, hence substantially reducing their risk of avascular necrosis.

Kinematics

Overview

Within 1 year after the announcement of the discovery of x-rays in 1895, Bryce published a report of a roentgenographic investigation of the motions of the carpal bones. This marked a turning point for basic mechanical investigations of the wrist. The number of published biomechanical investigations of the wrist have increased almost exponentially over the past three decades. As such, a review of all mechanical analyses of the wrist is well beyond the scope of this chapter. Rather, an overview of basic biomechanical considerations of the wrist is presented in the following categories: kinematics, kinetics, and material properties.

The global range of motion (ROM) of the wrist, measured clinically, is based on angular displacement of the hand about the "cardinal" axes of motion: palmar flexion/dorsiflexion and radioulnar deviation. The conicoid motion generated by combining displacement involving all four directions of motion is called *circumduction*. A functional axis of motion has also been described as the *dart-thrower's* axis, which moves the wrist–hand unit from an extreme of dorsiflexion/radial deviation to an extreme of palmar flexion/ulnar deviation. The magnitude of angular displacement in any direction varies greatly between individuals, but in "normal" individuals, it generally falls within the ranges of palmar flexion (65–80 degrees), dorsiflexion (65–80 degrees), radial deviation (10–20 degrees), ulnar deviation (20–35 degrees), forearm pronation (80 degrees), and forearm supination (80 degrees).

Several attempts to define the "functional" ranges of wrist motion required for various tasks of daily living, as well as vocational and recreational activities, have been performed using axially aligned electrogoniometers fixed to the hand and forearm segments of volunteers. Although some variability between results was found, the vast majority of tested tasks could be accomplished with 40 degrees of dorsiflexion, 40 degrees of palmar flexion, and 40 degrees of combined

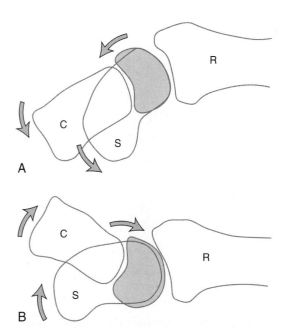

Figure 2-9 *Schematic of carpal bone motion during wrist palmar-flexion* **(A)** *and dorsiflexion* **(B).** *Note that all three bones essentially move in the same plane synchronously. C, Capitate; R, radius; S, scaphoid (lunate shown as shaded bone).*

radial and ulnar deviation. The concept of a "center of rotation" of the wrist has been tested by a number of techniques and widely debated. It is generally agreed, however, that an approximation of an axis of flexion–extension motion of the hand unit on the forearm passes transversely through the head of the capitate, as does a separate orthogonal axis for radioulnar deviation. It must be remembered that the global motion of the wrist is a summation of the motions of the individual carpal bones through the intercarpal joints as well as the radiocarpal and midcarpal joints. Thus, although easier to understand, the concept of a center of rotation of the wrist is at best an approximation and of limited basic and clinical usefulness.

Individual Carpal Bone Motion

The bones within each row display kinematic behaviors that are more similar than those observed between the two rows. Because the kinematic behaviors of the carpal bones are measurably different between palmar flexion/dorsiflexion and radioulnar deviation, these two arcs of motion are considered separately (Figs. 2-9 and 2-10). More recently, attention has been drawn to the importance of the "dart thrower's" axis of motion. This is a combination of the cardinal motions defined later on, in which the wrist passes from radial deviation and extension through flexion and ulnar deviation. This represents a more physiologic motion pattern than pure flexion–extension and radial–ulnar deviation. It is being analyzed extensively in the laboratory for possible implications in injury patterns and rehabilitation advantages.

Palmar Flexion/Dorsiflexion

The metacarpals are pulled through the range of palmar flexion and dorsiflexion by the action of the extrinsic wrist

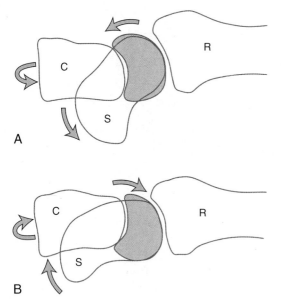

Figure 2-10 *Schematic of carpal bone motion during wrist radial devia-tion **(A)** and ulnar deviation **(B)**. Note that the scaphoid and lunate primarily palmar-flex during radial deviation and dorsiflex during ulnar deviation. This behavior is called* conjunct rotation. *C, Capitate; R, radius; S, scaphoid (lunate shown as shaded bone).*

motors attaching to their bases. The hand unit, made up of the metacarpals and phalanges, is securely associated with the distal carpal row through the articular interlocking and strong ligamentous connections of the second through fifth carpometacarpal joints. The trapezoid, capitate, and hamate undergo displacement with their respective metacarpals with no significant deviation of direction or magnitude of motion (see Fig. 2-9). Because of the strong interosseous ligaments, the trapezium generally tracks with the trapezoid but remains under the influence of the mobile first metacarpal. The major direction of motion for this entire complex is palmar flexion and dorsiflexion, with little deviation in radioulnar deviation and pronation–supination.

In general, the proximal row bones follow the direction of motion of the distal row bones during palmar flexion/dorsi-flexion of the wrist (see Fig. 2-9). However, the scaphoid, lunate, and triquetrum are not as tightly secured to the hand unit as are the distal row bones by virtue of the midcarpal joint. In addition, the interosseous ligaments between the proximal row bones allow for substantial intercarpal motion. Thus measurable differences occur between the motions of the proximal and distal row bones, as well as between the individual bones of the proximal carpal row. This is most pronounced between the scaphoid and lunate. From the extreme of palmar flexion to the extreme of dorsiflexion, the scaphoid undergoes substantially more angular displacement than the lunate, primarily in the plane of hand motion. Measurable "out-of-plane" motions occur between the scaph-oid and lunate as well because the scaphoid progressively supinates relative to the lunate as the wrist dorsiflexes. The effect of the differential direction and magnitude of displace-ment between the scaphoid and lunate is to create a relative separation between the palmar surfaces of the two bones as dorsiflexion is reached and a coaptation of the two surfaces

as palmar flexion is reached. The extremes of displacement are checked by the "twisting" of the fibers of the interosseous ligaments. Once this limit is reached, the scaphoid and lunate move as a unit through the radiocarpal and midcarpal joints. Similar, although of lesser magnitude, behaviors occur through the LT joint. In all, the lunate experiences the least magnitude of rotation of all carpal bones during palmar flexion and dorsiflexion. The radiocarpal and midcarpal joints contribute nearly equally to the range of dorsiflexion and palmar flexion of the wrist when measured through the capitolunate–radiolunate joint column. In contrast, when measured through the radioscaphoid–STT joint column, more than two thirds of the ROM occurs through the radioscaphoid joint.

Radioulnar Deviation

As with palmar flexion and dorsiflexion, the bones of the distal row move essentially as a unit with themselves as well as with the second through fifth metacarpals during radial and ulnar deviation of the wrist (see Fig. 2-10). However, the proximal row bones display a remarkably different kinematic behavior. As a unit, the proximal carpal row displays a "recip-rocating" motion with the distal row, such that the principal motion during wrist radial deviation is palmar flexion (see Fig. 2-10). Conversely, during wrist ulnar deviation, the proximal carpal row dorsiflexes. In addition to the palmar flexion/dorsiflexion activity of the proximal carpal row, a less pronounced motion occurs, resulting in ulnar displacement during wrist radial deviation and radial displacement during wrist ulnar deviation. Additional longitudinal axial displace-ments occur between the proximal carpal row bones, as they do during palmar flexion and dorsiflexion. Although of sub-stantially lower magnitude than the principal directions of rotation, these longitudinal axial displacements contribute to a relative separation between the palmar surfaces of the scaphoid and lunate in wrist ulnar deviation and a relative coaptation during wrist radial deviation, limited by the taut-ness of the SL interosseous ligament. Once maximum tension is achieved, the two bones displace as a single unit. As with palmar flexion and dorsiflexion, the lunate experiences the least magnitude of rotation of all carpal bones during radial and ulnar deviation. The magnitude of rotation through the midcarpal joint is approximately 1.5 times greater than the radiocarpal joint during radial and ulnar deviation.

Kinetics

Force Analysis

Force analyses of the wrist have been attempted using a variety of methods, including the analytical methods of free-body diagrams and rigid-body spring models and experi-mental methods using force transducers, pressure-sensitive film, pressure transducers, and strain gauges. Because of the intrinsic geometric complexity of the wrist, the large number of carpal elements, the number of tissue interfaces that loads are applied to, and the large number of positions that the wrist can assume, these analyses have been difficult and are riddled with assumptions. Thus relative changes and trends

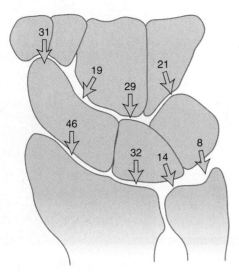

Figure 2-11 *Schematic of the wrist showing the approximate load percentages transmitted across the midcarpal joint and the percentages transmitted across the radiocarpal joint.*

in forces brought about by the introduction of experimental variables are generally more useful than absolute values.

Normal Joint Forces

Experimental and analytical studies of force transmission across the wrist in the neutral position are in general agreement that approximately 80% of the force is transmitted across the radiocarpal joint and 20% across the ulnocarpal joint space (Fig. 2-11). This can be further compartmentalized into forces across the UL articulation (14%) and the UT articulation (8%). In the neutral position, one study reported that 78% of the longitudinal force across the wrist is transmitted through the radiocarpal articulation, with 46% transmitted by the radioscaphoid fossa and 32% by the lunate fossa. Forces across the midcarpal joint in a neutrally positioned joint have been estimated to be 31% through the STT joint, 19% through the SC joint, 29% through the lunatocapitate joint, and 21% transmitted through the triquetrohamate joint. In general, it has been shown that forearm pronation increases ulnocarpal force transmission (up to 37% of total forces transmitted), with a corresponding decrease in radiocarpal force transmission. This has been theoretically linked to the relative distal prominence of the ulna that occurs in forearm pronation. The ulnocarpal force transmission increases to 28% of the total in ulnar deviation of the wrist,

whereas radiocarpal forces increase to 87% of the total in radial deviation. Wrist palmar flexion and dorsiflexion have only a modest effect on the relative forces transmitted through the radiocarpal and ulnocarpal joints.

Normal Joint Contact Area and Pressure

With use of pressure-sensitive film placed in the radiocarpal joint space, three distinct areas of contact through the radiocarpal joint have been identified: radioscaphoid, radiolunate, and UL. Overall, it has been determined that the actual area of contact of the scaphoid and lunate against the distal radius and TFCC are quite limited, regardless of joint position, averaging 20% of the entire available articular surface. The scaphoid contact area was greater than that of the lunate by an average factor of 1.5. The centroids of the contact areas shift with varying positions of the wrist, as do the areas of contact. For example, palmar flexion of the scaphoid results in a dorsal and radial shift of the radioscaphoid contact centroid and a progressive diminution of contact area. With externally applied loads, the peak articular pressures are low, ranging from 1.4 to 31.4 N/mm.[2] The midcarpal joint has been difficult to evaluate using pressure-sensitive film because of its complex shape. It has been estimated that less than 40% of the available articular surface of the midcarpal joint is in actual contact at any one time. The relative contribution to the total contact of the STT, SC, lunatocapitate, and triquetrohamate joints have been estimated to be 23%, 28%, 29%, and 20%, respectively. Thus it may be surmised that more than 50% of the midcarpal load is transmitted through the capitate across the scaphocapitate and lunatocapitate joints.

Summary

The wrist is a complex joint and truly a mechanical marvel. A thorough understanding of the anatomy and kinesiology of the wrist is required by all involved in any aspect of diagnosis, treatment, and rehabilitation of wrist disorders. This understanding provides the insight and foundation needed in the approach to conservative, operative, or rehabilitation management.

REFERENCES

The complete reference list is available online at www.expertconsult.com.

Anatomy and Kinesiology of the Elbow 📹

JULIE E. ADAMS, MD AND SCOTT P. STEINMANN, MD

BIOMECHANICS
ANATOMY
SUMMARY

CRITICAL POINTS

- A functional and stable elbow allows for the complex motions of flexion and extension and pronation–supination necessary for daily life.
- The functional range of motion of the elbow joint has been determined to be 30 to 130 degrees in the flexion extension arc and 50 degrees each of pronation and supination.
- The elbow joint is a trochleoginglymoid joint that has complex motion in flexion–extension and axial rotation difficult to reapproximate with implants or external fixators.
- Stability of the elbow is conferred by bony congruity, ligamentous structures, and dynamic action of muscular forces.
- A posterior utilitarian approach to the elbow is useful for addressing many conditions. Variations exist to deal with specific problems.
- An understanding and appreciation of the complex anatomy of the elbow joint, including the soft tissues and neurovascular structures, is essential to understand and treat pathology about this joint.

The elbow joint functions as a link between the arm and forearm to position the hand in space and allow activities of prehension; it transmits forces and it allows the forearm to act as a lever in lifting and carrying. A functional and stable elbow allows for the complex motions of flexion and extension and pronation–supination necessary for daily life.[1] Stability of the elbow is conferred by bony congruity, ligamentous restraints, and dynamic stabilization by muscular forces. Biomechanical aspects of the elbow are considered in the context of motion, function, and stability. An understanding of the anatomic features contributing to these roles is critical and is outlined in this chapter.

Biomechanics

It has been determined that although the normal arc of motion of the elbow is 0 to 150 or 160 degrees in the flexion extension arc and 75 to 85 degrees each of pronation and supination, a functional range of motion in which most activities of daily living can be accomplished is 30 to 130 degrees in flexion extension and 50 degrees each of pronation and supination.[2] When the elbow is affected by pathologic conditions, the ability to place the hand in space is diminished.

In full extension, 60% of axial loads are transmitted across the radiocapitellar joint while 40% of loads are transmitted across the ulnohumeral joint[3] (Fig. 3-1, online). With elbow flexion, the relationship is altered such that loads are equally shared between the ulnohumeral and radiocapitellar articulations.[4]

In the flexion–extension arc the elbow does not follow motion of a simple hinge joint; the obliquity of the trochlear groove and ulnar articulation results in a helical pattern of motion[1,5] (Fig. 3-2). The varus–valgus laxity over the arc of flexion–extension measures 3 to 4 degrees. The center of rotation in the sagittal plane lies anterior to the midline of the humerus and is colinear with the anterior cortex of the distal humerus. The axis of rotation runs through the center of the articular surface on both the anteroposterior and lateral planes (Fig. 3-3, online). Forearm rotation occurs through an axis oblique to both the longitudinal axis of the radius and the ulna, through an imaginary line between the radial head at the proximal radioulnar joint and the ulnar head at the distal radioulnar joint.[1] As described in the analogy by Kapandji, the distal and proximal radioulnar joints function as the hinges of a door. Disruption of either hinge results in loss of complete motion in pronation or supination.[1,6]

Anatomy

Osteology

Palpable bony landmarks about the elbow include the medial and lateral epicondyles, the radial head, and the olecranon[7] (Figs. 3-4 and 3-5).

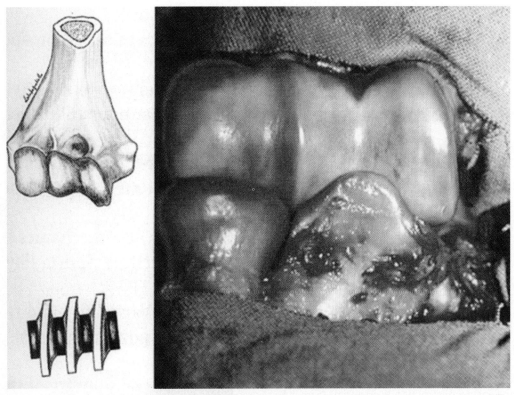

Figure 3-2 The olecranon moves on the articular surface of the trochlea like a screw tapping on it. (Celli A. Chapter 1: Anatomy and biomechanics of the elbow. In: Celli A, Celli L, Morrey BF, eds. *Treatment of Elbow Lesions: New Aspects in Diagnosis and Surgical Techniques*. Milan, Springer-Verlag Italia, 2008, pp. 1–11. Used with permission from Springer-Verlag.)

The prominent medial and lateral epicondyles serve as the attachment point for the medial collateral ligament (MCL), the flexor pronator group and lateral collateral ligament complex (LCL), and the common extensor tendon origin. The distal humerus articulates with the proximal ulna via the trochlea, a spool-shaped surface. The center of the medullary canal is offset laterally to the center of the trochlea. The olecranon, together with the coronoid process, forms the semilunar or greater sigmoid notch of the ulna (Fig. 3-6). This articulates with the trochlea of the humerus and confers stability and facilitates motion in the anteroposterior plane.[7] The lateral ridge of the trochlea is less prominent than the medial side, resulting in a 6- to 8-degree valgus orientation and creating the valgus carrying angle of the arm.[8] Laterally, the capitellum articulates with the proximal radius. The radius also articulates with the lesser sigmoid notch of the ulna. Together, the hinge motion at the trochlea–proximal ulnar articulation and the rotational motion at the radiocapitellar joint provide the complex motion at the elbow in flexion–extension and forearm rotation.

Anatomically, a transverse "bare area" devoid of cartilage is found at the midpoint between the coronoid and the tip of the olecranon. The unwary surgeon may inadvertently discard structurally significant portions of the olecranon if this is not considered when reconstructing a fracture.[9] The anterior portion of the sigmoid notch is represented by the coronoid, which has increasingly been recognized as an important contributor to stability of the elbow (Fig. 3-7, online). Posteriorly, the olecranon tip is the attachment site of the triceps. McKeever and Buck determined in the laboratory that one may excise up to 80% of the olecranon without sacrificing stability if the coronoid and anterior soft tissues are intact.[10,11] In addition, An and colleagues[12] noted increasing instability of the elbow with olecranon excision in a linear fashion, with laboratory data suggesting that loss of up to 50% of the olecranon may be associated with no instability. If anterior damage is present, instability results if too much proximal ulna is excised. Significant coronoid loss, such as occurs with untreated coronoid fractures, will lead

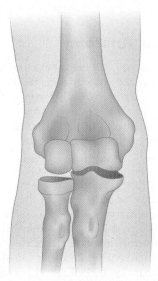

Figure 3-4 Anterior elbow osseous anatomy.

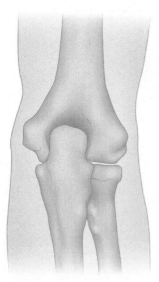

Figure 3-5 Posterior elbow osseous anatomy.

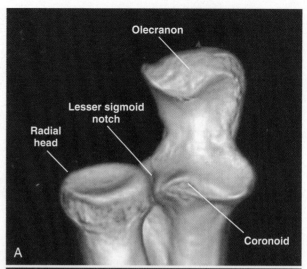

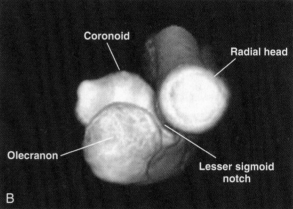

Figure 3-6 A, B, The proximal ulna and radius aspects with the bone landmarks (CT 3D reconstruction). (Celli A. Chapter 1: Anatomy and bio-mechanics of the elbow. In: Celli A, Celli L, Morrey BF, eds. *Treatment of Elbow Lesions: New Aspects in Diagnosis and Surgical Techniques.* Milan, Springer-Verlag Italia, 2008, pp. 1–11. Used with permission from Springer-Verlag.)

to instability.[13,14] The clinical importance is that severely comminuted olecranon fractures in the absence of anterior injury may be treated with partial excision, particularly in elderly or low-demand patients. However, if significant anterior damage is present, reconstruction is essential[9] (Fig. 3-8).

The articular surface of the radial head is oriented at a 15-degree angle to the neck away from the radial tuberosity[7] (Fig. 3-9). The radial head has been called a secondary stabilizer of the elbow. In the setting of a ligamentously intact elbow, fracture or removal of the radial head renders the joint unstable. However, in the setting of MCL deficiency, the radial head becomes crucial to stability against valgus forces[15] (Fig. 3-10, online). The portion of the radial head that articulates with the capitellum is an eccentric dish-shaped structure with a variable offset from the neck,[16] both of which factors have implications for fracture fixation or prosthetic replacement. Likewise, the portion of the radial head that articulates with the proximal ulna has clinically important features. The cartilage of the radial head encompasses an arc of about 280 degrees about the rim of the radius.

Ligamentous Anatomy

Ligamentous structures that contribute to the stability of the elbow joint include the collateral ligaments and the capsule both anteriorly and posteriorly.[17] Dynamic stability is conferred by the actions of the muscles crossing the joint.

Medially, the medial collateral ligament consists of the anterior oblique ligament (AOL), the posterior oblique ligament (POL), and the transverse ligament[7,17] (Fig. 3-11). The AOL of the MCL is the most important stabilizer to valgus stresses and should be preserved or reconstructed.[15,17–20] The AOL has two bands: an anterior band that is tight from 0 to 60 degrees and a posterior band that is tight from 60 to 120 degrees.[19] The AOL and POL arise from the central portion of the anterior inferior medial epicondyle[21] and insert near the sublime tubercle (AOL) and in a fan-shaped insertion along the semilunar notch (POL).[22] The transverse segment of the MCL appears to have little functional significance.[23]

The lateral ligament complex includes the radial collateral ligament, the lateral ulnar collateral ligament (LUCL), the annular ligament, and the accessory LCL (Fig. 3-12). The LUCL serves as the major lateral ligamentous stabilizer. It arises from the inferior aspect of the lateral epicondyle and inserts on the supinator crest. It has near isometry during the flexion extension arc.[7] The radial collateral ligament also arises from the lateral epicondyle and inserts on the radial head along the annular ligament. The annular ligament arises and inserts on the anterior and posterior margins of the lesser sigmoid notch. It functions to stabilize the radial head in contact with the ulna. Because of the eccentric dish-shaped nature of the radial head, the anterior leaf of the ligament becomes tight in supination and the posterior portion becomes tight in pronation.[23,24]

The joint capsule has been regarded as a passive stabilizer of the elbow; however, conflicting opinions exist regarding this point. Morrey and An suggest that it functions as a stabilizer to varus–valgus stresses and against distraction loading in extension but not flexion.[22] The maximal capacity of the joint exists at 70 to 80 degrees of flexion and is 25 to 30 mL.[25] This may be significantly decreased when the capsule becomes

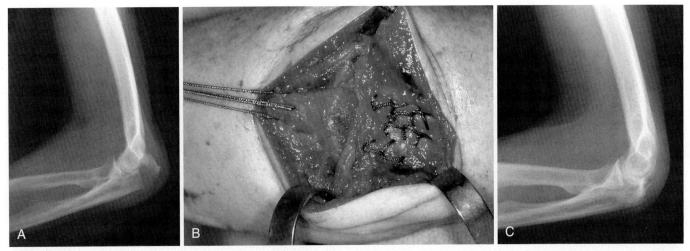

Figure 3-8 A, This 69-year-old man with poorly controlled type I diabetes fell sustaining this type IIA olecranon fracture. **B,** He was subsequently treated to excise fracture fragments, and the triceps was sutured down to the remaining distal fragment. **C,** At 4 years' follow-up, the patient had no complaints, no instability, and range of motion was pronation–supination 80–80, full flexion and a 25-degree extension lag. Radiographs were satisfactory. (Adams JE, Steinmann SP. Fractures of the olecranon. In: Celli A, Celli L, Morrey BF, eds. *Treatment of Elbow Lesions: New Aspects in Diagnosis and Surgical Techniques.* Milan: Springer-Verlag Italia, 2008, pp. 71–81. Used with permission from Springer-Verlag.)

contracted by post-traumatic changes or arthritic conditions. Clinically, this may make joint entry more difficult and dangerous during arthroscopy.[23,25]

Muscles Crossing the Elbow

The biceps serves as a flexor and supinator of the elbow and forearm. The brachialis originates from the distal half of the humeral shaft and inserts along the tuberosity of the ulna; it acts as a strong flexor of the elbow.[25]

The common extensor group and the mobile wad of Henry arise from the lateral epicondyle and humerus. The mobile wad of Henry, which comprises the brachioradialis, the

extensor carpi radialis brevis (ECRB), and extensor carpi radialis longus (ECRL), forms the radial-sided contour of the forearm and lateral border of the antecubital fossa (Fig. 3-13). The brachioradialis has a lengthy origin along the distal third of the humerus; it then has a broad insertion along the distal radial radius shaft and styloid. It is a strong flexor of the elbow. The ECRL and ECRB arise from the lateral epicondyle and insert on the base of the second and third metacarpals, respectively. These two muscles extend the wrist. The ECRB is covered by the ECRL proximally, which must be elevated to expose the diseased origin of the ECRB in open lateral epicondylitis procedures. Dorsally lie the extensor digitorum communis (EDC), extensor indicis

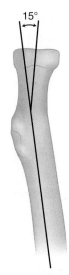

Figure 3-9 Proximal radius has a 15-degree angulation away from the radial tuberosity. (Morrey BF. Anatomy and surgical approaches. In: Morrey BF, ed. *Reconstructive Surgery of the Joints,* Vol. 1, 2nd ed. New York: Churchill Livingstone, 1996, pp. 461–487. Used with permission from Elsevier [Churchill Livingstone].)

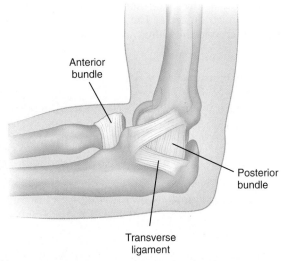

Figure 3-11 Medial aspect of the joint. The anterior and posterior bundles of the medial collateral ligament are consistently present and identifiable. (Morrey BF. Anatomy and surgical approaches. In Morrey BF, ed. *Reconstructive Surgery of the Joints,* Vol. 1, 2nd ed. New York: Churchill Livingstone, 1996, pp. 461–487. With permission from Elsevier [Churchill Livingstone].)

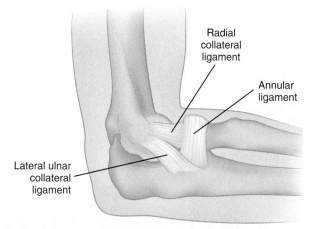

Figure 3-12 *Lateral ligament complex is composed of the radial collateral ligament, the annular ligament, and the less well-recognized ulnar collateral ligament. (Morrey BF. Anatomy and surgical approaches. In Morrey BF, ed. Reconstructive Surgery of the Joints, Vol. 1, 2nd ed. New York: Churchill Livingstone, 1996, pp. 461–487. With permission from Elsevier [Churchill Livingstone].)*

(EI), the extensor digiti quinti (EDQ or EDM), the humeral and ulnar attachments of the extensor carpi ulnaris (ECU), and the anconeus (Fig. 3-14, online).

At the ulnar side of the elbow, the flexor pronator group arises from the medial epicondyle and includes the flexor carpi ulnaris (FCU), the palmaris longus, the flexor carpi radialis (FCR), flexor digitorum profundus (FDP) and superficialis (FDS), and the pronator teres (Fig. 3-15, online). The pronator teres usually has two heads through which the median nerve passes: one from the medial epicondyle and a second from the coronoid. This can be a site of median nerve entrapment. The pronator inserts on the radius and acts as a strong pronator of the forearm and a weak flexor of the elbow. The FCR is a wrist flexor, and the palmaris longus is functionally insignificant but is useful as a graft donor for reconstructive procedures. The supinator originates from the lateral epicondyle, the LCL, and the proximal anterior ulna along the supinator crest. The muscle runs obliquely to finally wrap around the radius and end in a broad insertion

along the proximal radius. Like the biceps, it serves as a supinator of the forearm.[25]

The triceps posteriorly acts to extend the elbow. It arises from the posterior aspect of the humerus (lateral and medial heads) and from the scapula (long head).

Neurovascular Structures About the Elbow

Multiple neurovascular structures are at risk of injury with procedures or pathology about the elbow joint. An understanding of anatomy is crucial to avoiding iatrogenic injury and for anticipating possible problems as well as exploiting internervous planes during surgical approaches.[26]

The brachial artery traverses between the brachialis and biceps muscles in its course down the arm and lies lateral to the median nerve in the antecubital fossa. Typically, the radial artery arises at the level of the radial head, travels between the brachioradialis and the pronator teres, and sends a recurrent branch (radial recurrent branch) proximally. This anastamoses with the radial collateral and middle collateral arteries (from the profunda brachii) to form the radial-sided network of collateral circulation. The ulnar artery is the larger of the two branches and gives rise to the common interosseous artery and then posterior and anterior interosseous arteries. The ulnar artery, like the radial artery, gives off recurrent branches (the posterior and anterior recurrent arteries) that then anastamose with the superior and inferior ulnar collateral arteries arising from the brachial artery proximal to the elbow.[7] The basilic vein and cephalic vein drain the distal extremity and cross the elbow in a variable course.

Proximal to the elbow joint, the median nerve travels anteromedial to the humerus and lateral to the brachial artery. At the elbow joint, it crosses anterior to the artery to lie medial to the artery and the biceps tendon in the antecubital fossa (Fig. 3-16). No muscular branches arise from the median nerve in the arm.[27] At the antecubital fossa, the nerve is covered by the lacertus fibrosis as it crosses over the elbow joint. It then dips beneath the two heads of the pronator teres. The first motor branches from the median nerve arise laterally and are to the pronator teres and flexor carpi

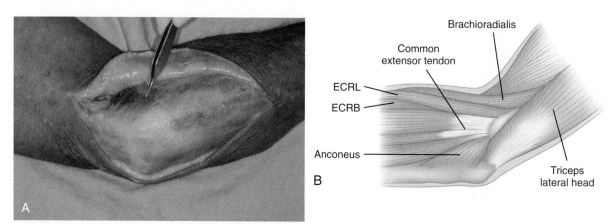

Figure 3-13 A, *Lateral elbow demonstrating extensor carpi radialis longus (forceps) and common extensor origin.* **B,** *Drawing of common extensor origin, lateral elbow. ECRB, extensor carpi radialis brevis; ECRL, extensor carpi radialis longus. (Murray PM. Elbow anatomy. In: Trumble TE, Budoff J, eds. Wrist and Elbow Reconstruction & Arthroscopy: A Master Skills Publication. Rosemont: American Society for Surgery of the Hand, 2006. Used with permission from American Society for Surgery of the Hand.)*

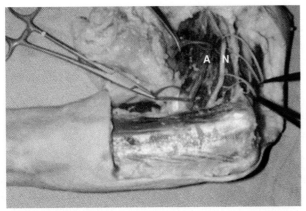

Figure 3-16 *The relationship of the median nerve (N) and brachial artery (A) proximal to the elbow joint. (Adams JE, Steinmann SP. Nerve injuries about the elbow.* J Hand Surg Am *2006;31A:303–313. Used with permission from Elsevier.)*

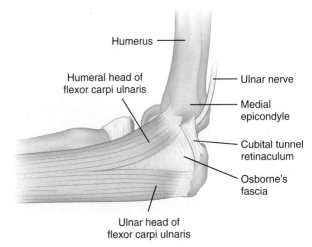

Figure 3-18 *Medial cubital tunnel anatomy.*

radialis. The nerve passes through the forearm along the dorsal surface of the FDS, which it supplies.[7,27]

The anterior interosseous nerve (AIN) arises from the median nerve 2 to 6 cm distal to the medial epicondyle.[28] This purely motor nerve travels down the forearm on the interosseous membrane.[27,29] The AIN may be injured in association with a (typically pediatric) supracondylar fracture as a result of contusion, traction, or both, particularly in the setting of irreducible, highly displaced or comminuted fractures.[28]

The ulnar nerve travels subcutaneously along the medial aspect of the arm between the coracobrachialis laterally and the long and medial heads of the triceps posteriorly (Fig. 3-17). Near the insertion of the coracobrachialis, the ulnar nerve passes through the medial intermuscular septum and the arcade of Struthers to enter the posterior compartment of the arm. The nerve then travels along the medial head of the triceps toward the medial epicondyle. It passes posterior to this structure, superficial to the joint capsule and the MCL, and through the cubital tunnel[30] (Fig. 3-18). The posterior

branch of the medial antebrachial cutaneous nerve passes over the ulnar nerve at a point between 6 cm proximal to 4 cm distal to the medial epicondyle.[30,31]

The ulnar nerve passes between the humeral and ulnar heads of the FCU as it enters the forearm. The first muscular branch is usually to the FCU, and multiple branches may arise anywhere from 4 cm proximal to 10 cm distal to the medial epicondyle. The muscular branch to the FDP usually arises 4 to 5 cm distal to the medial epicondyle.[30]

Because of its close proximity to the MCL of the elbow and its tethered location under the medial epicondyle, the ulnar nerve is often affected by pathology about the elbow joint. In addition to cubital tunnel syndrome, the nerve may be stretched during elbow dislocations, or injured as a result of fractures or during surgical procedures. In addition, the late sequelae of trauma, including deformities such as cubital varus or valgus or heterotopic ossification, may be problematic.[30] Trauma may promote adhesions and scarring, which can cause compression at classic locations of ulnar nerve entrapment, including the cubital tunnel, the arcade of Struthers, the medial intermuscular septum, or between the two heads of the FCU.[29,30] Typically, decompression and/or transposition is recommended when procedures such as total elbow arthroplasty or open reduction of significant distal humerus fractures is performed. Likewise, with contracture releases, the nerve is particularly vulnerable to stretch postoperatively if a large restoration of motion occurs; in this case the ulnar nerve may need to be assessed.[32]

The radial nerve exits the triangular space and travels along the posterior aspect of the humerus.[27,33] Distally, the nerve emerges from the spiral groove about 10 cm and 15 cm proximal to the lateral epicondyle and elbow joint, respectively[34,35] (Fig. 3-19). Above the spiral groove, a muscular branch to the medial head of the triceps is given off. This continues distally to supply the anconeus muscle. Surgical approaches can exploit this relationship to reflect the anconeus on a proximally based pedicle preserving its neurovascular supply.[7] Prior to piercing the lateral intermuscular septum to travel in the anterior aspect of the arm, two cutaneous branches are given off: the inferior lateral brachial cutaneous branch and the posterior antebrachial cutaneous

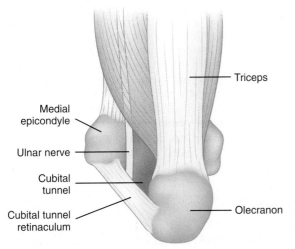

Figure 3-17 *Posterior cubital tunnel anatomy.*

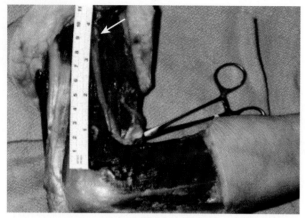

Figure 3-19 The radial nerve (*arrow*) as it pierces the intermuscular septum 9 to 10 cm proximal to the elbow joint. (Adams JE, Steinmann SP. Nerve injuries about the elbow. *J Hand Surg Am* 2006;31A:303–313. Used with permission from Elsevier.)

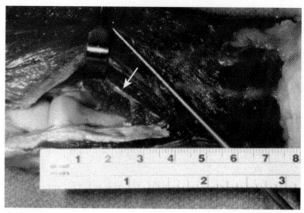

Figure 3-20 The posterior interosseous nerve (*arrow*) entering the supinator muscle distal to the radial head. (Adams JE, Steinmann SP. Nerve injuries about the elbow. *J Hand Surg Am* 2006;31A:303–313. Used with permission from Elsevier.)

nerve.[36] The radial nerve then pierces the lateral intermuscular septum and travels down the lateral column of the humerus over the lateral edge of the brachialis muscle.[33–37]

Muscular branches to the brachialis and ECRL are given off proximal to the elbow joint.[36,37] The nerve travels deep to the brachioradialis, ECRB, and ECRL muscles and passes directly over the annular ligament.[36] At the radiocapitellar joint level, the radial nerve bifurcates into a deep branch, which becomes the posterior interosseous nerve (PIN), and a superficial branch, which continues as the superficial radial nerve.[37–39] Innervation to the ECRB arises at the level of the bifurcation of the nerve and is variable.[36] The superficial branch of the radial nerve initially lies deep to the brachioradialis and superficial to the ECRL but distally emerges from the lateral edge of the brachioradialis to provide cutaneous sensation to the dorsoradial aspect of the hand.[36,38]

The PIN dips into the arcade of Frohse—a tunnel formed by fibrous bands of the brachialis and brachioradialis muscle, ECRB, and the superficial head of the supinator[36,39] (Fig. 3-20). The floor of the tunnel is formed by the anterior capsule of the elbow and the deep head of the supinator. The PIN then wraps about the lateral aspect of the radius, giving off branches to the supinator muscle.[36] At the distal border of the supinator, the PIN splits into two major branches: a short or recurrent branch, which supplies the ECU, EDC, EDM; and the long or descending branch, which innervates the abductor pollicis longus (APL), extensor pollicis longus (EPL), extensor pollicis brevis (EPB), and EI, and supplies sensation to the dorsal aspect of the wrist.[36,38,39]

Diliberti and colleagues[40] demonstrated in a cadaveric study the effect of pronation on the PIN. With full supination of the forearm, the PIN crossed the radial shaft at an average of 33 mm (range, 22–47 mm) from the radiocapitellar joint, whereas pronation caused the PIN to become more parallel to the long axis of the radius, and full pronation increased the distance to 52 mm (range, 38–68 mm).[40] The PIN is "tethered" by the supinator muscle and therefore is rotated with the radius during rotation.[41] Thus, during dorsal surgical approaches to the proximal radius, the forearm should be positioned in pronation to minimize risk of injury to the PIN.[41,42] Additional principles that may be helpful in avoiding

PIN injury include releasing the supinator close to its ulnar attachment rather than over the radius and using the bicipital tuberosity as a landmark to the region that may be safely exposed during surgery.[42]

Several cutaneous nerves are important to mention about the elbow. Inadvertent injury can cause a bothersome numb patch or a painful neuroma. The lateral antebrachial cutaneous nerve is the terminal sensory branch of the musculocutaneous nerve and pierces the brachial fascia approximately 3 cm proximal to the lateral epicondyle.[27,43] It then passes 4.5 cm medial to the lateral epicondyle. Anterior and posterior branches supply cutaneous sensation to the anterolateral and posterolateral surfaces of the forearm, respectively.[43] It is at risk during exposures of the distal humerus and should be identified in the interval between the brachialis and the biceps muscles and preserved.[27]

The medial antebrachial cutaneous nerve travels down the arm medial to the brachial artery.[31] It pierces the deep fascia in the mid or distal arm to become subcutaneous and has a variable relationship with the basilic vein.[31,44] At an average of 14.5 cm proximal to the medial epicondyle (range, 1–31 cm), the medial antebrachial cutaneous nerve gives off its anterior and posterior branches. The anterior branch crosses over the elbow joint between the medial epicondyle and biceps tendon.[31] The posterior branch gives off two to three additional branches, which have a variable course, crossing over the elbow usually proximal to the medial epicondyle, but between 6 cm proximal to 6 cm distal to it.[31,43] Injury of the medial antebrachial cutaneous branch of the median nerve or its branches may occur during cubital tunnel release. A more posterior incision, full-thickness flaps, and careful dissection and preservation of branches can lessen the risk of a bothersome hypoesthetic patch over the olecranon or symptomatic neuromas.[31,43,44]

Summary

An understanding of the complex anatomy and biomechanics of the elbow joint including the soft tissues and neurovascular structures is essential in treating pathology about this joint. Stability of the elbow is conferred by bony congruity, ligamentous structures, and dynamic action of muscular forces. Mobility of the elbow is critical for the accomplishment of a variety of activities of daily living. The functional ROM of the elbow has been determined to be 30 to 130 degrees in the flexion and extension arc and 50 degrees each of pronation and supination. The intimate relationship of the many neurovascular structures about the elbow make them vulnerable in elbow injuries, and they require protection during surgery.

REFERENCES

The complete reference list is available online at www.expertconsult.com.

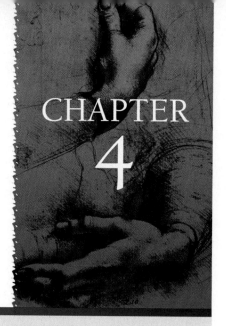

Anatomy and Kinesiology of the Shoulder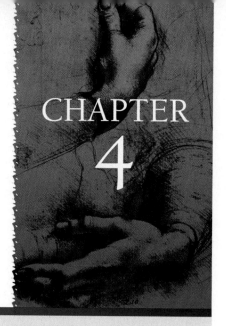

MARK LAZARUS, MD AND RALPH RYNNING, MD

RANGE OF MOTION	BIOMECHANICS OF THE SHOULDER COMPLEX
GLENOHUMERAL ANATOMY	THE COORDINATED MUSCLE ACTIVITY OF THE
GLENOHUMERAL BIOMECHANICS	SHOULDER
GLENOHUMERAL STABILIZERS	SUMMARY
THE CLAVICLE AND SCAPULA	

CRITICAL POINTS

- Shoulder motion is a result of the complex interactions of the individual joints and muscles of the shoulder girdle.
- Scapulothoracic motion significantly affects measurements of glenohumeral motion.
- Shoulder motion is measured and described in multiple planes of motion.
- Stability of the shoulder is conferred by dynamic and static constraints.
- The clavicle serves as a strut and suspension between the thorax and scapula
- Scapular motion is a complex interaction of motion in three planes.
- The coordinated movement of the clavicle, scapula, and humerus involves a complex interaction of more than twenty muscles.
- Scapulohumeral rhythm is a dynamic state adapting to varying speed, load, and stability.

The shoulder is the most mobile joint in the body. Motion occurs through complex interactions of the individual joints of the shoulder girdle, including the glenohumeral joint, the sternoclavicular joint, the acromioclavicular joint, and the scapulothoracic articulation. Together the coordinated interaction of these structures allows for an extraordinary freedom of movement and function.

Range of Motion

Measuring Normal Range of Motion

Traditionally, shoulder motion has been described by measuring the angle formed by the arm relative to trunk. Forward elevation, or flexion, of the shoulder is in the sagittal plane and may in some individuals reach 180 degrees. The normal range varies, but has been reported to be on average 165 to 170 degrees in men, and 170 to 172 degrees in women.[1] Posterior elevation or extension in the sagittal plane has been found to be on average 62 degrees.[2] Axial rotation of the arm is described by degrees of internal and external rotation. With the arm at the side an average external rotation is 67 degrees.[3] Estimates of total axial rotation (the sum of internal and external rotation) with the arm at the side range from 150 degrees to 180 degrees. Total axial rotation with the arm abducted to 90 degrees is reduced to about 120 degrees. In the horizontal plane, when the arm is perpendicular to the trunk, motion is commonly described as horizontal abduction and adduction (or horizontal extension and flexion).

Range of motion is influenced by several factors, including the determination of the end-point, the plane in which the motion is tested, and whether the scapula is stabilized.[3] By comparing the relative contribution of passive and active arcs of motion, McCully and colleagues concluded that scapulothoracic motion significantly influences glenohumeral range-of-motion measurements.[3]

Factors such as age, gender, and hand dominance also affect shoulder range of motion. Normal shoulder range of motion decreases with age. Boone and Azen reported on two

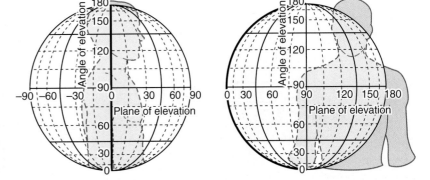

Figure 4-1 Range of motion of the shoulder is most similar to motion about a globe. (Reprinted from Rockwood CA Jr, Matsen FA III, *The Shoulder*. 3rd ed. Philadelphia: Saunders Elsevier, 2004.)

groups of males with an age difference of 12.5 years. The younger group averaged 3.4 degrees more flexion and internal rotation, 8.4 degrees more external rotation, and 10.2 degrees more extension.[4]

Codman's Paradox

Shoulder motion is rarely limited to one plane. Therefore, in describing the position of the arm in space it is necessary to use multiple planes of reference. The traditional methods of motion description are inadequate for complex motion because the final position of the arm is dependent on the motion sequence. This is illustrated by a concept known as the Codman's paradox.[5] If the arm is raised forward to the horizontal, then horizontally abducted, followed by a return adduction to the side, the final resting position of the arm is externally rotated axially 90 degrees, yet the arm was never specifically externally rotated. Serial angular rotations about orthogonal axes are not additive, but sequence-dependent. Rotation about the x-axis, followed by rotation about the y-axis results in a different end resting position from the reverse sequence.[6]

Three-Dimensional Joint Motion

A central feature to the understanding of joint kinematics is the ability to measure and describe motion in a consistent and reproducible manner. One method of describing complex joint kinematics is to use a system of vertical planes of elevation, similar to the degrees of longitude used to describe global positioning[6] (Fig. 4-1). Pure coronal abduction is defined as 0 degrees, and pure sagittal flexion as 90 degrees. At the horizontal, the maximum adduction is 124 degrees whereas the maximum abduction is −88 degrees, producing a total of 212 possible vertical planes of elevation.[7] Humeral elevation is measured by the angle formed between the elevated arm and the unelevated arm. Isolated forward flexion to 90 degrees in this coordinate system is described as (90,90), whereas isolated abduction to 90 degrees is described as (0,90). Finally, axial rotation is described in reference to the plane of elevation by an angle formed by the forearm with the elbow flexed to 90 degrees. If the forearm is perpendicular to the plane of elevation, the rotation is 0 degrees. External rotation is positive, internal rotation is negative. A classic military salute in this system would be described as (+30, +80, −406).[6]

Glenohumeral Anatomy

Glenoid

The glenoid arises laterally from the scapular neck at the junction of the coracoid, scapular spine, and lateral border of the scapular body. It is a pear-shaped structure forming a shallow socket that is retroverted on average 7 degrees with respect to the scapular plane, but maintains an overall anteversion of about 30 degrees with respect to the coronal plane of the body.[8] The glenoid also maintains a superior tilt of about 5 degrees in the normal resting position of the scapula. It is thought that this superior inclination contributes to inferior stability via a cam effect that is a function of the tightening superior capsular structures.[9]

The glenoid surface area is about one third that of the humeral head. The depth of the glenoid measures about 9 mm in a superoinferior direction, but only 5 mm in an anteroposterior direction, half of which is constituted by the labrum.[10] In addition, the glenoid cartilage is thicker peripherally than centrally, further deepening the socket. The glenoid socket is therefore significantly more concave and congruous with the humerus than the bony anatomy would suggest.

Humeral Head

The humeral head is oriented with an upward tilt of about 45 degrees from the horizontal, and it is retroverted about 30 to 40 degrees with respect to the intercondylar axis of the distal humerus. The articular surface forms approximately one third of a sphere. Utilizing stereophotogrammetric studies, Soslowsky and associates demonstrated that the glenohumeral joint congruence is within 2 mm in 88% of cases, with a deviation from sphericity of less than 1% of the radius.[11] Retroversion is greater in young children, with an average of 65 degrees between the ages of 4 months to 4 years.[12] By 8 years of age most of the derotation has occurred with a more gradual derotation continuing until adulthood.

Glenohumeral Biomechanics

Laxity

Glenohumeral laxity is a normal finding to varying degrees in all shoulders. In cadaveric shoulders, average passive humeral translation of 13.4 mm anteriorly and 10.4 mm

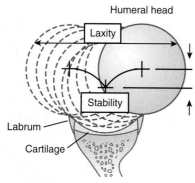

Figure 4-2 The difference between laxity and stability can be demonstrated graphically. Laxity is the translation permitted from one end of capsular tension to the other. Stability is the centered point of lowest potential energy and is related not only to capsular tension but also to joint congruency. [Modified from Lazarus MD, Sidles JA, Harryman DT 2nd, Matsen FA 3rd. Effect of chondral-labral defect on glenoid concavity and glenohumeral stability. A cadaveric model. *J Bone Joint Surg Am.* 1996;78A:94–102].

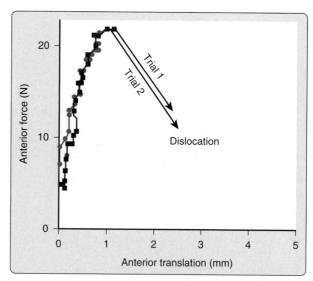

Figure 4-3 Even in older, cadaveric shoulders, in response to a translating force, humeral heads remain relatively well-centered until a threshold force is reached, resulting in sudden and explosive dislocation. [Modified from Lazarus MD, Sidles JA, Harryman DT 2nd, Matsen FA 3rd. Effect of chondral-labral defect on glenoid concavity and glenohumeral stability. A cadaveric model. *J Bone Joint Surg Am.* 1996;78A:94–102].

posteriorly has been demonstrated with a 20-N force.[13] In a study of healthy unanesthetized volunteers, passive humeral translation averaged 8 mm anteriorly, 9 mm posteriorly, and 11 mm inferiorly.[14] Far less translation occurs with normal glenohumeral kinematics. Radiographic analysis of normal volunteers demonstrates that the humeral head is maintained precisely centered in the glenoid in all positions except simultaneous maximal horizontal abduction and external rotation.[15] In this extreme position an average of 4 mm of posterior translation occurred. These studies demonstrate that despite the great potential for translational motion in the shoulder, the combined stabilizers of the glenohumeral joint act in concert to maintain centricity.

Laxity Versus Instability

Shoulder *laxity* is a normal property that varies widely within the general population.[16-19] It is often measured as increased passive translation of the humeral head on the glenoid and may be affected by several factors, including age, gender, and congenital factors.[20] *Instability* is a pathologic condition involving active translation of the humeral head on the glenoid (Fig. 4-2). Unlike laxity, instability is usually symptomatic. It represents a failure of static and dynamic constraints to maintain the humeral head precisely centered within the glenoid. Instability may occur in one direction, such as anterior instability following a traumatic anterior dislocation, or it may be multidirectional, occurring in any combination of anterior, posterior, or inferior directions. Patients with multidirectional instability often have asymptomatic laxity of the contralateral shoulder.[21] What distinguishes these shoulders from normally functioning shoulders is a complex interaction of muscular, neurologic, and structural factors.

Glenohumeral Stabilizers

Shoulder dislocations are the most common form of joint dislocation, with an average incidence of 1.7%, demonstrat-

ing the great potential for instability that exists in the shoulder.[22] The critical constraints for the control of shoulder stability may be divided into static and dynamic elements. The interaction of these constraining elements is complex. In the pathologic state, where one or more constraining factors is abnormal, instability may occur. Restoring these normal anatomic constraints is critical to the successful treatment and rehabilitation of the shoulder.

Static Stabilizers

Early investigators focused on the articular components of glenohumeral stability. The humeral head retroversion roughly matches the glenoid orientation on the chest wall. Saha emphasized the contribution of this articular version to stability, noting that individuals with congenital anteversion of the glenoid had a greater tendency for recurrent dislocation.[8] Subsequent studies have not confirmed this hypothesis, finding instead considerable variability in articular version and inclination.[23-25] In any position of rotation only about 25% to 30% of the humeral head surface is in contact with the glenoid. The glenohumeral index, calculated by measuring the diameter of the humeral head relative to the glenoid, has been measured. It was hypothesized that individuals with larger heads relative to their glenoid would be unstable; however, investigators have made no such correlation.[26]

The relatively smaller surface area of the glenoid relative to the humeral head emphasizes the importance of soft tissues surrounding the joint, including the labrum, capsular, and ligamentous structures. The labrum is composed of dense collagen fibers that surround and attach to the glenoid rim, creating a deeper and broader glenoid surface. Functionally the labrum increases the articular contact of the glenoid with the humerus to about one third and improves the articular conformity and thereby stability[27] (Fig. 4-3). Lippitt and Matsen demonstrated the contribution of the labrum to joint

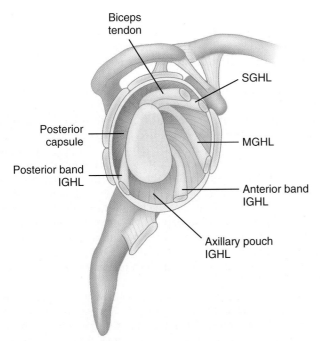

Figure 4-4 The glenohumeral joint is stabilized by discreet capsular ligaments, each of which has a separate role in maintaining stability. IGHL, inferior glenohumeral ligament; MGHL, middle glenohumeral ligament; SGHL, superior glenohumeral ligament.

stability in cadavers.[28] Excision of the labrum resulted in a 20% decrease in stability as measured using the stability ratio defined by Fukuda and coworkers.[29]

Slight mismatch of the articular surface diameter of curvature between the glenoid and humeral head may have a significant effect on glenohumeral stability. Saha initially described three types of glenohumeral articulations: type A had a shallow glenoid, type B had conforming surfaces, and type C had a humeral radius greater than that of the glenoid.[8] Soslowsky and associates, using stereophotogrammetric studies of fresh frozen cadaveric shoulders, found that 88% of glenohumeral articulations are perfectly congruent.[11] Kim and colleagues, however, recently analyzed MRI scans in patients with multidirectional instability (MDI) and compared them with normal MRIs. They determined that the diameter of curvature of the glenoid surface in the MDI patients was greater than the humeral diameter, suggesting that this loss of conformity may play a role in instability.[30]

A slightly negative intra-articular pressure of the glenohumeral joint also acts to maintain joint stability.[31] Normally the shoulder contains about 1 mL of synovial fluid, which is maintained at a lower atmospheric pressure by high osmotic pressures in the surrounding tissues. Warner and coworkers demonstrated that in normal shoulders an inferiorly directed force of 16 N generated an inferior translation of 2 mm; however, if the capsule of the same shoulder is vented, the same force generates an inferior translation of 28 mm.[32]

The conformity of the glenohumeral joint combined with the presence of synovial fluid generates adhesion and cohesion between the humeral head and the glenoid in much the same fashion as a moist glass sticks to a coaster. Adhesion is due to the material properties of the synovial fluid, but cohesion is due to the conformity of the joint. The compliant labrum further potentiates these stabilizing effects.

The glenoid geometry and labrum in concert with muscle contractions of the rotator cuff are responsible for stability in the midranges of motion.[3] The capsuloligamentous structures that remain lax during the midrange of motion are mainly responsible for stability at the end ranges of motion when all other stabilizing mechanisms have been overwhelmed.[33,34]

The Glenohumeral Ligaments

The superior ligaments comprise the coracohumeral ligament (CHL) and the superior glenohumeral ligament (SGHL) (Fig. 4-4). The CHL is broad, thin, extra-articular structure originating on the coracoid process and inserting broadly on the greater and lesser tuberosities, intermingling with the fibers of the supraspinatus and subscapularis. The SGHL, which lies deep to the CHL, is present in over 90% of cases, originating on the superior tubercle of the glenoid and inserting anteriorly just medial to the bicipital groove. Together these structures resist inferior translation with the arm in adduction.

The middle glenohumeral ligament (MGHL) has the greatest variation both in size and presence of all glenohumeral ligaments. It is absent in up to 30% of shoulders.[35] The morphology of the MGHL may be sheetlike or cordlike, and it usually originates along with the SGHL on the superior glenoid tubercle, inserting just medial to the lesser tuberosity. Although the MGHL limits inferior translation in the adducted and externally rotated shoulder, the ligament primarily functions to limit anterior translation of the humerus on the glenoid with the shoulder abducted 45 degrees.[36] In individuals with a more cordlike MGHL it may also function to limit anterior translation in the 60- to 90-degree abduction range with the arm externally rotated.[36,37]

The inferior glenohumeral ligament (IGHL) is likely the most important ligament complex of the glenohumeral joint. The IGHL is composed of thickened bands that form a sling, or "hammock," that cradles the humerus inferiorly in what is referred to as the axillary pouch. Typically, the IGHL originates broadly at the equatorial to inferior half of the anterior glenoid adjacent to the labrum and inserts just inferior to the MGHL medial to the lesser tuberosity. In a histologic and anatomic study by O'Brien and coworkers, they demonstrated that the posterior and anterior portions of the IGHL contain thickened bands of dense collagen fibers.[35] Gohlke and coworkers confirmed the existence of the anterior band, but found the posterior band to be present in only 62.8% percent of individuals.[38] The stabilizing function of the IGHL complex increases as the arm is elevated in abduction. With external rotation of the arm in 90 degrees of abduction, the anterior band broadens and tightens, forming a taut sling that prevents anterior translation. Similarly, with internal rotation of the abducted arm, the posterior band fans out and tightens.[39] The IGHL is also the primary restraint to inferior translation of the humerus with the arm in 90 degrees of abduction.

The Interplay Between Static and Dynamic Constraints

Ligaments only function under some degree of tension. However, during normal motion of the glenohumeral joint the ligaments remain under little to no tension. In addition a large amount of passive translation is commonly possible in multiple directions. Yet the humeral head remains perfectly centered in the glenoid during normal active motion. Therefore, it seems that factors other than the capsule and ligaments must be contributing to the lack of translation observed with normal motion. The factor responsible for maintaining the humeral head centered in the glenoid is therefore the interplay between the remaining static stabilizers (adhesion, cohesion, negative intra-articular pressure, and the congruency of the joint) and the dynamic stabilizers (the rotator cuff muscles, biceps brachii, the scapular rotators, and coordinated proprioceptive feedback) of the shoulder.

Despite the complex dynamic and static constraints that maintain the humeral head centered in the glenoid, pathologic translation of the humeral head does occur. In all but the most severe cases of laxity, shoulder dislocations result in tearing or fracturing of the glenohumeral architecture.[40] Selective cutting experiments have demonstrated the potential instability that may result from sectioning individual capsular and ligamentous structures of the glenohumeral joint.

Cadaveric experiments have demonstrated the primary ligamentous constraints to translation of the humeral head on the glenoid in the anterior, inferior, and posterior directions. The anterosuperior band of the IGHL is the primary ligamentous constraint to anterior translation with the arm abducted and externally rotated.[41] As abduction decreases, the MGHL is of increasing importance in resisting anterior translation.[42] The primary constraints to inferior translation in the adducted arm are the superior structures, particularly the SGHL which is maximized by external rotation.[36,43] With increasing abduction to 90 degrees, the IGHL becomes the primary constraint to inferior translation.[44] The primary constraint to posterior translation is the posterior band of the IGHL. Although resection of the posterior capsule increases posterior translation, it is not sufficient for a posterior glenohumeral dislocation to occur.[45] However, posterior dislocation is possible if the same shoulder is incised anterosuperiorly, cutting the SGHL and MGHL. Posterior translation increases with the arm in 30 degrees of extension if the anterior band of the IGHL is incised or detached from its glenoid insertion.[44,46]

Dynamic Stabilizers

The rotator cuff muscles improve joint stability by increasing the load necessary to translate the humeral head from its centered position in the glenoid. Lippitt and Matsen found that tangential forces as high as 60% of the compressive force were required to dislocate the glenohumeral joint in a cadaveric study,[28] finding also that joint stability was reduced with removal of a portion of the anterior labrum. Similarly, Wuelker and associates noted a nearly 50% increase in anterior displacement of the humeral head in response to a 50% reduction in rotator cuff forces.[47] The glenohumeral joint reaction force has been calculated in a cadaveric model to reach a maximum of 0.89 times body weight.[48] Glenohumeral joint contact pressures measure a maximum of 5.1 MPa in cadavers using pressure-sensitive film with the arm in 90 degrees of abduction and 90 degrees of external rotation.[49]

Joint reaction forces increase with increasing abduction angle and peak at 90 degrees abduction.[50] Increasing joint compression appears to increase the centering of the humeral head, thereby providing a stable fulcrum for arm elevation.[51,52]

Other factors may also contribute to dynamic glenohumeral stability. Ligament dynamization through attachment to the rotator cuff muscles has been postulated, whereby rotator cuff contraction may affect tensioning of the glenohumeral capsuloligamentous complex.[53] Similarly, Pagnani and colleagues hypothesized that biceps contracture may tension the relatively mobile labrum and thereby tension the associated SGHL and MGHL, potentially enhancing stability.[54] They also conclude that the long head of the biceps may itself stabilize the joint depending on shoulder position. Whether this is a true dynamic function is controversial. Yamaguchi and coworkers observed no biceps muscle activity with normal arm motion in both normal rotator cuffs and deficient cuffs.[55]

The capsuloligamentous structures may also provide proprioceptive feedback on joint position. Vangsness and associates found low-threshold, rapid-adapting pacinian fibers in the glenohumeral ligaments.[56] Others have found diminished proprioception in shoulders with instability, with subsequent improvement after repair.[57] Proprioceptive feedback likely helps not only to tension the rotator cuff muscles, but also to position the scapula and clavicle appropriately in space.

The Clavicle and Scapula

The glenoid socket is relatively unconstrained compared with the acetabulum of the hip. The added mobility that this confers requires the coordinated movement and function of the muscles that position the scapula and clavicle in space. The glenoid may therefore be placed in a variety of positions that allow it to effectively resist the joint reaction forces generated by the muscles that power and position the arm.

The Anatomy of the Clavicle

The clavicle is a double-curved bone that functions as a strut and suspension between the thorax and the scapula while also protecting the underlying neurovascular structures (Fig. 4-5). While carrying a load at the side, for example, the clavicle functions as a strut, giving the muscles that elevate the clavicle and scapula a fulcrum to carry the load away from midline. Each end of the clavicle forms a diarthrodial articulation with an intervening fibrocartilagenous meniscus. The shape and mobile articulations of each joint allows for more motion than is typically observed. Muscles that power the shoulder cause compression across the glenohumeral joint. The force is transmitted to the trunk via the acromioclavicular (AC) and sternoclavicular (SC) joints. The conoid, trapezoid, and AC ligaments strongly suspend the scapula and the remaining upper extremity from the clavicle.

Sternoclavicular Joint

The SC joint connects the axial skeleton to the upper extremity. The somewhat flattened bony articulation provides little

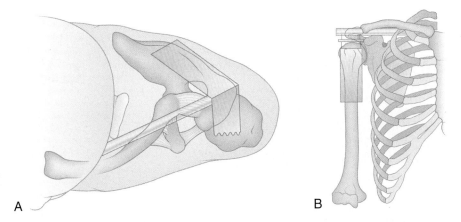

Figure 4-5 The clavicle serves as a strut (**A**) to position the scapula away from the thorax and as a suspension (**B**) for the shoulder girdle. (Reprinted from Lazarus MD. Fractures of the clavicle. In: Bucholz RW, Heckman JD, Court-Brown C, et al., eds. *Rockwood and Green's Fractures in Adults.* 5th ed. Philadelphia: Lippincott Williams & Wilkins, 2001.)

inherent stability. Instead ligamentous structures both anteriorly and posteriorly confer stability (Fig. 4-6). Early studies demonstrated that the SC capsule was responsible for stability of the joint, but they did not isolate individual ligaments or regions of the capsule.[58,59] Spencer and Kuhn demonstrated in a cadaveric selective cutting study that the posterior capsule is the primary restraint to both posterior and anterior translation;[60] however, the anterior capsule is also important, particularly for restraint on anterior translation. Their research also showed that the costoclavicular and interclavicular ligaments are not crucial stabilizers of the SC joint.

Acromioclavicular Joint

The AC joint is a diarthrodial joint that allows articulation of the medial acromion with the lateral clavicle. Similarly to the SC joint, the AC joint has little inherent stability, instead relying on ligamentous support (Fig. 4-7). A capsule surrounds the joint, thickening superiorly to form the AC ligament. The scapula is suspended from the clavicle by way of the conoid and trapezoid ligaments connecting the distal clavicle to the coracoid process. Early investigators observed only minimal motion at the AC joint. However, a cadaveric selective cutting experiment by Fukuda and colleagues measured the relative constraint provided by the AC capsule,

conoid, and trapezoid ligaments to small and large displacements.[61] They concluded that in small displacements (10 N of force) the AC capsule is the primary restraint on both superior and posterior translation. With large displacements (90 N of force) there is a shift to the conoid ligament with respect to restraint to superior translation; however, 90% of the restraint on posterior translation is still maintained by the AC capsule. The coracoclavicular ligaments, especially the trapezoid, resist most of the load transmission in axial compression. The individual contributions of the AC ligament to resisting translation were further clarified by Klimkiewicz and coworkers in a cadaveric-sectioning study.[62] They concluded that the posterior and superior ligaments are the most critical, resisting on average 25% and 56% of the posterior displacement, respectively. These results were confirmed by Debski and associates in a cadaveric study using in situ force measurements in three dimensions.[42] They concluded that the superior AC ligament is the primary restraint

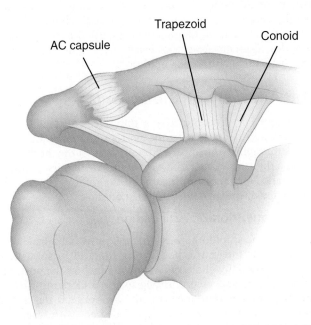

Figure 4-7 The ligamentous anatomy of the acromioclavicular joint. (Reprinted from *Gray's Anatomy,* 2007.)

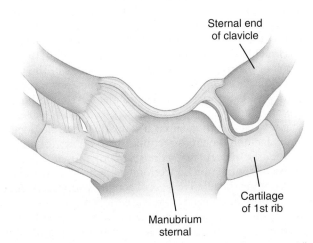

Figure 4-6 The sternoclavicular joint is stabilized by the strongest ligamentous complex in the body. (Reprinted from *Gray's Anatomy,* 2007.)

Table 4-1   Range of Motion at the
Sternoclavicular (SC) Joint
(in Degrees)[58]

Action at the SC Joint	Degrees of Motion
Upward rotation	35
Anterior rotation	35
Posterior rotation	35
Axial rotaion	45–50
Downward rotation	10
Upward rotation	45

on posterior translation and that the conoid is the primary restraint on superior translation. Moreover, they note that the constraints on the AC joint affect the resulting joint motion, but motion also affects the force on each ligament.

Clavicular Motion

Clavicular motion occurs in anteroposterior and superoinferior directions as well as rotating on its longitudinal axis. Inman noted that about 30 degrees of clavicular elevation occurs with about 130 degrees of forward elevation of the upper extremity with relatively more motion occurring at the SC joint than the AC joint.[63] Ten degrees of forward elevation also occurs with the first 40 degrees of elevation and an additional 15 to 20 degrees of forward elevation occurs with motion above 130 degrees of elevation.[64] DePalma summarized this elevation and forward rotation by describing the motion of the distal clavicle as forming an angular cone of about 60 degrees.[65]

Dempster originally described six discrete motions at the SC joint (Table 4-1).[58] The physiologic range of each type of motion has been defined by various studies.[63,66] Additionally, anteroposterior rotation is greater than superoinferior motion by a ratio of 2 to 1.[67] Motion at the AC joint is more limited than at the SC joint. The motion may be thought of as rotational, either axial (anterior and posterior) about the long axis of the clavicle, or hinging in an anteroposterior or superoinferior manner. Anteroposterior rotation is three times greater than superoinferior motion.[58]

The Anatomy of the Scapula

The scapula is predominately a thin sheet of bone loosely attached and congruent to the posterior chest wall, which serves to stabilize the upper extremity against the thorax. The scapula thickens along its borders at the site of muscle attachments and along its four projections: the spine of the scapula, the coracoid, the glenoid, and the acromion.

The Scapulothoracic Articulation

Although the scapulothoracic articulation is not a true joint, its motion is integral to positioning the arm in space. The scapula essentially glides over a muscle bed on the posterior chest wall, its shape conforming to the underlying ribs. At rest the scapula is rotated anteriorly about 30 degrees as viewed from above, upward about 3 degrees with respect to the sagittal plane, and tilted forward about 20 degrees as viewed from the side.

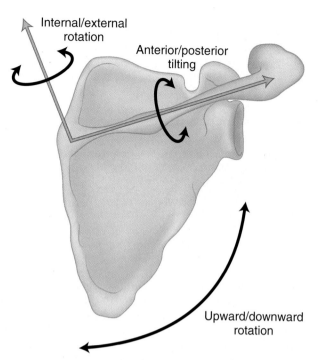

Figure 4-8 The definitions of scapular motion.

Scapular Motion

Although scapular motion has long been recognized as complex, descriptions of this motion have largely focused on elevation in the coronal or scapular plane. Using sensors attached to percutaneous pins McClure and associates demonstrated that scapular motion is three-dimensional and task-dependent.[68] With arm elevation in the scapular plane, the scapula rotates upward on average 50 degrees, posteriorly about a mediolateral axis about 30 degrees, and externally about 24 degrees about a vertical axis (Fig. 4-8).

Biomechanics of the Shoulder Complex

More than 20 muscles coordinate their function to move the shoulder joint complex. Several of these muscles have differing functional heads that further enhance shoulder function, including the three heads of the deltoid, the two heads of the biceps brachii, the three heads of the triceps brachii, the three portions of the trapezius, and the two portions of the pectoralis major. Based on these muscles' origins and insertions, they may be categorized as glenohumeral, scapulothoracic, or thoracohumeral.

The relative function of each individual muscle depends on three factors: the cross-sectional area, the vector angle of pull, and the percentage recruitment of muscle fibers (or intensity of contraction). Electromyography (EMG) is useful in determining the relative level of activity within a particular muscle group, but it cannot measure the force of contraction. To understand the forces generated requires a calculation of the moment arm of the muscle as well as the physiologic cross-sectional area, both of which are dynamic, making accurate calculations challenging. Anatomic studies have calculated the cross-sectional area of several muscles of the shoulder girdle.[69] Cross-sectional measurements and approximations of force vectors have been used to calculate glenohumeral joint reaction forces. Current research is focusing on in vivo calculations.

Active Arm Elevation

During active forward elevation of the arm, synchronous activity of the deltoid and rotator cuff muscles has been measured using a combination of stereophotogrammetry and EMG recordings. Inman and colleagues demonstrated that the deltoid and supraspinatus act synergistically during forward elevation of the arm.[64] Synchronous function of the remaining rotator cuff muscles provides the humeral head depression necessary to prevent superior migration of the humeral head.[52] The deltoid provides a substantial initial force nearly 90% of its total potential force.[67] In massive rotator cuff tears the force required of the remaining rotator cuff to keep the glenohumeral joint centered increases experimentally by as much as 86%.[70]

The supraspinatus is thought to initiate abduction; however, the deltoid and all four rotator cuff muscles are active throughout the full range of forward arm elevation. The specific contributions of each muscle have been studied using selective nerve blocks in healthy volunteers. Blocks of either the suprascapular nerve or the axillary nerve demonstrate that both the deltoid and supraspinatus are responsible for generating torque during active forward elevation of the arm. Full abduction has been shown to be possible with an axillary nerve block with a reduction of strength of about 50% of normal.[71] Similarly, suprascapular nerve block allowed full abduction with diminished strength. However, simultaneous axillary and suprascapular nerve blocks eliminated all active elevation, demonstrating that the deltoid, supraspinatus, and infraspinatus are essential for active shoulder elevation. With a suprascapular nerve block, strength is reduced about 50% at 30 degrees, 35% at 90 degrees, and 25% at 120 degrees of forward elevation.[67]

Classically the contributions to arm elevation are thought to be a 2:1 ratio of glenohumeral to scapulothoracic motion.[64] More recent investigations suggest a more complex interaction with motion during the first 30 degrees as mostly glenohumeral,[48,72,73] whereas the last 60 degrees comprises a near equal contribution by the glenohumeral and scapulothoracic joints. McClure and coworkers measured a ratio of 1.7 to 1 of glenohumeral motion to scapulothoracic motion with arm elevation in healthy volunteers.[68] The speed of arm elevation also affects the relative contribution of each joint, with predominance of glenohumeral motion at high speeds.[74] With age, the ratio of glenohumeral to scapulothoracic motion remains relatively constant; however, the range of motion is diminished.[75]

External Rotation of the Humerus

Maximal forward elevation of the arm requires external rotation of the humerus.[76] Early observers concluded that external rotation was necessary for the tuberosity to clear the acromion, but more recent clinical and cadaveric studies suggest other factors play a significant role. Maximal external rotation may confer greater stability to the glenohumeral joint in the elevated position.[77] Jobe and Iannotti conclude, based on a cadaveric range-of-motion study in three planes, that obligate external rotation makes more humeral head cartilage available for articulation with the glenoid.[78] A cadaveric study using magnetic three-dimensional tracking devices determined maximal elevation was associated with approximately 35 degrees of external rotation.[76] In vivo data suggest a greater amount of external rotation exists. Using a magnetic field around volunteers, Stokdijk and colleagues found an average external rotation of 55 degrees.[79]

The Coordinated Muscle Activity of the Shoulder

Scapulohumeral Rhythm

Codman understood the complex and dependent relationships of the structures of the shoulder when he coined the term *scapulohumeral rhythm* to describe the coordinated motion.[80] Inman noted the early phase of scapular motion as the *setting phase*, indicating the importance of positioning the scapula in an advantageous position for the rotator cuff muscles.[63] More recent dynamic studies have confirmed this dependent relationship,[68,81] defining more accurately the complex motion of the scapula in relation to the humerus in normal as well as pathologic states.[82] Even with a 3-kg weight held in the hand, the scapulohumeral rhythm remains unchanged except in the midrange of elevation where the position of the scapula compensates for the increased load.[81] These subtle coordinated adaptations in neuromuscular coordination contribute to the dynamic stability and unique function of the joint under a broad range of conditions.

Summary

Shoulder motion is a result of the complex interactions of the glenohumeral, acromioclavicular, sternoclavicular, and scapulothoracic joints. The shoulder is powered by the coordinated motion of more than twenty muscles interacting to confer stability under varying speeds and loads. Shoulder motion is measured and described in discrete planes of motion with motion at each joint affecting the measure of each other joint. The broad range of shoulder motion makes it vulnerable to instability and injury, including glenohumeral dislocation. Stability is maintained by the interaction of dynamic and static motion constraints. These include the bony anatomy, the soft-tissue constraints, and the dynamic coordinated muscle activity of the shoulder girdle.

REFERENCES

The complete reference list is available online at www.expertconsult.com.

Surface Anatomy of the Upper Extremity

NEAL E. PRATT, PhD, PT

CRITICAL POINTS

- The purpose of this chapter is to present the surface anatomy of the upper extremity that is most relevant and useful to the clinician.
- The upper limb is presented regionally, starting proximally and proceeding distally.
- Each region is presented as a unit and organized in a similar manner so the reader can follow the anatomy in a logical sequence.
- In each region the bony landmarks are used as the basic references for most other structures.
- Most of the chapter is devoted to the osteologic and muscular structures that are apparent through the skin.
- Because muscles are most readily palpable when they are active, the maneuvers necessary to produce specific muscle activity are included where appropriate.
- Nerve and vessel locations are included when they can be either palpated directly or specifically located relative to definitive landmarks.
- Much of the information contained in this chapter is derived from multiple sources. As a result specific references are not included in the text but sources for additional information are included in a bibliography at the end of the chapter.

The purpose of this chapter is to present the surface anatomy of the upper extremity that is most relevant and useful to the clinician. The upper limb is presented regionally, starting proximally and proceeding distally. Each region is presented as a unit and organized in a similar manner so that the reader can follow the anatomy in a logical sequence. The specific regions are the posterior cervical triangle, shoulder, arm and elbow, forearm and wrist, and hand. In each region, the bony landmarks are used as the basic references for most other structures.

Most of this chapter is devoted to the osteologic and muscular structures that are apparent through the skin. Because muscles are most readily palpable when they are active, the maneuvers necessary to produce specific muscle activity are included where appropriate. Nerve and vessel locations are included when they can be either palpated directly or specifically located relative to definitive landmarks. The names of structures appear in italics when their surface locations are described. Much of the information contained in this chapter is derived from multiple sources. As a result, specific references are not included in the text, but a variety of sources of additional information is included in a bibliography at the end of this chapter.

Posterior Cervical Triangle

The *posterior cervical triangle (posterior triangle of the neck)* (Fig. 5-1) is included because it houses the major neurovascular structures that supply the upper extremity and is the site of various clinical problems that can affect these structures and, potentially, the entire limb. The boundaries of this triangle are easily palpated and in most people can be identified visually. The base of the triangle is bony and formed by the *middle third* of the *clavicle*; the two sides are muscular and formed by the posterior border of the *sterno-cleidomastoid* and the superior border of the *trapezius*. The borders of these muscles converge as they are followed superiorly toward the *mastoid process*. These boundaries can be accentuated by hunching the shoulder anteriorly and superiorly (trapezius) and rotating the head to the opposite side (sternocleidomastoid).

The *floor* of the triangle is muscular and palpable deep in the triangle. The *subclavian artery* and *proximal part* of the *brachial plexus* (roots or trunks) pass through this floor and are palpable in the anteromedial corner of the triangle (i.e., where the sternocleidomastoid muscle attaches to the clavicle). In the triangle, the *subclavian artery* is positioned medially and inferiorly; its pulse can be felt in the angle formed

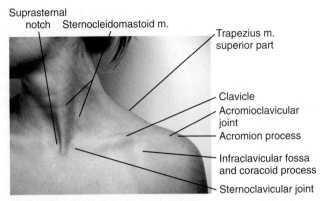

Figure 5-1 *Anterolateral view of the left posterior cervical triangle. To accentuate the sternocleidomastoid muscle, the head is rotated to the opposite side.*

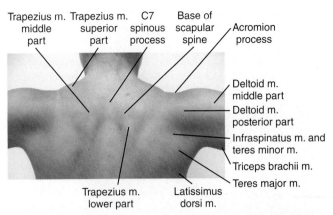

Figure 5-3 *Posterior view of the cervical and upper thoracic portions of the back and the scapular regions. Horizontal abduction of the abducted upper limbs is resisted to reveal certain of the intrinsic and extrinsic muscles of the shoulder. Because the upper limbs are moderately abducted, the scapulae are rotated somewhat superiorly.*

by the clavicle and sternocleidomastoid, just posterior to the clavicle where the artery passes superior to the first rib. The *superior trunk* of the brachial plexus is located approximately 2 to 3 cm superior to the clavicle at the posterior border of the sternocleidomastoid muscle. This structure feels like a strong cord or rope. Even though the *accessory nerve* is not palpable, its superficial course across the posterior triangle can be approximated because its course parallels a line between the earlobe and the acromion process.

Shoulder

The term *shoulder* (Figs. 5-2 through 5-5) is nonspecific because the areas and structures that can be included vary considerably. In this discussion, the "shoulder" includes the clavicle, the scapula, the proximal portion of the humerus, and all related articulations and soft tissues.

The *clavicle* is palpable throughout its length. In the midline, the *suprasternal (jugular) notch* is easily felt just superior to the manubrium of the sternum and between the medial ends of the clavicles. The *sternoclavicular joint* is located just lateral to the notch; its location can be verified by circumducting the arm and thereby moving the clavicle at the joint. From the joint, the shaft of the clavicle can be followed laterally; medially, it is anteriorly convex, and laterally, it is anteriorly concave. The clavicle ends laterally at the *acromioclavicular joint,* which is marked by either an eleva-

tion or a "step-off." The *infraclavicular fossa* is the depression inferior to the concavity of the clavicle; the *coracoid process* is palpable in the depths of that fossa.

The *acromion process* is the bony shelf just lateral to the acromioclavicular joint. The lateral border of this process ends abruptly and marks the most superior and lateral aspects of the *scapula.* The posterior aspect of the acromion continues medially and somewhat inferiorly as the *spine of the scapula.* The spine then ends medially, at its blunted *base,* at the *medial (vertebral) border* of the scapula. The base of the spine of the scapula typically is at the level of the spinous process of the third thoracic vertebra. From the base of the spine, the medial border of the scapula can be followed superiorly to the *superior angle* and inferiorly to the *inferior angle.* Most of the medial border is palpated through the trapezius muscle. From the inferior angle, the *lateral (axillary) border* can be followed superiorly to the glenoid fossa, which cannot be palpated.

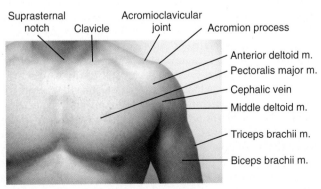

Figure 5-2 *Anterior view of the left shoulder, pectoral region, and proximal aspect of the arm.*

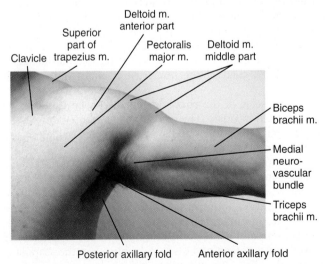

Figure 5-4 *Anterior and slightly inferior view of the left shoulder and axillary region. The arm is moderately abducted to reveal both the anterior and posterior axillary folds and the medial neurovascular bundle.*

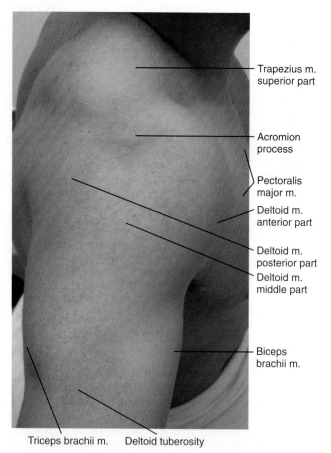

Trapezius m.
superior part

Acromion
process

Pectoralis
major m.

Deltoid m.
anterior part

Deltoid m.
posterior part

Deltoid m.
middle part

Biceps
brachii m.

Triceps brachii m.   Deltoid tuberosity

Figure 5-5 Superolateral view of the right shoulder.

Those aspects of the *proximal humerus* that can be palpated must be felt through the deltoid muscle around the edge of the acromion process. Because the head of the humerus articulates with the glenoid fossa of the scapula, it is positioned inferior to the acromion and therefore cannot be palpated. Even though the head of the humerus is not palpable, the tubercles surrounding it are. These are the *greater tubercle* laterally and posteriorly and the *lesser tubercle* anteriorly. These structures are separated by the *intertubercular groove,* which is positioned anterolaterally. The position of this groove can be verified by rotation of the humerus. The *deltoid tuberosity* is easily located on the lateral aspect of the shaft of the humerus, at about the midshaft level.

The muscles of the shoulder region can be classified as extrinsic and intrinsic. The *extrinsic muscles* interconnect the scapula, clavicle, or humerus with the axial skeleton and function to stabilize and move the shoulder girdle. Those that are palpable are the trapezius, pectoralis major, serratus anterior, and latissimus dorsi. The *trapezius* can be both visualized and palpated. The curvature of the neck between the head and the shoulder is formed by its superior part, and the middle and inferior parts extend laterally from the vertebral column and are superficial to most of the scapula. This muscle is prominent and easily palpable when the scapula is adducted. The *pectoralis major* forms the entire pectoral region, can be felt inferior to most of the clavicle, and forms the anterior axillary fold. It is active with horizontal adduc-

tion of the arm. The *latissimus dorsi* forms the most inferior part of the posterior axillary fold and can be palpated just lateral to the axillary border of the scapula, particularly when the arm is extended. The *serratus anterior* arises from the anterolateral aspects of most ribs and extends posteriorly and superiorly toward the vertebral border of the scapula. Because the muscle is largely deep to the scapula, only its anterior and inferior aspects can be felt. Forced scapular protraction (as during a push-up) makes these points of attachment easily identified. The *rhomboid major* and *minor* are located deep to the trapezius between the scapula and the vertebral column. Contraction of these muscles can be felt only when they are active and the trapezius is not, as when the scapula rotates inferiorly (i.e., during resisted extension of the arm). The *levator scapulae* also is deep to the trapezius, specifically its superior part, as it extends from the superior angle of the scapula to the upper cervical vertebrae. Even though this muscle is ropelike in shape, as opposed to the broader trapezius, it can be difficult to distinguish from the trapezius because both muscles elevate the scapula.

The *intrinsic muscles* of the shoulder extend from the scapula or clavicle to the humerus and function to stabilize the glenohumeral joint and move the humerus. The largest of these is the *deltoid,* which forms the entire contour of the shoulder. Its three parts are easily palpable: the *middle part* with abduction of the arm, the *anterior part* with flexion, and the *posterior part* with extension. The *teres major* extends from the inferior aspect of the axillary border of the scapula to the anterior aspect of the proximal humerus; posteriorly, it is superior to the latissimus dorsi and forms part of the posterior axillary fold. Resisted medial rotation or extension of the humerus makes this stout muscle easily visible and palpable. Palpation of the *rotator cuff muscles* is difficult because they are covered (at least partially) by larger muscles, specifically the deltoid and trapezius. The tendons of all four muscles can be located through the deltoid, where they insert on the tubercles of the humerus. The *subscapularis* inserts anteriorly on the lesser tubercle, the *supraspinatus* superiorly on the greater tubercle, and both the *infraspinatus* and *teres minor* posteriorly on the greater tubercle. When external rotation of the humerus is resisted, portions of the muscle bellies of both the infraspinatus and the teres minor can be felt on the posterior aspect of the scapula in the interval between the deltoid and the teres major.

The interval between the lateral aspect of the acromion process and the humerus, the *suprahumeral* (or *subacromial*) *space,* is important clinically because it is most often the site of pain associated with an impingement syndrome. The soft tissue structures in this interval and deep to the deltoid muscle are the *subacromial (subdeltoid) bursa,* the *tendon of the supraspinous muscle,* and the superior aspect of the *glenohumeral joint capsule.* Even though each of these structures is palpable, each is palpated simultaneously with the others. As a result, distinguishing them is difficult. The *tendon of the long head of the biceps brachii muscle* also passes through this space. It is positioned somewhat anteriorly and is largely under the acromion, so it is palpable only in the intertubercular groove of the humerus.

Most *neurovascular structures* in the shoulder region are difficult to palpate because they are separated from the surface by a variety of other structures. However, the main

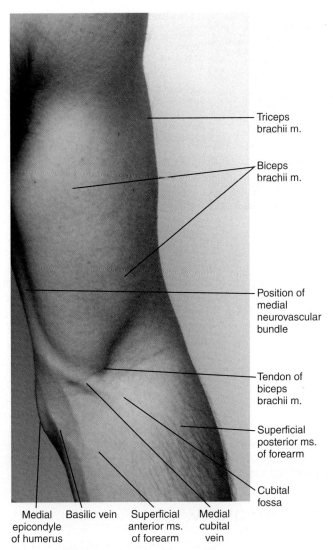

Triceps
brachii m.

Biceps
brachii m.

Position of
medial
neurovascular
bundle

Tendon of
biceps
brachii m.

Superficial
posterior ms.
of forearm

Cubital
fossa

Medial   Basilic vein   Superficial   Medial
epicondyle   anterior ms.   cubital
of humerus   of forearm   vein

Figure 5-6 Anterior view of the left elbow.

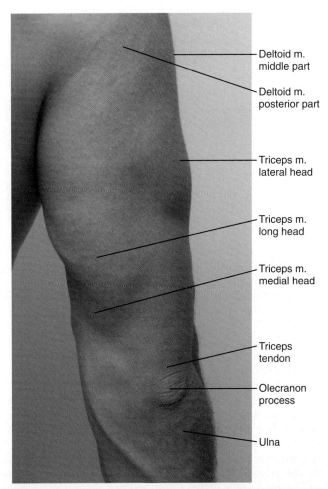

Deltoid m.
middle part

Deltoid m.
posterior part

Triceps m.
lateral head

Triceps m.
long head

Triceps m.
medial head

Triceps
tendon

Olecranon
process

Ulna

Figure 5-7 Posterior view of the right shoulder, arm, and elbow. Extension at the elbow is moderately resisted.

neurovascular bundle that supplies the upper limb passes through the axilla, where it can be palpated with the arm moderately elevated. This bundle consists of the *axillary artery* and the *median, ulnar, and radial nerves.*

Arm and Elbow

The bones of the arm (see Fig. 5-4) and elbow (Figs. 5-6 and 5-7) region consist of the *distal half* of the *humerus* and *proximal aspects* of the *radius* and *ulna.* Because the humerus widens significantly at its distal end, the *medial* and *lateral humeral epicondyles* are easily palpable as the most pronounced medial and lateral prominences at the elbow. The soft tissue masses associated with these epicondyles are the *common tendons of origin* of the *superficial flexor* (medial) and *superficial extensor* (lateral) *muscles* of the forearm. From each of these epicondyles, the *supracondylar ridges* can be followed proximally for approximately 4 or 5 cm. Posteriorly, the *olecranon process* of the ulna forms the point of the elbow. From this process, the *shaft of the ulna* can be followed distally because it is subcutaneous throughout its length.

The location of the *elbow joint* can be determined both medially and laterally. The *lateral joint line* is marked by a depression distal to the lateral epicondyle between the capitulum and the *head of the radius;* the location of the radial head can be confirmed by supination and pronation of the forearm. Just distal to the radial head, the *radial neck* narrows to the shaft, which is deep to the lateral forearm musculature. The depression formed by the joint line is less distinct laterally than either anteriorly or posteriorly because of a thickening of the lateral aspect of the joint capsule—the *lateral (radial) collateral ligament.* The *medial joint line* of the elbow is less distinct because the medial epicondyle is prominent. In addition, the posterior and distal aspects of the epicondyle are commonly sensitive because of the presence of the *ulnar nerve.*

The *muscles of the arm* are separated into *anterior* and *posterior groups* by medial and lateral intermuscular septa. The *lateral septum* extends from the deltoid tuberosity to the lateral humeral epicondyle, and the location of the *medial septum* is marked by the medial neurovascular bundle, which continues from the axilla. Although there are three muscles in the anterior compartment, the *biceps brachii* is the most superficial; therefore its belly is readily palpable, particularly with resisted forearm flexion and supination. The *triceps brachii* occupies virtually the entire posterior compartment

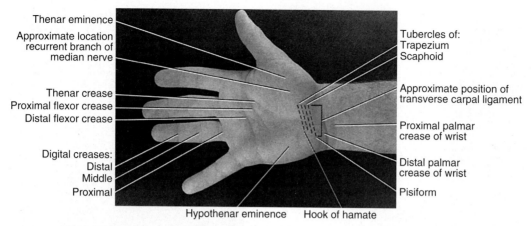

Thenar eminence
Approximate location
recurrent branch of
median nerve

Thenar crease
Proximal flexor crease
Distal flexor crease

Digital creases:
Distal
Middle
Proximal

Hypothenar eminence   Hook of hamate

Tubercles of:
Trapezium
Scaphoid

Approximate position of
transverse carpal ligament

Proximal palmar
crease of wrist

Distal palmar
crease of wrist

Pisiform

Figure 5-8 Ventral, or palmar, view of the right wrist and hand with the digits extended.

and is readily palpable throughout the posterior arm. Even its three heads can be identified (i.e., the *lateral head* proximally and laterally, the *long head* proximally and medially, and the *medial head* distally on either side of the triceps tendon).

The *muscles of the forearm* are separated into anterior and posterior groups even though their positions are not truly anterior and posterior. The *anterior muscles* are medial proximally and anterior distally; the *posterior muscles* are lateral proximally and posterior distally. Only a few of the forearm muscles can be palpated individually in the proximal forearm because they either have common tendons of origin or are deep to other structures. At the wrist, however, several of their tendons can be readily identified. Proximally and medially, the *pronator teres* can be palpated with resisted pronation; it feels like a distinct cord passing obliquely laterally from the medial epicondyle to the radius. It forms the medial boundary of the cubital fossa. Of the lateral muscles, the *brachioradialis* is most prominent. It is obvious when the forearm is flexed with the forearm midway between supination and pronation.

The *cubital fossa* is the triangular depression in front of the elbow. Its medial and lateral borders are the pronator teres and brachioradialis muscle, respectively; its proximal border is a line between the humeral epicondyles. With the exception of the *ulnar nerve,* which enters the forearm by passing posterior to the medial epicondyle, the major neurovascular structures of the forearm and hand pass through this fossa. The *tendon of the biceps brachii* disappears into the center of the fossa. From this tendon, a fibrous band, the *bicipital aponeurosis (lacertus fibrosus),* passes medially to blend with the investing fascia of the forearm. The sharp proximal border of this aponeurosis can easily be identified when forearm flexion is resisted. The *brachial pulse* can be felt on the medial side of the biceps tendon, and the *median nerve* is between the tendon and the artery. Both the nerve and artery pass deep to the bicipital aponeurosis. The *median cubital vein* is superficial to the aponeurosis as it passes obliquely across the front of the elbow. This vein interconnects the major superficial veins of the upper limb (i.e., the *cephalic vein* laterally and the *basilic vein* medially).

Forearm and Wrist

As mentioned, the *ulna* is palpable for its entire length, ending distally in the dorsomedially positioned *styloid process.* The *radius* cannot be palpated through most of the forearm, but at its distal end, it has two major landmarks. The most distal aspect of either forearm bone is the *styloid process of the radius,* which is easily felt on the lateral aspect of the wrist (Figs. 5-8 through 5-12). The *dorsal radial*

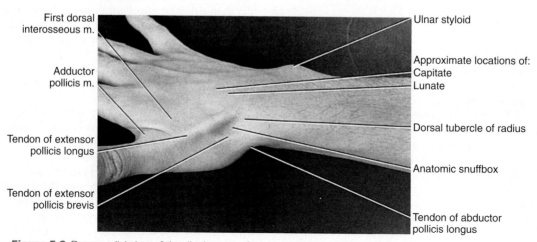

First dorsal
interosseous m.

Adductor
pollicis m.

Tendon of extensor
pollicis longus

Tendon of extensor
pollicis brevis

Ulnar styloid

Approximate locations of:
Capitate
Lunate

Dorsal tubercle of radius

Anatomic snuffbox

Tendon of abductor
pollicis longus

Figure 5-9 Dorsomedial view of the distal aspect of the right forearm, wrist, and hand, with the digits extended.

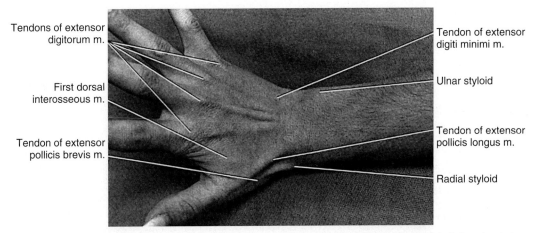

Tendons of extensor digitorum m.

First dorsal interosseous m.

Tendon of extensor pollicis brevis m.

Tendon of extensor digiti minimi m.

Ulnar styloid

Tendon of extensor pollicis longus m.

Radial styloid

Figure 5-10 *Dorsal view of the distal aspect of the right forearm, wrist, and hand, with the digits extended.*

(*Lister's*) *tubercle* is the most apparent dorsal prominence. This tubercle is easy to locate when the thumb is extended because the tendon of the extensor pollicis longus makes a turn around the ulnar side of the tubercle.

Dorsally, the *distal end of the radius* forms a transverse ridge that marks the junction with the carpus or the *radiocarpal joint*. This ridge becomes more prominent when the hand is slightly flexed. Because the distal surface of the radius is concave (dorsal to palmar) and the dorsal aspect extends considerably more distally than the palmar aspect, the more proximal carpal bones are somewhat hidden by this dorsal ridge of the radius when the hand is extended. With the hand in the neutral position or slightly flexed, a depression is apparent just distal to the radius approximately in line with the third ray. This depression marks the interval between the radius and the base of the third metacarpal and contains the *lunate* proximally and *capitate* distally. The *scaphoid* forms the floor of the anatomic snuffbox. Palpation of this bone commonly produces moderate discomfort.

On the palmar side, the junction of the forearm and carpus along with the location of the carpal tunnel can be determined. The radiocarpal joint is located at the level of the *proximal palmar skin crease* of the wrist. The *distal skin crease* approximates the proximal border of the carpal tunnel. All four major bony attachments of the *transverse carpal ligament* (*deep flexor retinaculum*) can be identified. The *pisiform* is just distal to the distal carpal crease on the ulnar side. The *hamulus* (*hook*) of the *hamate* is slightly distal and lateral to the pisiform; it also is deeper than the pisiform, and its palpation may produce some discomfort because of the proximity of the ulnar nerve. On the radial sides, the distal crease separates the *tubercles* of the *scaphoid* and *trapezium*; both tubercles are approximately in line with the tendon of the flexor carpi radialis.

On the *palmar aspect* of the *wrist* the tendons of three muscles are both constant and reliable landmarks. The *tendon of the flexor carpi radialis* is large, crosses the wrist just lateral to the center, and is clearly visible when flexion of the hand is resisted. On the extreme ulnar side, the *tendon of the flexor carpi ulnaris* is directly in line with the pisiform. This tendon becomes more apparent with resisted flexion and ulnar deviation of the hand. The *tendons of the flexor digitorum superficialis* (*sublimis*) occupy the interval between the tendons of the flexor carpi radialis and flexor carpi ulnaris muscles. These tendons are arranged side-by-side and occupy most of the interval.

The *tendon of the palmaris longus*, which is present in approximately 85% of the population, is the most superficial

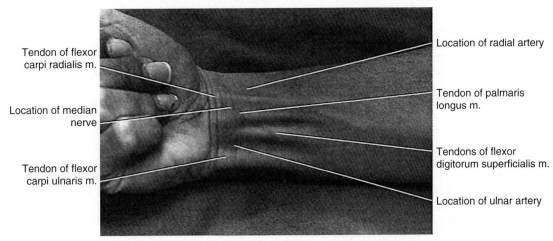

Tendon of flexor carpi radialis m.

Location of median nerve

Tendon of flexor carpi ulnaris m.

Location of radial artery

Tendon of palmaris longus m.

Tendons of flexor digitorum superficialis m.

Location of ulnar artery

Figure 5-11 *Palmar view of the distal right forearm, wrist, and hand. The fingers are flexed forcefully to reveal the tendons of certain forearm muscles.*

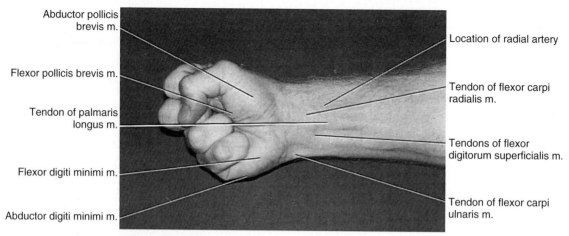

Abductor pollicis brevis m.

Flexor pollicis brevis m.

Tendon of palmaris longus m.

Flexor digiti minimi m.

Abductor digiti minimi m.

Location of radial artery

Tendon of flexor carpi radialis m.

Tendons of flexor digitorum superficialis m.

Tendon of flexor carpi ulnaris m.

Figure 5-12 Palmar view of the distal right forearm, wrist, and hand. The hand is clenched into a strong fist.

tendon on the palmar aspect of the wrist. It is located on the ulnar side of the tendon of the flexor carpi radialis and superficial to the lateral tendon(s) of the flexor digitorum superficialis. The tendon of the palmaris longus becomes more prominent when the hand is slightly flexed and "cupped."

On the palmar wrist, the *median nerve* is in a deep position between the tendons of the flexor carpi radialis and the palmaris longus. When the palmaris longus is not present, the nerve is just ulnar to the tendon of the flexor carpi radialis. A very small branch of the median nerve, the *palmar branch*, arises from the radial side of the main trunk in the distal third of the forearm. This branch enters the hand superficially (not through the carpal tunnel) in line with the radial side of the median nerve or the radial side of the middle finger. In the distal forearm, the *ulnar nerve* and *artery* are deep to the flexor carpi ulnaris muscle. At the wrist, the nerve is deep to this tendon and the artery is just radial. The two structures then pass radial to the pisiform and ulna to the hook of the hamate as they pass through Guyon's canal. Although the *radial artery* does not cross the palmar aspect of the wrist, its pulse is easily palpable 2 to 3 cm proximal to the wrist on the radial side of the tendon of the flexor carpi radialis.

The extensor tendons entering the hand cross both the radial and dorsal aspects of the wrist. The *tendons of the abductor pollicis longus* and *extensor pollicis brevis* typically occupy a common compartment as they cross the wrist. These two tendons are positioned superficial to the radial styloid as the most volar tendons on the radial aspect of the wrist. The *tendon* of the *extensor pollicis longus* muscle is apparent when the thumb is extended. This tendon crosses the wrist just ulnar to Lister's tubercle, then immediately turns radially as it passes toward the thumb. Along with the tendons of the abductor pollicis longus and extensor pollicis brevis, the tendon of the extensor pollicis longus forms the boundaries of the anatomic snuffbox. The *tendons of the extensor carpi radialis longus* and *brevis* muscles can be palpated just distal to the radius, in line with the index and middle fingers, respectively. Because both tendons are deep to other tendons, they are most apparent when extension of the hand is resisted while the fingers and thumb are relaxed. The *tendons* of the *extensor digitorum* are easily palpated after they are visualized; extension of the fingers makes them readily apparent. The most medial tendon is that of the *exten-

sor carpi ulnaris.* It is in line with the ulnar styloid and bridges the indentation between that prominence and the base of the fifth metacarpal.

Other than the more deeply positioned radial artery, the neurovascular structures crossing the dorsal aspect of the wrist all are found in the subcutaneous tissue. The *radial artery* passes through the anatomic snuffbox, deep to all of the bordering tendons. *Superficial veins* contributing to both the *cephalic* and *basilic* veins usually can be observed on the lateral and medial aspects of the wrist, respectively. The *superficial radial nerve* crosses the dorsolateral aspect of the wrist. It usually can be palpated about midway between Lister's tubercle and the metacarpophalangeal joint of the thumb, where it crosses the tendon of the extensor pollicis longus muscle.

Hand

Like the palmar wrist, the *palmar aspect of the hand* has skin creases that are consistently present and helpful in localizing deeper structures (see Figs. 5-8 through 5-12). The palm has three such creases, which usually appear to share a common point of origin at approximately the metacarpophalangeal joint of the index finger. The *distal volar flexor crease* extends across the palm from that point and marks the locations of the metacarpophalangeal joints. The *proximal volar flexor crease* is more oblique in position than the distal crease and ends at about the hypothenar eminence. The *thenar crease* outlines the border of the thenar eminence. The four fingers have three creases each. The *proximal digital crease* is located at the web space, and the *middle* and *distal creases* are at the proximal and distal interphalangeal joints, respectively.

The approximate locations of the two arterial arches in the palm can be determined in the following manner. The *superficial palmar arterial arch* is at about the level of the proximal flexor crease in the center of the palm; this location also corresponds to the distal surface of the fully extended thumb. The *deep palmar arterial arch* is approximately the width of a finger proximal to the distal arch.

The nerves of the palm are the median and ulnar nerves. The main trunk of the *median nerve*, at the distal end of the carpal tunnel, is aligned with the middle finger. At that point, it separates into terminal branches. The *motor (recurrent, thenar) branch* recurs into the thenar musculature and is located midway between the first metacarpophalangeal joint and the pisiform. The *digital branches* of the median nerve pass toward the first, second, and third web spaces.

The *ulnar nerve,* after passing radial to the pisiform and ulnar to the hook of the hamate, bifurcates into *superficial* and *deep branches.* The superficial branch continues distally toward the fourth web space. Another branch, a proper digital nerve, passes toward the ulnar side of the little finger. The deep branch of the ulnar nerve passes deep and accompanies the deep arterial arch.

The *proper palmar digital nerves* and *arteries,* branches of both the median and ulnar nerves, provide the major nerve and arterial supplies to the digits. These nerves and vessels are located on both the ulnar and radial sides of the palmar aspects of the digits.

Only a small number of the *intrinsic muscles* of the hand can be palpated. In the most radial aspect of the thenar compartment, the *abductor pollicis brevis* is apparent when abduction of the thumb is resisted. With flexion of the thumb, the *flexor pollicis brevis* can be felt in the thenar compartment, in line with the flexor surface of the thumb. The *abductor digiti minimi* and *flexor digiti minimi* are apparent with abduction and flexion of the little finger, respectively. Two muscles can be distinguished in the first web space. Dorsally, the *first dorsal interosseous* is easily palpated with abduction of the index finger. In the palmar aspect of that web space, the distal aspect of the *adductor pollicis* is visible when thumb adduction is resisted.

REFERENCES

The complete reference list is available online at www.expertconsult.com.

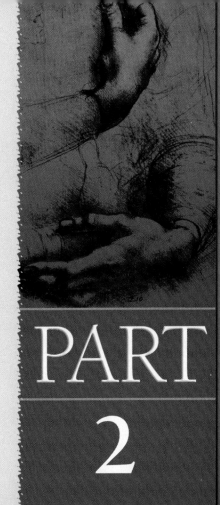

PART
2

Examination

CHAPTER 6

Clinical Examination of the Hand

JODI L. SEFTCHICK, MOT, OTR/L, CHT, LAUREN M. DETULLIO, MS, OTR/L, CHT, JANE M. FEDORCZYK, PT, PhD, CHT, ATC, AND PAT L. AULICINO, MD

HISTORY	VASCULARITY OF THE HAND
PHYSICAL EXAMINATION	MEDICAL SCREENING AND REVIEW OF SYSTEMS
NERVE SUPPLY OF THE HAND—MOTOR AND SENSORY	SUMMARY

CRITICAL POINTS

- Observation, visual inspection, and palpation provide information regarding the patient's general health status and present condition.
- Therapists and surgeons need to obtain a thorough patient history so that they can understand the patient's problem and how it affects the patient physically, psychologically, and economically.
- Perform a systematic examination, documenting and organizing the results well.
- Include medical screening and systems review with all patients.

Clinical examination of the hand is a basic skill that both the surgeon and the therapist should master. To do so, it is necessary to understand the functional anatomy of the hand. A thorough history, a systematic examination, and knowledge of disease processes that affect the hand minimize the examiner's diagnostic dilemmas. Radiographs, CT scans, MRI scans, electrodiagnostics, and specialized laboratory tests are ancillary tools that only confirm a diagnosis that has been made on a clinical basis (see Chapters 13 and 15).

An organized approach and clear and concise records are of paramount importance. Either line drawings of the deformities or clinical photographs should be prepared for each new patient examined. Digital photographs may be a more efficient means for storage with electronic medical records. Range of motion (ROM) of the affected parts should be recorded and dated, ideally in a table format. Any discrep-

ancy between active and passive motion, if present, also should be noted. A good hand examination is useless if the results are not recorded accurately.

This chapter outlines one approach to examination of the hand. The most important points already have been made: perform a systematic, organized clinical examination and record the results accurately and clearly.

History

Before a patient's hand is examined, an accurate history must be taken. The patient's age, hand dominance, occupation, and avocations are elicited. Another option for determining hand dominance is to administer the Waterloo Handedness Questionnaire (see Fig. 12-3).[1] If the patient has had an injury, the exact mechanism as well as the time and date of the injury and prior treatments are recorded. Prior surgical procedures, infections, medications, and therapy also are noted. After this background information is obtained, the patient is questioned specifically regarding the involved hand and extremity, including a pain interview. (See Box 114-1 and Chapter 114 for additional information on pain assessment.) Open-ended questions about the present signs and symptoms are included to determine what the patient is not able to do now that he or she could do before the injury or what brought the patient to the surgeon or therapist. Questions related to the history of present illness allow the clinician to develop a hypothesis about the level of irritability. Low irritability is defined as minimal to no pain at rest, transient pain with movement, and symptoms that are not easily provoked. Highly irritable conditions present with resting pain, higher pain levels with activity, and decreased mobility.

The level of irritability determines how vigorously the surgeon or therapist may perform the tests and measures during the physical examination and direct treatment goals.

What are the patient goals? This question is extremely important. The patient's reply assists the clinician in determining whether the patient has a realistic understanding of the true nature of the injury. Unrealistic expectations can never be fulfilled and result in both disappointment and frustration for both the patient and the therapist and surgeon. During this interview, it is also important to assess the effect that the injury or disease process has on the patient's family and economic and social life. Patients who have litigation pending or possible significant secondary gain may be poorly motivated and are not optimal candidates for elective hand surgery. Successful hand surgery requires precise surgical techniques followed by expert hand therapy in conjunction with a well-motivated, compliant patient.

The patient's pertinent medical history is obtained to determine general health status, especially regarding comorbidities that may affect the patient's recovery or increase surgical risks? Additional questions should be asked about current medications (prescription and nonprescription), allergies, and lifestyle choices (smoking, alcohol use, or substance abuse). Current practice trends require hand surgeons and therapists to do medical screening and review of systems.[2] This is a key component in medical education and training; however, it is a recent addition to the entry-level education for therapists, especially physical therapists. More information is provided later in this chapter.

The patient's social history should be obtained. What is his support system? How well do the patient and his family understand the injury and required care? What are his avocational interests? The patient's economic status may also influence ability to comply with therapy and follow-up care. What is his insurance coverage or co-pay amount? Does he have a limited number of authorized visits? Does his injury present a financial hardship or limit his ability to care for children or elderly parents?

If the patient is working, information should be gathered about his job description, physical demands, or essential functions, and the last date worked even if the injury is not work-related. This information may indicate the presence of risk factors associated with the injury. Therapists and surgeons can use these data to outline a plan of care that incorporates appropriate modified duty work, if available, and the use of work-oriented tasks in the clinic to keep the patient on track to return to full duty. Although it may be too early in the examination process to discern a return to work date, an experienced clinician can usually tell how motivated the patient is to return to his job based on the patient's answers regarding employment. Patient's who are receiving compensation for an injury or illness may be more difficult to treat, more likely to have a prolonged course of rehabilitation, and more likely to become disabled than patients with similar conditions who are not receiving compensation.[3]

Self-report health-related outcome measures such as Disabilities of the Arm, Shoulder, and Hand (DASH),[4] Carpal Tunnel Instrument,[5] or Michigan Hand Outcomes Questionnaire (MHQ)[6] can serve as valuable tools for gathering information on pain, function, activity participation, disability, and patient satisfaction.[7,8] These measures have all proven to be reliable and valid.[4-6] The Carpal Tunnel Instrument is a condition-specific measure, whereas the DASH and MHQ are region-specific. Global measures such as the SF-36 and patient-specific scales that contain no standardized questions may also be used.[7,8] These questionnaires can be invaluable in gathering information about problems with activities of daily living (ADL), such as toileting or sexual activity. Patients are not usually comfortable addressing these issues upfront. It is important for the examiner to become familiar with self-report health-related outcome measures to determine which would be most useful and clinically relevant for the patient. Chapter 16 discusses the measurement issues and use of outcome measurement in the upper extremity.

The history is completed only after the surgeon or therapist has a complete understanding of the patient's problem and how it affects the patient physically, psychologically, and economically.

Physical Examination

Observation, Inspection, and Palpation

Hands are used to interact with the surrounding environment and for communication. People "actively" use their hands for a variety of functional activities. "Passively" the hands communicate to clinicians about the health status of their patients. When examining a patient's upper extremity, one must be able to observe the shoulder, arm, forearm, and hand. Therefore, the patient's entire upper extremity should be exposed. The gross appearance of the entire extremity is inspected. Table 6-1 outlines the physical characteristics of the skin and musculoskeletal tissues that should be observed, inspected, and palpated during the physical examination to determine the presence of diseases such as arthritis, impairments such as edema and loss of motion, as well as level of irritability.

Skin and nail changes may be associated with chronic diseases of the kidney or liver as well as the respiratory system.[2] A review of systems and past medical history should determine the associated condition. These changes are chronic, and the patient should already be aware of the condition. Normally, with the hand resting and the wrist in neutral, the fingers are progressively more flexed from the radial to the ulnar side of the hand. A loss of the normal resting attitude of the hand can indicate a tendon laceration, a contracture, or, possibly, a peripheral nerve injury (Fig. 6-1).

Edema

Another important component of the clinical examination of the hand is to assess edema if noted on visual inspection. Edema may be assessed using circumferential or volumetric measurements. Volumetry is primarily used if the entire hand is edematous, but not for an isolated finger. Chapters 63 through 65 present detailed information on the examination and management of edema and lymphedema in the hand and upper extremity.

Table 6-1   Physical Characteristics of the Skin and Musculoskeletal Tissues That Should Be Observed, Inspected, and Palpated During the Physical Examination

General Observations	Clinical Significance
Hand relationship to the body How does the patient carry the arm? Is there spontaneity or ease of movement? What is the quality of the movement? Is the patient using substitution patterns with movement? Is the patient able to place his or her hand in a functional position?	Cradling the arm or guarded posture is a sign of patient apprehension to movement typically due to high levels of pain associated with a high level of irritability. Signs of muscle weakness or loss of motion that may be related to nerve injury, disuse, or joint contracture If not, the elbow and shoulder motion may be limited and should be examined. If the hand cannot be placed in a functional position, a brilliantly reconstructed hand is useless.

Visual Inspection	Clinical Significance
Muscle atrophy	Muscle weakness due to disuse or nerve injury
Blisters and small cuts	Sign of decreased cutaneous sensibility due to nerve injury
Needle marks	Indication of current or previous substance abuse or the use of injectable prescription medication for disease such as insulin-dependent diabetes
Wounds and scars	Scars indicate previous injuries or surgeries. Wounds may indicate decreased cutaneous sensibility.
Skin color, tone, moisture, and trophic changes	Sympathetic signs of nerve injury. Dry skin indication of peripheral nerve laceration. Increased sweating (hyperhidrosis) sign of increased sympathetic activity that may be related to complex regional pain syndrome (CRPS).* Color changes due to metabolic conditions or disease Skin that has been denervated has lost its autonomic input. The finger pulp becomes atrophic, smooth, and dry, with relative loss of dermal ridges. Denervated skin does not wrinkle when placed in warm water (the "wrinkle test").[31]
Normal skin creases or ridges	Diminished due to presence of edema or trophic changes of the skin associated with nerve injury
Are the nails ridged, pitted, or deformed? Is there correct rotational alignment of the nail plates?	Nail changes linked to chronic diseases of the kidney, liver, respiratory system. Spoon nails found in patients with iron deficiency. Changes may be related to peripheral nerve injury.
Edema, hematoma, ecchymosis	Indicates acute tissue injury and healing
Loss of resting attitude of the hand	Indicates a tendon laceration, a contracture, or peripheral nerve injury
Contractures	Loss of motion
Gross deformities	Congenital, acquired, traumatic
Preservation of hand arches	Flattening of the aches associated with intrinsic muscle atrophy due to nerve injury or disuse

Palpation	Clinical Significance
Temperature	Warm temperature is a sign of acute inflammation. Cool temperature is a sign of decreased blood flow; may be vasomotor instability.
Nodules, tumors	Likely benign lesions that may be associated with wrist instability, arthritis, Dupuytren's or other soft tissue conditions
Edema	Pitting edema leaves depressions with palpation. Brawny edema is immobile and hard to palpate.
Capillary refill	Skin should blanch when palpated and resume normal color when pressure removed.
Skin mobility	Lack of mobility due to fibrosis, scar, and edema
Scar	Painful to touch (tactile allodynia) indicates hypersensitivity.

*See Table 14-4 in archived Chapter 14 in the fifth edition located on companion Web site.

Range of Motion

The motion of the entire upper extremity and cervical region should be screened with hand injuries and compared with that of the opposite side for possible loss of motion and pain. Joints that demonstrate loss of active or passive motion (or both) should be measured with an appropriately sized goniometer.[9] Measurements have been shown to be relatively reliable within and between examiners; intrarater and interrater variability is in the range of 5 to 10 degrees.[10] If possible, the same examiner should take measurements.

Digital motion is typically assessed with the metal finger goniometer placed on the dorsal aspect of the phalanges (Fig. 6-2). If it is not possible to place the goniometer on the dorsal aspect of the digit, then a lateral goniometer placement may be used and this exception should be documented. When possible, active measurements of the finger joints are taken in a composite manner by asking the patient to make a fist for flexion and then straighten the hand for extension. Isolated motions may be performed for an individual joint, typically with stabilization of the proximal joint; however, this should be recorded (Fig. 6-3).

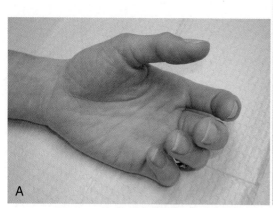

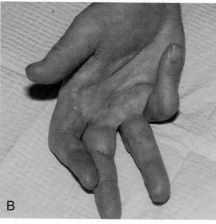

Figure 6-1 A, Normal attitude of the hand in a resting position. Notice that the fingers are progressively more flexed from the radial aspect to the ulnar aspect of the hand. **B,** This normal attitude is lost because of contractures of the digits as a result of Dupuytren's disease.

Total active motion (TAM) and total passive motion (TPM) measurements can be assessed for the individual digits. TAM is calculated by adding the composite flexion measurement of the metacarpophalangeal (MCP), proximal interphalangeal (PIP), and distal interphalangeal (DIP) joints and subtracting the sum of any extension deficits at these joints.[11] TPM is computed the same way, except passive measurements are used. Both TAM and TPM provide relevant data on composite motion of the finger and allow ease of comparison over time. This type of documentation is frequently used in research.

Goniometry manuals should be reviewed for detailed information on measuring joint motion of the hand and upper extremity.[12,13] When measuring carpometacarpal (CMC) motion of the thumb, some manuals describe the procedures differently. The starting angle for CMC extension or abduction is never 0 degrees; it is typically 25 to 30 degrees. Some manuals direct the clinician to measure the starting angle and subtract it from the measurements at the end of the available ROM. Some manuals just recommend that the examiner measure the end range motion. In terms of clinical relevance, only the end range motion is significant as it correlates with the patient's ability to open the first webspace. Therapists and surgeons working together should agree on a standard procedure for their patients to allow comparison of measurements.

If motion is lacking, the distance from the tip of the finger to the distal palmar crease (DPC) is measured. If the finger touches the palm but does not reach the crease, as occurs with profundus tendon disruption, this should be noted, and the distance from the tip of the finger to the DPC should be recorded; however, it should be stated that the finger did touch the palm but did not reach the DPC (Fig. 6-4).

After all active and passive motions have been examined; the wrist is flexed and extended to see if the normal tenodesis effect is present. In an uninjured hand, when the wrist is flexed, the fingers and the thumb extend, and as the wrist is extended, the fingers assume an attitude of flexion and the thumb opposes the fifth digit (Fig. 6-5). This is an automatic motion of the hand and requires only that the patient be relaxed. The alignment of the digits is then inspected. The nail plates all should be parallel to one another, and their alignment should be similar to that of the other hand. Each finger should point individually to the scaphoid tuberosity, and the longitudinal axis of all fingers when flexed should point in the direction of the scaphoid (Fig. 6-6).

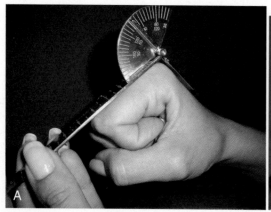

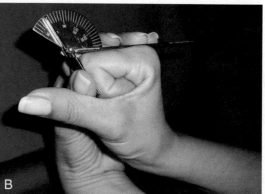

Figure 6-2 Digital motion is typically assessed with the metal finger goniometer placed on the dorsal aspect of the phalanges **A,** Measuring metacarpophalangeal flexion with the hand in composite flexion. **B,** Measuring proximal interphalangeal joint flexion with the hand in composite flexion.

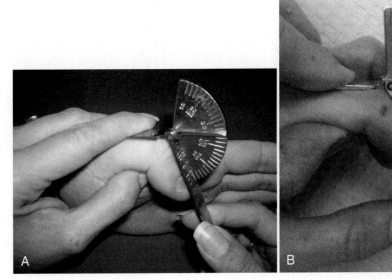

Figure 6-3 A, A finger goniometer is used to measure the range of motion (ROM) of the interphalangeal (IP) joint of the thumb. **B,** A finger goniometer is used to measure the ROM of the proximal IP joint of the index finger. Note proximal joint stabilization.

Muscle Testing

The hand is powered by intrinsic and extrinsic muscles. The extrinsic muscles have their origin in the forearm and the tendinous insertions in the hand. The extrinsic flexors are on the volar side of the forearm and flex the digits and the wrist. The extrinsic extensors originate on the dorsal aspect of the forearm and extend the fingers, thumb, and wrist. The intrinsic muscles originate and insert in the hand. These include the thenar and hypothenar muscles as well as the lumbricals and the interossei. The thenar and hypothenar muscles help position the thumb and the fifth finger and also aid in opposition of the thumb and with pinch. The interossei assist in abduction and adduction of the digits. The interossei flex the MCP joints and extend the interphalangeal (IP) joints along with the lumbricals.

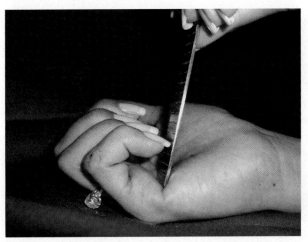

Figure 6-4 A ruler is used to measure the distance of the pulp of the finger from the distal palmar crease. Active and passive motions should be noted and recorded.

Extrinsic Muscle Testing—The Extrinsic Flexors

As each specific extrinsic muscle–tendon unit is tested, its strength should be graded and recorded (Table 6-2). The extrinsic muscles should be tested with respect to gravity, but this is not essential for the intrinsic muscles. Note tendon excursion during muscle contraction, which is reflected in ROM of the joints that the tendon acts on.

It is not necessary to test each hand muscle during examination. Key muscles for each nerve, radial, ulnar, and median, can be selected for screening. For each nerve, select one muscle that is innervated proximally ("high") and one muscle that is innervated distally ("low"). Table 6-3 provides examples. If nerve injury is present, all muscles innervated by the injured nerve should be assessed to determine the level of injury and to document return.

The flexor pollicis longus (FPL) long flexor of the thumb flexes the IP joint of the thumb. This muscle is tested by asking the patient to actively flex the last joint of his thumb (Fig. 6-7).

The flexor digitorum profundus of the fingers are then tested, in sequence, by having the patient flex the DIP joint of the finger being tested while the examiner holds the digit in full extension and blocks motion at the PIP joint and the MCP joint. During the testing of each profundus tendon, the other fingers may unintentionally flex due to the common muscle belly of the long, ring, and small finger profundus tendons, and this is permitted (Fig. 6-8).

The flexor digitorum superficialis of each finger is then tested. The examiner must hold the adjacent fingers in full extension. The PIP joint of the finger being tested is not blocked (Fig. 6-9). If the flexor system is functioning properly, the PIP will flex and the DIP joint will remain in extension. The fifth finger often has a deficient superficialis.[14] That is, it is not strong enough to flex the IP joint: on testing, the MCP joint flexes and the DIP joint and the PIP joint remain in extension. In the presence of a deficient superficialis tendon of the fifth digit, simultaneous testing of the fourth

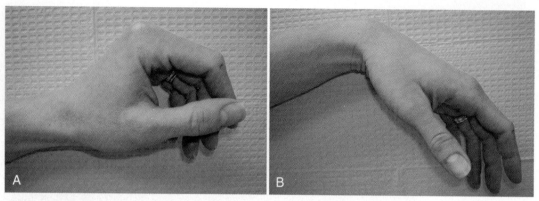

Figure 6-5 Tenodesis of the hand. In an uninjured hand **(A),** on wrist extension the fingers and thumb flex, and **(B),** on flexion of the wrist the thumb and fingers extend. In the presence of a tendon laceration, contractures of the joints, or adhesions of the flexor or extensor systems, the normal tenodesis effect is lost. This test can be performed actively by the patient or passively by the examiner.

and fifth digits often reveals normal superficialis function of the fourth digit.

The flexors of the wrist can be tested by having the patient flex the wrist against resistance in a radial and then in an ulnar direction while the examiner palpates each tendon. The flexor carpi radialis (FCR) is palpated on the radial side of the wrist, and the flexor carpi ulnaris (FCU) is palpated on the ulnar side of the wrist. The palmaris longus tendon can be palpated just ulnar to the FCR tendon.

Extrinsic Muscle Testing—The Extensors

As previously stated, the extensors of the digits and the wrist originate on the dorsal aspect of the forearm and pass through six discrete retinacular compartments at the dorsum of the wrist before their insertions in the hand.

The first dorsal compartment contains the abductor pollicis longus (APL) and the extensor pollicis brevis (EPB) tendons. The APL usually has multiple tendon slips and inserts on the base of the first metacarpal. It often has insertions on the trapezium. The EPB often runs in a separate compartment within the first dorsal compartment. The EPB and APL function in unison and are responsible for abduction of the first metacarpal and extension into the plane of

the metacarpals. The EPB is also an extensor of the MCP joint of the thumb. These musculotendinous units are tested by asking the patient to bring the thumb "out to the side and then back." Pain in the area of the first dorsal compartment and radial styloid is common and often a result of stenosing tenovaginitis of these tendons. This was first described by de Quervain in 1895 and now is a well-established clinical entity that bears his name. In 1930, Finkelstein stated that acute flexion of the thumb and deviation of the wrist in an ulnar direction produces excruciating pain at the first dorsal compartment, near the radial styloid, in patients who had stenosing tenovaginitis. This examination is now universally known as *Finkelstein's test*[15] (see Fig. 7-9). The extensor carpi radialis longus and brevis run in the second dorsal compartment. The longus inserts on the base of the second metacarpal and the brevis on the third. These are tested by asking the patient to make a tight fist and to strongly extend or dorsiflex the wrist. The two tendons are then palpated by the examiner.

The extensor pollicis longus (EPL) runs in the third dorsal compartment. This tendon both extends the IP joint of the thumb and adducts the first ray. The tendon passes sharply around Lister's tubercle and may rupture spontaneously after a distal radius fracture or in rheumatoid arthritis.[16] Its func-

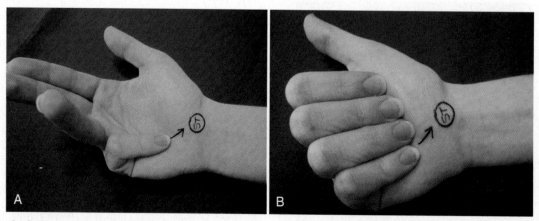

Figure 6-6 A, On flexion the tip of the fifth finger points directly to the scaphoid tuberosity, as do all the fingers when individually flexed. **B,** When all the digits are flexed simultaneously, the finger tips come together distal to the tuberosity, but the longitudinal axes of all fingers converge at an area proximal to the scaphoid tuberosity because of crowding of the adjacent digits. If there is a malunited fracture, the rotational alignment will be off and often there will be crossover of the digits.

Table 6-2 Manual Muscle Testing Grades for Hand Muscles

Numeric Grade	Result	Qualitative Grade
0	No evidence of contractility or tension	Zero
1	Slight evidence of contractility; no motion	Trace
2	Muscle action present; partial or full motion	Poor
	Gravity eliminated for extrinsic muscles	
3	Muscle action present; full ROM against gravity	Fair
4	Muscle action present; full ROM against gravity with moderate resistance	Good
5	Muscle action present; full ROM against gravity with maximum resistance	Normal

ROM, range of motion.

Table 6-3 Key Muscles to Screen for Peripheral Nerve Function

Nerve	Innervated Proximally ("High") or Distally ("Low")	Muscle
Radial nerve	High	Extensor carpi radialis longus and brevis
	Low	Extensor digitorum or extensor pollicis longus
Median nerve	High	Flexor carpi radialis or flexor digitorum superficialis
	Low	Thenar muscles
Ulnar nerve	High	Flexor carpi ulnaris or flexor digitorum profundus (ring, small)
	Low	Palmar or dorsal interossei

tion is tested by placing the patient's hand flat on the examining table and having him or her lift only the thumb off the table. The EPL can be visualized and palpated (Fig. 6-10A).

The area of the wrist just distal to the radial styloid and bounded by the EPL ulnarly and the APL and EPB radially is known as the *anatomic snuffbox* (Fig. 6-10B). In this area runs the dorsal branch of the radial artery. A sensory branch of the radial nerve also passes over this area. The scaphoid can be palpated in the base of the snuffbox. Tenderness in this area is suggestive of an acute scaphoid fracture or a painful scaphoid nonunion. However, strong pressure over this area results in pain in the normal individual caused by pressure on the sensory radial nerve and dorsal branch of the radial artery.

The fourth dorsal compartment contains the extensor indicis proprius (EIP) and the extensor digitorum communis (EDC). These tendons are responsible for extension of the MCP joints of the fingers. The EIP allows independent extension of the index MCP joint. The EIP is tested by having the patient extend the index finger while the other fingers are flexed into a fist. The mass action of the EDC tendons is tested by having the patient extend the MCP joints. This test is performed with the IP joints flexed because the PIP joints are

extended by the intrinsic muscles and not the long extensors of the hand. This may be a source of confusion to an inexperienced examiner. Patients with a high radial nerve palsy are still be able to extend the IP joints through the intrinsics.

The fifth dorsal compartment contains the extensor digiti minimi (EDM), which is responsible for independent extension of the MCP joint of the little finger. It is tested by having the patient extend the fifth finger while the others are flexed. Because the EDM and the EIP work independently of the communis tendons, most examiners test them simultaneously by having the patient extend the index and fifth fingers while the middle and ring fingers are flexed.

The sixth dorsal compartment contains the extensor carpi ulnaris (ECU), which inserts into the base of the fifth metacarpal and helps extend the wrist in an ulnar direction. This is tested by having the patient pull the hand dorsally and in an ulnar direction while the examiner palpates the tendon.

Intrinsic Muscle Testing

The intrinsic musculature of the hand consists of the thenar and hypothenar muscles and the lumbricals and the interossei. All of these muscles originate and insert within the hand. There is a delicate balance between the intrinsic and extrinsic muscles, which is necessary for normal functioning of the hand.

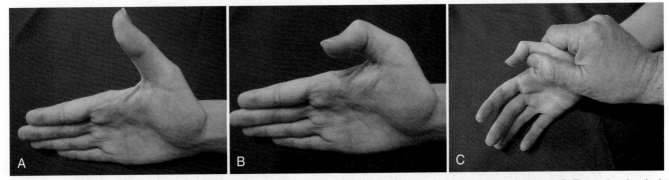

Figure 6-7 Testing the flexor pollicis longus. **A,** With the thumb in a position of full extension at the interphalangeal joint. **B,** The patient is asked to actively flex this joint. **C,** It is also important to note whether the motion is obtained with or without blocking of the proximal joint by the examiner. This applies not only to testing the flexor pollicis longus but also to testing all other flexor systems because more power and motion can be obtained when blocking is used.

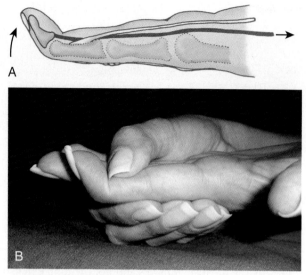

Figure 6-8 Profundus test. **A,** The flexor digitorum profundus tendon flexes the distal interphalangeal joint. **B,** With the metacarpophalangeal joint and the proximal interphalangeal joint held in extension by the examiner, the patient is asked to flex the distal interphalangeal joint. (Redrawn from Hoppenfeld S: *Physical Examination of the Spine and Extremities.* New York: Appleton-Century-Crofts, 1976.)

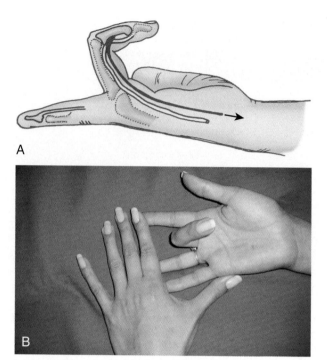

Figure 6-9 Superficialis test. **A,** The flexor digitorum superficialis tendon flexes the proximal interphalangeal (PIP) joint. **B,** The examiner must hold the adjacent fingers in full extension while asking the patient to flex the finger being tested. If the flexor system is functioning normally, the PIP joint will flex, while the distal interphalangeal joint remains in extension. (Redrawn by permission from Hoppenfeld S: *Physical Examination of the Spine and Extremities.* New York: Appleton-Century-Crofts, 1976.)

The thenar muscles consist of the abductor pollicis brevis (AbPB), the flexor pollicis brevis (FPB), the opponens pollicis (OP), and the adductor pollicis (AdP). These muscles position the thumb and help perform the complex motions of opposition and adduction of the thumb.[17] Opposition, according to Bunnell, takes place in the intercarpal, CMC, and MCP joints.[18] All three of these joints contribute to the angulatory and rotatory motions that produce true opposition. If one observes the thumb during opposition, it first abducts from the hand and then follows a semicircular path. The thumb pronates, and the proximal phalanx angulates radially on the first metacarpal. If the nail plate is observed, one can see that before beginning opposition, the thumbnail is perpendicular to the plane of the metacarpals. At the end of the opposition, the thumbnail is parallel to the plane of the metacarpals. During adduction, the thumb sweeps across the palm without following the semicircular path. The nail plate remains perpendicular to the plane of the metacarpals at all times. Because opposition is median nerve innervated and adduction is usually ulnar nerve innervated, one can easily see the difference between these two motions by comparing the hands of a patient with a longstanding low median nerve palsy on one side (Fig. 6-11).

Opposition is tested by having the patient touch the tip of the thumb to the tip of the little finger. At the end of opposition, the thumbnail should be perpendicular to the nail of the little finger and parallel to the plane of the metacarpals.

The AbPB, which is the most radial and superficial of the thenar muscles, is usually the first to atrophy with severe

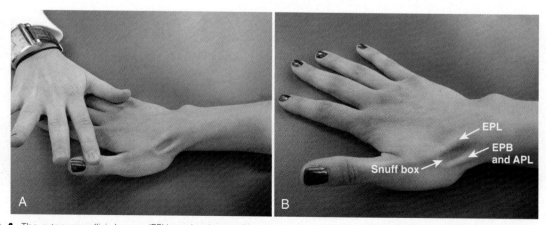

Figure 6-10 A, The extensor pollicis longus (EPL) tendon is tested by placing the patient's hand flat on the examining table and asking the patient to lift the thumb off the table. The EPL can then be visualized and palpated. **B,** Note that the EPL serves as the ulnar border to the anatomic snuff box and the extensor pollicis brevis and abductor pollicis longus create the radial border.

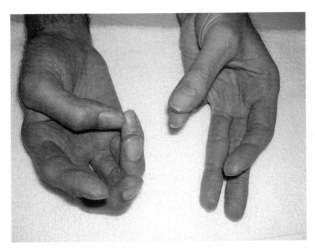

Figure 6-11 Hands of a patient with a low median nerve palsy on the right side, resulting from a longstanding carpal tunnel syndrome. Notice that in attempted opposition, the nail plate is perpendicular to the plane of the metacarpals on the affected side (right), while the nail plate is parallel to the plane of the metacarpals on the normal side (left). Tip-to-tip pinch is impossible on the side with the loss of opposition.

median-nerve dysfunction, such as that resulting from a longstanding carpal tunnel syndrome. This muscle can be tested by having the patient abduct the thumb while the examiner palpates the muscle.

Thumb adduction is performed by the adductor pollicis (AdP), which is an ulnar-nerve-innervated muscle. This muscle, in combination with the first dorsal interosseus, is necessary for strong pinch. The adductor stabilizes the thumb during pinch and also helps extend the IP joint of the thumb through its attachment into the dorsal apparatus. Thumb adduction can be tested by having the patient forcibly hold a piece of paper between the thumb and the radial side of the proximal phalanx of the index finger. When adduction is weak or nonfunctional, the IP joint of the thumb flexes during this maneuver; this is known as *Froment's sign*[19] (Fig. 6-12). Froment's sign is an indication of weak or absent adductor function. *Jeanne's sign* is hyperextension of the MCP joint of the thumb during pinch.[19]

The hypothenar muscles consist of the abductor digiti minimi, the flexor digiti minimi, and the opponens digiti minimi. The abductor and flexor aid in abduction of the fifth digit and in MCP joint flexion of that digit. The deeper oppo-

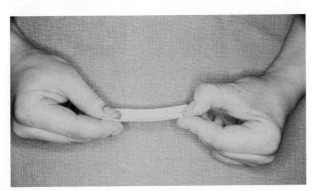

Figure 6-12 Patient with low ulnar nerve palsy on the right. Weakness of pinch is demonstrated by Froment's and Jeanne's signs on the affected side (right). (Photo courtesy of Mark Walsh, PT, DPT, MS, CHT, ATC.)

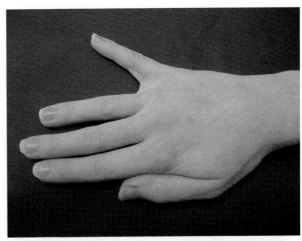

Figure 6-13 Testing function of the hypothenar muscles by having patient abduct the fifth digit.

nens digiti minimi aids in adduction and rotation of the fifth metacarpal during opposition of the thumb to the fifth finger. This helps cup the hand during grip and opposition. The hypothenar muscles are tested as one unit by having the patient abduct the little finger while the examiner palpates the muscle mass (Fig. 6-13).

The anatomy of the interossei is very complex, with much variation in their origins and insertions. There are seven interossei: four dorsal and three palmar. These muscles arise from the metacarpal shafts but have variable insertions. The palmar interossei almost always insert into the dorsal apparatus of the finger. The first dorsal interosseus almost always inserts into bone. The remaining dorsal interossei have varying insertions. Refer to the work of Eyler and Markee for a more detailed description of the anatomy.[20] The interossei are usually ulnar nerve innervated, with a few exceptions.

There are four lumbricals, which originate on the radial side of the profundus tendons and usually insert on the dorsal apparatus. Occasionally, a few fibers insert into the base of the proximal phalanges. Because these muscles are a link between the extrinsic flexor and extrinsic extensor mechanisms, they act as a modulator between flexion and extension of the IP joints.[21]

The interossei are much stronger than the lumbricals; however, both muscle groups work in conjunction. All of these muscle groups are of fundamental importance in extension of the IP joints and flexion of the MCP joints. The interossei also abduct and adduct the fingers. The dorsal interossei are the primary abductors, and the volar interossei are the primary adductors of the fingers.

The preceding statements are an oversimplification of the anatomy and functional significance of the interossei and the lumbricals. The clinical examination of these two groups of muscles is, however, rather easy.

To test interossei function, one should ask the patient to spread his or her fingers apart. This is best done with the hand flat on the examining table to eliminate the action of the long extensors, which can simulate the function of the dorsal interossei (Fig. 6-14). To supplement this test, one can have the patient radially and ulnarly deviate the middle finger while it is flexed at the MCP joint. This cannot be performed if the interossei are paralyzed; this test is known as *Egawa's sign*.[19]

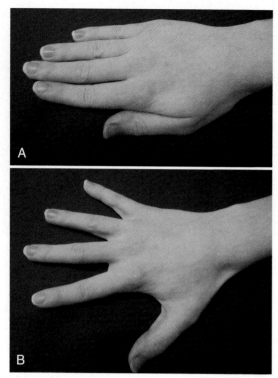

Figure 6-14 Testing function of the interossei. Abduction and adduction are assessed from the relationship of the digits to the axis of the third metacarpal. **A,** All fingers adducted toward the third metacarpal. **B,** All fingers abducted away from third metacarpal.

The first dorsal interosseus is a very strong radial abductor of the index finger and plays an important role in stabilizing that digit during pinch. It can be tested separately by having the patient strongly abduct the index finger in a radial direction while the examiner palpates the muscle belly (Fig. 6-15). The IP extension function of the lumbricals and interossei is tested by having the patient extend the IP joints of the digits while the examiner holds the MCP joints in flexion (Fig. 6-16).

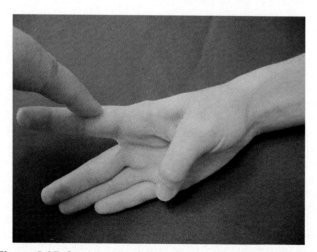

Figure 6-15 On abduction of the patient's index finger, the examiner can palpate the first dorsal interosseus. This is the last muscle to receive innervation from the ulnar nerve.

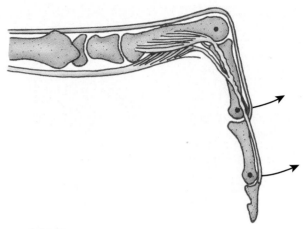

Figure 6-16 The intrinsic muscles, by means of their attachment into the lateral bands and proximal phalanges, produce flexion of the metacarpophalangeal (MCP) joints and extension of the proximal interphalangeal (PIP) joints. The function of the lumbricals and interossei is tested by having the patient extend the PIP joints of the digits while the examiner holds the MCP joints in flexion. (Redrawn from Tubiana R: *The Hand.* Philadelphia: WB Saunders, 1973.)

If all of the interossei and lumbricals are functioning properly, the patient will be able to put his or her hand into the "intrinsic-plus position"; that is, the MCP joints are flexed and the PIP joints are in full extension. James has recommended this as the position of immobilization for the injured hand to maintain the length of the collateral ligaments of the MCP joint and prevent joint contractures at the IP joints.[22]

Injuries to the median or ulnar nerves, or both, or a crushing injury to the hand can result in paralysis or contractures of the intrinsic muscles. A hand without intrinsic function is known as the *intrinsic-minus hand*.[23,24] This hand has lost its normal cupping. The arches of the hand disappear, and there is wasting of all intrinsic musculature. Clawing of the fingers is evident, as described by Duchenne in 1867.[19] The claw deformity is defined as hyperextension of the MCP joints and flexion of the PIP and DIP joints (Fig. 6-17). This is the result

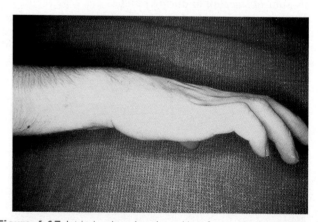

Figure 6-17 Intrinsic-minus hand resulting from a longstanding low ulnar palsy. Notice loss of normal arches of the hand and wasting of all intrinsic musculature between metacarpals. Notice hyperextension of the metacarpophalangeal joints and flexion of the proximal and distal interphalangeal joints because of an imbalance of the extrinsic flexor and extensor systems as a result of paralysis of the ulnar innervated intrinsic muscles. (Photo courtesy of Mark Walsh, PT, DPT, MS, CHT, ATC.)

of an imbalance between the intrinsic and extrinsic muscles of the hand.[25] The extrinsic extensors hyperextend the MCP joints, and the extrinsic flexors flex the PIP and DIP joints. The flexion vector, induced by the intrinsics, across the MCP joint is lost.[26] In time, the volar capsular–ligamentous structures stretch out, and the claw deformity increases in severity.[27]

Injury to the intrinsics, which can be caused by ischemia, crushing injuries, or other pathologic states (e.g., rheumatoid arthritis), can result in tightening of the intrinsic muscles. A test for intrinsic tightness was first described by Finochetto in 1920.[28] Later, Bunnell and then Littler redescribed this test.[29] The intrinsic tightness test is performed by having the examiner hold the patient's MCP joint in maximum extension (stretching the intrinsics) and then passively flexing the PIP joint. The MCP joint is then held in flexion (relaxing the intrinsics), and the examiner passively flexes the PIP joint again. If the PIP joint can be passively flexed more when the MCP joint is in flexion than when it is in extension, there is tightness of the intrinsic muscles[28-30] (Fig. 6-18). In patients with rheumatoid arthritis, intrinsic tightness is common and may result in a swan-neck deformity.[31] The swan neck is a result of the strong pull of the contracted intrinsics, through the lateral bands, which subsequently sublux dorsal to the axis of rotation of the PIP joint. The resultant deformity is one of hyperextension at the PIP joint and flexion at the DIP joint.

Occasionally, there is confusion as to the cause of limited PIP joint flexion. Is the condition a result of intrinsic tightness, of extrinsic extensor tightness (e.g., scarring of the long extensors proximal to the PIP joint), or of the joint itself (i.e., capsular and collateral ligament tightness)? Three simple tests clarify the situation. The intrinsic tightness test helps the examiner either rule out or identify intrinsic muscle problems. The extrinsic tightness test is just the opposite of the intrinsic test. Again, the examiner holds the MCP joint in maximum extension, passively flexes the PIP joint, and notes the amount of flexion. He or she then flexes the MCP joint and passively flexes the PIP joint again. If extrinsic extensor tightness (because the long extensors are scarred) is present, passive flexion of the PIP joint will be greater when the MCP joint is held in extension than when it is held in flexion. If the motion of the PIP joint is unchanged regardless of the position of the MCP joint, then the limitation is attributed to PIP joint capsular and collateral ligament tightness (Fig. 6-19).

Oblique Retinacular Ligament Test

Occasionally, a patient exhibits a lack of active flexion at the DIP joint. This may be caused by a joint contracture or a contracture of the oblique retinacular ligament.[32] The oblique retinacular ligament arises from the volar lateral ridge of the proximal phalanx and has a common origin with the distal A2 and C1 pulleys. It then traverses distally and dorsally to attach to the dorsal apparatus near the DIP joint (Fig. 6-20). As pointed out by Shrewsbury and Johnson, the tendon varies in its development and occurrence.[33] However, it is consistently made taut by flexion of the DIP joint, particularly with the PIP joint in extension. If this ligament is contracted, DIP motion will be limited. The oblique retinacular

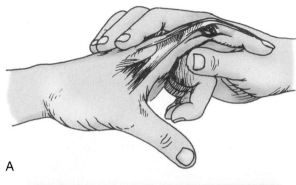

A

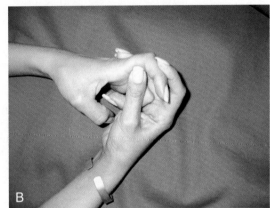

B

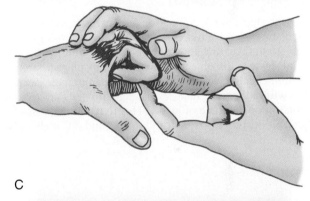

C

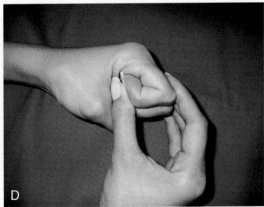

D

Figure 6-18 Intrinsic tightness test. **A, B,** The intrinsics are put on stretch by the examiner, who then passively flexes the proximal interphalangeal (PIP) joint. **C, D,** The intrinsics are then relaxed by flexing the metacarpophalangeal (MCP) joint. If the PIP joint can be passively flexed more with the MCP joint in flexion than when it is in extension, the intrinsic muscles are tight. (Redrawn from Hoppenfeld S: *Physical Examination of the Spine and Extremities*, New York: Appleton-Century-Crofts, 1976.)

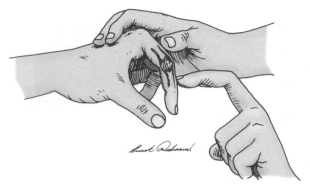

Figure 6-19 Proximal interphalangeal joint (PIP) contracture. Collateral ligament tightness limits PIP motion, regardless of the position of the metacarpophalangeal joint.

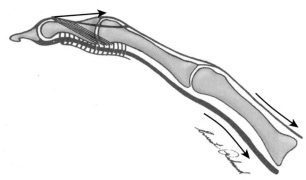

Figure 6-20 Oblique retinacular ligament. (Redrawn from Tubiana R: *The Hand*, Philadelphia: WB Saunders, 1981.)

ligament tightness test is performed by passively flexing the DIP joint with the PIP joint in extension and then repeating this with the PIP joint in flexion. If there is greater motion when the PIP joint is flexed than when it is extended, there is tightness of the ligament (Fig. 6-21). Equal loss of flexion indicates a joint contracture.

Grip and Pinch Strength

The next step after examination of intrinsic and extrinsic musculature of the hand is determination of gross grip and pinch strength of the injured versus the noninjured hand. Several devices for objective measurement of grip strength are commercially available. The grip dynamometer (see Fig. 12-4) with adjustable handle spacings provides an accurate evaluation of the force of grip.[34] This dynamometer has five adjustable spacings at 1.0, 1.5, 2.0, 2.5, and 3.0 inches. The

patient is shown how to grasp the dynamometer and is instructed to grasp it with his maximum force. The grip test position should be standardized. The forearm should be in neutral rotation and the elbow flexed 90 degrees. The shoulder should be adducted. The patient self-selects a wrist position with the gripping motion. O'Driscoll states that optimal grip strengths are achieved at 35 degrees of wrist extension.[35] Grip strength is measured at each of the five handle positions. The right and left hands are tested alternately, and the force of each grip effort is recorded. The test is paced at a rate to eliminate fatigue. If only one level is measured, an average of three trials is recommended for each hand.[11] According to Bechtol, there is usually a 5% to 10% difference between the dominant hand and the nondominant hand in normal subjects.[34] A graph of the grip measurements at the five handle positions forms a bell curve if the patient provides maximal effort and has not sustained a median or ulnar nerve injury;

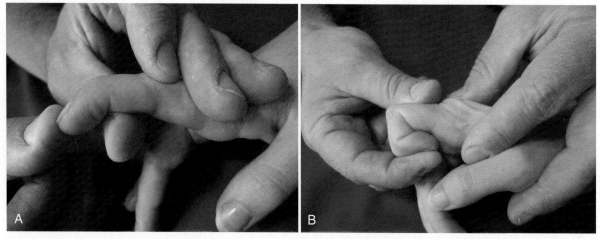

Figure 6-21 The oblique retinacular ligament tightness test. **A,** The distal interphalangeal (DIP) joint is passively flexed with the proximal interphalangeal (PIP) joint held in extension. **B,** The DIP joint is then passively flexed with the PIP joint flexed. If there is greater motion when the PIP joint is flexed than when it is extended, there is tightness of the ligament. Equal loss of DIP joint motion regardless of PIP joint position indicates a joint contracture.

grip strength is typically greatest at the middle handle position and weakest at each end resulting from the differential action of extrinsic and intrinsic muscles involved with grip at each handle position. At the widest handle position, extrinsic finger flexor muscle action is predominantly involved; at the most narrow handle position, intrinsic muscle action predominates. At the middle spacings there is a combination of both intrinsic and extrinsic muscle action, resulting in greater strength output and thus, the bell curve configuration of grip readings at all five handle positions. With generalized weakness of the hand, the bell curve pattern is usually still present (Fig. 6-22). However, patients with an intrinsic-minus hand are an exception to this rule. Their curve is flattened as their grip increases from level I to V because the extrinsic flexors are at a better mechanical advantage with the wider handle positions.[36] Other patients that may present with a "flattened" curve may be using submaximal effort;[34] however, it may be proportional to the amount of forced produced.[37,38]

For years, the rapid exchange grip (REG) test has been used to detect submaximal effort. The REG test is administered with a dynamometer at the setting that achieves maximum grip during static testing. During testing, the clinician holds the dynamometer in place. The patient is then instructed to maximally grip the dynamometer, alternating hands as rapidly as possible. Each hand grips the dynamometer 5 to 10 times. A positive REG test shows a significant increase in grip strength on the affected side compared with static scores. A positive REG test in the presence of a flat curve on static testing suggests inconsistent effort by the patient.[39,40] A more recent study has concluded that the REG is not a reliable or valid way to detect submaximal effort due to a lack of standardization in the procedures.[40]

There are three basic types of pinch: (1) chuck, or three-fingered pinch; (2) lateral, or key pinch; and (3) tip pinch (Fig. 6-23). These can be tested with a pinch meter (see Fig. 12-6). Many disease processes can affect pinch power: basilar arthritis of the thumb, ulnar nerve palsy, and anterior interosseus nerve palsy, to mention a few.

Additional information on grip and pinch functional strength measures is presented in Chapter 12 on functional tests.

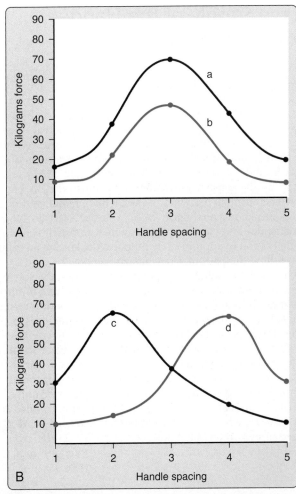

Figure 6-22 A, The grip strengths of a patient's uninjured hand *(a)* and injured hand *(b)* are plotted. Despite the patient's decrease in grip strength because of injury, curve *b* maintains a bell-shaped pattern and parallels that of the normal hand. These curves are reproducible in repeated examinations, with minimal change in values. **B,** If the patient has an exceptionally large hand, the curve will shift to the right *(d)*; with a very small hand, the curve shifts to the left *(c)*. Notice, however, that the bell-shaped pattern is maintained despite the curve's shift in direction.

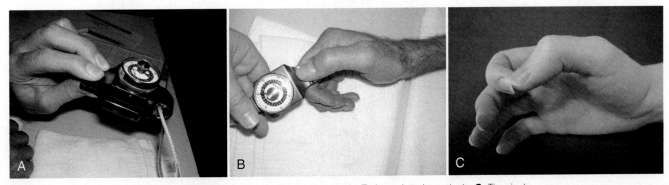

Figure 6-23 A, Chuck, or three point, pinch. **B,** Lateral, or key, pinch. **C,** Tip pinch.

Nerve Supply of the Hand— Motor and Sensory

Three nerves provide motor and sensory function to the hand: the median, radial, and ulnar nerves. The motor and sensory innervation of the hand also is subject to much variation, as pointed out by Rowntree.[41] The median, radial, and ulnar nerves are peripheral branches of the brachial plexus. The radial nerve is formed from the C6 and C7 nerve roots. The median and ulnar nerves are formed by branches of the C7, C8, and T1 nerve roots. The neurologic levels represented by the sensory dermatomes are illustrated in Figure 6-24. The terminal branches of the median, radial, and ulnar nerves are shown in Figure 6-25. It is necessary to have a fundamental knowledge of the branches and their sequence of innervation to appropriately pinpoint the level of an injury or to follow the path of a regenerating nerve.

The median, radial, and ulnar nerves enter the forearm through various muscle and fascial planes and have multiple potential sources of entrapment. These nerve conditions may be associated with traumatic injuries such as fractures of the elbow, forearm, or wrist. Entrapment of these nerves results in classic clinical presentations, with loss of motor function (in longstanding compression) and paresthesias in the distribution of each nerve.[42-46] Careful and systematic examination of cutaneous sensibility and motor function is required to determine the extent of the compression. The examination and management of these compression syndromes are discussed elsewhere in this book.

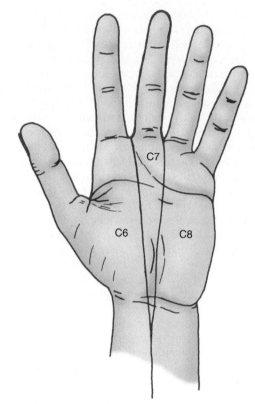

Figure 6-24 Sensory dermatomes of the hand, by neurologic levels. (Redrawn from Hoppenfeld S: *Physical Examination of the Spine and Extremities.* New York: Appleton-Century-Crofts, 1976.)

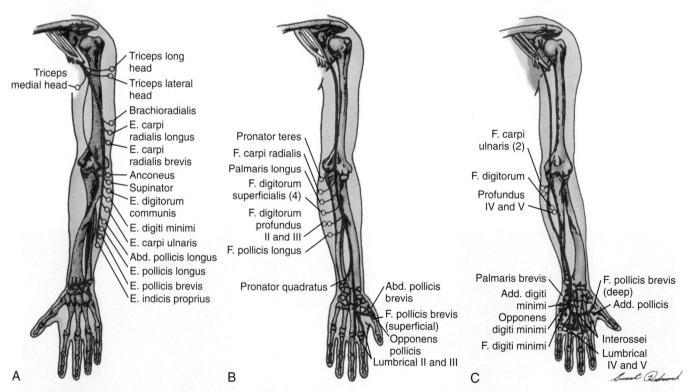

Figure 6-25 Terminal branches of the radial **(A)**, median **(B)**, and ulnar **(C)** nerves. (Redrawn from American Society for Surgery of the Hand: *The Hand, Examination and Diagnosis,* Aurora, Colo.: The Society, 1978.)

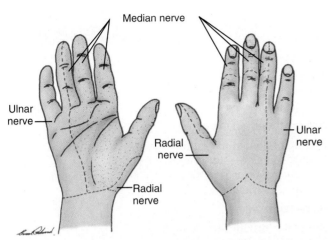

Figure 6-26 Sensory distribution of the median, radial, and ulnar nerves in the hand. (Redrawn from Weeks PM, Wray RC: *Management of Acute Hand Injuries: A Biological Approach*, St Louis: Mosby, 1973.)

Cutaneous Sensibility

Normal sensibility is a prerequisite to normal hand function. A patient with a median nerve injury has essentially a "blind hand" and is greatly disabled, even if all motor function is present. The assessment of sensibility is therefore an integral and important part of the examination of the hand. The distribution of sensory nerves is subject to as much variation as the distribution of the motor branches.[41] The classic distribution of the median, ulnar, and radial nerves is shown in Figure 6-26.

There are many ways to assess sensibility, including monofilaments, Moberg's Picking-up Test, Seddon's coin test, the moving two-point discrimination test described by Dellon, and Weber's two-point discrimination test.[49-51] Chapter 11 in this edition of the book and Chapter 14 from the fifth edition (located in the archived chapters section on the companion Web site) discuss sensibility testing in detail.

Vascularity of the Hand

The vascular supply of the hand is usually extensive; however, it should be examined carefully before any surgery on the hand. The primary blood supply to the hand is through the radial and ulnar arteries. In some individuals, the dominant blood supply to the hand can be from one artery. The ulnar artery gives rise to the superficial palmar arch, and the radial artery gives rise to the deep arch. These arches usually have extensive anastomoses.[52,53] The superficial palmar arch gives rise to four common digital arteries, which then branch to form the proper digital arteries. The superficial arch may supply blood to the thumb, or the thumb may be completely vascularized by a branch of the radial artery known as the princeps pollicis artery. To assess blood supply to the hand, one should check the color of the hand (red, pale, or cyanotic), digital capillary refill, the radial artery and ulnar artery pulses at the wrist, and perform Allen's test. In 1929, Allen described a simple clinical test to determine the patency of the radial and ulnar arteries in thromboangiitis obliterans.[54] This test is performed by having the patient open and close his or her hand to exsanguinate it while the examiner occludes the radial and ulnar arteries at the wrist with digital pressure. The patient then opens the hand, which is white and blanched. The examiner then releases either the ulnar or the radial artery and watches for revascularization of the hand. If the hand does not flush, the artery is occluded. This test is then repeated with the opposite artery (Fig. 6-27).

A modification of Allen's test can be performed on a single digit.[55] The steps are the same as just outlined, except that the examiner occludes and releases the radial and ulnar digital arteries.

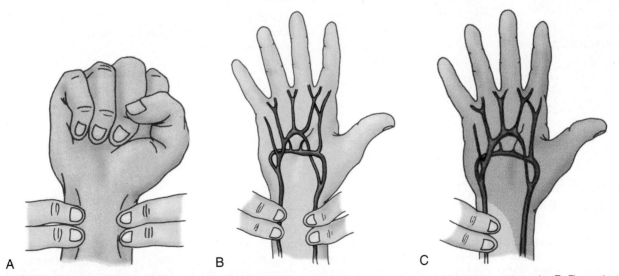

A   B   C

Figure 6-27 Allen's test for arterial patency. **A,** The examiner places her fingers over the ulnar and radial arteries at the wrist. **B,** The patient then forcibly opens and closes his hand to exsanguinate it while the examiner occludes the radial and ulnar arteries. **C,** Next the patient opens his hand, and the examiner releases one artery and observes the flushing of the hand. The steps are then repeated, and the other artery is tested for patency. (Redrawn from American Society for Surgery of the Hand: *The Hand, Examination and Diagnosis*, Aurora, Colo.: The Society, 1978.)

Box 6-1   Review of Systems (Selected Examples)

GENERAL QUESTIONS

Fever, chills, sweating (constitutional symptoms)
Fatigue, malaise, weakness (constitutional symptoms)
Vital signs: blood pressure, temperature, pulse, respirations
Dizziness, falls

INTEGUMENTARY (INCLUDE SKIN, HAIR, AND NAILS)

Recent rashes, nodules, or other skin changes
Increased hair growth (hirsutism)
Nail bed changes

MUSCULOSKELETAL AND NEUROLOGIC

Frequent or severe headaches
Paresthesias (numbness, tingling, "pins and needles" sensation)
Weakness; atrophy
Problems with coordination or balance; falling
Involuntary movements; tremors
Radicular pain

RHEUMATOLOGIC

Presence and location of joint swelling
Muscle pain, weakness
Skin rashes
Raynaud's phenomenon

CARDIOVASCULAR

Chest pain or sense of heaviness of discomfort
Limb pain during activity (claudication; cramps, limping)
Pulsating or throbbing pain anywhere, but especially in the back or abdomen
Peripheral edema; nocturia
Fatigue, dyspnea, orthopnea, syncope
High or low blood pressure, unusual pulses

PULMONARY

Shortness of breath (dyspnea, orthopnea)
Night sweats; sweats anytime
Pleural pain

PSYCHOLOGICAL

Stress levels
Fatigue, psychomotor agitation
Depression, confusion, anxiety
Irritability, mood changes

GASTROINTESTINAL

Abdominal pain
Diarrhea or constipation
Skin rash followed by joint pain (Crohn's disease)

HEPATIC AND BILIARY

Feeling of abdominal fullness, ascites
Changes in skin color (yellow, green)
Skin changes (rash, itching, purpura, spider angiomas, palmar erythema)

HEMATOLOGIC

Skin color or nail bed changes
Bleeding: nose, gums, easy bruising, melena
Hemarthrosis, muscle hemorrhage, hematoma

GENITOURINARY

Reduced stream, decreased output
Burning or bleeding during urination; change in urine color
Urinary incontinence, dribbling

GYNECOLOGIC

Pain with menses or intercourse
Surgical procedures
Pregnancy, birth, miscarriage, and abortion histories

ENDOCRINE

Fruity breath odor
Headaches
Carpal or tarsal tunnel syndrome
Periarthritis, adhesive capsulitis

CANCER

Constant, intense pain, especially bone pain at night
Excessive fatigue
Rapid onset of digital clubbing (10–14 days)

IMMUNOLOGIC

Skin or nail bed changes
Fever or other constitutional symptoms
Lymph node changes

Modified from Goodman CC: Screening for medical problems in patients with upper extremity signs and symptoms. *J Hand Ther.* 2010;23:105–125.

Medical Screening and Review of Systems

Direct access is the right of the public to obtain physical therapy services without a legal need for referral. It is now available in 45 states within the United States.[56] This legislation occurring in the past decade prompted the need to teach medical screening to professional physical therapy students. It became apparent that medical screening was needed by both physical and occupational therapists even without direct access because any patient may present with risk factors, precautions, or "red flags" to therapeutic interventions.

Current practice trends suggest that patients are discharged more quickly from the hospital and more likely to have outpatient same-day surgery. This means that patients are not monitored as closely as they used to be. If the patient is referred to therapy postoperatively, he or she may present with more medical issues or complications. The public is generally sicker, with almost 80% of patients over 70 years of age having at least one chronic disease.[2] Therapists need to identify these comorbidities. Patients are being referred to hand therapy clinics with a signed prescription, without an adequate medical screening, because they never saw the physician or ancillary medical personnel, and sometimes when they do see the doctor, they are not examined. Finally, knowledge related to screening for risk factors has increased significantly over the past decade for several medical conditions and diseases. For example, screening criteria have been developed for female patients with low bone mass (osteoporosis) that present in the clinic with an upper extremity fracture due to a fall. Screening tests for risk factors and balance following a wrist fracture have been developed so that therapists can serve as "gatekeepers" to address falls risk, balance impairments, or low bone mass.

Goodman created a five-step model for medical screening[2] that includes: (1) personal and family history; (2) risk factor assessment, (3) clinical presentation, (4) associated signs and symptoms of systemic diseases, and (5) review of systems.

Box 6-1 presents selected examples for review of systems pertaining to upper extremity patients.

Summary

Clinical examination is an art that improves with practice and experience. This chapter presents a systematic approach to clinical examination of the hand. Hand surgeons and therapists need to use valid and reliable tests and measures to collect impairment data to assess treatment outcomes. Diagnostic special tests used in clinical examination must be evaluated for their diagnostic accuracy and interpretation of results.[57] Research is needed to determine the sensitivity, specificity, and likelihood ratios of diagnostic tests used in hand and upper extremity clinical examinations.

REFERENCES

The complete reference list is available online at www.expertconsult.com.

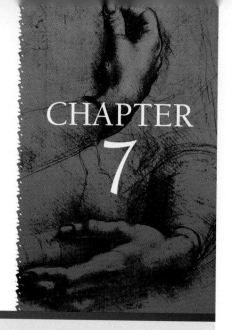

Clinical Examination of the Wrist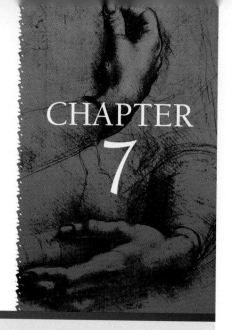

TERRI M. SKIRVEN, OTR/L, CHT AND A. LEE OSTERMAN, MD

HISTORY OF THE INJURY OR ONSET
INSPECTION OF THE WRIST
OBJECTIVE ASSESSMENTS
DIAGNOSTIC INJECTION

PHYSICAL EXAMINATION
GENERAL TESTS
SUMMARY

CRITICAL POINTS

- Successful clinical examination of the wrist requires a thorough knowledge of wrist anatomy, biomechanics, and pathology.
- The wrist examination includes a complete history, visual inspection, objective assessments, and a systematic physical examination, including palpation and provocative testing.
- The keys to a successful examination are to link the symptoms with the underlying palpable structures and to correlate the mechanism of the injury with the physical findings.
- Before the wrist is examined, a careful inspection of the entire upper extremity should be performed to rule out other extrinsic and more proximal causes for the wrist symptoms.
- The bony and soft tissue anatomy is systematically palpated to define areas of tenderness and to determine the area of maximum tenderness.
- The symptomatic wrist should always be compared with the uninvolved side.
- Starting the examination in an asymptomatic area helps the patient develop trust in the examiner and may reduce wrist guarding.
- By methodically examining each structure in each zone, the examiner can most effectively localize the patient's symptoms and develop a differential diagnosis.

The diagnosis of "wrist sprain" was at one time a common and acceptable diagnosis for the patient with wrist pain. More recently, however, as the understanding of wrist anatomy, mechanics, and pathology has evolved, more sophisticated clinical examination procedures have been developed, allowing more specific diagnosis of wrist problems.

The wrist is a highly complex joint in a very compact space. Successful clinical evaluation of the wrist requires a thorough knowledge of wrist anatomy, biomechanics, and pathology. Also required is knowledge of surface anatomy and the corresponding underlying structures. The keys to a successful examination are to link the symptoms with the underlying palpable structures and to correlate the mechanism of the injury with the physical findings. Some common conditions may be easily identified on the basis of the clinical examination, whereas others may require additional diagnostic studies, imaging, and repeat evaluations.

The components of the wrist examination include a thorough history, visual inspection, objective assessments, and a systematic physical examination, including palpation and provocative testing to identify tenderness and abnormal motion between bones. Before the wrist is examined, the entire upper extremity should be inspected to rule out other extrinsic and more proximal causes for the wrist symptoms.

History of the Injury or Onset

A detailed history can provide insight into the nature of the wrist problem and can help focus the subsequent physical examination. The patient's age, dominance, occupation, and avocations should be noted. The date of onset of the problem and the circumstances related to the onset need to be explored. If the wrist problem resulted from a single incident or injury, the mechanism of the injury should be reviewed thoroughly, including the position of the wrist at the time of injury and the subsequent degree and direction of stress. For example, an acute rotational injury to the forearm or a fall on the pronated outstretched upper extremity can result in a triangular fibrocartilage complex (TFCC) injury.[1] Mayfield[2] describes a progression of perilunar instability initiated radially or ulnarly, depending on the position of the wrist during loading. For example, dorsiflexion and supination usually produce radially initiated perilunate injuries, whereas palmar-flexion and pronation forces may result in ulnarly initiated perilunar injuries. Weber and Chao[3] found that load applied to the radial side of the palm with the wrist in extreme dorsiflexion produces scaphoid fracture.

If the wrist condition developed over time, and not as a result of a single injury, it is important to explore potential causes. Some patients have definite ideas about what caused their wrist to hurt, but others require careful questioning. New responsibilities at work or home that increase physical demands on the wrist, increased productivity requirements, an awkwardly configured workstation, and participation in a new hobby or sport are examples of factors that may precipitate symptoms.

The presence of symptoms such as pain; swelling; numbness and tingling; temperature and color changes; and abnormal sounds, such as clicks, grating, or clunks, should be noted. Their location, frequency, intensity, and duration should also be discussed. Some patients may present with very localized symptoms, whereas others report more diffuse discomfort. In the latter case, it is sometimes helpful to instruct the patient to point to the most painful spot or spots to attempt to localize the problem. Some patients may say they have pain all the time and have difficulty qualifying their symptoms. It is sometimes helpful to start by asking patients if they have pain at the present moment or "right now" as a way to help them begin to focus more specifically on when and how often their symptoms occur. The activities, positions, or conditions that aggravate the symptoms and the measures taken to obtain relief are discussed. It is important to review previous treatment interventions such as orthoses, anti-inflammatory medications, injections, and therapy, and to gauge the efficacy of the treatments. The effect the wrist condition has had on the patient's ability to work and perform his or her usual life tasks needs to be discussed to determine the degree of disability caused by the wrist problem.

Inspection of the Wrist

Visual inspection of the wrist and comparison to the uninvolved side can provide clues about the nature of the problem. As the patient enters the clinical setting, the examiner can observe the posture of the involved side and wrist. The posture of the neck, shoulder, and elbow should be noted because wrist symptoms may sometimes be referred from an extrinsic and more proximal site. Spontaneous use can be noted to give an indication of the extent of disability and to later correlate observations with the patient's report of disability. If the patient enters holding a heavy briefcase or bag with the involved side and then later reports inability to lift any weight at all, the reliability of their symptom report would be in question.

The wrist should be visually inspected and compared with the uninvolved side. On the dorsal side, the skin, nails, color, and muscle bulk should be observed. Any masses, such as a dorsal ganglion (Fig. 7-1) or traumatic or surgical scars are noted. The six extensor compartments can be inspected for any focal tubular swelling, as seen with tenosynovitis, or for

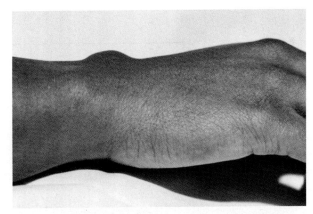

Figure 7-1 Dorsal wrist ganglion, the most common mass on the dorsum of the wrist.

any evidence of ruptures or extensor lags. Some predictable conditions involve the extensor tendons, and these should be kept in mind when examining the extensor compartments (Table 7-1, online).[4] The contour, alignment, and profile of the wrist are observed in comparison with the contralateral side. Characteristic examples of abnormalities include the post-traumatic deformity that occurs with radius shortening following a malunited distal radius fracture. Another example is the prominent distal ulnar head indicative of distal radioulnar joint (DRUJ) disruption (Fig. 7-2). The profile of the wrist is observed to detect any malalignment such as a volar sag, or carpal supination (Fig. 7-3, online), compared with the other side. On the palmar side, the fingertips can be observed for callusing or atrophy to determine extent of use. The thenar and hypothenar eminences are inspected for muscle bulk.

Objective Assessments

The active and passive range of motion (ROM) of all planes of wrist motion, as well as of supination and pronation, should be assessed. Compensatory maneuvers used by the patient when motion is limited need to be identified and eliminated. For example, the patient may elevate the elbow when attempting wrist flexion. When forearm rotation is

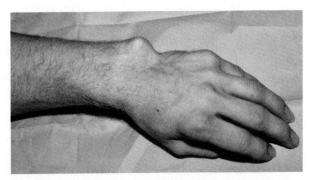

Figure 7-2 Prominence of the distal ulna, indicating distal radioulnar joint disruption.

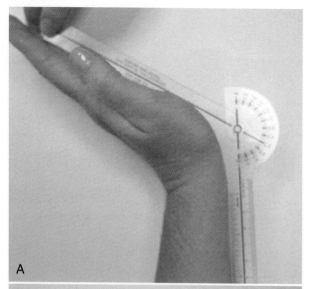

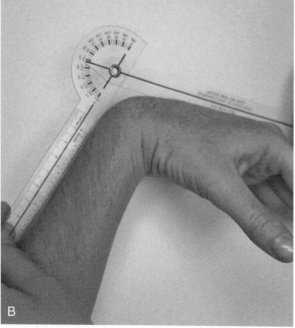

Figure 7-4 Range of motion measurement of wrist extension **(A)** and flexion **(B)**.

wrist motion is between 5 degrees of flexion and 30 degrees of extension, 10 degrees of radial deviation, and 15 degrees of ulnar deviation. Ryu and coworkers[8] found that 40 degrees of wrist extension, 40 degrees of wrist flexion, and a total of 40 degrees of radial and ulnar deviation are needed to perform most ADLs.

Swelling of the wrist and hand can be measured with a volumeter. Both involved and uninvolved sides are measured for comparison. The volumeter has been found by Waylett-Rendall and Seibly[9] to be reliable to within 1% of the total volume when one examiner performs the measurements. van Velze and associates[10] found that the left nondominant side was 3.3% smaller than the dominant right side with volume measurement in a study of 263 male laborers. She concluded that the volume of one hand could be used as a reliable predictor of the volume of the other. The measurement of bilateral wrist circumference may also be used as an indicator of swelling.

Grip strength testing is advocated by some as a reliable indicator of true impairment that deserves further investigation in cases of obscure wrist pain. Czitrom and Lister[11] found a significant correlation between decreased grip strength and positive bone scans and confirmed pathology with chronic wrist complaints. Submaximal effort was ruled out with the use of rapid-exchange grip testing and a bell curve with five-position grip testing using the Jamar dynamometer.[11]

LaStayo and Weiss describe the GRIT (i.e., the gripping rotatory impaction test), which is used to identify ulnar impaction using a standard dynamometer to test grip with the forearm in three positions: neutral, supination, and pronation.[12] The rationale for the test relates to the fact that ulnar impaction correlates with positive ulnar variance and gripping with pronation maximizes potential impaction and gripping with supination reduces it. The supination and pronation readings are calculated as a ratio, that is, supination/pronation, and the potential for impaction is considered high if the GRIT ratio is more than 1 on the involved and no different from 1 on the uninvolved side.

Sensibility examination is done to screen for possible nerve compressions. Semmes-Weinstein light-touch threshold testing has been found to be the most sensitive clinical test for detecting nerve compression.[13] The median, ulnar, and dorsal radial sensory nerve (DRSN) can become compressed or irritated at the level of the wrist and can be a source of wrist symptoms. Particular attention is paid to the cutaneous distribution of these nerves with sensibility testing.

Diagnostic Injection

Injections are utilized to assist diagnosis and predict surgical success. Shin and coworkers[14] recommend that injections should be performed in joints or along tendons that may be injured and that they can help to distinguish between intra-articular and extra-articular pathology. Bell and colleagues[15] suggest that midcarpal injection with lidocaine is a useful diagnostic test to determine the presence or absence of intracarpal pathology in patients with chronic wrist pain and normal routine radiographs by evaluating grip strength and pain relief after injection. They found that midcarpal

limited, the patient may substitute with shoulder motions. Measurement with a goniometer helps ensure an accurate assessment. The most reliable method for measuring wrist flexion and extension is the volar/dorsal technique[5] (Fig. 7-4). The examiner needs to determine whether any restrictions are the result of pain or a mechanical cause, such as capsular contracture or a malunited fracture. Normal ROM of the wrist and functional ROM should be considered when evaluating wrist motion. Normal maximum ROM of the wrist has been documented with the use of wrist goniometry.[6] However, there is some variation in normal values. Therefore the uninvolved side should be measured for comparison. Functional ROM (i.e., the motion of the wrist required to perform most activities of daily living [ADLs]) has also been documented. Palmer and colleagues[7] found that functional injection of lidocaine that resulted in a 28% improvement of grip strength had a statistically significant association with intracarpal pathology later diagnosed by wrist arthroscopy. These authors conclude that diagnostic injection can be an effective tool in the evaluation of the patient with chronic wrist pain. The authors point out limitations of their study, including the small sample size of normal subjects and uncertainty regarding penetration of the lidocaine into the radiocarpal joint, which would affect results if the TFCC or radiocarpal joint was the source of pathology. Freeland cautions that more study is needed to establish a reliable diagnostic test and threshold values.[16]

Green reported the results of a retrospective study that supports the value of carpal tunnel steroid injections as a reasonably accurate diagnostic test for carpal tunnel syndrome (CTS).[17] Ninety-nine wrists in 89 patients receiving carpal tunnel injection were subsequently treated surgically. Correlations between results of injections and subsequent operations indicate that a good response to injection is an excellent diagnostic and prognostic sign. On the other hand, poor relief from injection does not mean that the patient is a poor candidate for surgery. In a more recent review of published studies, Boyer reports that the predictive value of corticosteroid injection should be considered unproved at this time.[18]

Physical Examination

Palpation and provocative testing are the core of the examination. The goal is to define areas of tenderness by systematically palpating the bony and soft tissue anatomy and to determine the area of maximum tenderness. These tender areas are then related to a specific underlying structure, such as the bone, tendon, or joint. The provocative tests are performed to identify carpal instabilities. Patients with carpal instabilities often complain of pain, decreased motion, and "clicks or clunks" with motion of the wrist. The provocative tests may reproduce these sounds, which are the result of abnormal carpal movements. A painless click or clunk may be obtained in the asymptomatic wrist with lax ligaments and is not considered a sign of disease. The symptomatic wrist should always be compared with the uninvolved side. The sequence of the evaluation can be tailored to the patient's area of maximum tenderness. Starting the examination in an asymptomatic area will help the patient to trust the examiner and may reduce the tendency toward wrist guarding.

Torosian et al[19] describe a systematic approach to wrist examination. They divide the wrist into five zones: three dorsal and two volar. By methodically examining each structure in each zone, the examiner can most effectively localize the patient's symptoms and develop a differential diagnosis. Table 7-2 (online) lists common wrist conditions for each zone and the corresponding clinical signs and tests.

Radial Dorsal Zone

The structures to examine in the radial dorsal zone include the radial styloid, the scaphoid, the scaphotrapezial (ST) joint and trapezium, the base of the first metacarpal and the

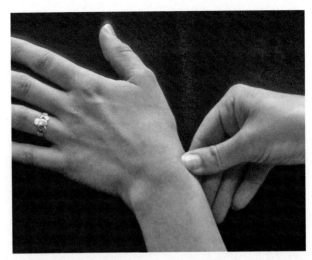

Figure 7-5 *Palpation of the radial styloid.*

first carpometacarpal (CMC) joint, the tendons of the first and third extensor compartments, and the DRSN.

The radial styloid is palpated on the radial aspect of the wrist proximal to the anatomic snuffbox with the wrist in ulnar deviation (Fig. 7-5). Tenderness of the styloid may indicate contusion, fracture, or radioscaphoid arthritis.[20] The last is common with longstanding scapholunate dissociation and scaphoid instability.[21] Tenderness may be aggravated by radial deviation.

The scaphoid is palpated just distal to the radial styloid in the snuffbox, which is formed by the tendons of the extensor pollicis longus (EPL) on the ulnar border and the extensor pollicis brevis (EPB) and abductor pollicis longus (APL) on the radial border. The scaphoid is most easily palpated when the wrist is in ulnar deviation because the proximal carpal row slides radially and the scaphoid assumes an extended or vertical position when the wrist is in ulnar deviation.[22] Tenderness of the scaphoid in the snuffbox may indicate scaphoid fracture, nonunion, avascular necrosis (Preiser's disease), or scaphoid instability.[23] The *clamp sign* refers to the patients grasp of the volar and dorsal aspects of the scaphoid when asked to indicate where the wrist hurts (Fig. 7-6).[24]

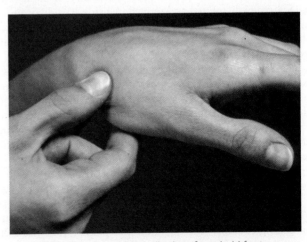

Figure 7-6 *Clamp sign indicative of scaphoid fracture.*

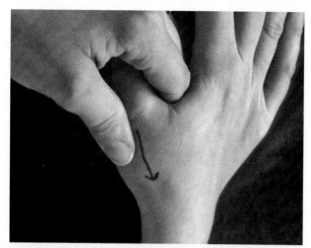

Figure 7-7 Grind test for arthritis of the carpometacarpal joint of the thumb is performed by applying axial pressure with rotation.

The ST joint and trapezium are palpated just distal to the scaphoid. Opposition of the thumb to the small finger and ulnar deviation of the wrist makes the trapezium more prominent and easier to palpate. Circumduction of the thumb while palpating facilitates differentiation between the base of the thumb metacarpal and the adjacent trapezium. Tenderness in this region may indicate ST arthritis, which may result from scaphoid instability.[25]

The base of the first metacarpal and the first CMC joint are localized by palpating in a proximal direction along the dorsal aspect of the flexed first metacarpal until a small depression can be felt. This depression represents the first CMC joint. Tenderness here is often caused by degenerative arthritis. The *grind test* has been described for CMC arthritis[26] and involves axial compression of the first metacarpal with rotation (Fig. 7-7). This clinical maneuver grinds the articular surfaces of the base of the first metacarpal and the trapezium. A positive test elicits pain, and crepitus may be felt. First CMC joint arthritis may be accompanied with radial subluxation of the base of the first metacarpal. If the subluxation is more than 2 to 3 mm, the outline of the thumb will form a step called the "shoulder sign"[27] (Fig. 7-8). Occasionally, CMC joint pain may be caused by laxity or instability. To test for CMC joint instability or laxity, the metacarpal is distracted and moved in a side-to-side or radioulnar direction while the trapezium is stabilized. Comparison with the opposite side allows determination of whether joint laxity or instability is present.

The EPB and APL tendons make up the first extensor compartment and form the radial border of the anatomic snuffbox. The thumb is extended and radially abducted to allow identification and palpation of these tendons. Fullness, tenderness, and nodularity may be indicative of de Quervain's tenosynovitis. *Finkelstein's test* is used to detect de Quervain's tenosynovitis.[28] This test involves flexion of the thumb combined with ulnar deviation of the wrist (Fig. 7-9). A positive test produces pain localized to the radial aspect of the wrist.

The EPL tendon forms the ulnar border of the snuffbox. With the palm facing down, the thumb is extended toward the ceiling to allow identification and palpation of the EPL. The excursion of the tendon should be noted and compared

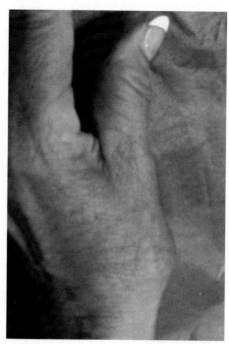

Figure 7-8 "Shoulder sign," indicating radial subluxation of the base of the first metacarpal seen with first carpometacarpal joint arthritis.

with the opposite side. The EPL tendon passes around Lister's tubercle on its path to the thumb and can rupture or become adherent after distal radius fractures, resulting in loss of or incomplete thumb extension.[4] EPL tendinitis, also referred to as *drummer's palsy,*[29] presents clinically as tenderness of the third extensor compartment just ulnar to Lister's tubercle.

Intersection syndrome refers to friction at the point where the muscle bellies of the EPB and the APL cross over the radial wrist extensor tendons proximal to the wrist, resulting in an inflammatory peritendinitis.[30] This condition may result from activities or sports that require forceful, repetitive wrist flexion and extension, such as rowing, weight lifting, and racquet sports. Friction and crepitus may be palpated 4 to 5 cm proximal to the radial styloid during wrist flexion and extension with radial deviation and has led to the name "squeaker's wrist"[31] (Fig. 7-10). The muscle bellies of the EPB and APL may be palpated proximally while the thumb is actively moving to further identify tenderness or crepitus.

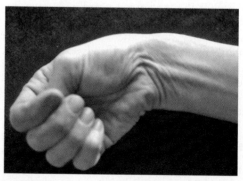

Figure 7-9 Finkelstein's test for de Quervain's tenosynovitis involves flexion of the thumb combined with ulnar deviation of the wrist.

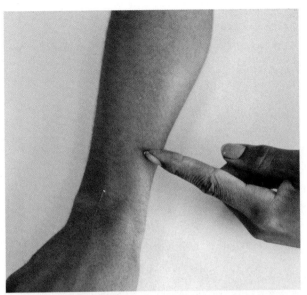

Figure 7-10 Location of symptoms of intersection syndrome 4 to 5 cm proximal to the radial styloid.

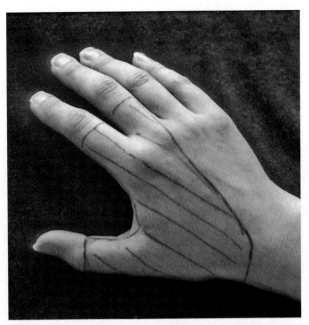

Figure 7-11 Cutaneous distribution of the dorsal radial sensory nerve.

The DRSN travels along the dorsal radial aspect of the wrist and can become implicated in a variety of radial-sided injuries. Irritation of the DRSN is referred to as *Wartenberg's syndrome* or *Wartenberg's neuralgia*.[32] Because of its superficial location, the DRSN is easily susceptible to any compressive forces, such as tight externally applied wrist straps. Forearm position can accentuate the discomfort of DRSN compression. When the forearm is supinated, the DRSN lies between the tendons of the brachioradialis and the extensor carpi radialis longus (ECRL) without compression from these two tendons. When the forearm is pronated, however, the ECRL tendon crosses under the brachioradialis tendon and in a scissor-like fashion creates compression of the DRSN.[33] Palmar, ulnar flexion of the wrist puts the nerve on stretch. When irritated, the DRSN causes numbness, tingling, burning, and pain over the dorsal radial aspect of the hand (Fig. 7-11). Percussion along the course of the nerve produces tingling and pain, and this may radiate distally. Sensibility over the dorsal web and dorsum of the thumb may be diminished and can be assessed with Semmes-Weinstein monofilaments.[32]

Central Dorsal Zone

The structures of the central dorsal zone include the dorsal rim of the distal radius, Lister's tubercle, the lunate, the scapholunate interval, the capitate, and the base of the second and third metacarpals. The soft tissue structures include the tendons of the second and fourth extensor compartments and the posterior interosseous nerve (PIN).

To locate the dorsal rim of the distal radius, the examiner should palpate the radial styloid and move dorsally. Tenderness in this area may be caused by impingement of the scaphoid on the distal radius. This condition may be caused by activities such as gymnastics in which repetitive contact of the scaphoid on the dorsal rim of the distal radius occurs

during wrist hyperextension. As a response to the repeated stress, the body forms a spur, or osteophyte, on the distal radius, which is painful with pressure or with hyperextension and radial deviation of the wrist.[34,35]

Lister's tubercle forms a bony prominence over the dorsal and distal end of the radius and can easily be palpated (Fig. 7-12, online). It is helpful to use as a landmark when localizing other structures.

The lunate is found just distal and ulnar to Lister's tubercle with the wrist flexed. In this position the lunate forms a rounded prominence (Fig. 7-13, online). Tenderness with palpation of the lunate can indicate Keinböck's disease—avascular necrosis of the lunate.[36]

The scapholunate interval is found just distal to Lister's tubercle between the third and fourth extensor compartments. Dorsal wrist ganglions are the most common mass on the dorsum of the hand and often arise from the scapholunate interval.[37] These ganglions are generally soft and freely moveable and are more easily palpable with the wrist flexed. Tenderness may be present with wrist flexion or extension secondary to compression of the ganglion. An occult ganglion is one that is suggested by patient history and complaints of pain with deep palpation but that is not detectable by clinical exam.[38,39] Sometimes confused with a ganglion is the muscle belly of the extensor manus brevis, which is a vestigial wrist extensor. The extensor manus brevis is an extra muscle–tendon unit for the index or long fingers found distal to the retinaculum.[40]

Tenderness or fullness in the scapholunate region may indicate scapholunate ligament injury, occult ganglion, or dorsal wrist syndrome, described by Watson[41] as localized scapholunate synovitis that occurs secondary to overstress of ligaments in this area. The finger extension test, used to demonstrate dorsal wrist syndrome, involves resisted long finger extension with the wrist in flexion (Fig. 7-14, online). The test is positive if pain is produced in the scapholunate region.[41] Kayalar and associates compared surgical findings with preoperative test results of the finger extension test in a series of patients diagnosed with occult dorsal wrist ganglion and found 92% diagnostic accuracy of the finger extension test for occult dorsal wrist ganglion.[42]

Scapholunate ligament injury can lead to scaphoid instability and rotary subluxation of the scaphoid. This involves dissociation of the scaphoid and the lunate and rotation of the scaphoid to a volar-flexed position. Watson[41] identified five clinical signs for rotary subluxation of the scaphoid. These include tenderness over the scaphoid in the snuffbox, scaphotrapezial-trapezoid (STT) joint synovitis and tenderness, dorsal scapholunate synovitis, a positive finger extension test, and an abnormal scaphoid shift test.[41]

The *scaphoid shift test* (SST), also referred to as the *Watson test* or the *radial stress test,* was described by Watson and coworkers[43] as a provocative maneuver to assess scaphoid stability (Fig. 7-15). To perform the SST, pressure is applied over the volar prominence of the scaphoid, found at the base of the thenar crease as the wrist is moved from ulnar deviation to radial deviation with slight flexion. Normally, with radial deviation, the scaphoid palmar flexes. With ligament laxity or disruption, and under pressure from the examiner's thumb, the proximal pole of the scaphoid shifts up onto the dorsal rim of the distal radius. When thumb pressure is withdrawn, the scaphoid returns with a clunk. A positive test is one that reproduces the patient's symptoms, usually a painful clunk. The test may be falsely positive in up to one third of individuals and is thought to be due to ligamentous hyperlaxity that permits capitolunate translation with similar findings.[44]

The validity of the SST has been studied by LaStayo and Howell.[45] They found a 69% sensitivity and a 66% specificity, indicating that approximately one third of the scapholunate injuries in their sample population were missed and that approximately one third of those individuals who did not have an injury tested positively.

Lane[46] has described the *scaphoid thrust test,* which involves pushing on the tubercle of the scaphoid in a dorsal direction. A dorsal shift of the scaphoid is apparent with scapholunate instability.

The scapholunate ballottement test may also be used to assess scapholunate instability.[47] This test involves grasping the scaphoid with the thumb and finger with one hand while stabilizing the lunate with the other. The scaphoid is then moved in a volar and dorsal direction on the lunate, and any pain or increased movement relative to the other side is noted.

Palpating in a proximal direction over the dorsal surface of the third metacarpal until a small depression is felt localizes the capitate. Tenderness here may be associated with scapholunate or lunotriquetral instability or with capitolunate degenerative disease, which occurs with scapholunate advanced collapse, or SLAC, wrist. The SLAC wrist has undergone a pattern of degenerative change that is based on and caused by articular alignment problems among the scaphoid, the lunate, and the radius.[21]

The base of the second and third metacarpals and the CMC joints are localized by palpating proximally along the dorsal surfaces of the index and long metacarpals to their respective bases (Fig. 7-16). Tenderness may indicate injury

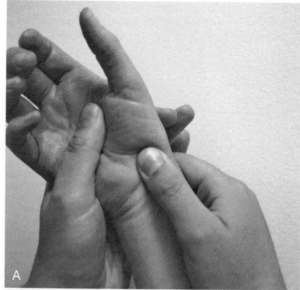

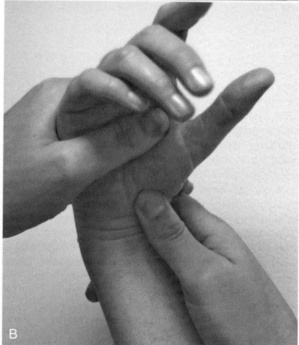

Figure 7-15 Watson's test for scaphoid instability. **A,** Starting position is with the wrist in ulnar deviation and slight wrist extension with the examiner's thumb over the volar prominence of the scaphoid. **B,** The wrist is moved to radial deviation with slight wrist flexion while maintaining thumb pressure over the scaphoid. A positive test produces a painful clunk, which reproduces the patient's symptoms.

to the CMC joints and ligaments, which can occur with forced palmar flexion of the wrist and hand.[48] A bony prominence at the base of the second and third metacarpal may be a carpal boss. A carpal boss is not necessarily a pathologic process, but rather a variation found in some individuals. It may represent hypertrophic changes of traumatic origin. These can occasionally cause pain and irritation of the local soft tissues.[49]

The *Linscheid test* is performed to detect ligament injury and instability of the second and third CMC joints.[50] This

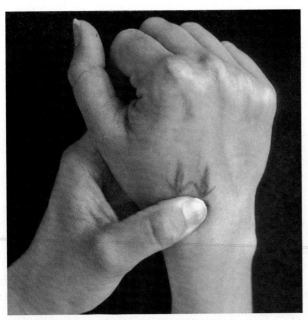

Figure 7-16 Palpation of the second and third carpometacarpal joints.

test is performed by supporting the metacarpal shafts and pressing distally over the metacarpal heads in a palmar and dorsal direction. A positive test produces pain localized to the CMC joints.

The *metacarpal stress test* involves fully flexing the metacarpophalangeal (MCP) joint and pronating and supinating the metacarpal (Fig. 7-17, online).[51] This test helps detect pain and injury at the CMC joint.

The ECRL and the extensor carpi radialis brevis (ECRB) travel radial to Lister's tubercle, insert at the base of the second and third metacarpals, and act to extend and radially deviate the wrist. The extensor digitorum communis (EDC) travels ulnar to Lister's tubercle and acts to extend the MCP joints of the digits. Tenderness, nodularity, and fullness of the tendons and pain with resisted motion may indicate tendinitis. The function of the EDC tendons should be assessed by having the patient extend at the MCP joints and then fully extend the digit. Incomplete excursion of a digital extensor tendon suggests tendon adherence or incipient rupture, which can occur at the level of the wrist with rheumatoid arthritis or after distal radius fractures that have had dorsal plate fixation.[52]

The PIN, which is mainly a motor nerve to the finger extensors, ends in the dorsal capsule of the wrist. This nerve may be a source of pain when a ganglion develops and distends the wrist capsule. Neuromas of the PIN after wrist surgery performed from a dorsal approach can be a reason for persistent postoperative pain. PIN neuritis is characterized by pain with palpation over the dorsal aspect of the wrist and proximal to Lister's tubercle.[53]

Ulnar Dorsal Zone

The structures of the ulnar dorsal zone include the ulnar styloid and the ulnar head, the DRUJ, the TFCC, the hamate, the triquetrum, the lunotriquetral (LT) interval, the fourth and fifth CMC joints, and the extensor carpi ulnaris (ECU).

The ulnar head forms a rounded prominence on the ulnar side of the wrist. It is easily palpated and most prominent with the forearm in pronation. The ulnar styloid is localized ulnar and slightly distal to the ulnar head. Tenderness in this region may be caused by an ulnar styloid fracture or nonunion.

The DRUJ is formed by the sigmoid notch of the radius and the ulnar head and is palpated just radial to the ulnar head (Fig. 7-18, online). Tenderness here may be caused by incongruity or instability with DRUJ arthritis. Prominence of the distal ulnar head is a sign of DRUJ instability and may be associated with a *piano key sign* (Fig. 7-19, online). Gentle downward pressure is applied to the distal end of the ulna with the forearm in pronation. The head moves volarly but springs back when pressure is released, resembling the action of a piano key. When this maneuver causes pain, the subject may vocalize a "note" of pain.[54]

A variation of the piano key sign, the *piano key test*, is also used to assess DRUJ instability[55] (Fig. 7-20, online). To perform this test, the distal ulna is grasped and moved passively in a volar and dorsal direction at the extremes of pronation and supination. Pain, tenderness, and increased mobility relative to the uninjured side suggest DRUJ instability.

The *ulnar compression test* involves the application of radially directed pressure on the ulnar head into the sigmoid notch of the radius. When combined with pronation and supination, compression of the DRUJ is painful in the presence of arthritis.[20]

The TFCC is the soft tissue and ligamentous support for the DRUJ and ulnar carpus. The components of the TFCC include the triangular fibrocartilage (TFC) proper or articular disk, the volar and dorsal radioulnar ligaments, the ulnocarpal ligaments, the ECU sheath, and the LT interosseous ligament.[56]

The TFCC is palpated between the head of the ulna and the triquetrum. By palpating the shaft of the ulna from proximal to distal along its lateral aspect, the examiner reaches the ulnar styloid. With continued palpation more deeply and in a palmar direction, the fovea can be detected (Fig. 7-21). The fovea is a groove at the base of the ulnar styloid that serves as an attachment point for the TFCC. Berger and Dobyns[57] describe the *ulnar fovea sign*, which is detected by the examiner pressing his or her thumb distally into the interval between the patient's ulnar styloid process and flexor carpi ulnaris (FCU) tendon, between the volar surface of the ulnar head and the pisiform. A positive sign is indicated by tenderness that replicates the patient's pain.[58] The ulnar fovea sign has been found to detect foveal disruptions of the distal radioulnar ligaments or ulnotriquetral (UT) ligament injuries with 95.2% sensitivity and 86.5% specificity.[58] The authors state that differentiation between the two conditions can be made clinically by the presence or absence of DRUJ instability, which is present with foveal disruptions of the radioulnar ligaments but not with UT ligament injuries.

Kleinman stresses the importance of testing the integrity of the palmar and dorsal fibers of the *ligamentum subcruentum*, which refers to the deep components of the TFCC inserting into the ulnar styloid fovea.[59] With the patient's forearm in full supination (dorsal fibers of the ligamentum subcruentum are under maximum tension), the examiner,

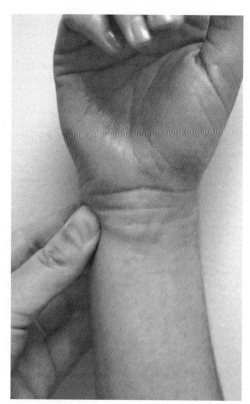

Figure 7-21 Palpation of the fovea, which is a groove at the base of the ulnar styloid. Tenderness may indicate triangular fibrocartilage complex injury.

sitting opposite the patient, applies a volarly directed pressure on the distal ulna while pulling the radiocarpal unit dorsally. If the deep dorsal fibers of the ligamentum subcruentum are injured this maneuver will result in pain and with greater injury, subluxation or gross instability. The test is repeated with the forearm in pronation (palmar fibers of the ligamentum subcruentum are under tension) and applying a dorsally directed pressure on the distal ulna and pulling the radiocarpal unit volarly. In this position, pain resulting is attributed to involvement of the palmar fibers of the ligamentum subcruentum.[59]

Ulnocarpal abutment, a condition involving abutment or impaction of the TFCC between the end of a long ulna (with positive variance) and the triquetrum, may also cause tenderness in this region.[60] The *TFCC load test* is performed to detect ulnocarpal abutment or TFCC tears (Fig. 7-22, online). It is performed by ulnarly deviating and axially loading the wrist and moving it volarly and dorsally or by rotating the forearm. A positive test elicits pain, clicking, or crepitus and reproduces the subject's symptoms.[55] Friedman and Palmer[61] describe the ulnocarpal stress test for the evaluation of ulnocarpal abutment. The test is performed by moving the forearm through supination and pronation with the wrist maximally deviated ulnarly, which increases the axial load on the ulnar wrist. A positive test reproduces ulnar wrist pain with rotation. Nakamura found that the test was sensitive but not specific for ulnar-sided pathology.[62]

Lester and colleagues describe the "press test," which is a simple provocative test to detect TFCC tears. The seated patient pushes up off the chair using the affected wrist, thus creating an axial ulnar load.[63] A positive test produces ulnar wrist pain that replicates the patient's presenting complaint. The authors report 100% sensitivity in a review of 14 patients comparing preoperative test results with surgical findings.

Ulnocarpal instability is caused by disruption of the ulnocarpal ligaments and the TFCC and is characterized by a volar sag and supination of the ulnar carpus (see Fig. 7-3, online). The *relocation test*, described by Prosser,[64] involves the combined movement of carpal pronation and anterior to posterior glide of the carpus on the ulna, which relocates the carpus into normal alignment (Fig. 7-23, online). The test is positive if the relocation of the subluxed ulnar carpus reduces the patient's wrist pain.[64]

The *pisiform boost test* is similar to the relocation test.[57] Dorsally directed pressure is applied over the palmar aspect of the pisiform, resulting in a lifting of the carpus. This test may result in pain, crepitus, or clicking, suggestive of involvement of the ulnar support structures of the wrist.

The hamate is palpable proximal to the base of the fourth and fifth metacarpals. Dorsal tenderness of the hamate may indicate fracture.[65]

The triquetrum is palpated just distal to the ulnar styloid in the "ulnar snuffbox," a term used by Beckenbaugh[50] to refer to the interval between the FCU and the ECU tendons. The wrist should be radially deviated to palpate the triquetrum because the proximal carpal row slides ulnarly with wrist radial deviation. Tenderness may indicate triquetral fracture or instability.

Pain, swelling, and tenderness in the dorsal triquetral-hamate area is suggestive of midcarpal instability.[66,67] This condition, which may be caused by ligament laxity or disruption, is characterized by a volar sag on the ulnar side of the wrist and a clunk that occurs as the wrist moves from radial to ulnar deviation. The *midcarpal shift test* (catch-up clunk test, pivot shift test) is performed by placing a palmarly directed load over the capitate and then ulnarly deviating the wrist with simultaneous axial load (Fig. 7-24).[68] A positive test is one that produces a painful clunk, which reproduces the patient's symptoms. The clunk represents the abrupt change in position of the proximal carpal row from flexion to extension as the head of the capitate engages the lunate and the hamate engages the triquetrum under compressive load as the wrist moves from radial to ulnar deviation. Lichtman and coworkers[68] have developed a grading system for the midcarpal shift test based on the degree of palmar midcarpal translation and the presence of a clunk. Feinstein and associates' quantitative assessment of the midcarpal shift test[69] confirmed its validity and usefulness as an indicator of midcarpal instability.

The LT interval is palpated just ulnar to the lunate in line with the fourth ray between the EDC and the extensor digiti quinti tendons. Tenderness and swelling in this region may be caused by LT instability. The *ballottement test* for LT instability is performed by stabilizing the lunate and attempting to displace the triquetrum volarly and dorsally with the other hand (Fig. 7-25). A positive test elicits pain, clicking, or laxity.[70]

LaStayo and Howell[45] found that the sensitivity of the ballottement test to discover a true injury was 64%; that is, approximately one third of LT injuries were missed with this test. The specificity was 44%, suggesting that more than half

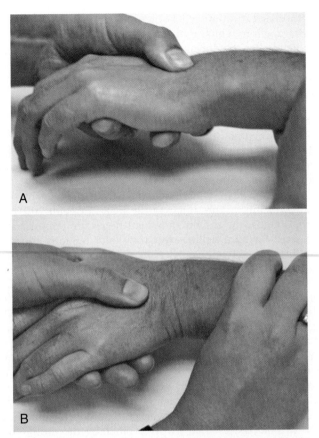

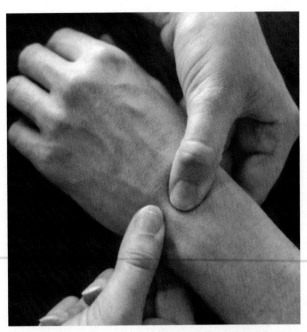

Figure 7-25 Lunotriquetral (LT) ballottement test to assess for LT instability. The lunate is stabilized with one hand while the other attempts to displace the triquetrum volarly and dorsally on the lunate. A positive test elicits painful clicking.

Figure 7-24 Midcarpal shift test. **A,** The palmarly directed load is placed over the capitate to achieve midcarpal palmar translation. **B,** This is followed by ulnar deviation with simultaneous axial load. A positive test produces a painful clunk, which reproduces the patient's symptoms.

of those who tested positively had no injury to the LT ligament.[45]

Kleinman has described a *shear test* for LT instability (Fig. 7-26). The examiner's fingers are placed dorsal to the lunate and the thumb is placed on the pisotriquetral complex. With the lunate supported, the pisotriquetral complex is loaded in the anteroposterior plane, creating a shear force across the LT joint. The wrist is then ulnarly and radially deviated. The test is positive if pain or clicking is produced.[71]

The *ulnar snuffbox test* involves lateral pressure on the triquetrum in the sulcus distal to the ulnar head formed by the ECU and FCU tendons (Fig. 7-27, online). A positive test reproduces the patient's pain, suggesting LT instability.[72]

The fourth and fifth CMC joints are localized by palpating proximally along the dorsal surfaces of the fourth and fifth metacarpals to their base. Tenderness in this region may indicate ligament injury or fracture.

The ECU tendon is palpated in the gap between the ulnar styloid and the base of the fifth metacarpal with the forearm in pronation and during active ulnar deviation. Tenderness and pain with resisted motion may indicate tendinitis. Ruland and Hogan describe the ECU synergy test as an aid to diagnose ECU tendinitis.[73] The test exploits an isometric contraction of the ECU during resisted radial abduction of the thumb with the wrist neutral and forearm supinated. During this maneuver the ECU and FCU fire synergistically to stabilize the wrist, which was confirmed by the authors electromyo-

graphically. The test is considered positive when the patient reports ulnar-sided wrist pain. The test minimizes loading of other ulnocarpal structures and allows differentiation between intra-articular and extra-articular pathology.

Pain and snapping with forearm rotation may be caused by ECU subluxation. The ECU tendon is normally held securely in the ulnar groove of the distal ulna by the ECU sheath. With disruption of the sheath, the ECU tendon subluxes and snaps during forearm rotation as it slides out of its

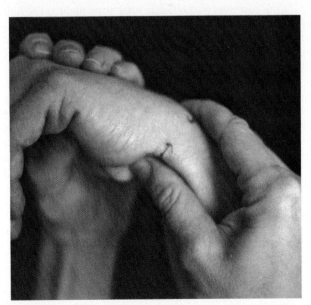

Figure 7-26 Shear test for lunotriquetral (LT) instability. Shear force is applied to the LT joint by loading the pisotriquetral complex in a dorsal direction with the lunate stabilized dorsally and then deviating the wrist in an ulnar and radial direction.

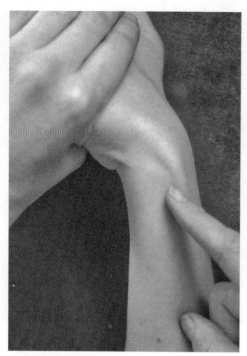

Figure 7-28 The extensor carpi ulnaris (ECU) tendon. To test for ECU subluxation, the forearm is supinated and the wrist ulnarly deviated; the tendon is then observed and palpated to assess for ulnar and volar subluxation.

groove and bowstrings ulnarly and volarly across the ulnar styloid[73,74] (Fig. 7-28). To test for ECU subluxation, the forearm is supinated and the wrist is ulnarly deviated while the tendon is observed and palpated to assess for ulnar and volar subluxation.[75]

Radial Volar Zone

Structures to assess in the radial volar zone include the radial styloid, the scaphoid tuberosity, the STT joint, the trapezial ridge, the flexor carpi radialis (FCR), the palmaris longus if present, the digital flexor tendons, the median nerve, and the radial artery.

The radial styloid is located at the base of the anatomic snuffbox. Palpate in a palmar direction to find its volar aspect (Fig. 7-29, online). Tenderness here may be caused by distal radius fractures or by radiocarpal ligament injury. Wrist extension and radial deviation accentuates discomfort in the case of extrinsic ligament injury.[55]

The scaphoid tuberosity can be found just distal to the volar aspect of the distal radius at the base of the thenar crease (Fig. 7-30, online). While palpating this area, the wrist can be moved from ulnar to radial deviation. The scaphoid assumes a flexed position and becomes more prominent and more easily identifiable in radial deviation. Tenderness over the volar scaphoid may indicate scaphoid disease.[52]

The STT joint can be found just distal to the scaphoid tuberosity. Tenderness here can be caused by STT arthritis, a common cause for radial volar wrist pain. As the wrist moves into radial deviation, the scaphoid is forced into a flexed position by the trapezium. With arthritis of the STT joint, radial deviation is often painful and restricted.[52]

Another cause for radial volar wrist symptoms is a volar wrist ganglion, which is the second most common mass of the hand after the dorsal wrist ganglion. The volar ganglion may arise from the radiocarpal or STT joints and manifests clinically as a swelling or soft mass at the base of the thumb to the distal third of the volar forearm.[52]

The trapezium is located just distal to the distal pole of the scaphoid. Tenderness over the trapezium may indicate trapezial fracture. Ulnar to the scaphoid tuberosity is the FCR tendon, which flexes and radially deviates the wrist. Tenderness and swelling of the tendon and pain with resisted movement are signs of tendinitis.

The digital flexor tendons and the palmaris longus, present in 87% of limbs,[76] are ulnar to the FCR. To define the palmaris longus, the thumb and small finger are opposed and the wrist flexed. Swelling over the flexor tendons and discomfort with active finger flexion are associated with flexor tenosynovitis.

The median nerve is deep and ulnar to the palmaris longus. *Tinel's sign* and *Phalen's tests* are clinical tests used to identify median nerve compression at the wrist—that is, CTS. To perform Tinel's test,[77] the median nerve is gently percussed at the wrist level (Fig. 7-31, online). A positive test produces pain and tingling that radiates to the fingers in the median nerve distribution. Phalen's test[78] involves passive flexion of the wrist for 15 to 60 seconds (Fig. 7-32). A positive test produces numbness and tingling in the distribution of the median nerve.[78] Smith and coworkers[79] described a modification of Phalen's test that involves pinching the thumb and index with the wrist flexed; they found that this was more reliable in young people. The Durkan carpal compression test involves application of direct pressure over the carpal tunnel.[80] MacDermid and Doherty, in a narrative review, reported that Phalen's test and the carpal compression test have the highest overall accuracy, whereas Tinel's nerve percussion test is more specific to axonal damage that may occur as a result of moderate to severe CTS. Sensory evaluation of

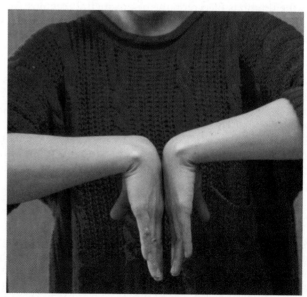

Figure 7-32 Phalen's test for median nerve compression at the wrist involves passive flexion of the wrist for 15 to 60 seconds. A positive test produces numbness and tingling in the distribution of the median nerve.

light touch and vibration can detect early sensory changes, but two-point discrimination and thenar atrophy indicate more advanced nerve compression.[81]

Graham and colleagues developed standardized clinical diagnostic criteria for CTS, which include numbness in the median nerve distribution, nocturnal numbness, weakness or atrophy of the thenar musculature, positive Tinel's sign, positive Phalen's test, and loss of two-point discrimination.[82] The authors assert that these criteria should lead to more effective treatment by improving the consistency of the diagnosis of CTS.

The radial artery lies radial to the FCR. *Allen's test* is used to assess the patency of the radial and ulnar arteries (Fig. 7-33, online).[83] To perform this test, the patient makes a tight fist and the examiner occludes both the radial and ulnar arteries. The subject opens and closes the hand until the skin is white and blanched. The radial artery is then released while compression of the ulnar artery is maintained, and the palm is observed for flushing, which indicates blood flow. If there is no flush or if flushing is delayed relative to the uninvolved side, occlusion may be present. The test is repeated to assess the ulnar artery. Symptoms of arterial occlusion include coldness and pain.

Gelberman and Blasingame introduced a variation, the timed Allen test, which records the time it takes for color to return to the hand after either the ulnar or radial artery compression is released.[84] He found the average time for radial artery refill was 2.4 seconds ±1.2 and 2.3 seconds ±1.0 for the ulnar artery in a study of 800 hands. The digital Allen test is performed by occluding both digital arteries at the base of the finger and having the patient flex and extend the finger several times to blanch the finger and then observe for return of color.[85]

Ulnar Volar Zone

The structures to assess in the ulnar volar zone include the pisiform, the hook of the hamate, the FCU, and the ulnar nerve and artery.

The pisiform is located at the base of the hypothenar eminence at the flexion crease of the wrist. It is a carpal sesamoid bone that overlies the triquetrum and lies within the fibers of the FCU. With the hand relaxed, the pisiform can be moved easily from side to side. Tenderness with palpation of the pisiform may indicate fracture or pisotriquetral arthritis, which can occur with impact loading on the ulnar side of the wrist and proximal palm, resulting in impaction of the pisotriquetral articular surface.[86]

The *shear test* for pisotriquetral arthritis involves pushing or rocking the pisiform into or across the triquetrum (Fig. 7-34, online). A positive test elicits pain or crepitus.[55]

The hook of the hamate is found in the hypothenar eminence radial and 1 to 2 cm distal to the pisiform. Tenderness may indicate hamate fracture. Pain may be accentuated with resisted flexion of the ring and small fingers with the wrist in ulnar deviation because the flexor tendons of the ring and small fingers rub against the fractured surface of the hamate during flexion.[87]

Thrombosis of the ulnar artery may cause ulnar-sided pain and coldness. This may result from repeated impact on the ulnar side of the palm when using the hand to substitute for a hammer. This is referred to as *ulnar hammer,* or *hypothenar hammer, syndrome.*[88] Allen's test, described previously, is used to detect occlusion of the ulnar artery.

Cyclist's palsy refers to ulnar-nerve compression within Guyon's canal. Long-distance cyclists often develop numbness and paresthesias in the small and ring fingers secondary to sustained compression of the ulnar nerve on the handlebars of their bicycle.[88,89]

The FCU is palpated on the ulnar, volar side of the wrist. This tendon is easily identified with wrist flexion, ulnar deviation, and fifth-finger abduction. Tenderness, fullness, and discomfort with resisted motion are signs of tendinitis.

General Tests

Additional tests for the assessment of wrist pain include the carpal shake test, the windmill test, and the sitting hands test. The *carpal shake test* is performed by grasping the distal forearm and "shaking" or passively extending and flexing the wrist. This is an "all or none" test; that is, lack of resistance or lack of complaint are significant, suggesting no pain at the wrist.[57]

The *windmill test* is performed by grasping the forearm and passively and rapidly moving the wrist in a circular pattern, simulating the rotation of a windmill.[57] This is also an all or none test.

The *sitting hands test* is used to gauge the severity of wrist involvement.[57] The subject places both hands on the seat of the chair and pushes off, attempting to hold himself or herself suspended using only hands. This maneuver produces great stresses in the wrist and is too difficult in the presence of significant synovitis.

Summary

Clinical examination of the wrist requires a thorough knowledge of wrist anatomy and pathology. The keys are to localize and identify the tender structures through systematic palpation and to reproduce the patient's symptoms and identify instability through provocative testing. Not all of the previously described tests need to be performed for every clinical wrist examination. In general, tests are selected for their relevance to the most symptomatic area or structures of the wrist, identified after a screening assessment. It is important to keep in mind that clinical findings must be interpreted with caution. This is because many of the tests described require a subjective response from the patient and their response can be influenced by factors such as motivation to magnify symptoms or limited comprehension. North and Meyer[90] correlated clinical and arthroscopic findings and concluded that it is possible to identify the region of injury based on a clinical examination, but not the specific ligament. Imaging and other diagnostic studies are needed to complete the evaluation of the wrist and to permit an accurate diagnosis.

REFERENCES

The complete reference list is available online at www.expertconsult.com.

CHAPTER 8

Clinical Examination of the Elbow

JOHN A. McAULIFFE, MD

HISTORY
PHYSICAL EXAMINATION
SPECIFIC DIAGNOSTIC MANEUVERS
ADDITIONAL DIAGNOSTIC MODALITIES
SUMMARY

particularly when the elbow is placed in extension and supination.
- Frank instability or subluxation can rarely be reproduced during physical examination, except under anesthesia; however, apprehension and pain during extension and supination stress to the elbow are suggestive.

CRITICAL POINTS

Valgus Instability

- Valgus instability is due to attenuation or rupture of the anterior bundle of the medial collateral ligament.
- Symptomatic medial collateral ligament injury is almost exclusively a problem of throwing athletes (e.g., pitchers or javelin throwers).
- Athletes usually present with the gradual onset of pain while throwing or an inability to throw with great force or velocity, although acute rupture of the ligament occasionally occurs.
- Due to the repetitive valgus stress of throwing, other medial elbow complaints may occur simultaneously, including medial epicondylitis, ulnar nerve irritation, and posteromedial elbow pain due to osteophyte impingement (valgus extension overload syndrome).
- Physical examination seldom reveals obvious gapping or instability, but relies on the reproduction of pain during a variety of valgus stress maneuvers.

Posterolateral Rotatory Instability

- Posterolateral rotatory instability is due to attenuation or rupture of the lateral ulnar collateral ligament.
- Posterolateral rotatory instability is usually a late result of elbow dislocation or subluxation.
- Iatrogenic injury to the lateral ligament complex, which usually occurs during surgery for lateral epicondylitis or radial head fracture, is another cause of posterolateral rotatory instability.
- Although patients may suffer recurrent dislocation or obvious subluxation, symptoms are often much more subtle, including pain, snapping, clunking, or locking,

A relatively limited number of symptoms prompt a patient with elbow dysfunction to seek medical attention. The most commonly voiced complaint is elbow pain that may arise from the joint itself or from any of the myriad surrounding soft tissues.[1] Although pain in or around a joint is usually the result of arthrosis, inflammation, or trauma of some sort, other, more subtle diagnostic possibilities must not be overlooked, including those of neurologic, metabolic, neoplastic, and even congenital origin. Complications related to prior surgical treatment or failed attempts at fracture fixation, specifically infection, nonunion, or malunion, may also be causes of pain.

Limitation of motion is the next most common elbow complaint. The elbow has the greatest functional range of motion of any joint in the upper extremity, and it has a great propensity for capsular contracture following even minor trauma or brief periods of immobilization.[2] The unfortunate association of these two circumstances in a single joint makes loss of elbow motion a significant problem.

Instability of the elbow is encountered much less frequently than either pain or loss of motion, and for this reason it has only recently begun to be more clearly understood. Instability can be the result of a single traumatic event, such as dislocation, often accompanied by fracture and, in these circumstances, may even rarely manifest as recurrent dislocation.[3] Although it seems counterintuitive, instability after major trauma to the elbow may cause significant pain, leading to stiffness and joint contracture. Instability may also result from chronic attritional injury to ligamentous structures as seen, for example, in throwing athletes.[4] Patients with elbow instability often do not appreciate "giving way," "clunking," or other more obvious mechanical symptoms, but instead complain that they cannot use their elbows with force in

Table 8-1   Recommended Questions to Ask During History Taking

1. When did symptoms first appear, and how have they changed over time?
2. Are the symptoms constant or intermittent?
3. Have you noticed any activity or circumstance that makes them better or worse?
4. Where are the symptoms? (I ask patients to "point with one finger" in an attempt to get as precise a localization as possible, although this is not always successful.)
5. If pain is present, can you describe it (aching, burning, stabbing) and rate its severity?
6. Does the pain radiate to other areas?
7. Have you taken medication for the pain? If so, what medication, how much, and how often?
8. Have you tried anything else that has helped, or worsened the symptoms?
9. Is there anything else you can think of that we have not yet talked about?

certain positions or cannot perform certain activities with the power to which they are accustomed.

Weakness associated with attempted use of the elbow may accompany other presenting symptoms. In the absence of more proximal neurologic injury, this complaint is usually the result of an underlying painful process causing reflex inhibition or instability leading to apprehension.[1]

History

Examination of the elbow begins with a thorough history of the presenting complaint. If a specific traumatic episode has occurred, an attempt should be made to define the mechanism of injury as accurately as possible. Such information often suggests subtle diagnoses or patterns of injury that may involve anatomic areas other than the elbow itself. In the absence of a specific traumatic event, it is often helpful to inquire about any new or different activities that the patient had engaged in during the days and weeks preceding the onset of symptoms.

It is best to allow patients a minute or two at the beginning of the interview to explain matters in their own words; they may provide information that we would not think to ask about. Careful questioning then leads to establishing a list of differential diagnostic possibilities, which can guide the physical examination. Table 8-1 contains recommended questions to ask your patient during the history. Especially when visiting a specialist, patients often neglect to volunteer information that they believe is unrelated to the current problem. Associated complaints, including involvement of other joints, fever, malaise, and related constitutional symptoms, should be specifically sought. An accurate understanding of the general medical history is another important prerequisite for appropriate diagnosis and treatment.

We should endeavor to understand not only the constellation of elbow symptoms that prompts the patient's visit, but also, and perhaps more importantly, how these symptoms interfere with vocational and avocational function.[1] Dynamic elbow instability may incapacitate an athlete, interfering with his or her livelihood, whereas it is often a minor annoyance that can be managed symptomatically in an older, more sedentary individual. Relatively minor joint contracture that might not even be considered for treatment in the average individual may occasionally prove disabling for certain musicians or skilled craftsmen.

When obtaining a history from an athlete with elbow complaints, detailed knowledge of the specific sport or activity can be of great benefit. For example, throwing athletes with ulnar collateral ligament insufficiency or other medial elbow disorders experience symptoms during the late cocking and acceleration phases of the throwing motion, whereas those with posterior elbow pathology more often complain of pain during deceleration and follow-through.[5,6] Pitching style, innings pitched, average pitch count, and even the timing of the appearance of symptoms during training or seasonal play may all be important variables to consider.

An understanding of the response to previous treatment is helpful in both establishing a diagnosis and making plans for further efforts. The details of surgical procedures are appreciated most clearly after reviewing the operative record. Such documentation may provide an invaluable firsthand description of the status of articular surfaces or supporting soft tissue structures. It is particularly helpful to know how the ulnar nerve has been handled during previous surgery: Has the nerve been transposed anteriorly? Is it subcutaneous or submuscular? Occasionally, it may be helpful to speak directly with prior caregivers if adequate records are unavailable.

Physical Examination

In our zeal to determine the cause of elbow pain we must not focus so narrowly on the elbow that we miss other associated or causative pathologic conditions. Injury around the elbow may be associated with fracture or dislocation throughout the length of the linked bones of the forearm, particularly the distal radioulnar joint.[7] An obvious fracture with significant deformity at the level of the elbow may draw our attention away from a more subtle, unrelated injury elsewhere in the limb. In athletes, shoulder dysfunction may alter throwing mechanics, resulting in secondary elbow pathology. It is imperative that the entire upper extremity be examined.[8] Radiculopathy may occasionally manifest as elbow pain, necessitating careful examination of the cervical spine.[9]

It is helpful to have access to the entire upper limb, including the shoulder, during examination of the elbow. Access to a standard orthopedic examination table may be necessary, as certain maneuvers, especially when evaluating elbow instability, may be more easily performed with the patient supine. It is advisable, especially for the novice, to establish a "routine" examination that can be performed the same way each time.[10] This helps to ensure that components of the examination are not omitted and makes follow-up more consistent and reliable. Normal or asymptomatic areas should be examined first, saving those areas that may be uncomfortable for the conclusion of the examination.[11] Subtle or questionable findings may be confirmed by reference to the contralateral, presumably normal, extremity.[12] Examination of the asymptomatic elbow first may help to relieve patient anxiety, making it more likely that subtle findings are elicited, particularly when evaluating elbow instability.[11]

All three of the major nerves in the upper extremity pass in close proximity to the elbow joint and can be injured or functionally impaired by elbow pathology. Careful documentation of neurologic function is necessary before any treatment is rendered. Supracondylar fractures of the humerus and, occasionally, elbow dislocation can result in critical vascular compression or disruption.[13] In certain individuals, collateral arterial flow is insufficient, and injury to the brachial artery results in dysvascularity of the distal extremity. Failure to promptly recognize such injury can result in devastating consequences, such as compartment syndrome, secondary ischemic contracture, or loss of limb.

Inspection

Any physical examination begins with careful observation. Obvious signs of trauma, including edema, ecchymosis, or cutaneous injury, are noted. In all but the most obese individuals, the bony prominences of the medial humeral epicondyle and tip of the olecranon are apparent unless masked by overlying edema. The most obvious swelling to occur around the elbow is associated with olecranon bursitis, which may be either inflammatory or infectious in origin.

Occasionally, the ulnar nerve or medial triceps muscle can be seen to snap over the medial epicondyle during active range of motion (ROM), although this finding is usually more apparent during palpation of the medial elbow.[14] The lateral humeral epicondyle may be visible in very thin individuals. There is normally a depression, the infracondylar recess, just distal and posterior to the lateral epicondyle, although it can sometimes only be appreciated by palpation. Hemarthrosis, joint effusion, or synovial proliferation may obliterate the recess, causing a visible bulge or swelling in this area.[1,15] Muscular atrophy or hypertrophy may be appreciated by comparison with the contralateral extremity; athletes may exhibit significant hypertrophy in their dominant arms.[10]

The integrity and adequacy of the soft tissue envelope should be noted. The location of wounds; healed surgical incisions; and scarred, adherent, or atrophic skin resulting from previous injury must be documented carefully. Cutaneous scarring owing to thermal burns often causes significant joint contracture. Poor-quality soft tissue surrounding this superficial joint may influence available management options or may have to be addressed as part of the treatment plan, particularly if surgery is contemplated.

The carrying angle of the elbow is evaluated with the joint in full extension and the forearm in full supination. Although measures vary greatly, the normal elbow is in modest valgus, which has been reported to average 11 to 14 degrees in males and 13 to 16 degrees in females.[1,16,17] The carrying angle may be 10 to 15 degrees greater in the dominant arm of throwing athletes due to adaptive remodeling of the bone as a result of repetitive stress.[10] This angle can be difficult to evaluate in the face of a flexion contracture, because the carrying angle normally changes gradually from valgus to varus as the elbow is flexed.[1]

Alteration of the carrying angle may be caused by malunion of fractures around the elbow or a growth disturbance resulting from childhood injury to the physeal mechanism. Cubitus varus is caused by a reversal of the normal valgus carrying angle and, when significant, is termed a *gunstock* deformity. Cubitus valgus is used to describe an exaggeration of the normal valgus carrying angle. This deformity may cause a traction neuropathy of the ulnar nerve, resulting over many years in what has been termed *tardy ulnar nerve palsy*.[18]

Palpation

Because the elbow is relatively superficial, deliberate and systematic palpation performed with an appreciation of the underlying anatomy can yield significant diagnostic information. The major osseous landmarks around the elbow are directly palpable beneath the subcutaneous tissue.

Posterior

When viewed from behind, the tips of the medial epicondyle, lateral epicondyle, and olecranon form an isosceles triangle when the elbow is flexed; in full extension, these three landmarks are collinear (Fig. 8-1, online). In the event of supracondylar fracture of the humerus, this triangular configuration is maintained, although its relationship to the proximal humerus will be altered. Disruption of the symmetry of the triangle indicates that the relationship between the olecranon and the epicondyles has been altered, suggesting ulnohumeral dislocation or distal humeral growth disturbance.[18]

Tenderness, thickening, and fluctuance over the tip of the olecranon are indicative of *olecranon bursitis*. These findings occasionally may be associated with a bony prominence at the tip of the bone or with fibrinous free-floating bodies within the bursa.[15] Infectious bursitis may present with marked increased warmth, tenderness, and blanching of the skin.

The broad insertion of the triceps can be palpated and defects recognized in cases of rupture of this tendon, although local swelling and hemorrhage may make this difficult following acute injury.[19] The posteromedial olecranon is a common site of tenderness, local articular cartilage injury, and osteophyte formation in throwing athletes[20] (see subsequent section on Specific Diagnostic Maneuvers). Pain to palpation directly over the tip of the olecranon in an adolescent may be caused by *apophysitis*.

Osteophyte formation on the most proximal extent of the olecranon is commonly seen in cases of primary osteoarthritis.[21] In thin individuals, tenderness in this area can be appreciated during deep palpation in the region of the olecranon fossa with the elbow flexed to approximately 30 degrees. In full extension, the proximal olecranon is contained within the olecranon fossa of the humerus and cannot be palpated; with elbow flexion beyond 30 degrees, the triceps becomes increasingly taut, prohibiting palpation of the proximal olecranon.

Lateral

The lateral supracondylar ridge of the humerus can be palpated, terminating at the prominence of the lateral epicondyle. Snapping of the lateral aspect of the triceps tendon over the epicondyle as the elbow is flexed has been described as a rare source of elbow symptoms.[22] Just distal and slightly posterior to the lateral epicondyle, a quadrant of the radial head can be felt, veiled only by the anconeus muscle and subjacent capsuloligamentous structures. As the forearm is

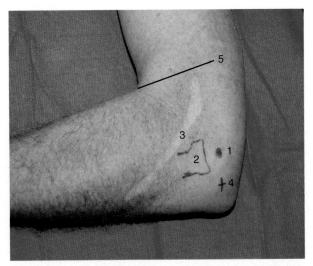

Figure 8-2 Clinical photograph of the lateral aspect of the elbow, showing (1) the lateral epicondyle, (2) the radial head, (3) the course of the radial/posterior interosseous nerve as it courses around the neck of the radius, (4) the infracondylar recess and the point at which aspiration is usually performed, and (5) the proximal extent of brachioradialis originating from the lateral supracondylar ridge.

rotated, the margin of the radial head passes beneath the examiner's fingers (Fig. 8-2). The lateral ligaments are located beneath the overlying musculature, and cannot be palpated directly. Disruption or incompetence of the lateral ligaments is seldom associated with local tenderness to palpation, except in the acute stage immediately following injury.

The infracondylar recess, located in the triangular area bounded by the lateral epicondyle, the radial head, and the tip of the olecranon, contains the most superficial and easily palpable extent of the elbow joint capsule. The earliest signs of hemarthrosis, synovitis, or joint effusion may be appreciated here.[15] This is also the preferred location for performing arthrocentesis of the elbow (Fig. 8-3, online).

The brachioradialis and extensor carpi radialis longus originate on the anterior edge of the lateral supracondylar ridge and are most easily appreciated when elbow flexion and wrist extension are resisted. These muscles, along with extensor carpi radialis brevis, whose origin lies deep to that of the longus, have been described by Henry as the "mobile wad of three," in recognition of the fact that they can be grasped and moved relative to the other musculature originating from the lateral epicondyle at the common extensor origin.[23] The most proximal extent of brachioradialis may be 8 cm or more proximal to the tip of the lateral epicondyle (see Fig. 8-2).

The degenerative process known as *lateral epicondylitis* (or colloquially, *tennis elbow*) most commonly involves the origin of the extensor carpi radialis brevis. In these cases, pain on palpation is located just distal or adjacent to the tip of the lateral epicondyle, and symptoms are exacerbated by resisted wrist extension, particularly when the elbow is fully extended, thereby placing the muscle on maximum stretch. Repeated corticosteroid injections utilized in the treatment of this disorder may result in dimpling of the overlying soft tissue due to subcutaneous fat atrophy and local skin depigmentation.

Although it lies deep to the overlying musculature and cannot be directly palpated, the posterior interosseous nerve

is most easily appreciated 4 to 5 cm distal to the lateral epicondyle as it courses around the proximal radius in the substance of the supinator muscle (see Fig. 8-2). Local tenderness in this area, not directly adjacent to the epicondyle, helps to distinguish posterior interosseous compression neuropathy from lateral epicondylitis, although the two may sometimes coexist. Motor palsy involving the digital extensors may result from compression of the nerve in this area, usually due to mass effect or local trauma. More commonly, entrapment of the posterior interosseous nerve in the proximal forearm presents as deep aching pain, sometimes with radiation to the wrist, and is known as *radial tunnel syndrome*.

Anterior

The anterior aspect of the elbow or cubital fossa is a triangular area bounded medially by pronator teres and laterally by brachioradialis. The median nerve, as its name implies, is the most medial structure in the fossa. Unusual tenderness to palpation of the nerve in this area may be a sign of local compression of the nerve, known as *pronator syndrome*; however, more distal median nerve compression at the level of the carpal tunnel may also be associated with tenderness to palpation of the nerve near the elbow. Compression of the median nerve near the elbow seldom causes distinct sensory or motor deficits in the distal distribution of the nerve, but is usually associated with deep, aching discomfort in the proximal forearm that is aggravated by activity and relieved by rest. The brachial artery is found directly lateral to the nerve. With the elbow in extension, both of these structures, which lie on the surface of brachialis, are thrust anteriorly. The arterial pulse can then be easily palpated and the position of the nerve inferred (Fig. 8-4).

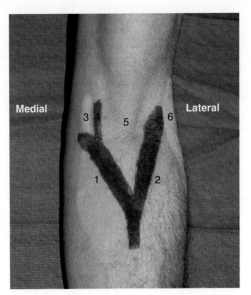

Figure 8-4 Clinical photograph of the anterior aspect of the elbow shows the cubital fossa bounded medially by (1) the pronator teres and laterally by (2) the brachioradialis. Also demonstrated are the courses of (3) the median nerve, (4) the brachial artery, (5) the biceps tendon, prominent here as flexion is resisted, and (6) the radial/posterior interosseous nerve.

The biceps tendon crosses the anterior elbow centrally and is readily palpated as elbow flexion is resisted (see Fig. 8-4). This is accomplished most easily by having the patient place his or her hand and wrist beneath the edge of the examining table and attempt to flex the elbow. As we begin to lose the feel of the tendon distally, it continues toward its insertion on the bicipital tuberosity of the radius, which is not directly palpable. A strong fascial continuation of the tendon, the bicipital aponeurosis, or lacertus fibrosus, continues medially to blend with the fascia overlying the flexor-pronator musculature.[9]

Rupture of the biceps tendon usually occurs in young or middle-aged men who experience an unexpected extension force to the elbow. Acutely, these injuries result in significant pain, swelling, and ecchymosis in the cubital fossa. If the patient does not seek medical attention until after the acute symptoms subside, some anterior elbow discomfort is usually still accompanied by a feeling of weakness, particularly involving activities that require forceful supination of the forearm. In either circumstance, the palpable absence of the biceps tendon in the cubital fossa is diagnostic. If the bicipital aponeurosis remains intact, the anterior tendon defect and the obvious proximal retraction of the muscle belly of the biceps with attempts at active elbow flexion are not quite as obvious, but usually can be appreciated by comparison with the contralateral extremity.[24] When the patient voices complaints of anterior elbow pain and weakness and the tendon is obviously palpable, consideration must be given to the possibility of partial tendon rupture.[25] Other less commonly encountered diagnostic possibilities include *cubital bursitis* and *bicipital tendonitis*.[24] It is generally not possible to distinguish these conditions by examination alone; imaging of the soft tissue is usually required.

The lateral antebrachial cutaneous nerve is the distal, purely sensory, continuation of the musculocutaneous nerve into the forearm. This nerve emerges from behind the lateral border of the biceps at the level of the interepicondylar line and becomes subcutaneous by piercing the deep fascia in this area, continuing distally into the anterolateral forearm.[26] Irritation or entrapment of the nerve in this area is another, albeit uncommon, cause of anterior elbow pain and is usually accompanied by paresthesias radiating down the anterolateral forearm.[27] Overzealous retraction of the nerve during anterior elbow surgery is the most common cause of these symptoms.

The brachialis muscle forms the floor of the cubital fossa and is intimately applied to the anterior capsule of the elbow. Snapping of a prominent medial tendinous portion of the brachialis muscle over the humeral trochlea has been reported as a cause of anterior elbow pain and swelling, also resulting in neuropathic symptoms in the distribution of the median nerve.[28]

Medial

The medial epicondyle is the most obvious landmark on the medial side of the elbow. The flexor-pronator muscle group originates here and from the distal 2 to 3 cm of the medial supracondylar ridge of the humerus (Fig. 8-5). Pain produced by palpation just distal to the tip of the medial epicondyle that is exacerbated by resisted wrist flexion is indicative

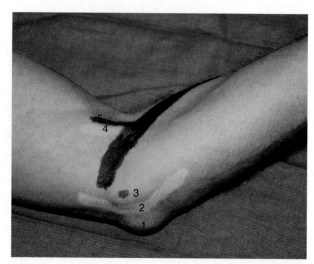

Figure 8-5 Clinical photograph of the medial aspect of the elbow showing (1) the tip of the olecranon process, (2) the ulnar nerve coursing posterior to (3) the medial epicondyle, and (4) the median nerve and (5) the brachial artery disappearing beneath the proximal extent of the flexor/pronator musculature.

of *medial epicondylitis (golfer's elbow)*. In adolescence, pain to palpation directly over the tip of the epicondyle may represent *apophysitis*. The epitrochlear lymph node is located approximately 4 cm proximal to the medial epicondyle, usually just anterior to the supracondylar ridge and the medial intermuscular septum, which arises from it. Normally not palpable, this node may occasionally be enlarged in the presence of severe hand infection and is often markedly inflamed and tender in cases of *cat-scratch disease* (*Bartonella* infection).

The ulnar nerve can be palpated immediately posterior to the medial epicondyle (see Fig. 8-5). Tinel's sign is said to be positive when percussion on the nerve causes lancinating pain or paresthesias in the distal distribution of the nerve and is found in cases of compression or traction neuropathy, known as *cubital tunnel syndrome*. Many normal nerves exhibit some element of sensitivity to percussion in this area. Maximal flexion of the elbow places the nerve on stretch and may also elicit symptoms in the ulnar nerve distribution.[29] An unusually broad distal triceps insertion sometimes may snap over the medial epicondyle as the elbow is flexed. This finding may be associated with varus malalignment of the humerus due to malunion at the supracondylar level or result from other bony deformities, including hypoplasia of the medial epicondyle.[30] The ulnar nerve itself may also subluxate anteriorly over the medial epicondyle.[14,31] Both of these conditions may cause neuropathic symptoms in the ulnar nerve distribution.

The medial ligamentous structures are not directly palpable because they lie deep to the overlying musculature. Pain or tenderness on deep palpation over the submuscular extent of these structures may be associated with ligament injury. Provocative testing that places the ligaments on stretch to determine their mechanical competence, and the presence of pain or patient apprehension, is usually a more reliable method of assessing the integrity of the ligaments[32] (see subsequent section on Instability).

Range of Motion

Simple goniometric measurement of elbow ROM has been shown to exhibit extremely high interexaminer and intraexaminer reliability. Even the simple expedient of obtaining the mean of multiple measurements is generally unnecessary, producing no improvement in measures of reliability.[33] Electrogoniometry and other more sophisticated forms of measurement may prove helpful in research situations during which multiple rapid observations must be recorded, but they are not necessary in the clinical setting.[2] Active ROM may provoke pain, crepitance, or other articular symptoms not present during passive ROM.[1]

Measurement of forearm rotation is best performed with the arm at the side and the elbow flexed to 90 degrees in an attempt to eliminate substitution by shoulder rotation. Having the patient grasp a pencil or similar object may assist in measuring rotation. When passive forearm rotation is being measured, care should be taken to ensure that rotatory force is not applied distal to the wrist, but at the level of the distal forearm. Certain loose-jointed individuals exhibit significant amounts of intercarpal pronation and supination that can sometimes confuse measurement. Although loss of forearm rotation may be associated with abnormalities of the radiohumeral articulation or proximal radioulnar joint, the cause may be located anywhere along the forearm axis, with common causes including fracture malunion and distal radioulnar joint derangement.[1]

Although reports of motion vary slightly, and minor differences are associated with age and sex, a flexion–extension arc of 0 to 140 degrees, plus or minus 10 degrees, is an acceptable approximation of normal. Normal supination tends to average 80 to 85 degrees, with pronation being slightly less, at 70 to 75 degrees.[1,34]

Functional elbow motion has been measured using an electrogoniometric technique, demonstrating that most activities can be performed with a 100-degree flexion–extension arc (from 30 to 130 degrees) and 100 degrees of forearm rotation (50 degrees of both pronation and supination).[2] Treatment of relatively minor amounts of joint contracture that fall beyond these limitations should be undertaken only after careful consideration. In contrast, severe contracture or ankylosis of the elbow causes greater functional limitation than similar loss of motion at any other articulation in the upper extremity. The inability of adjacent joint motion to compensate for the stiff elbow makes these functional limitations particularly problematic.[35]

Elbow extension is generally the first motion lost and the last to be recovered in cases of intrinsic elbow joint pathology, making this measurement a sensitive but nonspecific indicator of joint pathology.[12] Throwing athletes frequently lack 10 to 20 degrees of terminal elbow extension due to bony remodeling of the posterior medial olecranon caused by repetitive stress.[6] The capacity of the elbow joint capsule reaches a maximum at approximately 80 degrees of flexion. To reduce intra-articular pressure and resultant pain, joints with capsular distention resulting from synovitis or hemarthrosis tend to assume this position.[36]

Strength

Although sophisticated techniques are available for measuring strength around the elbow,[37] for the purposes of clinical evaluation, straightforward manual muscle testing is usually sufficient.[10] A strength difference of approximately 7% exists between dominant and nondominant limbs, although this cannot be appreciated in the clinical setting.[38] The strength of males has been shown to be nearly 50% greater than that of age-matched females.[38] Maximal elbow flexion force is exerted at 90 degrees of flexion.[39,40] For the sake of consistency, it is advisable to make all strength measurements with the elbow flexed 90 degrees.

Instability

The appropriate history of injury or activity, patient complaints, and clinical setting should arouse the clinician's suspicions regarding the possibility of elbow instability. Except in cases of chronic gross instability, which are usually apparent immediately, clinical demonstration of instability can be very difficult in the awake patient. Guarding manifested by contraction of the powerful musculature around the elbow, combined with the inherent osseous stability of the joint, may obscure subtle physical findings. Shoulder rotation may also confound examination of elbow instability, as it can be difficult to stabilize the humerus during examination.[11] Occasionally, instillation of a local anesthetic into the joint may make it possible to demonstrate instability, but examination under anesthesia may be required. Although gapping or instability may not be appreciated during physical examination in the clinic, patient apprehension or pain during stress examination is often a valuable clue indicating ligament pathology.[32]

The anterior bundle of the medial collateral ligament, which originates at the base of the medial epicondyle and inserts onto the sublime tubercle of the ulna, is the critical stabilizing structure on the medial aspect of the elbow.[41,42] The anterior bundle has been further anatomically and functionally defined into anterior and posterior bands, the former providing stability from 30 to 90 degrees of flexion, and the latter from 60 to 140 degrees (Fig. 8-6).[43] When this portion of the ligament is disrupted or attenuated, valgus stress produces opening on the medial side of the joint, often accompanied by pain. This stress should be applied with the joint flexed a minimum of 20 to 30 degrees to relax the anterior capsule and to eliminate the osseous constraint of the olecranon process of the ulna being "locked" into the olecranon fossa, as occurs in full extension. Valgus stress is applied most easily with the shoulder in full external rotation to stabilize the humerus[32] (Fig. 8-7B). This may be accomplished in a number of ways with the patient and examiner standing or seated, or even with the patient supine and the shoulder abducted and externally rotated so the elbow is near the edge of the exam table (Fig. 8-8, online).

Incomplete injuries to the medial collateral ligament may not result in frank instability but may cause significant symptoms in high-demand patients, such as throwing athletes. Only a millimeter or two of medial joint opening may be sufficient to cause symptoms in these patients, making demonstration of instability by physical examination nearly

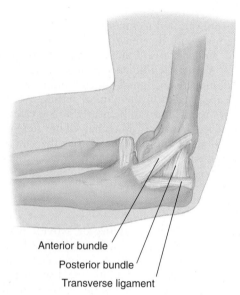

Anterior bundle
Posterior bundle
Transverse ligament

Figure 8-6 *The anterior bundle of the medial collateral ligament, originating from the undersurface of the medial epicondyle and inserting on the coronoid process of the ulna at the sublime tubercle, is the major stabilizing structure on the medial aspect of the elbow. The anterior bundle is further divided into anterior and posterior bands, each of which contributes variously to stability throughout the range of elbow flexion. (From Green DP, Hotchkiss RN, Pederson WC, et al, eds. Green's Operative Hand Surgery. 5th ed. Philadelphia: Elsevier Churchill Livingstone; 2005.)*

impossible. Veltri and coauthors have described the "milking maneuver," during which the patient places the opposite hand beneath the affected elbow to grasp the thumb of the fully supinated forearm.[44] A valgus stress is placed on the elbow, which is flexed approximately 90 degrees, stressing the posterior band of the anterior bundle of the medial collateral ligament in a position of elbow flexion that more nearly approximates that in which the athlete tends to experience symptoms during the throwing motion (Fig. 8-9). Although this maneuver may help to elicit pain or apprehension, laxity and gapping has been shown to be greatest in neutral forearm rotation throughout the full range of elbow flexion in a cadaver study.[45] O'Driscoll and colleagues have more recently described the "moving valgus stress test" for the throwing athlete in which moderate valgus torque is applied to the fully flexed elbow while the elbow is rapidly extended. Reproduction of medial elbow pain between 120 and 70 degrees was shown to be a highly sensitive indicator of medial collateral ligament injury when compared with assessment by surgical exploration or arthroscopic valgus stress testing.[46] Although physical examination maneuvers may reproduce pain in the throwing athlete, in order to demonstrate the very small amount of medial joint opening that may be problematic in these instances, more sophisticated diagnostic methods, including arthroscopic examination, are often required (Fig. 8-10, online).[47]

The lateral or radial collateral ligament (Fig. 8-11) resists varus stress and may be similarly evaluated. Full internal rotation of the shoulder serves to stabilize the humerus for this examination[32] (see Fig. 8-7A). Isolated injuries to this

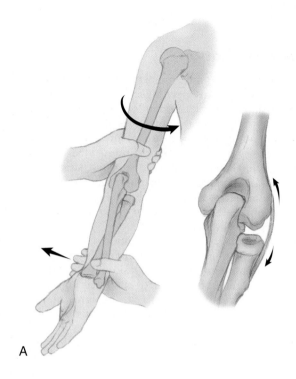

A

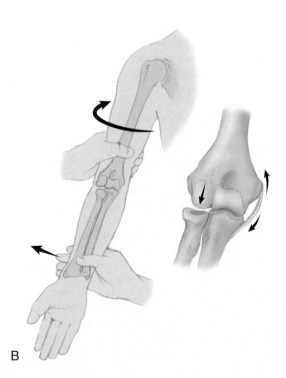

B

Figure 8-7 A, *Laxity of the radial collateral ligament (varus instability of the elbow) is examined with the humerus in full internal rotation while varus stress is applied to the joint.* **B,** *Laxity of the medial collateral ligament (valgus instability of the elbow) is evaluated with the humerus in full external rotation as valgus stress is applied to the joint. In both instances, rotation helps stabilize the humerus, allowing ligament laxity to be more easily appreciated. (From Morrey BF, ed. The Elbow and Its Disorders. 3rd ed. Philadelphia: WB Saunders; 2000.)*

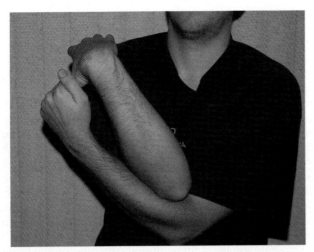

Figure 8-9 The "milking maneuver" applies valgus force to the elbow via traction on the thumb. As demonstrated here, it is performed by the patient, according to its original description. The examiner can also use this method to apply valgus force to the elbow.

ligament resulting in pure varus instability are exceedingly rare. Long-term crutch use occasionally results in attritional rupture of the radial collateral ligament.

The most common lateral ligament injury involves the lateral ulnar collateral ligament, which passes from the lateral epicondyle to a raised area on the lateral aspect of the proximal ulna, called the crista supinatoris (see Fig. 8-11). Injury to this ligament results in the phenomenon known as *posterolateral rotatory instability* of the elbow. In this circumstance, the proximal radius and ulna, which maintain their normal relationship at the proximal radioulnar joint, supinate away from the lateral aspect of the distal humerus, hinging on the intact medial collateral ligament.[48] In the

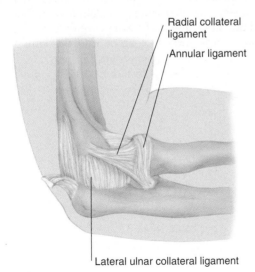

Radial collateral ligament

Annular ligament

Lateral ulnar collateral ligament

Figure 8-11 The lateral ligament complex of the elbow. The radial collateral ligament, originating on the lateral epicondyle and inserting on the annular ligament, resists pure varus stress and is seldom injured in isolation. Injury to the lateral ulnar collateral ligament, which inserts on the crista supinatoris of the ulna, is far more common, resulting in posterolateral rotatory instability of the elbow. (From Morrey BF, ed. *The Elbow and Its Disorders.* 3rd ed. Philadelphia: WB Saunders; 2000.)

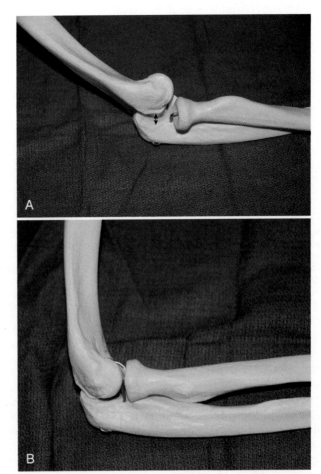

Figure 8-12 Lateral photograph of the elbow skeleton. In cases of posterolateral rotatory instability, the radial head lies posterior to the capitellum and the lateral aspect of the ulnohumeral articulation is widened (arrow). Supination, valgus, and compressive force applied to the elbow in slight flexion cause this pattern of subluxation following injury to the lateral ulnar collateral ligament **(A).** Further flexion of the joint results in reduction of the radius and ulna onto the humerus **(B).**

subluxated position, the radial head lies posterior to the capitellum and the lateral aspect of the ulnohumeral articulation is widened (Fig. 8-12). This form of instability is often not present at rest, occurring only dynamically or with provocation. It has recently been recognized that long-standing cubitus varus deformity alters the mechanical axis of the elbow so as to significantly increase the risk of tardy posterolateral rotatory instability.[49]

Posterolateral rotatory instability is demonstrated by using the pivot shift test in which the examiner subjects the elbow to supination, valgus, and compressive stress.[48] This maneuver is best performed with the humerus locked in full external rotation. As the elbow is extended from a semiflexed position, posterior subluxation of the radial head can be appreciated and often causes a dimpling in the skin on the lateral aspect of the joint; maximum subluxation usually occurs at about 40 degrees of flexion.[48] Further flexion of the elbow results in a sudden reduction of the radius and ulna onto the humerus. This maneuver may be most easily performed with the patient supine on the exam table with the arm overhead (Fig. 8-13). Examination under anesthesia is almost always required to demonstrate this finding.

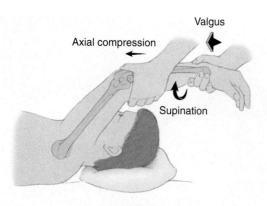

Subluxation

Figure 8-13 Examination for posterolateral rotatory instability is most easily performed with the patient supine and the arm overhead. Valgus force and axial compression is applied to the maximally supinated forearm. Subluxation occurs most readily with the elbow in 20 to 40 degrees of extension; further flexion results in visible and palpable reduction. (Reprinted with permission from The Journal of Bone and Joint Surgery, Inc. From O'Driscoll SW, Bell DF, Morrey BF: Posterolateral rotatory instability of the elbow. *J Bone Joint Surg (Am)*. 1991;73:440-446.)

Forearm supination, valgus stress, and compression across the elbow joint can also be produced by asking the patient to push off with his hands from the examining table.[1] Visible instability may only be appreciated in the most unstable joints; however, patient apprehension during the performance of this maneuver or an inability to bear weight on the elbow in this position is suggestive of posterolateral rotatory instability (Fig. 8-14, online).

Specific Diagnostic Maneuvers

Discomfort associated with lateral epicondylitis during resisted wrist extension is evaluated easily by asking the patient to stand and to extend his or her elbow, to fully pronate the forearm, to grasp the back of a chair, and to attempt to lift it off the ground. Medial epicondylitis is similarly evaluated by having the patient place the supinated palm beneath the examining table with the elbow fully extended and attempting to lift the table.

The *valgus extension overload* test is used to simulate forces applied across the elbow during the acceleration phase of throwing. While stabilizing the humerus with one hand, the examiner pronates the forearm with his or her opposite hand and applies a valgus force while quickly maximally extending the elbow. A positive test causes posteromedial pain as the osteophyte and locally inflamed synovium that form in response to the chronic stress of throwing are compressed against the medial wall of the olecranon fossa (Fig. 8-15).[5,10] Chronic valgus extension stress can cause injury other than posteromedial impingement and degeneration, including ulnar neuropathy and medial collateral ligament strain.[50,51] The close proximity of these injured structures on the medial side of the elbow can make diagnosis challenging.

The radiocapitellar chondromalacia test is essentially a "grind" test involving the radiohumeral articulation. It is positive in the event of disease involving either the radial head (arthrosis) or capitellum (osteonecrosis). Forearm rotation accompanied by valgus stress and lateral compression of the elbow produces crepitance or pain in the event of a positive test.[10]

Additional Diagnostic Modalities

A thorough history and physical examination of the elbow is usually followed by diagnostic imaging, beginning with plain radiographs. Details regarding imaging of the elbow may be found in Chapter 14. Even after detailed clinical and radiographic evaluation, unanswered questions may remain. Arthrocentesis for aspiration or injection may be helpful in these circumstances. The question of infection following prior surgery or open injury is definitively answered by examination and culture of a sample of synovial fluid. Instillation of a local anesthetic agent into the joint may help

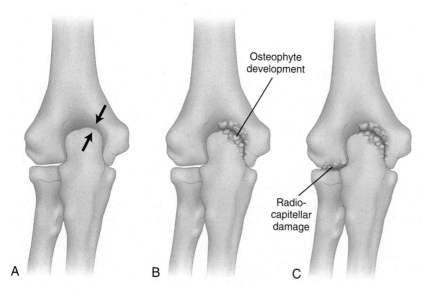

Figure 8-15 Drawing depicting the effects of valgus extension overload on the elbow of the throwing athlete. (From Green DP, Hotchkiss RN, Pederson WC, et al, eds. *Green's Operative Hand Surgery.* 5th ed. Philadelphia: Elsevier Churchill Livingstone; 2005, Fig. 26-8, p. 961.)

determine whether intra-articular or extra-articular pathology is the source of reported pain. Arthrocentesis or injection of the elbow is commonly performed posterolaterally through the infracondylar recess (see Fig. 8-3), although an alternative direct posterior approach through the triceps tendon, which positions the tip of the needle in the olecranon fossa, may occasionally be useful.[52]

Arthroscopy of the elbow may provide additional information. The magnitude of articular cartilage injury is best evaluated under direct vision. When symptoms of locking or catching persist despite normal imaging studies, arthroscopy may be used as the definitive diagnostic and therapeutic modality.[53] Incomplete ligament injury or subtle instability in the competitive athlete may sometimes require intra-articular evaluation that can be performed only arthroscopically.[54]

Elbow Scoring Systems and Self-Report Measures

No single, well-accepted elbow scoring system is used commonly in the clinical setting. Several composite impairment scales assign point values based on observations of pain, motion, and strength; some also include assessments of stability, function, and deformity. The maximum number of possible points assigned to the various measured parameters varies considerably among these systems. The total score, out of a possible of 100, is used to assign a categorical rank (excellent, good, fair, poor), although the score required to achieve a given rank also varies from system to system. A review of five observer-based impairment scales found remarkably little agreement among the categorical rankings assigned to patients by these systems. Good correlations among the various systems were observed when raw scores were compared, leading to the recommendation that raw scores, not rank scores, should be reported when these scales are utilized.[41] Unfortunately, comparisons between studies based on different scoring systems are not possible.

The Mayo Elbow Performance Index (MEPI) is arguably the most commonly used of these observer-rated scales, although others have been reported and compared.[41] The MEPI assigns points for pain,[15] motion,[54] stability,[5] and five functional tasks.[20,55] A recent study has noted that 66% of the variability in MEPI scores is accounted for by pain alone,

with other observer-based rating systems exhibiting similar findings.[56] These authors suggest that the psychosocial aspects of illness related to pain may be overvalued by these scales and propose that it may be advisable to evaluate pain separately from other objective measures of elbow function.[56]

Another concern with the currently available observer-based impairment scales is that even the numerical raw scores generated by the various systems demonstrated only moderate correlation with patient-reported function on a visual analog scale.[41] Outcome questionnaires completed by the patients, including the Disabilities of the Arm, Shoulder, and Hand (DASH) questionnaire[57] and the Modified American Shoulder and Elbow Surgeons (ASES) patient self-evaluation form,[58] showed much better correlation with patients' perception of function.[41] The Patient-Rated Elbow Evaluation (PREE) is another available self-report measure of pain and function that has been shown to be reliable and valid.[59] The PREE has demonstrated high correlation with the ASES patient self-evaluation form, has a more patient-friendly format, and has the added advantage of allowing computation of a single combined score.[60] Additional information on self-report questionnaires can be found in Chapter 16.

A complete evaluation of the result of elbow treatment requires the use of a patient-reported functional evaluation (self-report questionnaire), together with the more traditional clinical measures of motion, strength, stability, and deformity, as well as an assessment of pain.[41]

Summary

A thorough history, a detailed physical examination, and readily available imaging studies provide an accurate diagnosis of most elbow complaints. Only rarely are more advanced techniques, such as magnetic resonance imaging, or invasive diagnostic modalities, including arthroscopy, required. Evaluation of the results of treatment requires a patient-completed outcome questionnaire designed to assess function, in addition to documentation of more commonly measured clinical parameters, such as motion, strength, and stability, and an assessment of pain.

REFERENCES

The complete reference list is available online at www.expertconsult.com.

9

Clinical Examination of the Shoulder

MARTIN J. KELLEY PT, DPT, OCS AND
MARISA PONTILLO PT, DPT, SCS

PATIENT CHARACTERISTICS
POSTOPERATIVE EVALUATION
PHYSICAL EXAMINATION
SUMMARY

CRITICAL POINTS

Characteristics of Pain

When assessing pain:
- Use a visual analog scale (VAS) or outcome tool.
- Determine if pain is constant or intermittent.
- Night pain is very common with most shoulder disorders.
- Correlate pain with functional activities and position.
- Ask the patient what relieves pain.

Physical Examination

- Examination progresses from least to most provocative activities.
- The authors recommend starting with observation, perform physical testing, and end with palpation.
- Determining a patient's irritability level does not always establish the extent of the pathology but helps the clinician to develop an appropriate therapeutic plan.
- Reassessment must be frequent to determine the response to treatment.

Contractile Versus Noncontractile Tissue

- Contractile tissue is generally evaluated through resisted testing.
- Noncontractile tissue is generally evaluated through passive motions.

Scapular Muscle Strength Testing and Special Tests

- Using an evaluating scapular muscle algorithm helps identify the cause of scapular dyskinesis.

Passive Range of Motion

- A capsular end-feel is considered normal at all shoulder end-ranges; however, muscle guarding may mimic a capsular end-feel in patients with frozen shoulder.

Special Tests

- The external rotation lag sign is valuable when determining if a patient has a full-thickness supraspinatus tear.
- Negative impingement signs help to rule out rotator cuff pathology due to their high sensitivity.

Palpation

Areas of the shoulder that are normally tender:
- Biceps groove
- Coracoid process
- Inferior posterior deltoid fibers
- Lesser tubercle

Clinical examination of the shoulder is important for determining pathology, irritability level, and functional status. A proper examination requires a systematic approach involving a complete history, observational skills, and the assessment of signs and symptoms. The ability to interpret examination findings derives from the examiner's knowledge of anatomechanics and pathology. An important goal of the examination is establishing baseline signs and symptoms. Treatment efficacy and outcomes are determined by comparing baseline findings with subsequent findings. Reexamination is incorporated into each subsequent treatment visit through manual and visual feedback. Although questioning during the history taking often leads to a diagnosis well before a hand is laid on the patient, the curtailment of a complete examination and "diagnosis prejudging" should be avoided.

The examination visit is the initial contact between patient and clinician and therefore creates a lasting impression for the patient. The patient should feel comfortable and trust the clinician. If the clinician conducts a thorough, organized evaluation, and if he or she demonstrates a sound knowledge of current orthopedic concepts and practices by answering the patient's questions regarding incidence, etiology, pathophysiology, and prognosis, the clinician–patient relationship will be strengthened.

94

Table 9-1 Irritability Classification

High Irritability	Moderate Irritability	Low Irritability
High pain (≥7/10)	Moderate pain (4–6/10)	Low pain (≤3/10)
Consistent night or resting pain	Intermittent night or resting pain	No resting or night pain
High disability on DASH, ASES	Moderate disability on DASH, ASES	Low disability on DASH, ASES
Pain prior to end ROM	Pain at end ROM	Minimum pain at end ROM with overpressure
AROM < PROM, secondary to pain	AROM ~ PROM	AROM = PROM

AROM, active range of motion; ASES, American Shoulder and Elbow Surgeons score; DASH, Disabilities of the Shoulder, Elbow, and Hand score; PROM, passive range of motion; ROM, range of motion.

Patient Characteristics

Age

Patient age helps categorize shoulder pathology. The two most common conditions, rotator cuff disease and glenohumeral instability, are both age-dependent. Rotator cuff tendonopathy can occur at any age due to trauma or overuse. However, there is a high incidence of rotator cuff lesions of a degenerative nature in individuals older than 40 years of age due to tendon attrition,[1,2] reduced vascularity,[3,4] mechanical impingement,[1,5,6] and decreased tendon tensile strength.[7-9]

The diagnosis of glenohumeral instability, both primary and recurrent, is found most commonly in patients younger than 30 years of age. Although instability can occur in the population older than 40, the recurrence rate is significantly lower than in those younger than 30.[10-12]

Irritability is used to describe the inflammatory status of joints and surrounding soft tissue structures. Irritability categories are mild, moderate, and severe (Table 9-1). Determining a patient's irritability level does not always establish the extent of the pathology but it does help the clinician to develop an appropriate therapeutic plan. For example, Patient A may present with mild irritability and have full active and passive range of motion (AROM, PROM, respectively), slight pain at end range, resisted motions that are painful only in abduction, and slight pain elicitation with impingement signs. Patient B, presenting with severe irritability, may have considerably painful restrictions of AROM and PROM; significant pain and weakness on resisted abduction, external rotation, and flexion; and an exceedingly painful impingement sign. Patient A may have only mild supraspinatus tendinitis, patient B may have a large rotator cuff tear, or both patients may have the same relative tissue involvement yet each appears to be at a different stage of inflammation or healing. Their irritability level determines whether pain-relieving modalities and techniques are used versus more intense stretching and strengthening.

History

The patient's history often defines pathology prior to clinical examination because it fits a certain "pattern" consistent with a particular pathology. A pattern that is not recognized or is different may reflect the examiner's *developing* experience or result from an unusual pathology. Information about the patient's age, occupation, and activities are essential to commencing diagnostic categorization. Although rotator cuff pathology is related to tendon degeneration and osseous spur formation, occupations that involve heavy lifting or repetitive or sustained overhead use of the arm are correlated with increased rotator cuff incidence.[13] A patient's general health and other joint involvement may influence symptoms through a systemic or referred mechanism; therefore, details regarding general health and other joint involvement should be outlined. In addition, information on hand dominance, medications, and recreational activities should be obtained. Determining the patient's activity goals assists in guiding treatment. Table 9-2 lists the subjective information that should be relayed during history taking.[14]

Chief Complaint

Establishing the chief complaint is imperative. Is pain, weakness, parasthesia, or difficulty performing activities of daily living (ADL) the reason for seeking medical attention? The chief complaint may be isolated or, more typically, a combination of symptoms. Onset and chronology should be investigated and clarified. A specific event, such as a fall, may be easily identified as the precipitating episode.

Insidious onset is characteristic of some conditions, such as primary frozen shoulder. Asking about specific, activity-related questions can "jog" the patient's memory into identifying the initiating incident. Commonly a new activity or change of environment such as beginning a new job, starting a workout routine, acquiring a new tennis partner, or painting a bedroom, is identified. If the episode was traumatic, such as a high-velocity, uncontrolled fall or a motor vehicle accident, details regarding the direction of forces on the upper extremity are clarified. If the injury was related to a specific sporting event, replication or breakdown of the specific athletic stroke or technique is performed. Mechanisms of injuries are similar for specific pathologies; for example, a fall on the superior aspect of the shoulder is consistent with an acromioclavicular (AC) joint separation. Frequently, disabling rotator cuff inflammation can result from relatively innocuous activities such as reaching behind the car seat to lift a briefcase or opening a jammed window. The clinician must elucidate the relationship between pertinent shoulder anatomy and biomechanics, the mechanism of injury, and pathogenesis of common shoulder conditions. During this process, relevant faulty tissue can be identified.

Characteristics of Pain

Location

The area of perceived pain helps distinguish the problematic structure. In general, primary pain experienced over the neck, upper shoulder, or scapula indicates cervical spine-related tissue, possibly nerve root, dura mater, outer annular disk fibers, or facet joint. Pain can originate from muscles either specific to the cervical spine or those sharing shoulder function responsibility. Commonly, the levator scapulae and

Table 9-2 History

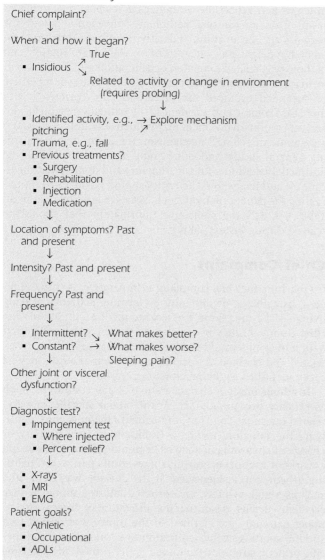

ADLs, activities of daily living; EMG, electromyography; MRI, magnetic resonance imaging. (From Kelley MJ: Evaluation of the shoulder. In: Kelley MJ, Clark WA, eds. *Orthopedic Therapy of the Shoulder.* © 1995. Philadelphia: J.B. Lippincott Company.)

upper and middle trapezius develop spasm, trigger points, or overuse soreness, primarily or secondarily, in response to primary shoulder or cervical pathology. Knowledge of dermatomal, myotomal, scleratomal (Fig. 9-1, online), and trigger point reference zones is crucial to the correct interpretation of pain.[15]

Pain around the deltoid, typically laterally, is consistent with dysfunction of the glenohumeral joint or associated soft tissue structures. This region encompasses the C5 dermatome but symptoms can refer into the C6 dermatomes. A patient with a diagnosis of a supraspinatus tendon tear or tendinitis usually reports referred pain over the lateral deltoid, not over the tendon. Referred pain can be explained by cerebral and limb bud embryologic development. The supraspinatus tendon is a deep member of the C5 dermatome. A lesion of this structure stimulates the corresponding C5 cerebral cortex, thereby producing a diffuse, often lateral perception of pain. Pain perceived over the AC and sternoclavicular joints is characteristic of dysfunction in that corresponding joint, although other portions of the C4 dermatome also can be stimulated.

Intensity and Frequency

Pain intensity and frequency characteristics provide further status of tissue irritability. Considerable inflammation has a high correlation with increased symptoms and tissue reactivity. A VAS can be valuable in providing objective information about pain intensity.[16] Whether pain is constant or intermittent is important in further deciphering symptom features. Prolonged, constant, unyielding pain is unusual for glenohumeral joint or soft tissue pathology, excluding tumors. Even patients who have experienced acute injury or surgery find relief from constant pain within several days or by appropriate positioning of the arm. Neural irritation or damage can produce uninterrupted pain.

Intermittent pain can vary in frequency and intensity. Night pain is quite common with shoulder dysfunctions; most patients with rotator cuff pathology find it difficult to sleep on the involved side. The eventual ability to sleep on the involved shoulder is a sign of recovery and reduced irritability. The relationship between activity and position requires exploration. Intermittent pain may occur following aggressive activity, overhead use, or the routine performance of ADL. Discovering what relieves the pain is also vital information. Patients with a C7 radiculopathy may find relief by placing the arm overhead, yet this position is provocative in those having rotator cuff pathology or instability. Prior utilization and efficacy of the medical intervention such as corticosteroid injections, exercise, thermal agents, and medication(s) also should be determined.

Diagnostic Tests

The physical therapist without special radiographic training typically does not have the ability to interpret radiographs and must therefore rely on a radiologist or an orthopedic surgeon for interpretation of plain radiographs, MRIs, ultrasonography, CT scans, and bone scans. Electromyographs (EMGs) usually are performed and interpreted by a specialist. The clinician should learn and appreciate the appropriate use, limitations, sensitivity, and specificity of diagnostic equipment and results. This knowledge will improve the clinician's evaluative abilities and enables him or her to recommend or suggest further testing when appropriate.

Postoperative Evaluation

In addition to typical history, information gathered postoperatively should include presurgery ROM and function status. Regardless of whether a specific diagnosis is provided by the referring physician or if the patient presents following a surgical procedure, a detailed history may provide additional information to the therapist that was not appreciated previously.

To provide a safe and informative postoperative evaluation, the clinician should understand operative procedures and the associated possible and common complications. Clinicians and surgeons should interact frequently during the treatment of a postoperative patient. It is a disservice to the patient if the surgeon does not disclose surgical nuances, surgical modifications, or patient tissue idiosyncrasies to the treating therapist. Although surgeons do not always express relevant details to the therapist, therapists also need to acquaint themselves with surgical procedures. A communicative surgeon and a an informed therapist decrease the possibility of patient complications and increase optimal outcomes.

Information regarding tissue quality, tear size, tendon lateral mobilization, chronicity, and the presence of synovitis is important when examining a patient following rotator cuff repair. Significant preoperative supraspinatus muscle belly atrophy with fatty infiltration is related to a higher incidence of retearing following rotator cuff repair.[17] If the repair was for a large chronic retracted cuff tear, discretion regarding adduction and force application is necessary since a high retear rate has been associated with tears greater than 3 cm that have been repaired arthroscopically.[18,19] Significant weakness and unresolved ROM deficits prior to surgery have been shown to depreciate postoperative results.[20]

Patients who are seen following a reconstructive procedure for instability also require special attention. It should be determined if their injury was traumatic or atraumatic. Information regarding the quality of labral, tendinous, and capsular tissue fixation is essential. Assessment of generalized hypoelasticity and hyperelasticity may be the clinician's greatest guide to examination and treatment progression. If a patient with significant hyperelasticity is evaluated at 4 weeks after surgery and demonstrates 50 degrees of true glenohumeral joint external rotation with the arm adducted and 150 degrees of elevation, care should be taken to deemphasize ROM because stability may be sacrificed over time as a result of the individual's collagen tissue pliability.

Tissue fixation and healing principles must be followed when assessing ROM and strength. Typically, 4 to 6 weeks is sufficient for capsular and tendinous tissues to achieve adequate physiologic healing (depending on tissue quality and degree of tension). Controlled, gentle tension can be administered to patients at 2 weeks following a capsular plication and Bankart procedures.

The examination of the postoperative patient is defined by the time period from surgery. Regardless of the procedure, an examination performed on the first day after surgery differs from one performed 4 weeks postoperatively. Strength assessment requiring significant resistance should be avoided until the relevant tissue can maintain its integrity. The time varies depending on factors previously discussed. Necessary information regarding muscular, structural, and neurovascular intactness usually can be gained with a submaximal contraction within the first 2 weeks. Corroborating evidence to determine whether neurovascular integrity is present should be an early goal of all evaluations, but especially following multiple traumas, humeral head fractures, and any surgical procedure.[21] Typically, at 6 weeks, a full shoulder examination can be performed, although prudence is always required

following a rotator cuff repair pertaining to strength assessment.

Outcome Forms

Using patient-oriented outcome forms to document the patient's response to treatment is becoming a necessity in today's health care market. These forms can provide information about the effectiveness and appropriateness of treatment. Several generic outcome forms have been developed. The SF-36 has gained popularity as a generic health status measure. However, to evaluate greater sensitivity over time, some investigators advocated using condition-specific forms.[22] Several shoulder outcome forms have been developed over the recent years.[22-26]

The clinician should consider using an outcome form as part of the examination. The form is filled out by the patient at the initial visit and then again at intervals, including discharge. The form may ask patients about pain, satisfaction, and function; in addition, some include objective data, such as ROM, strength, and clinical test measurements. The clinician should investigate the shoulder-specific outcome forms to decide which best fits the needs.

Physical Examination

Skill, experience, and a systematic approach are required to gather and interpret signs and symptoms correctly. A consistent examination must be done on each patient regardless of history so that the clinician can appreciate "normal" abnormalities, concomitant lesions, and commonly associated lesions (i.e., rotator cuff disease and AC joint arthritis). The patient's history and physical examination findings should correlate; if they appear to be unrelated, further questioning is required. The possibility of a catastrophic cause should be ruled out early if suggestive signs and symptoms emerge.

The goal of the physical examination is to determine the source of the chief complaint by reproducing symptoms. The patient must understand that the purpose of particular techniques and positions is to reproduce or change the patient's chief complaint, whether it is pain, stiffness, or parasthesia. Typically, the evaluation process progresses from least to most provocative. As Cyriax[27] discussed, point palpation should be done last because it can only bias and confuse the clinician and prematurely irritate the patient if it is done early in the examination. The patient should be warned that his or her symptoms may worsen following the examination; therefore, the patient should be given appropriate pain relief guidelines to follow.

The order of the physical assessment presented here is based on our preferred performance.

Observation

An enormous amount of information is gained by general and detailed observations of the patient. General observations regarding upper extremity posturing as well as normal movement patterns, such as taking a shirt off, provide a gauge of irritability and functional impairment. A patient experiencing pain characteristically protects the upper extremity by

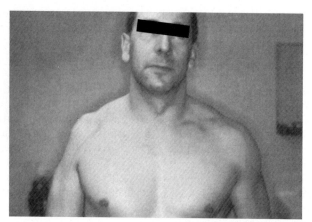

Figure 9-2 Significant right deltoid atrophy due to axillary nerve palsy. (From Kelley MJ. Evaluation of the shoulder. In: Kelley MJ, Clark WA, eds. *Orthopedic Therapy of the Shoulder.* © 1995 J.B. Lippincott Company.)

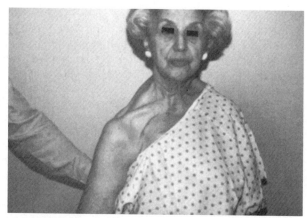

Figure 9-3 Patient 11 years after complete and unresolved spinal accessory nerve palsy caused by radiation therapy following a radical mastectomy. Note the inferior clavicular orientation. (From Kelley MJ. Evaluation of the shoulder. In: Kelley MJ, Clark WA, eds. *Orthopedic Therapy of the Shoulder.* © 1995 J.B. Lippincott Company.)

maintaining an internally rotated and adducted position. Consistency of motion should always be noted. If a patient can easily place his or her arm overhead while disrobing but then can barely elevate the extremity while AROM is being assessed, the clinician notes an inconsistency. A physiologic reason for such a discrepancy must be found; if it cannot be found, secondary gains or psychosis should be considered as motivators.

Detailed observations to assess soft tissue and osseous deformity or asymmetry then follow. The patient should be properly exposed; males disrobe from the waist up, and females should wear a gown that allows the appropriate visualization of the complete shoulder girdles and middle to upper thoracic spine. Bony prominences, particularly of the AC and sternoclavicular joints, should be viewed for symmetry. A squared appearance of the lateral shoulder, exposing the lateral acromion, may indicate deltoid wasting or anterior glenohumeral dislocation (Fig. 9-2). Clavicular orientation should be appreciated from the anterior view; in the presence of a chronic spinal accessory nerve injury or facioscapulohumeral muscular dystrophy, the clavicle and associated shoulder girdle may be significantly depressed and protracted due to lost upper trapezius suspensatory function (Fig. 9-3).

Muscle contour inspection to determine atrophy or hypertrophy is critical. Complete lesions of the nerve or musculotendinous unit produce conspicuous muscle mass changes, whereas subtle bulk disparity such as in infraspinatus atrophy of a throwing athlete may be more difficult to appreciate. The infraspinatus and supraspinatus fossae and scapular spine should be viewed posteriorly and superiorly (Fig. 9-4). Fossa hollowing indicates pathology of the musculotendinous unit, cervical nerve root, peripheral nerve, or upper plexus. Tendon rupture produces noticeable muscle contour changes, as in the "popeye" muscle that results from long head of the biceps tendon rupture. Detection of muscle bulk changes in unconditioned or obese individuals requires visualization enhanced by active contraction or palpation.

Posture

A formal postural assessment is performed to determine scapular and spinal misalignment. Postural alignment should

be viewed with the patient both sitting and standing and correlated with provoking activities. Spinal alignment directly influences shoulder girdle orientation and function.[28-30] A sedentary individual sitting or standing in a posterior pelvic tilt, lumbar flexion, increased thoracic flexion, and a forward-head position is obliged to anteriorly displace the shoulder girdles. Prolonged chronic placement in this orientation may cause adaptive shortening and stretch weakness of associated spinal, trunk, and shoulder musculature.[29] Attempted arm elevation in this position restricts scapular rotation and retards trunk and rib expansion, thereby limiting motion (Fig. 9-5, online).[28,30] Repetitive shoulder level or overhead use of the arm while maintaining this posture could predispose the shoulder to soft tissue overload resulting in trigger point formation or rotator cuff impingement.

Both sitting and standing posture should be viewed posteriorly, laterally, and anteriorly to recognize and correlate postural faults. Particular attention should be directed toward scapular alignment. Posteriorly, the scapular inferior angle should be level with the T7 spinous process; the vertebral border should be 5 to 9 cm, depending on the size of the

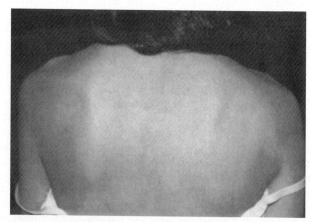

Figure 9-4 Atrophy of the supraspinatus and infraspinatus muscles demonstrated by hollowing of the spinati fossae. (From Kelley MJ. Evaluation of the shoulder. In: Kelley MJ, Clark WA, eds. *Orthopedic Therapy of the Shoulder.* © 1995 J.B. Lippincott Company.)

individual, from the spinous processes.[31] Bilateral comparisons should be made and although hand dominance affects scapular orientation, left-handed individuals are inconsistent because they tend to perform many activities with the right hand. The greater the unilateral activity, the greater the asymmetry; this is particularly true of pitchers and tennis players who tend to have a depressed and protracted shoulder girdle.[32]

Scapular orientation has two characteristic presentations: (1) The scapula is abducted and inferiorly displaced relative to the nondominant side, and (2) the scapula is elevated, medially rotated, and forward, yet the acromion is lower than the uninvolved side (Fig. 9-6, online). In the second scapular position described, the coracoid is pulled forward, elevating and anteriorly tilting the relatively flat scapula over the curved posterior thoracic wall, thereby displacing the acromion forward and down. The tilting causes the inferior angle to migrate posteriorly away from the thoracic wall; this is often mistaken for scapular "winging." In both the aforementioned scapular orientations, the middle and lower trapezius muscles are elongated, tending to be weak, and the pectoralis minor is tight.[33] Excessive scapular deformity has been described as the SICK (Scapula Infera and Inferior angle, Coracoid and Clavicular dysKinesis) scapula.[32]

Cervical Range of Motion

Any time the upper quadrant is involved, the cervical spine requires a screening examination to rule out primary or associated pathology. Active cervical motions are performed in flexion, extension, both side bendings, and rotations. ROM and symptom reproduction are assessed and correlated with the chief complaint. Frequently, a patient reports upper trapezius or cervical pain or pulling of the stretched side when rotating or laterally flexing away. The patient must distinguish the normal sensation of a stretch from the pain for which he or she seeks medical attention.

A simple technique that helps determine true, full passive cervical ROM and also helps distinguish between painful trapezius limitation and restriction from a spinal structure (i.e., disk, facet, ligament, or paravertebral muscle) is to compare cervical range while the patient is sitting or standing and while supine. While sitting and standing, the shoulder girdle is depressed by gravity and upper extremity weight, prestretching the upper trapezius muscle, which results in limited contralateral cervical side bending and rotation. Repeating this motion while supine and while manually elevating the shoulder opposite to the head direction allows the upper trapezius to slacken, thus enabling full assessment of true cervical side bending and rotation. To accept cervical side bending and rotation motion as true motion when performed in the sitting or standing position is equivalent to accepting hip flexion motion with the knee extended.

Cervical Spine Special Tests

Spurling Test

The Spurling test is a nonspecific yet excellent test for determining cervical involvement. The head is extended, laterally flexed, and rotated to the ipsilateral side. Overpressure is

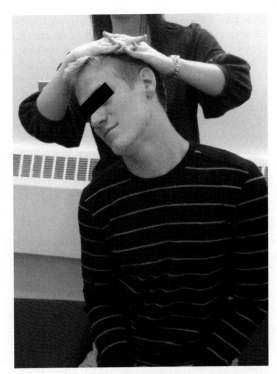

Figure 9-7 Spurling test.

then applied, which further compresses the posterolateral disk, facet joint, and foraminal space on the side of motion. This test does not always isolate a particular cervical level or structure, but if scapular or upper extremity pain is generated, cervical involvement is strongly suggested (Fig. 9-7).

Compression and Distraction Test

Compression and traction with the head in a neutral position also assist in determining cervical involvement. Compression is applied by an axial load through the head and neck, which then compresses the disk, nerve root, or facet. Distraction is performed to increase foraminal opening and remove cranial weight, thereby arresting compression. Distraction can relieve peripheral nerve or dura mater mechanical pressure at the disk level. By expanding the foraminal space, pain due to nerve root compression can be alleviated. Distraction is reported to have sensitivity, specificity, and a positive likelihood ratio of 44%, 90%, and 4.40, respectively.[34] A positive compression or distraction test indicates cervical pathology related to radiculopathy or mechanical compression.

Further cervical examination is indicated if there is positive cervical test findings. These techniques are not described in this text, but a myriad of literature exists regarding indepth discussion of cervical examination and related pathologies.

Contractile Versus Noncontractile Tissue

The tissues surrounding the glenohumeral joint are described as either contractile or noncontractile tissue.[27] Before discussing physical examination, further distinction between contractile and noncontractile tissue needs to be reviewed.

Contractile tissue includes muscle belly, tendon, and tendon insertion to bone (tenoperiosteal junction).

Noncontractile tissue includes the capsule, ligaments, subchondral bone, labrum, bursa, and nerves.[27] In general, these two groups are evaluatively distinguished by employing static resisted contractions, referred to as *resisted motions*, and by assessing PROM. A lesion within the contractile chain promotes pain when force is translated by muscle activity from muscle, tendon, then to bone. Noncontractile tissue can be grossly assessed by PROM. If passive motion is limited, a correlation is drawn between the motion (i.e., external rotation or abduction), tissue stretched during the motion, pain, and end feel. The clinician also must consider that passive motion can elicit a painful response from a contractile lesion when stretched opposite to its action, for example, supraspinatus elongation during functional internal rotation (reaching up the back).

When a double lesion exists, one affecting a contractile element and the other affecting a noncontractile element, confusion can arise. A common example of this is primary instability and secondary supraspinatus tendinitis.

A third mechanism of eliciting pain from either contractile or noncontractile tissue is compression. For instance, the supraspinatus tendon and bursa are both compressed or impinged when forcing the humerus into elevation and stabilizing the scapula. This is the position for the "impingement sign." Full external rotation at 90 degrees of abduction or full arm elevation also can result in contractile and noncontractile tissue compression. In both positions, the supraspinatus tendon can impinge against the glenoid rim.[6,35,36]

Active Range of Motion

AROM, although nonspecific with respect to distinguishing contractile and noncontractile tissue, does yield valuable information. AROM provides degrees of motion assessment and the ability to complete a fair grade, giving the clinician information regarding irritability status, symptom location, painful arc presence, and appropriate scapulohumeral rhythm.

AROM is estimated or measured in all cardinal planes and then is compared with the uninvolved side. Elevation, whether flexion, abduction, or scapular plane abduction, is performed to assess ROM and the ability to complete the motion against gravity. External rotation at 90 degrees of abduction and neutral can be assessed quickly in the standing position, as can functional internal rotation (glenohumeral internal rotation, extension, and adduction). Frequently, pain, weakness, or structural restriction produces dysfunctional motion compared with the uninvolved side. Pain and speed of motion help define tissue irritability.

Location of pain may provide further insight about pathology. The glenohumeral joint and its associated soft tissues usually refer pain laterally over the deltoid, but pain also can be focused more posteriorly or anteriorly. Discomfort associated with biceps tendinitis is commonly felt anteriorly over the groove. The AC joint and sternoclavicular joint are implicated when discomfort exists over either joint. Frequently, concomitant pathology of the rotator cuff, biceps tendon, and AC joint exists, although the superseding area of pain commonly correlates with the rotator cuff. Active trigger points can further confuse the issue because of characteristic referred pain zones.

Although the Academy of Orthopaedic Surgeons[37] no longer distinguishes flexion from abduction, preferring instead to use the term *elevation*, further information is provided by evaluating elevation in multiple planes. Pain may be present in flexion but not abduction, or vice versa. The correlation between pathology and planar motion cannot be drawn. However, further insight into the mechanical nature of the subacromial space components and the capsuloligamentous complex (CLC) is elucidated. Mechanical properties can be examined further by changing physiologic motion, for example, by combining flexion while maintaining external rotation, as opposed to allowing the obligatory internal rotation. At times, a patient experiences pain with normal flexion yet is pain-free when external rotation is attempted and elevation is performed in the sagittal plane. During the modified flexion movement, the greater tuberosity and adjoining rotator cuff avoid their journey, and imminent compression, beneath the anterior acromion and coracoacromial ligament. Functional internal rotation is a simple active task that demonstrates the patient's ability to perform glenohumeral internal rotation, extension, and adduction in conjunction with elbow flexion and pronation. A clinician should be aware that the supraspinatus and infraspinatus are elongated during this activity and can result in a painful stretch if a tendinous lesion exists. Functional internal rotation as well as coronal plane abduction are almost always limited in a patient presenting with a frozen shoulder.

Painful Arc

The painful arc has been described during active elevation. The classic painful arc occurs between 60 and 120 degrees, correlating to the rotator cuff/bursal complex traveling beneath the coracoacromial arch (Fig. 9-8).[38] If the rotator cuff/bursal complex is inflamed or if abnormal superior migration occurs during elevation, the tissue is painfully compressed. After approximately 120 degrees of elevation, the rotator cuff/bursal tissue clears the coracoacromial arc, thereby relieving symptoms. The painful arc has high specificity (>80.5) in patients with all grades of subacromial impingement syndrome (SIS) related to rotator cuff tear.[39,40]

Variations of the painful arc have been described in which pain occurs at the end of motion. Both AC joint pathology and the rotator cuff/bursa can produce end-range pain.[6,38] Recently, Pappas and colleagues[6] revealed that end-range elevation causes compression of the supraspinatus against the superior glenoid rim. Often, a painful arc occurs only when descending the arm from shoulder elevation. This may occur because of the eccentric contraction of the rotator cuff or the increased load across the intratendinous structures. A second explanation is based on reduced contribution of the scapular lateral rotators, particularly of the serratus anterior. Many individuals demonstrate early release of scapular lateral rotation or "dumping," when returning from elevation, which causes the coracoacromial arch to "clamp down" on subacromial structures (Fig. 9-9). This scapular dumping has also been appreciated in many individuals who have no shoulder symptoms. The authors have observed that individuals who have performed years of push-ups or bench pressing tend to show a greater tendency to have scapular dumping when descending from the elevated position. If the patient is told to reach forward and slightly up while

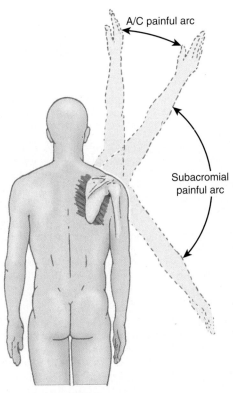

Figure 9-8 *Painful arcs arising due to subacromial and acromioclavicular pathology. (From Kessel L, Watson M. The painful arc syndrome. Clinical classification as a guide to management.* J Bone Joint Surg *1977;59B: 166–172.)*

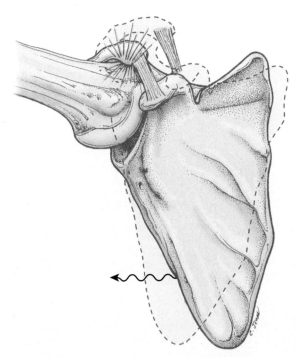

Figure 9-9 *Subacromial tissue compression caused by weak or dysfunctional scapular rotators. (From Kelley MJ. Evaluation of the shoulder. In: Kelley MJ, Clark WA, eds.* Orthopedic Therapy of the Shoulder. *© 1995 J.B. Lippincott Company.)*

lowering, thereby activating the serratus anterior, the painful arc may disappear due to improved scapular lateral rotation.

Scapulohumeral Rhythm

Scapulohumeral rhythm is the coordinated and synchronous movement of the shoulder's osseous structures driven by the muscular and ligament systems. Literature has been published on normal subjects and symptomatic individuals in attempts to quantify the movement.[41-46] McClure and associates[42] described three main scapular movements during elevation: posterior tilting, upward (lateral rotation), and external rotation. However, controversy still remains regarding the scapulohumeral ratio. Abnormal scapulohumeral rhythm has been noted in patients with anterior glenohumeral joint instability and rotator cuff tendonopathy.[41,47-49]

Abnormal scapulohumeral rhythm or scapular dyskinesis is an alteration in the normal position or motion of the scapula during coupled scapulohumeral movements.[50] Measuring scapulohumeral rhythm in the clinic has proven difficult because the equipment used to attain these measurements is not clinically applicable. The clinician is left with visual inspection and linear measurements that have low reliability.[51] Kibler[52] advocates the lateral slide test to objectively determine abnormal scapular asymmetry in different degrees of elevation. Obvious dyskinesis is easier to detect, whereas subtle variations may not be noticed. In either case the clinician is left with the task of identifying the cause of the dyskinesis and intervention. Further discussion regarding the etiology of scapular dyskinesis can be found under

the section Scapular Muscle Strength Testing and Special Tests.

Strength Testing

Strength testing can be performed manually or by a device such as a dynamometer. Manual strength assessment or manual muscle testing (MMT) has been found to be subjective and have questionable reliability and validity.[53,54] However, MMT remains the most common form of strength assessment used in the clinic. In its purest form MMT requires the patient to be specifically positioned and move against gravity. Using antigravity test positions in the orthopedic population can be provocative and painful, and therefore impractical to use. For example, it is unwise and yields invalid information to evaluate external rotation strength in the prone position of 90 degrees of abduction and full external rotation in an individual 2 weeks after anterior dislocation. This position could cause an instability event or apprehension resulting in reflex inhibition of the external rotators. Although a full description of MMT positions is not presented, Table 9-3 lists the shoulder muscles and gives a brief description of testing technique.

The more practical way to assess strength of the glenohumeral muscles is sitting or standing with the arm at the side or in slight abduction and with the elbow bent to 90 degrees. Testing the rotators and elevators in varying degrees of elevation and rotation may be beneficial. Recognizing position-based weakness is extremely valuable so treatment can be position-focused.

The strength assessment should combine an upper quarter screen (evaluating each myotome including the elbow, wrist,

Table 9-3 Manual Muscle Testing

Muscle	Nerve Supply	Root Level	Technique
Trapezius Upper	Spinal accessory n.	CN XI, C3–C4	Patient upright; place into cervical extension, ipsilateral SB, and contralateral rotation. Patient elevates scapula while resistance is over distal acromion into depression and at posterior cranium into flexion and contralateral SB.
Middle	Same		Patient prone; set scapula; arm is brought into 90 degrees; patient lifts into glenohumeral horizontal abduction and ER, scapular adduction without elevation. Resistance is over the distal scapular spine into scapular abduction.
Lower	Same		Patient prone; set scapula; arm is brought into 135 degrees of glenohumeral elevation and ER. Patient lifts into scapular depression and lateral rotation. Resistance is over the distal scapular spine into scapular elevation and abduction.
Sternocleidomastoid	Spinal accessory n.	CN XI, C3–C4	Patient supine; patient lifts head into cervical flexion and contralateral rotation. Resistance is over forehead.
Serratus anterior	Long thoracic n.	Pretrunk, C5, C6, C7	Patient supine; patient arm at 90 degrees of flexion with elbow flexed. Patient pushes arm anteriorly. Resistance is over the olecranon pushing posteriorly.
Rhomboids/levator scapulae	Dorsal scapular n.	C4–C5	Patient prone; set scapula; patient adducts, elevates, and medially rotates the scapula. Resistance is over the distal scapular spine into abduction and depression.
Pectoralis minor	Medial pectoral n.	Medial cord, C8–T1	Patient supine; patient lifts shoulder girdle forward (protract clavicle). Resistance is over the anterior humerus into retraction.
Pectoralis major Sternal	Medial and lateral pectoral n.	Lateral and medial cord, C5–T1	Patient supine; arm is brought into 135 degrees of coronal abduction; patient lifts arm into extension and horizontal adduction. Resistance is over the distal humerus opposite the above.
Clavicular	Lateral pectoral n.	Lateral cord, C5–C7	Patient supine; arm is brought into 60 degrees of coronal abduction; patient lifts arm into flexion and horizontal adduction. Resistance is over the distal humerus opposite the above.
Latissimus dorsi	Thoracodorsal n.	Posterior cord, C5–C8	Patient prone; patient lifts arm from neutral into extension and adduction. Resistance is over the distal humerus opposite the above.
Teres major	Lower subscapular n.	Posterior cord, C5–C6	Patient prone; patient lifts arm from neutral into extension, adduction and IR. Resistance is over the distal humerus opposite the above.
Deltoid Anterior	Axillary n.	Posterior cord, C5–C6	Patient upright; patient lifts arm into elevation 30 degrees posterior to the sagittal plane and some ER. Resistance is over the distal humerus into adduction and extension.
Middle	Same		Patient upright; patient lifts arm into coronal plane abduction and neutral rotation. Resistance is over the distal humerus into adduction.
Posterior	Same		Patient prone; arm is brought into 90 degrees of coronal plane abduction; patient lifts into horizontal abduction in neutral rotation. Resistance is over the distal humerus into horizontal adduction.
Supraspinatus	Suprascapular	Upper trunk, C5–C6	Patient upright; patient lifts arm into scapular plane abduction in IR. Resistance is over the distal humerus into adduction.
Infraspinatus	Suprascapular	Upper trunk, C5–C6	Patient prone; arm is brought into 90 degrees of abduction with forearm off the table edge; patient lifts into ER. Resistance is over distal forearm into IR.
Subscapularis	Upper and lower subscapular n.	Posterior cord, C5–C8	Patient as above; patient lifts into IR. Resistance is over the distal forearm into ER.
Teres minor	Axillary n.	Posterior cord, C5–C6	Same as for infraspinatus.
Coracobrachialis	Musculocutaneous n.	C4, C5, C6, C7	Patient upright; patient flexes and horizontally adducts the arm. Resistance is over the distal humerus opposite the above.
Biceps brachii	Musculocutaneous n.	C4, C5, C6, C7	Patient upright; patient supinates and flexes elbow. Resistance is over the distal forearm into extension.
Triceps	Radial n.	C5, C6, C7, C8	Patient prone; arm is brought into 90 degrees of abduction with forearm over the table edge; patient extends the elbow. Resistance is over the distal forearm into flexion.

CN, cranial nerve; ER, external rotation; IR, internal rotation; n., nerve; SB, side bend. (From Kelley MJ: Evaluation of the shoulder. In: Kelley MJ, Clark WA, eds. *Orthopedic Therapy of the Shoulder.* © 1995, Philadelphia: J.B. Lippincott Company.)

and hand), as the examiner considers the contractile tissue being "isolated" by resistance. A break test is performed by having the patient perform an isometric contraction as directed by the examiner. The examiner gradually increases the force, attempting to provoke symptoms or overcome the patient's resistance, thereby assessing strength. Additionally, the scapula should be observed to determine how well it is being stabilized on the thoracic wall. If scapular destabilization occurs, then further scapular muscle examination is required. Resisted abduction, external rotation, internal rotation, flexion, extension, adduction, elbow flexion, and elbow extension are performed in addition to completing the upper quarter screen by testing wrist extension, wrist flexion, and finger adduction.

If neurologic involvement is suggested, the primary muscles (or tendons) should be palpated to determine their activity. Neurologic involvement following multiple shoulder trauma, contusions, or surgery often can be missed if specific muscle palpation is not performed; this is particularly true of the deltoid. Full active elevation may be possible in the presence of a partial or even full deltoid palsy because the rotator cuff and scapulothoracic muscles are capable of achieving functional arm elevation. In this case, injury to the deltoid may not be considered if it is not properly palpated. Simple palpation of the deltoid while asking the patient to lift the arm slightly from an elevated position of 45 degrees can determine neurologic intactness.

Quantitative Strength Testing

Various forms of quantitative devices are currently used to measure muscle strength and endurance. These include hand-held dynamometers (HHDs), tension dynamometers, isokinetic dynamometers, spring-loaded devices, and free weights. Each device offers advantages and disadvantages. For instance, the isokinetic dynamometer can provide valuable dynamic and isometric data yet is very expensive and requires an involved setup. Compare this with a hand-held dynamometer, which is relatively inexpensive, easy to use, and reliable, yet only yields isometric data. Whether MMT, HHD, isotonics, or isokinetics are utilized, all testing methods must be standardized in such a fashion as to maximize reliability, validity, and safety. The examiner must determine what information is desired from quantitative testing. If a strength value is all that is needed, then using a HHD may be all that is required. Leggin[55] described a reliable assessment for shoulder muscle strength using a HHD. Research has shown quantified isometric activity to correlate well with isokinetic values.[56] When requiring muscle performance throughout a ROM in a specific position, an isokinetic device is indicated. Muscle performance guidelines have been suggested in the literature and are summarized by Sapega and Kelley.[57] When assessing healthy individuals, a less than 10% interextremity difference is normal, a 10% to 20% difference may be abnormal (consider normal values of 15% greater strength in unilateral sport-specific muscles), and a greater than 20% difference is abnormal. If the individual has been injured or is postoperative, a bilateral comparison where a 10% to 20% difference is found may be abnormal and greater than 20% is abnormal. It is generally accepted that an athlete or laborer who achieves 80% to 90% return in muscle performance may be ready to return to functional activity,

however, the performance and tolerance for the sport-specific activity is the ultimate test.

Resisted Motions

As stated earlier, strength assessment should be considered part of the upper quarter examination and achieve several goals: (1) Assess strength of the primary muscle(s). (2) Determine central or peripheral neurologic involvement. (3) Identify the musculotendinous structure causing pain or weakness. (4) Assist in determining the tissue irritability level. The term *resisted motions* is somewhat confusing because an isometric contraction is performed. Cyriax[27] believed that resisted motions helped to identify the symptomatic contractile structures (muscle, tendon, and tenoperiosteal junction) by assessing weakness and pain. If a lesion exists within a muscle's contractile chain, pain is caused when resistance is applied in a specific direction that isolates that particular muscle's action. True contractile element isolation is usually ensured by negating any joint motion. There are exceptions to this rule, such as resisted internal rotation causing pain in the presence of glenohumeral joint osteroarthritis.

Cyriax[27] emphasized placing the joint near or at midrange when performing resisted motions. Whenever possible, resistance should be applied over the distal bone to isolate muscle function at a single joint. The exception to this rule is rotation that requires resistance at the distal forearm, thus crossing the elbow. Resisted motions can be performed at various arcs of motion so that the mechanical nature of the involved tissue is clearly illustrated. For example, resisted abduction may be moderately painful when performed with the arm at the side, slightly painful when performed at 45 degrees of abduction, and significantly painful when performed at 90 degrees of abduction. The explanation for this scenario is that in the presence of a supraspinatus tendon lesion, the adducted position places a significant degree of tension on the tendon that is further magnified by muscle contraction. At 45 degrees, the tendon is slackened, resulting in less passive tendon tension and pain even though forces are transmitted through the tendon. At 90 degrees, the resisted motion, combined with possible impingement of the tendon against the coracoacromial arch, results in increased discomfort.

Weakness or Pain

The presence or absence of pain or weakness is of great importance when assessing resisted motions. Five general presentations can occur: strong and painless, strong and painful, weak and painful, weak and painless, and all painful.[27]

If a particular resisted motion elicits no pain even when strong resistance is produced, there is no abnormality of the muscle complex responsible for that motion. Either repetitive resisted motions or an examination after a known aggravating activity may be required for symptom provocation in certain individuals, particularly athletes or those patients with mild reactivity.

A strong and painful presentation upon a resisted motion typically indicates a lesion within a specific muscle, tendon, or tenoperiosteal region. Definition of a lesion can range from simple tendinitis to minimal macro fraying of the tendon, to a partial- or even small full-thickness tear. The problematic musculotendinous unit is identified by being most painful when tested in its primary direction of action. The degree of irritability usually correlates well with associated pain.

A weak and painful response is commonly seen in cases of moderate to high tissue irritability or with a reactive or significant tear of the musculotendinous unit. Weakness and pain demonstrated on resisted abduction or external rotation can occur in patients with painful tendonopathy or large rotator cuff tears. Other pathologies that present in this manner are tubercle fractures or neoplasms. Certainly, following any acute trauma, such as a dislocation, a weak and painful response to resisted motions may be encountered.

If more than one resisted motion is painful or weak, it becomes difficult to determine the primary structure at fault. Lesions involving shoulder musculature other than the rotator cuff are somewhat easier to identify because muscle-specific localized pain is produced during resistance of the muscle's primary motion. For example, pain associated with a pectoralis major tendon tear is felt along the distal portion of the muscle. It is more confusing to sort out which portion of the rotator cuff harbors a lesion since the four tendons create a confluent dynamic envelope about the glenohumeral joint (Fig. 9-10, online). A lesion in the anterior supraspinatus may be influenced by resisted internal rotation because some of the subscapularis fibers are connected to the supraspinatus.[58] Likewise, pain may also occur with resisted external rotation since the infraspinatus fibers are interlaced with the supraspinatus.[9,58]

If the patient presents with no pain but has weakness, a massive or chronic large rotator cuff tear may be present. Whenever painless weakness is encountered, neurologic involvement must be investigated to determine whether the lesion is located at the cord, cervical root, plexus, or peripheral nerve level; a thorough evaluation by manual muscle, sensation, and reflex testing is essential.

When all resisted motions are painful, an acute inflammatory condition probably exists, as in acute calcific bursitis or tendinitis, progressive glenohumeral joint degeneration, or rotator cuff arthropathy. If all clinical and diagnostic tests are negative, a psychogenic disorder or malingering should be considered.

Resisted Abduction

Resisted abduction isolates the deltoid and supraspinatus musculotendinous units. The deltoid can be a source of pain in the patient having a minideltoid split or open rotator cuff repair. Occasionally, poor-quality tissue or premature return to activity results in deltoid tearing. Primary or secondary deltoid trigger points can cause pain.

Pain on resisted abduction is usually caused by a supraspinatus tendon lesion. Differentiating between tendinitis, partial-thickness cuff tear, and a small full-thickness cuff tear is very difficult. The degree of pain may depend on the tissue irritability; weakness may or may not be present. A significantly reactive tendinitis may be more painful than a mildly reactive partial- or full-thickness supraspinatus tear. Many individuals have partial-thickness, small full-thickness, and even massive tears and function quite well without significant symptoms.[59] Abduction weakness is often the result of a full-thickness rotator cuff tear.[27,39,40] Other causes are a C5

nerve root compression, upper plexus lesion, suprascapular nerve palsy, or axillary nerve palsy.

To assess abduction, resistance is applied at the distal humerus at 0, 45, and 90 degrees of coronal plane or plane of the scapula (POS) elevation. The effect of position on pain is examined to help determine reactivity and mechanical effect on soft tissue (Fig. 9-11, online).

Resisted Flexion

Although the supraspinatus is thought to be a primary abductor, 50% of flexion torque output is attributed to the supraspinatus and infraspinatus.[60] Therefore, it is not surprising that a supraspinatus tendon lesion often causes pain during resisted flexion. Although the biceps is not considered a primary flexor, pain is occasionally provoked during resisted shoulder flexion testing. Location of pain over the biceps groove helps identify the biceps as the culprit. The clavicular fibers of the pectoralis major and anterior deltoid are also humeral flexors. Shoulder flexion weakness is often related to a full-thickness rotator cuff tear or axillary nerve palsy. A palsy of the anterior branch of the axillary nerve can occur, possibly due to extended surgical retraction of the deltoid when a deltopectoral incision is required. This is seen after glenohumeral joint arthroplasty of open reduction internal fixation following a proximal humeral fracture.

Resistance is applied at the distal humerus to isolate the glenohumeral joint and associated shoulder flexor muscles. The test can be performed in the sagittal plane at 0, 45, and 90 degrees.

Resisted External Rotation

The infraspinatus, supraspinatus, teres minor, and posterior deltoid all contribute to external rotation, but 80% of this force is attributed to the posterior cuff.[61] The most common reason for pain or weakness during resisted external rotation is a supraspinatus lesion.[27,39,40] Isolated infraspinatus tendonopathy can infrequently occur, causing pain or weakness, but more often profound weakness is the result of complete tearing of the supraspinatus and infraspinatus.[62] The infraspinatus may house primary active trigger points that are painful during resisted external rotation and palpation. Commonly, an infraspinatus trigger point refers pain to the anterior shoulder.[15] Other causes are a C6 nerve root compression, upper plexus lesion, or suprascapular nerve palsy.

It is essential to isolate external rotation during the resisted external rotation test. Resistance should be placed at the distal forearm, not the hand. As the patient attempts to externally rotate, the clinician should stabilize the distal arm, but not to the point of encouraging abduction. Some patients attempt to substitute by either abducting the shoulder or extending or flexing the elbow. This substitution allows the external rotators to appear stronger. If elbow flexion or extension substitution is detected, the dorsal aspect of the examiner's second and third middle phalanx is placed against the dorsal wrist. If the patient is employing elbow substitution, the wrist slips off the examiner's fingers (Fig. 9-12, online).

The examiner should assess the effect of scapular stabilization during resisted motion testing. For example, if the patient experiences pain when resisting external rotation, the clinician should have the patient slightly retract (stabilize with trapezius and rhomboid muscles) then retest. If pain vanishes or is significantly reduced, further examination of the scapular muscles should be made. In addition, this finding indicates that scapular muscle integration should be used during rotator cuff strengthening exercises. Tate and coworkers[63] reported increased strength in patients with impingement by stabilizing the scapula using the scapular repositioning test.

Resisted Internal Rotation

The internal rotators are the subscapularis, pectoralis major, teres major, and latissimus dorsi muscles. Pain with resisted internal rotation may indicate subscapularis involvement. Isolated tearing of the subscapularis has been reported to occur during anterior dislocation events or when the arm is forcefully externally rotated in adduction.[64-66] Significant internal rotation weakness noted after an open anterior capsular reconstruction procedure (Bankart's or capsular shift) in which the subscapularis was incised and repaired is a prognosticator for possible subscapularis rupture. Significant weakness has been reported following shoulder arthroplasty and may be associated with rupture or subscapularis tendon alterations.[67] Further examination is required by performing the lift-off test, internal rotation lag sign, and belly press test. Another indicator of subscapularis rupture is increased passive external rotation with the arm in adduction.[64,65] If the subscapularis has ruptured, it should immediately be brought to the referring physician's attention.

Trigger points also can cause pain with resisted internal rotation.[15] A supraspinatus tear extending to the rotator cuff interval (RCI) also may elicit pain with resisted internal rotation due to the pull of the subscapularis on the associated torn fibers.[66,68]

Pain and weakness have been reported during isolated internal rotation in patients with frozen shoulder.[69-71] The subscapularis tendon is intimate with the anterior capsule since it serves as an attachment region (Fig. 9-13).[68] Tension may translate from the subscapularis to the inflamed capsu-

loligamentous complex, producing pain. Resisted internal rotation may also be painful in patients with biceps tendinitis since the subscapularis tendon fortifies the medial wall of the biceps groove and is anatomically intimate with the biceps synovial lining. The relationship of the long head of the biceps and subscapularis can be fully appreciated by the frequent incidence of biceps tendon dislocation/subluxation noted when the subscapularis tendon has ruptured.[64-66,72]

Assessment of the internal rotators is performed at neutral, elbow bent to 90 degrees, and with resistance applied over the distal wrist. Strain or tearing of the latissimus dorsi, pectoralis major, and teres major can occur, but because these muscles are multiaction, prestretching them or altering shoulder position to accentuate their activity magnifies tension on the involved fibers and assists in identifying the source of pain.

Resisted Extension

The shoulder extensors are the posterior deltoid, teres major, latissimus dorsi, and long head of the triceps. Typically, resistance to shoulder extension performed at neutral is painless, even in the presence of significant shoulder pathology. Therefore, information to help identify the source of pain is minimal, although weakness should be appreciated if present. Whenever significant weakness of shoulder extension is noted, an axillary nerve palsy should be considered.

Resistance is applied over the distal arm with the arm at the side or in shoulder extension.

Resisted Elbow Flexion

Elbow flexion isolates the biceps, brachialis, and brachioradialis; however, only the biceps long and short heads extend to the scapula.

Pain may occur with resisted elbow flexion in the presence of long head of the biceps tendinitis. We have found this to be an unreliable test position in reproducing pain, even in moderately reactive biceps tendon inflammation. Provoking biceps tendon pain sometimes can be accomplished if resistance is applied when the shoulder and elbow are placed in extension in addition to forearm pronation, thereby increasing passive and active tension through the inflamed tendon. Combining humeral external rotation with elbow and shoulder extension further stretches the long head tendon and compresses it against the lesser tuberosity.

Resistance is applied to the distal wrist with the arm adducted, forearm supinated, and elbow flexed to 90 degrees.

Resisted Elbow Extension

The elbow extensors are the triceps. If pathology exists, commonly of the long head insertion into the infraglenoid rim, pain may be experienced with this test. Tendinitis of the triceps long head can occur in throwing, spiking, or racquet sport athletes. As with elbow flexion, different positions of elevation should be explored to place more tension across the long head and provoke symptoms.

Resistance is applied to the distal wrist with the arm adducted, forearm neutral, and elbow flexed to 90 degrees.

The wrist and finger extensors and flexors as well as the intrinsics of the hand should be evaluated by resisted motions to determine distal muscle weakness either from neurologic

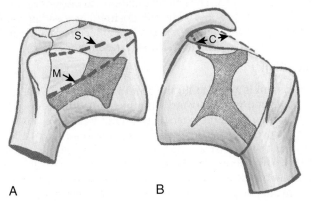

Figure 9-13 Zones of rotator cuff adherence to the capsuloligamentous complex. Regions of tendinous attachment are shaded lightly. Areas of muscle fiber attachment are shaded darker. **A,** Anterior view. **B,** Posterior view. C, margins of the coracohumeral ligament; M, axes of middle glenohumeral ligament; S, axes of superior glenohumeral ligament. (From Clark JC, Sidles JR, Matzen FA III: The relationship of the glenohumeral joint capsule to the rotator cuff. *Clin Orthop* 1990;254:29–34).

A   B

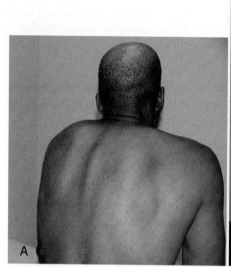
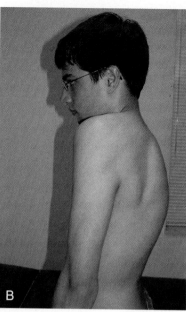

Figure 9-14 Serratus anterior isolation test. **A,** Positive. **B,** Negative.

or intrinsic musculotendinous involvement, thereby completing the upper-quarter screen.

Scapular Muscle Strength Testing and Special Tests

An alteration in the normal position or motion of the scapula during coupled scapulohumeral movements is called scapular dyskinesis.[50] Scapular dyskinesis can be caused by multiple reasons.[73] Scapular winging may be considered a type of scapular dyskinesis characterized by significant scapular medial border displacement during shoulder motion. Kelley[74] and Leggin and Kelley[75] described special tests and muscle testing used in an evaluative scapular muscle algorithm. We describe examination tests to assist in determining if the cause of scapular dyskinesis is from a nerve palsy, glenohumeral instability, or poor motor control.

The patient is first observed in standing for resting winging or scapular displacement and obvious atrophy. If resting winging is noted, the patient is checked for a scoliosis demonstrated by a thoracic rib hump during trunk flexion. Resting medial winging can be caused by an increased thoracic rib angle since the flat scapula's medial border is displaced. AROM of both shoulders is assessed in the standing position by elevating in the sagittal and coronal planes. Significant scapular winging that normalizes beyond 90 degrees during sagittal plane flexion elevation is typically related to poor motor control of the serratus anterior. If medial winging persists beyond 90 degrees, a long thoracic nerve palsy or posterior glenohumeral instability is suggested. Often, normal scapular motion occurs while elevating, but dyskinesis is seen on descent of the arm (usually below 90 degrees). As mentioned earlier, "eccentric dumping" is a common finding among many individuals, especially those who performed years of bench pressing or push-ups.

Eccentric dumping is a common finding and may or may not be related to shoulder pathology.

Long Thoracic Nerve Palsy

Serratus Anterior Isolation Test

This test activates the serratus anterior without glenohumeral motion. The patient places the arms at the side and in external rotation. The patient actively protracts and slightly elevates the scapula (Fig. 9-14). A positive test is the inability to fully protract equal to the uninvolved side. The examiner can apply resistance by placing a hand on the patient's back medial to the scapula and the other over the coracoid process and anterior shoulder. The examiner attempts to push the scapula posteriorly. A positive test is the ability to significantly displace the scapula posteriorly. The patient's inability to move the scapula into a protracted and elevated position or easy posterior scapular displacement upon the examiner's resistance indicates neural involvement to the serratus anterior.

Plus Sign

The patient is asked to lift the arm to 90 degrees in the sagittal plane and reach forward without rotating the body while maintaining humeral external rotation. A positive plus sign is indicated when medial winging increases (Fig. 9-15). A positive test almost always indicates a long thoracic nerve (LTN) palsy; however, the possibility of posterior glenohumeral subluxation must be considered. Setting the scapula into protraction and elevation before shoulder elevation can eliminate the posterior instability and winging if related to instability.

Resisted Functional Flexion Test

The patient is asked to place the arm at approximately 135 degrees of sagittal plane flexion. The examiner resists

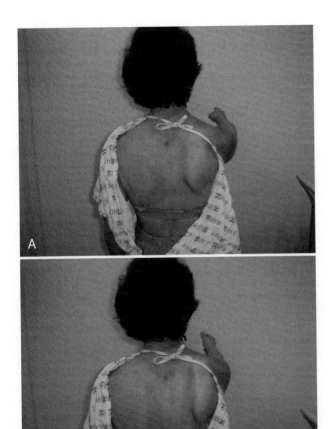

Figure 9-15 Plus sign. **A,** The patient demonstrates medial scapular winging with shoulder flexion. **B,** The plus sign is positive since the winging increases as she attempts to reach forward. (From Leggin B, Kelley MJ. Disease-specific methods of rehabilitation. In: Iannotti JP, Williams GR, eds. *Disorders of the Shoulder: Diagnosis and Management.* Philadelphia: Lippincott Williams & Wilkins, 2005.)

shoulder flexion while palpating the inferior scapular angle. The patient should be able to maintain the inferior angle fixed on the thoracic wall during resistance.[29] Significant inferior angle or medial border displacement with minimal forces indicates an LTN palsy. If part of the serratus anterior has been reinnervated, less displacement occurs. Performing a plus maneuver before resisting flexion inhibits lower trapezius substitution.

Posterior Instability

Scapular medial winging has been associated with posterior instability resulting from abnormal shoulder girdle muscle activation.[76,77] In some patients it appears that immediate posterior subluxation on elevation may inhibit serratus activation. To help determine if posterior instability is the cause, the external rotation stabilizing maneuver (ERSM) can be performed along with a full instability examination. Stability gained by ERSM is thought to result because humeral external rotation tightens up the RCI and activates the posterior cuff, both of which improve posterior stability.[78] Additionally, elevating the arm in external rotation has been found to maximally recruit the serratus anterior.[79]

External Rotation Stabilizing Maneuver

If scapular winging occurs during sagittal plane elevation, the patient is asked to repeat elevation with the arm maintained in humeral external rotation. The verbal cue is "turn your palm up." Elimination of scapular winging helps to confirm posterior instability. At times the patient may need to initially protract and slightly elevate the scapula before elevating the arm.

Poor Motor Control

Poor serratus anterior motor control can result in subtle dyskinesis and occasionally dramatic medial scapular winging on arm elevation. To determine if serratus anterior motor control is the cause of dyskinesis, the serratus anterior isolation position can be used. The patient is asked to protract and slightly elevate the scapula followed by arm elevation in the sagittal plane. If scapular dyskinesis or symptoms are eliminated, poor serratus anterior control is suggested.

An LTN palsy or posterior instability is ruled out in patients demonstrating significant medial winging if the following are present: (1) negative serratus anterior isolation test, (2) negative plus sign (scapula moves forward on thoracic wall), (3) full resistance is applied with no or minimal displacement of the inferior angle during the resisted functional flexion test. Commonly, this type of patient has bilateral winging and appears to voluntarily activate the pectoralis minor, thereby inhibiting the serratus anterior.

Spinal Accessory Nerve Palsy

Associated signs and symptoms of spinal accessory nerve palsy (SANP) affecting the trapezius have been reported.[80-82] Kelley and colleagues[80,82] also described the scapular flip sign as a simple test to determine the presence of a SANP. In a case series ($n = 20$) all patients having a positive scapular flip sign were unable to elevate beyond 90 degrees in the coronal plane, and had 0/5 muscle grade of the middle and lower trapezius.

Scapular Flip Sign

The scapular flip sign is evaluated by resisting the shoulder external rotators (Fig. 9-16). The patient's arm is placed at the side in neutral rotation. The examiner stands at the patient's side so that the scapula can be observed. The patient is asked to push their wrist into the examiner's hand (external rotation).[82] A positive scapular flip sign occurs when the medial border of the scapula lifts (flips) from the thoracic wall. This occurs because the middle and lower trapezius normal tethering effect is lost secondary to an SANP.

Middle Trapezius Testing

The patient is placed prone, and the examiner manually lifts the scapula into anatomic position. The patient's arm is placed at 90 degrees full horizontal abduction and external rotation. The patient is instructed to hold the arm in this position with the thumb up. The middle trapezius fibers should be palpated. Resistance is given at the posterior angle of the scapula or at the wrist. The examiner attempts to push the scapula into abduction or the arm to the ground.[29] Substitution by the rhomboid is seen in Figure 9-17.

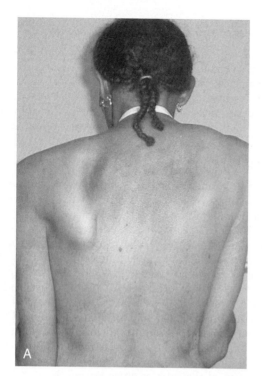

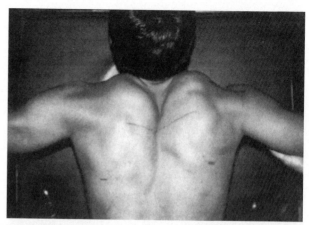

Figure 9-17 Manual muscle testing position for the middle trapezius in a patient with right spinal accessory nerve palsy. Note the correct adducted position of the left scapula. The right scapula is elevated and adducted by substitution of the rhomboids and levator scapulae. (Reprinted, with permission, from Kelley MJ. Evaluation of the shoulder. In: Kelley MJ, Clark WA, eds. *Orthopedic Therapy of the Shoulder.* © 1995 J.B. Lippincott Company.)

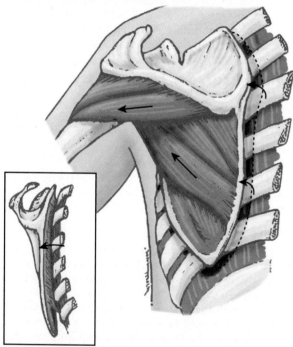

Figure 9-16 A, A positive scapular flip sign occurs when the medial scapular border "flips" off the thoracic wall when glenohumeral external rotation is resisted. **B,** Schematic demonstrating the unopposed pull of the external rotators causing the scapular flip sign. (From Kelley MJ, Kane TE, Leggin BG. Spinal accessory nerve palsy associated signs and symptoms. *J Orthop Sports Phys Ther.* 2008;38(2):78–86.)

Lower Trapezius Testing

The patient is placed prone, and the examiner manually lifts the scapula into anatomic position. The examiner places the arm in approximately 135 degrees of elevation. The patient is instructed to hold the arm with the thumb up. The lower trapezius fibers are palpated. Resistance is given at the posterior angle of the scapula or at the wrist. The examiner attempts to push the scapula into abduction and elevation or the arm to the ground.[29]

Summary

Resisted motions are of critical value when differentiating contractile from noncontractile tissue and identifying the involved musculotendinous unit. Completion of the upper-quarter screen by strength testing below the elbow is essential to correlate or confirm neurologic involvement.

The examiner must be consistent in positioning, hand placement, and direction of force application yet must explore various positions out of the neutral to gain additional information about the mechanical nature of the soft tissue, osseous structures, and their mutual relationship.

Scapular dyskinesis can result from a palsy, poor motor function, or primary instability. Performing a scapular algorithmic examination can help determine the cause of the dyskinesis.

Passive Range of Motion

Assessment of PROM, as opposed to resisted motion, primarily determines the status of noncontractile tissue, particularly the CLC. Lesions or adhesions of the CLC typically lead to restrictions in all planes, although limitations may predominate in one or several planes. Cyriax[27] describes two patterns of general restriction characteristics of all synovial joints: capsular and noncapsular.

The capsular pattern of the shoulder is described as having the greatest restriction in external rotation, followed by abduction and the least in internal rotation. Although the capsular pattern is considered a characteristic of adhesive capsulitis or primary frozen shoulder it has not been consistently found when objectively measured.[83] The noncapsular pattern exists if the proportional limitations differ from the

Table 9-4 Goniometry

Plane of motion	Excursion (Degrees)	Movable Arm	Stationary Arm	Axis	Primary Capsuloligamentous Complex Area Stretch	Substitution
Flexion	160–180	Humeral shaft to lateral epicondyle	Lateral trunk	Halfway between the posterolateral acromion and axilla	Posterior and inferior	Excessive scapular rotation and/or elevation Lumbar extension Thoracic elevation (rib expansion) Thoracic lateral flexion
Abduction (coronal plane)	160–180	Humeral shaft to medial epicondyle	In line with sternum	Center of axilla	Anterior and inferior	As above
Abduction (POS)	160–180	As above	As above	Approximately 1 in lateral to the coracoid process	Inferior	As above
Hyperextension	50–65	Greater tuberosity to lateral epicondyle	Lateral trunk	Greater tuberosity	Anterior and superior	Scapular anterior tilting and elevation
External rotation 90 degrees (coronal plane)	90–100	Shaft of forearm to ulnarstyloid process	The vertical or horizontal	Olecranon	Anterior and inferior	Scapular posterior tilting and depression
External rotation (0 degrees)	50–76	As above	As above	As above	Anterior and superior	Scapular adduction
Internal rotation 90 degrees (coronal plane)	40–60	As above	As above	As above	Posterior and inferior	Scapular anterior tilting and elevation
Horizontal adduction	125–140	Greater tuberosity to lateral epicondyle	Coronal plane	Superior acromion	Posterior	Scapular adduction and lateral rotation
Horizontal abduction	40–45	As above	As above	As above	Anterior	Scapular adduction

POS, plane of the scapula. (From Kelley MJ: Evaluation of the shoulder. In: Kelley MJ, Clark WA, eds. *Orthopedic Therapy of the Shoulder.* © 1995, Philadelphia: J.B. Lippincott Company.)

capsular pattern. Three pathology categories can result in a noncapsular pattern:

1. Isolated capsuloligamentous lesions
2. Internal derangement
3. Extra-articular limitations

Examples of each at the shoulder include an isolated lesion of the anterior capsule leading to limited external rotation, displaced labral tissue, and acute subdeltoid bursitis causing greater restrictions of abduction.

Four parameters are assessed during passive movement:

1. Range of motion
2. Presence of pain
3. Relationship between pain onset and end-range pain
4. End-feel

Range of Motion

Goniometry is performed to determine PROM. Table 9-4 lists the technique and common substitutions to detect end-range. Standardization of technique is absolutely essential in opti-

mizing measurement reliability. Although some clinicians find goniometry unnecessary, we believe that it defines a baseline to gauge progress or regression.

Pain

The second parameter important in PROM assessment is pain; in particular, when does pain occur? Does pain occur near end-range, at end-range, or when overpressure is applied following end-range arrival? The clinician also needs to determine whether a passive painful arc is present. On occasion, pain causing apparent limited motion abates only if further motion is pursued. Varying humeral rotation and plane of elevation can allow further range by mechanically relieving tissue compression.

Pain occurring before true end-range, whether full or limited, signifies an inflammatory condition. This is commonly noted in acute bursitis, reactive rotator cuff pathology, and the early stages of reactive adhesive capsulitis. Pain arises from stretching irritated synovium, capsuloligamentous tissue, inflamed or torn tendon, or by soft tissue compression of structures such as the bursa and rotator cuff. The earlier pain is encountered in the ROM, the greater the inflammatory intensity or reactivity. Caution is required when evaluating and treating individuals in the early, or "freezing," stage of adhesive capsulitis because forcing end-range by stretching usually intensifies the condition. Pain present as end-range is reached indicates moderate irritability as seen in patients with the stage 3 frozen shoulder. Stretching should still be approached with caution. Pain sensed after achieving a premature end-range demonstrates mild irritability due to stretching constricted connective tissue. This is noted in stage 4 frozen shoulder in the presence of dense connective tissue fibrosis without synovitis.

End-Feel

In conjunction with ROM and pain, the end-feel at end-range should be scrutinized. *End-feel* is the restrictive sensation perceived by the examiner when end-range is attained. This tactile impression is valuable in determining the tissue status and treatment approach. Six end-feels have been identified[27]:

1. Soft tissue approximation
2. Bone to bone
3. Springy
4. Capsular
5. Spasm (muscle guarding)
6. Empty

The former three are uncommon at the shoulder.

Soft tissue approximation is normally met at several joints, such as the elbow and knee, when full flexion is available and only the soft tissue mass prevents further motion. A normal bone-to-bone end-feel is felt at full terminal elbow extension when a hard, abrupt feel is noted. A springy block end-feel results from internal derangement, which is best appreciated at the knee having a displaced meniscal tear. Overpressure at end-range engages the derangement between the articular surfaces, producing a "springy" effect.

A capsular end-feel is considered normal at all shoulder end-ranges. The actual tactile sense has been described as stretching a piece of leather—firm yet pliable. The literature typically incriminates the CLC as being responsible for normal capsular feel. However, recognizing the intimate relationship between the rotator cuff tendons and the CLC, tendinous tissue also must participate in the end-feel. Turkel and colleagues[84] found that by incising the subscapularis, external rotation ROM increased by 18 degrees when performed with the arm at the side. Obviously, this tendon primarily limits external rotation and thus is also responsible for the end-feel. It is difficult to rationalize that passive motion is not limited to some degree, whether in the normal or pathologic condition, by the rotator cuff tendons or surrounding shoulder musculature.

Cyriax[27] uses the term *spasm* to describe an end-feel characterized by involuntary protective muscle activity reflexively initiated by pain. Because spasm has a confusing connotation, we choose the term *muscle guarding*. Two types of muscle guarding have been described: fast and slow.[85] Fast muscle guarding occurs as twinges of protective muscle activity when the arm is moved through the ROM or at end-

range. Slow muscle guarding is more controlled yet prevents further motion. The clinician can be fooled by slow muscle guarding because, at some point, undetectable muscle activity limits the motion, mimicking a capsular end-feel. This phenomenon can be appreciated if a patient with a stiff and painful shoulder is examined before and after anesthesia. Often a capsular end-feel is appreciated while awake yet under anesthesia 10 degrees or more of motion is achieved. One can only conclude the increased motion occurs because pain and muscle guarding is eliminated.

An empty end-feel is sometimes encountered in the presence of acute calcific tendinitis; here, pain is so significant that reflexive inhibition of the shoulder muscles occurs. A sense of mechanical limitation is absent at an early end-range, with motion limited only by pain. An empty end-feel also can be encountered in patients with scapular or acromial fractures or nondisplaced humeral head fractures.

Accessory Motions (Joint Play)

PROM can indicate the general hypermobility or hypomobility status of noncontractile tissue. Assessment of accessory motion provides specific information concerning joint CLC contracture or hyperelasticity. All of the joints encompassing the shoulder complex can be evaluated and treated using accessory motions. *Accessory motions* are movements not under voluntary control but essential for normal joint function.[86,87] At the glenohumeral joint, these include anterior, posterior, and inferior humeral head gliding, as well as distraction. All except distraction are considered component motions, defined as necessary for full active motion.[86,87]

Stability Testing

Stability testing utilizes specific techniques and positions to determine whether the glenohumeral joint is unstable. Conceptually, these tests are similar to assessing accessory joint motions to determine mobility. Some tests are similar to joint play assessment except that they are performed out of the loose pack position (LPP) or encompass humeral rotation to further provoke signs and symptoms.

Stability testing is beneficial in patients who describe a history of instability or joint "looseness" or who are athletic. However, clinical judgment should determine the necessity of instability testing. For example, performing an anterior apprehension sign may not be required in a patient who incurred a documented anterior dislocation 2 weeks previously. Commonly, the history helps determine the presence of instability. In many instances, the diagnosis of rotator cuff tendinitis or impingement is often applied to a patient when symptoms are in fact secondary to a primary instability problem. Bilateral comparison is essential to determining asymmetry. In the patient with multidirectional instability (MDI), capsuloligamentous laxity may be symmetrical, but symptoms may be present on only one side.

A word of caution is needed regarding humeral translation assessment. Accessory motions and laxity testing are subjective and gain credence when performed in the symptomatic,

Table 9-5 Instability Tests: Sensitivity, Specificity, and Likelihood Ratios

Test	Specificity (%)	(+) Likelihood Ratio	Sensitivity (%)	(−) Likelihood Ratio	Reference
Posterior Glenohumeral Instability Tests					
Kim test	94	12.00	80	0.21	94
Jerk test*	98	36.50	73	0.28	94
Posterior load and shift	100	1.70	0	0.99	113
Anterior Glenohumeral Instability Tests					
Anterior release test*	89	8.40	92	0.09	91
Apprehension test*	50	1.80	88	0.23	113
Relocation test*	87	6.50	85	0.18	113
Anterior release test	87	6.50	85	0.17	113
Apprehension test— apprehension (+)	100	68.00	68	0.32	90
Relocation test— apprehension (+)	100	57.00	57	0.43	90
Apprehension test—pain (+)	44	0.96	54	1.05	90
Anterior load and shift	78	2.50	54	0.59	113
Relocation test—pain (+)	58	1.20	30	1.21	90
Inferior Glenohumeral Instability Tests					
Sulcus	89	2.80	31	0.78	113

*Original description of test.
From Uhl TL. Rehabilitation of Scapular Dysfunction. In: *APTA Combined Section Meeting*. San Diego, CA, 2006.

grossly unstable patient, particularly if excursion findings are asymmetrical; however, when attempting to quantify excursion in the subtly unstable patient, validity is questionable. Patient relaxation is absolutely essential. Only with standardization of technique and experience is this testing meaningful. See Table 9-5 for instability testing sensitivity, specificity, and likelihood ratios.[88]

Hyperelasticity or Hypoelasticity

Assessing gross connective tissue hyperelasticity or hypoelasticity at other joints is essential to aide in diagnosis and treatment. The metacarpophalangeal joints, wrist, elbows, and knees should all be evaluated for mobility (Fig. 9-18, online). Typically, the patient with MDI demonstrates hypermobility of other joints. Determining general connective tissue elasticity can be valuable in assessing and progressing ROM exercises in the postoperative patient. Those with hyperelastic joints are monitored so that motion does not return too quickly. This contrasts with hastening the rehabilitation in a patient with hypoelastic connective tissue characteristics who demonstrates early postoperative tightness.

Special Tests

Apprehension Maneuver

Apprehension refers to the sensation that a patient with recurrent glenohumeral instability experiences when his or her arm is placed in the position that provokes instability. Apprehension is most often associated with anterior instability. The apprehension maneuver can be performed with the patient in both the upright and supine positions. The arm is passively elevated to 90 degrees in the scapular plane, with the elbow bent to 90 degrees. The examiner gradually and simultaneously brings the humerus posterior to the scapular plane and externally rotates the humerus using one hand (Fig. 9-19). The thumb of the examiner's other hand can be placed at the posterior aspect of the glenohumeral joint and used as a fulcrum. During testing in the supine position, the palm of the examiner's other hand is placed behind the glenohumeral joint and used as a fulcrum. As external rotation and extension are applied, the patient with recurrent anterior dislocations becomes very anxious that a dislocation is about to occur. Most patients with recurrent subluxation rather than dislocation, however, experience pain instead of apprehension with this maneuver. It is important to distinguish between pain and apprehension with this maneuver because pain is a much less specific and sensitive indicator for recurrent instability than apprehension.

Relocation Test

The relocation test is a modification of the anterior apprehension maneuver. The relocation test is performed with the patient in the supine position, using the edge of the examination table as a fulcrum, rather than the examiner's free hand. The patient may perceive pain or apprehension in this position. If the pain or apprehension is relieved with a simultaneously applied, posteriorly directed force on the shaft of the humerus, anterior glenohumeral instability or internal glenoid impingement may be present[36,89,90] (Fig. 9-20). Like the apprehension maneuver, when the symptom elicited by this test is pain, rather than apprehension, it is much less sensitive and specific for instability.[90]

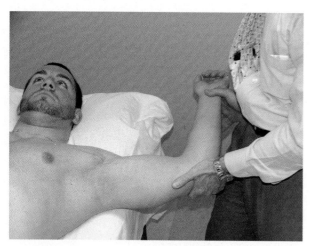

Figure 9-19 Apprehension maneuver.

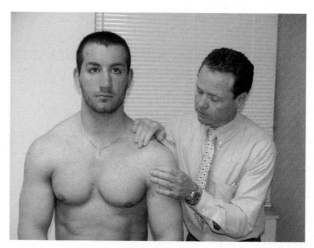

Figure 9-21 Anterior drawer test.

Anterior Release Test

The anterior release test was developed to diagnose occult anterior instability by reproducing the mechanical action that causes the patient's symptoms. The patient starts supine with the affected arm over the edge of the examining table. The examiner abducts the patient's arm to 90 degrees while using his or her hand to direct a posterior force on the patient's humeral head. While maintaining the posterior force, the patient's arm is brought into terminal external rotation, and then the posterior force is released. This test can be performed immediately after a positive relocation test and uses a mechanism that removes the force directed to relocate the humeral head. The test is considered positive if the patient experiences sudden pain, a distinct increase in pain, or symptom reproduction.[91]

Anterior and Posterior Laxity Testing

The anterior–posterior drawer test is performed with the patient in the seated position with the muscles as relaxed as possible. The head of the humerus is grasped in one hand by the examiner, and the scapula is stabilized on the rib cage using the other hand and forearm. The humeral head is compressed into the glenoid fossa slightly to center the head on the glenoid. The humeral head is then shifted anteriorly, and the amount of anterior translation is estimated (Fig. 9-21); the head is then returned to the center of the glenoid fossa, and this test is repeated in the posterior direction.

The load and shift test differs from the anterior–posterior drawer test in two ways: first, it is performed with the patient in the supine position, and second, translation is tested in three positions: (1) arm at the side (i.e., 20 degrees abduction, neutral humeral rotation); (2) arm at 90 degrees of elevation in the scapular plane, neutral humeral rotation; and (3) arm at 90 degrees of elevation in the scapular plane, maximal humeral external rotation and then maximum internal rotation (Fig. 9-22). In each position, the patient's arm is supported with one hand and the humerus is grasped in the other. An axial load is placed along the humeral shaft to provide a centering force, and the humerus is displaced anteriorly. This is repeated with the force directed posteriorly. The amount of anterior and posterior translation is quantified and compared with that on the opposite side. The degree of translation exhibits significant individual variability, and the

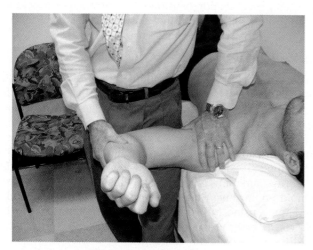

Figure 9-20 Relocation test.

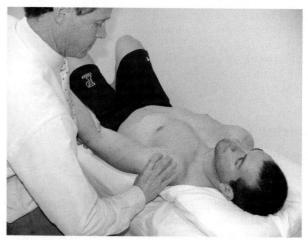

Figure 9-22 Supine anterior load and shift test.

ability to sublux the humeral head over the glenoid rim is a normal variant; therefore, comparison with the opposite side is critical. In a normal shoulder, the greatest amount of translation in both directions is appreciated in position 1 as this is the loose-pack position of the shoulder, where the capsule displays the most laxity. Although no specific degree of translation can confidently rule in instability, a variety of grading systems have been described, with the modified Hawkins' rating appearing to have the most clinical relevance (Fig. 9-23, online). The rating system is graded as follows: grade 0 has no or little motion; grade I is the translation of the humeral head onto the glenoid rim; grade II is the dislocation of the humeral head that can be spontaneously relocated; grade III is a dislocation that does not relocate when the pressure is removed.[92] These tests are primarily used to assess laxity and not elicit symptoms.

Sulcus Test

Inferior instability refers to symptomatic increased inferior translation of the humerus with the arm at the side. It is most often present as a component of MDI. The mere presence of increased inferior translation with the arm at the side, without symptoms, is insufficient for a diagnosis of inferior instability. Inferior translation of the humerus with the arm at the side is primarily resisted by the RCI (i.e., the superior glenohumeral ligament and the coracohumeral ligament). Therefore, laxity or deficiency of the RCI may result in increased inferior translation during sulcus testing.

The sulcus test is performed with the patient in the seated or the supine position. The patient may be most relaxed in a seated position with both hands in the lap; this also allows the examiner to test both extremities simultaneously to examine for symmetry. The humerus is placed in neutral rotation and an inferiorly directed force is applied to the shaft of the humerus. Inferior translation of the humerus at the glenohumeral joint is observed as a dimpling effect just below the anterior acromion and is quantified by measuring the sulcus in centimeters (Fig. 9-24). The humerus is returned to the resting position, and the test is repeated with the arm at the side in maximal external rotation. In the normal shoulder, any inferior translation with the humerus in neutral rotation should be substantially reduced or eliminated in

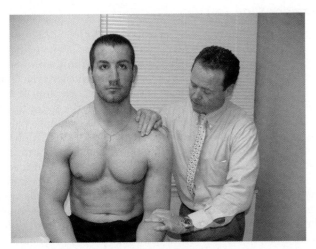

Figure 9-24 Sulcus sign.

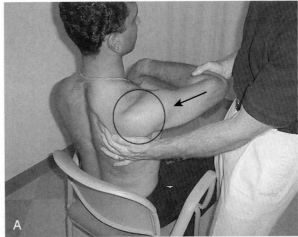

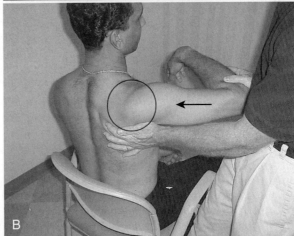

Figure 9-25 Jerk test. Subluxed (**A**) and reduced (**B**).

external rotation because this tightens the RCI. In the presence of RCI injury, the sulcus is either not reduced in external rotation or the amount of external rotation required to reduce the inferior translation is markedly increased compared with the opposite side. For the sulcus sign to truly be positive for inferior or MDI, it must reproduce the patient's symptoms of instability. The sulcus sign has a high specificity when the sulcus is 2 cm or more.[92]

Jerk Test

The jerk test is useful for diagnosing posteroinferior instability. It is most easily performed with the patient upright (Fig. 9-25). The examiner places the arm in 90 degrees of elevation in the scapular plane with the humerus in slight internal rotation. With one hand, the scapula is stabilized against the thorax. With the other hand, the patient's flexed elbow is grasped, an axial load is applied to the humeral shaft, and the arm is simultaneously adducted across the body and maximally internally rotated. A click or jerk is felt as the humeral head rides over the posterior glenoid rim. The humerus is then externally rotated and returned toward the coronary plane. A more pronounced click or jerk is felt as the humerus passes back over the posterior glenoid rim to return to the glenoid fossa. For this test to have clinical significance, it must reproduce the patient's symptoms and differ from the opposite, normal side. In addition, there is a correlation between pain with this test and failure with non-operative treatment;[93] pain occurring as the humeral head is subluxed over the posterior glenoid rim often signifies a structural defect.

Kim Test

The Kim test[94] is a modified version of the jerk test and was designed to detect posteroinferior labral lesions of the shoulder. The test is performed with the patient sitting with the arm abducted to 90 degrees. The examiner places one hand on the elbow and the other on the lateral upper arm and applies a strong axial force. The examiner then elevates the arm 45 degrees diagonally and applies a force downward and backwards to the proximal arm. Applying a strong posterior force is necessary for an accurate test, thus having the patient sit on a supportive surface such as a chair with a back is preferable. Sudden posterior shoulder pain with or without a clunk is considered a positive test. It has been further suggested that pain indicates a posterior labral lesion, whereas pain with a clunk implies posterior instability with a labral lesion. Combining this test with the jerk test increases the sensitivity for detecting posteroinferior labral lesions.[94]

Multidirectional Instability

The tests for MDI are the same as those used for unidirectional instability. The challenge for the examiner is to differentiate between multidirectional laxity and MDI. Laxity without symptoms is not pathologic. Symmetrical laxity, even in the presence of symptoms, may not be the cause of the symptoms. Once the diagnosis of MDI seems accurate, the challenge then becomes determining which direction is the most symptomatic. An examiner's ability to make the correct diagnosis improves with experience. Multiple examinations of the same patient at different times may also help.

Summary

Accessory motion and stability testing assesses the restrictive status and capabilities of the capsuloligamentous soft tissue surrounding the shoulder joint by determining whether excessive or reduced motion is allowed. To gain valid information from this portion of the evaluation, the clinician must (1) possess knowledge of positional influence on the static restraints, (2) stabilize the proximal segment when able to, and (3) compare findings with the uninvolved side. Experience and correlation with the history and diagnostic tests are absolutely vital.

Special Tests for Superior Labrum Anterior–Posterior Lesions

Active Compression Test (O'Brien's Sign)

The active compression test is used to determine the presence of a superior labral anterior–posterior (SLAP) lesion or AC joint pathology (Table 9-6).[95] The examiner places the arm in 10 degrees medial to the sagittal plane with the thumb down (Fig. 9-26). The patient is asked to resist the downward force of the examiner. A positive test is indicated by a painful click, which is eliminated if the arm is externally rotated (palm up). The first position creates a high pressure in the joint as the greater tuberosity loads the AC joint and bicipital–labral complex is tensioned; the second position clears the greater tuberosity from under the AC joint and relieves bicipital–labral complex tension, thus testing in this position relieves symptoms.[95] This test can be used to clinically detect both labral and AC joint abnormalities, assuming that both the examiner and the patient can distinguish between pain or symptoms at the AC joint ("on top") versus pain or clicking deep inside the shoulder, the latter indicating labral pathology.

Biceps Load Test I

The biceps load test is used to detect SLAP lesions in patients with recurrent anterior dislocations. With the patient in the supine position, the examiner grasps the patient's wrist and elbow, abducts the patient's affected shoulder to 90 degrees, and supinates the forearm (Fig. 9-27). With the patient relaxed, an anterior apprehension test is performed; external rotation is stopped at the point where the patient becomes apprehensive. At this point, the patient is asked to flex the elbow while the examiner resists elbow flexion. The patient is asked if apprehension has changed. If the patient experiences less apprehension or pain, the test is negative. If apprehension remains unchanged or the pain increases, the test is positive.[96] It is important to realize that the test was developed for patients specifically with anterior instability, thus stability testing should precede this test to determine its appropriateness.

Biceps Load Test II

The biceps load test II is used to detect isolated SLAP lesions and is most useful for the detection of type II lesions, distinct for their biceps anchor detachment. The test starts with the patient supine and the examiner sitting adjacent. The examiner grasps the patient's affected arm by the wrist and elbow, abducts the shoulder to 120 degrees, flexes the elbow to 90 degrees, and fully externally rotates the shoulder and supinates the forearm (Fig. 9-28). The patient is asked to flex the elbow while the examiner resists this motion. The test is considered positive if this maneuver elicits pain, or if the patient experiences an increase in pain from the resisted elbow flexion.[97]

Anterior Slide Test

The anterior slide test was developed to test for SLAP lesions in athletes who may or may not have concurrent pathologies.[52] The patient may start sitting or standing with his or her hands on the hips, thumbs pointing posteriorly (Fig. 9-29). The examiner places one hand on the top of the patient's shoulder, pointing posteriorly, with the index finger extending over the anterior acromion. The examiner places his or her other hand behind the elbow and forward, applying a slightly superior force to the elbow and upper arm; the patient pushes back against this force. The test is considered positive if pain is elicited in the front of the shoulder under the examiner's hand, or a click or pop is felt in the same area. This test stresses mainly the anterior labrum in the region of the biceps anchor, but unlike other provocative testing for SLAP tears, does not require end-range positioning and may be more comfortable for patients who are highly irritable.[52]

Table 9-6 Special Tests for Superior Labrum Anterior–Posterior (SLAP) Lesions

Test	Specificity (%)	(+) Likelihood Ratio	Sensitivity (%)	(–) Likelihood Ratio	Reference
Labral Tests					
Active compression (O'Brien's test)*	98	21.00	100	0.01	95
Crank test*	93	13.00	.91	0.10	108
Biceps load test II*	96	26.00	90	0.10	97
Biceps load test I*	98	29.00	83	0.09	96
Resisted supination–external rotation test*	82	4.55	83	0.21	98
Anterior slide test*	92	8.30	78	0.20	52
Active compression test	11	0.88	78	2.00	98
Active compression test	73	2.33	63	0.51	109
Active compression test	25	0.84	63	1.48	Michener LA et al., JOSPT, 2004 (Abstract)
Crank test	83	3.40	56	0.50	Michener LA et al., JOSPT, 2004 (Abstract)
Active compression test	31	1.60	54	0.31	110
Anterior slide test	90	5.10	51	0.50	Michener LA et al., JOSPT, 2004 (Abstract)
Active compression test	55	1.04	47	0.96	114
Crank test	56	1.10	46	1.00	110
Crank test	73	1.50	40	0.80	111
Crank test	70	1.15	35	0.93	98
Crank test	76	1.00	24	1.00	114
Anterior slide test	83	0.50	8	1.00	114
Speed's test—Biceps plus labral tear	14	1.10	90	0.70	115

*Original description of test.
From Uhl TL. Rehabilitation of Scapular Dysfunction. In: *APTA Combined Section Meeting.* San Diego, CA, 2006.

Crank Test

The crank test is used to diagnose labral tears and is particularly useful for patients with stable shoulders. With the patient in the upright position, the examiner elevates the patient's arm to 160 degrees in the scapular plane. The examiner applies a joint load along the axis of the humerus with one hand while the other hand internally and externally rotates the humerus in an effort to catch the labrum. Pain during the maneuver (with or without a click) or reproduction of symptoms indicate a positive test. Symptoms are most often noted with external rotation. If the patient is unable to relax in the seated position, the test may be performed also in the supine position.

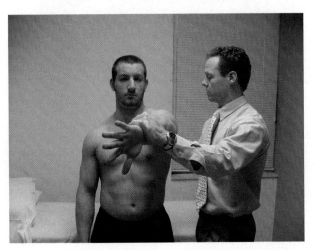

Figure 9-26 Active compression sign.

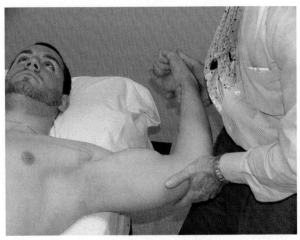

Figure 9-27 Biceps load test I.

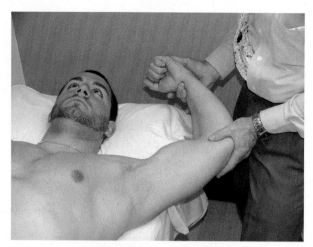

Figure 9-28 Biceps load test II.

Resisted Supination External Rotation Test

In the abducted, maximally externally rotated position, the biceps tendon may transfer a torsional force to the superior labrum, which, in turn, rotates the posterior superior labrum medially away from the glenoid, resulting in a SLAP tear. This is referred to as the "peel-back" mechanism. The resisted supination external rotation test is used to identify superior labral lesions by attempting to recreate this peel-back mechanism by which SLAP tears occur. The test is performed with the patient supine and the affected shoulder near the edge of the examination table. The examiner abducts the shoulder to 90 degrees, flexes the elbow 60 to 70 degrees, and places the forearm in neutral or slight pronation. The patient's scapula is stabilized by the table. The patient is asked to supinate the forearm with maximal effort; the examiner resists this motion while externally rotating the shoulder to end-range. The test is considered positive if the patient experiences anterior or deep shoulder pain, clicking or catching in the shoulder, or usual symptom reproduction. Posterior shoulder pain, apprehension, or no pain are considered a negative test.[98]

Summary

Unfortunately, the accuracy of labral testing varies widely based on the examiner and is confounded by the fact that patients with labral pathology often have concurrent pathologies in the affected shoulder. A thorough history and clinical examination are crucial tools for the clinician. A patient history with either a distinct trauma or repetitive provocative motions (perhaps most commonly pitching) may lead the clinician to consider labral pathology, along with complaints of mechanical symptoms, such as popping, clicking, or catching. These patients may have pain in the classic apprehension position, but further instability testing is negative. Physical examination using a battery of tests has been found to be more sensitive than MRI in diagnosing labral pathology;[99] however, arthroscopy remains the gold standard.

Rotator Cuff and Biceps Special Tests

Neer's Impingement Sign

Impingement of the supraspinatus tendon or biceps against the anterior acromion and coracoacromial ligament may result in anterior shoulder pain. Neer[5] described the impingement sign as a means of reproducing pain associated with subacromial impingement. The sign is elicited by passively elevating the arm in a plane that is slightly anterior to the scapular plane (Fig. 9-30). As the arm is brought into the final degrees of elevation, contact occurs between the coracoacromial arch and the supraspinatus tendon, and subacromial bursa and biceps. However, recent in vivo evidence reveals that supraspinatus impingement occurs on the superior glenoid rim not the arch.[6] Regardless of the site of

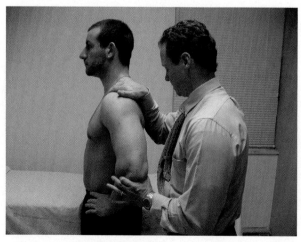

Figure 9-29 Anterior slide test.

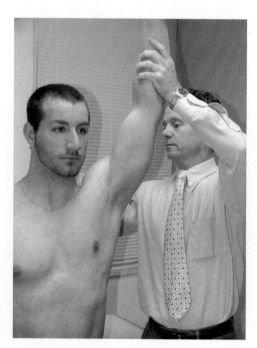

Figure 9-30 Neer's impingement.

Table 9-7 Rotator Cuff and Biceps Special Tests

Test	Specificity (%)	(+) Likelihood Ratio	Sensitivity (%)	(−) Likelihood Ratio	Reference
Impingement Tests					
Hawkins'*	44	1.64	92	0.18	111
Hawkins'	25	1.23	92	0.32	112
Painful arc*	81	3.89	74	0.32	40
3/6 Combined positive	44	1.50	84	0.36	112
Neer's	31	1.28	89	0.37	112
Hawkins'	66	2.12	72	0.42	40
4/6 Combined positive	67	2.12	70	0.45	112
Neer's	69	2.19	68	0.46	40
Neer's	48	1.44	75	0.52	111
Speed's	56	1.55	69	0.56	112
Neer's and Hawkins' combined	51	1.45	71	0.57	111
Supraspinatus muscle test (empty can)	90	4.40	44	0.62	40
Infraspinatus strength test	90	4.20	42	0.64	40
Cross-body adduction	28	1.13	82	0.65	112
Yeargson's	86	2.66	37	0.73	112
Speed's	83	2.24	38	0.75	40
Drop arm	88	2.25	27	0.83	40
Painful arc	81	1.69	33	0.83	112
Cross-body adduction	82	1.28	23	0.94	40
Drop arm	97	2.86	8	0.95	112
Rotator Cuff Tears					
External rotation lag sign (supraspinatus and infraspinatus)*	100	94.00	94	0.06	62
Supraspinatus FT tears—Empty can (pain and/or weakness)	50	1.78	89	0.22	102
Hawkins'	43	1.54	88	0.28	111
Supraspinatus FT tears—Full can (pain and/or weakness)	57	2.00	86	0.25	102
Neer's and Hawkins' combined	56	1.89	83	0.30	111
Neer's	51	1.69	83	0.33	111
Internal rotation lag sign (subscapularis)*	96	19.20	80	0.21	62
Supraspinatus FT tears—Full can (weakness)	74	2.96	77	0.31	102
Supraspinatus FT tears—Empty can (weakness)	68	2.41	77	0.34	102
Painful arc	62	2.00	76	0.39	40
Hawkins'	48	1.33	69	0.65	40
Lift-off test	100	62.00	62	0.38	62
Neer's	47	1.11	59	0.87	40
Supraspinatus empty can test	82	2.94	53	0.57	40
Infraspinatus muscle test	84	3.19	51	0.58	40
Speed's	75	1.60	40	0.80	40
Drop arm test	88	2.92	35	0.74	40
Cross-body adduction	81	1.21	23	0.95	40
Drop arm test	100	11.00	21	0.95	62

*Original description of test.
FT, full-thickness.
From Uhl TL. Rehabilitation of Scapular Dysfunction. In: *APTA Combined Section Meeting.* San Diego, CA, 2006.

impingement, this sign has very good sensitivity but poor specificity (Table 9-7). This means that if a patient does not have pain with this test they probably do not have pathology of the rotator cuff, biceps, or subacromial bursa. The sensitivity of the impingement sign can be improved by repeating the maneuver after the subacromial space has been infiltrated with local anesthetic. If the impingement sign is no longer painful, subacromial impingement syndrome is strongly indicated. The combination of the impingement sign with subacromial local anesthetic is referred to as the *impingement test.*[5]

Hawkins' Sign

The Hawkins' sign or impingement reinforcement sign is based on the concept that elevation of the humerus to 90 degrees in the scapular plane brings the rotator cuff tendons, biceps, and bursa into close approximation to the coracoacromial arch. In this position the arm is passively

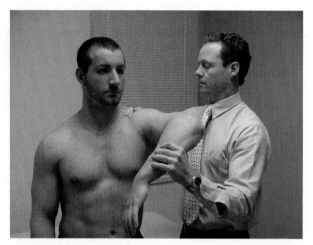

Figure 9-31 Hawkins' impingement.

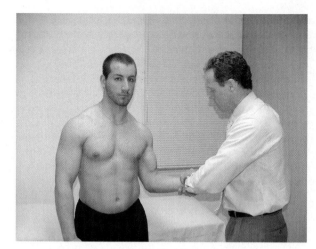

Figure 9-32 Modified Yergason's sign.

internally rotated, thereby compressing the supraspinatus tendon, biceps, and bursa against the coracoacromial arch (Fig. 9-31). This is painful in patients with impingement syndrome.[100]

Biceps Provocative Signs

Tendinitis of the long head of the biceps can be a difficult diagnosis to make unless the biceps is primarily involved. Palpation of the bicipital groove is not a reliable test. Moreover, many of the commonly described maneuvers or tests to elicit pain in patients with bicipital tendinitis are also painful in other pathologic conditions affecting the shoulder. Two such signs are Yergason's and Speed's signs. Yergason's sign is present if pain is elicited by resisted supination with the elbow flexed and slightly externally rotated. Speed's sign is performed by asking the patient to place the arm at or near shoulder height (approximately 60 degrees) in the scapular plane with the elbow extended. The patient is then asked to attempt to further elevate the arm in the scapular plane against resistance supplied by the examiner. This maneuver is thought to elicit pain in patients with biceps tendinitis and had good specificity.[40]

A useful refinement of Yergason's sign may improve the specificity of biceps testing. Combined elbow flexion to 90 degrees and neutral humeral rotation places the long head of the biceps in a position of relative laxity. Resisted supination of the forearm in this position causes little stress on the biceps. If the humerus is then maximally externally rotated, the biceps is forced against the medial wall of the bicipital groove (Fig. 9-32). Resisted forearm supination in this position of greater biceps tension is painful in patients with biceps tendinitis. This biceps provocative sign is considered positive if resisted supination in the first position is nonpainful or mildly painful and becomes markedly painful in the second position.

Supraspinatus Isolation Test

The test position was initially advocated by Jobe and Moynes,[101] who found that the position increased activity of the supraspinatus. The arm is placed at 90 degrees in the POS with the thumb down, which maintains internal rotation (Fig. 9-33). The examiner then resists by pushing

into adduction. A painful or weak response is elicited if a supraspinatus tendon lesion exists.[102] The test is more specific for a rotator cuff full-thickness cuff tear if weakness is present.[40,102] Kelly and Speer[103] found maximal activity of the supraspinatus with the arm in external rotation at 90 degrees in the POS. This position was also found to be more comfortable because it tends to avoid painful compression of the tendon–bursal complex. Another way to avoid subacromial impingement yet still isolate the supraspinatus is to place the arm at 45 degrees in the POS with either internal or external rotation.

External Rotation Lag Sign and Drop Sign

The external rotation lag sign (ERLS) and drop sign are tests recently published by Hertel and colleagues[62] to further evaluate the integrity of the supraspinatus and infraspinatus tendons or nerve involvement. Two positions are performed. The first is to passively place the arm in *full* external rotation with the arm 20 degrees abducted in the POS (Fig. 9-34A, B). Care should be taken not to over-rotate, which can result in elastic recoil. The examiner instructs the patient to maintain the arm in this position and releases at the wrist but supports the elbow. A patient with an intact supraspinatus

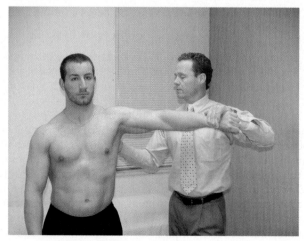

Figure 9-33 Supraspinatus isolation test.

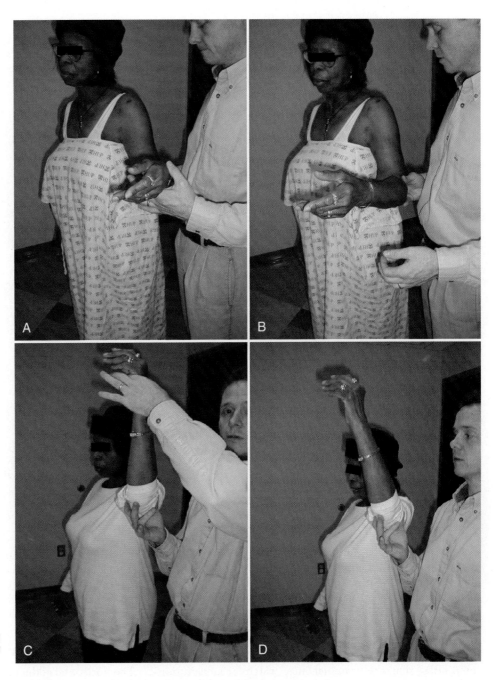

Figure 9-34 A, B, External rotation lag sign. **C, D,** Drop sign (external rotation lag performed in the elevated position).

and infraspinatus can maintain the arm in this position. If the arm lags or falls toward internal rotation, the test is positive. The degree of lag is related to the size of tendon tear or severity of nerve involvement. A lag of 5 to 10 degrees was found to indicate a supraspinatus tear, and a lag of greater than 10 degrees was associated with a supraspinatus and infraspinatus complete tearing.[62] Significant lagging may also occur with a severe *complete* suprascapular nerve palsy. This test can be extremely valuable postoperatively when assessing cuff integrity. As with all resisted motion testing, this test is most appropriately used after 6 weeks in a patient after rotator cuff repair.

The drop sign is performed in elevation. The patient's arm is passively placed at 90 degrees of POS abduction and near full external rotation (Fig. 9-34C, D). The patient is instructed to maintain the arm in this position as the wrist is let go but the arm supported. The magnitude of drop into internal rotation is recorded. This test is designed to assess primarily infraspinatus function. A patient with a positive lag in the 90-degree position is believed to have a full-thickness tear of both the supraspinatus and infraspinatus.

Lift-Off Test

The lift-off test is performed with the patient sitting or standing.[64] The patient is asked to place the dorsal aspect of the hand on the lower back and lift it away (Fig. 9-35). The test is positive if the patient cannot remove the hand from the back or only do so partially. This position places all of the internal rotators in their shortened position but primarily isolates the subscapularis.[104] For this test position to be valid,

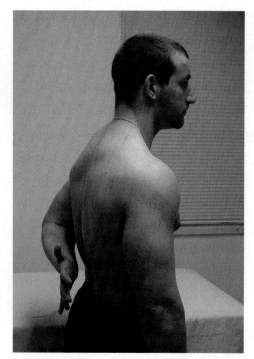

Figure 9-35 Lift-off test.

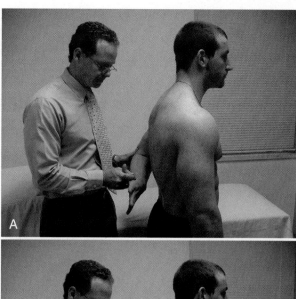

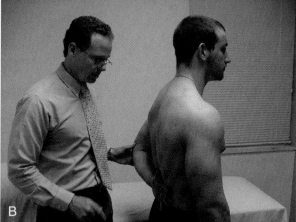

Figure 9-36 Internal rotation lag sign (**A**) lift-off and (**B**) demonstrates positive test.

the patient must have the available pain-free motion. Many individuals who have rotator cuff tears not involving the subscapularis have difficulty placing their arm in the lift-off position because of pain or contracture.

Internal Rotation Lag Sign

This test can help to determine if the subscapularis is torn.[62] If full motion is available, the internal rotation lag sign can be performed. The examiner passively places the patient's arm into internal rotation behind the back and lifts the dorsum of the hand from the back (essentially the completed lift-off position) (Fig. 9-36A). Care must be taken not to rotate beyond available range. The elbow is supported, and the patient is asked to maintain this position as the hand is released. A positive test is when the hand falls toward or onto the back (Fig. 9-36B). In both the lift-off test and internal rotation lag sign, the examiner must watch for substitution of shoulder extension and elbow extension.

Belly Press Test

The belly press test is useful in the patient who cannot be placed into the lift-off or lag sign position because of pain or contracture.[64] However, it still isolates the subscapularis. The patient is asked to place the hand flat against the stomach and to place the elbow out to the side and slightly forward (Fig. 9-37). The patient is instructed to push into the stomach while keeping the elbow out to the side. A positive test is indicated when the elbow cannot be maintained out to the side and forward (the arm adducts). To further appreciate the degree of weakness, the examiner may also attempt to pull the hand from the stomach. With rupture or insufficiency of the subscapularis, the hand is easily pulled from the stomach.

Miller and coworkers[67] reported on patients with positive signs for subscapularis rupture following a total shoulder replacement or hemiarthroplasty. It is doubtful that these people have ruptured their subscapularis, but weakness may be caused by mechanical insufficiency of the subscapularis or tendon alterations.

Horizontal (Cross-Body) Adduction Test

The horizontal adduction test is useful in patients thought to have AC arthritis or derangement of the intra-articular disk. The test is performed by passively elevating the arm to 90 degrees in the POS. The arm is then forced into adduction by passively bringing the arm across the body. Patients with AC arthritis or derangement of the intra-articular disk complain of pain localized to the AC joint. The test may be even more painful if adduction is performed with the arm elevated slightly above shoulder height. The patient should be carefully examined for posteroinferior capsular contracture. Horizontal adduction in these patients tightens the posterior capsule prematurely and may result in a feeling of pain or stretching in the posterior aspect of the shoulder. Anterior shoulder pain may also be elicited under these circumstances because of obligate anterior translation into the coracoacromial arch (impingement). In addition, superior labral tears may also be symptomatic with this maneuver. The specificity

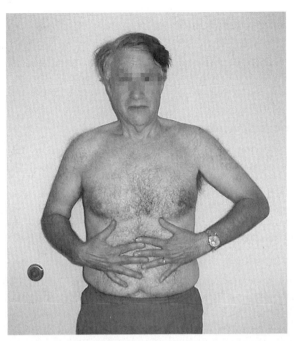

Figure 9-37 *Belly press sign positive on the right.*

of the horizontal adduction test for AC pathology is strengthened if the patient has localized tenderness over the AC joint. In addition, combining the test with an AC injection of local anesthetic determines the joint involvement.

A patient complaining of pain medial to the glenohumeral joint may experience a reproduction of symptoms by performing horizontal adduction. Patients with coracoid impingement experience pain with this maneuver as the coracoid bursa or subscapularis is compressed against the coracoid process. The examiner must also be aware that horizontal adduction places the glenohumeral joint into a provocative position in patients with posterior instability.

Neural Tests

Sensation and Reflexes

Sensation testing is critical to determining neurologic involvement demonstrated by cutaneous disruption. Light touch, pinprick, and thermal discrimination should be determined in all dermatomes correlated with the nerve root level or peripheral nerve. As previously stated, Spurling's test can be useful in determining whether the cervical spine is involved. Reflexes need to be examined bilaterally at the biceps (C5), brachioradialis (C5–C6), and triceps (C7). Altered or absent reflexes are recorded and correlated with other findings. Although the vascular tests are considered positive when changing vascular flow is noted, they also provoke the adjoining structure to the vessels, the brachial plexus. As Rayan and Jensen[105] demonstrated, healthy subjects can have neurologic symptoms with vascular test positioning, therefore, caution is required in interpreting the results.

Upper Limb Tension Test

The upper limb tension test can provide the clinician with information about the neural tissue extending from the cervical nerve roots to the peripheral nerves.[106] The test itself is not considered positive or negative but is used to help confirm a diagnosis when coordinated with the rest of the examination. This test should be performed in stages, with careful monitoring of the patient. Testing can be biased toward the median, ulnar, or radial nerve. Elvey[106] emphasizes that the examiner focus on the "feel" of tension imparted to the examiner's hand as the patient's extremity is moved. Symptoms should not be encouraged. The technique for this test is described fully in Chapter 118.

Tinel's Sign

Tinel's sign has been described as eliciting tenderness from a neuroma.[107] In fact, paresthesia caused by compression of neural tissue is augmented when assessing this sign's presence. The test can be performed anywhere along the nerve path, but the sign is best elicited over the more superficial areas of neural tissue. Areas the Tinel's sign is best assessed are Erb's point, the medial arm, the ulnar groove, medial to the common flexor tendon origin, the middle of the volar aspect of the wrist, and over the pisiform. The test is performed by tapping over the chosen area; if paresthesia or pain is produced at the region or, more typically, within the involved nerve sensory distribution, the sign is considered positive. This indicates involvement of the nerve at that level or somewhere proximal along the neural track. For example, a positive Tinel's sign is commonly elicited at the ulnar groove, yet the lesion may be in the brachial plexus.

Vascular Tests

The clinical diagnosis of vascular compromise is suggested by provocation or relief of signs and symptoms by selective anatomic positioning and alteration of tissue tensions.

The examiner must attempt to evaluate changes induced in the arterial, venous, and nervous systems during each diagnostic maneuver. Three or more distinct anatomic sites in the shoulder girdle region can be involved in the production of thoracic outlet syndrome (TOS). The classic diagnostic maneuvers attempt to provoke neurovascular disturbances by introducing mechanical forces at these specific sites.

Test maneuvers and general examination for vascular compromise are performed with the patient seated and well stabilized. All tests are performed bilaterally and compared. The examiner should begin with observation of the hands, resting palms up on the thighs. Notation of color is made in the dependent position and observed for change when in the test position. Skin temperature and moisture are noted. With the palms down and forearms pronated and resting on the thighs, the radial pulse is monitored at the wrist. The pulse volume or strength is assessed bilaterally in the rest position. Bilateral brachial blood pressures can be taken and compared. A difference of more than 30 mm Hg is significant.

Symptom reproduction or intensification is one objective of the provocative testing. The patient is asked to report the location, nature, and intensity of symptoms before each diagnostic maneuver while in the rest position and provide commentary on perceived changes during and immediately following each test. Common tests are described in Chapter

54. To more accurately diagnose vascular compromise in the clinic, performance of a battery of these tests is recommended.

Difficulties in Testing

Diagnostic accuracy can prove difficult for several reasons. The list of signs and symptoms attributed to TOS is extensive, and they are typically intermittent in nature. Changes in the radial pulse volume occur in many asymptomatic individuals; the absence of change in the radial pulse suggests the lack of significant arterial compression but does not rule out venous or neurologic involvement. Inflamed nerves are sensitized to stretch or compression distal to the site of the lesion, and more than one lesion can coexist. Paresthesias can also occur with TOS testing in asymptomatic individuals; using pain or symptom attenuation reduces the incidence of false positives with this testing.

Palpation

Palpation is performed to detect temperature changes, pain, atrophy, and swelling and to identify bony landmarks and structures such as muscle bellies and tendons. Temperature change can indicate inflammation or reduced circulation. Warmth commonly exists following surgery as the healing process continues. In severe to moderate reactive rotator cuff irritation, warmth may be noticed about the greater tuberosity.

Subtle swelling or atrophy may be palpated by symmetrically "smoothing" with the fingers the areas around the deltoid and scapular fossae for contour asymmetry. Crepitus and clicking are palpated for during both AROM and PROM. Crepitus can indicate articular or rotator cuff deficits, whereas clicking about the shoulder can be quite normal. Tracing clicking to soft tissue, labral, or articular origin can be challenging because of the ability of bones to transmit vibration. Symptomatic clicking should be noted and entered into examination data. Painless clicking, such as that which occurs at the biceps tendon when throwing, can become painful with repetitive mechanical irritation.

The examiner needs to gain appreciation for normal tender areas responding to deep palpation. These include the biceps groove, coracoid process, inferior posterior deltoid fibers, and lesser tubercle. Without prior knowledge of vulnerable tenderness or if palpated without contralateral comparison, significant erroneous information can be gathered. Knowledge of referred pain zones and trigger points is invaluable in establishing a diagnosis and treatment plan. The clinician may become frustrated when palpation is performed over the reference pain area because the lesion lies elsewhere.

Last, accurate palpation can be performed only if the clinician has appropriate knowledge of anatomy and biomechanics. Anatomic visualization is essential to strip away the overlying tissue, and biomechanical principles are required to fully expose the underlying structures. For example, although the supraspinatus insertion to the greater tuberosity lies anterior to the acromion in the resting position, full exposure is gained through humeral internal rotation, extension, and adduction.[27,84]

Sternoclavicular Joint

The sternoclavicular joint can be found easily just lateral to the sternal notch. Movement is felt as the shoulder girdle is elevated, depressed, protracted, or retracted. Abrupt joint motion occurring as the arm is elevated could indicate subluxation.

Acromioclavicular Joint

The AC joint is found at the distal lateral clavicle junction with the acromion. Point tenderness could indicate pathology, and contralateral comparison is required. Following a grade II or grade III separation, the scapula depresses as a consequence of coracoclavicular and AC ligament tearing. This results in a noticeable prominence of the distal clavicle compared with the uninvolved side (Fig. 9-38, online).

Supraspinatus

Belly. The supraspinatus muscle belly can be difficult to isolate because the upper trapezius blankets it superiorly. Commonly, in a chronic condition such as a large rotator cuff tear or a suprascapular nerve injury, atrophy is appreciated by hollowing of the fossa. Atrophy may not be present in a recent injury, and palpation to determine supraspinatus contraction during active elevation is frustrating because of the trapezius obligatory activity. To better palpate the supraspinatus muscle belly, the patient is placed in a side-lying position on the uninvolved side; this places the trapezius in a relatively gravity-eliminated position for arm elevation. The examiner then passively places the patient's involved upper extremity into abduction to approximately 60 degrees, and then, while palpating over the supraspinatus belly, the patient is asked to maintain this position. The supraspinatus belly can be felt to contract through the relatively inactive trapezius. If no contraction is felt, interruption of the muscle–tendon unit or innervation is suggested.

Musculotendinous Junction. Cyriax[27] describes palpation of the supraspinatus musculotendinous junction just posterior to the distal clavicle and anterior to the suprascapular spine. Pain at this location could indicate the lesion location.

Tendon. Full exposure of the supraspinatus tendon insertion should be gained by placing the patient's arm into functional internal rotation (Fig. 9-39, online). This position completely exposes the tenoperiosteal junction and tendon.[27] Using the anterolateral acromion as a reference, the examiner moves approximately 2 cm inferiorly; this is where the tendon and tenoperiosteal junction are palpated. The subacromial bursa also can be palpated in this position. The clinician should recognize that palpation is performed to determine if these sites are painful versus differentiating the rotator cuff tendons. Because the rotator cuff tendons are flat confluent structures and because the deltoid lies over the tendon, one can rarely "feel" the tendon.

Infraspinatus

Belly. The infraspinatus muscle belly is readily palpated in the infraspinatus fossa because no overlying musculature is present (Fig. 9-40, online).

Tendon. The patient can be placed prone or seated with the arm at 90 degrees of flexion, slight horizontal adduction, and external rotation. This displaces the infraspinatus insertion posteriorly and inferiorly to the acromion. The examiner must identify the posterior lateral acromion and palpate inferiorly approximately 1 cm. The tendon can be found distal to the muscle belly.

Subscapularis

Belly. The subscapularis muscle belly is difficult to palpate because its origin is on the ventral surface of the scapula. A position has been described for trigger point assessment in which the patient is placed supine with the arm abducted to 90 degrees, causing lateral rotation of the scapula.[15] The examiner identifies the anterior latissimus dorsi border and palpates deep into the exposed subscapularis muscle belly. Trigger points of the subscapularis are believed to be a source of pain and potentially restrict shoulder ROM.

Tendon. The subscapularis tendon and insertion into the lesser tubercle can be a source of pain. To palpate, the patient is placed upright or supine and the lesser tubercle is located by using the anterolateral acromion as a landmark. The examiner palpates inferiorly approximately 2 cm, and the arm is rotated internally and externally beneath the thumb. Movement of the tuberosities and groove is appreciated underneath the thumb. In external rotation, the lesser tuberosity is palpated; as the arm is internally rotated, the finger falls into the groove and then onto the anterior greater tuberosity. To gain greater exposure of the insertion and tendon, the humerus should be externally rotated approximately 50 degrees.

Biceps

Tendon. This structure is intra-articular and extra-articular. Trauma to the tendon has been described as commonly occurring as it wraps laterally around the lesser tuberosity. This is an area of friction, which, over time, can cause fraying and eventual rupture. The intra-articular component also can be traumatized by impingement against the overlying coracoacromial arch.

Groove. This is a normally tender area even in the asymptomatic shoulder, and bilateral comparison is essential. The patient's arm is placed at approximately 10 degrees of internal rotation, placing the groove anteriorly. The examiner finds the groove position relative to the tuberosities, as discussed under subscapularis tendon palpation (Fig. 9-41, online). The actual tendon cannot be appreciated because it lies tight in the groove and is covered by the anterior deltoid. Many clinicians mistakenly "palpate" the biceps tendon in the groove, but further discrimination reveals the septum between the anterior and middle deltoid heads. The intra-articular component can be identified over the humeral head as it runs an oblique course to the supraglenoid tubercle. This is best palpated in a very thin individual or in the presence of marked deltoid atrophy.

Deltoid

The deltoid can harbor trigger points, particularly in a patient with a chronically painful shoulder. The deltoid heads require palpation for tenderness and comparison with the uninvolved side. Commonly, the symptomatic trigger point is found in the distal anterior portion of the middle deltoid. We have found the inferior fibers of the posterior deltoid to be normally tender, possibly due to the axillary nerve superficial location.

Evaluative Friction Massage or Acupressure

Once a tender region of the contractile element has been identified, friction massage can be performed to determine the effect on signs and symptoms. The patient is initially examined and painful ranges and resisted motions determined. Friction massage or acupressure is then performed for 3 to 5 minutes to the suspected soft tissue element. The patient is then reassessed and the percentage reduction of pain reported. In essence, this is a noninvasive equivalent to the impingement test. This is more appropriate in the less reactive patient. If an area is exquisitely tender, particularly if the examination determines a high degree of reactivity, evaluative friction massage or acupressure should be deferred.

As discussed previously, palpation should be performed last to prevent premature irritation of the involved structures as well as avoiding "diagnosis prejudging." Palpation assessment quite literally places the "finishing touches" on the evaluation process. Results should confirm the history and previously gathered information regarding symptom etiology and diagnosis.

Summary

A thorough examination of the shoulder can be an integral part when assessing the upper extremity. In this chapter, we described shoulder examination in the authors' preferred order. Patient characteristics can provide insight into shoulder pathology and help aid diagnosis and classify irritability. A thorough history is critical in gaining information about the patient and his or her diagnosis, including the chief complaint and the attributes of the pain. When appropriate, information about the patient's specific surgery is essential.

The physical examination should be performed systematically, respecting the irritability of the patient and possible healing structures. Observation, postural assessment, and examination of proximal joints are invaluable for differential diagnosis and identifying possible confounding factors. An integrated examination includes testing of contractile and noncontractile tissues and, often, a myriad of special testing to confirm accurate diagnosis and create a complete picture of the patient's present status. Again, we recommend palpation as the final stage of the examination to prevent possible irritation of involved structures. In the end, fastidious examination and attention to detail maximizes the clinician's ability to form a diagnosis and prognosis and ultimately to treat the patient.

REFERENCES

The complete reference list is available online at www.expertconsult.com.

Upper Quarter Screen

PHILIP McCLURE, PT, PhD, FAPTA

INSPECTION	SENSORY SCAN
CERVICAL SPINE	PALPATION
JOINT SCAN	DEEP TENDON REFLEXES
MYOTOME SCAN	SUMMARY

CRITICAL POINTS

- The upper quarter screen is appropriate when the diagnosis is unclear or when there is potential for referred pain from more proximal structures.
- The purpose of the upper quarter screen is to determine which anatomic region of the upper quarter is contributing to the patient's symptoms and to rule out gross sensory or motor neurologic deficits.
- The examiner should observe for reproduction of the patient's chief complaint of pain or symptoms, and, when identified, a more thorough examination of that region is necessary.
- The screening examination is performed bilaterally. This is especially true for reflex testing since results in normals can vary widely.

Anatomically, the upper quarter includes the cervical spine, upper thoracic spine, and the upper extremity. Because the source of a patient's symptoms is often unclear, a screening examination can be helpful in providing an efficient mechanism for determining more precisely which region(s) may be contributing to the symptoms.[1] The upper quarter screening examination is designed to achieve two basic purposes: (1) determine which anatomic region of the upper quarter is contributing to the patient's symptoms and therefore needs to be examined in greater detail, and (2) rule out gross sensory or motor neurologic deficits consistent with a cervical radiculopathy or other source.[2,3]

A screening examination is often unnecessary when the source of a patient's symptoms or dysfunction is very clear from the history, such as with postsurgical problems or when some isolated traumatic injury has occurred to the upper extremity. The screening examination is most appropriate when the diagnosis is unclear or when there is a potential for referred pain, typically emanating from more proximal structures.

Referred pain can be simply defined as pain perceived in an area other than its source. A complete discussion of referred pain is beyond the scope of this chapter, but understanding some general characteristics of referred pain can be very helpful clinically. First, deeper, more proximal structures are most likely to refer pain.[4,5] Therefore, the majority of the upper quarter screening examination focuses on the cervical spine and shoulder. These areas are known to be potential sources able to refer pain to multiple sites in the upper extremity.[6-8] However, it is rare that distal structures in the upper extremity refer pain proximally. Referred pain is also typically described as a poorly localized, dull aching sensation.[4,5] Therefore, the patient who rubs the entire lateral aspect of the arm while describing a dull aching pain is more likely to have referred pain than a patient who, for example, complains of a sharp localized pain on the lateral aspect of the elbow.

While performing the examination, the goal is to reproduce the patient's chief complaint of pain or other symptoms. Occasionally, patients have mild restrictions in cervical range of motion (ROM) or complaints of discomfort or pulling sensations during cervical spine testing. Painless restrictions in motion or symptoms that are not part of the patient's chief complaint should not be interpreted as positive tests but more likely represent normal variations.

What is included in the screening examination varies greatly; however, a suggested format is given in the form shown as Figure 10-1. As a general rule, the vigor and extent of the examination should be based on the patient's history. The goal is to gain enough information to proceed intelligently without exacerbating the patient's symptoms

To view a companion video on this topic, please access ExpertConsult.com.

Patient Name: _____

Date: _____

Upper Quarter Screening Examination Form

Inspection:

☐ Forward head posture
☐ Asymmetry
☐ Muscle atrophy
☐ Deformity

Cervical Spine (AROM + Passive overpressure)

	Pain	↓ ROM
Flexion	☐	☐
Right rotation	☐	☐
Left rotation	☐	☐
Right Side Bend	☐	☐
Left Side Bend	☐	☐
Extension	☐	☐
Distraction	☐	
Compression	☐	
Left Spurling's	☐	
Right Spurling's	☐	

Joint Scan (AROM + Passive overpressure)

	Pain	↓ ROM
Shoulder Elevation	☐	☐
Elbow Flexion (pron/sup)	☐	☐
Elbow Extension (pron/sup)	☐	☐

Deep Tendon Reflexes

	Left	Right
Biceps	+ 1 2 3 4	+ 1 2 3 4
Brachioradialis	+ 1 2 3 4	+ 1 2 3 4
Triceps	+ 1 2 3 4	+ 1 2 3 4

Myotome Scan

	Weakness	Pain
Shoulder Shrug (C2,3,4)	☐	☐
Shoulder Abduction (C5)	☐	☐
Elbow Flexion (C5–6)	☐	☐
Elbow Extension (C7)	☐	☐
Wrist Extension (C6)	☐	☐
Wrist Flexion (C7)	☐	☐
Thumb Abduction (C8)	☐	☐
Finger Abduction/adduction (T1)	☐	☐

Sensory Scan (light touch)

	Diminished
Supraclavicular (C4)	☐
Anterolateral arm (C5)	☐
Lateral forearm/thumb (C6)	☐
Middle finger (C7)	☐
Ulnar hand (C8)	☐
Medial forearm (T1)	☐
Apex of axilla (T2)	☐

Neural Tension

	Symptoms
Shoulder abduction/external rotation + elbow extension + wrist/finger extension	☐

Palpation/Neural Compression

	Symptoms
Brachial Plexus	☐
Radial tunnel	☐
Cubital tunnel	☐
Carpal tunnel	☐

Figure 10-1 Upper quarter screening form. (This figure is available as a PDF at ExpertConsult.com)

unnecessarily. Therefore, for patients with very severe symptoms the exam should be more limited. Also, tests or motions that are anticipated to most likely provoke symptoms should be saved for the end of the examination whenever possible so as to avoid clouding the remaining tests.

The screening examination includes inspection, progressively vigorous cervical spine testing, a brief systematic scan of the peripheral joints, myotome testing for motor weakness, sensory testing for diminished light touch sensation, reflex testing, and special tests related to neural tension and palpation of common entrapment sites.

Inspection

Inspection includes observation from the side as well as anterior and posterior views. Any asymmetry should be noted as well as gross postural abnormalities. Careful attention should be given to normal soft tissue contours to observe for muscle wasting in key areas such as the supra- and infraspinous fossa (rotator cuff atrophy), and the upper trapezius and deltoid musculature (Fig. 10-2A). Anteriorly, the supraclavicular area should be inspected for any swelling (loss of normal concavity), which could represent swelling associated with brachial plexus injury as well as the potential for an upper lung tumor (Fig. 10-2B). Asymmetrical shoulder heights are

somewhat common, with the dominant side being lower than the nondominant side. However, an elevated shoulder girdle could represent protective guarding associated with a cervical spine or neural tension problem, and a low shoulder may provoke neural tension problems.

Cervical Spine

The cervical spine is probably the most common source of referred pain to the upper extremity. If the problem is from direct compression of a nerve root or spinal nerve (cervical radiculopathy), the symptoms will include either sensory disturbances or motor weakness.[3,10] More commonly, the cervical somatic tissues (ligaments, facet joints, disk, muscle) can refer pain to the upper extremity without direct neural compression.[4,5,9,11-13] In either case, the goal of the examination is to reproduce the chief complaint symptoms with ROM tests or special tests. ROM testing is done in each direction, first actively, then with passive overpressure applied at the end range if the active motion was pain-free (Fig. 10-3). Generally, cervical extension is the most provocative motion and should be performed last. If standard motions do not provoke symptoms, special tests can be performed. These include cervical distraction, the Spurling test, shoulder abduction test, and the upper limb tension test (Figs. 10-4 to 10-7). For

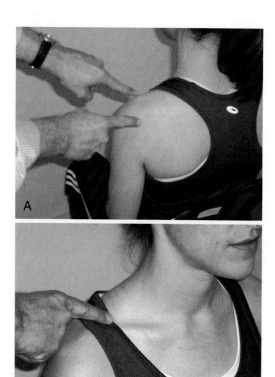

Figure 10-2 A, Normal soft tissue contours for the upper trapezius, supraspinatus, and infraspinatus muscles. **B,** Normal concavity in supraclavicular area.

cervical distraction (see Fig. 10-4A, B), patients must be relaxed, which is best accomplished by having them supine and applying traction by pulling on the occiput and mandible.[3] A positive test is diminished symptoms during distraction. Distraction may also be accomplished with the patient

seated while leaning back slightly on the chair or directly on the examiner.[14,15] Spurling's maneuver[16] as originally described involves passive sidebending with overpressure and axial loading (see Fig. 10-5); although, several authors have described the test to include ipsilateral rotation and extension. A positive test requires reproduction of the patient's chief complaint symptoms, because many patients feel some local neck discomfort during the maneuver that is not part of their symptom complex. The basis for this test is that this position maximally narrows the intervertebral foramina on the side being tested.[17] The shoulder abduction test is performed by the patient resting the hand on top of the head for approximately 30 seconds, and a positive test is when the chief complaint symptoms are reduced or eliminated (see Fig. 10-6). The upper limb tension test has many variations, but all utilize a combination of extremity movements performed sequentially to produce tension in the neural tissues.[18] Specific tests for adverse neural tension within the upper quarter are discussed more completely in Chapter 118. A simple screening maneuver for the upper quarter is the combined active motions of full shoulder abduction in the frontal plane plus elbow, wrist, and finger extension. Generally, the elbow, wrist, and fingers are extended first, and shoulder abduction is the final motion. If the chief complaint symptoms are reproduced, or shoulder abduction is appreciably reduced when combined with elbow, wrist, and finger extension, the possibility of adverse neural tension must be more fully evaluated. Wainner and colleagues[3] studied the upper limb tension test (ULTT, part A), which was performed passively with the patient supine in a sequential fashion as follows: (1) scapular depression, (2) shoulder abduction, (3) forearm supination with wrist and finger extension, (4) shoulder lateral rotation, (5) elbow extension, and (6) contralateral and ipsilateral cervical sidebending. The patient is questioned regarding reproduction of chief complaint symptoms during the entire procedure. The criteria for a positive response were any of the

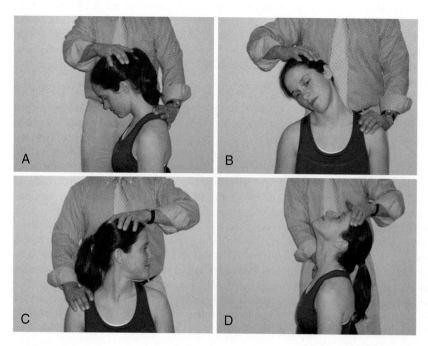

Figure 10-3 Cervical range-of-motion testing. The patient first moves to the end range actively. If no symptoms are elicited, passive overpressure is added. **A,** Flexion. **B,** Sidebending. **C,** Rotation. **D,** Extension.

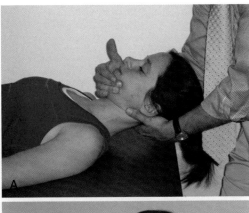

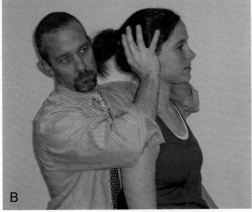

Figure 10-4 Cervical distraction. **A,** The supine position is best for relaxation and application of force but may not be efficient during a screening examination. **B,** In seating, the force is applied superiorly via the occiput. The patient must be completely relaxed which is best achieved by asking her or him to lean back on the chair or against the examiner.

following: (1) reproduction of the chief complaint symptom, (2) greater than a 10-degree difference between sides with elbow extension, (3) chief complaint symptoms increased with contralateral sidebending and decreased with ipsilateral sidebending.

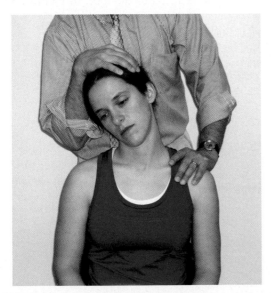

Figure 10-5 Spurling's maneuver is performed by combining cervical sidebending and axial compression to the cervical spine.

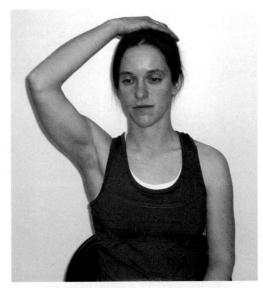

Figure 10-6 Shoulder abduction test.

A few studies have provided data regarding the ability of these special clinical tests to detect cervical radiculopathy.[2,3,15,19-21] In these studies, cervical radiculopathy was generally confirmed using needle electromyography or imaging findings as an appropriate gold standard. However, positive electromyographic or imaging findings would not necessarily be expected with referred pain from the cervical somatic tissues (i.e., disks, ligaments, facet joints, muscles), which could occur with or without direct irritation of a cervical nerve root (radiculopathy). Therefore, these studies are relevant only to screening for cervical radiculopathy and not for any referred pain emanating from the cervical spine. The findings of these studies are summarized in Table 10-1. Of particular relevance to a screening examination are the sensitivity and specificity of these tests. For screening purposes, tests with high sensitivity are most valuable because a highly sensitive test is least likely to miss a positive case (i.e., a low rate of false negatives) and is therefore useful for "ruling out." In contrast, tests with high specificity are useful for "ruling in" a specific condition, which is not the goal of a screening examination. Based on the available data, the ULTT is the most valuable screening test because of its high sensitivity. Although other tests may be useful in diagnosing radiculopathy, they are less useful as screening tests because of their generally low sensitivity. However, given generally acceptable specificity, when they are positive, patients should be examined in greater detail for a probable cervical spine-related problem.

Joint Scan

Having tested the cervical spine, the joint scan is designed to quickly ascertain whether the shoulder or elbow joints may be a source of symptoms. The idea here is to take the glenohumeral and elbow joints through full passive motion and then apply overpressure. If no symptoms are produced, this is reasonable evidence that these joints are not the source of

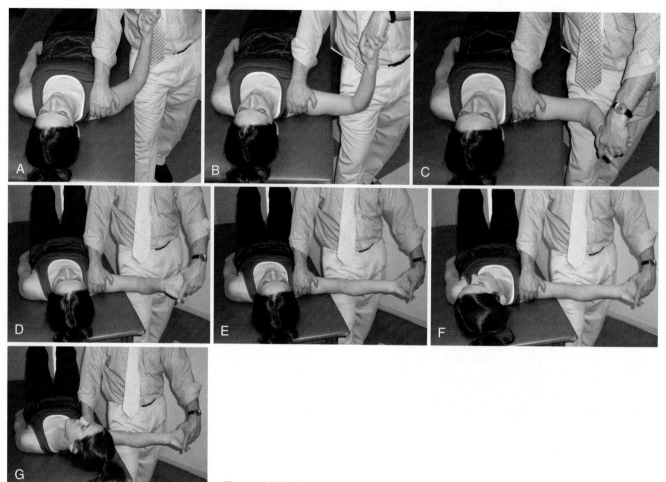

Figure 10-7 (**A–G**) Upper limb tension test (version A with median nerve bias).[3,17]

symptoms. For glenohumeral testing, the scapula must be blocked from gliding or rotating superiorly, so the stress is focused on the glenohumeral joint (Fig. 10-8). Full elbow flexion and extension are combined with pronation and supination.

Myotome Scan

During the myotome scan (Fig. 10-9), muscles that correspond to particular spinal segments are tested for the presence of weakness, as listed in the form in Figure 10-1. The

Table 10-1 Sensitivity and Specificity of Special Tests to Detect Cervical Radiculopathy*

Test and Author	Gold Standard Used for Diagnosis	Subjects with Disease	Subjects Without Disease	Sensitivity	Specificity	+LR	−LR
Distraction							
Viikari-Juntura et al.[15]	Myelography	9	35	0.44 (0.14–0.79)	0.97 (0.85–1.0)	14.7	0.58
Wainner et al.[3]	Needle EMG/NCS	19	63	0.44 (0.21–0.67)	0.90 (0.82–0.98)	4.4	0.62
Spurling's							
Shah and Rajshekhar[21]	MRI and operative findings	29	21	0.93 (0.77–0.99)	0.95 (0.76–1.0)	18.6	0.07
Tong et al.[19]	EMG	20	172	0.3 (0.12–0.54)	0.93 (0.88–0.96)	4.29	0.75
Wainner et al.[3]	Needle EMG/NCS	19	63	0.50 (0.27–0.73)	0.86 (0.77–0.94)	3.6	0.58
Shoulder Abduction							
Davidson[22]	Myelography	18	4	0.78 (0.52–0.94)	0.75 (0.19–0.99)	3.1	0.29
Viikari-Juntura et al.[15]	Myelography	13	13	0.46 (0.19–0.75)	0.85 (0.55–0.98)	3.1	0.64
Wainner et al.[3]	Needle EMG/NCS	19	63	0.17 (0.0–0.34)	0.92 (0.85–0.99)	2.1	0.90
Upper Limb Tension Test							
Quintner[23]	Plain-film radiography of the cervical spine	18	27	0.83 (0.59–0.96)	0.11 (0.02–0.29)	0.93	1.5
Wainner et al.[3]	Needle EMG/NCS	19	63	0.97 (0.90–1.0)	0.22 (0.12–0.33)	1.2	0.14

EMG/NCS: electromyography/nerve conduction study.
*Downloadable form available at ExpertConsult.com.

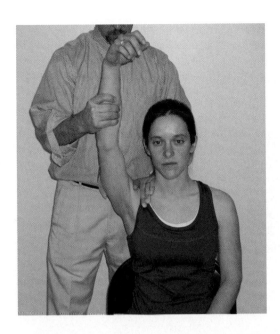

Figure 10-8 Passive stress to the glenohumeral joint is accomplished by blocking upward scapular motion with one hand while passively elevating the arm.

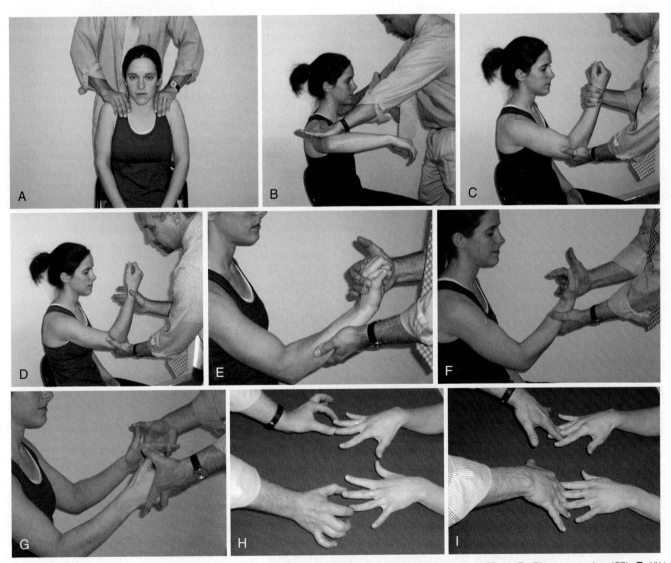

Figure 10-9 Myotome scan. **A,** Shoulder shrug (C2–4). **B,** Shoulder abduction (C5). **C,** Elbow flexion (C5–6). **D,** Elbow extension (C7). **E,** Wrist extension (C6). **F,** Wrist flexion (C7). **G,** Thumb abduction (C8). **H,** Finger abduction. **I,** Finger adduction (T1).

patient should be instructed to "hold, don't let me move you" while the examiner slowly increases the applied force in a controlled fashion. Because the primary goal here is to detect weakness associated with neurologic compromise, strength should be judged normal or diminished relative to the uninvolved side. If both sides are symptomatic, the examiner must use judgment based on past experience. The results of manual muscle testing must be interpreted cautiously because the reliability of these tests is generally poor to moderate.[3] If the strength of the muscle is questionable, some type of instrument should be used to document muscle performance more precisely. Resistance that is initially strong but then is easily broken because of pain does not represent neurologic compromise but more likely some irritation of the muscle–tendon unit itself. Painless weakness is most suggestive of neurologic compromise or a complete tear within the muscle-tendon unit.

Sensory Scan

During the sensory scan (Fig. 10-10), dermatomes that correspond to particular spinal segments are tested for the presence of diminished sensitivity to light touch as listed in the form. A cotton ball or a brush of the examiner's fingertip may be used bilaterally while the patient is asked "Do these feel the same or different?" If the patient responds "different," the examiner asks "more or less?" The examiner should be careful not to lead the patient by saying something like "Does this feel less here?"

Palpation

If the history suggests the possibility of peripheral nerve entrapment, the more common sites of entrapment may be

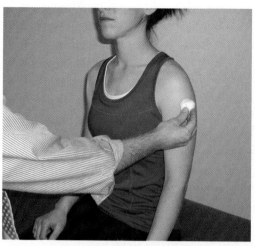

Figure 10-10 *Sensory scan shown for C5 dermatome using a cotton ball.*

palpated in an effort to reproduce the symptoms (Fig. 10-11). These sites include the brachial plexus in the supraclavicular fossa, the posterior interosseous nerve in the radial tunnel as it pierces the supinator muscle, the ulnar nerve in the cubital tunnel, and the median nerve in the carpal tunnel.

Deep Tendon Reflexes

Reflex testing (Fig. 10-12) may be helpful in determining if there is neurologic compromise; however, hyporeflexia is rather common, so care must be taken to compare reflexes bilaterally.[1,10] Hyporeflexia represents lower motor neuron compromise, which may be at the nerve root, spinal nerve, or at a more distal level. If hyper-reflexia is observed, upper

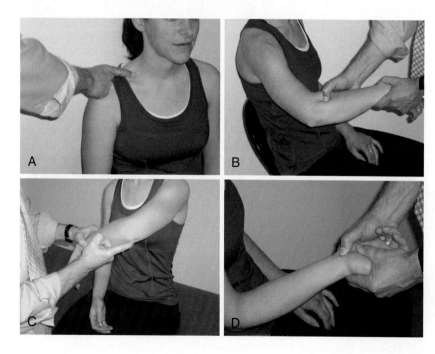

Figure 10-11 Palpation of common entrapment points. **A,** Brachial plexus. **B,** Radial tunnel. **C,** Cubital tunnel. **D,** Carpal tunnel.

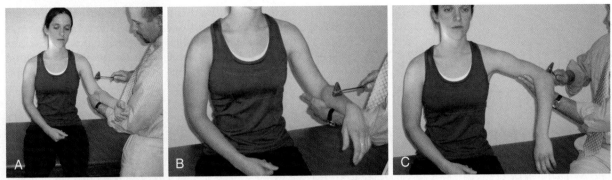

Figure 10-12 Deep tendon reflex testing. **A,** Biceps (C5). **B,** Brachioradialis (C6). **C,** Triceps (C7).

motor neuron compromise is suggested, such as might occur with spinal stenosis in the cervical region.

Summary

The upper quarter screening examination is designed to provide a quick (5–10 minute) method of (1) determining the region(s) that should be examined in greater detail and (2) ruling out serious neurologic deficits. The screen is most useful in patients whose history suggests the possibility of cervical spine involvement, referred pain, or those for whom the source of symptoms is unclear.

REFERENCES

The complete reference list is available online at www.expertconsult.com.

Sensibility Testing: History, Instrumentation, and Clinical Procedures

JUDITH A. BELL KROTOSKI, MA, OTR/L, CHT, FAOTA*

CRITICAL POINTS

- Accurate sensibility tests are useful for early recognition of peripheral nerve problems and allow early intervention and monitoring.
- Screening of touch threshold perception according to the zones and areas of peripheral nerve innervations and illustrating the results using a color-coded hand map is possible using Semmes–Weinstein-style monofilaments.
- Other sensibility tests, such as those for two-point discrimination, may add to the overall assessment of patient status.
- Assessments of sensory and motor nerve conduction velocity along with sensibility tests form a crucial basis for treatment decisions in patients with peripheral nerve problems.

Neurophysiologists are interested in "normal" sensory function.[1-6] Clinicians are interested in accurately assessing abnormal sensibility and detection thresholds.[7-12] The examiner of sensibility must determine how a client's performance on the spectrum of sensibility tests compares with a normal baseline and, if abnormal, be able to quantify the degree of change in measurable increments. In this chapter, abnormal results for sensibility measured by clinicians via various tests are referenced against normal values so that degrees of loss can be accurately assessed and monitored.

Test Instrument Considerations

Sensibility measurement instruments must have *instrument integrity* before test results can be considered *valid in clinical studies*.[8,13-16] Instrument accuracy can only be as good as the quality of stimulus input the instrument provides. For example, a sensibility test instrument that is not repeatable in force of application lacks the needed accuracy, does little to clarify, and can actually be misleading in results.

In any given skin area of 10 mm^2 there are more than 3000 sensory end organs.[3] Sensibility tests are intended to measure the physiologic function of the peripheral nerves by assessing response of their respective end-organ mechanoreceptors in the skin. All force and pressure tests used to excite sensory mechanoreceptor nerve endings in the skin (which respond to stretch or deformation) should be in repeatable force or pressure units defined by the National Institute of Standards and Technology (NIST).

Pathomechanics and Degrees of Injury

The examiner of sensibility should be aware of the normal patterns of sensory nerve innervation in the hand and upper

*I gratefully acknowledge Bill Buford, bioengineer, University of Texas at Galveston, formerly at the Paul W. Brand Research Laboratory, Gillis W. Long Hansen's Disease Center, Carville, Louisiana, for his help in reviewing the monofilament calculations, in developing instrument measurements, and collaborating on sensibility test design.

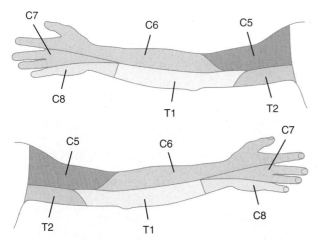

Figure 11-1 Cutaneous dermatomes of the upper extremity.

extremity as well as the typical sensory signs and symptoms that result from different levels of lesions along nerve pathways[17-20] (Figs. 11-1 and 11-2). The prognosis for recovery of function of the sensory nerves depends on which nerve structures are involved, and their degree of damage (axons, endoneurium, perineurium, or epineurium). Modes of nerve injury are mechanical, thermal, chemical, or ischemic. Swelling and inflammation can exacerbate internal and external nerve compression and compromise vital nutrition to nerve axons, particularly where the nerves must pass through tight structures. Direct injury can result in a nerve lesion in continuity (axonal conduction disruption) or in complete transection.[21,22]

Observation and interview before testing may help to identify apprehensive patients, those with exaggerated symptoms, and those whose intention is secondary gain from an injury. Often, patients provide clues as to their condition by how they hold their arms, sign papers, manipulate objects, and present themselves. If patients have a history of symptoms suggestive of peripheral nerve involvement, but test within normal limits, the examiner may use certain provocative positions, or otherwise stress the nerve in question in order to provoke symptoms that can then be measured. Stress testing can be static (e.g., sustained wrist flexion or extension at end range for 1 minute), or dynamic (e.g., putty squeezed for 5 minutes, or provocative work and activity), with sensibility measurement before and after stress.[15,21,23-25]

Nerve Conduction Velocity: A Companion Assessment

The objective of nerve conduction velocity (NCV) assessment is to determine the speed of neural conduction and, if slowed or abnormal, to determine whether more than one nerve or site is involved.[25-27] NCV does not determine if and how much a patient can and cannot actually "feel." In order to determine a subject's touch threshold detection and discrimination, tests of sensibility need to be done along with

NCV.[28,29] It is important for clinicians to understand how NCV test results fit in with sensibility test results to enable an overall interpretation of peripheral nerve status.

A common peripheral nerve condition in the upper extremity is median nerve compression at the level of the wrist, thus the median nerve is frequently initially targeted for NCV testing when numbness or tingling occur in a patient's fingers. But the astute clinician is aware that other peripheral nerves can be involved and more than one level of involvement, referred to as a "double-crush" syndrome. Furthermore, there can be, and frequently is, bilateral involvement. Patients can have nerve lesions in continuity at all segments of upper extremity nerves, including brachial plexus and thoracic outlet.[30-32] Sensory involvement usually precedes motor. Hunter and others maintain that high-level traction neuropathies commonly result from high-speed vehicular trauma, falls on the outstretched arm, repetitive assembly work (lateral abduction or overhead lifting), overuse (when heavy work exceeds physical capacity), and poor posture.[18,33,34] NCV testing from the neck to the fingers bilaterally is recommended when the initial history and physical do not readily suggest the level, type, and degree of involvement. Although valuable, NCV testing is known to vary according to the time of day, temperature of the extremity, size of the electrodes, placement of the electrodes, and instrument. In skilled hands using correctly calibrated machines, NCV testing can be accurate and repeatable.[26,33] Results of NCV and sensibility tests do loosely correlate but do not always directly correlate as evidence of peripheral nerve involvement.[14,27] "Slowing" of sensory NCV, or abnormal amplitude, along with abnormal sensibility testing, help confirm abnormal nerve function.

When NCV examination results show a "slowed" nerve conduction response, and light touch threshold tests such as the Semmes–Weinstein monofilament test demonstrate results that are "within normal limits," the clinician can assume that there is not yet a detectable change in sensory threshold detection. NCV can be reported as "absent," while the heaviest monofilaments, or a pinprick, can still be detected in some instances, signaling the nerve does have residual viable function that could potentially improve if treated. *These differences in the test results do not mean that one is more sensitive or objective, but that they are different tests and measurements of neural physiologic function.*[7,35] See Chapter 15 for a detailed discussion of nerve conduction studies.

Hierarchy and Categories of Sensibility Tests

Five hierarchal levels of sensibility testing have been described by Fess[15] and LaMotte.[2] They include the following: autonomic/sympathetic response, detection of touch, touch discrimination, quantification, and identification.

Callahan[15] divides sensibility tests into four categories: threshold tests, functional tests, objective tests and provocative or stress tests. Selected tests from these categories are discussed in the following sections. *For another perspective and more details, the reader is referred to Callahan's archived chapter on sensibility assessment on the companion Web site of this text.*

Note: Usual composition shown.
Prefixed plexus has large C4
contribution but lacks T1.
Postfixed plexus lacks C5 but
has T2 contribution.

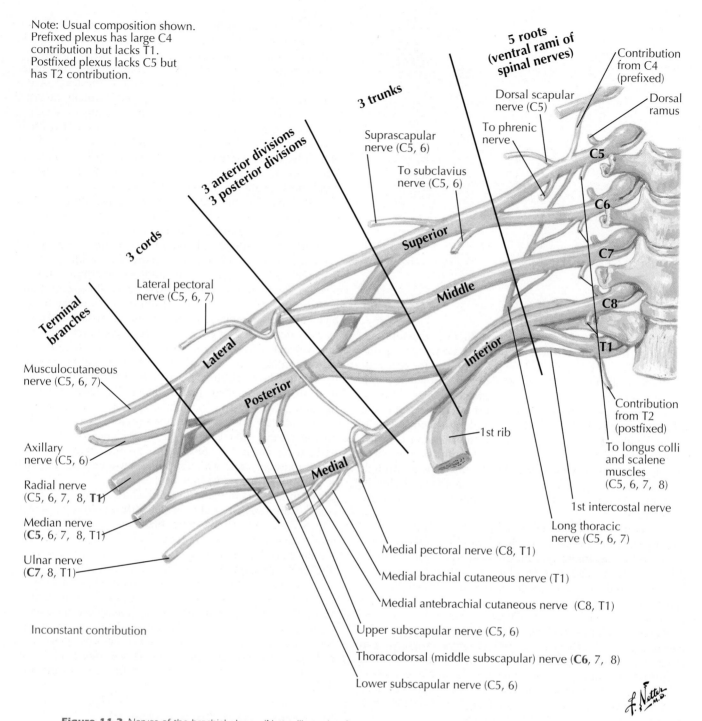

5 roots
(ventral rami of
spinal nerves)

Contribution
from C4
(prefixed)

Dorsal scapular
nerve (C5)

Dorsal
ramus

3 trunks

To phrenic
nerve

Suprascapular
nerve (C5, 6)

C5

To subclavius
nerve (C5, 6)

C6

3 anterior divisions
3 posterior divisions

C7

Superior

3 cords

C8

Lateral pectoral
nerve (C5, 6, 7)

Middle

T1

Terminal
branches

Lateral

Inferior

Contribution
from T2
(postfixed)

Musculocutaneous
nerve (C5, 6, 7)

Posterior

To longus colli
and scalene
muscles
(C5, 6, 7, 8)

Axillary
nerve (C5, 6)

1st rib

Radial nerve
(C5, 6, 7, 8, **T1**)

Medial

1st intercostal nerve

Median nerve
(**C5**, 6, 7, 8, T1)

Long thoracic
nerve (C5, 6, 7)

Ulnar nerve
(**C7**, 8, T1)

Medial pectoral nerve (C8, T1)

Medial brachial cutaneous nerve (T1)

Medial antebrachial cutaneous nerve (C8, T1)

Inconstant contribution

Upper subscapular nerve (C5, 6)

Thoracodorsal (middle subscapular) nerve (**C6**, 7, 8)

Lower subscapular nerve (C5, 6)

Figure 11-2 Nerves of the brachial plexus. (Netter illustration from www.netterimages.com. © Elsevier Inc. All rights reserved.)

Touch–Pressure Threshold Testing (Semmes–Weinstein-Style Monofilaments)

Touch–pressure threshold testing involves the use of nylon monofilaments of *standard length and increasing diameters* that provide controlled gradients of force to the mechanoreceptors in the skin to determine light-touch to deep-pressure detection thresholds (Fig. 11-3). The advantage of monofilament testing is that it provides clear, quantified, and repeatable information about the patient's detection of touch. The *pattern* of sensibility loss reflected by the monofilament testing helps to identify pathology.

It is important to note any changes in touch–pressure detection thresholds with repeated testing, but this requires the clinician's interpretation to guide the course of further treatment. Improvement in light-touch to deep-pressure

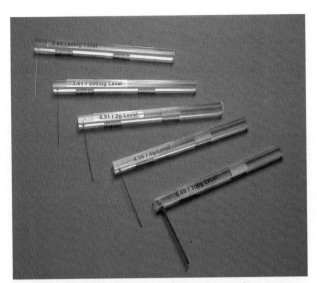

Figure 11-3 Semmes–Weinstein-style monofilaments: Hand/body screen monofilament set (5 of 20 available in full set). Critical monofilaments for monitoring in the reduced set needed for most evaluations—marking numbers 2.83, 3.61, 4.31, 4.56, and 6.65.

thresholds may be seen even in chronic conditions, episodes of worsening may occur, and the course of recovery following nerve release or suture can be predictable or complicated by scar and fibrosis. All of these occurrences can be reflected with repeat testing of touch–pressure thresholds.

The monofilament form of testing is used in patients with neuropathies, entrapment or compression syndromes, lacerations, and other abnormalities, including patients with diabetes.[36-38] The test can reveal sensibility losses in patients with Hansen's disease (HD), in which early changes are often superficial, and with worsening of the disease process, changes can mimic other peripheral nerve lesions or compression. Early testing in this situation can lead to prevention, reversal, or improvement of neural damage with timely use of steroids and other anti-inflammatory medications.[39-41]

Monofilament testing is easy to perform yet profound in the information it provides. Results are understood by the examiner, physician, insurance provider, health care gatekeeper, the patient, and others involved in treatment and employment. The versatile monofilament form of testing can be used in a 10-minute screen or for a full map showing clearly and completely in detail the area and degree of abnormality. Screening examinations are used to evaluate the autonomous areas of cutaneous innervation of the median, ulnar, or radial nerves or other sites of potential or suggested involvement.

Monofilament test results are mapped to identify the area and degree of abnormality, and repeat testing reflects changes over time. *For normative studies*, it is critical to include a lighter, above-threshold monofilament from the set of 20 so the study includes above-threshold sensitivities. Szabo[7,42] and others use all of the lighter monofilaments in the within-normal-limits functional level, along with the hand screen monofilament sizes when testing patients with possible compression or entrapment, considering it important to use the most sensitive possible. This is an accepted variation of the test when time allows, which adds additional data to the hand

screen. See studies by Szabo,[43] Gelberman,[44] and Lundborg[45] for their protocols.

Examiners sometime include additional monofilaments in the heavy range with the hand screen monofilaments. The 5.07, 10-g level monofilament is most frequently added, specifically for testing of the diabetic foot for measuring gross protective sensation of the plantar surface.[46,47] Some prefer 4.56, 4-g level monofilament (already included in the hand screen kit) for screening protective sensation of the foot.[7,13]

It is important to consider that the patient's activities immediately prior to testing can influence the testing results. For example, if the patient has had a relatively stress-free morning, after sleeping late, having a good breakfast, and a more quietly paced and lighter-duty work schedule than is normal routine, the results of testing may be better than after heavy-duty work of a few hours' duration. Hunter terms this condition *transient stress neuropathy* and recommends monofilament testing after activities and positions that reproduce their symptoms.[33]

Sensitivity

Monofilament testing can detect abnormal sensory threshold responses all over the body, even on the face, where sensitivities exceed that of the hand, and on the plantar contact area of the foot, where slightly heavier detection thresholds allow for callus.[7,48,49] The force range of the monofilaments in available diameter sizes is 4.5 mg, for the lightest, to over 300 g for the heaviest. Semmes and Weinstein[50] and Weinstein[51,52] found that within normal subjects, differences can be found between men and women, the left- and right-handed, and among age groups. *For most clinical testing, however, it is not as important to use the very lightest above-threshold monofilaments as it is to determine if the patient is normal or not.* The 2.83 marking number (50-mg level monofilament) is then the most important of the monofilaments available. It is the last of the lightest monofilaments falling within normal limits for screening of men and women and right and left hands.[50-53]

Nylon monofilament force of application was examined by Bell-Krotoski and Buford at the Paul W. Brand Research Laboratory.[7,13,54-56] Nylon material was obtained, tested, and used for sets researched and produced at the former Gillis W. Long Hansen's Disease Center (GWLHDC), Carville, Louisiana, in 1989. All sets were made to Weinstein's original specifications for *diameter size and length of 38 mm*. Bell-Krotoski provided these original specifications for sets first produced by North Coast Medical (NCM). Both the GWLHDC sets and NCM sets were then used in a normative study by six examiners who tested 131 subjects (262 hands, 520 tests; 182 feet, total 364 tests).[48] In this study, *which used the standard protocol detailed in this chapter and included all of the lighter monofilaments*, the 2.83 (marking number) 50-mg level monofilament was confirmed as the optimal size for within-normal-limits screening for males and females, right and left hands, and all over the body, except the plantar contact area of the foot where the 3.61 (marking number) 200-mg level was found to be a better predictor of normal[57] (Fig. 11-4, online).

A normal person is not expected to detect the 2.83, 50-mg level monofilament 100% of the time, but a normal person can detect this level of monofilament force of application most of the times it is applied. The correlation of monofilament sizes with functional levels of detection was developed by von Prince and Butler, Werner and Omer, and as used today by Bell (Bell Krotoski).[7,58,59] Those who detect a 3.61-size monofilament (but not lighter) also have difficulty in discerning textures and symbols drawn on the fingertips (*"diminished light touch"*) (Table 11-1).

In repeated measurements over time using standard specifications for this size monofilament (7 mil diameter, and 38-mm length) the 3.61 monofilament size was found to measure a more sensitive 200-mg level, not actually reaching the 400-mg level shown in Weinstein's original calculated forces[13,57,60–62] (Table 11-2). Both 200- and 400-mg forces fall in the diminished-light-touch functional level of detection. It is important that manufacturers of the monofilaments appreciate the fact that *if the length or diameter of a monofilament is changed from that used in the normative and clinical studies according to Weinstein's original specifications, these studies no longer apply for interpretation* of test results with the changed monofilaments for accuracy and reliability. It is recommended that the force of application for each monofilament should remain that of the original design with the standard 38-mm length and specified diameters.[13,63]

Table 11-1 Interpretation Scale for Monofilaments

		Filament Markings*	Calculated Force (g)
Green	Normal	1.65–2.83	0.0045–0.068
Blue	Diminished light touch	3.22–**3.61**	0.166–0.408
Purple	Diminished protective sensation	3.84–**4.31**	0.697–2.06
Red	Loss of protective sensation	**4.56–6.65**	3.63–447
Red-lined	Untestable	>6.65	>447

*Minikit monofilaments are in **bold**. Descriptive levels based on other scales of interpretation and collapse of data from 200 patient tests.
Force data, used with permission, from Semmes J, Weinstein S: *Somatosensory Changes After Penetrating Brain Wounds in Man*, Cambridge, Mass.: Harvard University Press, 1960.

Touch–pressure detection thresholds increase to gram levels with more severe degrees of nerve loss.[63-65] Hand screening determines magnitude of response in established functional sensibility levels, beginning with within-normal limits and progressing to diminished light touch, "diminished protective sensation," "loss of protective sensation," "deep pressure sensation," or unresponsive.

Table 11-2 Monofilament Marking Numbers, Force Comparisons, and Diameters

MN	CF (g)	S-WF (g)	LMF (g)	B-TMMAF (g)	ASD (g)	Diameters (inches)	Diameters (mm)
1.65	0.0045	0.0045	0.0040	0.0081	0.000	0.0025	0.064
2.36	0.0229	0.0230	0.0094	0.0146	0.002	0.003	0.076
2.44	0.0276	0.0275	0.034	0.0346	0.004	0.004	0.102
–2.83	0.068	0.0677	0.091	0.0798	0.007	0.005	0.127
3.22	0.166	0.1660	0.112	0.1722	0.012	0.006	0.152
–3.61	0.408	0.4082	0.213	0.2171	0.025	0.007	0.178
3.84	0.693	0.6968	0.562	0.4449	0.030	0.008	0.203
4.08	1.20	1.194	0.977	0.7450	0.060	0.009	0.229
4.17	1.48	1.494	1.58	0.9765	0.082	0.010	0.254
–4.31	2.05	2.062	1.85	2.35	0.16	0.012	0.305
–4.56	3.64	3.632	2.81	4.19	0.33	0.014	0.356
4.74	5.51	5.500	3.14	4.64	0.62	0.015	0.381
4.93	8.53	8.650	10.60	5.16	0.81	0.016	0.406
5.07	11.80	11.7	17.0	7.37	0.86	0.017	6.432
5.18	15.20	15.0	18.6	12.50	1.17	0.019	0.483
5.46	28.90	29.0	22.3	20.90	1.68	0.022	0.559
5.88	76.00	75.0	73.2	46.54	3.67	0.029	0.711
6.10	126.00	127.0	86.5	84.96	7.92	0.032	0.813
6.45	283.00	281.5	—	164.32	15.33	0.040	1.016
–6.65	448.00	447.0	—	279.40	21.75	0.045	1.143

	Filament Index	Application Force Mean, Minikit Filaments from Standard Kit (g)	Application Force Mean, Previous Minikit Test Results (g)
Minikit Screen filaments	–2.83	0.080	0.072
	–3.61	0.213	0.205
	–4.31	2.35	2.35
	–4.56	4.19	4.91
	–6.65	279.00	192.22

One tester, seven complete testing kits.
The range of forces for all filaments can be read as the mean plus or minus the SD value. Note in offset the comparison of means of filaments in the minikits and minikit filaments tested in the long kits.
ASD, average standard deviation; B-TMMAF, Bell-Tomancik measured mean application force; CF, calculated force based on buckling equation; LMF, Levin Pearsall, and Ruderman measured force; MN, marking number derived from log scale; S-WF, Semmes–Weinstein force.
Reprinted, with permission, from Table V, Bell JA, Tomancik E. Repeatability of testing with Semmes–Weinstein monofilaments. *J Hand Surg.* 1987;12A:155.

Instrument Integrity

The monofilaments clearly have been shown to be accurate and their results repeatable if the instrument is calibrated correctly.[65] The monofilaments bend when the predetermined threshold for that size is applied to the patient and cannot go beyond if applied correctly.[13] The elastic properties of the nylon monofilament material provides the instrument with the unique ability to dampen the vibration of the examiner's hand that occurs with hand-applied devices that do not control for this vibration.[63] In extensive materials testing, characteristics of the nylon used to manufacture the monofilaments was found to be important.[35] Additives during manufacture can change nylon's physical properties, that is, the force of application. Nylon fishing line is beginning to be used by some manufacturers of the filaments, but it is extruded on rolls instead of in straight lengths. Any rolled nylon when extruded does not hold repeatable calibration, even if artificially heat-straightened and, thus, cannot be recommended. Clinicians should recognize and replace any nylon monofilament that is bent and stays bent.

Straight-length, extruded nylon holds calibration, even if curved slightly, until damaged, because nylon has an indefinite shelf life.[57] The elasticity of straight-length nylon monofilament and its bending and recovery at a specific force means the force it can apply is limited and controlled, thus *the monofilament form of testing with pure straight nylon is force-controlled.*

Some of the monofilaments in the full set of 20 have been found to be so close in force of application that they occasionally overlap and represent the same force[62] (see Table 11-2). Those examiners concerned with losing test sensitivity because they are not using all 20 monofilaments need to consider that sensitivity is better using the hand screen set where the forces never overlap, rather than the full set, where some overlap is possible.

Sidney Weinstein and his physicist son Curt Weinstein developed the Weinstein Enhanced Sensory Test (WEST) following review and discussion with Bell Krotoski and Fess regarding abnormal functional levels, and the Hand Screen set.[57,66] The Weinsteins improved on Bell Krotoski's "pocket filament" prototype of the Hand Screen monofilaments in one handle, by rounding monofilament tips, and designing a less fragile handle[35,57,66] (Fig. 11-5). The Weinsteins certify the WEST monofilament force of application, and do slightly adjust the lengths toward Weinstein's original calculated forces. The WEST monofilament set is recommended for research (available through Connecticut Bioinstruments, Connecticut) but the difference in stimulus needs to be considered when attempting to compare the WEST with threshold and functional scales of interpretation developed from Weinstein's standard style monofilaments. The tip geometry has changed, and force of application differs slightly from standard sets used. Although the instruments are very close in stimuli, additional clinical testing is needed to determine how the WEST compares with the original standard monofilament design in test stimuli and if the interpretation scales are applicable for the WEST.

Instrument handle variations may not affect the specified monofilament force of application if the nylon is maintained at a 90-degree angle to the handle, and force of the monofilament

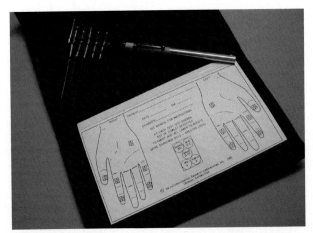

Figure 11-5 Weinstein Enhanced Sensory Test (WEST). Hand screen/ body screening monofilaments in one handle, and rounded application tips.

applied to the skin is correct and at a distance from the examiner's hand. These two criticisms of Semmes–Weinstein-style monofilaments have been addressed in a new handle design: the examiner's difficulty in seeing the tip of the lightest monofilaments on application, and the monofilaments' breaking at the point it leaves the handle. The new handle design extends over the monofilament where it exits from the handle and includes a light to illuminate the skin being tested, while keeping the 90-degree orientation of the monofilament to the rod handle. This new handle design prevents the monofilament from being sheared off by a neighboring monofilament, from being laid down upon itself, and from damage when inadvertently dropped[55] (available at timely-neuropathytesting.com) (Fig. 11-6).

Calibration

If made of pure nylon, and the diameter size and length are correct, the standard Semmes–Weinstein-style monofilament instrument stimulus has been found to be repeatable within a small specified standard deviation.[13,65] The monofilament length can be checked to be 38 mm with a millimeter ruler.

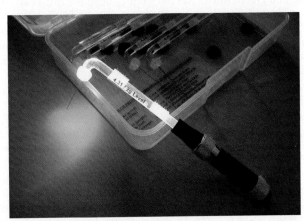

Figure 11-6 BK CLEAR Lighted Monofilaments. Bell-Krotoski JA. Device for evaluating cutaneous sensory detection, notice of publication of application, United States Patent and Trademark Office, US-2009-0105606-A1, 2009.

Diameters can be checked with a micrometer. Because the monofilaments are not always perfectly round, diameters are taken three times and averaged. (See diameters in Table 11-2).

Clinicians either need to request actual monofilament calibration measurements on test sets they use or measure their sets to confirm calibration. Monofilaments are applied 10 times and averaged for application force measurement. Nevertheless, it is most accurate to use the same set for retesting.[57] It is not enough just to state in studies that a calibrated instrument was used, or say sets used are made to specifications based on a published calculated table of application force.[50]

A known problem in measurement of monofilament application force is the use of top-loading balance scales in an attempt to measure monofilament force of application. For most who attempt monofilament calibration, these scales are inaccurate in measuring the monofilament "dynamic" force of application because the instruments are intended for measuring static weight, and depend on an internal spring mechanism that works against the elasticity of the nylon.[13]

Bell and Buford specifically engineered an instrument measurement system to be sensitive enough to measure dynamic force application and range of the monofilaments, in addition to any other hand-held sensory testing instruments (Fig. 11-7). The signature of a monofilament repeatedly applied was accurately displayed in real time on an oscilloscope, measured, and examined for spikes in force, vibration of the tester's hand, or subthreshold application.[13,65] The lightest monofilaments were applied to a calibrated strain gauge accurate to less than 1 g. If applied too quickly (less than 1.5 seconds) and "bounced" against the skin, the monofilament force of application will spike, overshoot, and exceed intended force of application, thus technique of application is important.[65] A spectrum analyzer (not shown) was used in the measurement system to detect the force frequency of application. Frequency signal outputs from the lightest to the heaviest monofilament were detected throughout the available frequency spectrum, negating claims that the monofilaments only test low- or high-frequency (slowly or quickly adapting) end-organ response.[13,63]

In recent years, mechanical engineer researchers James Foto and Dave Giurintano have reproduced the earlier strain-gauge transducer design and engineered the force output to be read directly on a computer. This system, like the original, can measure any hand-held sensibility testing device, but allows former analog measurements to be digital in real time. Computer calculations of force of application and standard deviation help eliminate potential examiner error in calculations of average force (developed in Labview scientific program, National Instruments, Austin, Texas). A still more recent development adds a motorized attachment to apply the monofilament to the measurement system (Fig. 11-8). All variations in hand-held application are thus eliminated for measurement. Foto and Giurintano initiated this automation in a project between Louisiana State University and the Paul W. Brand Research Laboratory, National Hansen's Disease, Programs (NHDP) now in Baton Rouge, Louisiana.

Clinical Validity

Three applications of the lightest monofilaments are used in clinical testing even though the patient usually responds to

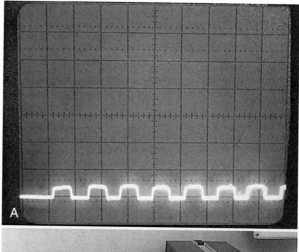
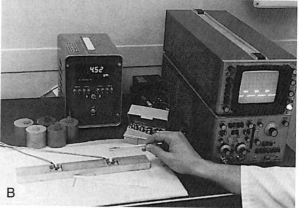

Figure 11-7 A, Oscilloscope screen showing force on repeated application of the 2.83 (marking number) within normal limits Semmes–Weinstein monofilament (250 mg/division). The instrument application force is highly repeatable within a very small range if the lengths and diameters of the monofilaments are correct. **B,** Sensory Instrument Measurement System used to measure any hand-held instrument "dynamic" force of application.

the first application. It was found in instrument testing that one touch of these extremely light monofilaments may not reach the required threshold, but one out of three always reaches intended threshold.[13,66,68] Clinical studies and papers *that require two out of three, three out of five, or one out of five,*

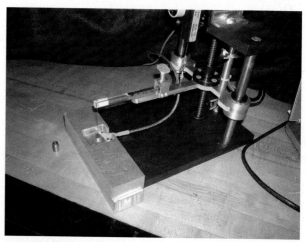

Figure 11-8 Automated application to Sensory Instrument Measurement System for elimination of any hand-held variable in force measurement.

and so forth for a correct response are incorrect, as this is not the test protocol used in normative studies and clinical studies for functional levels (which requires one correct response out of three trials).[50,52,57,61]

When calibrated and applied correctly, the monofilaments are a valid test for determining sensibility detection thresholds. Studies have clearly demonstrated their ability to accurately detect intended clinical conditions.[15,21,27,44,69] Used in standard consistent protocols, the monofilament test is able to compare patient data in individual and multicenter studies and is providing information regarding peripheral nerve changes with treatment not previously available with less sensitive and uncontrolled instruments.[9,40,41,70] When calibrated correctly, it is one of the few, if not the only, sensibility measurement instrument that approaches requirements for an objective test.

Comparison with Other Tests of Sensibility

Weinstein found that the normal detection threshold for touch pressure does not vary widely over the entire body.[51] The relative consistency is what makes light-touch/deep-pressure threshold mapping of the cutaneous innervation of the peripheral nervous system possible. This is in contrast to point localization and two-point discrimination thresholds.

Depending on the question, one may need more than one test of sensibility to obtain an adequate picture of neural abnormality. *The monofilaments do not measure end-organ innervation density.* Once monofilament threshold is screened or mapped to establish areas of abnormality, other tests such as two-point discrimination and point localization can be focused in abnormal areas to help further qualify and quantify abnormal sensibility as to innervation density and localization of touch.

It is known that monofilament testing can sometimes reveal peripheral nerve compression before conventional two-point discrimination tests and reveal return of innervation long before two-point discrimination is measurable at the fingertips.[57] Authors and clinicians have traditionally championed one or more methods of sensibility testing, and clinicians should understand that to determine the relative control and validity of another instrument versus the monofilaments, a comparison study requires a valid protocol with direct comparison of instrument stimulus and results, not just opinion.

The first sign of nerve return after laceration and repair is not the heaviest monofilament but a positive Tinel's test distal to the site of repair.[71] A positive Tinel's test—in which there is perception of shocking and shooting electrical sensations—is a valuable, albeit subjective, indicator of returning nerve physiologic response after laceration concurrent with or before the heaviest touch–pressure threshold can be measured. Since peripheral nerve return occurs from proximal to distal, Tinel's test, like the monofilament test, shows improvement proximally to distally over time.

Background Needed for Understanding

Von Frey[72] was the inventor of the monofilament form of testing using horsehairs only capable of producing light thresholds. Weinstein first invented the 20 nylon monofilaments, added heavier levels of detection, and did normative studies.[50] The range of forces of the monofilaments occur simply from available diameter sizes of nylon. In studies, they

cannot be treated as occurring at equal mathematical increments as some researchers have done. Today the monofilament log numbers are primarily used as marking numbers for ordering and specifying diameter size[35,63-65] (see Table 11-1).

Von Prince[58] was greatly influenced by Moberg's emphasis on sensibility and hand function.[73] She began investigating the residual function of patients who had sustained a variety of peripheral nerve injuries from war wounds. She observed that *of two patients who could not tell a difference in testing between one and two points, one could feel a match that would burn his finger, and the other could not.* She thus described the all important *"level of protective sensation"* that was not being measured by the Weber[74] two-point discrimination test frequently used in practice. She also noticed that of two patients who responded to a pinprick, one would have the ability to discriminate textures and one would not. Thus she first described a "level of light touch sensation" that could be equated with the patient's ability to discriminate textures. As she searched for tests that would be able to discern these differences in patients, she found the answer in Weinstein's monofilament test. Von Prince published her findings but was transferred overseas before fully completing her investigation. Omer realized the value of the monofilament test and insisted it be continued by Werner.[59]

James M. Hunter, originator of the Hand Rehabilitation Center, Ltd., in Philadelphia, realized the value of monofilament testing in producing information on patient neural status that was not forthcoming from other examinations. He insisted on this form of testing for his patients, many of whom came to him with previously longstanding unresolved peripheral nerve problems. But the test originally took 2 hours when included with other sensory tests and was confounded by inconsistent coding and the inclusion of other tests for interpretation.

Working with Hunter in 1976, Bell (later Bell-Krotoski) made changes to the test to make consistent peripheral nerve mappings and eliminate variables. Changes included (1) a constant scale of interpretation for the entire upper extremity rather than the interpretation scale changed for thumb, fingers, and palm, (2) eliminating two-point discrimination as a requirement for light touch, (3) eliminating point localization as a requirement for a "yes" response," and (4) adding consistent colors from cool to warm for quick recognition of increase in force required for detection of touch–pressure. Results of mappings serially compared for changes in neural status could then be easily recognized in seconds numerically and visually for extent and severity of peripheral nerve abnormality. The mappings were found to predict the rate of neural return or diminution, as well as of the quality of neural return or severity of diminution (Figs. 11-9 to 11-11).

After 2 years of testing with the revised test in a battery of other sensibility tests, it was found that not all of the monofilaments were needed to obtain results in functional levels of sensibility[7] (Fig. 11-12). This work was based on over 200 tests of patients with nerve compressions and lacerations at the Hand Rehabilitation Center, Ltd, Philadelphia, PA. The interpretation scale and test protocol were later used in still other studies, becoming the standard in monofilament testing.[7]

At the time this work was published in the first edition of this text, the scale of interpretation was found to largely agree

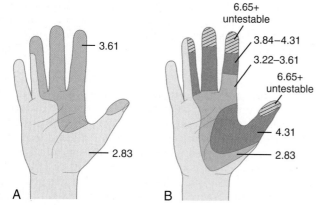

Figure 11-9 A, Monofilament mapping showing a median nerve compression as measured in a woman with a history of numbness for 2 years and no corrective intervention. **B,** Same patient as measured 4 months later. Touch–pressure recognition has become worse from diminished light touch to untestable with monofilaments in fingertips.

with threshold studies of von Prince and colleagues, and that of Omer and Werner in levels of "functional discrimination and recognition." These independent works are significant in their similar agreement corroborating the relative relationship of monofilament threshold detection with functional discrimination. The hand screen monofilaments evolved from the standard scale of interpretation by selecting the

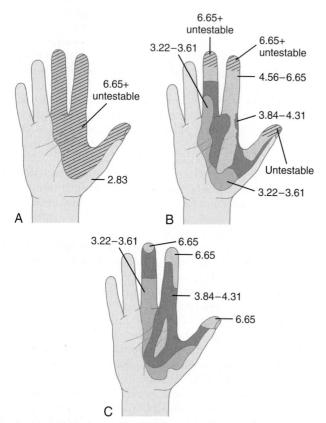

Figure 11-10 A, Monofilament mapping showing a median nerve laceration before surgery. Two-point untestable. **B,** Same patient 3 months after surgery. Two-point untestable. **C,** Same patient 7 months after surgery. Two-point untestable, fingertips now testable with monofilaments.

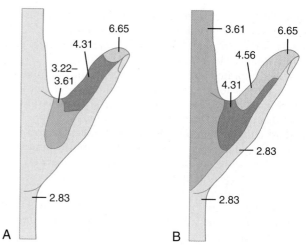

Figure 11-11 A, Two years after incomplete amputation of right thumb. Digital nerves were not resutured. Small centimeter pedicle of dorsal skin was intact. **B,** Same patient after injection of lidocaine around median nerve to determine whether innervation was radial nerve or median. Notice that although the volar thumb sensation was downgraded, it and the palmar area of the median nerve did not become asensory. This finding brings into question the blocking of the contralateral nerve in testing. Such blocks may be incomplete and lead to false conclusions.

heaviest monofilament falling within normal limits, and one monofilament corresponding with each functional discrimination level.[7]

Test Protocol

Quiet Room

All sensibility testing is best performed in a quiet room that has good light and normal room temperature. A quiet testing area is mandatory. The hand/extremity being tested is extended by the patient and comfortably relaxed resting on a rolled towel. A folder or screen is used to block the patient's line of vision from the site tested. (Theraputty as an anchor and blindfolds are not recommended.)

History

A thorough patient history helps focus testing where most needed. Unless a higher lesion is suggested, it is often necessary to examine only the hands with the monofilaments, although it is possible to test the entire body when indicated.

Reference Area

Using the 2.83 monofilament it is important to *establish a reference area that is within normal limits that the patient always responds to.* This can be done while demonstrating the monofilaments and reassuring the patient that they do not hurt. An area more proximal on the extremity or alternate extremity usually suffices, but the back, or face, can also be used. *This reference area helps the clinician to eliminate guessing and ensure attention.* If the patient does not respond in a test area, then the reference area is revisited in order to ensure there is still a response in the reference area used as

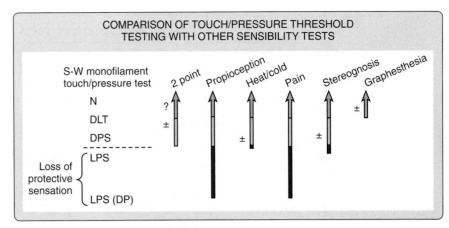

Figure 11-12 Comparison of monofilament touch–pressure detection testing with other sensibility tests.

a control. Then the test area can be rechecked to confirm that what the patient does not detect in the test area can be detected in the reference area.

Consistent Colors

On the hand map, colors from cool to warm are used to document the monofilament level detected for each area tested. Each color corresponds with force of application detected and its corresponding functional sensibility level.

Application

Monofilament testing begins with filaments in the normal threshold level and progresses to filaments of increasing force/pressure until the patient can identify touch. The filaments 1.65 to 4.08 are applied three times to the same test spot, with *one response out of three considered an affirmative response.*

All the filaments are applied in a perpendicular fashion to the skin surface in 1 to 1.5 seconds, continued in pressure in 1 to 1.5 seconds, and lifted in 1 to 1.5 seconds. The filaments 1.65 to 6.45 should bend to exert the specific pressure. The 6.65 filament is relatively stiff and found most repeatable if applied just to bending.

On initial patient testing, the patient's baseline detection level is established. On subsequent testing, the previous test serves as a comparison to establish the direction of change and improvement or worsening, if any. It is most accurate for the same examiner to repeat successive evaluation, if possible. But if instrument specification, protocol, and technique are kept standard, testing can be repeatable among examiners, whether in Japan or California. Testing by other examiners is often used in a double-blind design for studies.

Hand Screen

A hand screen examination facilitates more frequent testing and monitoring of patients over time with treatment. The hand screen monofilament sizes include normal, 2.83 (marking number) 50-mg level; diminished light touch, 3.61 (marking number) 200-mg level; diminished protective sensation 4.31 (marking number) 2-g level; and loss of protective sensation. Two filaments are included for the loss of protective sensation level, the lightest of these is 4.56

(marking number) 4-g level, important to define loss of protective sensation versus lighter diminished protective sensation, and the heaviest 6.65 (marking number) over 300-g level, needed for determining residual sensation or returning nerve function.

Test sites specific to the median nerve are the tip of the thumb, index, and proximal index. (The radial base of the palm is avoided to eliminate innervation from the recurrent branch of the median nerve.) Test sites specific to the ulnar nerve are the distal little finger, proximal phalanx, and ulnar base of the palm. The test site specific for the radial nerve is the dorsal aspect of the thumb webspace. These represent the minimum critical consistent data points for monitoring the peripheral nerves (Fig. 11-13A, B).

The test protocol for the hand screen (can also screen any area of the body) is the same as for mapping, except that fewer test sites are used. Usually monofilaments always used are the five most critical, although sets of six monofilaments are becoming available [including the 5.07 (marking number) 10-g level]. Predetermined, consistent sites are recorded for monofilament response for that site. Because there are limited test sites in a screen test versus a mapping, *an examiner revisits a nonresponsive test site at least three times to ensure a monofilament is not detected at that site.*

Mapping

Note and draw on a recording form any unusual appearances on the hands, including sweat patterns, blisters, dry or shiny skin, calluses, cuts, blanching of the skin, and so on.

1. Draw a probe across the area to be tested in a radial-to-ulnar and proximal-to-distal manner. Ask the patient to describe where and if his or her feeling changes. Do not ask for numbness because the patient's interpretation of numbness varies. Draw the area described as "different" with an ink pen (Fig. 11-14). The examination is easier if the patient can identify the gross area of involvement as a reference; if the patient cannot, proceed the same way on testing but allow more testing time.

2. Establish an area of normal sensibility as a reference. Familiarize the patient with the filament to be used and demonstrate it in a proximal control reference area.

Program Name:		**HAND SCREEN RECORD**		Initial F/U — —	Date:
Patient's Name *(Last, First, Middle)*:			Date of Birth:	SS No.	ID No:
Patient's File No.	Medications:			Date Diagnosis:	Date Onset:

Section I. **SENSORY TESTING:** Use first filament (A) at site indicated *(apply three times)*: If no response, use next heavier filament to determine level of loss.

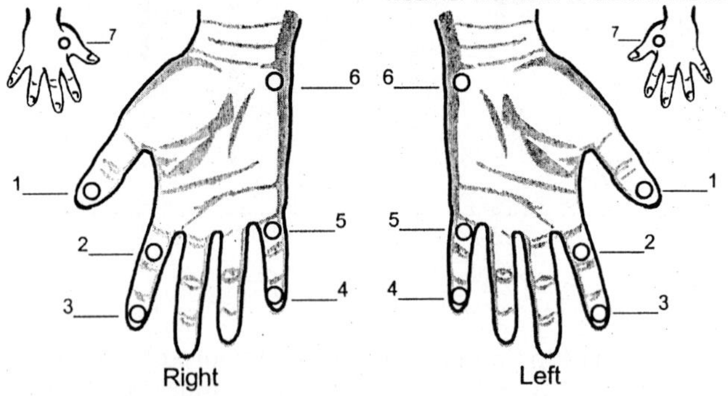

Right   Left

Filament	Force, gms	Interpretation	(Grade Pts.)
A Green (2.83)	0.05	Normal	(5)
B Blue (3.61)	0.20	Residual Texture	(4)
C Purple (4.31)	2.00	Residual Protective Sensation	(3)
D Red (4.56)	4.00	Loss of Protective Sensation	(2)
E Orange (6.65)	300.00	Residual Deep Pressure	(1)

Section II. **SKIN INSPECTION:** Draw and label *(above)*: **W** - Wound, **C** - Callus, **S** - Swelling, **R** - Redness, **D** - Dryness, **T** - Temperature, **M** - Missing, **J** - Contracture, **O** - Other

Section III. **MUSCLE TESTING:**   Mark *(below)*: **S** = Strong, **W** = Weak, **P** = Paralysis   *(or Grade 5 to 0)*

(Ulnar Nerve)   (Median Nerve)   (Radial Nerve)

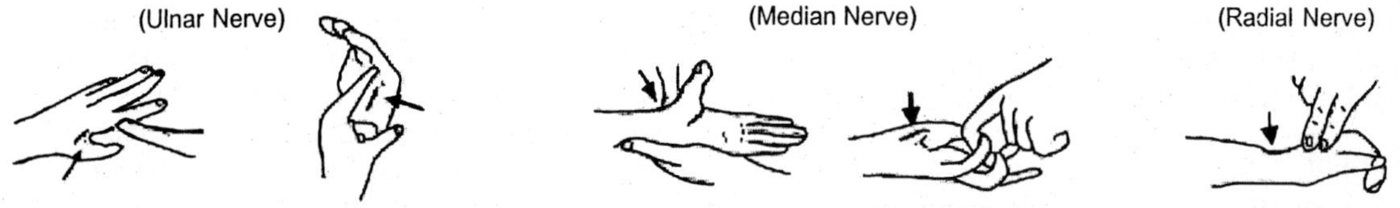

R__ L__   R__ L__   R__ L__   R__ L__   R__ L__

1) Index finger
Abduction (FDI)   2) Little Finger
MP Joint Flex. (L)   3) Thumb Abduction
Out of Palm (APB)   4) Thumb to Little
Finger (OP)   5) Radial Wrist
Extension (ECR)

Section IV. **PERIPHERAL NERVE RISK:** Mark: **U** = Ulnar, **M** = Median, **R** = Radial, (or **UM**)

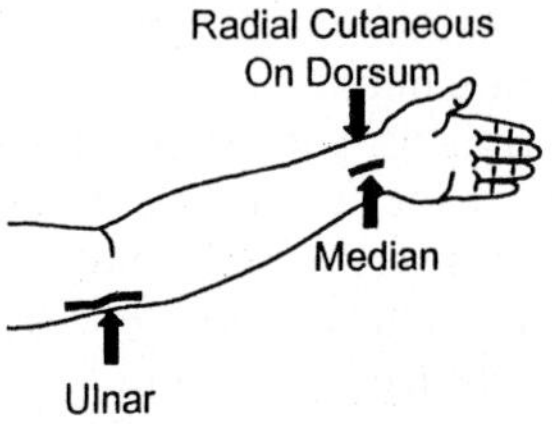

Radial Cutaneous
On Dorsum

Median

Ulnar

1) Enlarged or swollen nerve   R ___   L ___
2) Tender / painful on stretch or compression   R ___   L ___
3) Sensory change in the last 12 months   R ___   L ___
4) Muscle change in the last 12 months   R ___   L ___

High Risk *(acute or changing nerve)*   Yes ___   No ___
(refer to physician / therapist)

Section V. **DEFORMITY RISK:** *(Check if present)*

1) Loss of Protective Sensation   R ___   L ___   4) Injuries *(wounds, blisters, etc.)*   R ___   L ___
2) Clawed but Mobile Hand   R ___   L ___   5) Contracted or Stiff Joints   R ___   L ___
3) Fingertip Absorption (Mild___ Severe___) R ___   L ___   6) Wrist Drop *(radial nerve)*   R ___   L ___

High Risk *(any of the above)*:   Yes ___   No ___
(refer for appropriate treatment)

Has there been a **change in the hand since last exam**?   Yes ___ No ___

Examined by:_____

A

Figure 11-13 A, Hand screen record.

Program Name:	PERIPHERAL NERVE MONITORING			
Patient's Name *(Last, First, Middle)*:		Date of Birth:	SS No:	ID No:
Patient's File No.	Other Diagnoses:		Date Diagnosis:	Date Onset:

Right

1 FDI ___ 4 OP ___
2 L ___ 5 ECR ___
3 APB ___

1) Enlarged Nerve ___
2) Tender Nerve ___
3) Sensory Change ___
4) Muscle Change ___

1) Protective Loss ___
2) Clawed/MobileJts ___
3) Absorption:
Mild ___ Severe ___
4) Injuries ___
5) Contracted/Stiff Jts ___
6) Wrist Drop ___

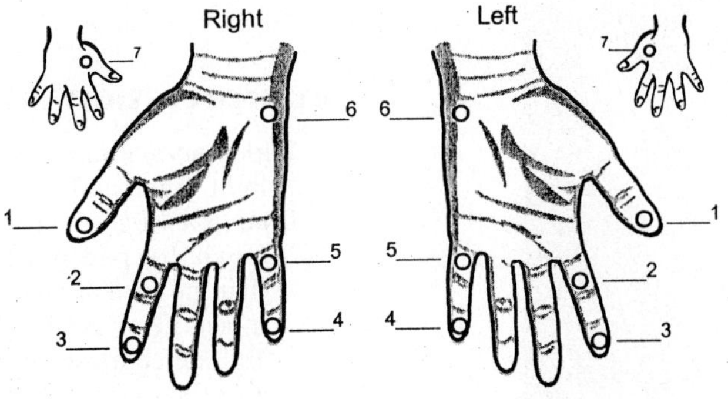

Left

1 FDI ___ 4 OP ___
2 L ___ 5 ECR ___
3 APB ___

1) Enlarged Nerve ___
2) Tender Nerve ___
3) Sensory Change ___
4) Muscle Change ___

1) Protective Loss ___
2) Clawed/MobileJts ___
3) Absorption:
Mild ___ Severe ___
4) Injuries ___
5) Contracted/Stiff Jts ___
6) Wrist Drop ___

Comment: ______________________ **Date:** ________

Medication: ______________________ **Examined by:** ________

1 FDI ___ 4 OP ___
2 L ___ 5 ECR ___
3 APB ___

1) Enlarged Nerve ___
2) Tender Nerve ___
3) Sensory Change ___
4) Muscle Change ___

1) Protective Loss ___
2) Clawed/MobileJts ___
3) Absorption:
Mild ___ Severe ___
4) Injuries ___
5) Contracted/Stiff Jts ___
6) Wrist Drop ___

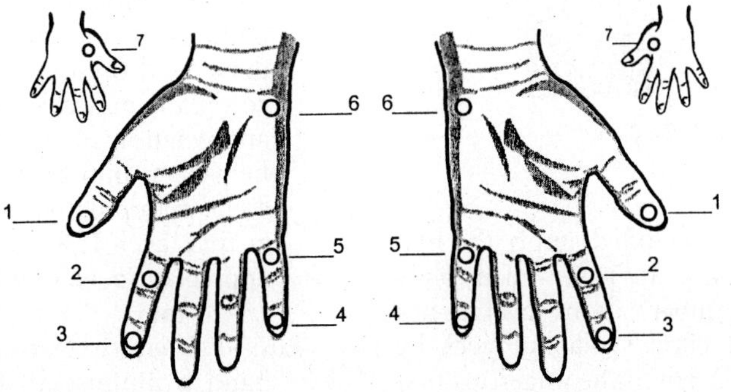

1 FDI ___ 4 OP ___
2 L ___ 5 ECR ___
3 APB ___

1) Enlarged Nerve ___
2) Tender Nerve ___
3) Sensory Change ___
4) Muscle Change ___

1) Protective Loss ___
2) Clawed/MobileJts ___
3) Absorption:
Mild ___ Severe ___
4) Injuries ___
5) Contracted/Stiff Jts ___
6) Wrist Drop ___

Comment: ______________________ **Date:** ________

Medication: ______________________ **Examined by:** ________

1 FDI ___ 4 OP ___
2 L ___ 5 ECR ___
3 APB ___

1) Enlarged Nerve ___
2) Tender Nerve ___
3) Sensory Change ___
4) Muscle Change ___

1) Protective Loss ___
2) Clawed/MobileJts ___
3) Absorption:
Mild ___ Severe ___
4) Injuries ___
5) Contracted/Stiff Jts ___
6) Wrist Drop ___

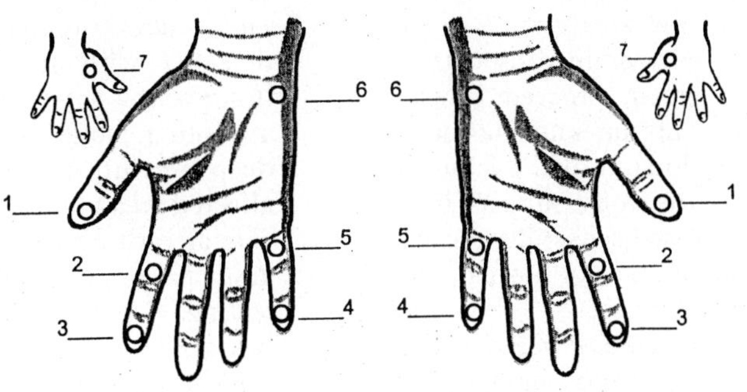

1 FDI ___ 4 OP ___
2 L ___ 5 ECR ___
3 APB ___

1) Enlarged Nerve ___
2) Tender Nerve ___
3) Sensory Change ___
4) Muscle Change ___

1) Protective Loss ___
2) Clawed/MobileJts ___
3) Absorption:
Mild ___ Severe ___
4) Injuries ___
5) Contracted/Stiff Jts ___
6) Wrist Drop ___

Comment: ______________________ **Date:** ________

Medication: ______________________ **Examined by:** ________

NHDP FORM 131
PERIPHERAL NERVE MONITORING

B

Figure 11-13—cont'd B, Peripheral nerve monitoring.

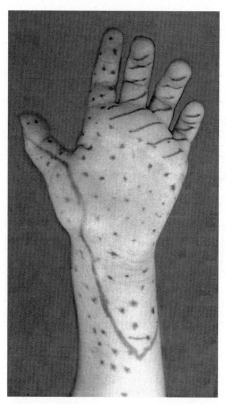

Figure 11-14 Peripheral nerve mapping.

Then, with the patient's eyes occluded, apply the filament in the reference area until the patient can easily identify the 2.83 (marking number) 50-mg level monofilament. Test the involved hand (volar surface) by applying the same filament (2.83) to the fingertips first and working proximally. Dot the spots correctly identified with a *green* felt-tip pen. (Explain to the patient that one touch is a marking of the pen.) In general, the patient is tested distally to proximally, but a consistent pattern is not used to avoid patient anticipation of the area to be touched. When all the area on the volar surface of the hand that can be identified as within normal limits is marked in green, proceed to the dorsum of the hand and test in the same fashion. Because the sensibility on the dorsum of the hand is not always as well defined as the volar surface, it is easier to establish areas of decreased sensibility on the volar surface first. Now the gross areas of normal and decreased sensibility have been defined.

3. Return to the volar surface of the hand. Proceed to the filaments within the level of diminished light touch (see Tables 11-1 and 11-2, and color maps Figs. 11-9 to 11-11), but change the color of the marking pen for this level to *blue*. Test as discussed earlier in the unidentified areas remaining, working again first on the volar surface and then on the dorsum.

4. If areas remain unidentified, proceed to the filaments in the diminished protective sensation level (*purple*) and then loss of protective sensation level (*red*) and continue testing until all the areas have been identified.

5. Record the colors and filament numbers on the report form to produce a sensory mapping. (Color and mark hands on the form.) Note any variations and unusual responses, especially delayed responses. Delayed responses (more than 3 seconds) are considered abnormal and should be noted. Note the presence and direction of referred touch with arrows.

Interpretation and Levels of Function

Within normal limits is the level of normal recognition of light touch and therefore deep pressure.[64]

Diminished light touch is diminished recognition of light touch. If a patient has diminished light touch, provided that the patient's motor status and cognitive abilities are intact, he or she has fair use of the hand; graphesthesia and stereognosis are both close to normal and adaptable; he or she has good temperature appreciation and definitely has good protective sensation; he or she most often has fair to good two-point discrimination; and the patient may not even realize he or she has had a sensory loss.

Diminished protective sensation is diminished use of the hands, difficulty manipulating some objects, and a tendency to drop some objects; in addition, the patient may complain of weakness of the hand, but still have an appreciation of the pain and temperature that should help keep him or her from injury, and the patient has some manipulative skill. Sensory reeducation can begin at this level. It is possible for a patient to have a gross appreciation of two-point discrimination at this level (7–10 mm).

Loss of protective sensation is compromised use of the hand; a diminished, if not absent, temperature appreciation; an inability to manipulate objects outside line of vision; a tendency to be injured easily; and potential danger for the patient with sharp objects and around machinery. Instructions on protective care are needed to prevent injury.

Deep-pressure sensation is a rudimentary deep pressure detected with the heaviest monofilament. Patients describe this as a sensation of heavy weight, but without any other tactile discrimination. The patient still has deep pressure recognition, which does not make the affected area totally asensory. Instructions on protective care are critical to prevent injury.

Untestable is no response to monofilament threshold testing. A patient may or may not feel a pinprick but has no other discrimination of levels of feeling. If a patient feels a pinprick in an area otherwise untestable, it is important to note that some potential nerve response is still present. Instructions on protective care are critical to prevent the normally occurring problems associated with the asensory hand.

Further interpretation of the effect that a decrease or loss of sensibility has on patient function depends on the area and extent of loss and whether musculature is diminished. Light-touch/deep-pressure threshold measurements can be used to consider the need for treatment, changes in treatment, and the success of treatment.

Protective Sensation

Maintenance of protective sensation is a major goal for preventing injury from loss of sensory feedback. Patients with loss of protective sensation are injured easily and experience repetitive injuries, which can lead to lifelong psychological stress, as well as deformity and disability[48,56,68,75,76] Certainly, when it comes to sensory abnormality and functional discrimination or recognition, whether or not protective sensation is present is a defining factor in patient treatment because it determines if the patient is still relatively safe with sharp or hot objects, or conversely, in danger of wounds and amputations from complications of burns and injuries that could be incurred through use of everyday objects.

Hand Screen Coding

A computer coding method was developed in 1984, for monitoring large numbers of HD patients in the United States and for overseas projects.[61] This relatively simple method is available for coding patient peripheral nerve status. Data can be digitized for computer analysis by giving each filament a weighted score similar to muscle testing, where 5 = normal, 4 = fair, 3 = good, 2 = poor, and 1 = trace. In sensibility coding, green, 2.83 (marking number) = 5; blue, 3.61 (marking number) = 4; purple, 4.31 (marking number) = 3; red, 4.56 (marking number) = 2; red-orange, 6.65 (marking number) = 1; no response equals zero. Scores can be totaled for each nerve and overall. A normal hand then would have a score of 15 for the median nerve, 15 for the radial nerve, and 5 for the radial, for a total of 35 points.[39] Computer entry and grading can be done in Microsoft Excel or Access programs to record and analyze hand screen site response.

Computerized Touch–Pressure Instruments

The optimally designed computerized instrument automatically applies and controls the stimulus with a built-in limit on how much force is applied.[9,15,69,77,78] Computerized instruments reported to be accurate and sold for clinical testing of patients—just as hand-held instruments—need to have their forces of application measured and these measurements made available along with other instrument specifications.[63]

If the instrument still depends on a hand-held application of the stimulus, it is still subject to the same limitations of any hand-held instrument.[13,79-81] Computer averaging of force stimuli can hide peaks of higher force and examiner hand vibration[79,80,82] (Fig. 11-15).

Two-Point Discrimination

Application

Two-point discrimination is a classic test of sensibility used by hand surgeons over several decades.[83-85] The test is believed by many to be a test of innervation density. Some think two-point discrimination a good predictor of patient function and manipulation. It does follow that once normal two-point discrimination has returned to the fingertips after nerve repair, the quality of sensibility is good. The test overall

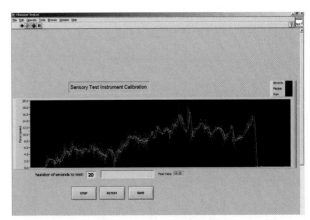

Figure 11-15 Variable force versus time application—significantly variable force which results from holding a probe from any hand-held instrument without force control.

has yet to be related to the presence or absence of protective sensation.

At one time it was popular to use a paper clip to test two-point discrimination, but this is not recommended. The probe tips should be blunt, of the same geometry, and not so sharp that pain is elicited. Commonly available hand-held two-point discrimination test instruments range from the relatively light Disk-Criminator (P.O. Box 16392, Baltimore, Maryland),[14] to a heavy Boley Gauge (Boley Gauge, Research Designs, Inc., Houston, Texas) (Fig. 11-16).

Sensitivity

In addition to touch–pressure thresholds, Weinstein published a table for two-point discrimination thresholds all over the body (Fig. 11-17). The widely variable pattern for two-point discrimination does not correlate with touch detection threshold (0.17), but does correlate and is almost identical to that for localization of touch (0.92).[51] With common scoring methods, two-point discrimination testing is most accurate at the fingertips. The clinician should know that studies have found subjects with entrapments and compressions in which two-point discrimination is normal, but monofilament and nerve conduction testing are abnormal.[27,70]

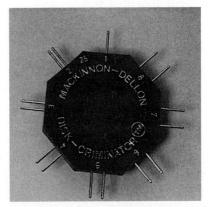

Figure 11-16 Disk-Criminator. The weight of the instrument improves control on force of application but does not totally eliminate variable force from hand-held application.

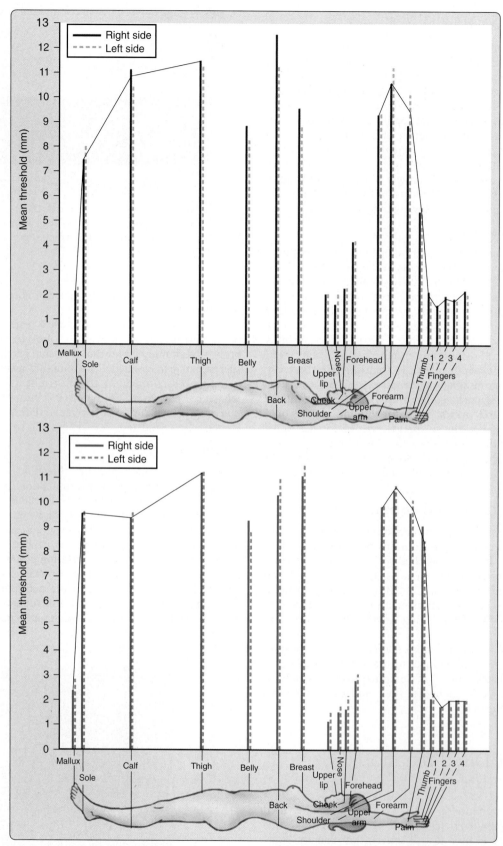

Figure 11-17 Weinstein's two-point discrimination body thresholds. (Reprinted, with permission, from Bell-Krotoski JA. Advances in sensibility evaluation. *Hand Clin.* 1991;7:534, Figure 11-3; and Weinstein S. Intensive and extensive aspects of tactile sensitivity as a function of body part, sex, and laterality. In: Kenshalo DR, ed. *The Skin Senses.* Springfield, Ill, Charles C Thomas. 1968; pp 195–222.)

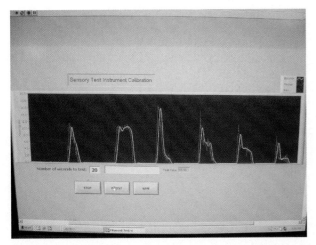

Figure 11-18 Variable force from conventional two-point discrimination instruments. Six applications to Sensory Instrument Measurement System.

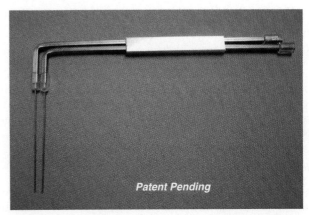

Figure 11-19 Design for controlled monofilament two-point discrimination instrument, showing that force control design for two-point discrimination is possible and could potentially improve the test. (Bell-Krotoski JA: Device for evaluating cutaneous sensory detection, notice of publication of application, United States Patent and Trademark Office, US-2009-0105606-A1, 2009.)

Instrument Integrity

The known uncontrolled variable in two-point discrimination testing is the unspecified force at which all of the hand-held two-point discrimination instruments are applied. Unless the instruments are force-controlled for hand-held application, they are relatively incapable of producing repeatable application force. Different instruments vary in weight and configuration, and the test probes vary. For this reason the examiner should always use the same instrument for repeated testing.

Calibration

Many think the two-point discrimination test is objective and calibrated because it can be numerically adjusted to repeatable distances at its probe tips for measurement.[63] Two-point discrimination may be a very good test if force-controlled, but most hand-held instruments do not provide the opportunity to produce consistent repeatable data[13,63] (Fig. 11-18). Specifying the stimulus in pressure (pressure being force/unit area) is no more accurate than force calculation. The "moving" two-point discrimination test is more uncontrolled in force of application (or pressure) because of the varying topography of the finger as the test probes are moved across the joints and fingertip. Both "static" and moving forms of testing need limits on the force applied, or at a minimum to show that clinical results from testing are not different when applied with various force/pressures and instruments.

A prototype controlled two-point discrimination instrument has been designed using heavier monofilaments that hold their distance when on a sliding scale (available at timelyneuropathytesting.org; patent pending) (Fig. 11-19). This is a force-controlled two-point discrimination design which can apply 5 g, 10 g, or 30 g of force.

Clinical Validity

Two-point discrimination testing has been clinically useful despite the lack of control of the application force. The potential for greater usefulness depends on the development of instruments that are designed with the force of application controlled.[71,86]

Background Needed for Understanding

Weber invented the two-point discrimination test.[74] Moberg and others have advocated that the test is closely related to "tactile gnosis" and functional ability of the patient to use the hand for fine motor and skilled tasks.[73,87] Dellon introduced the moving two-point discrimination test.[83] His objective and rationale is that fingertip sensibility is highly dependent on motion.

Moberg agreed with the need for force control of two-point discrimination instruments after hearing a critique of the force-control weaknesses in two-point discrimination instruments, suggesting a design for a prototype instrument that would use 5- and 10-g weights.[71,86]

Test Protocol

Static Two-Point

Usually only the fingertips are assessed in static two-point discrimination testing, as norms vary widely farther up the extremity. The patient's hand should be fully supported on a towel. The examiner should take care not to touch the patient's hand with anything except the instrument, as touch by the examiner adds extraneous touch stimuli and may confuse the patient. A very light application of two versus one point of the instrument is used. Vision is occluded—usually by obscuring the line of vision with a folder rather than a blindfold. Results can be recorded on a hand screen form or hand drawing.

Testing begins with 5 mm of distance between the two points in a random sequence with one point applied in a longitudinal orientation to avoid overlapping the innervation zones of the digital nerves. The point of blanching has been suggested as a control for force of application, but this is problematic as blanching has been found to occur at different forces on different fingers and tissue areas, somewhat dependent on condition of the skin.[13] Seven of 10 responses is necessary to be considered accurate. If there is no response or an inaccurate response, the distance between the ends is increased by increments of 1 mm, until 7 of 10 responses are accurate. Testing is stopped at 15 mm.

Interpretation

Normal two-point discrimination is considered less than 6 mm, fair is 6 to 10 mm, and poor is 11 to 15 mm (see guidelines of the American Society for Surgery of the Hand,[7] and International Federation of Hand Surgery Societies).[75,88]

Dellon Moving Two Point

In the moving two-point discrimination test, testing is begun with an 8-mm distance between the two instrument tip points.[83] The instrument is moved parallel to the long axis of the finger (testing ends side by side). Testing begins proximal to distal toward the fingertip. For a correct response, the patient has to respond accurately to 7 of 10 stimuli of one or two points, before the distance is narrowed for testing with a smaller distance. Testing is stopped at 2 mm, which is considered normal.

Interpretation

The moving two-point stimulus is more easily detected than the static two-point. Several authors have reported correlation between moving two-point discrimination and object recognition.[11,83]

Computerized Two-Point Discrimination Instruments

Dellon recommends the pressure-specified sensory device (PSSD) as optimal for two-point and moving two-point discrimination testing (PSSD, Post Office Box 16392, Baltimore, MD).[79,80,89] For the specific testing technique for the PSSD, the reader is referred to literature available with the instrument.[80,89] Dellon, based on two-point discrimination research with the PSSD, reports finding that clinical results can be quite different at various thresholds of pressure (force) of application.[80,89] Other computerized force and pressure-controlled devices have been tried experimentally.[69,90] Used for research, these may help determine optimum target thresholds for two-point discrimination testing.[13,81,91-93]

Point or Area Localization

Application

The objective of using a point localization test after nerve injury or repair is *to determine the accuracy of localization of a touch stimulus* and when inaccurate *to determine and record the direction and distance in centimeters to another point, area, or finger to which the touch is referred.* The regenerating peripheral nerve after laceration or suture does not always find and innervate the same mechanoreceptor end organs in the skin, and until a certain density of endings has returned, insufficient data is available for a patient to accurately determine localization. Localization generally improves over time as nerve healing and regeneration progresses, but localization also requires an integrated level of perception and cortical interpretation by the patient (Fig. 11-20).

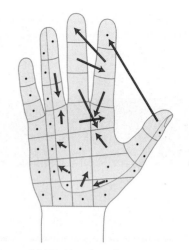

Figure 11-20 Mapping of touch localization.

Sensitivity

Weinstein tested normal subjects and published a table for localization of touch sensitivities all over the body. The variable pattern for localization in normal subjects is quite different from that found for touch detection threshold, but very similar to that found for two-point discrimination. The ability to localize in 48 normal adults was found to have a high correlation with two-point discrimination thresholds (0.92), but did not have high correlation with light-touch threshold (0.28).[51]

Instrument Integrity/Calibration

Types of test instruments used have varied from dowels, used by Werner and Omer, to monofilaments. The monofilaments do provide a repeatable force of application and therefore are recommended for a stimulus probe. Whatever instrument is used, it should be reported and used consistently for the same and subsequent patients in order to be the most meaningful.

Clinical Validity

Localization early after nerve repair is poor and generally improves with time and use of the affected part. Poor localization after nerve repair can seriously limit function. Localization may vary with the cognitive ability of a patient to adapt to new sensory pathways more than as a result of the actual level of return of the nerve and its response to touch stimuli.

Shortly after a lacerated nerve begins to show a Tinel's[94] sign distal to the suture line, a touch with a probe or heaviest monofilament may be detected by the patient (pressure recognition), but is not usually correctly localized. When asked, a patient may refer to another finger or area. Some patients never regain normal point localization, but most regain area localization.[59] Few would contest that improvement in point localization is faster and better if the affected area is used for grasp and manipulation, and in the reverse, is slower, and of poor quality if not frequently used after repair.

Errors in localization can frequently be reduced in one treatment session with reeducation, indicating that the change is in part relearning, rather than a physiologic change in the nerve. The research of Rosen and Lundborg regarding the plasticity of the brain supports this concept.[95]

Comparison with Other Tests of Sensibility

Localization can easily be tested and recorded on a hand screen form after other sensibility tests such as monofilament testing to help further determine the quality of sensibility for patients who have had nerve lacerations.[96] Localization should be tested separately and not used as a requirement with other tests of sensibility. This was once the procedure with monofilament testing but it confounded the results of testing and their interpretation.[7,16]

As the repair matures, that skin area initially reinnervated subsequently tends to improve toward lighter touch threshold detection. As touch–pressure recognition improves, the distance the touch is referred tends to lessen and can be recorded in millimeters.

Background Needed for Understanding

Werner and Omer described differences in both area and point localization, with area localization being the first to return. In area localization, after being touched, the patient responds by indicating the area that was touched. In point localization, the patient responds by covering the point touched with a wooden dowel within a centimeter.

Test Protocol

In a recommended test protocol by Callahan, the lightest Semmes–Weinstein monofilament perceived is used for testing localization over the involved area.[15] A grid divided into zones is used for recording the results of this test on standard hand or arm recording forms.[16,97] With the patient's vision occluded, the monofilament is applied. Patients are instructed to open their eyes and point to the exact spot touched. If inaccurate, the distance from the correct spot is measured in millimeters. Arrows are drawn on the recording form from the correct stimulus point to the incorrect point indicated by the patient. If the stimulus is correctly localized, a dot is marked on the recording form. Nakada[96] provides a method to more objectively document and score errors by using a 4.17 (marking number) Semmes–Weinstein monofilament and measuring errors in localization with a vernier caliper.

Vibration Testing

The objective of a test for vibration is *to determine frequency response of mechanoreceptor end organs.* Some neurologists believe that vibration as a separate sense does not exist, but is rather the perception of variable changes in stimuli.[82] Dellon has advocated 30- and 256-Hz tuning forks for measuring patient response to vibration.[63] However, the vibratory stimulus with the tuning forks is not controlled and the stimulus varies with the examiner's technique and force of application.

Computerized Instruments

Szabo,[98] and Gelberman,[27] have investigated vibratory sensory testing with computerized instruments, but these are not sufficiently controlled in force of application and vibration to be recommend for clinical use. Horch developed a computerized instrument with control of applied force of its probe that has been used by Hardy and coworkers, and Lundborg has reported results with a force-controlled computerized instrument, but these are not yet commercially available[9,69,90,99]

Functional Tests

Application

Monofilament threshold detection levels can predict patient function and thus are a first-order functional assessment. Results of testing can help focus reeducation on what is realistic relative to the degree of physiologic nerve return.[7,54,55,58,59,100] For example, light touch is necessary for the epicritic quality of sensibility. In addition, protective sensation, at a minimum, is especially important to prevent injury to hands during use. Instruction in protective techniques to prevent injury to the skin is needed until protective sensation has returned to the fingertips in the affected area. But touch–pressure threshold testing does not include measurement of secondary skill and adaptation.[12,70] Human brains adapt very quickly after injury, and even without nerve return patients exhibit varying adaptations and use of extremities.

Sensitivity, Instrument Integrity, and Calibration

The classic Moberg pickup test[87] is an observational object recognition test requiring motor participation and is most appropriate for median or combined median and ulnar nerve lesions. The Functional Performance Sensory Test (FPST) is standardized, but is not specific for nerve change.[56] *A still relatively untapped frontier for clinicians is the development of standardized functional skill assessments.*

Clinical Validity

Functional skill tests are particularly indicated when the objective of testing is to determine an injured individuals' potential for return to life activity and work.[101,102] These can indicate the need for sensory reeducation and training or retraining (as long as the test used for reeducation is not also used for the primary assessment in the same patient).[83,92,93,103]

Comparison with Other Tests of Sensibility

Disagreement among clinical investigators about which instrument best tests patient function frequently results from the fact that they are considering both patient physiologic function (which needs to be measured without cortical reasoning and accommodation) and patient adaptation (which includes coping and learned skill). Whereas a patient's level of physiologic function can often predict tactile gnostic function, which correlates in general with patient functional performance, his or her ability to cope with change and the degree of adaptation cannot be used as direct measurement of neural status.[56] Both physiologic function and adaptive function are important, but they need to be clearly defined and considered separately.

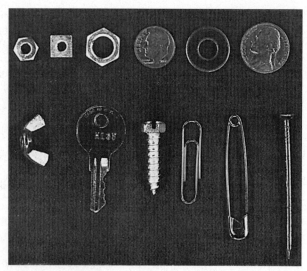

Figure 11-21 Dellon modification of Moberg's pickup test.

Background Needed for Understanding

Moberg highlighted the need for the hand to be used after injury, referring to the hand without median and ulnar nerve sensibility as "blind."[84,87,104] He considered a loss in sensibility to be greatly underestimated and argued to rate the total loss of sensibility in the palm of the hand as 100% disability. He spoke of sensibility as a tactile "gnosis," with the hand being the "eye" for the body and touch.

Test Protocols

Moberg's Pickup Test

The now classic Moberg pickup test uses an assortment of common office objects placed on a table (paper clip, piece of cotton, etc.). The patient is instructed to quickly pick up the objects and place them into a box, first with the involved hand, then with the uninvolved, while the examiner times and observes. This process is repeated with the patient's eyes closed. With eyes closed, the patient tends not to use the fingers or other sensory surfaces with poor sensibility. Ng and colleagues[105] and others have proposed a standard protocol using standard objects for administering the test. Dellon[86] modified the pickup test by standardizing the items used and requiring object identification (Fig. 11-21). No more than 30 seconds is permitted to identify the object, which is presented twice. King correlated the results of Semmes–Weinstein-style monofilament testing in carpal tunnel syndrome patients with their response times for texture and object recognition and found a significant association between level of touch perceived and time required to identify the test items.[106]

Waylett and the Flinn Functional Performance Sensory Test

Waylett designed a standard tactile discrimination test.[107] The Flinn Functional Performance Sensory Test (FPST) is a standard and objective test of functional performance that is sensitive but not specific for sensory abnormality.[56,75,101]

Other Useful Tests

Sudomotor Function

Onne[108] and Richards[109] describe vasomotor and nutritional aspects of peripheral nerve function. Sudomotor function is important for hydrating and lubricating the skin and maintaining its normal pliability. When examined, the skin in an area with abnormal sensibility also often has changes in sweat and vascularity. Affected skin that does not receive specific care is dry to the touch and can crack easily, leading to infection. Soaking of the skin and applying an oil before drying is an effective way of maintaining suppleness and skin condition.[68]

Ninhydrin Sweat Test

The objective of using Moberg's ninhydrin sweat test is to *help document sweat and indicate change in sensibility* in early injury.[50,110,111] Moberg scored ninhydrin test results on a scale of 0 to 3, with 0 representing absent sweating and 3 representing normal sweating.[21] Perry[112] and Phelps[97] describe a commercially available ninhydrin developer and fixer. The patient's hand is cleaned, rinsed, and wiped with ether, alcohol, or acetone with a minimum of a 5-minute waiting period during which nothing contacts the fingers. Then the fingertips are placed against the bond paper for 15 seconds and traced with a pencil. The paper is sprayed with ninhydrin spray reagent (N-0507) (Sigma Chemical Company, St. Louis, Missouri) and dried for 24 hours or heated in an oven for 5 to 10 minutes at 200°F (93°C). After development, the prints are sprayed with the ninhydrin fixer reagent (N-0757). In a normal print, dots representing sweat glands can be clearly seen, and the lack of dots indicates a lack of sweating.

Wrinkle Test

The objective of O'Riain's wrinkle test is *to demonstrate a lack of wrinkling.*[113] It was observed that a denervated hand placed in warm water (40°C; 104°F) for 30 minutes does not wrinkle. This test is rated using a 0 to 3 scoring system. It is most useful for determining areas of denervation from lacerations in adults who cannot be responsive and in young children. Phelps noted that wrinkling can return without return of sensibility, so this should be used early after injury.[97]

Temperature Recognition

The objective of thermal testing is *to demonstrate temperature recognition.* Temperature sensibility, like pain, is difficult to quantify precisely.[114] Normal discrimination between hot and cold temperatures has been reported to be within 5°C, but hot and cold test tubes as used by clinicians greatly exceed this range. Diminished temperature recognition can be shown to occur when touch–pressure detection thresholds are at the diminished and loss of protective sensation levels.[115] Most forms of temperature testing are relatively gross, however, and not capable of revealing small changes, which may better correlate with lighter levels of touch–pressure change. Controlled and sensitive laboratory instruments that can measure temperature and pain are available to neurophysiologists and other researchers, but these are expensive and primarily used experimentally. Instrument reliability in these would need to be improved before clinical use, as some have been found to change in stimulus with various electrical voltages or change with the charge of their battery.[66]

Test Battery Recommendations

Early detection of developing nerve problems offers the best opportunity for improvement.[48,58,116,117] At a minimum, Semmes–Weinstein-style monofilament testing using hand screen size monofilaments (for hand and body) is recommended. The following battery is recommended after obtaining a thorough patient history. The tests should be administered in a manner designed to minimize variables, and they should be knowledgeably interpreted. Optimally, testing is done both before and after treatment intervention, including surgery, in order to clearly show the direction of change, whether improvement, the same, or worsening. Testing is repeated using a standard protocol at intervals specific to the individual case.

For Nerve Lesions in Continuity

- NCV to help define site of involvement and severity of slowed or absent conduction
- Semmes–Weinstein-style monofilament hand screen or mapping to determine the touch–pressure threshold in the involved areas
- Static and moving two-point discrimination (optional for comparison)
- For patients with intermittent symptoms, stress testing with provocative activity or positioning (in coordination with referring physician) followed with repeat NCV or Semmes–Weinstein-style touch–pressure threshold tests
- Functional and other tests as indicated by need

For Nerve Lacerations

- Examination of the hand for evidence of sympathetic dysfunction
- Tinel's test distal to the repair to determine distal progression of regenerating axons
- Semmes–Weinstein-style monofilament hand screen or mapping to assess level and area of touch–pressure return and to reveal changes over time

- Pinprick test if tested areas are unresponsive to the thickest diameter (6.65 marking number), 300-g+ level Semmes–Weinstein-style monofilament
- Static and moving two-point discrimination tests on the fingertips (if indicated)
- Touch localization testing distal to nerve repair
- Dellon modification of the Moberg pickup test for median or median and ulnar nerve dysfunction
- Functional tests and use assessment of the hand in activities of daily living (FPST where available)[101]

Note: For a child younger than 4, the wrinkle test, possibly the ninhydrin sweat test, and the Moberg pickup test may provide the best information.

Summary

The clinician needs to be a peripheral nerve detective and begin an evaluation with screening of all of the peripheral nerves of the upper extremity, even when a referral has been made to test a specific nerve and level. Accurate testing and common understanding of the need for thorough evaluation among the surgeons, therapists, and others involved in the peripheral nerve assessment facilitates early diagnosis and accurate resolution of developing nerve problems. Data from consistent tests can be numerically quantified and compared among measurements, following treatment, and among patient groups. Semmes–Weinstein-style monofilament screening or mapping of detection thresholds enables the examiner to "see" what is otherwise invisible. Hand-held instruments without sufficient control on their application do not produce repeatable results and are therefore invalid in clinical testing. Many of our traditional hand-held tests need to have a means of control developed for their test stimulus. Computerized test instruments could help to eliminate the uncontrolled variables of hand-held tests. But computerized instruments must also meet sensitivity and repeatability requirements for objective testing. NCV and sensibility tests together hold the potential to improve patient outcome by enabling earlier recognition of developing problems and intervention at a point before nerve damage is irreversible.

REFERENCES

The complete reference list is available online at www.expertconsult.com.

Functional Tests

ELAINE EWING FESS, MS, OTR, FAOTA, CHT*

"Rule #1: When you get a bizarre finding, first question the test."[†]

INSTRUMENTATION CRITERIA
FUNCTIONAL ASSESSMENT INSTRUMENTS
SUMMARY

CRITICAL POINTS

- Standardized functional tests are statistically proven to measure accurately and appropriately when proper equipment and procedures are used.
- In order for a test to be an acceptable measurement instrument, it must include all of the following elements: reliability, validity, statement of purpose, equipment criteria and administration, and scoring and interpretation instructions.
- Hand and upper extremity assessment tools fall at varying levels along the reliability and validity continuum and therefore must be selected based on satisfying as many of the required elements as possible.

Objective measurements of function provide a foundation for hand rehabilitation efforts by delineating baseline pathology against which patient progress and treatment methods may be assessed. A thorough and unbiased assessment procedure furnishes information that helps match patients to interventions, predicts rehabilitation potential, provides data from which subsequent measurements may be compared, and allows medical specialists to plan and evaluate treatment programs and techniques. Conclusions gained from functional evaluation procedures guide treatment priorities, motivate staff and patients, and define functional capacity at the termination of treatment. Assessment of function through analysis and integration of data also serves as the vehicle for professional communication, eventually influencing the body of knowledge of the profession.

The quality of assessment information depends on the accuracy, authority, objectivity, sophistication, predictability, sensitivity, and selectivity of the tools used to gather data. It is of utmost importance to choose functional assessment instruments wisely. Dependable, precise tools allow clinicians to reach conclusions that are minimally skewed by extraneous factors or biases, thus diminishing the chances of subjective error and facilitating more accurate understanding. Functional instruments that measure diffusely produce nonspecific results. Conversely, instruments with proven accuracy of measurement yield precise and selective data.

Communication is the underlying rationale for requiring good assessment procedures. The acquisition and transmission of knowledge, both of which are fundamental to patient treatment and professional growth, are enhanced through development and use of a common professional language based on strict criteria for functional assessment instrument selection. The use of "home-brewed," functional evaluation tools that are inaccurate or not validated is never appropriate since their baseless data may misdirect or delay therapy intervention. The purpose of this chapter is twofold: (1) to define functional measurement terminology and criteria and (2) to review current upper extremity functional assessment instruments in relation to accepted measurement criteria. It is not within the scope of this chapter to recommend specific test instruments. Instead, readers are encouraged to evaluate the instruments used in their practices according to accepted instrument selection criteria,[1] keeping those that best meet the criteria and discarding those that do not.

Instrumentation Criteria

Standardized functional tests, the most sophisticated of assessment tools, are statistically proven to measure accurately and appropriately when proper equipment and procedures are used. The few truly standardized tests available in hand/upper extremity rehabilitation are limited to instruments that evaluate hand coordination, dexterity, and

---

*The author receives no compensation in any form from products discussed in the chapter.
†Weinstein, S. 50 Years of somatosensory research. *J Hand Ther*. 1993;6(1): 113.

work tolerance. Unfortunately, not all functional tests meet all of the requirements of standardization.

Primary Requisites

For a test to be an acceptable measurement instrument, it must include all of the following crucial, non-negotiable elements:

Reliability defines the accuracy or repeatability of a functional test. In other words, does the test measure consistently between like instruments; within and between trials; and within and between examiners? Statistical proof of reliability is defined through correlation coefficients. Describing the "parallelness" between two sets of data, correlation coefficients may range from +1.0 to −1.0. Devices that follow National Institute of Standards and Technology (NIST) standards, for example, a dynamometer, usually have higher reliability correlation coefficients than do tests for which there are no governing standards. When prevailing standards such as those from NIST exist for a test, use of human performance to establish reliability is unacceptable. For example, you would not check the accuracy of your watch by timing how long it takes five people to run a mile and then computing the average of their times. Yet, in the rehabilitation arena, this is essentially how reliability of many test instruments has been documented.[2]

Once a test's instrument reliability is established, inter-rater and intrarater reliability are the next steps that must be confirmed. Although instrument reliability is a non-negotiable prerequisite to defining rater reliability, researchers and commercial developers often ignore this critical step, opting instead to move straight to establishing rater reliability with its less stringent, human performance-based paradigms.[3] The fallacy of this fatal error seems obvious, but if a test instrument measures consistently in its inaccuracy, it can produce misleadingly high rater reliability scores that are completely meaningless. For example, if four researchers independently measure the length of the same table using the same grossly inaccurate yardstick, their resultant scores will have high inter-rater and intrarater reliability so long as the yardstick consistently maintains its inherent inaccuracies and does not change (Fig. 12-1). Unfortunately, this scenario has occurred repeatedly with clinical and research assessment tools, involving mechanical devices and paper-and-pencil tests alike.

Validity defines a test's ability to measure the thing it was designed to measure. Proof of test validity is described through correlation coefficients ranging from +1.0 to −1.0. Reliability is a prerequisite to validity. It makes no sense to have a test that measures authentically (valid) but inaccurately (unreliable). Validity correlation coefficients usually are not as high as are reliability correlation coefficients. Like reliability, validity is established through comparison to a standard that possesses similar properties. When no standard exists, and the test measures something new and unique, the test may be said to have "face validity." An example of an instrument that has face validity is the volumeter that is based on Archimedes' principle of water displacement. It is important to remember that volumeters must first be reliable before they may be considered to have face validity. A new functional test may be compared with another similar

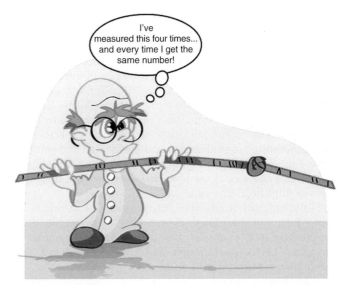

Figure 12-1 If an inaccurate assessment tool measures consistently and does not change over time, its intrarater and inter-rater reliabilities can be misleadingly high. Despite these deceptively high rater correlations, data collected from using the inaccurate test instrument are meaningless. (Courtesy of Dr. Elaine Ewing Fess.)

functional test whose validity was previously established. However, establishing validity through comparison of two new, unknown, tests produces fatally flawed results. In other words, "Two times zero is still zero." Unfortunately, it is not unusual to find this type of error in functional tests employed in the rehabilitation arena.

Statement of purpose defines the conceptual rationale, principles, and intended use of a test. Occasionally test limitations are also included in a purpose statement. Purpose statements may range from one or two sentences to multiple paragraphs in length depending on the complexity of a test.

Equipment criteria are essential to the reliability and validity of a functional assessment test instrument. Unless absolutely identical in every way, the paraphernalia constituting a standardized test must not be substituted for or altered, no matter how similar the substituted pieces may be. Reliability and validity of a test are determined using explicit equipment. When equipment original to the test is changed, the test's reliability and validity are rendered meaningless and must be reestablished all over again. An example, if the wooden checkers in the Jebsen Taylor Hand Function Test are replaced with plastic checkers, the test is invalidated.[4]

Administration, scoring, and interpretation instructions provide procedural rules and guidelines to ensure that testing processes are exactly conducted and that grading methods are fair and accurate. The manner in which functional assessment tools are employed is crucial to accurate and honest assessment outcomes. Test procedure and sequence must not vary from that described in the administration instructions. Deviations in recommended equipment procedure or sequence invalidate test results. A cardinal rule is that assessment instruments must not be used as therapy practice tools for patients. Information obtained from tools that have been used in patient training is radically skewed, rendering it invalid and meaningless. Patient fatigue, physiologic adaptation, test difficulty, and length of test time may also influence results. Clinically this means that sensory testing is done before assessing grip or pinch; rest periods are provided appropriately; and if possible, more difficult procedures are not scheduled early in testing sessions. Good assessment technique should reflect both test protocol and instrumentation requirements. Additionally, directions for test interpretation are essential. Functional tests have specific application boundaries. Straying beyond these clearly defined limits leads to exaggeration or minimization of inherent capacities of tests, generating misguided expectations for staff and patients alike. For example, goniometric measurements pertain to joint angles and arcs of motion. They, however, are not measures of joint flexibility or strength.

Although, not a primary instrumentation requisite, a bibliography of associated literature is often included in standardized test manuals. These references contribute to clinicians' better appreciation and understanding of test development, purpose, and usage.

Secondary Requisites

Once all of the above criteria are met, data collection may be initiated to further substantiate a test's application and usefulness.

Normative data are drawn from large population samples that are divided, with statistically suitable numbers of subjects in each category, according to appropriate variables such as hand dominance, age, sex, occupation, and so on. Many currently available tests have associated so-called normative data, but they lack some or, more often, all of the primary instrumentation requisites, including reliability; validity; purpose statement; equipment criteria; and administration, scoring, and interpretation instructions. Regardless of how extensive a test's associated normative information may be, if the test does not meet the primary instrumentation requisites, it is useless as a measurement instrument.[5]

Tertiary Options

Assuming a test meets the primary instrumentation requisites, other statistical measures may be applied to the data gleaned from using the test. The optional measures of sensitivity and specificity assist clinicians in deciding whether evidence for applying the test is appropriate for an individual patient's diagnosis.

Sensitivity, a statistical measure, defines the proportion of correctly identified positive responses in a subject population. In other words, sensitivity tells, in terms of percentages, how good a test is at properly identifying those who actually have the diagnosis (Fig. 12-2).[6] The mnemonic "SnNout" is often associated with *Sensitivity*, indicating that a Negative test result rules *out* the diagnosis.[7] As an example, out of a population of 50, if a test correctly identifies 15 of the 20 people who have the diagnosis and who test positive (TP), the sensitivity of the instrument is 75.0% (TP/[TP + FN] = sensitivity %).*

Specificity, also a statistical measure, defines the proportion of negative results that are correctly identified in a subject population. Specificity, in the form of a percentage,

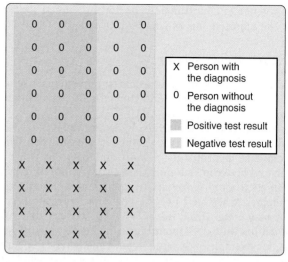

Figure 12-2 Hypothetical population (*n* = 50) used to compute sensitivity, specificity, and predictive values. (Adapted from Loong TW. Understanding sensitivity and specificity with the right side of the brain. *BMJ.* 2003;327[7417]:716–719.)

tells how good a test is at correctly identifying those who do not have the diagnosis (see Fig. 12-2).[6] "SpPin," the mnemonic associated with *Sp*ecificity, designates that a *P*ositive test result rules *in* the diagnosis.[7] If out of the same example population of 50 subjects, the test correctly identifies 12 of 30 people who do not have the diagnosis who test negative (TN), the specificity of the test is 40.0% (TN/[TN + FP] = specificity %).†

Predictive values define the chances of whether positive or negative test results will be correct. A *positive predictive value* looks at the true positives and false positives a test generates and defines the odds of a positive test being correct in terms of a percentage.[6] Using the examples previously mentioned, 18 of 33 positive test results were true positives (pink), resulting in a positive predictive value of 54.5%. Conversely, a *negative predictive value* specifies, in terms of percentage, the chances of a negative test result being correct by looking at the true negatives and false negatives it generates. In the previous example, 12 of 17 negative test results were true negatives (blue), for a 70.6% negative predictive value. The advantage of predictive values is that they change as the prevalence of the diagnosis changes. Loong's 2003 article, "Understanding sensitivity and specificity with the right side of the brain" is an excellent reference for students and those who are new to these concepts.[6]

It is important to remember that sensitivity, specificity, and predictive values have higher accuracy when test instruments meet the primary instrumentation requisites addressed earlier in this section. If a test measures inconsistently or inappropriately, or if instrumentation equipment or procedural guides are disregarded, the test's respective sensitivity, specificity, and predictive value percentages are compromised.

Additional Considerations

Scale and range of test instruments are also important when choosing measurement tools.

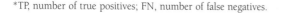

*TP, number of true positives; FN, number of false negatives.

†TN, number of true negatives; FP, number of false positives.

Scale refers to the basic measurement unit of an instrument. Scale should be suitably matched to the intended clinical application. For example, if a dynamometer measures in 10-pound increments and a patient's grip strength increases by a half a pound per week, it would take 20 weeks before the dynamometer would register the patient's improvement. The dynamometer in this example is an inappropriate measurement tool for this particular clinical circumstance because its scale is too gross to measure the patient's progress adequately.

Range involves the scope or breadth of a measurement tool, in other words, the distance between the instrument's beginning and end values. The range of an instrument must be appropriate to the clinical circumstance in which it will be used. For example, the majority of dynamometers used in clinical practice have a range from 0 to 200 pounds and yet, grip scores of many patients in rehabilitation settings routinely measure less than 30 pounds. Furthermore, the accuracy of most test instruments is diminished in the lowest and highest value ranges. This means that clinicians are assessing clients grip strength using the least accurate, lower 15% of available dynamometer range. With 85% of their potential ranges infrequently used, current dynamometers are ill suited to acute rehabilitation clinic needs. However, these same dynamometers are well matched to work-hardening situations where grip strengths more closely approximate the more accurate, midrange values of commercially available dynamometers.

Standardized Tests Versus Observational Tests

Through interpretation, *standardized tests* provide information that may be used to predict how a patient may perform in normal daily tasks. For example, if a patient achieves *x* score on a standardized test, he may be predicted to perform at an equivalent of the "75th percentile of normal assembly line workers." Standardized tests allow deduction of anticipated achievement based on narrower performance parameters as defined by the test.

In contrast, *observational tests* assess performance through comparison of subsequent test trials and are limited to like-item-to-like-item comparisons. Observational tests are often scored according to how patients perform specific test items; that is, independently, independently with equipment, needs assistance, and so forth. "The patient is able to pick up a full 12-ounce beer can with his injured hand without assistance." Progress is based on the fact that he could not accomplish this task 3 weeks ago. Observational information, however, cannot be used to predict whether the patient will be able to dress himself or run a given machine at work. Assumptions beyond the test item trial-to-trial performance comparisons are invalid and irrelevant. Observational tests may be included in an upper extremity assessment battery so long as they are used appropriately.

Computerized Assessment Instruments

Computerized assessment tools must meet the same primary measurement requisites as noncomputerized instruments. Unfortunately, both patients and medical personnel tend to assume that computer-based equipment is more trustworthy than noncomputerized counterparts. This naive assumption is erroneous and predisposed to producing misleading information. In hand rehabilitation, some of the most commonly used noncomputerized evaluation tools have been or are being studied for instrument reliability and validity (the two most fundamental instrumentation criteria). However, at the time of this writing, none of the computerized hand evaluation instruments have been statistically proven to have intrainstrument and interinstrument reliability compared with NIST criteria. Some have "human performance" reliability statements, but these are based on the fatally flawed premise that human normative performance is equivalent to gold-standard NIST calibration criteria.[2-3,5] Who would accept the accuracy of a weight set that had been "calibrated" by averaging 20 "normal" individuals' abilities to lift the weights? Human performance is not an acceptable criterion for defining the reliability (calibration) of mechanical devices, including those used in upper extremity rehabilitation clinics.

Furthermore, one cannot assume that a computerized version of an instrument is reliable and valid because its noncomputerized counterpart has established reliability. For example, although some computerized dynamometers have identical external components to those of their manual counterparts, internally they have been "gutted" and no longer function on hydraulic systems. Reliability and validity statements for the manual hydraulic dynamometer are not applicable to the "gutted" computer version. Even if both dynamometers were hydraulic, separate reliability and validity data would be required for the computerized instrument.

The inherent complexity of computerized assessment equipment makes it difficult to determine instrument reliability without the assistance of qualified engineers, computer experts, and statisticians. Compounding the problem, stringent federal regulation often does not apply to "therapy devices." Without sophisticated technical assistance, medical specialists and their patients have no way of knowing the true accuracy of the data produced by computerized therapy equipment.

Instrumentation Summary

Although many measurement instruments are touted as being "standardized," most lack even the rudimentary elements of statistical reliability and validity,[8,9] relying instead on normative statements such as means or averages. These norm-based tests lack even the barest of instrumentation requisites, meaning they cannot substantiate their consistency of measurement nor their ability to measure the entity for which they were designed. Because relatively few evaluation tools fully meet standardization criteria, instrument selection must be predicated on satisfying as many of the previously mentioned requisites as possible.[10] Hand/upper extremity assessment tools vary in their levels of reliability and validity according to how closely their inherent properties match the primary instrumentation requisites.

As consumers, medical specialists must require that all assessment tools have appropriate documentation of

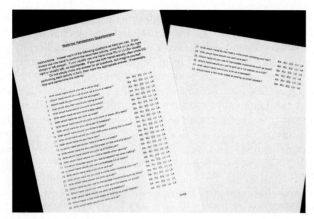

Figure 12-3 The Waterloo Handedness Questionnaire (WHQ) provides a more accurate definition of handedness than does the traditionally used self-report.

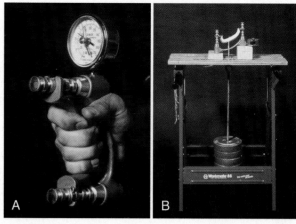

Figure 12-4 A, The hydraulic Jamar dynamometer has excellent reliability when calibrated correctly. **B,** A calibration testing station is easy to set up and will pay for itself over time. The most expensive components of the testing station are the F-tolerance test weights. The hook-weight combination is drill-calibrated to match the other weights, eliminating the need to subtract the weight of the hook.

reliability and validity at the very least. Furthermore, "data regarding reliability [and validity][†] should be available and should not be taken at face value alone; just because a manufacturer states reliability studies have been done, or a paper concludes an instrument is reliable, does not mean the instrument or testing protocol meets the requirements for scientific design."[11] *Purchasing and using assessment tools that do not meet fundamental measurement requisites limits potential at all levels, from individual patients to the scope of the profession.*

Functional Assessment Instruments

Handedness

Handedness is an essential component of upper extremity function. Traditionally, the patient self-report is the most common method of defining hand preference in the upper extremity rehabilitation arena. Although hand preference tests with established reliability and validity have been used by psychologists to delineate cortical dominance for several decades,[12,13] knowledge of these tests by surgeons and therapists is relatively limited. Recent studies show that the Waterloo Handedness Questionnaire (WHQ),[13-15] a 32-item function-based survey with high reliability and validity, more accurately and more extensively defines hand dominance (Fig. 12-3) than does the patient self-report.[16-17] The WHQ is inexpensive, simple and fast to administer, easy to score, and patients respond positively to it, welcoming its user-friendly format and explicitness of individualized results. Better definition of handedness is important to clinicians and researchers alike, in that it improves treatment focus and outcomes on a day-to-day basis, and, through more precise research studies, it eventually enhances the professional body of knowledge. (Also see the Grip Assessment section of this chapter.)

Hand Strength

Grip Assessment

Grip strength is most often measured with a commercially available hydraulic Jamar dynamometer (Fig. 12-4), although other dynamometer designs are available.[18-22] Developed by Bechtol[23] and recommended by professional societies,[24-26] the Jamar dynamometer has been shown to be a reliable test instrument,[27] provided calibration is maintained and standard positioning of test subjects is followed.[28-34]

In an ongoing instrument reliability study, of over 200 used Jamar and Jamar design dynamometers evaluated by the author, 51% passed the requisite +0.9994 correlation criterion compared with NIST F-tolerance test weights (government certified high-caliber test weights). Of these (0.9994 and above), 27% needed minor faceplate adjustments to align their read-out means with the mean readings of the standardized test weights. Of 30 brand new dynamometers, 80% met the correlation criterion of +0.9994. Interestingly, two Jamar dynamometers were tested multiple times over more than 12 years with less than a 0.0004 change in correlation, indicating that these instruments do maintain their calibration if carefully used and stored.[35]

Test procedure is important. In 1978 and 1983, the American Society for Surgery of the Hand recommended that the second handle position be used in determining grip strength and that the average of three trials be recorded.[24,36] In contrast to the recommended mean of three grip trials, one maximal grip is reported to be equally reliable in a small cohort study.[37] Deviation from recommended protocol should be undertaken with caution in regard to the mean-of-three-trials criterion, which is commonly utilized in research studies. More information is needed before adopting the one-trial method.

Of importance is the concept that grip changes according to size of object grasped. Normal adult grip values for the five consecutive handle positions consistently create a bell-shaped curve, with the first position (smallest) being the least advantageous for strong grip, followed by the fifth and fourth

---

[†]Author insert.

positions; strongest grip values occur at the third and second handle positions.[23,38] If inconsistent handle positions are used to assess patient progress, normal alterations in grip scores may be erroneously interpreted as advances or declines in progress. Fatigue is not an issue for the three-trial test procedure, but may become a factor when recording grip strengths using all five handle positions (total of 15 trials with 3 trials at each position).[39] A 4-minute rest period between handle positions helps control potential fatigue effect.[40] Although a 1-minute rest between sets was reported to be sufficient to avoid fatigue, this study was conducted using a dynamometer design instrument whose configuration is different from that of the Jamar dynamometer.[41] Percent of maximal voluntary contraction (MVC) required is also important in understanding normal grip strength and fatigue.[42] For example it is possible to sustain isometric contraction at 10% MVC for 65 minutes without signs of muscle fatigue.[43] Although Young[40] reported no significant difference in grip scores between morning and night, his data collection times were shorter compared to those of other investigators who recommend that time of day should be consistent from trial to trial.[23,44]

Better definition of handedness directly influences grip strength. Using the WHQ, Lui and Fess found a consistent polarization pattern with greater differences between dominant and nondominant grip strengths in normal subjects with WHQ classifications of predominantly left or right preference versus those who were ambidextrous or with slight left or right preferences. This polarization pattern was especially apparent in the second Jamar handle position.[45]

Norms for grip strength are available,[46-49] but several of these studies involve altered Jamar dynamometers or other types of dynamometers.[50-54] Independent studies refute the often cited 10% rule for normal subjects,[55] with reports finding that the minor hand has a range of equal to or stronger than the major hand in up to 31% of the normal population.[54,56,57] The "10% rule" also is not substantiated when the WHQ is used to define handedness.[45] Grip has been reported to correlate with height, weight, and age,[23,54,56,58] and socioeconomic variables such as participation in specific sports or occupations also influence normal grip.[59,60] Grip strength values lower than normal are predictive of deterioration and disability in elderly populations.[61-67] It is important to note that the Mathiowetz normative data reported for older adults[48] may be "up to 10 pounds lower than they should be."[68] A 2005 meta-analysis by Bohannon and colleagues that combined normative values from 12 studies that used Jamar dynamometers and followed American Society of Hand Therapists (ASHT) recommended testing protocols may be the most useful reference for normative data to date.[69] In a 2006 study, Bohannon and coworkers also conducted a meta-analysis for normative grip values of adults 20 to 49 years of age.[70]

Although grip strength is often used clinically to determine sincerity of voluntary effort, validity of its use in identifying submaximal effort is controversial, with studies both supporting[71-76] and refuting its appropriateness.[77-82] Niebuhr[83] recommends use of surface electromyography in conjunction with grip testing to more accurately determine sincerity of effort. The rapid exchange grip test,[84,85] a popular test for insincere effort, has been shown to have problems with procedure and reliability;[86,87] and even with a carefully standardized administration protocol, its validity is disputed due to low sensitivity and specificity.[86,88,89]

Hand grip strength is often an indicator of poor nutritional status. Unfortunately, the majority of these studies have been conducted using grip instruments other than the Jamar or Jamar-like dynamometers.[90-93] Furthermore, very few of these studies address calibration methods, rendering their results uncertain.

Bowman and associates reported that the presence or absence of the fifth finger flexor digitorum superficialis (FDS) significantly altered grip strength in normal subjects, with grip strength of the FDS-absent group being nearly 7 pounds less than the FDS-common group, and slightly more than 8 pounds less than the FDS-independent group.[94]

The Jamar's capacity as an evaluation instrument, the effects of protocol, and the ramification of its use have been analyzed by many investigators over the years with mixed, and sometimes conflicting, results. Confusion is due in large part to the fact that the vast majority of studies reported have relied on nonexistent, incomplete, or inappropriate methods for checking instrument accuracy of the dynamometers used in data collection. A second and more recent development is the ability to better define handedness using the WHQ. Scientific inquiry is both ongoing and progressive as new information is available. Although past studies provide springboards and directions, it is important to understand that all grip strength studies need to be reevaluated using carefully calibrated instruments and in the context of the more accurate definition of handedness provided by the WHQ.

Other grip strength assessment tools need to be ranked according to stringent instrumentation criteria, including longitudinal effects of use and time. Although spring-load instruments or rubber bulb/bladder instruments (Fig. 12-5) may demonstrate good instrument reliability when compared with corresponding NIST criteria, both these categories of instruments exhibit deterioration with time and use, rendering them inaccurate as assessment tools.

Pinch Assessment

Reliability of commercially available pinchometers needs thorough investigation. Generally speaking, hydraulic pinch

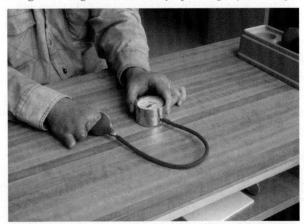

Figure 12-5 Rubber or spring dynamometer components deteriorate with use and over time, rendering the dynamometers useless as measurement devices.

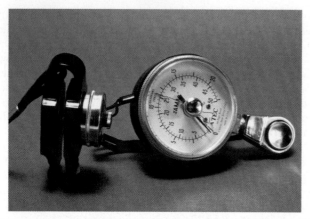

Figure 12-6 A hydraulic pinchometer (*right*) is consistently more reliable than the commonly used, elongated-C-spring design pinchometer (*left*). This is because the C-spring design pinchometer (*left*) is actually one large spring that is compressed as a patient pinches its two open ends together.

instruments are more accurate than spring-loaded pinchometers (Fig. 12-6). A frequently used pinchometer in the shape of an elongated C with a plunger dial on top is, mechanically speaking, a single large spring, in that its two ends are compressed toward each other against the counter force of the single center C spring. This design has inherent problems in terms of instrument reliability.[95]

Three types of pinch are usually assessed: (1) prehension of the thumb pulp to the lateral aspect of the index middle phalanx (key, lateral, or pulp to side); (2) pulp of the thumb to pulps of the index and long fingers (three-jaw chuck, three-point chuck); and (3) thumb tip to the tip of the index finger (tip to tip). Lateral is the strongest of the three types of pinch, followed by three-jaw chuck. Tip to tip is a positioning pinch used in activities requiring fine coordination rather than power. As with grip measurements, the mean of three trials is recorded, and comparisons are made with the opposite hand. Better definition of handedness via the WHQ improves understanding of the relative value of dominant and nondominant pinch strength. Cassanova and Grunert[96] describe an excellent method of classifying pinch patterns based on anatomic areas of contact. In an extensive literature review, they found more than 300 distinct terms for prehension. Their method of classification avoids colloquial usage and eliminates confusion when describing pinch function.

Sensibility Function

Of the five hierarchical levels of sensibility testing ([1] autonomic/sympathetic response, [2] detection, [3] discrimination, [4] quantification, and [5] identification),[97,98] only the final two levels include functional assessments. (See Chapter 11 for details regarding testing in the initial three levels.) At this time no standardized tests are available for these two categories although their concepts are used frequently in sensory reeducation treatment programs. However, several observation-based assessments are used clinically.

Quantification is the fourth hierarchical level of sensory capacity. This level involves organizing tactile stimuli according to degree. A patient may be asked to rank several object variations according to tactile properties, including, but not

limited to, roughness, irregularity, thickness, weight, or temperature. An example of a quantification level functional sensibility assessment, Barber's series of dowel rods covered with increasingly rougher sandpapers requires patients to rank the dowel rods from smoothest to roughest with vision occluded. For more detail, the reader is referred to Barber's archived chapter on the companion Web site of this text.

Identification, the final and most complicated sensibility level, involves the ability to recognize objects through touch alone.

The Moberg Picking-Up Test is useful both as an observational test of gross median nerve function and as an identification test. Individuals with median nerve sensory impairment tend to ignore or avoid using their impaired radial digits, switching instead to the ulnar innervated digits with intact or less impaired sensory input, as they pick up and place small objects in a can. This test is frequently adapted to assess sensibility identification capacity by asking patients, without using visual cues, to identify the small objects as they are picked up. A commercially available version of the Moberg Picking-Up Test is available. Currently, the Moberg is an observational test only. It meets none of the primary instrumentation requisites, including proof of reliability and validity; and for most of the noncommercial versions that are put together with a random assortment of commonly found small objects, it lacks even the simplest of equipment standards.

Daily Life Skills

Traditionally, the extent to which daily life skills (DLS) are assessed has depended on the type of clientele treated by various rehabilitation centers. For example, facilities oriented toward treatment of trauma injury patients required less extensive DLS evaluation and training than centers specializing in treatment of arthritis patients. However, with current emphasis on patient satisfaction reporting, it is apparent that more extensive DLS evaluation is needed to identify specific factors that are individual and distinct to each patient and patient population.

The *Flinn Performance Screening Tool* (FPST)[99] is important because of its excellent test–retest reliability (92% of the items: Kendall's $\tau > 0.8$ and 97% agreement); and because it continues to be tested and upgraded over time (Fig. 12-7). The FPST allows patients to work independently of the evaluator in deciding what tasks they can and cannot perform. The fact that this test is not influenced by the immediate presence of an administrator is both important and unusual. Busy clinicians may prejudge or assume patient abilities based on previous experience with similar diagnoses; and some patients hesitate to disclose personal issues. With the FPST, the potential for therapist bias is eliminated and issues such as patient lack of disclosure due to social unease is reduced. Patients peruse and rank the cards on their own without extraneous influence. The FPST consists of three volumes of over 300 laminated daily activity photographs that have been tested and retested for specificity and sensitivity of task. Volume 1 assesses self-care tasks; volume 2 evaluates home and outside activities; volume 3 relates to work activities. This test represents a major step toward defining function in a scientific manner.

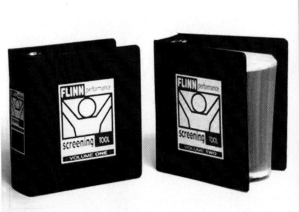
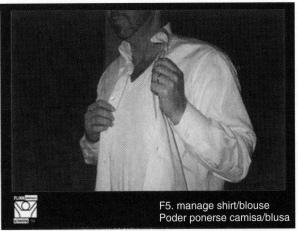

F5. manage shirt/blouse
Poder ponerse camisa/blusa

Figure 12-7 With a high reliability rating, the Flinn Performance Screening Tool (FPST) consists of a series of laminated photographs of activities of daily living and instrumental activities of daily living tasks from which patients identify activities that are problematic. Patients work independently, thereby avoiding potential evaluator bias or inhibiting societal influence. **A,** Volumes 1 and 2. **B,** One of more than 300 laminated photo cards contained in volumes 1–3.

Manual Dexterity and Coordination

Tests that assess dexterity and coordination are available in several levels of difficulty, allowing selection of instruments that best suit the needs and abilities of individual patients. As noted earlier, when using a standardized test instrument, it is imperative not to deviate from the method, equipment, and sequencing described in the test instructions. Test calibration, reliability, and validity are determined using very specific items and techniques, and any change in the stipulated pattern renders resultant data invalid and meaningless. Using a standardized test as a teaching or training device in therapy also excludes its use as an assessment instrument, due to skewing of data.

Jebsen Taylor Hand Function Test

Of the tests available, the *Jebsen Taylor Hand Function Test*[100] requires the least amount of extremity coordination, is inexpensive to assemble, and is easy to administer and score. The Jebsen consists of seven subtests: (1) writing, (2) card turning, (3) picking up small objects, (4) simulated feeding, (5) stacking, (6) picking up large lightweight objects, and (7) picking up large heavy objects. Originally developed for use with patients with rheumatoid arthritis,[100,101] the Jebsen has been used to assess aging adults,[102] hemiplegic persons,[103] children,[104] and patients with wrist immobilization,[105] among others. Jebsen norms are categorized according to maximum time, hand dominance, age, and gender.[106] Rider and Lindon[4] report a statistically significant difference in times with substitution of plastic checkers for the original wooden ones, and a trend of faster times with use of larger paper clips than originally described, invalidating the test. Equipment for standardized tests cannot be substituted or altered from that of the original test unless the test is restandardized completely with the new equipment. Capacity to measure gross coordination makes the Jebsen test an excellent instrument for assessing individuals whose severity of impairment precludes use of many other coordination tests, which often require very fine prehension patterns. The Jebsen is commercially available, but, before being used, this commercial format must be assessed thoroughly to ensure that it meets the original equipment standards and procedures.

Minnesota Rate of Manipulation Tests

Based on placing blocks into spaces on a board, the *Minnesota Rate of Manipulation Tests* (MRMT) include five activities: (1) placing, (2) turning, (3) displacing, (4) one-hand turning and placing, and (5) two-hand turning and placing. Originally designed for testing personnel for jobs requiring arm–hand dexterity, the MRMT is another excellent example of a test that measures gross coordination and dexterity, making it applicable to many of the needs encountered in hand/upper extremity rehabilitation. Norms for this instrument are based on more than 11,000 subjects. Unfortunately, some of the commercially available versions of the MRMT are made of plastic. Reliability, validity, and normative data were established on the original wooden version of the test and are not applicable to the newer plastic design. Essentially, the plastic MRMT is an unknown whose reliability, validity, and normative investigation must be established before it may be used as a testing instrument.

Purdue Pegboard Test

Requiring prehension of small pins, washers, and collars, the *Purdue Pegboard Test*[107] evaluates finer coordination than the two previous dexterity tests. Subcategories for the Purdue are (1) right hand, (2) left hand, (3) both hands, (4) right, left, and both, and (5) assembly. Normative data are presented in categories based on gender and job type: male and female applicants for general factory work, female applicants for electronics production work, male utility service workers, among others. Normative data are also available for 14- to 19-year-olds[108] and for ages 60 and over.[109] Reddon and colleagues[110] found a learning curve for some subtests when the Purdue was given five times at weekly intervals, reinforcing the concept that standardized tests should not be used as training devices for patients.

In terms of psychomotor taxonomy, all of the previously described tests assess activities that are classified as skilled movements, with the exception of the Jebsen's task of picking up small objects with a spoon. Skilled movements involve picking up and manipulation of objects using finger–thumb interaction. At this level, tool usage is not involved in the testing process. In contrast, compound adaptive skills, the next higher psychomotor level, incorporates tool use, a more difficult proficiency.

Crawford Small Parts Dexterity Test

Evaluating compound adaptive skills, the *Crawford Small Parts Dexterity Test* adds another dimension to hand function assessment by introducing tools into the test protocol. Increasing the level of difficulty, this test requires patients to control implements in addition to their hands and fingers. The Crawford involves use of tweezers and a screwdriver to assemble pins, collars, and small screws on the test board. It relates to activities requiring very fine coordination, such as engraving, watch repair and clock making, office machine assembly, and other intricate skills.

O'Connor Peg Board Test

The *O'Connor Peg Board*[111] test also requires use of tool manipulation to place small pegs on a board.

Nine-Hole Peg Test

Although frequently used in clinics, the *Nine-Hole Peg Test* lacks all the primary instrumentation requisites, including the critical elements of proof of reliability and validity. This "test" does have reported normative values but without the presence of primary instrumentation criteria, it is therefore useless as a measurement tool.

With the exception of the Nine-Hole Peg Test, all of the previously mentioned dexterity and coordination tests meet all of the primary and secondary instrumentation requisites. Other hand-coordination and dexterity tests are available. Before being used to assess patients, these tests should be carefully evaluated in terms of the primary, secondary, and optional instrumentation requisites discussed earlier in this chapter to ensure they have been proved to measure appropriately and accurately.

Work Hardening

Work-hardening tests span a wide range in terms of meeting instrumentation criteria, with many falling into the category of specific item or task longitudinal tests designed specifically to meet the needs of an individual patient.

Valpar Component Work Samples

On the sophisticated end of the continuum, the *Valpar Work Sample* consists of 19 work samples, each of which meets all the criteria for a standardized test. The individual tests may be used alone or in multiple groupings depending on patient requirements. The work samples may also be administered in any order. With the exception of the Valpar Work Samples, many work-hardening tests are not standardized.

Baltimore Therapeutic Equipment Work Simulator

The *Baltimore Therapeutic Equipment Work Simulator* (BTEWS) employs static and dynamic modes to produce

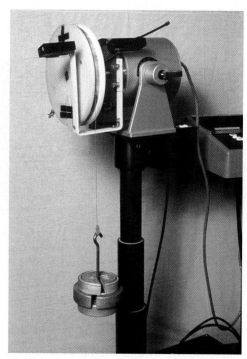

Figure 12-8 Designed by engineers, this method of testing the consistency of resistance of the Baltimore Therapeutic Equipment Work Simulator dynamic mode is more appropriate and more accurate than static weight suspension or human performance data. With the Work Simulator dynamic mode resistance set at 92% of the applied weights, when the pin is pulled, the wheel begins to rotate one revolution against the preset Simulator resistance and the weights are lowered to the floor in a controlled descent. If the resistance remains constant, the timed descent of the weights remains constant both within and between weight drop trials. If, however, the resistance fluctuates, the timed descent of the weights is inconsistent within and between trials. In many of the Work Simulators, resistance surges produced by the Simulator were sufficiently strong to halt the descent of 20 to 40 pounds of weight in midair. Other times the weights crashed unexpectedly to the floor when Simulator resistance suddenly decreased. (Coleman EF, Renfro RR, Cetinok EM, et al. Reliability of the manual dynamic mode of the Baltimore Therapeutic Equipment Work Simulator. *J Hand Ther.* 1996;9[3]:223–237.)

resistance to an array of tools and handles that are inserted into a common exercise head. Although the basic concept of this machine is innovative and the static mode has been shown to be accurate with high reliability correlation coefficients, the dynamic mode has problems producing consistent resistance. Coleman and coworkers found the dynamic mode resistance to vary widely both within machines and between machines, making the Work Simulator inappropriate for assessment when consistent resistance is required (Fig. 12-8).[112-114] Because of the fluctuating and unpredictable dynamic mode resistance changes, which are not accurately reflected by the computer printout (Figs. 12-9 and 12-10), caution should be used in allowing patients with acute injuries, geriatric patients, pediatric patients, patients with inflammatory problems such as rheumatoid arthritis, patients with unstable vascular systems, or patients with impaired sensibility to exercise on this machine. Longitudinal pre-BTEWS and post-BTEWS volumetric measurements may be helpful in identifying patients whose inflammatory response to working in the Work Simulator dynamic mode may be progressively increasing.

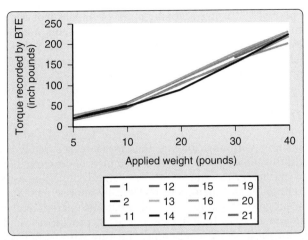

Figure 12-9 A composite of the Work Simulators tested, these are the reports generated by the Work Simulator dynamic mode printouts of the resistance (torque) produced by Simulator dynamic modes. The Simulator printouts reported output data that closely mirrored the input resistance set by the engineer researchers. (Coleman EF, Renfro RR, Cetinok EM, et al. Reliability of the manual dynamic mode of the Baltimore Therapeutic Equipment Work Simulator. *J Hand Ther.* 1996;9[3]:223–237.)

Interestingly, a review of reliability studies involving the Work Simulator identifies a pattern that is all too often found with mechanical rehabilitation devices, in that multiple studies were conducted and reported using human performance to establish its reliability as an assessment instrument.[115-121] Human performance is not an appropriate indicator of accuracy or calibration for mechanical devices using NIST criteria. Furthermore, the recommended method for "calibrating" Work Simulators involves a static process of weight suspension that is incongruous with assessing dynamic mode resistance. Later, when a team of engineers evaluated the consistency of resistance of the dynamic mode

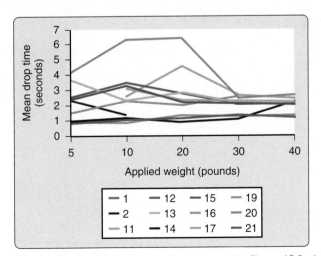

Figure 12-10 In contrast to the printout reports in Figure 12-9, the timed weight drops against Simulator-produced resistance indicate large inconsistencies in resistances created by the various dynamic modes of the Work Simulators. Furthermore, Simulator-generated printout reports did not accurately reflect the actual resistances produced by the Simulator dynamic modes. (Coleman EF, Renfro RR, Cetinok EM, et al. Reliability of the manual dynamic mode of the Baltimore Therapeutic Equipment Work Simulator. *J Hand Ther.* 1996;9[3]:223–237.)

according to NIST standards and employing an appropriate dynamic measurement method, reliability and accuracy of the dynamic mode were found to be seriously lacking.[113]

A second-generation "work simulator," the BTE Primus, is currently on the market, along with similar machines from other companies. The Primus drops the terminology of "static" and "dynamic" modes, opting instead for isometric, isotonic, and isokinetic resistance and continuous passive motion modes. No NIST-based reliability information for the modes in which patients work against preset resistances is available for any of these second-generation machines including the Primus.[122-125] Before the Primus may be used as an assessment instrument, or for that matter, a treatment tool, the Coleman and associates[113] engineering methods used to evaluate the BTEWS should be employed to fully identify the consistency of resistance produced by its resistance modes. Unfortunately, the Coleman and associates NIST-based engineering study of the BTEWS is not included in the Primus operator's manual bibliography.

Assessment of a patient's potential to return to work is based on a combination of standardized and observational tests, knowledge of the specific work situation, insight into the patient's motivational and psychological resources, and understanding of the complexities of normal and disabled hands and upper extremities in general. Although its importance has been acknowledged in the past, vocational assessment of the patient with an upper extremity injury is now given a higher priority in most of the major hand rehabilitation centers throughout the country. Treatment no longer ends with achievement of skeletal stability, wound healing, and a plateau of motion and sensibility. This shift in emphasis has been the result, in large part, of the contributions of the Philadelphia Hand Center.

Patient Satisfaction

Testing *patient satisfaction* has become an integral part of rehabilitation endeavors.[126,127] Just as other test instruments must meet primary instrumentation requisites, so too must patient satisfaction assessment tools,[128-130] which are often in the format of patient self-report questionnaires.

Current symptom or satisfaction tools used in evaluating patients with upper extremity injury or dysfunction include the *Medical Outcomes Study 36-Item Health Survey* (SF-36), the *Upper Extremities Disabilities of Arm, Shoulder, and Hand* (DASH),[131-150] the *Quick DASH*, and the *Michigan Hand Outcomes Questionnaire* (MHQ).[151,152] In contrast to the DASH instruments, the MHQ takes into consideration the important factors of hand dominance and hand/upper extremity cosmesis.[151-160] These assessment tools have been extensively tested and meet all the primary instrumentation requisites. They are also available in many languages.

Diagnosis-Specific Tests of Function
Rheumatoid Arthritis

Arthritis literature is replete with dexterity and coordination tests, due in no small part to the numerous research studies involving outcomes of pharmacologic interventions. Some of the more frequently used assessments include the *Sequential*

Occupational Dexterity Assessment (SODA), the *Sollerman Test of Hand Grip,* the *Arthritis Hand Function Test,* the *Grip Ability Test,* the *Keitel Function Test,* and the previously mentioned *Jebsen Taylor Hand Function Test.*

In contrast to these sophisticated coordination tests is the ubiquitous use of *sphygmomanometers* to assess grip strength. Despite a 1999 engineering report by Unsworth and colleagues[161] that found "bags of different diameter and volume were seen to give statistically different pressure readings when squeezed by the same subjects," the blood pressure cuff remains a common tool for evaluating grip strength in contemporary rheumatoid arthritis literature.

Stroke

The *Wolf Motor Function Test* (WMFT)[162-171] assesses motor function in adults with hemiplegia due to stroke or traumatic brain injury. Although the original WMFT had 21 tasks, the adapted WMFT is shortened to 15 functional tasks and "includes items that cover a range of movements that can be evaluated within a realistic time period for both clinical and research purposes." Ranging from 0.86 to 0.99, the WMFT-15 has good inter-rater, intrarater agreement, internal consistency, and test–retest reliability. A video demonstration of the WMFT may be found at *www.youtube.com/watch?v=SIJK88NdZM.*

Used in constraint-induced movement therapy, the original *Motor Activity Log* (MAL)[172-176] was designed as a structured interview to assess how hemiparetic poststroke individuals use their more involved upper extremity in real-world activities. The MAL is divided into two components: amount of use (AOU) and quality of movement (QOM), during activities of daily living. The MAL is "internally consistent and relatively stable in chronic stroke patients not undergoing intervention." However, its longitudinal construct validity is in doubt. The Motor Activity Log-14, a shortened version of the MAL, corrects many of the inconsistencies of the original MAL.[174]

Carpal Tunnel Syndrome

The *Severity of Symptoms and Functional Status in Carpal Tunnel Syndrome questionnaire* is an outcomes tool that was developed specifically to assess carpal tunnel syndrome symptoms[177-183] using a combination of impairment assessment tools, patients' self-reports of their symptoms, and their abilities to accomplish a few specific functional tasks that are problematic for those suffering from median nerve compression at the wrist.

Summary

Evaluation with instruments that measure accurately and truthfully allows physicians and therapists to correctly identify hand/upper extremity pathology and dysfunction, assess the effects of treatment, and realistically apprise patients of their progress. Accurate assessment data also permit analysis of treatment modalities for effectiveness, provide a foundation for professional communication through research, and eventually influence the scope and direction of the profession as a whole. Because of their relationship to the kind of information obtained, assessment tools should be chosen carefully. The choice of tools directly influences the quality of individual treatment and the degree of understanding between hand specialists. Criteria exist for identifying dependable instruments for accurate measurement when used by different evaluators and from session to session. Unless the results of a "home-brewed" test are statistically analyzed, the test is tried on large numbers of normal subjects, and the results are analyzed again, it is naïve to assume that such a test provides meaningful information. In the future, currently utilized tools may be better understood through checking their reliability and validity levels with bioengineering technology,[176] and statisticians may be of assistance in devising protocols that will lead to more refined and accurate information. We as hand specialists have a responsibility to our patients and our colleagues to continue to critique the instruments we use in terms of their capacities as measurement tools. Without assessment, we cannot treat, we cannot communicate, and we cannot progress.

REFERENCES

The complete reference list is available online at www.expertconsult.com.

CHAPTER 13

Diagnostic Imaging of the Upper Extremity

JOHN S. TARAS, MD AND LEONARD L. D'ADDESI, MD

RADIOGRAPHY
CLINICAL APPLICATIONS
SUMMARY

CRITICAL POINTS

- Plain radiography is the standard imaging technique. It provides the vast majority of information needed in many hand and wrist disorders.
- Advanced imaging is necessary when disorders cannot be adequately assessed through routine measures.
- A bone scan is a minimally invasive technique that provides information about blood flow, soft tissue elements and bone pathology. Anatomic resolution is poor, yet bone scanning is an important adjunct to other imaging modalities. Bone scanning is useful especially when the diagnosis is enigmatic.
- Arteriography is a minimally invasive technique to accurately visualize arterial anatomy and integrity and may be necessary when considering vascular surgery or to view the vascularity of musculoskeletal lesions.
- Ultrasound is a noninvasive modality for viewing and differentiating masses within the musculoskeletal system, especially between solid and cystic masses. Ultrasound can provide a dynamic account of tendon excursion as well, and look for tendon injury.
- Computed Tomography (CT) is a noninvasive modality, but exposes patients to ionizing radiation. Benefits include the ability to observe occult fractures within the carpus, identify displacement of fracture fragments, and evaluate for bone healing and nonunion. CT is especially useful for looking at the distal radioulnar joint for subluxation or dislocation.
- Magnetic Resonance Imaging (MRI) is a noninvasive imaging technique that has become the gold standard in viewing and differentiating soft tissue lesions, identifying lesions of the carpal ligaments, triangular fibrocartilage, and occult fractures of the hand and wrist. Flexor tendon injuries and tenosynovitis is easily identified. MRI is contraindicated in patients with pacemakers and cochlear implants.

The diagnosis of upper extremity disorders relies on information obtained in the history, physical examination, and views of the region acquired through one or more imaging techniques. Plain radiography provides adequate visualization of most problems and, for that reason, is a standard part of the initial evaluation. Excellent depiction of fractures, fracture alignment, fracture healing site, dislocation, soft tissue calcification, foreign bodies, and bony detail can be obtained by this readily available, cost-effective, and noninvasive means. In certain cases, however, the problem cannot be properly assessed by routine measures; thus, other imaging modalities are needed to provide further diagnostic information. In this chapter, radiography and advanced imaging techniques are discussed in relation to the diagnosis of hand and wrist disorders.

Radiography

Routine Studies

Routine studies of the hand consist of posteroanterior (PA), lateral, and oblique views, which are evaluated for bone density, bony lesions, fractures and dislocations, integrity of the articular surfaces and joint spaces, and irregularities of the soft tissue (Fig. 13-1).[1]

Bone density, which is evaluated grossly, may be normal, less than normal (osteopenia), or greater than normal (osteosclerosis). Osteopenia is most often encountered in the elderly and is known as senile osteoporosis when associated with advanced age. Osteosclerosis occurs in conditions such as avascular necrosis (AVN) (Fig. 13-2), fracture healing, and metabolic bone disease.[2] Plain films may reveal discrete or diffuse bone lesions, including primary or metastatic bone tumors, infection, and metabolic bone disease (Fig. 13-3). The cortical integrity is carefully inspected for evidence of acute fracture (Fig. 13-4) and the joint alignment evaluated for subluxation or dislocation.[3] Abnormalities of the articular

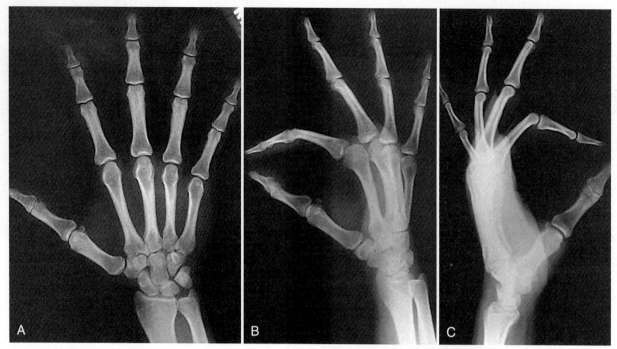

Figure 13-1 Routine views of the hand. **A,** Posteroanterior. **B,** Oblique. **C,** Lateral.

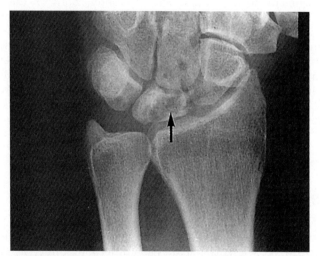

Figure 13-2 Avascular necrosis (AVN) of the lunate, or Kienböck's disease. Coned-down posteroanterior views of the wrist demonstrate two manifestations of AVN: bony sclerosis, seen in the ulnar aspect of the lunate, and osteopenia, seen in the radial side of the lunate *(arrow)*. The latter is due to increased blood flow as the bone attempts to heal.

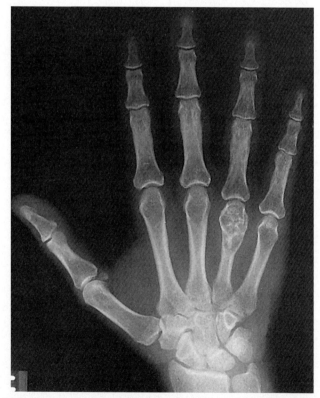

Figure 13-3 An enchondroma is demonstrated in this posteroanterior view. Note the decreased bone density of the fourth metacarpal head and shaft, which also are increased in size. Within the area of decreased bone density are stippled calcifications—a classic finding in this type of lesion.

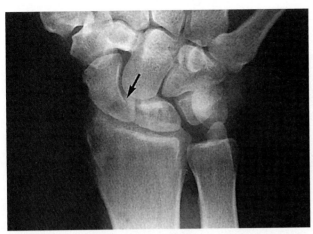

Figure 13-4 This posteroanterior view of the wrist shows a fracture of the proximal third of the scaphoid *(arrow)* with an associated cyst.

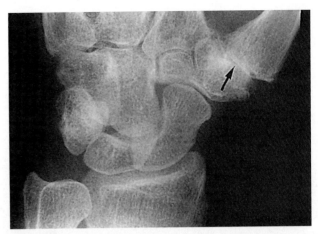

Figure 13-6 Osteoarthritis. Oblique view of the wrist showing decreased height of the articular cartilage at the first metacarpal joint *(arrow)*. The disease also has resulted in increased bone density on both sides of the joint.

surface and cartilage joint space also are documented. Narrowing of the cartilage space may indicate arthritis, resulting from degeneration, inflammation, infection, or trauma (Figs. 13-5 and 13-6).[4] Finally, the soft tissue shadows are evaluated for irregularities. Any evidence of calcification (Fig. 13-7), foreign bodies (Fig. 13-8, online),[5] or soft tissue masses must be correlated with the clinical findings.

Special Views

If the history and physical examination indicate a localized problem, a coned-down view of the area can be obtained. This magnified spot film focuses on a specific area of the wrist, which is especially useful for isolated disease of the carpal bones because fractures and abnormalities in this region often cannot be seen on plain views (Fig. 13-9, online). Special positioning and maneuvers also are used to allow more complete visualization of a possible pathologic condition. For example, stress views may demonstrate joint malalignments that are not evident on routine films. Tears of the ulnar collateral ligament of the thumb metacarpophalangeal (MCP) joint are a case in point because these can become apparent by applying a force to this joint in radial deviation (Fig. 13-10).[5] A special maneuver is often needed to demonstrate damage to the scapholunate ligament complex. This complex is important in stabilizing the scaphoid and preventing rotatory subluxation. When it is injured, the

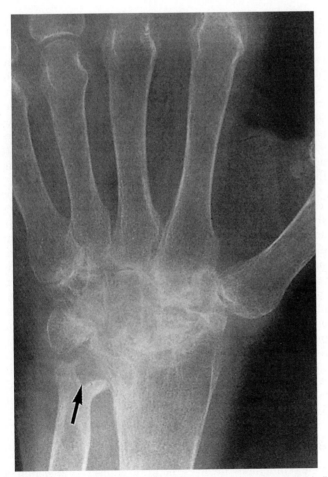

Figure 13-5 Posteroanterior views of the wrist demonstrating the hallmarks of rheumatoid arthritis: osteopenia, which may be the earliest sign of the disease (compare with normal bone density in Fig. 13-1, **A**), loss of articular cartilage, and erosions. In this patient, erosion is evident at the ulnar styloid *(arrow)*.

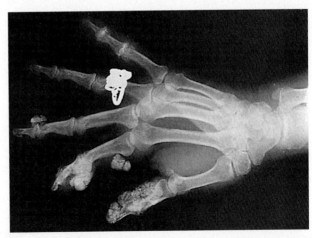

Figure 13-7 Oblique view of the hand demonstrating extensive calcification in the soft tissues of the digits.

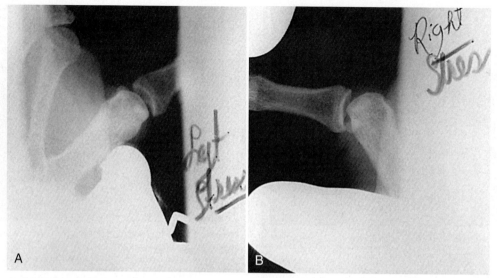

Figure 13-10 Thumb dislocation. **A,** This patient's left thumb appears normal under radial stress. **B,** The right thumb, which had a disruption of the ulnar collateral ligament, shows subluxation of the first metacarpophalangeal joint when subjected to the same stress.

scapholunate interval may appear completely normal on a routine view, but it widens when a compression load is applied by clenching the fist in supination (Fig. 13-11). Recently, a modified clenched-fist view, called the "clenched-pencil" view, was described.[6] This view allows the appropriate amount of pronation of the wrist to view the scapholunate interval most favorably. Special views, such as those of the trapezial ridge (Fig. 13-12) and hook of the hamate (Fig. 13-13), also are useful in demonstrating the bony anatomy of the carpal tunnel and certain fractures.

Advanced Imaging Techniques

When a diagnosis cannot be made on the basis of the routine clinical examination and plain radiographs, more advanced imaging techniques can be used to visualize the bone and soft tissue anatomy more completely. The decision to use another technique must consider the invasiveness and cost of the procedure (Table 13-1, online) as well as its specificity.

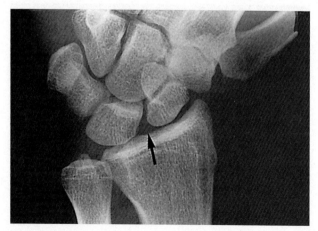

Figure 13-11 When this patient clenched the fist in supination, subluxation of the scaphoid (arrow) occurred.

Tomography

Plain tomography is capable of visualizing healing bone and fracture nonunion better than routine radiographs, especially in cases involving the scaphoid and hook of the hamate. This examination is noninvasive and relatively inexpensive. Computed tomography has largely replaced plain tomography in most centers. CT is more clinically useful than conventional tomography because it can obtain multiple contiguous sections with high resolution in a short time, multiplanar image reconstruction is possible, and additional information about adjacent soft tissues can be obtained. 3D reconstructions are now also available to help in planning surgery.[7] CT remains the best modality for demonstrating bony architecture.[8]

CT is useful in evaluating complex fractures and bony lesions, providing superior detail of cortical invasion, marrow abnormalities, and matrix calcification.[5,9,10] It is also an excellent means of depicting subluxations and dislocations of the distal radioulnar joint.[11] In patients with metallic hardware, significant scatter often overlays the image of the bony segment. Image techniques can be manipulated to minimize this beam-hardening artifact to fine-tune visualization of the bony anatomy. The advantage of CT over conventional radiography lies in its ability to obtain transaxial images and provide excellent contrast resolution for evaluating soft tissues. This modality is also noninvasive, unless used in conjunction with contrast agents. CT exposes patients to potentially harmful ionizing radiation. With the advent of fast CT scanners, availability has led to increased radiation doses to patients.

Bone Scintigraphy

Bone scintigraphy involves the intravenous (IV) injection of ^{99m}Tc-labeled monodiphosphonate (MDP), which is preferentially taken up by bone. Flow images are generated after 60 seconds, and a nuclear medicine angiogram is obtained. Delayed images are generated after 3 hours. Areas of

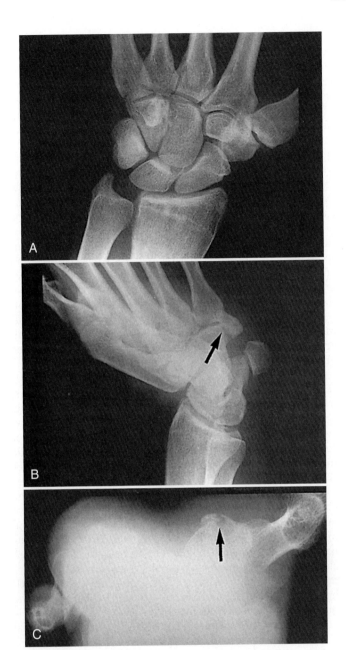

Figure 13-12 Fracture of the trapezial ridge. **A,** This routine postero-anterior view of the wrist is normal. **B,** A supinated oblique view shows a fracture of the trapezial ridge *(arrow)*. **C,** A carpal tunnel view in the same patient also demonstrates this type of fracture *(arrow)*.

abnormal blood flow and bone turnover can be detected on the scan, making it useful in the evaluation of infection, AVN of the lunate, tumors, and reflex sympathetic dystrophy. It also is used to screen patients who have unexplained wrist pain (Fig. 13-14).[12]

The examination is minimally invasive and moderately expensive. The poor anatomic resolution of the scan is its primary drawback. The test also is nonspecific, making it impossible to distinguish various processes that can cause increased uptake.[13] The results must be carefully correlated with the clinical findings to be properly interpreted. Today, MRI has largely replaced scintigraphy in most centers in musculoskeletal imaging.[14]

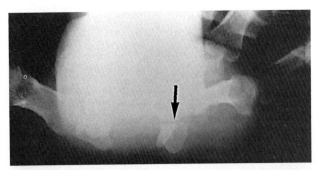

Figure 13-13 Carpal tunnel view showing a fracture of the hook of the hamate *(arrow)*.

Arteriography

Arteriography is the most specific means of evaluating vascular anatomy and pathology; it is used to evaluate aneurysms, arteriovenous malformations, tumors of vascular origin, traumatic vessel injuries, and solid tumor vascularity (Fig. 13-15).[8,15] The examination is performed by threading a catheter into the brachial artery using a femoral approach, injecting contrast material, and then taking multiple radiographs. The procedure is often painful, even with the use of new nonionic contrast material. Complications include bleeding hematoma, pseudoaneurysm formation, dissection, and thrombosis. The contrast medium may cause arterial spasm, although this can be controlled with the use of vasodilators. Anaphylaxis is another potential complication when iodinated contrast material is used, but severe episodes are rare, occurring in only 1 of 40,000 cases.

In the diagnosis of bone and soft tissue tumors, conventional angiography has largely been replaced with MRI and magnetic resonance angiography (MRA) to avoid potential complications.[8]

Arthrography

Arthrography is used to evaluate the integrity of the carpal ligaments and triangular fibrocartilage (TFC) (Fig. 13-16,

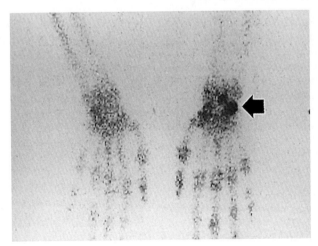

Figure 13-14 This bone scan demonstrates increased uptake in the right lunate, the right pisiform/triquetral area, and the first carpal metacarpal joint *(arrow)*. Such findings are nonspecific. Avascular necrosis of the lunate was demonstrated on other imaging studies.

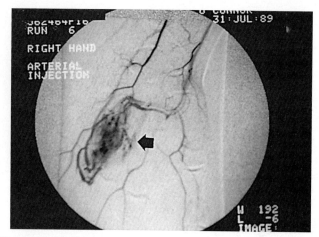

Figure 13-15 Contrast arteriogram of the wrist showing a hemangioma (arrow) in the ulnar aspect of the palm.

online). The examination involves injecting dye into the radiocarpal, radioulnar, and midcarpal compartments, so it must be performed carefully.[1] The injection of contrast material into the joint can highlight intra-articular soft tissue structures such as ligaments and fibrocartilaginous structures.[16] Communication of dye between the compartments of the wrist can be caused by a clinically unimportant perforation and does not necessarily indicate pathology.[17] Thus, the test results must be correlated with the clinical examination and interpreted with a great deal of caution. The examination is invasive but can be administered with minimal discomfort to the patient.

The role of arthrography had declined because of the excellent visualization of intra-articular structures by MRI.[18,19] Arthrography has also been found to be only 60% accurate in detecting tears in the triangular fibrocartilage complex (TFCC), scapholunate ligament, or lunotriquetral ligament.[20] Arthrography is currently used as a complement to MRI and CT to enhance the diagnostic accuracy.[21]

Cineradiography

Continuous radiographic imaging has many applications such as arthrography, tenography, bursography, arteriography, and percutaneous bone and soft tissue biopsy.[21] Evaluation of the wrist in motion is a useful method for detecting the rigidity of a freshly fixed fracture or for dynamic carpal instability. This noninvasive and inexpensive technique is the diagnostic imaging procedure of choice for determining and documenting the presence of dynamic rotatory subluxation of the scaphoid.[22] The role of MRI in this capacity is evolving but remains problematic. Dynamic MRI is a newer technique that may yield more comprehensive clinically relevant information with regard to wrist kinematics than conventional MRI.[23,24]

Magnetic Resonance Imaging

MRI visualizes tissue by applying a strong magnetic field with radiofrequency pulses to record differences in tissue signal intensity. A variety of magnet strengths are available from 0.2 to 3 T, with higher strengths providing greater contrast

resolution.[13,25] MRI provides high resolution and high-contrast tissue segmented information about the integrity of joint and soft tissue structures. It also is completely noninvasive, involves no ionizing radiation, and is able to obtain images through cast and fiberglass materials that limit the resolution of conventional radiography and CT.[8] Among its minor drawbacks are its contraindications in patients with pacemakers, cochlear implants, or ferromagnetic aneurysm clips. Implanted metallic objects create "holes" and distort the images of tissues hoped to be visualized.[8,21] In addition, the examination is performed with the patient lying in a narrow cylinder within the bore of a magnet, a closed space that may cause some individuals to become claustrophobic. In the event of such anxiety, IV benzodiazepam may be administered to the patient, provided that the patient can be monitored properly during sedation. Open MRIs have evolved and are advantageous in this setting. The diagnostic accuracy of low-field open scanners has been found to be comparable to that of high-field scanners.[26] Evaluating a suggested pathology with MRI involves the use of multiple sequences, including T1, T2, short tau inversion recovery (STIR), and spin echo; for this reason, close communication between the orthopedist and radiologist is essential.

MRI is of great value in defining soft tissue abnormalities (Figs. 13-17 to 13-19, all online). In the evaluation of tumors, it cannot provide a specific diagnosis, but it can define the size of the lesion and the extent of involvement of marrow and neurovascular structures (Fig. 13-20, online).[27] Other soft tissue abnormalities diagnosed more easily by MRI include ganglions, ligament tears, and cartilage abnormalities (Fig. 13-21).[28,29] Dorsal wrist pain can be attributed to hypertrophy of the dorsal capsule as well as ganglions that may be occult and not palpable. Patients with dorsal wrist pain of unknown origin are therefore candidates for MRI evaluation. MRI is especially helpful in diagnosing tears of the scapholunate and lunotriquetral ligaments, particularly when dissociation of the scapholunate is not evident on plain films.[30] Excellent depiction of the TFC can be achieved with MRI, but the image must be interpreted carefully; thinning of the disk occurs in many patients, but a tear of this structure is not diagnosed unless an avulsion from the ulnar or radial insertion can be observed.[31-33]

MRA is another tool that can easily demonstrate vascular abnormalities. MRA provides detailed information about the anatomy of the small vessels that constitute the carpal arches.[23] MRA is noninvasive because it does not require the use of IV contrast material (Figs. 13-22 and 13-23, both online). Rather, it relies on the property of blood flow, and special pulsed sequences are used to enhance the fluid within the vessels.[21]

Conventional radiography is still considered the first-line means of examining the wrist. More recently, CT has been used, especially for examining fractures. However, MRI has revolutionized the manner in which the orthopedic surgeon approaches diagnosis and decision making,[23] although the gold standard for assessment of the wrist for pathology is arthroscopy.

Ultrasound

Ultrasound (US) uses high-frequency sound waves to produce images. The images produced are a reflection of the

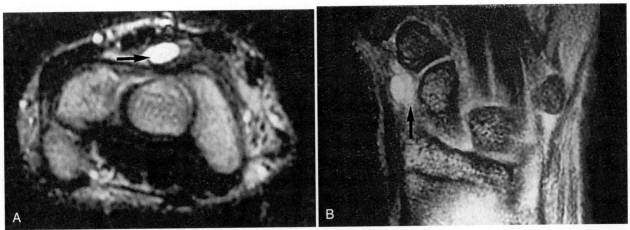

Figure 13-21 Ganglion. **A,** This axial magnetic resonance image demonstrates a dorsal mass *(arrow)* that was not palpable on clinical examination. **B,** Coronal magnetic resonance image in another patient showing a mass in the abductor canal *(arrow)*.

echogenicity of a structure, which determines its brightness on the ultrasound. Cysts and tendons have low echogenicity, whereas solid masses have high echogenicity and appear white on ultrasound. Doppler US can image motion and has been used routinely for imaging blood vessels.[13,25]

US is noninvasive, does not emit ionizing radiation, is readily available, and has high patient acceptance.[18] The two major indications for US are muscle injuries and tendon lesions. Joint effusions, ganglia, and ruptures of larger ligaments (not interosseous carpal ligaments) can be observed. Dynamic US can be used to view tendon movements. Nonorthogonal scanning, however, can produce hyperechoic zones mimicking partial tendon tears or tendinitis.[7]

The use of US has been limited mainly because of the inability to penetrate bone and view osseous pathology. US is also operator-dependent, involves long examination times, and produces static images that may be incomprehensible when viewed at a later time.[18,25] The accuracy and reliability of US for detecting ganglions, solid lesions, tenosynovitis, and tendon lesions are limited.[34,35]

Clinical Applications

Extensor Tendons

The extensor tendons are contained in six dorsal compartments numbered from the radial (I) to ulnar (VI) sides of the wrist. Lister's tubercle separates compartments II and III. Extensor disorders outside of compartments I or VI are rare; thus, fluid in multiple compartments usually represents synovitis and is often a marker for an inflammatory arthritis such as rheumatoid arthritis.

More commonly, the tendons of compartment I (abductor pollicis longus and extensor pollicis brevis tendons) are affected with stenosing tenosynovitis. This disorder is termed de Quervain's disease and is related to overuse. It is more common in women and also may occur as a complication of pregnancy. Patients typically present with pain radiating from the radial styloid to the thumb and proximally into the forearm. Pain is increased with passive movement of the thumb and swelling or tenderness over the first dorsal compartment of the wrist. This disorder usually is diagnosed

clinically. On MRI, fluid within the tendon sheath is increased, and the tendons themselves, which may show increased intrasubstance signal, are enlarged. On coronal images, there is focal obliteration of the adjacent subcutaneous fat and intense synovial enhancement following gadolinium administration. This stenosing tenosynovitis is analogous to adhesive capsulitis in the shoulder.

Compartment VI contains the extensor carpi ulnaris (ECU) tendon, which is another common site for disorders such as synovitis or tenosynovitis. ECU subluxation may occur, which can lead to synovitis or intrasubstance tears; thus, dynamic imaging may be performed to confirm the diagnosis. It should be recognized that artifactual increased signal within the ECU is commonly seen, which may represent subclinical degeneration or normal fascicular anatomy.

Ligament Injuries and Carpal Instability

The ligamentous anatomy of the wrist is complex because of the stabilization required for the numerous carpal bones and extensive range and axes of motion in this joint. The intrinsic carpal ligaments connect the carpal bones to each other, and the extrinsic ligaments connect the carpus to both the radius and ulna and to the metacarpals. The extrinsic ligaments are more important for overall carpal stability and have a complex nomenclature. In general, tears of the extrinsic ligaments are less common and more difficult to diagnose than intrinsic ligament tears. Ligaments can be injured by trauma or by inflammatory processes such as rheumatoid arthritis (RA).

The two main intrinsic ligaments of the wrist are the scapholunate (SL) and lunatotriquetral (LT) ligaments. SL ligament tears may be spontaneous, secondary to a fall on an outstretched hand, or associated with the subtypes of carpal instability. LT ligament tears also can be spontaneous or posttraumatic. LT tears are not uncommonly associated with instability patterns of the wrist and also have a high association with TFC tears.

Mechanically, both the SL and LT ligaments are divided into three portions: dorsal, volar, and central. The central or membranous portion is thin, whereas the dorsal and volar portions are thicker with individual fascicles usually visible.

Membranous tears can cause pain but are biomechanically unimportant. The dorsal and volar aspects of these ligaments are more important to the mechanical stability of the carpus. The dorsal SL ligament is the more significant portion that helps prevent dorsal intercalated segment instability (DISI), whereas the volar portion of the LT ligament is vital to prevent volar intercalated segment instability (VISI).

The carpal ligaments are best visualized on thin-section 3D gradient recalled echo (GRE) MR sequences in the coronal and axial planes. They appear as signal voids bridging the carpal bones. Ligament strains can be diagnosed if the signal is abnormal or the structure is attenuated. Discontinuity, complete absence, and increased intercarpal distances are findings compatible with ligament tears. The best finding for an intrinsic tear is fluid violating the space extending from the radiocarpal to the midcarpal joints. Normally, the ends of the lunate, scaphoid, and triquetrum should appear smoothly rounded. The presence of osteophytes is abnormal and often is caused by biomechanically incompetent ligaments, usually resulting from partial dorsal or volar aspect tears. The presence of marrow edema, subchondral sclerosis, or other signs of focal articular disease should suggest ligament dysfunction. Focal offset of two adjacent carpal bones and the lack of the normal articular parallelism also are signs suggestive of ligament dysfunction. Remember that perforation of the SL or LT ligament occurs with aging; thus, in a patient older than 35 to 40 years, a tear should be diagnosed only if the ligament is morphologically abnormal.

The diagnosis of many patterns of carpal instability can be established by routine radiographic findings. The lateral projection is useful in evaluating both DISI and VISI. In DISI, the lunate is tilted dorsally, with the scaphoid displaced vertically. The angle of intersection between the main longitudinal axis (along the radius, lunate, capitate, and third metacarpal) and the long axis of the scaphoid is greater than 60 degrees where it should normally be 30 to 60 degrees. The radioscapholunate ligament should be evaluated for tears. This injury is typically degenerative in origin and is thought to be the sequela of trauma to the outstretched hand in a young adult. In VISI, the lunate is flexed toward the palm, and the angle between the two longitudinal axes is less than 30 degrees. Note that this finding may be normal if bilateral and in a young female patient. VISI is less common than DISI overall. Most cases are thought to be degenerative in origin, although there is an association with RA. These patterns must also be carefully interpreted on sagittal MRI as the lunate may appear more dorsally tilted, mimicking a DISI pattern in otherwise normal wrists.[36]

The evaluation of these ligaments for abnormalities has been challenging. In the past, evaluation was limited to conventional arthrography. Proponents state that wrist arthrography has the potential to provide an equivalent diagnostic evaluation to arthroscopy, provided the technique is meticulously followed and the operator possesses fundamental knowledge regarding anatomy and age-related changes of the wrist.[16] With advanced imaging techniques, such as MRA, the extrinsic and intrinsic ligaments can easily be seen.[37]

Advanced cases of carpal instability are obvious on routine radiographic studies. Subtle instability may require advanced imaging. Yet there has been a discrepancy in the literature about the sensitivity and specificity of MRI in detecting intrinsic ligament tears.[19,38,39] Recently, CT arthrography was found to have high sensitivity and specificity in detecting interosseous ligament injuries.[40,41] Schmid and colleagues[41] compared CT arthrography with MRI and found the sensitivity, specificity, and accuracy of MRI to detect palmar and central tears of the SL and LT ligaments to be less than 80%. The volar portion of the ligament had a sensitivity and specificity of 0 and 100, respectively. CT arthrography was better at detecting these ligament injuries. Accurate visualization of the interosseous ligaments has also been established with MR arthrography.[37,42] Haims and coworkers[43] discovered improved sensitivity in detecting SL ligament tears with indirect MR arthrography over unenhanced MRI.

Carpal Fusion

Carpal fusion or coalition is clinically important because it places the patient at a somewhat higher risk for carpal instability and secondary SL ligament tears. There are three types of carpal fusion:

1. Congenital: Isolated fusions involve bones of the same carpal row, whereas syndrome-related fusions may affect bones in different rows (both proximal and distal). LT and capitate–hamate are the most common types of isolated fusion, although fusion may occur in almost any combination. LT fusion may be asymptomatic, but widening of the scapholunate interosseous space may be seen radiographically. Partial fusions may be associated with pain and cystic changes in the adjacent bones. Massive carpal fusion, which affects both carpal rows, is associated with congenital syndromes and chromosomal anomalies (e.g., Turner's, Holt–Oram, Ellis–van Creveld).
2. Surgical or post-traumatic.
3. Inflammatory: Pericapitate fusions are seen in adult Still's disease.

Triangular Fibrocartilage Complex

The most common internal derangement of the wrist involves the TFCC, which consists of the triangular fibrocartilage, the meniscal homologue, the ulnolunate and ulnotriquetral (volar ulnocarpal) ligaments, and the extensor carpi ulnaris tendon. The TFC is a biconcave fibrocartilage band that normally appears dark on all MRI sequences and is surrounded by higher-signal synovial fluid or hyaline cartilage. Its function is similar to that of the menisci in the knee. The TFC arises from the ulnar aspect of the distal radius and extends to the junction between the ulnar head and styloid process, adjacent to the meniscal homologue. The meniscal homologue at the ulnar edge of the TFC is made up of fibrofatty tissue that appears as high signal on T1-weighted and proton-density images in contrast to the low-signal TFC. Many authorities currently believe that the homologue is not a fibrofatty structure, but rather fat interposed between the extrinsic ligaments at the ulnar aspect of the wrist. The meniscal homologue should never appear similar to fluid on T2-weighted images.

The TFC is best demonstrated on coronal images, especially on thin-section 3D-GRE sequences. A suggested tear of the TFC is a common indication for MRI examination of the wrist. These tears are divided into degenerative and traumatic types.[44]

Degenerative tears are much more common and are often termed *central tears*. These occur in the thinnest portion of the TFC, which is central but slightly eccentric toward the radial aspect of this structure. Traumatic tears occur after a discrete injury and usually are located at the ulnar or radial side of the TFC. Traumatic tears tend to be perpendicular to the long axis of the TFC and are associated with fluid in the distal radioulnar joint (DRUJ) and, to a lesser degree, with excessive fluid in the radiocarpal joint. TFCC tears can be partial or full thickness. Ulnar-sided tears may be in the region of the meniscal homologue. It is these traumatic TFC tears that are most easily missed on MRI. High-signal intensity in this region on T2-weighted sequences is the most reliable finding (Fig. 13-24, online). Any fluid at the periphery of the TFCC on T2-weighted images that is not in the prestyloid recess or ECU tendon sheath should be described as a peripheral tear. TFCC tears are typically associated with LT, and less frequently, SL ligament tears.

Although the TFC is usually low in signal on all pulse sequences, increased internal signal may sometimes be seen on GRE or T1-weighted images. This represents degeneration of the TFC and not a true tear. This degenerative signal is globular, is hypointense to cartilage, and does not extend to both sides of the TFC. Another diagnostic pitfall is the line of high-signal hyaline cartilage seen at the insertion of the TFC onto the radius, which can be mistaken for a tear. True radial-sided tears are rare. They usually are caused by acute trauma and consist of a radial avulsion of the TFC with increased signal intensity on T2 images. Furthermore, TFC slit-like communicating lesions can be found in asymptomatic wrists.[45] Tears should be seen on at least two pulse sequences.

Multiple reports have emerged on the accuracy of current modalities in imaging the TFCC. MRI has been found in one report to have limited utility in imaging the peripheral attachment of the TFCC, with sensitivity and specificity of 17% and 79%, respectively.[43] A high signal intensity at the ulnar insertion was found to have low sensitivity and specificity as a marker for a peripheral tear. Blazar and associates[46] discussed the fact that MRIs coming in to most hand surgeons' practices are heterogeneous and not obtained in a standardized fashion, having been done at various locations. Less experienced radiologists also were found to have lower sensitivity, specificity, and accuracy in predicting a tear and its location. Potter and colleagues[47] found higher accuracy rates, but images were obtained using a standardized protocol. MR arthrography has also been evaluated as a potential modality to increase the prediction of TFCC injury. Haimes and coworkers[48] compared indirect MR arthrography with unenhanced MRI and found no improvement in the ability to evaluate central tears of the TFCC. Direct MR arthrography, on the other hand, found improved sensitivities, specificities, and accuracy over unenhanced MRI and conventional arthrography, and the highest rates when combining MR arthrography with conventional arthrography.[49] In another study, CT arthrography was highly accurate in detecting central TFC tears but not peripheral tears.[40]

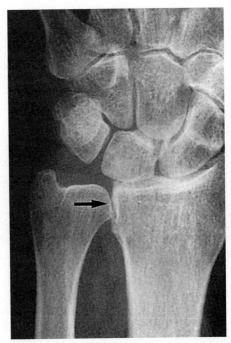

Figure 13-25 Incongruity of the distal radioulnar joint. Narrowing of the normal cartilage space *(arrow)* demonstrates loss of the articular cartilage.

Distal Radioulnar Joint: Instability, Ulnar Variance, and Impaction Syndrome

There are four types of problems affecting the DRUJ: incongruity, instability, impaction, and isolated tears of the TFC.[50] The presence or absence of each can be confirmed by using the various imaging techniques in a logical sequence.

Joint incongruity is evaluated on plain PA radiographs, which can demonstrate irregularity, sclerosis, spurs, and erosions of the articular surface of the sigmoid notch of the radius and ulnar head (Fig. 13-25). Instability is caused by a deficiency of the fibrocartilaginous support structure of the DRUJ, which can be determined on the basis of the clinical examination. Plain radiographs taken with the patient properly positioned will confirm the diagnosis if subluxation or dislocation of the ulnar head within the sigmoid notch of the radius is shown (Fig. 13-26). CT or MRI also can confirm the subluxation or dislocation by demonstrating the orientation of the DRUJ in the axial plane.[11,51]

Ulnar variance refers to the relationship between the distal ulna and radius, excluding their respective styloid processes. Normally, the articular surfaces of these bones are aligned. Changes in the length of the ulna relative to that of the radius alter the compressive forces across the wrist. In positive ulnar variance, the ulna is longer than the adjacent articular aspect of the radius, and with negative variance the ulna is shorter. Any variance greater than 2.5 mm is biomechanically significant. Ulnar variance can be viewed with conventional radiography using both neutral rotation and pronated grip PA radiographs.[52] Ulnar variance may be difficult to accurately assess on MRI, other than to describe the relationship between the ulna and the sigmoid sulcus of the radius. Negative ulnar

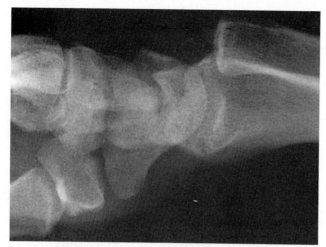

Figure 13-26 *Lateral view of the wrist showing dorsal subluxation of the ulna after trauma.*

variance is weakly associated with Kienböck's disease. Positive ulnar variance is associated with degenerative type TFC tears due to mechanical erosion.

Positive ulna variance can eventually lead to impaction of the lunate by the ulna with or without a degenerative TFC tear (Fig. 13-27). This is known as *ulnalunato abutment syndrome,* or *ulnar impaction syndrome.* This also may affect the triquetral bone of the carpus. On MRI, abutment is manifested by cartilage loss of the lunate with resultant marrow edema, subchondral cysts and eventual subchondral sclerosis. Cartilage defects are best seen on high-resolution images, whereas the sclerosis is seen as low signal on T1- and T2-weighted sequences. GRE sequences often accentuate this

dark signal. Characteristic focal signal changes are seen at the proximal ulnar aspect of the lunate, and often the triquetrum.[53]

Avascular Necrosis

AVN is common in the wrist. It may be the result of overuse, occur spontaneously, or be secondary to local trauma or systemic disease. Examples of systemic processes that can lead to AVN include steroid usage and systemic lupus erythematosus (SLE).

An example of AVN related to overuse occurs in the lunate and is termed *Kienböck's disease.* Repetitive microtrauma is thought to be the major cause, although it may occur after a single major traumatic event. The dominant extremity is usually affected, and young males are more commonly affected than females. The blood supply to the lunate is tenuous because most of this bone is covered with hyaline cartilage. The proximal aspect of the lunate is most vulnerable to injury, and if AVN involves only one part of the bone, it affects the radial side. Kienböck's disease also is associated with negative ulnar variance. The MR staging of Kienböck's disease (modified from plain film staging) is as follows:

Stage 1: Normal contour of the lunate, with a radiolucent or radiodense line representing the compression fracture; fracture is seen as a zone of decreased T1 signal

Stage 2: Resorption of bone along the fracture line

Stage 3: All of the changes of stages 1 and 2, plus sclerosis of the bone; necrotic bone has variably decreased T1 signal

Stage 4: Fragmentation or flattening of the lunate

Stage 5: Secondary osteoarthritis of the radiocarpal and intercarpal joints; fragmentation and decreased T1 signal of the lunate combined with osteophyte formation, subchondral sclerosis, or edema involving the adjacent articular surfaces; often an associated joint effusion

Because of its anatomic specificity, MRI is capable of demonstrating marrow abnormalities caused by AVN, and it can reveal these changes earlier than is possible with bone scintigraphy (Fig. 13-28).[29,54-57] Bone islands have a similar

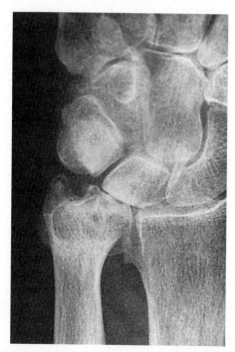

Figure 13-27 *Positive ulnar variance of the distal radioulnar joint seen in this posteroanterior view has resulted in impaction of the ulna into the lunate. The sclerosis indicates a chronic bone reaction to this trauma. Loss of the articular cartilage also is evident.*

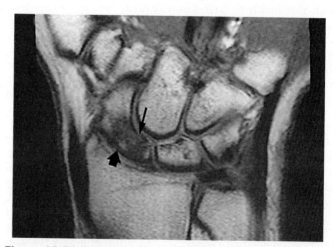

Figure 13-28 *Magnetic resonance image demonstrating a scaphoid fracture (disruption in the black cortical line at the thin arrow). The marrow of the scaphoid is relatively darker (thick arrow), indicating edema from the fracture.*

appearance on MR images, so the results must be correlated with plain films. The imaging findings of Kienböck disease show marrow replacement, best assessed on the T1-weighted images as decreased signal.[29,54-57] The T2 appearance varies somewhat but usually shows increased signal. As with all cases of AVN in the wrist, the classic "double-line" sign is rarely seen. The surrounding soft tissues are usually normal, and a joint effusion is variably present.

Post-traumatic AVN may be seen in any carpal bone; however, it is most common in the scaphoid. The proximal pole of the scaphoid is affected by AVN secondary to a disruption in the blood supply. The proximal pole is fed from the terminal branches of the artery entering the distal pole and passing through the middle segment of the scaphoid. A scaphoid waist fracture may disrupt this supply, and AVN may result in up to 60% of cases. The risk of AVN increases as the fracture becomes more proximal. Fractures that have a visible step-off also have a higher risk of AVN. On MRI, the proximal pole of the fractured scaphoid may show decreased bone marrow signal on T1 images. The contour of the cortex may become indistinct and irregular subsequent to collapse. MRI also can show reactive changes in the distal fracture fragment, with AVN rarely occurring here. Again, the double-line sign on T2 images is rarely seen. An acutely "negative" MR for scaphoid AVN is unreliable because false-negative results can occur up to 1 to 2 months. Gadolinium-enhanced MRI may better assess the proximal pole vascularity and is currently considered the best technique.[58] The proximal pole can appear hypointense on a T1-weighted image and hyperintense on a proton-density–weighted fat-suppressed image, resembling a necrotic proximal pole; but a gadolinium-enhanced T1-weighted fat-suppressed MRI can show some vascularized tissue within the fragment. This could represent spontaneous revascularization, or may be some unspecific reactive inflammatory tissue originating from the nonunion site. Also, if the fatty content of the proximal pole appears normal, then the absence of enhancement with gadolinium does not indicate AVN.

Spontaneous or idiopathic AVN occurring in the scaphoid is termed *Preiser disease.* Preiser disease demonstrates complete marrow replacement on T1-weighted images, with typical edema on T2-weighted images. Associated ligamentous injury is uncommon, as is collapse. The capitate bone is the third most common carpal bone to undergo AVN, but this occurs rarely, and when it does, is usually spontaneous in origin.

Carpal Tunnel Syndrome

The carpal tunnel is bounded by the concave volar surface of the carpus in continuity with the flexor retinaculum, which extends from the trapezium to the hook of the hamate. It consists of the eight flexor digitorum tendons [flexor digitorum superficialis (FDS) and flexor digitorum profundus (FDP)], the flexor pollicis longus tendon, and the median nerve.

Carpal tunnel syndrome (CTS) is a common syndrome characterized by pain, paresthesias, and weakness in the distribution of the median nerve. It is bilateral in 50% of cases and may be associated with repetitive mechanical activity, such as typing. Other causes of CTS include tenosynovitis,

RA, amyloidosis, infection, mass (intrinsic or extrinsic), pregnancy, or developmental anomalies. Diagnosis is usually made clinically and confirmed with electromyography (EMG) examinations.

MRI plays a limited role in the examination of patients with possible carpal tunnel disease. By and large, the diagnosis of this problem should be reached clinically, but MRI may be used occasionally if the symptoms derive from a soft tissue mass or an infection within the carpal tunnel.[59,60] Indications for wrist MRI include atypical symptoms, a lack of EMG findings, high clinical suspicion for a mass, young patient age (possible congenital anomalies), and recurrent symptoms in postoperative patients.

On MRI, the flexor retinaculum is normally taut to minimally convex, the median nerve is of uniform size (4 × 2 mm) and ovoid in shape with signal isointense to muscle, and the flexor tendons are not distinguishable from one another on T2-weighted sequences. MRI findings of CTS include volar bowing of the flexor retinaculum, synovitis of the tendon sheaths within the carpal tunnel, focal enlargement of the median nerve at the level of the pisiform, and increased signal of the nerve itself. The median nerve may alternatively appear flattened. Note that these findings are nonspecific in the absence of symptoms. High signal within the median nerve is the least reliable sign and is often seen in asymptomatic individuals. Mild bowing of the flexor retinaculum may be physiologic; thus, CTS should not be suggested unless this finding is marked. Masses rarely cause CTS, but the search for masses must be diligent. Ganglion cysts, lipomas extending from the thenar or hypothenar eminences, or focal amyloid deposition may be causative lesions. A dedicated extremity MRI may be a cost-effective way to make this diagnosis.

In postoperative patients, it is important to check for incomplete lysis of the flexor retinaculum. Although the retinaculum may have been completely incised at surgery, it may regrow and appear intact. Assessment for recurrent or residual masses or recurrent synovitis also should be performed. Postoperatively, the flexor tendons migrate volarly, and the median nerve usually regains normal size and signal.

Ulnar Nerve Compression (Guyon's Canal)

Compression of the ulnar nerve also may occur at the wrist, resulting in tingling and pain along the hypothenar region and ulnar side of the fourth and fifth fingers. The ulnar nerve, along with the ulnar artery and vein, travels within Guyon's canal. This space lies superficial to the retinaculum of the carpal tunnel, adjacent to the hook of the hamate. Processes that affect or extend into this space may cause the characteristic symptoms.

Guyon's canal is formed on the medial side by the pisiform and flexor carpi ulnaris muscle and on the lateral side by the hook of the hamate. The splitting of the flexor retinaculum forms the roof of Guyon's canal. Within the canal lies the ulnar nerve, ulnar artery, and vena comitans.[61] Pain in the ulnar aspect of the palm may be caused by a pathologic condition in the canal and may involve the hook of the hamate, pisiform, ulnar artery or vein, or ulnar nerve. A tumor such as a lipoma or ganglion that extends into or arises within the canal also may cause symptoms by compressing any of these structures.

Fractures involving the hamate or pisiform may be difficult to visualize on plain films and are best evaluated on a carpal tunnel view or CT scan. An anteroposterior oblique view also should be obtained to assess the possibility of pisotriquetral arthritis. Pisotriquetral arthritis may be idiopathic or the result of a fracture. MRI is the best option for examining vascular and other soft tissue structures. Routine MRI and MRA can definitively establish vessel patency noninvasively.

As with CTS, MRI may reveal masses, most commonly ganglion cysts or inflammatory changes within Guyon's canal. Compression of the ulnar nerve most commonly results from fibrous bands, which may not be visualized on MRI. Beware of looped ulnar vessels, which may mimic ganglia in this region.

Arthritis

Several types of arthritis affect the wrist, including osteoarthritis (OA), RA, crystal deposition diseases (most notably gout and calcium pyrophosphate deposition disease), and hemochromatosis. The presence of cysts and the specific distribution of disease can be helpful in differentiating the various types of arthritis.

Because the wrist is a non-weight-bearing joint, OA is usually secondary to other processes, such as prior trauma, inflammatory arthritides (RA), or infection. The radial distribution of OA is well recognized, with changes usually confined to the first carpometacarpal joint and the trapezioscaphoid space of the midcarpal joint. Clinical symptoms include pain, restricted movement, and instability. Increasing radial subluxation of the metacarpal base, narrowing of the interosseous space, sclerosis and cystic change of the subchondral bone, and osteophytosis is seen radiographically. Changes of OA on MRI are characterized by joint space loss, subchondral cyst or geode formation, and bony production manifested by subchondral sclerosis and osteophyte formation.

Focal arthritis also may occur secondary to a type II lunate or in the scapholunate advanced collapse (SLAC) wrist. OA at the base of the first metacarpal often demonstrates marked proliferative change, with large osteophyte production and synovial cysts that can sometimes mimic masses on MRI. This form of OA also can mimic a subluxation because the osteophytes may appear to displace the base of the first metacarpal radially. OA about the scaphoid is common and is not usually related to instability; however, this type of OA can be the sequela of a ligament tear or instability, particularly if the arthritis is focal. Usually, this focal type of arthritis occurs as the result of an SL or LT ligament tear.

The SLAC wrist may occur as a complication in patients with long-standing SL ligament tears and secondary widening of the SL interval. Proximal migration of the capitate is present, leading to focal arthritis at the capitoscaphoid and capitolunate joints. On MRI, the SLAC wrist demonstrates cartilage loss and subtle marrow edema at the distal central SL joint and the proximal capitate. The SLAC wrist may lead to CTS because of the shortening of the carpal tunnel with an infolding of the median nerve.

The last subtype of OA occurs in patients with a type II lunate. In this variant, an extra facet of the lunate articulates with the hamate. This is a common finding, occurring in approximately half of affected individuals. Accelerated cartilage loss with underlying marrow edema may be seen as the sequelae of the type II lunate. Frank OA may appear at the lunatohamate junction. The edema from the cartilage loss in this entity may mimic AVN or stress fractures of the hamate.

The next most common type of arthritis to affect the wrist is RA. RA has certain characteristic sites of involvement in the wrist, including the ulnar styloid (secondary to extensor carpi ulnaris synovitis) and the first and second MP joints. The cartilage loss in RA presents as diffuse, symmetrical joint space loss in contrast to the focal changes seen in OA. Joint effusions are common, with marked synovial proliferation (pannus) often seen. This pannus mimics fluid on T2-weighted images but may also demonstrate low signal secondary to ferritin deposition. The number and size of erosions, as well as the volume of pannus, are good markers for rheumatoid activity. These findings may be used to assess the effectiveness of medical intervention in this disease.

Calcium pyrophosphate deposition disease (CPPD) often affects the wrist. Usually, calcification is seen in the TFC, but it also may affect the SL and LT ligaments. Capsular calcification also can occur, but this type of calcification is usually senile or related to hyperparathyroidism caused by renal failure. On MRI, it may be difficult to see the calcifications of CPPD. This is because the TFC is normally low in signal intensity; therefore the signal void of calcification does not show up against it. Occasionally, the calcifications may appear bright, particularly on intermediate-weighted images. Calcifications may mimic a TFC, SL, or LT ligament tear because of the artifactual junction between the low signal calcification and the higher signal of a degenerated, but not torn, ligament.

The urate crystal deposition of gout tends to be low in signal on T1- and T2-weighted images. Sharply marginated erosions usually are seen, and pancarpal involvement often occurs, with variably sized lesions of high signal on T2-weighted images. Diseases with similar signal characteristics include amyloidosis, synovial chondromatosis, and pigmented villonodular synovitis (PVNS). All of these entities also show variable, but often significant, susceptibility artifact. Of note, some types of productive OA can occasionally have a peculiar appearance, which may mimic gout or PVNS. Last, the arthritis resulting from silicone implants also can have a similar appearance to this group of disorders.

Fracture

Most displaced wrist fractures can be adequately assessed by plain film. Frontal and lateral views are routine projections, with radiographs obtained during radial and ulnar deviation helpful in the evaluation of the carpal bones. In addition to evaluation for carpal fracture, the orientation of the carpal rows and the intercarpal relationships are important in the assessment of carpal instability. Fractures of the scaphoid are most common, with classification and prognosis for healing or complications based on the location of the fracture line and displacement of the fracture. Isolated fractures of the triquetrum (dorsal surface), lunate, and hamate are less common but also are seen.

The most commonly suggested occult fracture of the wrist involves the scaphoid. In the clinical setting, advanced imaging is often required because scaphoid fractures are difficult to visualize on routine radiographs. Proper radiographic evaluation of the scaphoid has been proposed as requiring four views: a PA in ulnar deviation with fist position, a lateral view, and oblique views with 60 degrees of pronation and supination.[62] In the past, scintigraphy, routine tomography, and CT had been used to examine occult fractures, but even in cases with negative CT or tomographs, patients often were treated as if a true fracture were present, if the clinical suspicion was high enough. Treatment was withdrawn if follow-up radiographs remained negative.

More recently, MRI has become the test of choice to assess for the presence of a scaphoid fracture, having been found to have sensitivity and specificity of 95% to 100%, with 100% interobserver agreement.[63] In patients in whom scaphoid fractures are clinically suggested, MRI can clearly demonstrate the abnormality, which appears as a dark, linear fracture line on T1-weighted images. It also has the advantage of showing other associated occult fractures, usually involving the triquetrum or distal radius. The MRI protocol should include coronal T1 and STIR images. If the STIR images are negative, a fracture can be confidently excluded. Many patients with suggested scaphoid fractures have only soft tissue injuries, including collateral ligament tears, peripheral TFCC tears, radial TFCC avulsions, and SL or LT ligament tears.

Other imaging modalities used to detect scaphoid fractures, such as scintigraphy and CT, are also used and may be necessary in patients who are unable to have an MRI. CT and conventional radiography have been compared in detecting displacement of scaphoid fractures greater than 1 mm.[64] Radiography had low sensitivity (52%) because of its inability to detect volar/dorsal displacement. Likewise, CT had difficulty detecting radial/ulnar displacement (sensitivity 49%). Scintigraphy was found to detect bony abnormalities more frequently than CT, although patients preferred CT since there is less of a time requirement.[65] The sensitivities and specificities of MRI compared with scintigraphy in detecting occult scaphoid fractures at 19 days from injury have been found to be 100% and 100% for MRI, respectively, and 83% and 95%, respectively, for scintigraphy.[66] Finally, when MRI is compared with CT, MRI is better able to detect trabecular involvement, whereas CT more reliably detected cortical involvement.[67]

Occult fractures may occur elsewhere in the wrist, but they are much less common and have infrequent complications. Triquetral fractures are the second most common carpal fracture, but they rarely require advanced imaging for diagnosis. The third most common carpal bone fracture involves the hamate. Hamate fractures usually occur either dorsally or involve the hook, with both areas often difficult to visualize radiographically. Thin-section axial CT images through this area may be required to diagnose a fracture. On MRI, hook of the hamate fractures are best evaluated on axial images, and they are clinically important because of the proximity to Guyon's canal and the possibility of ulnar nerve impingement. Even though lunate fractures are rare, AVN is a common complication (similar to the scaphoid). Some cases of Kienböck's disease likely result from this post-traumatic scenario. Occasionally, cysts in the lunate may mimic fractures.

Bone bruises are intimately related to occult fractures, and differentiating the two by MRI alone can be difficult. Bone bruises should be diffuse, have little articular or cortical extension, and show no obvious fracture line. In the wrist, however, occult fractures may be present with these findings alone. Bone bruises, although they may be symptomatic, heal spontaneously in 8 to 10 weeks without treatment and have no known sequelae. Occult fractures, on the other hand, are true fractures and may go on to nonunion and the other typical complications. It is our philosophy that in the hand and wrist, abnormalities seen on both T1 and STIR (or fat-suppressed T2 images) represent true fractures. Those injuries with abnormalities on STIR sequences only should be termed *bone bruises*.

Lunate fractures, proximal capitate fractures, and hook of hamate fractures may occur because of stress injuries; however, stress fractures are much less common in the upper extremity than the lower extremity. The differentiation of an acute traumatic fracture from a stress fracture is made on the basis of time. An acute traumatic fracture occurs at one specific episode of time, but a stress fracture has no discrete episode leading to it. In general, stress fractures are more common in the lower extremities, but they can occur in the wrist, especially in active sports participants. Before a stress fracture occurs, there is the normal physiologic response of the bone to attempt to remodel (Wolff's law). This remodeling might be visible on MRI as subtle areas of marrow edema. The stress response may be painful and can show uptake of moderate intensity on bone scintigraphy. The stress response can be thought of as a bone bruise, which can be a self-limited condition that heals spontaneously once the causative activity is stopped. If this activity continues, a fatigue-type stress fracture may result. This occurs in normal bones undergoing abnormal stresses. In older individuals, insufficiency-type fractures may occur when injury is due to normal stresses applied to abnormal underlying bone (usually as a result of osteoporosis).

Nonunion

Nonunion or delayed union occurs when a fracture does not heal within the first 6 months following the injury. *Delayed union* refers to complete healing occurring after a significant time interval, but healing never occurs in nonunion. Systemic diseases such as alcoholism, pancreatitis, cirrhosis, and malnutrition all contribute to delayed union. Nonunion is usually related to the type and location of the fracture and whether it was immobilized adequately or not. In particular, scaphoid fractures have a relatively high incidence of nonunion. Scaphoid nonunion may be fibrous, cartilaginous, or synovial (pseudoarthrosis).

Untreated occult fractures of the scaphoid that become nonunions can develop cystlike defects seen on conventional radiographs, often misreported as plain cysts.[68] Advanced imaging is appropriate for patients with persistent wrist pain and negative plain radiographs in whom an occult scaphoid fracture is suggested. On MRI, a fibrous nonunion demonstrates low signal on T1- and T2-weighted images. Because this appearance is similar to the MRI characteristics of some united fractures, only the presence of motion on physical examination can definitely define nonunion. Evaluation with thin-section CT may be a helpful adjunct in evaluating for subtle bony bridging. Motion at a site of nonunion is indirectly visible on MRI as high T2 signal about the fracture. This perifractural edema is either a sign of healing or abnormal motion, and distinguishing between the two can be difficult. In small bones, this edema is more likely secondary to pathologic motion. Cartilaginous nonunion shows intermediate T1- and T2-weighted signal and also can demonstrate motion or edema around the fracture line. The presence of synovial fluid in the fracture line after 6 months indicates a pseudoarthrosis or synovial nonunion. To diagnose a pseudoarthrosis on MRI, the fluid at the fracture site should be differentiated from the perifractural edema of healing by using heavily T2-weighted images. The granulation tissue of normal fracture healing fades on these long TE (time to echo) images.

Masses

The most common mass in the wrist is a ganglion. Occasionally, these can extend intraosseously, typically into the lunate. Ganglia are often signs of an internal derangement and may be a cause of pain if occult. The second most common wrist mass is a lipoma, characteristically located in the thenar or hypothenar eminence. Within the hand, tendon sheath fibromas and giant-cell tumors of the tendon sheath may occur. Distally, masses may occur in the tuft of the digits. These include glomus tumors, foreign body granulomas, paronychia, or felons. MRI is the preferred modality for imaging soft tissue masses in the extremities.[69]

Dorsal Wrist Pain

Dorsal wrist pain may be caused by pathology in the extensor tendon compartment, dorsal wrist capsule, or bony structures.

Bony Structures

Evaluation of the bony structures begins with routine plain views. If the bone density is increased, advanced Kienböck's disease is a possibility; otherwise, early AVN of the lunate must be ruled out. Bone scintigraphy is then performed and, in Kienböck's disease, may show decreased uptake within the first 48 hours and then increased uptake as the bone repairs. Bone scintigraphy is nonspecific, however, and demonstrates increased uptake wherever bone turnover is increased, such as in joints with synovitis. It also provides poor anatomic resolution and does not effectively distinguish between the joint space and the bone. MRI provides far greater resolution than bone scintigraphy in the evaluation of AVN. It also can

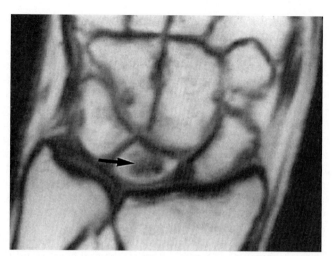

Figure 13-29 Avascular necrosis of the lunate *(arrow)*. Coronal magnetic resonance image shows a dark area in the marrow. The corresponding nuclear medicine scan is seen in Figure 13-14.

reveal pathology of the bone vascularity earlier than any other imaging techniques (Fig. 13-29).

Dorsal Capsule

Hypertrophy of the synovium of the dorsal capsule may be clinically indistinguishable from other causes of dorsal wrist pain, but MRI can provide a definitive diagnosis because of its excellent resolution of soft tissue structures (Fig. 13-30, online).

Summary

Disorders of the hand and wrist can be complex. Plain radiography is a standard imaging technique for many disorders, yet advanced imaging with bone scan, computed tomography, and magnetic resonance imaging may be necessary for evaluation. Advanced imaging provides the ability to identify painful conditions such as occult fractures and avascular necrosis in a more timely fashion. Accurate assessment of fracture alignment and healing is possible. Visualization of important soft tissue structures can also be detected. Cost–benefit aspects should be considered as well to prevent unnecessary use of more costly imaging modalities. Finally, imaging modalities provide information that allow health care workers to have knowledgeable discussions with patients and help provide direction for appropriate treatment options.

REFERENCES

The complete reference list is available online at www.expertconsult.com.

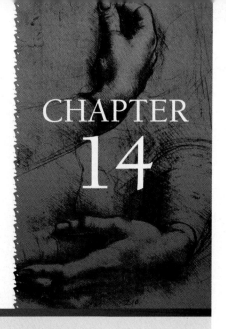

Diagnostic Imaging of the Shoulder and Elbow

CONOR P. SHORTT, MB, BCh, BAO, MSc, MRCPI, FRCR, FFR RCSI
AND WILLIAM B. MORRISON, MD

IMAGING MODALITIES
IMAGING OF SHOULDER PATHOLOGY

IMAGING OF ELBOW PATHOLOGY
SUMMARY

CRITICAL POINTS

Shoulder Ultrasound Applications

- Rotator cuff integrity assessment (especially post arthroplasty)
- Evaluation and fenestration of rotator cuff calcific tendinosis
- Evaluation of rotator cuff muscle atrophy
- Dynamic imaging of impingement
- Assessment of glenohumeral effusion
- Guided subacromial-subdeltoid bursal or joint injection

Elbow Ultrasound Applications

- Evaluation and treatment of medial and lateral epicondylitis
- Dynamic assessment of medial and lateral collateral stabilizers
- Ulnar and posterior interosseous nerve impingement assessment

MRI Contraindications*

Absolute

- Cardiac pacemaker/implantable cardiac defibrillators
- Ferromagnetic CNS clips
- Orbital metallic foreign body
- Electronically, magnetically, and mechanically activated implants

Relative

- Prosthetic heart valves
- Foreign bodies in non-vital locations
- Infusion pumps/nerve stimulators
- Cochlear and stapedial implants

Shoulder MRI Applications

- Rotator cuff pathology
- Labral/capsular injury (best using direct MR arthrography)
- Rotator cuff interval lesions
- Muscle and other tendon tears

- Occult fracture/bone bruise
- Osseous and soft tissue neoplasms
- Infection

Elbow MRI Applications

- Occult fracture/bone bruise
- Cartilage injury
- Osteochondritis dissecans—evaluation of stability
- Medial and lateral collateral ligament injury
- Muscle and tendon tears around the elbow including epicondylitis
- Osseous and soft tissue neoplasms
- Infection

*This is not intended as a complete list, but rather as a guide to MR contraindications. In individual cases, specific queries should be discussed directly with the radiology department before consideration for MR.

Diagnostic imaging is an invaluable adjunct to clinical examination in the assessment of many upper extremity disorders. Knowledge of available imaging modalities is essential to determining the most appropriate and cost-effective imaging test to be performed for a given clinical question. Some modalities, although perceived as superior to others, may be inappropriate in a particular clinical setting. For example, ultrasound in the assessment of rotator cuff tears after shoulder arthroplasty is, in most cases, superior to MRI.[1] Ordering the correct testing with pertinent clinical details in the appropriate setting yields maximum information and facilitates optimum patient treatment.

Radiography of the shoulder and elbow should be considered in all cases, because it provides useful information about the bony anatomy and a baseline for comparison with follow-up studies as well as acting as a complementary test to advanced imaging techniques. Advanced imaging techniques, such as US, CT, MRI, and nuclear medicine, are invaluable

177

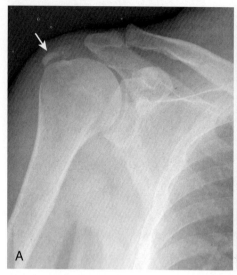
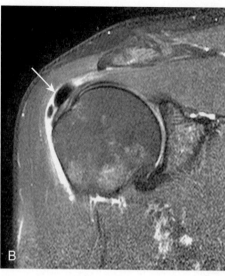

Figure 14-1 Calcific tendinosis of the rotator cuff and associated bursitis. **A,** Anteroposterior radiograph of the shoulder demonstrates calcific foci at the distal supraspinatus tendon consistent with calcific tendinosis or hydroxyapatite deposition disease (HADD). **B,** Coronal fat-saturated T2-weighted image of the shoulder in the same patient demonstrates foci of low (*black*) signal in the distal supraspinatus tendon (*arrow*) extruding into the adjacent subacromial/subdeltoid bursa with associated reactive bursitis (*fluid bright signal*).

in the appropriate clinical setting, providing clinicians with state-of-the-art radiologic assessment. This chapter first describes the modalities used in shoulder and elbow imaging, and then focuses on how imaging aids diagnosis with respect to specific shoulder and elbow pathologies.

Imaging Modalities

Radiography

Basic radiography has evolved from film-screen radiography, which is still in use today, to increasingly available digital and computed radiography techniques, which are more amenable to manipulation, image transfer and storage, and viewing on workstations.

Standard radiographic projections of the shoulder include an AP (anteroposterior) and lateral view (Y-view). Correctly performed AP and lateral views allow assessment of glenohumeral and acromioclavicular alignment as well as of osseous structures at the shoulder. Radiographs are of particular value in the initial assessment of trauma where fracture or dislocation is suspected, and in the assessment of arthritis, but they are also useful in other cases such as tumor evaluation and calcific rotator cuff tendinosis with hydroxyapatite deposition disease (HADD; Fig. 14-1). Further views of the shoulder are also of value in certain instances; for example, a transthoracic lateral view and axillary (axial) view.

Standard views of the elbow include AP and lateral radiographs. Oblique AP views may be of value in assessing for suspected radial head fractures not seen on conventional views.

Arthrography

Shoulder arthrography still has a role in the assessment of rotator cuff tears and adhesive capsulitis, although recently it is rarely used in isolation, being more often combined with MRI (direct MR arthrography) or sometimes CT arthrography. MR arthrography is usually performed when labral pathology is suspected and is of particular use in patients with instability signs and symptoms.[2]

For shoulder arthrography, a spinal needle (20–22 gauge) is used to gain access to the shoulder joint, using an anterior or posterior approach under fluoroscopic guidance (Fig. 14-2). The intra-articular position is confirmed with injection of a small amount of iodinated contrast medium, which is typically followed by 14 mL of dilute gadolinium when performing MR arthrography. Undiluted iodinated contrast material is injected when performing CT arthrography. Arthrography of the elbow, usually in association with MR (direct MR arthrography), is used in the assessment of medial and lateral stabilizing ligament integrity and in the assessment of cartilage loss and intra-articular bodies.

Computed Tomography

The latest generation CT scanners use multiple detector row arrays. Multidetector CT (MDCT) is a major improvement

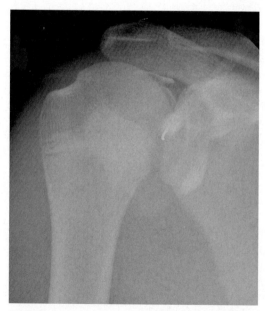

Figure 14-2 Shoulder arthrogram. For shoulder arthrography a 20- or 22-gauge spinal needle is used to gain access to the glenohumeral joint. High-density iodinated contrast material is seen flowing easily away from the needle tip into the joint, confirming intra-articular position.

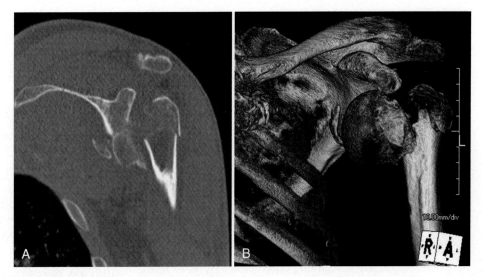

Figure 14-3 Comminuted intra-articular fracture. **A,** Coronal 2D CT image of a comminuted intra-articular right humeral head and glenoid fracture. **B,** Reconstructed 3D CT image in the same patient improves appreciation of fracture extent and pattern, assisting in operative planning.

in CT technology because the activation of multiple detector rows positioned along the patient's longitudinal axis allows for simultaneous acquisition of multiple slices. This also enables acquisition of thinner slices than were previously possible, allowing generation of exquisite multiplanar reformats (Fig. 14-3). In the setting of orthopedic prosthetic hardware, this technology results in decreased artifact.

CT allows precise characterization of fractures at the shoulder and elbow, defining degree of comminution and displacement, and identifying intra-articular osseous bodies if present. CT arthrography is an alternative to MR arthrography, allowing assessment of rotator cuff tears (especially full-thickness), labral tears, and cartilage loss at the glenohumeral joint (Fig. 14-4).[3] CT may also be used for image-guided intervention.

Ultrasound

US is the medical imaging modality used to acquire and display the acoustic properties of tissues. A transducer array (transmitter and receiver of US pulses) sends sound waves into the patient and receives returning echoes, which are converted into an image.

For musculoskeletal imaging of more superficial structures (tendons, ligaments), a high-frequency beam with a smaller wavelength provides superior spatial resolution and image detail. Thus, use of an appropriate transducer is of critical importance in performing shoulder and elbow imaging. Higher-frequency transducers are now available, ranging from 7.5 MHz up to as much as 15 MHz.

The acquisition of high-quality US images depends on operator experience, but in the right hands US can be a powerful tool in the assessment of a wide range of shoulder[4-6] and elbow[7-9] pathologies. US has shown increased utility for diagnostic and therapeutic procedures and for specific clinical concerns by providing more infrastructural detail more cost-effectively through improved transducer technology.[10,11] US is best used when a clinical question is well formulated and the condition is dichotomous (e.g., Is there a full-thickness rotator cuff tear or not?). US is also excellent for assessment of injuries that are only observed during certain

motions or in certain positions. For example, ulnar nerve subluxation can be documented during flexion and extension. Performing percutaneous interventions with US ensures accurate needle tip placement and helps direct the needle away from other regional soft-tissue structures and neurovascular bundles.[12] Applications of US at the shoulder and elbow are depicted in Boxes 14-1 and 14-2.

Magnetic Resonance Imaging

MRI is the workhorse of musculoskeletal imaging throughout the body, including the shoulder and elbow. MRI relies on the magnetic properties of the proton and does not involve ionizing radiation. It utilizes a strong magnetic field (most commonly 1.5 T) to align these protons. Their energy level is altered by a transmitted radiofrequency (RF) pulse, after which they are allowed to relax back to their original state,

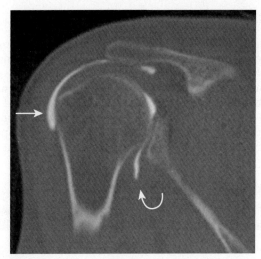

Figure 14-4 CT arthrogram of the shoulder. In patients for whom MRI is contraindicated, valuable information can be obtained with CT arthrography. In this instance iodinated contrast medium is seen to fill the inferior axillary recess of the glenohumeral joint as expected (*curved arrow*). However, contrast material is also seen to fill the subacromial/subdeltoid bursa (*straight arrow*), secondary to a full-thickness rotator cuff tear (tear not shown).

Box 14-1 Applications of Shoulder Ultrasound

Rotator cuff integrity assessment (especially after arthroplasty)

Evaluation and fenestration of rotator cuff calcific tendinosis and hypervascularity

Evaluation of rotator cuff muscle atrophy

Dynamic imaging of impingement

Assessment of glenohumeral effusion

Guided subacromial/subdeltoid bursal or joint injection

Box 14-3 MRI Contraindications*

ABSOLUTE

Cardiac pacemaker or implantable cardiac defibrillators

Ferromagnetic CNS clips

Orbital metallic foreign body

Electronically, magnetically, and mechanically activated implants

RELATIVE

Prosthetic heart valves

Foreign bodies in nonvital locations

Infusion pumps and nerve stimulators

Cochlear and stapedial implants

*This is not intended as a complete list, but rather as a guide to MRI contraindications. In individual cases, specific queries should be discussed directly with the radiology department before considering MRI.
CNS, central nervous system.

releasing energy. This energy is used to formulate an image based on the different relaxation properties of tissues. Various "sequences" are prescribed to focus on the different relaxation properties of the tissues in question. The main components of an MRI system include a strong magnetic field, coils (to transmit and receive RF signals), and gradients to localize signals quickly. MRI technology continues to evolve, with recent developments focusing on higher field strength magnets (3 T) and improved coils and gradients. Limitations of MRI include patient contraindications (Box 14-3), metallic susceptibility artifact from hardware, and patient intolerance secondary to claustrophobia.

The principal applications of MRI of the shoulder and elbow are show in Boxes 14-4 and 14-5. Direct MR arthrography is the favored technique for examination of possible shoulder labral tears. It involves direct injection of dilute gadolinium under fluoroscopic guidance as described earlier. It is also of value in assessing the rotator cuff and the stabilizing structures of the elbow. Indirect MR arthrography of the shoulder and elbow involves an IV injection of gadolinium, which diffuses into the joint cavity causing an "arthrographic" effect.

Nuclear Medicine

In nuclear medicine a radiopharmaceutical (radioactive isotope coupled with a pharmaceutical) is administered (usually intravenously), and subsequent gamma ray emissions are detected by a gamma camera. An isotope whole-body bone scan is used to detect areas of increased bone turnover, which may indicate pathology depending on the site and degree of activity (Fig. 14-5). The main application in the shoulder and elbow is in the evaluation of

neoplasia (particularly to assess for metastatic disease) and osteomyelitis.[13]

The most significant recent advancement in nuclear medicine is positron emission tomography (PET) and combination PET CT scanners with important implications for oncology. (^{18}F) fluorodeoxglucose (FDG) is a metabolic tracer most widely used in clinical PET oncology. PET applications are evolving, but it is currently approved for the diagnosis, staging, and restaging of many common malignancies and has shown efficacy for the detection of osseous metastasis from several malignancies, including lung

Box 14-4 Shoulder MRI Applications

Rotator cuff pathology

Labral or capsular injury (best using direct MR arthrography)

Rotator cuff interval lesions

Muscle and other tendon tears

Nerve pathology and impingement

Osseous and soft tissue neoplasms

Infection

MR, magnetic resonance.

Box 14-2 Applications of Elbow Ultrasound

Evaluation and treatment of medial and lateral epicondylitis

Dynamic assessment of medial and lateral collateral stabilizers

Ulnar and posterior interosseous nerve impingement

Box 14-5 Elbow MRI Applications

Occult fracture or bone bruise

Cartilage injury

Osteochondritis dissecans—evaluation of stability

Medial and lateral collateral ligament injury

Muscle and tendon tears around the elbow including epicondylitis

Nerve pathology and impingement

Osseous and soft tissue neoplasms

Infection

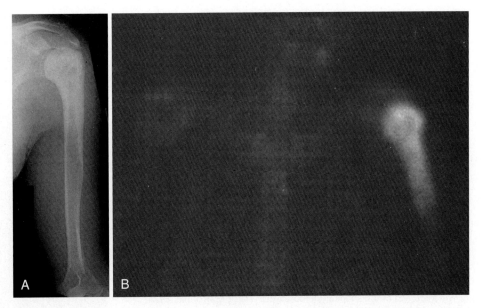

Figure 14-5 Paget's disease. **A,** Anteroposterior radiograph of the left humerus demonstrates bony expansion and trabecular and cortical thickening proximally extending to the glenohumeral joint, consistent with Paget's disease. **B,** Frontal image from an isotope whole-body bone scan shows marked tracer accumulation in the proximal humerus as expected in Paget's disease.

carcinoma, breast carcinoma, and lymphoma.[14] Such metastatic disease may be seen at the shoulder, but less commonly at the elbow and rarely more distally.

Other Modalities

Other modalities used rarely at the shoulder and elbow include fluoroscopy, which is used to assess joint stability, and arteriography, which is used in the assessment and sometimes treatment (embolization) of vascular lesions such as hemangiomas and pseudoaneurysms.

Imaging of Shoulder Pathology

Impingement

Although shoulder impingement is a clinical diagnosis, it has imaging manifestations that are helpful in guiding treatment. Radiography plays a role in the initial examination of impingement. Subacromial spurs, glenohumeral joint osteoarthritis, and evidence of chronic rotator cuff tear with a high riding humeral head may be identified with radiographs,[5] which may further influence management decisions (Fig. 14-6). Noncontrast shoulder MRI is frequently employed in the assessment of impingement. Manifestations of impingement, such as subacromial spur, subacromial/subdeltoid (SASD) bursitis, and rotator cuff tears, are all easily demonstrated on MRI.[15-17] Features of a rotator cuff tear that can be assessed on MRI include tear type (full vs. partial thickness), tear location, tear dimensions, tear morphology, tear gap/degree of tendon retraction, and the presence of rotator muscle atrophy (Fig. 14-7).

US is also a valuable tool in the assessment of impingement[18] and is useful for the evaluation of rotator cuff pathology (Fig. 14-8) although it cannot give a global assessment including labral, capsular, cartilage, and marrow pathology. US is useful in the setting of rotator cuff repair

and is particularly useful in shoulder arthroplasty where susceptibility artifact from the metallic prosthesis on MRI would limit interpretation of the adjacent cuff.[19] In addition, calcific tendinosis of the rotator cuff is well demonstrated on US[20] and is often amenable to SASD bursal injection of steroid and anesthetic or needling in refractory cases.

Instability

Radiography is useful in defining osseous alignment at the glenohumeral joint and may demonstrate a Hill–Sachs or

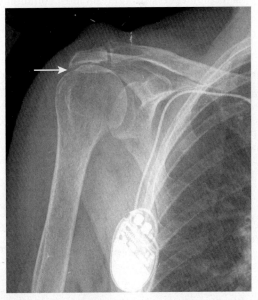

Figure 14-6 Chronic rotator cuff tear. Anteroposterior radiograph of the shoulder demonstrates severe narrowing of the acromiohumeral distance (arrow), indicating chronic rotator cuff tear. Marked subacromial spur formation is also seen. An MRI was contraindicated in this patient due to the presence of a cardiac pacemaker.

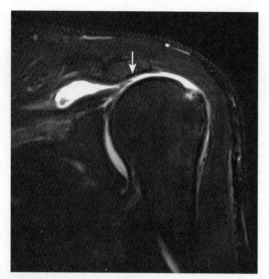

Figure 14-7 Full-thickness rotator cuff tear. Coronal fat-suppressed T2-weighted MRI of the shoulder demonstrates a large tear of the supraspinatus tendon. The tendon is torn, frayed, and retracted back, almost to glenohumeral joint level (*arrow*).

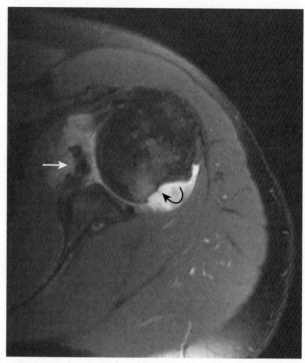

Figure 14-9 Bankart's and Hill–Sachs lesions. Axial T1 fat-saturated MRI after administration of intra-articular gadolinium (direct MR arthrogram) demonstrates sequelae of anterior shoulder dislocation. The anteroinferior labrum and bony glenoid has been disrupted (*white arrow*) consistent with a bony Bankart lesion. A bony defect is also seen at the posterior humeral head (*curved black arrow*) consistent with a Hill–Sachs lesion.

bony Bankart's lesion. CT also has utility in the assessment of osseous structures after subluxation/dislocation, particularly in evaluation of a subtle Bankart's fracture with an equivocal MRI or intra-articular osseous fragments.[21] CT is useful as a preoperative exam to assess fragment size and displacement. MR arthrography is the most sensitive test for evaluation of most of the causes, manifestations, and sequellae of glenohumeral instability.[22-24] It allows for precise evaluation of the capsulolabral and ligamentous complex. Labral tears are diagnosed when intra-articular contrast material tracks into or underneath the labrum. Noncontrast MRI is also very sensitive, although use of a high-field scanner (≥ 0.7 T) is recommended. Labral tears most commonly associated with instability are anteroinferior or posterior (Fig. 14-9). Superior labral tears that track anterior to posterior

(SLAP tears) are well seen with MR arthrography but are not usually associated with instability[25,26] (Fig. 14-10). Tendon tears that can be associated with instability, including tears of the long head of the biceps tendon or subscapularis, are also well seen by MR arthrography and noncontrast MRI.

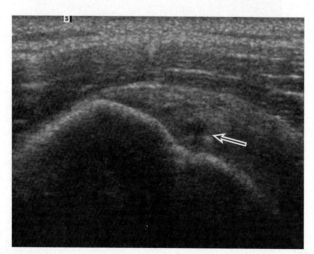

Figure 14-8 Partial-thickness rotator cuff tear. Ultrasound along the long axis of the distal supraspinatus tendon adjacent to its insertion on the greater tuberosity demonstrates a focal partial undersurface tear (*arrow*) as indicated by a hypoechoic (*dark*) defect.

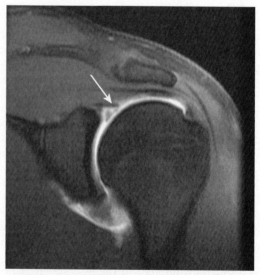

Figure 14-10 Superior labral anterior to posterior (SLAP) lesion. Coronal fat-suppressed T1-weighted image of the shoulder after intra-articular gadolinium injection (direct MR arthrogram) demonstrates abnormal tracking of contrast material into the superior labrum (*arrow*) consistent with a SLAP tear.

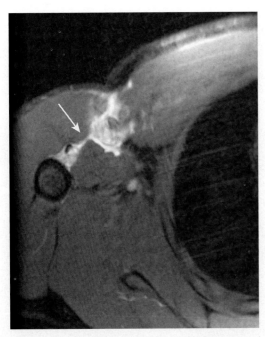

Figure 14-11 Pectoralis major muscle tear. Axial short tau inversion recovery (STIR) image of the right chest wall and proximal upper extremity acquired on a low field strength open magnet (0.3 T) demonstrates a complete (grade 3) tear of the right pectoralis major muscle with intervening bright hemorrhagic fluid (*arrow*)

Multidirectional instability typically shows no abnormality on imaging modalities, although capacious recesses may be observed.

Adhesive Capsulitis

Adhesive capsulitis, or frozen shoulder, has a variety of possible causes. Imaging features are usually nonspecific, but findings suggestive of adhesive capsulitis include a low joint capacity at arthrography, capsular thickening, and rotator cuff interval synovitis on MRI.[27]

Trauma

Radiography should always be the initial modality utilized in cases of trauma to the shoulder to evaluate for fracture or dislocation. Thereafter CT or MRI may be appropriate to assess for lesions occult on radiographs or for further characterization of fractures. CT with 2D and 3D reformats are excellent for preoperative planning (see Fig. 14-3). The excellent inherent soft tissue contrast afforded by MRI allows for assessment of injury to soft tissue structures such as tendon and muscle (Fig. 14-11).

Arthritis

Radiography is the mainstay for initial assessment of shoulder arthritis. MRI may be helpful in equivocal cases, particularly for identifying synovitis in inflammatory arthritides.[28]

Radiography is routinely employed in the assessment of joint prostheses. Septic arthritis and osteomyelitis of the glenohumeral and acromioclavicular joints are uncommon and may not demonstrate radiographic findings in the early stages. Radiographic findings seen in septic arthritis and osteomyelitis include soft tissue swelling, joint space narrowing, and articular erosions. MRI is a more sensitive test for evaluation of septic arthritis and osteomyelitis demonstrating a joint effusion, subchondral edema, and fatty marrow replacement in the setting of osteomyelitis. Osteomyelitis is also seen on whole-body isotope bone scan, with increased activity being seen on all three phases. In reality, if a septic arthritis is suspected, it should be confirmed by joint aspiration.

Masses

Evaluation of soft tissue masses at the shoulder invariably requires advanced imaging, namely ultrasound or MRI. A variety of benign and malignant soft tissue masses, including lipomas, liposarcomas, desmoids, malignant fibrous histiocytoma (MFH), and synovial sarcoma, may occur at the shoulder. MRI prior to and following administration of IV gadolinium contrast material is recommended by most authors. US may not provide a complete characterization of the lesion if osseous involvement is present but does allow for image-guided sampling. Radiographs are essential in the initial characterization of osseous tumors. MRI frequently aids in narrowing the differential diagnosis, especially with regard to solid versus cystic nature (requiring IV contrast). MRI is also useful for documentation of extent. CT is excellent for evaluation of cortical destruction and pathologic fracture and improves characterization of calcified matrix over radiographs.

The role of whole-body bone scan in the assessment of bone tumors is primarily for the evaluation of multiplicity of osseous lesions.

Imaging of Elbow Pathology

Tendon Injury

Lateral epicondylitis, or "tennis elbow," is a chronic tendinopathy of the common extensor origin and is a frequent cause of lateral elbow pain. On MRI, abnormal high signal is seen at the common extensor origin on fluid-sensitive sequences, sometimes with associated partial tears, which are fluid-bright.[29] In more severe cases, associated subtendinous bone marrow edema may be present at the lateral epicondyle, but this is not required for radiologic diagnosis. US is a valuable modality for examining the lateral epicondyle.[30,31] Sonographic features include common extensor origin thickening, heterogeneous echogenicity, calcific deposits, partial tears, and hypervascularity on Doppler imaging (Fig. 14-12). US may also be used to guide steroid or anesthetic injections and tendon fenestration.[32] Medial epicondylitis has similar MRI and US findings at the common flexor origin. Both of these entities may be associated with injury to the adjacent medial and lateral stabilizing structures.[33] Evaluation of the other tendons, including the biceps, triceps, and brachialis, is optimized with MRI. US is also useful for directed examination of tendon pathology at the elbow.

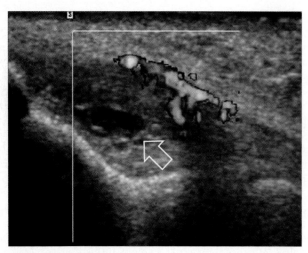

Figure 14-12 Lateral epicondylitis or common extensor tendinosis with partial tear. Ultrasound image demonstrates thickening of the common extensor origin consistent with tendinosis/epicondylitis with an associated hypoechoic (*black*) defect within the extensor tendon origin consistent with an interstitial partial tear (*arrow*). Power Doppler imaging demonstrates hypervascularity (orange areas), often seen with lateral epicondylitis/common extensor tendinosis.

Injury to Medial and Lateral Stabilizing Ligaments

Direct MR arthrography is most useful in detecting suggested injury to the medial and lateral stabilizing ligaments. The medial (ulnar) collateral ligament, for example, is frequently injured in baseball pitchers and can be assessed accurately with MR arthrography[34-36] (Fig. 14-13). US is also useful in assessing the elbow ligaments but has an advantage over MRI

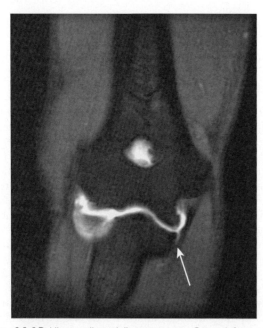

Figure 14-13 Ulnar collateral ligament tear. Coronal fat-suppressed T1-weighted image of the elbow after intra-articular gadolinium injection (direct MR arthrogram) demonstrates abnormal tracking of contrast (*arrow*) between the anterior bundle of the ulnar collateral ligament and the coronoid process of ulna at the sublime tubercle, indicating a distal partial thickness undersurface tear.

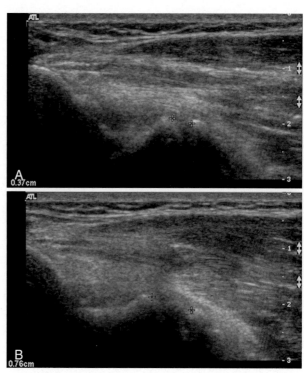

Figure 14-14 Ulnar collateral ligament (UCL) instability. **A,** Ultrasound at rest. Medial elbow joint demonstrates minimal gapping between the trochlea of humerus and ulna measured by crosshairs. **B,** When manual valgus stress is applied this gap increases significantly (difference of 3.9 mm) consistent with UCL instability. The difference between rest and stress measurement should be less than 2 mm. Multiple measurements (e.g., 3) should be taken and the average calculated. It is also useful to compare with the asymptomatic elbow.

with its ability to assess ligamentous laxity in real time with dynamic imaging[37,38] (Fig. 14-14). For example, during valgus stress for assessment of the medial collateral ligament, a difference in 2 mm between sides is diagnostic of abnormal ligamentous laxity.

Trauma

Like the shoulder, radiographs are indicated in the assessment of acute trauma at the elbow to determine the presence of fracture or malalignment. A useful sign on lateral radiographs is the visualization of a posterior fat pad or elevation on the anterior fat pad, indicative of elbow joint effusion[39] (Fig. 14-15). In the setting of acute trauma the presence of such an effusion suggests an occult radial head fracture. CT is also useful in the setting of complex acute bony injury, facilitating accurate assessment of fracture fragments and degree of displacement before surgical intervention. MRI is of value in the assessment of suggested occult osseous trauma due to its high sensitivity for detection of bone marrow edema and associated fractures. MRI is also warranted where soft tissue injury is suggested, such as in cases of distal biceps tendon or triceps tendon injury.

Neuropathy

US is particularly useful in the assessment of possible neuropathy at the elbow.[40-42] The ulnar nerve is the most

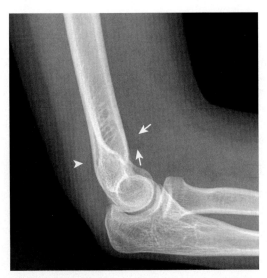

Figure 14-15 Elbow effusion. Lateral radiograph of the elbow shows abnormal elevation of the anterior fat pad forming a "sail" shape (*arrows*). A faint posterior fat pad is seen (*arrowhead*). Elevation of the anterior fat pad as shown or the mere visualization of a posterior fat pad indicate an elbow joint effusion. Elbow effusion is often associated with occult fracture with otherwise normal radiographs in the setting of trauma.

frequently involved. Neuropathy manifests as focal nerve enlargement at or proximal to the site of impingement at the cubital tunnel and is demonstrated by altered echogenicity. US also allows dynamic imaging of ulnar nerve subluxation or dislocation out of the cubital tunnel on elbow flexion[43] (Fig. 14-16). The median nerve may also be compressed at the elbow by a number of structures, most commonly the pronator teres muscle. The radial nerve may be injured above the elbow secondary to trauma or more distally at the supinator, compressing its posterior interosseous nerve branch. Similar to the ulnar nerve, US is useful in assessing focal neural dilatation and altered echogenicity.

Although lacking a dynamic component, MRI can identify nerve enlargement and edema and may also identify the specific site of impingement.[40] In addition, MRI may demonstrate neurogenic muscle edema (early sign) or muscle fatty atrophy (late sign) in the muscle groups supplied by nerves that are impinged.

Arthritis

Arthopathies that affect the elbow include rheumatoid arthritis (Fig. 14-17), osteoarthritis, crystal deposition diseases (gout and calcium pyrophosphate deposition disease), synovial osteochondromatosis, and septic arthritis. As with the shoulder, radiographs should be performed first, followed by advanced imaging if warranted. CT or CT arthrography is useful for assessing intra-articular osseous bodies. MRI and MR arthrography are also useful in this instance and are superior for assessing synovitis in inflammatory arthropathies.

Osteochondrosis and Osteochondritis Dissecans

In general, cartilage lesions are best evaluated using MRI or MR arthrography.

Panner's disease (osteochondrosis of the capitellum in children) is best assessed by MRI. It manifests as focal T2 hyperintensity of the subchondral bone of the capitellum with T1 marrow replacement. Osteochondritis dissecans of the capitellum is common and is best assessed with MR arthrography for determining lesion instability. Unstable lesions are characterized by a rim of fluid surrounding the osteochondral fragment, which may be associated with disruption of overlying cartilage and underlying cyst formation. Stable lesions with intact overlying cartilage may respond to conservative therapy.

Summary

Diagnostic imaging is an invaluable adjunct to clinical examination in the assessment of many shoulder and elbow disorders. Radiography of the shoulder and elbow should be considered in all cases, especially if there is a history of

Figure 14-16 Ulnar nerve subluxation. **A,** Transverse ultrasound image at the cubital tunnel on elbow extension shows ulnar nerve (*arrow*) in normal position. **B,** On elbow flexion, the ulnar nerve (*arrow*) is seen to sublux medially, lying perched on the medial epicondyle.

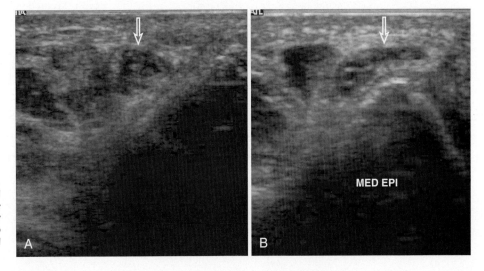

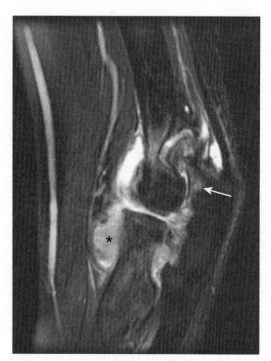

Figure 14-17 *Rheumatoid arthritis of the elbow. Sagittal short tau inversion recovery (STIR) sequence of the elbow demonstrates intermediate signal extensive pannus/synovitis (asterisk) with high-signal subchondral edema (arrow) in a patient with rheumatoid arthritis.*

trauma. Radiography provides useful information about bony anatomy and a baseline for comparison with follow-up studies, as well as providing a complementary test to advanced imaging techniques. Techniques such as US, CT, MRI, and bone scans are invaluable in providing state-of-the-art radiologic assessment and as a complement to radiography. Ordering the correct modalities with pertinent clinical details will yield maximum information and facilitate optimum patient management.

REFERENCES

The complete reference list is available online at www.expertconsult.com.

Clinical Interpretation of Nerve Conduction Studies and Electromyography of the Upper Extremity

GLENN A. MACKIN, MD, FRAN, FACP

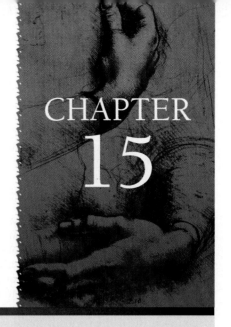

NERVE CONDUCTION STUDIES
ELECTROMYOGRAPHY

SUMMARY: QUALITY ASSURANCE AND PATIENT AND
CLINICIAN SATISFACTION

CRITICAL POINTS

- Nerve conduction studies (NCS) and electromyography (EMG) provide objective, localizing, prognostically important data about clinically suspected lesions.
- NCS and EMG also provide peripheral nerve system context about concurrent mononeuropathies, polyneuropathy, myopathy, and other neuromuscular disorders.
- NCS are generally more important in diagnosing nerve entrapments and injuries, but needle EMG is necessary to most studies for the complementary information it provides.
- Both NCS and EMG measure electrical potentials generated by nerves and muscles.
- Optimal neurophysiologic consultation is a process that calls for excellent communication between neurophysiologist and referring clinician before and after the study, as well as between patient and neurophysiologist during the study.

NCS and EMG rank second in importance only to obtaining a careful history and performing a neurologic examination for accurate and localizing diagnosis of nerve entrapments and disorders of the peripheral nervous system (PNS). Unlike clinical tests, such as Phalen's sign, that focus on specific nerve entrapments such as carpal tunnel syndrome (CTS),[1,2] well-designed NCS and EMG provide not only objective, localizing, prognostically important data about the clinically suspected lesion but also indispensable PNS *context* about concurrent mononeuropathies, polyneuropathy, myopathy, and other neuromuscular disorders. Neurophysiologists should provide prompt, understandable, "bottom line" answers that define PNS *lesion and context* in terms of the referral question and neurologic exam. The optimal neurophysiologist is a *physician*, fellowship-trained and board-certified in electrodiagnostic medicine, adept in sophisticated

examination and neuromuscular pattern recognition, and flexible enough to consistently perform studies tailored to each patient's circumstance.[3] This chapter develops a practical framework to enable referring clinicians and hand therapists to correlate clinical results and judge the quality of NCS and EMG reports.

Clinicians ordering studies seek pragmatic answers that will help their patients. Is CTS or another entrapment present? How severe is it? What is the precise localization? Are there atypical features or concurrent disorders such as radiculopathy or polyneuropathy? Do the neurophysiologic findings explain the patient's symptoms and signs, or are they at least consistent with them? Do they indicate additional or unsuspected diagnoses, or reveal a need for radiologic or other testing? Do the study design and results support the final interpretation logically and scientifically? Numerous textbooks, reviews, and courses are available with background information on neurophysiologic theory and techniques. Patients are best served when referring clinicians and neurophysiologists communicate on the basis of mutually understood interpretative principles, including what NCS and EMG actually test, their limitations, and timing considerations crucial to meaningful conclusions. The purpose of this chapter is to elucidate that indispensable conceptual framework.

Nerve Conduction Studies

General Principles

NCS are generally more important in diagnosing nerve entrapments and injuries, but needle EMG is necessary to most studies for the complementary information it provides. Both tests measure electrical potentials generated by nerves and muscles. In sensory and motor NCS, a square-wave stimulus in milliamps (mA) is delivered, usually percutaneously, to test points along the nerve, causing it to depolarize. The patient feels an instantaneous shock but usually not the wave of induced depolarization as it travels up and down the nerve itself. NCS measure voltage potential differences between two electrodes, the first recording over a nerve or muscle at an informative site at some distance from the stimulation point, the second a "neutral" reference. Recording electrodes are placed for sensory NCS over the nerve, and for motor NCS mostly over compact, usually distal superficial muscles. NCS parameters include *amplitude* (μV for sensory, mV for motor), *distal latency* (DL, in msec) from the most distal point of stimulation, and *conduction velocity* (CV, in m/sec) calculated in nerve segments demarcated by the selected points of stimulation. Although exceptions occur after nerve injury (to be discussed later), as a rule of thumb, the *size* (amplitude or area) of the NCS response is proportional to the quantity (not number) of measurable axons, and the *speed* (CV, DL) may provide insight into the integrity of myelin over the nerve segment tested.

Templates for Interpretation of Nerve Conduction Studies

The primary objectives of NCS are to localize the nerve lesion, characterize it as predominantly caused by axon loss (AL) or demyelination, determine the severity and prognosis, facilitate surgical planning when appropriate,[4] and monitor the pace of nerve regeneration.[5]

In normal nerve, the DL, amplitudes, and segmental CV are normal (Fig. 15-1A). With loss of large sensory or motor axons (AL), the amplitude of proximal and distal responses is reduced and CV may be normal or mildly slowed, but not more than 20% below the lower limit of normal (Fig. 15-1B). Examples of conditions with AL include focal mononeuropathies and most polyneuropathies. Demyelinating patterns include significant *synchronous slowing* (SS) occurring diffusely or focally (Fig. 15-1C–E); *conduction block* (CB) or "neurapraxia," which may be partial or complete (Fig. 15-1F, G), in which the proximally elicited response is smaller than distal; and *temporal dispersion* (TD), in which the proximal response has significantly longer duration and an often irregular shape (Fig. 15-1H). Examples of demyelination include SS across the wrist in CTS and across the elbow in ulnar neuropathy, CB at or near the elbow in some ulnar neuropathies and radial nerve compression at spiral groove, and TD in acquired demyelinating polyneuropathies such as Guillain–Barré syndrome (GBS) and chronic inflammatory demyelinating polyneuropathy (CIDP).[3,6,7] In entrapments, sensory fibers may show one pattern (e.g., AL), and motor fibers another (e.g., SS).

Conduction Slowing, Demyelination, and Remyelination

NCS patterns suggesting primary demyelination include significant SS, TD, and CB that meet published criteria.[1] All may be seen in acquired demyelinating neuropathies, but only SS is seen in hereditary acquired polyneuropathies such as Charcot–Marie–Tooth disease, type 1. Primary *demyelinating-range slowing* is not necessarily seen in a nerve segment with TD, unless SS also is present among the conducting fibers. As a rule of thumb, when amplitudes are normal or nearly so, slowing suggests primary demyelination when DL

(or long latency motor "F waves" to and from the spinal cord) is prolonged 30% or more above the upper limit of normal, or CV is reduced 30% or more below the lower limit of normal. (A common interpretive error, based on ignoring these criteria, takes *any* slowing of CV to be evidence of demyelination). CB and AL are more likely to correlate with symptoms than SS or TD, especially in motor axons. SS and TD may be asymptomatic, although mild degrees of both may be seen with AL of large myelinated axons over long nerve segments. (A common example is CTS with motor AL; median forearm CV is decreased due to large-fiber AL.) Muscles supplied by nerves showing TD are not weak, unless significant AL or CB is also present.

Demyelination may be the first effect of a pathologic process such as nerve entrapment that can progress to AL. Primary demyelination may be reversible and AL mitigated or avoided if the focal entrapment receives timely decompression or if acquired generalized GBS or CIDP is treated effectively with immunotherapy. By contrast, other mechanisms of injury and intrinsic disorders of axons cause primary AL, which disrupts the axon–myelin interface, resulting in secondary myelin loss. Although most nerve lesions have elements of both AL and demyelination, and NCS evidence is not as certain as biopsy evidence, clinicians should expect neurophysiologists to try consistently to specify the *predominant* pathologic process in most neuropathic cases. (Neurophysiologists equivocate unnecessarily when they habitually report "demyelination and axon loss" in all cases.)

Precise localization requires *focal SS* or *CB over a short nerve segment*.[8–10] The classic example is CTS, for which current practice guidelines stress sensitivity of sensory NCS over short nerve segments (median nerve stimulating in the palm, recording proximal to the wrist). Recent literature favors *internal comparison studies* between adjacent nerves over identical distances to mitigate the effects of cold on DL and CV (below 32°C in hand). Typical internal comparison studies in CTS include sensory comparisons (median vs. ulnar nerve palm to wrist and wrist to ring finger, and median vs. radial wrist to thumb)[11] and motor comparisons (median vs. ulnar wrist to lumbrical-interosseus).[12] Sensory internal comparisons are useful in avoiding false positive CTS due to borderline DL measured from wrist to fingers. When one internal comparison is borderline (e.g., median vs. ulnar palm to the wrist, normal difference < 0.4 msec), adding three comparisons to calculate a "combined sensory index" improves sensitivity and specificity (normal < 0.9 msec).

Slowing in many nerves suggests a generalized polyneuropathy, making it difficult to be sure that any focal slowing seen is disproportionate enough to attribute to superimposed entrapment (e.g., CTS in diabetic polyneuropathy, where motor internal comparisons may help). Focal slowing may confirm demyelination (or not meet criteria) and may occur in a symptomatic or asymptomatic location (e.g., ulnar slowing across the elbow). Focal slowing demonstrable across multiple points of entrapment, common and uncommon, symptomatic or not, suggests the autosomal dominant hereditary neuropathy with liability to pressure palsies (HNPP), for which a genetic test is available.

Conduction block is present when amplitude and area of waveforms obtained by stimulating proximal to the lesion is at least 20% less (ideally 50%) than the waveform obtained

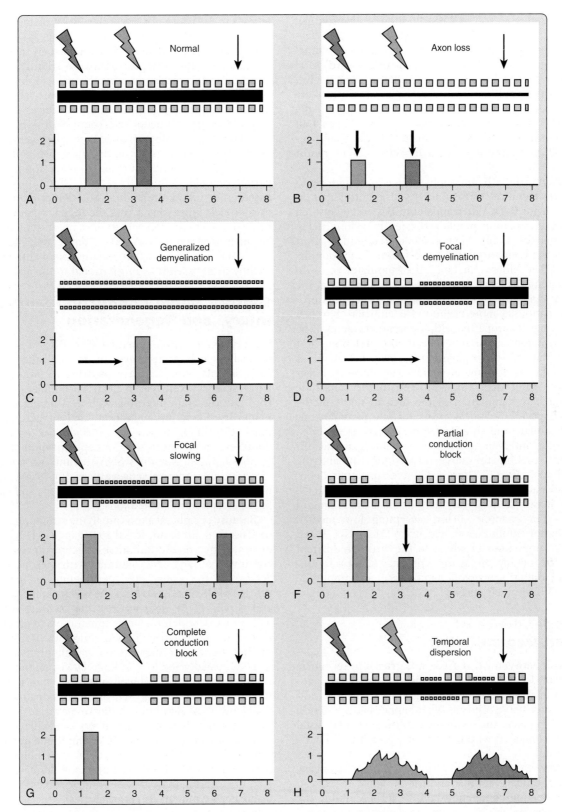

Figure 15-1 Schematic peripheral nerves illustrate "nerve conduction study (NCS) templates" in text. In all nerves, the *black horizontal bar* reflects the proportion of large sensory or motor axons, and *rows of small squares* reflect the myelin sheath on large sensory and motor fibers, available for testing. The *black down arrow* indicates the recording electrodes placed distally over a named sensory nerve or over the motor point and reference site for a motor NCS. The *blue "lightning bolt"* reflects the more distal point of stimulation along the nerve tested, and the *blue rectangle* reflects the recorded waveform amplitude, area, and morphology as a function of time. The *red "lightning bolt"* and *rectangle*, respectively, reflect the more proximal point of stimulation and recorded waveform. Arbitrary numbers on the *y*-axis for amplitude and *x*-axis for time of the recorded response are provided to facilitate visual comparison between normal and the different nerve injury patterns. **A,** Normal nerve. **B,** Axon loss (AL). **C,** Generalized demyelinating synchronous slowing (SS), as in Charcot–Marie–Tooth polyneuropathy, type 1. **D,** Focal, distal, demyelinating synchronous slowing (SS), as in carpal tunnel syndrome. **E,** Focal, proximal, demyelinating synchronous slowing (SS), as in ulnar neuropathy across the elbow. **F,** Focal, partial, demyelinating conduction block (CB), shown proximally as in ulnar neuropathy at elbow. **G,** Focal, complete, demyelinating CB, proximally. **H,** Temporal dispersion (TD), as in Guillain–Barré syndrome, chronic inflammatory demyelinating polyneuropathy, and some entrapments.

stimulating distal to it, provided the duration of the proximal response does not exceed the distal by more than 15%. *Temporal dispersion* is present when the duration of the proximal waveform exceeds the distal by more than 15%, regardless of any amplitude change. Like the velocity criteria for demyelination, these rules apply only when response amplitudes are near normal. Larger amplitude drops are required proximally to confirm CB when distal amplitudes are low. Given that motor responses are orders of magnitude larger than sensory ones, it is technically easier to show CB in motor conductions.

Before diagnosing CB, neurophysiologists should rigorously exclude technical errors and trivial abnormalities to minimize false positives. When apparent CB is noted between two standard stimulation points separated by a long nerve segment, it may be useful, when possible, to stimulate short segments in between to pinpoint the lesion. For example, with ulnar CB at elbow, "inching" the stimulator in 1- to 2-cm steps along the nerve may precisely localize CB at the humeroulnar aponeurosis or retrocondylar space, thus providing information far more useful to the clinician than just reporting "ulnar neuropathy with neurapraxia across the elbow."[13,14] Anatomic variants affect interpretation. For example, a Martin–Gruber anastomosis may mimic ulnar motor CB in the forearm, manifested by a significantly larger ulnar wrist-to-hand than elbow-to-hand motor amplitude and confirmed by stimulation of the median nerve at the antebrachial space[15] Technical errors include percutaneous stimulation too far from an intended deep nerve target (e.g., obesity, edema, intervening muscles), resulting in insufficient current reaching the nerve (mimicking CB) and the "virtual cathode" effect (CV errors due to an uncertain depolarization site and inaccurate distances). When very distal CB is possible, it may help to stimulate distal to the standard distal sites. For example, before accepting low median sensory or motor amplitudes as evidence of AL in CTS, based on standard stimulation proximal to the wrist, midpalmar stimulation or inching across the wrist may show a significantly larger digital sensory or motor response amplitude consistent with focal CB instead.

Time Dependence of Wallerian Degeneration

To distinguish between AL and CB, it is crucial to recognize that Wallerian degeneration (WD) after AL (including axonotmesis) is an active, time-dependent process. The key indicator of AL after nerve injury is what happens as a function of time after injury to the response amplitude elicited distal to the lesion compared with the response amplitude elicited proximal to it.

Immediately after nerve injury before WD has taken place, the distal amplitude is normal and the proximal is reduced or absent, reflecting conduction failure and resembling the CB pattern (see Fig. 15-1F, G). If pure demyelinating CB is present, axon continuity is preserved through the lesion and the CB pattern persists until remyelination occurs. If pure AL is present, the distal stump undergoes WD, and the distal amplitude declines to match the already low proximal amplitude, resulting in an AL pattern (see Fig. 15-1B). Although the time to WD is similar for motor and sensory axons, it

takes 3 to 4 days to observe a decline in distal motor amplitudes after AL lesions versus 10 to 12 days for distal sensory amplitudes. The difference is explained by neuromuscular junctions (NMJs) interposed between stimulated nerve and muscle. Axonotmesis disrupts axonal trophic support of muscle mediated by slow axon transport, so NMJ failure precedes WD, causing motor amplitude drop. WD is a stump length-dependent process, seen sooner in lesions near muscle.

When NCS are done immediately after nerve injury and before WD occurs, particularly when nerve transection is suggested, nerve conduction across the lesion proves *at least partial continuity*. Immediate NCS after injury provides a baseline for follow-up studies, but cannot define the status of *nonconducting* axons across the lesion, whether caused by AL, CB, or both. Repeat studies are essential after WD becomes apparent in NCS (10–12 days) and EMG (3 weeks). In general, the amount that serially documented amplitudes decline from baseline is proportional to the amount of AL.[5]

Sensory Nerve Conduction Studies, Injury, and Regeneration

Sensory nerve action potential (SNAP) is a summation of normally synchronous waves of depolarization traveling in large sensory axons as they pass the recording electrodes. Large sensory axons carry electrical impulses to the spinal cord that the brain interprets as touch, proprioception, two-point discrimination, vibration, and higher-order perceptions. Conventional sensory NCS do not record encoded impulses, actual perceptions, or depolarization of *small* axons (c-nociceptors). Nor does SNAP count the sensory axons. (Separate quantitative sensory tests [QST] are available to measure vibratory thresholds in large axons and thermal and pain perception in small axons.)

Because peripheral axons are living structural components of sensory neurons in dorsal root ganglia (DRG) located in or near spinal neural foramina, a recordable SNAP confirms continuity of large DRG neurons with their peripheral processes. In the arms, the "peripheral," or *postganglionic*, process of DRG cells traverses the brachial plexus and peripheral nerves. SNAP does not test the "central," or *preganglionic*, process, which traverses spinal roots to enter the spinal cord. A reduced or absent SNAP amplitude is not a localizing finding, because it suggests postganglionic AL at or distal to DRG, usually the loss of large DRG peripheral processes (mononeuropathies, polyneuropathies), but sometimes the loss of parent DRG cells (sensory neuronopathy). An abnormally low SNAP amplitude indicates partial loss of large DRG processes or cells, assuming delivery of adequate (supramaximal) stimulation. A normal SNAP amplitude proves there are "enough" large sensory axons, defined by published norms. A low-normal SNAP in a symptomatic dermatome or nerve territory calls for a side-to-side comparison, because a twofold or greater asymmetry is abnormal.

SNAPs are fraught with potential technical and interpretive pitfalls. First, with side-to-side comparisons, both sides may be affected (e.g., CTS). Second, although SNAP amplitudes usually are more prominently affected than motor potentials after axonotmesis, testing in the 5- to 9-day window after postganglionic AL is confusing because a reduced compound motor action potential (CMAP) but normal SNAP amplitude falsely suggests a preganglionic lesion. Third, a postganglionic lesion (e.g., plexopathy) does not exclude a concurrent preganglionic lesion (e.g., radiculopathy), especially when the injury may involve both (e.g., motorcycle traction injury to arm). Finally, when neurophysiologists approach injured nerves with an inflexibly preconceived notion of what they will find, they may erroneously accept a reduced or absent *sensory* response as confirmatory. Common examples include an absent ulnar sensory response stimulating wrist recording from the small finger in *suspected* ulnar neuropathy at elbow, and an absent median sensory response stimulating wrist recording from the middle finger in *suspected* CTS. The most circumspect interpretation of each of these isolated findings, respectively, would be a partial AL lesion at or distal to the C8 and C7 DRGs in either brachial plexus or peripheral nerves. Particularly in ulnar neuropathy, for which there are many potential sites of focal injury from axilla to its terminal branches, the burden of localization shifts from low SNAP to *motor* NCS and EMG.

Clinicians approach sensory symptoms thinking of the cutaneous distributions of spinal roots (dermatomes) and peripheral nerves. To understand what SNAP actually tests, it is crucial to recall that dermatomal symptoms can arise from preganglionic axons, postganglionic axons, or both. For example, C8 radiculopathies and lower-trunk plexopathies may cause similar distributions of distal sensory symptoms. With preganglionic C8 radiculopathies, postganglionic C8 axons are intact, so SNAPs are normal when recorded in the C8 dermatome, however numb the skin (e.g., ulnar nerve recording of the small finger, or dorsal ulnar cutaneous nerve recording of the dorsomedial hand). With lower-trunk plexopathies, similar sensory symptoms on the medial forearm or small finger could correspond with SNAP amplitudes that are absent, reduced in absolute terms, low-normal but less than half contralaterally, or *normal* if symptoms arise from irritation of large C8 postganglionic processes without AL or selective irritation or injury to c-nociceptor axons in the C8 dermatome.

Sensory nerve injuries recover through remyelination (over weeks to months) or regeneration of cut axons (1 inch/month or 1–2 mm/day). Reduced sensory amplitudes mean either that stimulation and recording distal to the point of actual partial CB is technically impossible or that the nerve is not there. As CB lesions remyelinate or large axons regenerate, SNAP amplitudes increase. However, sensory (and motor) axon sprouts may not reach their original target due to neuroma formation, blockage by scar, misdirection (aberrant regeneration), or regeneration failure (e.g., certain toxic neuropathies).

Motor Nerve Conduction Studies, Injury, and Regeneration

Interpretation of CMAPs uses similar principles and "templates" as for SNAPs, but several differences should be recognized. Even though both test living peripheral nerve systems, the proximal anatomy of the "motor unit" differs from the large DRG and peripheral process sensory system *in diagnostically important ways*. First, different sites of lower motor neurons (LMN) and DRG neurons aid in localization. LMN (anterior horn cells) are clustered in the spinal cord ventral horn, *proximal to both spinal roots and sensory neurons* located in the DRG at or near the spinal neural foramina. SNAPs do not reflect sensory root injury in cervical radiculopathies. For both motor NCS and needle EMG, neurophysiologic testing of the living "motor unit" includes LMNs, motor root and axons, NMJ, muscle membrane, and muscle fibers. Significant motor AL at LMN or root levels may be reflected as abnormal motor NCS (see Fig. 15-1B), EMG, or both. Because muscles are supplied by more than one motor root, acute AL in a single root must be severe to reduce CMAP amplitudes recorded distally, although side-to-side CMAP comparisons may be helpful. Second, given the rather different locations of anterior horn cells (AHC) and DRG, abnormalities in CMAP or EMG together with normal SNAP from the same spinal segment define a *preganglionic* lesion. Although interpretations should pass the test of reasonableness, mutually reinforcing CMAP, EMG, and SNAP findings that align to suggest a preganglionic rather than an expected postganglionic lesion should be taken quite seriously. When clinical and neurophysiologic localization appear to disagree, the neurophysiologist has a responsibility to consider the timing of the study relative to WD, additional testing (side-to-side, specialized, and serial), unexpected concurrent lesions, and even neuromuscular diseases. Occasional patients with painless thenar atrophy with suspected CTS show expected low-amplitude of the abductor pollicis brevis, but on EMG are found to have generalized motor neuron disease.

Although the rates of WD and axon regeneration are similar for sensory and motor axons, the distal anatomy of the "motor unit" and recording site for CMAP relative to it differ significantly from the sensory system as reflected in SNAP. First, unlike SNAP, which amounts to a "snapshot" of a traveling wave of depolarization passing under the recording electrodes over a "named" nerve, the CMAP represents the potential difference between a recording electrode on a muscle's "motor point" and a reference electrode off muscle. Although most reduced CMAPs recorded in patients with hand problems are caused by AL or demyelination related to focal mononeuropathies, it is important to recall that the motor unit reflected in CMAP tests more structures than just nerves. Thus, reduced or absent CMAP may reflect disorders of LMNs, roots (compressive and infiltrative), plexus, peripheral nerves, NMJ, muscle membranes, and muscles. Second, reinnervation after motor AL underlies increasing CMAP amplitudes and areas (but different wave shapes) by two distinct mechanisms: collateral sprouting and regeneration. Since sensory axons do not branch, sensory reinnervation proceeds by the sole mechanism of regeneration—the distal advance of growth cones. By contrast, after partial AL motor axons in continuity with muscle undergo collateral sprouting by 3 to 6 months to reinnervate disconnected muscle fibers. In addition, cut axons may regenerate at similar rates as sensory axons to grow back into muscle, provided they are not blocked or diverted. Muscle NMJs accept connections with ingrowing regenerating motor axons for a finite period, a year or possibly longer, depending on patient age and various strategies to prolong that receptivity. Because the CMAP (but not SNAP) is recorded from an end organ (muscle), and because there are two motor but only one sensory mechanism for reinnervation, a normal CMAP amplitude recorded in both the acute phase after nerve injury and chronic phase after reinnervation may misleadingly imply a normal number of motor axons. Further study with EMG would show reinnervation.[3,5,14,16]

Electromyography

It is beyond the scope of this chapter to discuss the diagnostic power of EMG in the evaluation of neuromuscular diseases. Even in the evaluation of focal peripheral mononeuropathies, EMG plays an indispensible role by demonstrating unsuspected PNS lesions, showing partial motor continuity that might not be clinically apparent after nerve injury, providing insight into the acuity of motor denervation and the cumulative extent of chronic denervation, and documenting reinnervation. Well-designed, skillful EMG studies provide such crucial information complementary to NCS that test requisitions stipulating "NCS only" (to spare the patient needles) do the patient a disservice.

In standard EMG, a sterile concentric or monopolar needle electrode is inserted into a muscle to record electrical activity on needle insertion, spontaneous activity in the resting muscle, and motor unit potentials (MUP) with voluntary contraction.

Insertional activity in the resting muscle on EMG needle insertion is often overinterpreted, but when markedly increased it suggests muscle membrane irritability immediately after axonotmesis before spontaneous activity appears or an underlying disorder of muscle membrane or muscle. (Clinicians should be wary of EMG diagnoses based exclusively on "increased insertional activity.")

Spontaneous activity in the resting muscle includes *fibrillations* and *positive sharp waves*, which reflect "acute" AL in denervating disorders and muscle fragmentation or necrosis in myopathies. Fibrillations and positive sharp waves are seen in neuropathic disorders when the EMG needle tip is near viable muscle fibers disconnected from axons and emerges in an axon stump length-dependent pattern. In acutely denervated muscles with short stumps, such as cervical paraspinals after radiculopathies and nerve transactions near muscle, these discharges may appear in 7 to 10 days. Usually, however, the muscle of interest is well distal to the injury site, such as an ulnar innervated intrinsic hand muscle after acute AL at the elbow. In such cases, fibrillations and positive waves appear after WD has occurred, requiring 3 to 4 weeks to appear. They persist until "silenced" by muscle reinnervation by collateral sprouting, nerve regeneration, or fibrosis of muscle isolated too long from axonal trophic support. Fasciculations are spontaneous discharges in resting muscle that reflect irritability of motor axons in continuity anywhere from LMN to muscle, as seen in motor neuron diseases, radiculopathies, mononeuropathies, polyneuropathies, and myopathies. Fasciculations can be observed by visual inspection of muscles; fibrillations require needle EMG.

Voluntary activity generates an "interference pattern" on the EMG oscilloscope that ideally reflects graded patient effort from slight to full contraction. Analysis includes MUP amplitude, duration and morphology (generally larger and more polyphasic after reinnervation), and firing patterns.

MUP recruitment analysis judges firing rates of single MUPs relative to the number of MUPs firing. In normal muscle, no MUP should fire excessively fast; as more force is required, more MUPs recruit. In denervating processes, recruitment is decreased, meaning that a reduced number of MUPs are seen firing at excessive rates. Immediately after nerve injury and before WD, before CMAP amplitudes decline and fibrillations and positive waves emerge, EMG recruitment is reduced in weak muscles whether the lesion is AL, CB, or both. Reduced recruitment in early demyelinating processes (e.g., soon after "Saturday night palsy" or Guillain–Barré symptoms) may be "downstream" evidence of proximal neurapraxic CB, which carries a good prognosis with remyelination. Neurophysiologists should always provide a semiquantitative severity estimate for recruitment abnormalities because, together with NCS, such estimates can greatly assist in decision making.[3,14]

"Positive" Sensory Symptoms and Test Sensitivity

Patients with nerve problems seek help for *negative* symptoms (a lack of sensory or motor function) or *positive* symptoms (excess or ectopic function). Negative sensory symptoms include numbness, whereas positive sensory symptoms include tingling and burning. Negative motor symptoms include weakness, whereas positive motor symptoms include cramps and fasciculations. Negative sensory and motor symptoms from the PNS correlate well with NCS and EMG abnormalities. Likewise, positive motor symptoms and signs often correlate with specific discharges on resting EMG and abnormalities on motor NCS or EMG during muscle contraction.

By contrast, positive sensory symptoms are elusive and sometimes frustrating for referring clinicians and neurophysiologists alike.[17] The SNAP correlate of *tingling* from large sensory axons may be a normal study, a nonlocalizing AL pattern, or localizing demyelinating SS, CB, or TD if recorded over a suggestive short nerve segment. The SNAP correlate of *burning* from small sensory axons may be a normal study, unless there are measurable large-fiber NCS abnormalities. The words "this study provides neurophysiologic *evidence* of" should precede every list of conclusions because, strictly speaking, a normal study does not "rule out" a PNS basis for paresthesias. It is crucial to recall the tradeoff between the sensitivity and specificity of diagnostic tests in general[18] and of neurophysiologic tests for specific nerve entrapments. In early CTS, some 10% to 15% of patients with "classic" sensory symptoms have normal NCS, a level of sensitivity sometimes criticized because it allows for too many false negatives. Some clinicians respond by using clinical test batteries and stress tests for entrapments with sensitivities said to rival NCS, though the precise clinical definitions and NCS norms used can be self-fulfilling. Some neurophysiologists respond by doing many specialized NCS variations to detect any abnormality, or they stress borderline changes. Such strategies risk high false positives, particularly in entrapments like CTS and ulnar neuropathy in which standard NCS and common internal comparison studies are sensitive. Neurophysiologists should comment when NCS of an entrapment is inherently insensitive (e.g., pronator syndrome).

The approach recommended herein recognizes the relative scarcity of natural history studies of very mild clinical entrapments, the illusion of the perfectly sensitive and specific test,[19] and the strengths of properly performed neurophysiologic consultation (objectivity, context, prognosis). It is important that neurophysiologists remind referring clinicians routinely in their reports that conventional sensory NCS do *not* test pain-sensitive structures that, when irritated, may underlie paresthesias arising from "named" peripheral nerves, myofascial structures, sensory roots, or the central nervous system. However, normal results in cases of possible entrapment for which NCS are highly sensitive provides reassurance that conservative management may be justified.

Summary: Quality Assurance and Patient and Clinician Satisfaction

Published neurophysiologic guidelines delineate professional, technical,[20] and *ethical*[21] standards for physicians providing electrodiagnostic consultation. Although clinicians look first for responsive "bottom line" results on NCS and EMG reports and may lack the experience to evaluate study design, certain markers of reliability should be apparent on the face of each report.

Hallmarks of *careful studies tailored to the patient* include (1) pertinent departures from routine to confirm borderline changes, (2) circumspect interpretation of minor deviations from normal, (3) routine adjectives that estimate the severity of NCS[22] and EMG abormalities, (4) the "fit" between referral issues and anatomic scope of study, (5) substantive clinical correlations, and (6) interpretations that suggest alternative diagnoses based on the objective data recorded. *External indicators of technical quality on reports* include (1) specification of the predominant pathologic process in neuropathic cases, (2) reported NCS normal values and temperature measures, (3) "internal comparison" studies, (4) side-to-side NCS comparisons for borderline results (especially in brachial plexopathies), (5) repetition and careful verification of difficult subtests, (6) actual NCS waves included with the report, and (7) patient satisfaction.

The importance of establishing confidence with the patient by using a reassuring manner and a thoroughness of approach cannot be overemphasized, given the discomfort inherent in NCS and EMG and the necessity of patient cooperation and relaxation for best results. Optimal neurophysiologic consultation is a process that calls for excellent communication not only between neurophysiologist and referring clinician before and after the study, but also between patient and neurophysiologist during the study. The optimal neurophysiologist puts the interests of the patient first, which includes a willingness to treat them with kindness, talk to them, and even say "I'm sorry that hurt" after a painful procedure.

REFERENCES

The complete reference list is available online at www.expertconsult.com.

CHAPTER 16

Outcome Measurement in Upper Extremity Practice

JOY C. MACDERMID, BScPT, PhD

WHAT IS A HEALTH OUTCOME MEASURE?

HOW CAN CLINICIANS USE OUTCOME MEASURES?

WHAT ARE THE IMPORTANT MEASUREMENT PROPERTIES OF OUTCOME MEASURES?

WHAT DO I NEED TO KNOW BEFORE USING OUTCOME TOOLS?

HOW DO I FIND OUTCOME MEASURES THAT ARE SUITABLE FOR ME?

HOW DO I ADMINISTER THE OUTCOME MEASURE TO MEASURE CHANGE IN MY PATIENTS?

HOW DO I ANALYZE OUTCOME SCORES?

HOW DO I INCORPORATE PREDICTORS OF OUTCOME?

HOW DO I SET UP A PROCESS TO MEASURE OUTCOMES IN MY PRACTICE?

SUMMARY

CRITICAL POINTS

- Outcome measures need to be both reliable and valid.
- Therapists should perform outcome evaluation using procedures that incorporate currently accepted standardized methods both in the clinical setting and in manuals or research paper(s).
- Outcome measures are typically used for evaluation over time, but they can also be used to discriminate between patient groups and predict future status such as return to work.
- The implementation of outcome measures within clinical practice requires information that may require purchase or permissions from developers and always requires knowledge about proper scoring and interpretation of scores.
- Selecting the appropriate outcome starts with determining the purpose and scope of measuring and then requires matching the patient's problem, level of difficulty, and communication capacity with these properties of the tool.

What Is a Health Outcome Measure?

A health outcome measure is any measurement of a patient's health status. That view of health status can be broad, such as when we measure overall health or quality of life. We can also focus on very specific aspects of health. Pain and function are specific aspects of health that are of particular interest to hand therapists. Health can change over time as a result of time, treatment, or disease. Patients' perceptions of their health status can change because of anatomic and physiologic changes that alter body functions, psychological changes that affect perception, or calibration of health or social changes that alter the experience of living with a specific health status. For this reason, measuring outcomes can be complex and requires a theoretical foundation, as well as different instruments to account for different perspectives and purposes.

The most internationally accepted standard of health is proposed by the World Health Organization. This organization produces both The International Classification of Diseases (ICD) (*www.who.int/classifications/icd/en/*) and an International Classification of Functioning, Disability and Health (ICF) (*www.who.int/classifications/icf/en/*). The latter is increasingly being used as a framework by which outcome measures are classified[1-6] (Fig. 16-1).

Body functions are physiologic or psychological functions of body systems.[7] *Body structures* are anatomic parts of the body, such as organs, limbs, and their components. *Impairment* is the loss or abnormality of psychological, physiologic, or anatomic structure or function. Examples of impairments that hand therapists typically measure include hand size, appearance, strength, range of motion (ROM), volume, sensory threshold, and pain. Methods and interpretation for measuring impairments of the hand are the traditional focus of hand therapy and are detailed in many of the chapters in this book discussing evaluation.

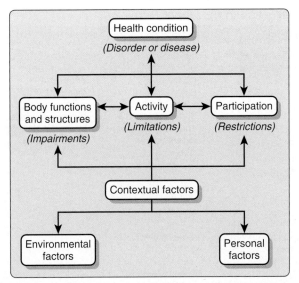

Figure 16-1 The conceptual model for the International Classification of Functioning. (Adapted from *www.who.int/classifications/icf/en/*.)

Activity is the execution of a task or action by an individual. *Participation* is involvement in a life situation. Inability in these areas can be termed activity limitations or participation restrictions. Tests that measure performance of specific tasks include tests such as the TEMPA (Test d'Evaluation des Membres Supérieurs de Personnes Agées),[8] Jebson Test of Hand Function,[9] Purdue Pegboard,[10] Minnesota Rate of Manipulation Test,[11] the RNK dexterity test,[12,13] and other "hand function tests" can measure activity limitations. Activity limitations can also be measured by self-report by asking individuals whether they can perform a specific activity like lifting a grocery bag. Indicators that focus on resuming roles, like returning to work, reflect participation and can be considered as measures of actual status or by self-report. Many self-report functional scales contain both activity and participation type of items. In fact, a number of studies have now classified items of specific upper extremity scales[14,15] or hand problems[16-18] using the ICF. However, moving ICF into practice has been slow. Recently, *core* and *brief core measures* were developed for hand conditions using an international evidence-based consensus process. These codes are available for all to use (*www.icf-research-branch.org/research/Hand. htm*).

In this chapter, we discuss principles that apply to all outcome measures, but emphasize self-report because many of the chapters in this book have focused on impairment measures.

How Can Clinicians Use Outcome Measures?

The basic functionalities about the measure's scores include evaluation of change over time, discrimination between groups of patients, and prediction of future status.[19] Hand therapy is characterized by development of advanced evaluative measures of hand impairment. Publication of *Clinical Assessment Recommendations* was one of the first accomplish-

ments of the American Society of Hand Therapists, and the second edition remained in print for 20 years.[20] This guide has traditionally focused on measuring hand impairments. However, increasingly it is becoming standard practice to include functional measures—particularly those involving self-report. In fact, some payers now mandate this practice. A new expanded version of the *Clinical Assessment Recommendations* is expected in 2010 and will include self-report measures and information on ICF.

A standardized outcome measure is one that has specific properties: it is published; there are detailed instructions on how to administer, score, and interpret the test; it has a defined purpose; it was designed for a specific population; and there are published data indicating acceptable reliability and validity. Standardization in clinical measurement is essential to ensure that outcome measures are capable of providing valid information about a patient's health status.

Evaluation over Time

The most common application in clinical practice is evaluation over time.[19] Optimally, evaluation over time includes using outcome measures to set goals and then determining whether detectable important changes have occurred.

When designing a treatment plan, hand therapists typically determine which pathologic processes or physical impairments are contributing to the patient's complaint or compromised health. Treatment programs are then designed to allow optimal recovery and to minimize any residual impairment or functional limitation. Before and after intervention, examination is required to determine the effectiveness of the selected intervention. For example, if a therapist evaluates a tendon repair and is concerned about tendon gliding, then active range of motion (AROM) is appropriate to measure. Treatment for this patient might include a variety of interventions that are expected to improve tendon glide. It is essential that hand therapists evaluate impairment measures that are expected to change, such as AROM in this case. However, AROM may not be relevant to function for all patients, problems, or stages of recovery. Therapists should avoid "rote" use of any measure without considering the context and whether the measurement is able to provide useful information. If we think about a flexor tendon patient who achieves improved glide as result of hand therapy, the goal should be concomitant to improving the patient's ability to perform activities such as gripping a handle and more successful participation in work. These effects can be measured using standardized outcome instruments. However, a review of outcome measures used when assessing patients with tendon and nerve repairs indicates a primary focus on impairments, particularly range of motion.[21]

The first step in using outcome measures to evaluate change over time begins at the initial assessment. The therapist must select an appropriate measure that is both relevant to the patient's problem and also has capacity to detect change. (See Table 16-1 and companion Web site for examples.) A short-term goal for improvement is then set using evidence from the literature about the minimal detectable change (MDC). Short-term goals are set to exceed the minimal detectable change so that you can be confident that

Text continues on p. 200

Table 16-1 Examples of Self-Report Scales Used on Outcome Evaluation in the Upper Extremity

Measure	Purpose	Format	Reliability	Validity	Responsiveness
Visual Analogue Scales (VAS)—Pain[81-86]	To measure quantity of pain	10-cm line in a variety of formats; requires careful instruction; score is distance from 0 (no pain) to end (worst pain imaginable); commonly used for pain but has been adapted to other constructs (revalidated)	Can vary, but high test–retest has been demonstrated[82,87]	High correlation between VAS and numeric pain-rating scale,[83] finger dynamometer,[86] and a verbal description of pain[86]	Able to detect 21 levels of just noticeable differences[85] some believe that it is less sensitive to change in acute pain than in chronic pain[81]
Numeric Rating Scales (NRS)—Pain	To measure quantity of pain	0–10 scale for pain, administered verbally or on paper; typically 0 = no pain and 10 = worst pain imaginable; has also been applied to other constructs and used as a rating scale within questionnaires	Not specifically reported but high when used as a subscale in other measures[52]	High correlation with VAS,[83] finger dynamometer,[86] and other outcome measures	High in distal radius fractures as subscale[53]
Sickness Impact Profile (SIP)[88-90]	Health status across demographic and cultural groups	136 items that are divided into two dimensions (physical and psychosocial) and 12 categories	Internal consistency, test–retest and inter-rater reliability (interview) are all high	Construct, concurrent validity reported;[89] has not been widely used for upper extremity	Not as responsive as regional measures in upper extremity conditions[91]
(Medical Outcomes) Short-Form SF-36[39,40]	Health status across demographic and cultural groups	36 items; 8 subscales (physical function, physical role, vitality, bodily pain, general health, social function, emotional role, and mental health and vitality); two summary component scales are calculated (physical and mental), which standardize the patient's score to the U.S. population norms	Has been reported to be high[39,40]	Numerous validity studies and normative data abundant[39,40] instrument well supported by Medical Outcomes Trust; may be preferable to SIP;[92] authors suggest that for upper extremity it should be combined with a more specific instrument[93]	Less responsive than the DASH or PRWE in evaluating wrist fractures;[53] most commonly used generic measure
(Medical Outcomes) Short-Form SF-12[94]	Health status across demographic and cultural groups	12 items; two summary component scales are calculated (physical and mental), which standardize the patient's score to the U.S. population norms	Has been reported to be high[39,40]	Numerous validity studies and normative data abundant;[39,40] instrument well supported by Medical Outcomes Trust; may be preferable to SIP[92]	Summary scores less responsive than the DASH or PRWE in evaluating wrist fractures[75-79]

Table 16-1   Examples of Self-Report Scales Used on Outcome Evaluation in the Upper Extremity—cont'd

Measure	Purpose	Format	Reliability	Validity	Responsiveness
Musculoskeletal Function Assessment (MFA)[95-99]	Health status instrument for use with a broad range of musculoskeletal disorders; to complement SF-36	100 items; subscales include self-care, sleep/rest, hand/fine motor, mobility, housework, employment/ work, leisure/ recreation, family relationships, cognition/ thinking, emotional adjustment	High[99]	Appropriate correlations with other instruments and other clinical measures;[58,96,98,99] normative and comparison data reported[95]	Moderate to large effect sizes reported
Disabilities of the, Arm, Shoulder and Hand (DASH)[35,37,50,52,82,100]	Upper extremity disability	30 items rated 1–5; majority of questions assess upper extremity function		Construct validity has been demonstrated[50,101]	More responsive than generic measures for patients with upper extremity pathology; shown to be reliable, valid, and responsive for a variety of upper extremity problems[49,50]
Quick Disabilities of the, Arm, Shoulder and Hand (QuickDASH)[37,49,50,52,82,100]	Upper extremity disability	11 items rated 1–5; derived from the original DASH[56] addresses regional symptoms and function of the upper extremity	Reliability has exceeded 0.90 for both the common 0–5 and VAS rating scales[58,60]	Construct validity has been demonstrated[56-62]	More responsive than generic measures for patients with upper extremity pathology and equivalent to full DASH[57-59,61,62]
Upper Extremity Function Scale (UEFS)[102]	To measure effect of upper extremity disorders on function	8 items scored 0–10	Internal consistency high	Excellent convergent and discriminative validity when compared with measures of symptom severity[102]	More responsive than grip and pinch in CTS[102]
Shoulder Pain and Disability Index (SPADI)[91,93,103,104]	Shoulder pain and disability	Pain and disability scored as 50% each; items scored on a visual or numeric analog scale; 5 pain questions, 8 function; a numeric (0–10) version has been shown to be highly correlated with VAS version[104]	High internal consistency and moderate test–retest[105]	Construct and criterion validity have been evaluated[44,104-111]	More responsive than regional or generic measures[54,91,104]
Shoulder Rating Questionnaire[112]	Severity of symptoms and functional status of the shoulder	21 questions in total, including 1 global rating on a VAS and 18 questions in a Likert format; 4 pain, 5 activities daily living (ADL), 3 recreation, 4 work, 1 satisfaction	High internal consistency and test–retest reliability[112]	Moderate to high validity coefficients compared with arthritis effect measurement scales[112]	Responsive[112]

Continued

Table 16-1   Examples of Self-Report Scales Used on Outcome Evaluation in the Upper Extremity—cont'd

Measure	Purpose	Format	Reliability	Validity	Responsiveness
Western Ontario Rotator Cuff WORC[113]	Quality of life in patients with rotator cuff pathology	21 questions on visual analog scales; sections on physical symptoms, sports/ recreation, work, lifestyle, and emotions	High	Moderate correlation with strength and range of motion in patients with rotator cuff pathology[114]	Manuscript in progress; presented but not published
Western Ontario Instability Index (WOSI)[115]	Quality of life in patients with shoulder instability	21 questions on VAS; sections on physical symptoms, sports/ recreation, work, lifestyle, and emotions	High[115]	Correlated appropriately with other instruments[115]	More responsive than 5 other instruments (DASH, ASES, UCLA, Constant score, and Rowe Rating)[115]
American Shoulder and Elbow Surgeons (ASES) Shoulder Form[116]	Patient-rated pain and disability for a wide variety of shoulder problems	1 pain question (VAS); 10 function questions (0–3)	Shown to have high reliability and internal consistency[117]	Construct, content, and discriminative validity demonstrated[117]	Insufficient data available
Shoulder Pain Score[118]	For assessing pain in patients with shoulder pathology	7 questions; 5 on a 4-point Likert scale and 1 VAS for global rating of pain	Not published	Factor analysis used to determine that question; addresses two factors considered passive and active situations by authors[118]	Not published
Constant Shoulder Score (patient component)[71]	Used for a variety of shoulder problems, including instability	Pain rated 0–4; function (work, recreation, sleep position of arm, work)		Has been validated in a number of studies, and some aspects of the validity question such as the appropriateness of age correction, standardization of test methods and strength rating processes	
Shoulder Disability Questionnaire[119]	Functional disability in patients with shoulder disorders	16 yes/no questions on pain, related disability	Not published		Responsive in 349 primary care patients with shoulder disorders[119]
Subjective Shoulder Rating Scale[120]	To briefly measure subjective shoulder complaints	Multiple-choice question; 1 pain, 1 motion, 1 stability, and 1 activity	Not published	Highly correlated to Constant–Murley score but much faster to complete[120]	Not published
Simple Shoulder Test[105]	To assess shoulder function	Yes/no responses; 2 pain, 7 function, 3 motion questions		Discriminant in patients with rotator cuff pathology;[114] appears to be more discriminative than other shoulder measures	Acceptable responsiveness in a number of shoulder studies
American Shoulder and Elbow Surgeons (ASES) Elbow Form[121]	To measure pain, disability, and patient satisfaction in patients with elbow pathology	Patient rating scales for pain ranked 0–10 for 5 pain items, 0–3 for 12 function items, and 0–10 for 1 satisfaction question	High[122]	Appropriate (high) correlation with PREE[53]	Not published

Table 16-1   Examples of Self-Report Scales Used on Outcome Evaluation in the Upper Extremity—cont'd

Measure	Purpose	Format	Reliability	Validity	Responsiveness
Patient-Rated Tennis Elbow Evaluation[123] (PRTEE)	To measure pain and disability in patients with lateral epicondylitis	5 pain questions scored 0–10; 10 function questions scored 0–10	Reliability coefficients exceed 0.90[124]	Appropriate (High) correlation with ASES elbow form[122]	More responsive than variety of other measures including ones devised for tennis elbow[124]
Patient-Rated Elbow Evaluation (PREE)[122]	To measure pain and disability in patients with elbow pathology	5 pain questions scores 0–10; 15 function questions scored 0–10	High[122]	Appropriate (high) correlation with ASES elbow form[122]	Not published
Patient-Rated Ulnar Nerve Evaluation	For patients with symptoms of ulnar nerve compression	Pain, sensory/motor scale, and function subscales	Not published	Not published; format similar to previous questionnaires by same author[122]	Not published
Patient-Rated Wrist Evaluation[38,52,53] (PRWE) and Patient-Rated Wrist/Hand Evaluation[51] (PRWHE)	To measure pain and disability in patients with wrist pathology	Items scores 0–10; 5 pain items; 6 specific function tasks; 4 items on usual ability in personal care, work, household work, and recreation	High test–retest[38,52]	Content based on expert survey/patient interviews construct and criterion validity evaluated;[38,52] has been validated in a variety of wrist and hand conditons[125-127]	More responsive than DASH or SF-36 for wrist fractures;[53] equally appropriate for wrist or hand pathology and formatted as PRWHE[51]
Carpal Tunnel Symptom [CTS] Severity Scale and Functional Scale[34]	To measure severity of symptoms in patients with CTS; to measure functional problems in patients with CTS	5-point Likert score questions in 2 subscales; symptom severity scale has 11 items; function subscale has 8 items	High in original format and a modified Swedish version[34,128]	Symptom severity scales differentiated between patients with CTS and without CTS;[129] a modified version added 2 items on palmar pain, 8 items on satisfaction, and 4 items on patients opinions on satisfaction with surgery; this scale was translated into Swedish and shown to be valid[128]	More responsive than generic measures or impairment scores;[130] responsive in Swedish version;[128] more responsive than the Michigan Hand Questionnaire in patients with CTS;[131] more responsive than other self-report sacles, a clinically important difference indicated by a change of one point[132]
Michigan Hand Questionnaire[133]	Health domains in patients with hand disorders	37 items: domains overall hand function, activities of daily living, pain, work performance, aesthetics, and patient satisfaction	Substantial test–retest reliability[133]	Factor analysis supported subscales; appropriate correlations between subscales and with SF-12; discriminant validity demonstrated[133]	Appropriate responsiveness;[134,135] responsive in patients with rheumatoid arthritis[136]
Patient-Specific scale[137]	To measure severity of problems in patients self-selected items	Patients select up to 5 items and rates these on a scale of 0–10	Acceptable; insufficient data for hand conditions	Has been validated for a number of different musculoskeletal conditions; has been associated with time to return to work in injured workers;[138] some concerns around the interpretability of patient specific measures[138,139]	Shown to be responsive when compared to the Michigan Hand Questionnaire and DASH for conditions like hand tumor, finger contracture, for CTS;[134] likely to be most responsive in individual patients because the items are ones which the person has difficulty with and are important

the patient has improved beyond the amount that might occur due to random fluctuation in patient status. Longer-term goals can be set using your clinical experience about reasonable targets for that patient population or surgical procedure, with assistance from published outcome studies that provide scores for different patient subgroups and stages of recovery. Using MDC helps us determine whether patients have changed in subsequent reassessments. Using published outcome data we can determine if patients have met acceptable targets.

Discrimination

Discrimination between groups is required when the purpose is to discern different subgroups within a population.[19] For example, the Katz hand diagram[22] discriminates between individuals having carpal tunnel syndrome (CTS) and those who do not. Others have developed a diagnostic scale to assess the probability of CTS.[23] Diagnostic tests are not outcome measures, but rather are designed to differentiate different groups (e.g., those having a pathology versus those who do not). In general, measures designed for diagnosis are not useful for evaluating change over time. For example, Phalen's test is useful for diagnosing CTS but not for assessing treatment effectiveness or outcome. Discrimination can also be performed for other purposes than diagnosis. It can be important to differentiate among clinical subgroups that do not require different treatment approaches or have a different prognosis. For example, with constructs like readiness or capability to return to work, safety during mobility, or return to home, determining if illiteracy is a factor can help in deciding how best to optimize treatment planning and patient outcomes. Increasingly, we are seeing a move toward differentiating patient subgroups that require different treatment approaches. Scales (or clinical prediction rules) devised for this purpose are an example of discriminative measures.

Prediction

Finally, outcome measures can be used to predict future outcomes. What will be the final strength 1 year after a fracture? Who will return to work? Who will require surgery for median nerve compression? These are prediction questions that might interest clinicians. When we predict outcomes, we use scores on rating scales at some preliminary stage to predict future scores or outcomes. For example, we demonstrated that patients presenting for conservative management of carpal tunnel that subsequently proceeded to have a surgical release had higher initial symptom severity scores[24] than those whose conditions were successfully managed conservatively (3.3 vs. 2.9). Similarly, high baseline scores after a distal radius fracture were indicative of patients less likely to return to work at 6 months.[25] In fact, baseline score is commonly a predictor of final status, suggesting that patients presenting with unusually poor scores are usually at higher risk of poor outcomes.

Outcome measures have specific measurement properties that determine how well they function in evaluating change, discriminating, or predicting. These measurement properties can be competing; therefore, an instrument designed for one

purpose may not be suited to others.[19] Generally, hand therapists are most interested in evaluative measures. Unfortunately, in some cases, clinicians use measures designed for discrimination as evaluative outcome measures without realizing they may not be appropriate for this purpose. For example, hand diagrams are useful for assessment, but not for evaluating treatment. Similarly, evaluative measures may not be predictive. For example, AROM may be used to evaluate a change in tendon glide over time, but does AROM predict the ability to return to work? We demonstrated that physical impairments were less predictive of time to return to work following distal radius fracture than were self-report measures.[25] Although there is some evidence in the clinical literature on the evaluative aspects of AROM as an outcome measure, we really do not have much evidence on its predictive or discriminative properties. It is clear that it is important to "pick the right tool for the job."

What Are the Important Measurement Properties of Outcome Measures?

The three measurement properties fundamental to how a tool can be used for clinical measurement are reliability, validity, and responsiveness (ability to detect clinical change over time).

Reliability

Reliability is the consistency or repeatability of a measurement. Reliability is fundamental to other measurement properties because without stability, the utility of any measure is compromised. However, high reliability, in itself, does not ensure that other measurement properties are also acceptable. Therefore, both the reliability and validity of outcome measures should be documented before clinicians use them to make decisions.

Measurements can be repeated by the same therapist (intrarater), by different therapists (inter-rater), or on different occasions (test–retest). Generally, intrarater reliability is higher than other forms of reliability analysis because the measurement error attributable to differences between testers and occasions is not considered. However, for evaluating patients over time, it is important to know that a measure remains constant over time if the patient remains stable (i.e., test–retest reliability). When we expect to share our measurements with others through clinical assessment notes, progress reports, or research studies, it is important to note that the status we report is consistent with what others would have determined (i.e., inter-rater reliability). Some clinicians mistakenly assume that impairment measures are more reliable than self-report measures because they consider the latter subjective. Certainly, patient perceptions of their status have some random fluctuation based on factors like recent functional demands and mood. However, in general, self-report measures have higher reliability coefficients than many impairment measures.[26,27]

Furthermore, a variety of factors affect measured impairments like grip strength. These include consistency of instructions and positioning, and interaction effects with the tester, time of day, fatigue, nutritional status, mood, and motivations. Hand therapists should be aware of methods to make their measurements more comparable to that described in the literature and consistent over time. Standardization, including elements like consistent technique, landmarking instructions, positioning, and instrument calibration, is used by hand therapists to reduce measurement error. It has been demonstrated that certain clinical measures such as ROM can be performed reliably by both novice and experienced therapists when a standardized method is used.[28] By using methods described in reliability studies, therapists can be more confident of comparing their results with those of others.

Reliability can be assessed using different statistics. Basic understanding of these statistics is important for clinicians because it helps them comprehend how to use published reliability studies to improve clinical expertise. The intraclass correlation coefficient (ICC)[29] is commonly used in the hand therapy literature to describe the relative reliability (the ratio between variability observed on repeated measurements within individuals compared with the variability between individuals). Reliability coefficients can be compared with benchmarks. Various benchmarks have been proposed. Fleiss suggested that less than 0.40 indicates poor reliability, that 0.40 to 0.75 is moderate, and that greater than 0.75 is excellent reliability.[30] The problem with this approach is that it suggests that reliability is a pass/fail criterion that measures should achieve. However, a better way for hand therapists to think about measurement error is that it exists for all measures and it is more important to understand the extent to which it affects a given assessment. Statistics like the standard error of measurement (SEM), or mean error, allow therapists to view measurement error in more quantitative terms.[31] For example, it has been shown that ROM measurements of elbow flexion and extension vary 3 to 5 degrees on average for the same tester and 5 to 8 degrees for different testers.[28] SEM is important because it can be used to calculate the MDC. Minimal detectable change is a useful target for short-term improvement as it represents the amount of change that is likely to indicate a real change in status. MDC has been established for many self-report measures. Exemplars of how to apply these principles to setting goals and evaluating change are available in the hand therapy literature.[31,32]

Validity

Validity is the extent to which the measure accurately portrays the aspect of health status that it was intended to describe. It can be thought of as the "trueness" of the measure.[33] Validity is difficult to ascertain because in many concepts of interest to hand therapists, such as pain or disability, there is no single or measurable true answer. A measure may be valid for one purpose, but not for other purposes. For example, a general health instrument may be a valid indication of overall health but may not be valid when assessing change in upper extremity function after certain hand injuries. Therefore, validity needs to be assessed by a variety of methods and in various situations. Validity is the cumulative evidence provided to support the use of outcome instruments in specific situations to perform specific analytic

functions. For this reason, various forms of validity are recognized.

Content validity is the extent to which a measure represents an adequate sampling of the concept being measured. This can be measured in the development of patient questionnaires by using focus groups or patient surveys to determine which items should contribute to the outcome scale. It can be determined through consensus reviews or expert panels that review existing items. For example, we expect a carpal tunnel instrument to include questions about classic symptoms of CTS, such as numbness, tingling, and waking at night. By looking at the items of the Symptom Severity Scale,[34] we make a judgment that it has content validity.

Construct validity is the extent to which scores obtained agree with the theoretical underpinnings of that scale. Testing constructs derived from the theoretical underpinnings of an instrument requires that relationships be investigated. Does the instrument relate to other instruments the way one would expect? Scales measuring similar constructs should be correlated (convergent validity); whereas dissimilar constructs should not demonstrate a significant relationship (divergent validity). Another type of construct that is tested is evaluating whether subgroups expected to be different based on the theoretical construct or existing evidence demonstrate this difference on the outcome measure being evaluated (known groups validity). For example, do people with more severe fractures score more poorly? Do patients in a nursing home have lower scores than patients living independently?

The process of demonstrating whether an instrument is valid and reliable is ongoing and requires multiple studies to ensure that measurement scales can be applied to different clinical populations and examination needs. Clinicians are often tempted to devise their own instruments or modify existing instruments to make something that is directly applicable to their own clinical situation. This is not advisable as the new instrument is not validated, nor comparable to other scores.

Responsiveness

The ability to detect change over time is critical to determining whether patients improve with treatment or deteriorate over time. *Responsiveness* is the measurement property that reflects this. Numerous studies in the hand therapy literature compare the responsiveness of different self-report and impairment measures. It is important for hand therapists to know about the relative responsiveness of different tools they might use in their practice. If an instrument is not able to pick up change, then insurers, patients, or members of the health-care team may not believe that the treatment efforts are effective. As a first step, therapists should consult the literature to find out about the relative responsiveness of different tools. As a general rule, the more specific the measure is to the problem or condition that is being treated, the more responsive the tool usually is. As an example, the Short-Form 36 (SF-36) is the common and important indicator of general health status. However, it is generally not very responsive in hand conditions. This might be expected when looking at the items since few of them relate to upper extremity function. However, therapists must also consider whether an instrument will be responsive in specific patients. A common example is patients with higher levels of functioning (younger, healthier patients) or higher demands (athletes, musicians, workers) who are unable to perform their normal roles but generally do not have difficulty with the lower-level items of many common functional scales. As a general rule, if a patient scores near the upper or lower range of a score, therapists should think about the potential for "ceiling" or "floor" effects. If the score is at a range where a MDC could not be achieved, then the tool is not appropriate for that patient. A different tool or a patient-specific tool might be indicated in these cases.

What Do I Need to Know Before Using Outcome Tools?

It is important to select an outcome measure that is reliable and valid for the purpose and clinical examination. A thorough search of the literature for a measure that meets your clinical examination needs is advisable since many recently developed impairment and disability measures are available. Then literature on the measurement properties of potentially useful instruments should be reviewed to determine which ones have acceptable measurement properties.

Once a measure with acceptable measurement properties has been identified, the clinician needs to investigate issues of practicality. Some patient questionnaires require permission from the authors or payment (or both) before being used. The time required to complete the test, language requirements, cost, data analysis requirements, and training requirements must be determined. Issues around whether a measure is feasible for your clinical setting are important considerations. Standards for the use of measures were described in 1991 by the American Physical Therapy Association's Task Force in their *Standards for Tests and Measurements in Physical Therapy*.[35] Other sources of information on standardization are the Advisory Group on Measurement Standards of the American Congress of Rehabilitation Medicine and a variety of publications that focus on outcome measures.[36] The general standards for use of measures discussed here are also addressed elsewhere.[33,35,36]

Users of measures should know the technical aspects of the instrument; that is, they should have documentation about the test's scoring, interpretation, reliability, and validity. For impairment-based measures, details on calibration and test positioning and procedures are key. Self-report measures have specific scoring metrics. Some instruments, such as the Disabilities of the Arm, Shoulder, and Hand (DASH)[37] or the Patient-Rated Wrist Evaluation (PRWE),[38] can be easily scored by the therapist at the time of examination. Others, such as the SF-36, have more complicated scoring algorithms.[39,40]

Measures should be used by the individuals who have the necessary training, experience, and professional qualifications. Certain types of examinations tend to fall in the domain of specific professionals. For example, certain psychometric examinations are performed only by licensed psychologists. Some aspects of hand examination require the expertise of a trained hand therapist. However, a number of outcomes can be evaluated by other professionals or even support staff. One purpose of reliability studies is to define what level of training and experience is required to administer a measure. Some assessments may not be technically demanding, and, thus, both inexperienced and experienced testers may achieve highly reliable results. For example, elbow flexion and extension and forearm rotation have been shown to be reliably measured when the tester is an experienced orthopedic surgeon, an experienced hand therapist, or an inexperienced physical therapist.[28] Some physical assessments may require greater technical skill. For example, passive movement characteristics of the shoulder have been measured reliably when the tester is an experienced manual therapist.[41] Knowledge of the technical skills required to perform specific measures may help determine appropriate delegation.

Therapists should make themselves aware of the training procedures required to properly administer a test and ensure that they adhere to the procedures. Sometimes the detail on how to perform the test or train personnel to perform the test is not provided or is incomplete. Dexterity tests such as the Jebson Hand Function Test are widely used to assess patient outcomes. However, the detail on how the test is performed is insufficient, resulting in variations in how different clinicians perform it. Therapists can find details about how to perform a test in a manual or in reliability studies. When the details of how to perform a test are absent or incomplete, it is the tester's responsibility to locate detailed instructions and to use these in clinical practice.

Having normative data or comparative data is required to interpret outcome scores objectively. For example, when commenting on a patient's strength, it is advisable to compare the patient's injured hand with the best estimate of that particular patient's normal strength (i.e., his or her uninjured side) and to also compare that patient's strength against scores considered normal values for patients of a similar size, age, and sex. Conclusions about the extent of strength recovered during rehabilitation or the ability to perform strength-based tasks can be made using these comparative data. For health status questionnaires like the SF-36, normative data and data for pathologic conditions are available for comparison.[40] Normative data for upper extremity self-report measures is less common, but comparative data for clinical populations is readily available from clinical research.

Therapists should know the proper environmental conditions and equipment requirements for completing the outcome evaluation. For example, examination of sensory thresholds requires specific equipment and environmental conditions. The patient must be positioned properly, and the surroundings must be quiet if an accurate measurement is to be achieved. Instruments must be sensitive to small increments in pressure and they must be calibrated to ensure that they remain consistent over time. Environment can also affect self-report measures. Patients may feel uneasy about expressing dissatisfaction to their doctor or therapist, but they can be more frank when an independent assessor administers the questions. Telephone administration or the use of interpreters may be necessary to obtain self-report information, but might influence how people respond. The optimal approach to administering self-report measures is to have them administered by an independent person, such as the clinic receptionist providing the forms.

How Do I Find Outcome Measures That Are Suitable for Me?

The first step in identifying an appropriate instrument is to decide which concepts are important to measure based on the problem being treated and the expected effects of the intervention. As previously stated, the ICF framework is increasingly being used as a conceptual framework. Outcome measures can be found by searching the literature or textbooks for information addressing their psychometric properties. For impairment measures, search (using Boolean operators) for the type of measure (e.g., grip, strength, motion) AND (reliability OR validity) in PubMed or the Cumulative Index to Nursing and Allied Health Literature (CINAHL). You should retrieve numerous articles addressing clinical measurements. For self-report measures, there is no standard term, so using synonyms for a self-report outcome measure like "self-report" OR "questionnaire" OR "outcome measure" can be a good search strategy, combined with the psychometric terms (reliability OR validity) to identify appropriate clinical studies. Sometimes you will be fortunate to find a systematic review of an outcome measure like ones published for the neck disability index,[42] shoulder outcome measures,[43,44] hand measures,[45] or measures specific to hand osteoarthritis.[46] Often, the actual forms required must be obtained from the developers as they may not appear in studies. Another source for locating outcome instruments are Web sites specific to the measures. Searching *"outcome measure database"* in a search engine takes you to a number of databases that contain information about different outcome measures. Many of these are by professional groups affiliated with rehabilitation. Searching using the name of the scale you wish to find and PDF (or using an advanced search to limit your retrieval to PDF files) can help you locate downloadable forms available on the Internet.

Data extraction forms, critical appraisal forms, and guides are available to assist in critically appraising the outcomes scales themselves.[32,47,48] However, in most circumstances, hand therapists are interested in using a measure that has acceptable psychometric properties, is clinically feasible, and is used by others in the profession.

Two commonly used self-report measures are the DASH and the PRWE. The DASH is a 30-item scale that focuses on disability of the upper extremity, but also contains items on symptoms.[49-51] The items are summated using a simple equation. The PRWE has 15 items; 5 addressing pain and 10 addressing disability (6 standardized specific activities and 4 inquiring about the patient's usual preinjury activity). Both have high reliability and have been validated for a variety of hand and wrist conditions, have been translated into multiple languages, and are used by a variety of hand therapy practices.[31,38,52] The DASH has the advantage of being useful for conditions of the upper extremity and being widely recognized. It is slightly less responsive than the PRWE for hand and wrist conditions, but substantially more responsive than generic measures.[53-55] Recently, the QuickDASH[56] was introduced. It contains 11 items from the original DASH, and in early studies has shown equivalent psychometric properties.[57-62] Any of these measures are appropriate for routine use in a hand therapy clinic as a supplement to relevant impairment measures. However, in some patients, traditional standardized self-report forms may not be adequate. Examples include patients with high demands (e.g., workers or athletes), unique skills (e.g., musicians), unique conditions (e.g., congenital problems, instability), or a mild spectrum of disease in an otherwise healthy patient. In these cases, scales specifically designed for the higher-level functioning may be an alternative. However, in many cases these are not available. Another alternative can be patient-specific scales. This option allows patients to select items that are of importance to them and for which they are currently experiencing difficulty. Therefore, the level of difficulty is determined by the patient. A brief form of this is the Patient-Specific Functional Scale,[63,64] in which three to five items are selected by the patient and rated on subsequent examinations. A more detailed clinician-administered instrument is the Canadian Occupational Performance Measure,[65-68] which identifies occupational performance issues in different domains and rates them according to performance and satisfaction. Both measures are suitable for hand therapy practice, although the latter is more time-consuming to use. Patient-specific scales can be very useful in clinical practice since they are by nature client-centered and tend to be most responsive in picking up clinical change. One drawback is that scores cannot be compared across patients because the items are different. But since most therapists are interested in change over time, this does not affect their usefulness in treating individual patients.

When a clinical condition has unique features and is common, a condition-specific tool may be developed. The most commonly used example in hand therapy is the Symptom Severity Scale.[34] This tool goes by several names, but addresses symptoms specific to CTS, such as waking at night, numbness, and tingling. It has been shown to be more responsive than functional scales and generic scales in detecting recovery following treatment for CTS.[69]

A number of scales combine measures of impairments, such as ROM and strength, with measures of functional ability, which is usually evaluated by the clinician. Examples of such scales are the Mayo Elbow Performance Index (MEPI)[70] and the Constant–Murley score.[71] Scores from these scales are often rated as *excellent, good, fair,* or *poor* so that the number of patients falling into each category can be reported in case series or outcome studies. Clinicians should be aware that these scales have limitations. The subjective categories are not meaningful because they have not been validated, are not consistent between scales, and are not reliable.[72] These scales tend to be developed by clinicians based on their personal opinion of items to include and weighting of subcomponents and, hence, have not been developed through the optimal clinimetric process. Of greater concern is that the reliability and validity of these scales tends to be poorly addressed. The most studied of this type of scales is the Constant-Murley scale developed for the shoulder. A recent systematic review of this measure highlighted some strengths and limitations of this scale.[73] Given that impairment and disability are separate constructs, it is advisable for therapists to track and interpret these separately in clinical practice. Where these clinician-based scales are used, the actual score—not subjective ratings like" good" and "fair"—should be reported.

How Do I Administer the Outcome Measure to Measure Change in My Patients?

When using outcome tools to assess change in individual patients, a number of practical details must be considered. Who will administer the questionnaire? Some therapists like to introduce the questionnaire themselves to their patients as a way to facilitate their subjective evaluation of them. Other therapists prefer the questionnaire to be administered by an independent person to minimize the opportunity for bias. Therapists need to work collaboratively with others in their clinic to determine which process is optimal for their clinic.

The way in which the questionnaire is administered may depend on the patient's capacity. The effect of illiteracy is grossly underestimated. When patients ask a spouse or family member to fill out forms, refuse to cooperate, or ask to take questionnaires home, illiteracy may be the underlying reason. Others may try to mask their illiteracy by completing the forms, but their answers will be nonsensical. By offering to read questions to patients in a circumspect way, or allowing them to complete it with a spouse, you can provide these patients the opportunity to convey their opinions on their status without compromising their dignity.

It is important to plan how often outcome instruments will be administered. A baseline and final status evaluation are the minimum requirements for determining the effect of treatment. However, when instruments are used throughout a treatment program, they can help assess the course of recovery. In this case, they must be applied at intervals over which an MDC is expected to occur. Some developers recommend 2 weeks, but clearly this depends on the rate of change of the problem. Instruments are not usually completed twice within the same week because patients may be relatively stable within this time frame.

Some clinical examinations are performed for research or program evaluation and require a postdischarge or long-term evaluation. This should be performed when surgical and rehabilitation efforts have been maximized. Long-term follow-up can also be performed to gauge deterioration in patients with chronic disease or to gauge the effects of late complications (e.g., joint arthoplasty failure). In these cases, it may be necessary to use multiple types or occasions of contact to get adequate responses. A combination of mail, phone, or Internet surveys of status can be useful for determining longer-term status with adequate response rates so that the information is considered valid.

How Do I Analyze Outcome Scores?

Treatment effects are assessed by evaluating the change in score from baseline to post-treatment. The MDC is the amount of change that exceeds measurement error. The clinically important difference (CID) is the amount of change that has been shown to make a difference to patients. These two concepts are determined differently, but a discussion of those methods is beyond the scope of this chapter. It is important to be aware of these two indicators because they help with interpretation of outcome measure scores. MDC and CID can sometimes be found in clinical measurement studies. Individual scores can be interpreted using these two concepts in combination with their clinical skills about expected outcomes and data from normal patients. MDC is a useful benchmark for short-term goals since it is the amount of change that provides us confidence that the person's ability has actually changed. Longer-term goals should exceed CID since we know that this amount of improvement should indicate a true benefit to the patient.

When introducing a new impairment or disability measure into your clinical practice, you must ensure that it is used as designed by the developers. Sometimes, because of the space limitations in scientific journals, the methodology description for tests has been abbreviated and the detail is insufficient to allow replication. In these cases, the user is obligated to contact the authors of the new methodology to provide more thorough instructions.

How Do I Incorporate Predictors of Outcome?

When measuring outcome and describing it to others, it is important to know and document important predictors of outcome. Unfortunately, we are at a preliminary stage in our understanding of how impairment translates into disability. Understanding this relationship is important in providing an accurate prognosis for patients, determining who is likely to benefit from treatment, and designing treatment programs that focus on the critical components of the disability and handicap. Certain factors, such as age, job demands, and comorbidity, may affect outcome in a predictable fashion; others, like gender, may have variable effects depending on the pathology or construct.

Severity of injury is an important consideration in evaluating outcome. Therapists need to understand how severity of injury affects prognosis and treatment response. For example, it has been suggested that conservative management is most effective for mild CTS. Our outcome data on distal radius fractures suggest that patients with more severe fractures (i.e., those with more radial shortening) experience more pain and disability in their long-term outcome.[74-77] On the other hand, patients with severe limitation at a baseline assessment have the most "room for improvement" and may experience the greatest change in raw scores.

Patient characteristics can also be powerful predictors of outcome. Further research is required to fully understand which patient characteristics affect outcome in upper extremity conditions. When patient characteristics and injury characteristics present at baseline examination of distal radius fractures are assessed, the most important predictor of the extent of pain and disability at 6 months after fractures was the presence of injury compensation (legal or worker's compensation).[75,77-79] Level of education was also shown to be predictive of outcome. It is important to recognize that these are associations and not necessarily causes. Injury compensation may be related to the level of difficulty of the job or to motivation. Educational level may relate to a number of factors, such as ability to modify job demands, ability to acquire less demanding employment, ability to understand home programs, and compliance.

How Do I Set Up a Process to Measure Outcomes in My Practice?

In studying the implementation of outcome measures into practice, key elements have been determined.[31,32,80] These include spending some initial time evaluating why the measures might be useful and how they might be used. Therapists need to determine how "high-tech" or "low-tech" their clinics' process will be, based on practical issues such as computer accessibility or funding. Hand therapists still predominantly use paper and pencil self-report measures in practice, although a customized computerized database system designed for hand therapists will soon be available. Regardless of the system, practical issues about who, when, and how the measures will be administered must be resolved—when several people work together in the clinic, this needs to be a group process. Some time reviewing research studies to identify different types of instruments is needed. At this point clinicians may benefit from attending workshops about outcome measures. Some time needs to be allocated to finding outcome measures and identifying their correct scoring and standardized administration. It is important to establish a realistic and incremental process for building outcome measure administration into routine practice. Making forms easily accessible and staff responsibilities clear and agreed upon is essential. Frequently, a trial of two different outcome measures can be useful to help therapists evaluate which works better for their practice. Once familiar with the basics of how to administer outcome scales, therapists should deepen their knowledge about how to interpret scores, use them to set goals, and write more definitive medical records.

Summary

Hand therapists assess their patients to determine how pathology of the upper limb has affected impairment, activity, and participation. They formulate treatment plans to mitigate related problems and assess the treatment's effectiveness by using standardized outcome evaluations. The foundations of hand therapy rest on standardized outcome measures used to improve the ability to diagnose impairment, assess change in patient status, predict future outcomes, conduct clinical research, and institute continuous quality improvement.

REFERENCES

The complete reference list is available online at www.expertconsult.com.

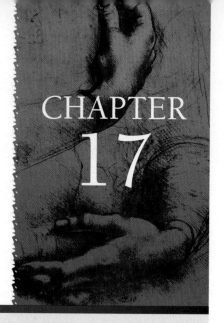

Impairment Evaluation

DAVID S. ZELOUF, MD AND LAWRENCE H. SCHNEIDER, MD

EXTENT OF THE PROBLEM	LIMITATIONS OF THE GUIDES
HISTORY OF IMPAIRMENT EVALUATION	SUMMARY
IMPAIRMENT EVALUATION	

CRITICAL POINTS

- The definition of what constitutes impairment is an evolving process, with the most recent attempt (*AMA Guides to the Evaluation of Permanent Impairment*, 6th edition, 2008) representing a paradigm shift compared with prior attempts.
- An impairment evaluation is performed once the patient has reached maximum medical benefit.
- *Impairment* should not be used synonymously with *disability*.
- The impairment rating requires a comprehensive medical evaluation, which includes a history and physical examination using objective measures.
- The 6th edition *Guides* now follow the International Classification of Functioning, Disability and Health (ICF) as developed by the World Health Organization (WHO).
- Diagnoses for the upper extremity are now defined in three major categories: *soft tissue, muscle–tendon, and ligament–bone–joint*. There are now five defined impairment classes, ranging from class 0 (no objective findings and thus no impairment), to class 4 ("very severe" problem with an upper extremity impairment range from 50%–100%).
- The 6th edition does account for inconsistencies during the physical examination, and using the Diagnosis-Based Impairment rating technique, less weight is given to the physical examination and functional status in the setting of significant inconsistencies.

Extent of the Problem

In the United States, disorders of the upper extremities are widespread and cause associated disability and considerable economic consequences.[1] Injuries and arthritic conditions are the most common disorders of the upper extremity, and musculoskeletal problems involving the upper and lower extremity and the spine are the most common cause of work-related disability.[2] As documented by Kelsey and colleagues,[3] approximately 18 million acute upper extremity injuries occur per year, and at any given time, approximately 31 million people have arthritis, many with upper extremity involvement. Twenty-four million visits are made to physicians' offices each year for upper extremity problems, at a cost of almost $19 billion in 1995. In 2004 the sum of the direct expenditures in health care costs for bone and joint health and the indirect expenditures in lost wages has been estimated to be $849 billion dollars, or 7.7% of the national gross domestic product. In a survey from the National Center for Health Statistics published in 2005, it was reported that chronic joint pain (defined as joint pain lasting longer than 3 months) was reported by 58.9 million adults aged 18 or older (26.4 of 100). These statistics illustrate the current significance of these problems.

Currently, musculoskeletal disorders and diseases are the leading cause of disability in the United States and result in the greatest number of total lost work days in the United States relative to other major medical conditions. For more information, the reader is directed to Jacobs and coworkers' informative text, *The Burden of Musculoskeletal Diseases in the United States*.[4] This text is an update of two prior works entitled *Musculoskeletal Conditions in the United States* published in 1992 and 1999 by the American Academy of Orthopedic Surgeons and is a joint project of the AAOS, American Academy of Physical Medicine and Rehabilitation, American College of Rheumatology, American Society for Bone and Mineral Research, Arthritis Foundation, National University of Health Sciences, Orthopedic Research Society, Scoliosis Research Society, and the United States Bone and Joint Decade. This text is available free of charge online at <*www.boneandjointburden.org/*>.

History of Impairment Evaluation

The need for impairment and disability evaluation became apparent with the development of entitlement programs and workers' compensation awards (private or public programs for the disabled).[5] Evidence indicates that some of these systems existed in ancient times, and in the Middle Ages, merchant and craft guilds organized to protect their members.[5,6]

Many guidelines developed in Europe in the 19th century[7] showed great variability in assigning value to the same impairment because of a lack of established standards. Rating was a conglomerate of many factors, and the physician was in a weak position to defend his opinion because of a lack of definitive criteria. In 1927, Kessler[7] proposed that medical decisions be based on measurable factors. McBride[8,9] then developed a complex system of medical measurements in disability evaluation. The first rating system for the American orthopedic surgeon, authored by McBride,[9] was published in 1936 and focused on workers' compensation laws. It was an attempt to standardize ratings on a more scientific basis. Unfortunately, problems remained because of the degree of subjectivity involved. Slocum and Pratt[10] offered a schedule based on function, which when reviewed today appears rudimentary. In response to the problem of impairment evaluation, the American Medical Association (AMA) appointed a Committee on Medical Rating of Physical Impairment in September of 1956 that was authorized to establish guidelines for a rating system. Kessler and McBride served as consultants on this committee. The first of these Guides was published as a special edition of the *Journal of the American Medical Association* on February 15, 1958;[11] its three sections covered the upper and lower extremities and the back. The upper extremity section, "a unit of the whole man" was divided into four categories: hand, wrist, elbow, and shoulder. The hand was further subdivided into the five digits and the digits into their respective joints.[11] Impairments were then rated based on loss of motion or ankylosis at the joints or secondary to amputation of a part as assigned by the committee and given on a provided chart. A functional value was derived for the deficit and then applied from the digit to the hand and the hand to the upper extremity and from there onto the whole person.

An attempt to give guidelines for standardization of evaluations done by the orthopedic surgeons also was developed and published in 1962 by the AAOS Committee on Disability Evaluation chaired by McBride.[12] This 30-page pamphlet was intended to standardize orthopedic evaluations. Despite the use of the term *disability* in the committee's name, this paper makes it clear that a disability rating is an administrative and not a medical responsibility. This effort was soon superseded by the *AMA Guides*.

In 1970, Kessler[7] pushed for more objectively obtained measurements. In his volume, published in 1970, he also stressed loss of function over anatomic loss. He refers to the fact that there were varying opinions on the AMA Committee to which he and Dr. McBride consulted.

Subsequent to the first attempt in 1958, the AMA Committee's scope was broadened, and from 1958 to 1970 it published 13 separate "Guides to the Evaluation of Permanent Impairment" in the *Journal of the American Medical Association*. A second edition of these guides was published as separate chapters in a single volume in 1971 entitled "Guides to the Evaluation of Permanent Impairment." These *AMA Guides*, now in a 6th edition (2008, with updates), are an "attempt to estimate the severity of human impairments based on accepted medical standards."[11] The concept here is that a loss of function could be translated to a percentage loss of the whole person. Although the *Guides* are needed, the complexity of issues in impairment evaluation makes them imperfect.[13] This is recognized by most experts, including the framers, who are cautious in their choice of language, stating, "this is an attempt to standardize these evaluation proceedings."[11] Frequent updates in response to inconsistencies will gradually further improve their utility. The section of the *Guides* devoted to the upper extremity was updated and developed by Alfred Swanson and coworkers,[14,15] and we are indebted for their work in this difficult area.[16] They also have provided the section on impairment evaluation in prior editions of this text. This chapter does not attempt to serve as a substitute for the *AMA Guides*, but rather as a help to the reader in the application of the *Guides*, pointing out the pitfalls and adding some opinions on their use.

The Impairment Evaluation

When is an impairment evaluation indicated? Impairment evaluation is not undertaken early, but rather is done after the patient's condition has stabilized for some time and thus has reached what is known as maximum medical improvement. Impairment, to be evaluated, must be permanent; that is, the patient's condition should be stabilized and unlikely to change either with time or further treatment.[17,18] When performing a rating examination, the rating physician should understand the use of the terms *impairment* and *disability*.

Impairment Versus Disability

Impairment is a deviation from normal in a body part and its functioning. It marks the degree to which an individual's capacity to carry out daily activities has been diminished. Impairment can be determined and thus is a medical decision made with the use of the *Guides* after a thorough review of the medical history and a medical examination conducted in combination with appropriate laboratory tests and diagnostic procedures. Physical impairment involves an anatomic or physiologic loss that interferes with the subject's ability to perform a certain function. After evaluation an impairment rating can be assigned. This impairment rating can the used to determine *disability*, which is a decrease in, or the loss of, an individual's capacity to meet personal, social, or occupational demands, or activities that the individual cannot accomplish because of the impairment. Many people exhibit an impairment but with adaptation do not have a disability. An example would be an elevator operator or 'a surgeon[19] who loses an index finger; although each has a 20% impairment of the hand, he or she has no disability.

It was originally intended that the medically determined impairment rating would be taken to a legal entity, such as a workers' compensation board or some other administrative body, that would then award the disability rating, but today it appears that these organizations more frequently rely on examining physicians to make the disability determination. This is in spite of the *Guides* telling us that impairment percentages derived according to *Guides* criteria should not be used to make direct estimates of disabilities. These impairment examinations are most often performed by physicians who specialize in occupational medicine or disability rating and specialists who, in some states, take a course and are then certified to perform such evaluations. Again, an impaired person is not necessarily disabled, and all impairments do not result in the same degree of disability in all cases. The impairment rating is a medical determination and directly related to the medical status of the individual, whereas disability can be determined only within the context of the personal, social, or occupational demands that the individual is unable to meet as a result of the impairment.[5] Ideally, impairment evaluation should provide only one element of the disability rating.

The Medical Evaluation

The medical evaluation is based on the clinical findings from a physical examination after a detailed history has been obtained. The examiner must recognize that the patient is heavily invested in the result of the examination, which consequently is often adversarial in nature. Despite this, the examiner should always present a neutral demeanor. The complaints and findings should be reasonably relatable to the nature of the injury or condition. The examiner should be cognizant of the difficulties inherent in this evaluation and search for objective findings that will correlate with the subjective symptoms. Psychological overlay, symptom magnification, and possible malingering should be noted and attention called to them in the final report with terms that point out such inconsistencies. These issues should not be confronted at the time of the examination, with the examiner maintaining an impartial attitude. On subjective testing, the experienced and sophisticated patient can present findings that may invalidate the meaning of a particular test.

Medical History

The examination should be preceded by a review of the available records, which the examiner should *insist* be made available. A detailed history of the present illness is then taken along with the current complaints and the examinee's reported functional difficulties. In trauma, it is useful to understand the details of the initial injury. This information may help the examiner judge whether the incident is likely to have led to the current complaints. The history of

treatment is developed along with the patient's perceived response to that treatment.

The patient's health history may be significant because certain medical conditions predispose to or explain certain conditions or symptoms. Prior trauma should be elucidated along with its possible relation to present symptoms. Knowledge of current medications and treatment bring out any concurrent problems. The use of inappropriate medications should be known. For example, the use of narcotics to treat a less than major problem greatly influences that patient's response and reporting of pain symptoms. In our experience, many of these patients who are on inappropriate narcotics for long periods would ideally benefit from withdrawal of their medication as part of their treatment and before their evaluation. A patient's social history may indicate a healthy or unhealthy lifestyle and reveal issues that may be adding undue stress to his or her life. A work history often reveals much about the patient. A job that requires heavy manual effort may explain symptoms. Other jobs, in which the worker perceives mental stress, can explain symptoms, the origin of which is otherwise obscure. Diffuse, poorly localized symptoms, vague chronic pain, intolerance of treatment, worsening with every treatment modality, excessive drug use, and poor compliance in treatment should all be noted.

Physical Examination

The physical examination should include the usual elements of a complete physical. Required instruments include a goniometer, a tape measure, and devices that allow measurement of sensation, including Semmes–Weinstein monofilaments and two-point discrimination. It is also helpful to have on hand a Jamar dynamometer and a pinch gauge. A current copy of the *Guides* is necessary to complete the report generated by the evaluation procedures, and software, in the form of a *Guides* impairment calculator, is available for purchase from the AMA. We have found this software useful; it can definitely aid in the calculation process.

The appearance of the upper extremity is noted, including obvious deformities, amputations, scars, masses, atrophy of muscles or finger pulps, trophic changes, skin discoloration, or sweat pattern abnormalities. The extremity, especially the hand, is palpated to determine temperature and sweat pattern. Range of motion (ROM) is measured at all joints in the involved area. Limb circumference is measured at specified locations above and below the elbow and compared with measurements of the contralateral limb. A sensory evaluation is carried out using monofilaments and a device that measures static two-point discrimination. All data are recorded on the multitude of forms and outlines available for this purpose. Appropriate imaging studies and neurodiagnostic testing should be reviewed. All of this is collated in a comprehensive report.

It is good discipline to conclude the physical examination with a usable diagnosis that is consistent with the current ICD-9 code. This diagnosis should be responsive to the findings and considered very carefully because it can, to a great degree, become a label that, if inaccurate, is difficult to eradicate. At times a clear-cut diagnosis cannot be made. The use of the nonjudgmental diagnostic code 729.5 for "pain— upper extremity" is an excellent tool when the diagnosis is not confirmable. It is useful for a patient without recognizable objective justification for his or her pain and is superior to assigning arbitrary terms such as "fibromyalgia syndrome, cumulative trauma disorder, or chronic pain syndrome."[20,21] Much confusion is created when patients, reporting wrist pain, are labeled as having "tendonitis" or "tenosynovitis" when, in fact, these easily confirmable inflammatory conditions are not truly present.[22] The use of the 729.5 code then serves to point out the lack of an objective or rational explanation for the symptoms and avoids a confirmatory label that confuses the issues. In such cases, the examiner should give the reasons for the offered opinion in the discussion section of the report. After the examination, the history and measurements and the subsequent diagnosis are then used with the *Guides* to estimate the impairment, which should be backed by the rationale that went into the rating assignment.

Using the Guides for Evaluation of Upper Extremity Impairment[23]

Chapters 1 and 2 of the *Guides* deal with general information, definitions, and how to apply the information derived through the *Guides*. The upper extremity is covered in the section on the musculoskeletal system, Chapter 15. Substantial changes have been made between the 5th and 6th editions, and it is highly recommended that the reader review all three chapters prior to performing an impairment rating evaluation that will be based on this newest edition to the *Guides*. The *Guides* now follow the ICF as developed by the World Health Organization (WHO).[24] The ICF framework is intended for describing as well as measuring health and disability both at the level of the individual and for population levels. Its three components include alteration in body function and body structure, activity limitation, and participation restrictions. The changes made in the 6th edition represent an ongoing evolution and introduces a paradigm shift to the assessment of impairment. Essentially, the *Guides* have become more *diagnosis and functionally based* and stress conceptual and methodologic congruity within and between organ system ratings. The reader is strongly encouraged to study the 6th edition, including the introductory chapters as well as the chapter on the upper extremities. A brief overview of the changes follows, but these changes are difficult to fully grasp without a careful study of the new *Guides*, including the provided examples found in Chapter 15.

Diagnoses for the upper extremity are now defined in three major categories; *soft tissue, muscle–tendon, and ligament–bone–joint,* and there are now five defined impairment classes, ranging from class 0 (no objective findings and thus no impairment), to class 4 (very severe problem with an upper extremity impairment range from 50%–100%) (Table 17-1). Most impairment values for the upper limb are now calculated using the diagnosis-based impairment (DBI) method. The impairment class is determined by the diagnosis once maximum medical improvement has been reached. The class can be modified based on non-key factors, such as functional history, physical findings, and clinical studies. Regional grids are now utilized once the diagnosis has been established, which allow the appropriate impairment rating to be determined for any allowable diagnosis, impairment class, and grade. To evaluate functional history, the 6th edition specifies that physicians should include a self-reported orthopedic functional assessment tool as part of the impair-

Table 17-1 Definition of Impairment Classes

| Class | Problem | Impairment Range | |
		Upper Extremity (UEI) (%)	Whole Person (WPI) (%)
0	No objective findings	0	0
1	Mild	1–13	1–8
2	Moderate	14–25	8–15
3	Severe	26–49	16–29
4	Very severe	50–100	30–60

Reprinted, with permission, from *The Guides to the Evaluation of Permanent Impairment,* 6th ed. Chicago: American Medical Association, 2008.

ment rating examination and recommends the use of the shorter version of the Disabilities of the Arm, Shoulder, and Hand (DASH) Questionnaire, the QuickDASH, for upper limb impairment.[25] The DASH Questionnaire was developed through a cooperative effort of the AAOS, ASSH, AAHS, and the Canadian province of Ontario Institute for Work and Health.[26]

Both the DASH and the QuickDASH, which is a subset of DASH questions and which has similar validity, are available at <http://www.dash.iwh.on.ca/outcome_quick.htm>. There is no charge for their use. The result of the QuickDASH should be compared with an activities of daily living questionnaire to evaluate for consistency. Depending on the result, it may or may not be used to modify the default impairment rating. Though it initially seems that the changes are cumbersome, after one reviews the introductory chapters along with the upper extremity chapter, the logic of the changes becomes apparent.

Peripheral nerve impairment is now similarly rated by class based on the nerve involved, along with the level of involvement. Variability within a class depends on the severity of the deficit. Entrapment–compression neuropathy is also rated differently and includes modifiers based on nerve conduction study data, history, physical findings, and functional scale (Table 17-2). Impairment due to amputation has also been modified in the 6th edition, and though largely based on the level of the amputation, the grade can be modified up or down from the default "C" based on other "adjustment factors" (Table 17-3).

The material in the *Guides* on the upper extremity is covered as follows:

1. Diagnosis-Based Impairment, 15.2
2. Peripheral Nerve Impairment, 15.4
3. Complex Regional Pain Syndrome Impairment, 15.5
4. Amputation Impairment, 15.6
5. Range-of-Motion Impairment, 15.7

Although nerve problems and vascular deficits in the upper extremity are covered in Chapter 15, one may need to refer to Chapter 13 on the nervous system and Chapter 4 on the cardiovascular system. Chapter 14, which covers mental and behavioral disorders, and Chapter 3, on pain, also may need to be referenced. When pain is a factor, the percentage of impairment designated in the various sections makes allowance for the pain that may accompany the primary impairing condition.

Each section of the *Guides* includes a discussion of measurement techniques; tables of relative impairment due to

Table 17-2 Entrapment–Compression Neuropathy Impairment

Clinical	Grade Modifier 0	Grade Modifier 1	Grade Modifier 2	Grade Modifier 3	Grade Modifier 4
Test findings	Normal	Conduction delay (sensory and/or motor)	Motor conduction block	Axon loss	Almost dead nerve
History	Mild intermittent symptoms	Mild intermittent symptoms	Significant intermittent symptoms	Constant symptoms	NA
Physical findings	Normal	Normal	Decreased sensation	Atrophy or weakness	NA
Functional scale	Normal (0–20) 0 Mild (21–40) 1 Moderate (41–60) 2	Normal (0–20) 0 Mild (21–40) 1 Moderate (41–60) 2	Mild (21–40) 1 Moderate (41–60) 2 Severe (61–80) 3	Mild (21–40) 1 Moderate (41–60) 2 Severe (61–80) 3	NA
UE impairment	0	1 2 3	4 5 6	7 8 9	NA

NA, not applicable; UE, upper extremity.

Table 17-3 Amputation Impairment

Diagnostic Criteria (key factor)	Class 0	Class 1					Class 2					Class 3					Class 4				
Impairment Ranges (UE %)	% UE	1%–13% UE					14%–25% UE					26%–49% UE					50%–100% UE				
Grade		A	B	C	D	E	A	B	C	D	E	A	B	C	D	E	A	B	C	D	E
Thumb, at:							18	18	18	20	22	36	36	36	38	40					
IP joint																					
MCP joint												37	37	37	39	41					
Half metacarpal												38	38	38	40	42					
Metacarpal at CMC																					
Index or middle finger, at:		8	8	8	9	10	14	14	14	16	18										
DIP joint																					
PIP joint							18	18	18	20	22										
MCP joint							19	19	19	21	23										
Half metacarpal							20	20	20	22	24										
Metacarpal at CMC																					
Ring or little finger, at:		5	5	5	6	7															
DIP joint		7	7	7	8	9															
PIP joint		9	9	9	10	11															
MCP joint		11	11	11	12	13															
Half metacarpal		12	12	12	13	13															
Metacarpal at CMC																					
Hand, at:																	54	54	54	58	58
All fingers at MP joints except thumb																	90	90	90	92	94
All digits at MP joints																	92	92	92	94	96
Distal to biceps insertion to transmetacarpophalangeal loss of all digits																					
Arm, at:																	92	92	92	94	96
Distal to deltoid insertion to bicipital insertion																	100	100	100	100	100
Deltoid insertion and proximally																					
Shoulder, at:																	100	100	100	100	100
Shoulder disarticulation																					

CMC, carpometacarpal; DIP, distal interphalangeal; IP, interphalangeal; MCP, metacarpophalangeal; PIP, proximal interphalangeal; UE, upper extremity.

restriction of motion, ankylosis, and amputations; and methods for combining and relating various impairments.[11]

Limitations of the Guides

In this section, we discuss the relevant sections of the *Guides* and offer our advice and comments on the strengths and weaknesses of each. There are, however, some obvious overall limitations that should be noted first. These include the following:

1. Age-related changes are difficult to separate from those related to an injury, but an attempt should be made to do so.
2. Some measurements lack reliability and validity.
3. Many of the clinical tests are subjective.
4. Psychosocial factors can greatly affect the patient's presentation. Psychogenic overlay, symptom magnification, and malingering may make it difficult to obtain an accurate estimate of impairment.
5. It is not possible to rate pain in a meaningful manner, especially with conditions such as complex regional pain syndrome, arthritis, wrist conditions, and incomplete nerve recovery, which may be unresolved.

These limitations are not the fault of the *Guides*, but they may never be totally resolvable. This was recognized by Swanson and colleagues,[15] who clearly warned us that there would be patients whose "complaints are not justified by objective findings or whose responses to testing are not felt to be justified by the diagnosis or the nature of the condition or whose response to testing varies widely from time to time." They went on to say that such patients should put the examiner on guard.

Unfortunately, many of the standardized and provocative tests done on a physical examination are by their nature subjective, that is, under the control of the patient. This includes such time-honored tests as Tinel's sign or Phalen's test for carpal tunnel syndrome. This applies particularly for most of the clinical tests for patients who present with upper extremity pain often attributed to thoracic outlet syndrome or brachial plexopathy. Many patients have had multiple examinations and become sophisticated enough to learn to supply the expected answers. The evaluation in those cases can test the ingenuity of the examiner. The 6th edition does account for inconsistencies during the physical examination, and using the DBI rating technique, less weight is given to the physical examination and functional status in the setting of significant inconsistencies. This is discussed in detail in section 15.3.

Conditions and Commentary Regarding Appropriate Use of Guides in Determining Impairment Rating

The following is a commentary concerning relevant sections of the *Guides*, including a discussion of strengths and weaknesses.

Amputation

Standard percentage values have been assigned to the various amputation levels in the upper extremity. When these percentages are learned, it is a relatively simple matter to assign

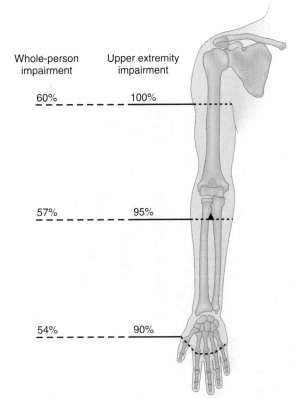

Figure 17-1 Impairment estimates for upper extremity amputation at various levels. (Redrawn from Swanson AB. Evaluation of impairment of function in the hand. *Surg Clin North Am.* 1964;44:925-940.)

impairment to the extremity resulting from amputation. Impairment of the entire upper extremity is equivalent to 60% of the whole person; therefore total amputation, or 100% loss of the limb, is evaluated as a 60% impairment of the whole person. Amputation of the upper extremity from the level of the biceps insertion to the level proximal to the metacarpophalangeal (MCP) joints is equivalent to a 95% loss of the upper extremity or 57% of the whole person (Fig. 17-1). Amputation at the MCP joints is rated as a 90% loss of the upper extremity. In regard to the hand, individual digits have been assigned values in relation to the whole hand: The thumb is evaluated as 40%, index and long fingers 20% each, and ring and little fingers 10% each (Fig. 17-2).

In turn, each portion of an amputated digit is given a value in relation to the entire digit. Amputation of the digit at the MCP joint is equal to a 100% loss of that digit; amputation at the proximal interphalangeal (PIP) level is 80% loss of the digit, and distal interphalangeal (DIP) amputation is equal to a 45% loss of the digit (Table 17-4). Determinations for amputations at intervals between the joints are adjusted proportionately. If all fingers and thumb are amputated at the MCP joints, it is equivalent to 100% loss of the hand, which is equal to 90% of the upper extremity or 54% of the whole person. Learning these simple rules helps keep the relative values for amputation in perspective. The total impairment assigned for a nonamputated finger with, for example, restricted motion or nerve damage should not exceed that given for amputation of that finger. Knowing the value of each finger in amputation sets a boundary for estimating impairment for other less definitive injuries.

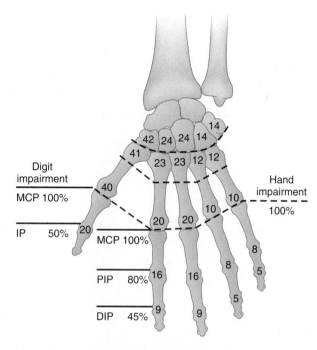

Digit impairment

MCP 100%

IP   50%

MCP 100%

PIP   80%

DIP   45%

Hand impairment 100%

MCP = metacarpophalangeal
PIP = proximal interphalangeal
DIP = distal interphalangeal

Figure 17-2 Impairment of the digits and the hand based on amputation level. (Redrawn from Swanson AB. Evaluation of impairment of function in the hand. *Surg Clin North Am.* 1964;44:925-940.)

Range of Motion

Diminished ROM of the joints of the upper extremity is a measurable factor used in the evaluation of loss of function.[27] The arc of motion (angular measurement) of the finger joints, for example, is represented by two numbers, one at the extreme of extension and the other at the extreme of flexion. Therefore, each joint is assigned a numerator and a denominator. Obtaining these measurements (14 in all just for the thumb and fingers) is cumbersome and time-consuming, but no better method is available.[28] The use of glove-embedded sensors or an electronic goniometer may help gather these data in the future. For now, a simple goniometer is used. ROM measurements are rounded off to the nearest 10 degrees. The goniometer, as placed over the dorsum of the finger or wrist joint, is not perfect. Swelling or deformity of the finger skews the measurement. The examiner and the *Guides* should recognize that this technique for measurement is somewhat of a compromise and that for the measurement to be truly accurate, it would have to be obtained via longitudinal lines drawn through the midaxis of the adjacent phalanges at the joints. Although use of the goniometer is required, an experienced examiner often can reproduce the measurements using an estimate obtained with a straight edge alongside the joint. If a patient demonstrates active motion that is short of the expected, in view of the patient's history, examination findings, and radiograph studies, then the examiner should try to determine whether maximum effort is being exercised. The examinee's active ROM should be consistent with the pathologic signs and the medical evidence. If possible, gentle passive ROM is tested. If there is a discrepancy between active and passive motion inconsistent

with the disease process, ROM testing can be discarded based upon the Diagnosis-Based Impairment system. If ROM testing is felt to be reliable, it can be used along with the functional history and clinical studies to modify the grade up or down within an impairment class.

In general, if there is a question of abnormal motion, one can compare the ROM in question to the contralateral unimpaired joint. This is generally reliable, except in the thumb, where ROM is not as consistent bilaterally.

Impairment Caused by Peripheral Nerve Disorders

Sensory Deficits. The *Guides* tell us that any sensory loss or deficit that contributes to permanent impairment must be unequivocal and permanent.[23] It must be remembered that there is no perfect, objective test for determination of sensory loss, and the examiner depends on the patient's input. Sudomotor function is an objective reflection of sensory integrity, but except for the clinical observation of a sweat pattern, it is not a practical test for everyday use. The ninhydrin test[29] has not been widely used but can occasionally be useful in cases that have no other solution. Neurodiagnostic testing is helpful for documenting the presence or absence of nerve deficiency. For sensory evaluation, the *Guides* recommend using either two-point discrimination testing or Semmes–Weinstein monofilament testing. In the hand, when two-point discrimination exceeds 15 mm, the area is said to be totally deficient in sensation or to have a 100% sensory impairment. Six-millimeter two-point discrimination and below is regarded as normal sensibility. Percentage impairment of the finger is then assigned (Fig. 17-3). Confirmatory findings in significant sensory deficit are loss of sudomotor function manifested by dryness of the finger pulps, which also may be atrophic. Because the two-point discrimination test, when done correctly, is a complex undertaking requiring an experienced and patient examiner, in critical cases the use of a certified hand therapist with training and experience is advised for this examination.[30] We do not advocate the use of the pin to test for sensory function and have not used it for many years because we have found that when a nerve is completely nonfunctional, the patient is left with bloody pinholes in that nerve's distribution. Alternatively, when the nerve is intact the examination can become very unpleasant for the patient. Neither is a happy situation. The sensory picture obtained should concur with anatomy and correlate with the patient's history and other findings. To calculate the impairment resulting from sensory loss in the thumb and fingers, the examiner can refer to Tables 17-5 and 17-6.

Motor Deficits. In cases of total denervation of a muscle, the problem is relatively simple to rate, but in cases of weakness or partial paralysis, detailed muscle testing may be required. This necessitates a knowledgeable examiner skilled in this examination. A standardized rating system, adapted by the *Guides*, for rating muscle power applies a rating of 5 for a full range of active motion against full resistance and at the other end of the scale, 0 for complete paralysis.

In relation to nerve problems, the framers of the *Guides* agreed on certain guidelines. There is also an established maximum value to be assigned as a result of any particular nerve dysfunction. For example, a completely nonfunctional median nerve injured in the proximal forearm, which has complete sensory and motor implications, is given a 44%

Table 17-4 Impairment for Upper Limb Amputation at Various Levels

Amputation Level	Digit	Impairment %		
		Hand	Upper Extremity	Whole Person
Thumb at:				
IP joint	50	20	18	11
MCP joint	100	40	36	22
Half metacarpal		41	37	22
Metacarpal at CMC		42	38	23
Index or Middle Finger at:				
DIP joint	45	9	8	5
PIP joint	80	16	14	9
MCP joint	100	20	18	11
Half metacarpal		21	19	11
Metacarpal at CMC		22	20	12
Ring or Little Finger at:				
DIP joint	45	5	5	3
PIP joint	80	8	7	4
MCP joint	100	10	9	5
Half metacarpal		12	11	7
Metacarpal at CMC		13	12	7
Hand:				
All fingers at MP joints except thumb	—	60	54	32
All digits at MP joints	—	100	90	54
Forearm/Hand:				
From distal to bicipital insertion to transmetacarpophalangeal loss of all digits	—	—	94–90	56–54
Arm/Forearm:				
From distal to deltoid insertion to bicipital insertion	—	—	95	57
Arm:				
Deltoid insertion and proximally	—	—	100	60
Shoulder disarticulation	—	—	100	60
Scapulothoracic (forequarter)	—	—		70

CMC, carpometacarpal; DIP, distal interphalangeal; IP, interphalangeal; MCP, metacarpophalangeal; PIP, proximal interphalangeal.

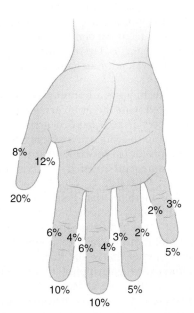

Figure 17-3 Hand impairment for sensory loss. (Redrawn from Swanson AB. Evaluation of impairment of function in the hand. *Surg Clin North Am.* 1964;44:925-940.)

impairment of the upper extremity. The ulnar nerve at a similar level is equivalent to a 46% impairment of the upper extremity. These guidelines give the examiner a reference to aid in rating nerve impairment in the upper extremity.

It is noted that the evaluator is instructed not to use impairment values from more than one section because this overlap will result in too high an impairment rating. When multiple areas of impairment are involved because of injury to the peripheral nerves, they are combined using the combined values chart.

Pain

Evaluation of chronic pain in impairment examination is a difficult problem. Chapter 3 of the *Guides* provides an excellent discussion of pain entities and refers the reader to other appropriate sections when chronic pain is the presenting symptom. In general, pain should be explainable by some underlying and definable problem. If it is not and thus cannot be rated by the DBI method, a pain-related impairment can be given as shown in Table 17-7. As is evident, the numbers are quite low.

Reflex Sympathetic Dystrophy. Reflex sympathetic dystrophy (RSD), now referred to as complex regional pain syndrome (CRPS), has been divided into two types: type 1,

Table 17-5 Digit Impairment for Sensory Loss of the Thumb and Small Finger

Percent of Digit Length	Percent of Digit Impairment					
	Transverse Loss		Longitudinal Loss			
	Both Digital Nerves		Ulnar Digital Nerve		Radial Digital Nerve	
	Total	Partial	Total	Partial	Total	Partial
100	50	25	30	15	20	10
90	45	23	27	14	18	9
80	40	20	24	12	16	8
70	35	18	21	11	14	7
60	30	15	18	9	12	6
50	25	13	15	8	10	5
40	20	10	12	6	8	4
30	15	8	9	5	6	3
20	10	5	6	3	4	2
10	5	3	3	2	2	1

From Swanson AB, de Groot Swanson G, Hagert CG. Evaluation of impairment of hand function. In: Hunter JM, Mackin E, Callahan AD, eds. *Rehabilitation of the Hand. Surgery and Therapy.* 4th ed. St Louis: CV Mosby, 1995.

where no known nerve injury has occurred, and type 2, with a recognizable peripheral nerve injury. Type 2 is what was referred to as *causalgia* in the older literature.[31] The 6th edition has further defined specific diagnostic criteria and includes the following:

1. Other differential diagnoses have been ruled out
2. Present for more than 1 year and confirmed by more than one physician
3. Objective findings present, such as hyperalgesia, allodynia, vasomotor changes, sudomotor changes, and motor or trophic changes

If the diagnostic criteria are met, an impairment rating can be given taking into account functional compromise,

Table 17-6 Digit Impairment for Sensory Loss of the Index, Middle, and Ring Fingers

Percent of Digit Length	Percent of Digit Impairment					
	Transverse Loss		Longitudinal Loss			
	Both Digital Nerves		Ulnar Digital Nerve		Radial Digital Nerve	
	Total	Partial	Total	Partial	Total	Partial
100	50	25	20	10	30	15
90	45	23	18	9	27	14
80	40	20	16	8	24	12
70	35	18	14	7	24	11
60	30	15	12	6	18	9
50	25	13	10	5	15	8
40	20	10	8	4	12	6
30	15	8	6	3	9	5
20	10	5	4	2	6	3
10	5	3	2	1	3	2

From Swanson AB, de Groot Swanson G, Hagert CG. Evaluation of impairment of hand function. In: Hunter JM, Mackin E, Callahan AD, eds. *Rehabilitation of the Hand. Surgery and Therapy.* 4th ed. St Louis: CV Mosby, 1995.

Table 17-7 Pain-Related Impairment

Degree of Pain-Related Impairment	Pain Disability Questionnaire Score	Whole-Person Impairment (%)
None	0	0
Mild	1–70	0
Moderate	71–100	1
Severe	101–130	2
Extreme	131–150	3

physical findings, and clinical studies (Table 17-8). It is recommended that the examiner not label a patient reporting chronic pain as having CRPS without the indicated findings. Because impairment evaluation is a late procedure in an injury or illness, the impairment examiner may not see the acute stage of CRPS but should recognize the late ravages of the condition, which may manifest with joint restriction and ongoing peripheral nerve problems. It is important not to use the diagnosis casually but only when a strong history and clinical picture supports it as this diagnosis carries many legal implications with it. Ensalata[32] presents an excellent discussion of the difficulties in the evaluation of these conditions and brings to our attention the great amount of work that still needs to be done in this area.

Grip Testing. One of the parameters on which hand function is based is the evaluation of grip strength in the hand.[33,34] Quantification of grip strength is said to be measurable and repeatable by the use of the Jamar dynamometer.[33] Unfortunately, the subjectivity of this evaluation when used under impairment evaluation conditions greatly reduces the value as a reliably measurable parameter. Swanson and coworkers[35] tell us that many factors determine the strength of grip, including age, handedness, pain, finger amputations, and restricted motion among others. Not the least is the compliance of the patient in the test and his or her willingness to put effort into the examination. When obvious deficiencies are present, they may be used to determine a percentage of impairment. In our opinion, it is rarely valid to register the loss of strength as a factor in the evaluation in the absence of confirmatory deficiencies. Despite this, we always measure grip strength on an evaluation to gain additional information about the patient.

Some standard techniques are applicable to grip testing.[15,36] The patient is seated with the arm carried at the side of the trunk and the elbow flexed at 90 degrees. Grip testing is generally done using the Jamar dynamometer at the second and third handle positions. In weak arthritic hands, one can use a blood pressure cuff inflated to 50 mm Hg, and the change in pressure with grip is recorded as strength.[35] Also suggested are two methods that help detect those who are not exerting their maximal strength on grip testing:

1. Testing at all five handle positions of the Jamar dynamometer and plotting the measurements should show a bell curve rather than a flat line.[35]
2. Using rapid exchange gripping, that is, using one hand and then the other for at least five repetitions, helps show who are not compliant because they exert much higher levels than on the routine tests, and when they realize this, their performance drops precipitously.[14]

Table 17-8 Complex Regional Pain Syndrome Impairment

Diagnostic Criteria (key factor)	Class 0	Class 1	Class 2	Class 3	Class 4
Impairment Ranges (UE %)	0% UE	1%–13% UE	14%–25% UE	26%–49% UE	50%–100% UE
Objective Findings (points threshold)		≥4 points	≥6 points	≥8 points	≥8 points
Severity		Mild	Moderate	Severe	Very severe
Grade	0; CRPS diagnosis not supportable	A B C D E 1 3 7 11 13	A B C D E 14 17 20 23 25	A B C D E 26 32 38 44 49	A B C D E 50 60 70 80 90

UE, upper extremity; CRPS, complex regional pain syndrome.
Note: Prior to using table, examiner must review Section 15.1 and 15.5. The diagnosis of CRPS must be defined by Table 15-24, Diagnostic Criteria for Complex Regional Pain Syndrome, and specified points threshold must be met as defined by Table 15-25, Objective Diagnostic Criteria for Complex Regional Pain Syndrome. The default value for impairment is grade C and modified by reliable findings and use of adjustment grids.
Cross references are to sections and tables in the *AMA Guides*.

Although it has been our observation that many people are stronger by approximately 10% on their dominant side, Swanson and associates,[15] in their study of unimpaired subjects, found a remarkable bilateral similarity of strength in a wide range of subjects; however, manual workers were usually stronger on their dominant side.

Pinch strength is also measurable using a pinch gauge. Key pinch is usually used, but again, is also of little value as a measurement in adversarial situations. In this test the noncompliant individual is able to directly view the measurements on the gauge and may consciously or subconsciously adjust his or her pinch pressure. In this setting, it is often useful to turn the device over during the second trial to prevent the patient from viewing the force generated.

Overall, we agree that when there is a possibility or evidence that the subject is exerting less than maximal effort during grip testing, the measurements become invalid for impairment evaluations. This is supported by Swanson and associates,[15] who do not assign a large role to grip and pinch values in an evaluation system based on anatomic impairment.

Functional Capacity Evaluation

One of the weaknesses of impairment and subsequent disability evaluation is the lack of ability to look at the patient's functional capacity—the ability to actually perform work. The entities we are able to measure may not correlate with the ability to perform a function.[15,16,37] Today, the difference between impairment and disability rating seems to be blurring, and examining physicians are frequently called on to fill out work evaluation certificates.[5] These forms may be for general work restrictions or for specific jobs, our knowledge of which may be rudimentary. Even with expertise in impairment evaluation we are at a disadvantage.[37] The ability to perform work is directly related to the person's physical capacities, but in addition, philosophic and psychological issues are involved. The ability and desire to perform work has numerous determinants, both conscious and subconscious. Illness behavior can pervade the evaluation. The use of a functional capacities evaluation performed by an upper extremity therapist trained in the administration of these studies is of great assistance to the physician performing an impairment evaluation.

Functional capacity evaluation (FCE) can be subdivided into physical capacity evaluation and work capacity evaluation.[38] Physical capacity evaluation examines isolated parts of the body or functional units. Work capacity evaluations assess performance involving several functional units.

These studies essentially were designed to assist the worker getting back to work after an injury but also could be of value in a permanent impairment situation. These evaluations are especially pertinent because the Americans with Disabilities Act prohibits exclusion of qualified persons with disabilities from employment,[16] and some mechanism is needed to evaluate the worker with a permanent impairment. The FCE can assist in the determination and validity of occupational disability. On the negative side is the fact that the examination is not standardized and there is a need for better validity testing if it is to have real value. The evaluator needs to be trained and skilled to make these evaluations pertinent. We have seen situations in which the findings were in great excess to the objective impairment, thereby creating considerable confusion. Although their value in cases with difficult patients is questionable,[16] we believe these evaluations could have great value in the process and would hope that better validity standards would make them even more useful.

Combining Impairments

When more than one impairing factor is to be considered in a part, the *Guides* tell us to combine them before converting to the next unit. To combine impairments in the upper extremity, the rater must first determine the impairments of each region (hand, wrist, elbow, and shoulder joints) if multiple regions are impaired. Combining is done using the combined values chart at the back of the *Guides*. When multiple areas within a unit contribute to impairment (e.g., in a finger), these impairments, such as restriction of motion and sensory loss, are combined before conversion to impairment of the hand. In the case of digit and hand impairments, convert to impairment of the upper extremity before regional impairments can be combined. After combining, the impairment can then be converted to whole-body impairment using the appropriate table.

Rule: When a unit has several impairments, they must be combined before going to the next unit. It must be remembered that one should not assign an impairment value that exceeds that for amputation of that part.

Summary

When an impairment evaluation is needed, a thorough examination is performed and a diagnosis is formulated. Assuming the patient has reached maximum medical improvement, an impairment rating can be issued. The 6th edition of the *Guides* has incorporated a new direction into this process. Most conditions involving the upper extremity can be assigned a class based on the specific diagnosis. Latitude within each class is determined by functional status, physical findings, and clinical studies. If one encounters a nonphysiologic test or an inconsistent QuickDASH score, the examination and functional status can be discounted maintaining the "default" grade. The use of the regional grid system seems cumbersome at first, but once one becomes familiar with concepts, it is soon apparent that this rating system is a significant improvement over prior methods. The methodology also allows for higher or lower rating based on a reliable functional status. We believe this new DBI method is a step forward in the ever-evolving process of upper extremity rating.

REFERENCES

The complete reference list is available online at www.expertconsult.com.

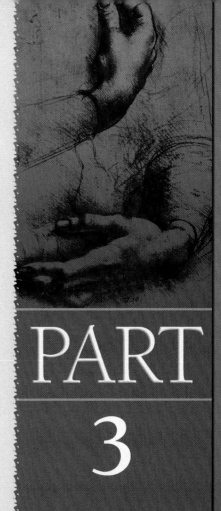

PART
3

Skin and Soft Tissue Conditions

Wound Classification and Management

REBECCA L. VON DER HEYDE, PhD, OTR/L, CHT AND
ROSLYN B. EVANS, OTR/L, CHT

STAGES OF WOUND HEALING	WOUND MANAGEMENT
ADVANCES IN BASIC SCIENCE	SCAR MANAGEMENT
WOUND ASSESSMENT	SUMMARY

CRITICAL POINTS

- Wound healing occurs in three stages and is characterized by changes in cellularity as different cell types migrate into and out of the wound bed.
- Recent advances in the bioregulation of normal wound repair include means for decreasing adhesion formation, the use of growth factors as a strategy for increasing early repair strength, and tissue engineering for the creation of replacement tissues.
- Wounds are evaluated in terms of risk factors for altered healing, the presence or absence of infection, physical location, size, appearance, and the stage of healing.
- The key issue in wound management is understanding the physiologic effect of such treatment steps as debridement, cleansing, disinfection, dressing, or the use of modalities of motion on the natural response of wound healing.

Comprehensive treatment of the patient with an upper extremity injury is often initiated within days following injury or surgery. Knowledge of the biology of the wound-healing process is an integral component of successful hand therapy practice. The purpose of this chapter is to review both seminal literature that has stood the test of time and offer current evidence as a means of advancing therapeutic intervention in the treatment of the healing wound.

Stages of Wound Healing

Knowledge of wound biology and the physiology of tissue repair is the basis of clinical decision making in the treatment of the simple, complex, or multilayered wound.

Wound healing is a cellular event. Each phase of wound healing is characterized by changes in cellularity as different cell types, primarily neutrophils, monocytes, macrophages, fibroblasts, and endothelial cells, migrate into and out of the wound bed[1-5] (Fig. 18-1). This cellular activity, initiated by tissue and platelet disruption, is regulated by a complex interaction of biochemical exchanges that orchestrate the events of phagocytosis, neovascularization, and biosynthesis of reparative collagen.[6-11]

The dramatic changes in wound-healing activity usually are divided into three overlapping stages.[11-17] In the first stage of repair, the inflammatory or exudative stage, the neutrophil and macrophage are responsible for clearing the wound of debris to set the stage for subsequent repair.[16,18,19] The macrophage is the most important regulatory cell in the inflammatory stage because it is critical to bactericidal control and is chemotactic to the fibroblast.[11,20-23] Secretory products of the macrophage can enhance fibroblast proliferation and collagen synthesis.[24] The macrophage also may be important in the normal process of angiogenesis—the formation of new blood vessels in granulation tissue.[19,25,26] A non-mitogenic chemoattractant for endothelial cells, possibly derived from macrophages, has been isolated from wound fluid.[27]

The migration of epithelial cells, the process known as *epithelialization*, is initiated within hours of injury, sealing the cleanly incised and sutured wound within 6 to 48 hours.[28] Epithelial cell movement is stimulated by an apparent loss of cellular contact that occurs with wounding and is stimulated by the process of contact guidance.[28] This cellular migration is terminated when advancing cells meet similar advancing cells by the phenomenon known as *contact inhibition*.[15] Epidermal cells migrate toward the area of cell deficit, following the predictable pattern of mobilization, migration, mitosis, and cellular differentiation.[15] The cells maintain their numbers by mitosis, both in fixed basal cells away from the wound edges, and in migrating cells, with the net result being a resurfacing of the wound and thickening of the new epithelial layer.[28,29] This reepithelialization process is

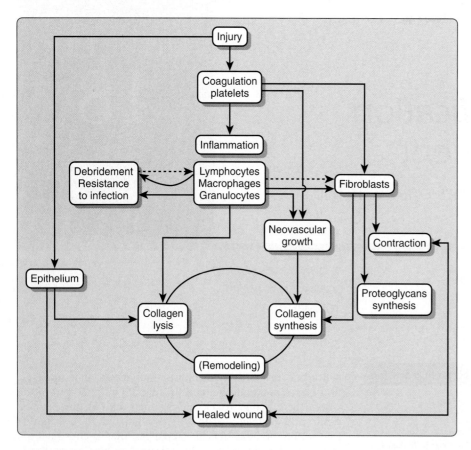

Figure 18-1 Schematic concept of wound healing. (From Hunt TK, Heppenstall RB, Pines E, Rovee D, eds. *Soft and Hard Tissue Repair*, New York, 1984, Praeger, an imprint of Greenwood Publishing Group, Westport, Connecticut.)

influenced and possibly directed by a bath of cytokines arising from cells in the wound environment and in distant tissues.[28]

In the second stage of healing, the fibroblastic or reparative stage, the fibroblast begins the process of collagen synthesis.[30,31] The fibroblast, signaled by the macrophage, growth factors, or other mononuclear cells, initially secretes the elements of ground substance, protein polysaccharides, and various glycoproteins, and at approximately the fourth to fifth day after wounding, collagen synthesis begins.[10,21,29,32]

The myofibroblast, a highly specialized form of fibroblast, is thought to be responsible for the phenomenon of wound contraction.[33] This contractile fibroblast has the characteristics of both the smooth muscle cell and the fibroblast and is found in open granulating wounds, whereas fibroblasts are found in closed incised wounds.[33] Researchers have suggested that the histologic existence of myofibroblasts is related to a transitional state of fibroblasts in granulation tissue, wherein they prepare to migrate from a healed wound.[33]

Endothelial cells form the new blood vessels in granulation tissue, which provide oxygen and nutrients to the wound site.[34] These nutrients are necessary for the synthesis, deposition, and organization of the extracellular matrix.[23] Angiogenesis is thought to be directed chemically by growth factors and macrophage-secreted angiogenic peptides.[19,23,26,27,35-37]

The third stage of wound healing is characterized by the maturation and remodeling of scar tissue or extracellular matrix manufactured during the second or reparative stage.[11,15,38] This phase is typically observed after the 21st day, terminating months and perhaps years after the wound has occurred.[39] As the healing tissues demonstrate decreased elasticity, a heightened awareness to stress at the wound site reduces the risk of skin breakdown during the reparative stage.[39]

Age is an important factor to consider in the analysis and management of the healing wound. Increased elasticity and strength of connective tissue facilitates both resilience and healing in the young patient.[39] As aging occurs, a decrease in collagen elasticity and fat deposition hinder protective capabilities, resulting in skin that is more easily damaged.[39] Chronic diseases, such as diabetes mellitus and renal failure, can confound the wound-healing process, leading to an increased risk for infection and amputation.[40,41]

Inasmuch as evidence of the cellular sequence of wound healing is abundant and consistent, histologic research has progressed to analyses of molecular events during the healing process. In the specialty of hand surgery, basic science research in the past two decades has focused on modulation of wound healing and adhesion formation, primarily in the healing flexor tendon.

Advances in Basic Science

Histologic research in wound healing has significantly evolved over the past three decades. Early studies manipulated the microenvironment of the wound and attempted to enhance cellular activity.[42-51] Experimental modalities were pursued for the control or stimulation of wound healing[21,37,51-58] and included peptides, cytokines, growth factors, and wound fluids.[21,50,59-63] More recent advances in the bioregulation of normal wound repair include means for decreasing adhesion formation, the use of growth factors as a strategy for increasing early repair strength, and tissue engineering for the creation of replacement tissues.

Modulation of Adhesion Formation

Collagen is the most abundant protein in the human body, significantly contributing to the integrity of connective tissue structures. Despite the integral role of collagen synthesis in wound healing, excessive proliferation of collagen can limit excursion and, ultimately, the function of healing tissues in the upper extremity. Collagen synthesis has been associated with fibroblastic activity,[10,21,29,32] and, as such, the chemical modulation of fibroblasts has been experimentally pursued.

Decreased synovial thickening and adhesion formation were observed following intraoperative application of 5-fluorouracil (5FU) in a chicken model.[64] In a subsequent study, adhesion reduction did not result in significant differences in excursion, maximal load, or work of flexion compared with results in normal controls.[65] 5FU has been suggested to have a preferential effect on fibro-osseous fibroblasts,[66] and these cells have been specifically targeted as highly responsible for adhesion formation.[67] Other chemical inhibitors, including those targeting proteinase and prostaglandin, have been noted to decrease adhesions in animal models.[68-71]

Hyaluronic acid is a glycosaminoglycan found in the extracellular matrix of skin, cartilage, and synovial fluid. Noted to decrease scar formation and promote healing[72-75] this carbohydrate has also been found in human amniotic fluid.[76] Injection of human amniotic fluid coupled with tendon sheath repair resulted in fewer adhesions and a higher tensile strength in a rabbit model.[76]

Human amniotic fluid also contains growth factors, naturally occurring proteins that stimulate growth.[76] Because research in adhesion modulation has offered limited clinically observable results, the tensile strength as afforded by growth factors has facilitated a transition toward the cellular repair processes that might accelerate tendon healing.

Acceleration of Healing

Vital to the process of wound healing, the differentiation of cell types in the intrasynovial flexor tendon has increased comprehension of both adhesions and tensile strength. Previously differentiated as extrinsic versus intrinsic, the analysis has expanded to consider the catalysts for collagen production at three distinct sites: the tendon sheath, epitenon, and endotenon.[77] The delicate balance of scar tissue necessary for tendon integrity as opposed to adhesion formation has guided the careful analysis of growth factors and cell regulation.

The healing process of the intrasynovial flexor tendon has been studied using both in vitro and in vivo animal models. Using a rat model in vivo, Oshiro and colleagues[78] demarcated the following sequence: superficial repair, initiation of collagen degradation at day 7, near completion of collagen degradation at day 21, synthesis of new collagen with remodeling, and neovascularization. In this study, preexisting endotenon fibroblasts were observed as the primary reparative cells when no gapping occurred.[78] This concurred with seminal work by Gelberman and coworkers,[79] who contrasted the role of epitenon fibroblasts in gapped tendons with endotenon fibroblasts in those tendons in which gapping had not

occurred.[79] In their study, Oshiro and colleagues[78] also identified matrix metalloproteinases (MMPs) involved in collagen degradation and remodeling.

An in vitro study of normal rabbit tendons addressed the role of lactate in collagen production.[77] Lactate was noted to stimulate both collagen and growth factors and to affect all cell types. Tendon sheath fibroblasts, however, exhibited the greatest proliferation and collagen production.[77] Tendon sheath cells were also analyzed in a rat model to determine their presence in the healing flexor tendon.[80] These cells were observed at 24 hours, increased in number through the fifth postoperative day, and decreased by day seven.[80]

The influence of vanadate added to drinking water was studied in two rat models. Following medial collateral ligament repair, vanadate yielded a significant increase in collagen fiber diameter, promoted collagen organization,[81,82] and significantly increased biomechanical stiffness and ultimate force.[82]

Basic fibroblast growth factor (bFGF) has been detected in both normal and injured intrasynovial tendons[83] with increased levels in the epitenon and tendon sheath cells during the first eight weeks of healing.[84] This growth factor has been extensively studied, with implications toward increased proliferation of tenocytes for collagen production.[85] Using a normal rabbit model in vivo, bFGF was observed to increase expression of nuclear factor κB (NF-κB), a cell proliferation regulator.[85] NF-κB has been suggested as a possible signaling pathway among growth factors, cell proliferation, and collagen synthesis,[85,86] yet clear cause and effect has not been established.[87] The delivery of bFGF to the healing tendon has also been studied. Adeno-associated viral vectors (AAV2) significantly increased expression of bFGF in vitro,[88] and bFGF-coated nylon suture increased strength and epitenon thickening in vivo.[89]

Transforming growth factor beta (TGF-β) has been noted to increase fibroblast recruitment and collagen production,[90] producing significant increases in collagen observed in epitenon, endotenon, and tendon sheath cells in response to all isoforms.[91] These proliferative characteristics spurred the research of TGF-β antibodies, found to decrease adhesions and increase range of motion after repair[92] and generally reduce the profibrotic effects in all three types of cells.[93]

In vitro animal models have established the presence of vascular endothelial growth factor (VEGF) in the healing flexor tendon. This protein has been observed as more prevalent in intrinsic tenocytes than in epitenon cells,[94] peaking between 7 and 10 days after repair and returning to baseline by day 14.[95] An in vivo rat Achilles tendon repair study attributed increased tensile strength to VEGF.[96] Platelet-derived growth factor (PDGF) has been differentially established as present in healing versus normal canine tendons.[83] This protein is commercially available for use in chronic wound management, with improved rate of healing being documented in clinical trials.[97,98]

As understanding of the influence of growth factors has increased, comparative studies have helped to establish their individual roles. An in vitro rat tendon model comparing VEGF and PDGF identified the former as less favorable.[99] VEGF was noted to significantly increase TGF-β, leading to adhesions, and the collagen produced was three times weaker than that stimulated by PDGF.[99] PDGF and bFGF were also preferable to VEGF and bone morphogenetic protein 2

(BMP-2) in a normal canine model, with increased cell proliferation and collagen production comparatively.[100]

Engineering of Tissues

The concept of tissue engineering has been the focus of much study in the past decade. Woo and associates[51] define *tissue engineering* as the manipulation of biochemical and cellular mediators to effect protein synthesis and to improve tissue remodeling. The new biologic therapies being developed from this basic science research include the application of growth factors to cutaneous wounds and the use of polymer scaffolds, cells, and growth factors to create replacement tissues.

Growth factors have been marketed primarily via products that interact with biologic tissues, often through impregnation in biologic dressings. These dressings are often referred to as skin substitutes, dermal matrix products, or scaffolds, and function as a vascularized dermis for subsequent split-thickness skin grafting.[101]

Current clinical expectations for these dressings include the following: the dressings must be safe, not cause an immunogenic response, not transmit disease, not be cytotoxic, and not cause excess inflammation.[102] Additional properties of interest include biodegradability, ample stability to support tissue reconstruction, sufficiently long shelf life, availability, and ease in handling.[102] Integrated sheets, carriers, and sprays have been implemented successfully as dermal substitutes.[101-103]

Integra (Integra LifeSciences, Plainsboro, NJ) is a well-known dermal substitute that has been specifically reviewed following use in the hand.[103] This collagen-based wound repair biomaterial was initially approved as a defect filler for the treatment of severe burns, allowing coverage of large full-thickness wounds to allow delayed split-thickness skin grafting.[103] In a case study offered by Carothers and coworkers,[103] Integra was sutured in a wound bed following tumor excision in the proximal palm. It is of note that both the median nerve and flexor tendons were exposed following tumor removal.[103] The patient was discharged home 1 day postoperatively and encouraged to complete digital motion as a means of decreasing adherence of the exposed structures on the skin substitute.[103] The patient underwent subsequent layering of Integra and split-thickness skin grafting 7 weeks after the initial coverage, resulting in full functional use without tendon adhesions.[103]

Four major challenges have been identified in the study of dermal replacement: safety, substitution for split-thickness skin grafting, improvement of angiogenesis in replacement tissue following graft, and increased ease of use.[101] One identified benefit is that tissue-engineered skin could optimally decrease the use of animals in pharmaceutical testing.[101]

Growth factors have also been studied for direct application to healing bone and ligament. The use of BMP-2 has yielded successful results in human studies of spinal fusion.[104-106]

The interdisciplinary field of regenerative medicine includes the sciences of biology and engineering. Procedures in this field are enabled by the use of scaffolds, cells, and growth factors. Polymer scaffolds are the structural base on which tissues are grown.[107] The ideal scaffold as described by Chong and associates[107] is a biocompatible mechanism that demonstrates the integrity and ability to house cells until new tissue regenerates.[107] Currently, the size of scaffolds has proved problematic in the maintenance of living cells,[107] and technology for injectable systems is under study.[108] Bioreactors have been employed for cyclic loading, a procedure that mimics stress and establishes desired physical and biochemical properties.[44,109,110]

The use of stem cells for tissue engineering has created notable public and scientific controversy. The ethical considerations associated with acquisition of embryonic stem cells and the possibilities of cloning are sources of heated debate. The plasticity of multipotent adult stem cells has been suggested as comparable to embryonic stem cells and is certainly less controversial.[109] Adult mesenchymal stem cells can be harvested from bone marrow and fat,[110] and these cells are capable of all types of differentiation, including osteogenesis, myogenesis, neurogenesis, and angiogenesis.[109] In a rabbit model, epitenon tenocytes, tendon sheath cells, bone marrow–derived stem cells, and adipoderived stem cells all contributed to the successful engineering of flexor tendons; however, use of stem cells hastened proliferation.[111]

Growth factors are applied to facilitate collagen synthesis and subsequent accrual of strength in the engineered tissues. Despite continued research of growth factors, questions remain regarding necessary concentrations and optimal transfer techniques.[110] A complete understanding of cell differentiation and signaling pathways for such differentiation has not been established.[110]

The successful engineering of a flexor tendon was reported by Cao and colleagues in 2002,[112] and Wang and coworkers[113] have quite recently engineered an extensor tendon complex using human fetal extensor tenocytes in an ex vivo rat model. Bone marrow–derived stem cells implanted via hydrogel scaffold have also contributed to cartilage formation in the subcutaneous tissue of mice.[108]

Continued experimental advances in wound healing and tissue engineering will predictably alter clinical management of repaired tendon, nerve, and the complex wound. The integration of biotechnology and the biochemical aspects of wound research may have tremendous relevance to our specialty because many of these new treatments will serve to regulate cellular activity. The application of a more scientific approach to wound healing may alter scar deposition and speed healing, decreasing the associated factors of morbidity: delayed healing, pain, excess fibrosis, longer treatment time, and increased expense. Treatment that may be helpful but not critical for the uncomplicated wound may be obligatory for the complex wound.

This new technology will most likely alter future treatment techniques,[51,53,54,114] but these new techniques do not have much clinical application for the hand clinician as of this writing. For the most part, management of the upper extremity cutaneous wound by the hand surgeon or hand therapist is not an issue. The cleanly incised and sutured wound epithelializes within 6 to 48 hours,[28] and the noninfected wound allowed to heal by secondary intention is expected to contract at a predictable pace.[11,33] The normal phases of wound healing usually proceed without difficulty when the wound is managed with careful debridement of nonviable tissue, physiologic repair, and routine wound care with cleansing and dressing.[115] The hand clinician, in most cases, focuses attention on the schedules for healing, immobilization, and mobilization for the deeper injured and repaired tissues. However, with complications of infection or dehiscence, and healing altered by malnutrition, irradiation, medication, immunosuppression, or a poor local blood supply, wound management becomes more of an issue and the significance of scientific clinical management becomes more apparent.[29,115-123] Depressed healing associated with vasculitis, venostasis, diabetes, immunosuppression, and burn care has inspired much of the work produced by multidisciplinary specialties that has produced the new clinical treatments with biologic dressings, oxygen therapy, and growth factors.[14,124,125] Cancer research has had a significant effect on the body of wound-healing knowledge, providing the early analysis of peptide growth factors.[10,36]

The next section addresses clinical decision making in wound evaluation and the effects of therapeutic management techniques on the cellular events in the different stages of wound healing.

Wound Assessment

Traditional wound assessment is well described in the literature.[30,35,63,126-133] Wounds are evaluated in terms of risk factors for altered healing, the presence or absence of infection, physical location, size, appearance, and the stage of healing. Wound edema, presence of hematoma, vascular perfusion, and the status of the deeper tissues are noted. The rate of healing in relation to the date of injury or surgery and the duration of previous treatment or chronicity of the wound are important factors in treatment planning.

Assessment of infection includes a review of risk factors for the individual case, visual inspection, and tissue cultures.[134-136] Before surgery or medical management, the surgeon will have established the factors that are predictive of susceptibility to infection or an altered rate of healing. This information determines timing of technique for wound closure or surgical management. Risk factors are determined based on an accurate history, including information concerning the mechanism of injury, the environment in which the injury occurred, the patient's medical and immunosuppressive state, systemic or local nutritional status, and previous medical treatment with medication or radiation.[18,115-118,121-123,134,137-139] These risk factors should be known to the hand therapist and the surgeon because the therapist in most cases is monitoring the wound more intensively than the surgeon. Patients at high risk for infection may need to be seen more often than those who will predictably experience benign wound healing.

Visual inspection helps determine whether a wound is healing with a normal inflammatory response or if, in fact, it has become infected. The cardinal signs of inflammation, redness, swelling, pain, and heat, accompany the biochemical and fluid aspects of the early inflammatory stage of wound healing and are not to be confused with infection.[11,16] The therapist should understand that purulence does not always represent the presence of infection.[29,140] If the inflammatory response is exaggerated or if the drainage is purulent, then bacterial counts must be obtained to determine the level of wound contamination.[141]

Clinical measurements of wound sepsis are determined by wound culture. The U.S. Institute of Surgical Research defines wound sepsis caused by bacterial overgrowth as bacterial counts exceeding 10^5 organisms per gram of tissue.[57,142] Traumatic wounds with multiple layers of injury to skin, muscle, and bone are difficult to evaluate because the colony count may vary at each level.[143]

One must understand that wound healing in the clinical situation occurs in the presence of bacteria; it is the quantity of and not the mere presence of bacteria that alters the reparative process.[29] Acceptable levels of endogenous, nonpathogenic microflora, as opposed to frank infection, determine the rate of wound healing and may actually stimulate tissue repair.[137] Favorable microflora in the wound bed may stimulate epidermal cell migration and healing.[144,145] Wound fluid monocyte and macrophage counts have been found to be markedly elevated and collagen deposition increased in wounds inoculated with 10^2 organisms.[145] Lower bacterial counts or well-controlled infection have been found to enhance chemotactic and bactericidal activity.[29]

However, in the presence of significant infection (greater than 10^5 organisms per gram of tissue), impaired leukocyte function, decreased chemotaxis, impaired cellular migration, epithelialization, and intracellular killing are noted.[29,146] Superficial infection may damage new epithelium through the release of neutrophil proteases,[147] and bacterial counts greater than 10^5 may retard wound contraction.[29] Infected wounds are affected adversely by the formation of thicker connective tissue and excessive angiogenesis, which is associated with prolific scar formation.[29,30,36,119,145] Robson and colleagues,[29] in a review of studies on the effect of bacterial count on fibroplasia, found the results to be inconsistent, but noted that collagen and hydroxyproline contents were consistently higher in infected wounds. Thus, infection control is important not only to the rate of healing but also to the management of scarring, which ultimately can interfere with tissue gliding and excursion for tendon, nerve, ligament, joint, and skin.

The wound healing by primary intention is usually simple to evaluate and treat. Attention in these cases is usually directed to protection of the deeper structures, the status of suture or staples, tension at the suture line, quality or quantity of drainage, and viability of the tissue. These wounds are described in terms of periwound edema, inflammation, infection, wound tension, viability, and rate of epithelialization.

If the wound closed by primary intention develops complications and dehisces, it becomes a wound healing by secondary intention.[134] Wounds left to heal by secondary intention, or the chronic or infected wound, pose more complex questions and require more clinical problem-solving and decision-making skills of the health-care practitioner. The following section attempts to simplify decision making and treatment planning for the hand therapist who may be confused by the many issues surrounding the management of the complex wound.

The Three-Color Concept

A universal classification system introduced by Marion Laboratories in the late 1980s continues to be the standard with which open wounds are characterized. Their approach uses

Table 18-1 Clinical Decision Making for Open Wounds

	Black Wound	Yellow Wound	Red Wound
Description	Covered with thick necrotic tissue or eschar	Generating exudate, looks creamy, contains pus, debris, and viscous surface exudate	Uninfected, properly healing with definite borders, may be pink or beefy red, granulated tissue and neovascularization
Cellular activity	Autolysis, collagenase activity Defense, phagocytosis Macrophage cell	Immune response, defense Phagocytosis Macrophage cell	Endothelial cells: Angiogenesis Fibroblast cells: collagen and ground substance Myofibroblast: wound contraction
Debridement	Surgical, preferred Mechanical, whirlpool, dressings Chemical, enzymatic digestion	Separate wound debris with aggressive scrubs, irrigation, or whirlpool	Not applicable: avoid any tissue trauma or stripping of new cells
Cleansing	Whirlpool Irrigation Soap and water scrubs	Use no antiseptics Soap and water Surfactant-soaked sponge Polaxmer 188, Pluronic F-68	No antiseptics Ringer's lactate Sterile saline, sterile water
Topical treatment	Topical antimicrobials with low white blood cell count or cellulitis	Topical antimicrobials to control bacterial contamination Silver sulfadiazine, bactroban, neomycin, polymixin B, neosporin	N/A for simple wounds Vitamin A for patients on steroids Antimicrobials for immunosuppressed
Dressing	Wet-to-dry for necrotic tissue Proteolytic enzyme to debride Synthetic dressing, autolysis Dress to soften eschar	Wet-to-dry—wide mesh to absorb drainage Wet-to-wet—saturated with medicants Hydrocolloid or semipermeable foam dressings, hydrogels	Occlusive or semiocclusive dressings; semipermeable films Protect wound fluids and prevent dessication
Desired goal	Remove debris and mechanical obstruction to allow epithelialization, collagen deposition to proceed Evolve to clean, red wound	Light debridement without disrupting new cells Exudate absorption Bacterial control Evolve to red wound	Protect new cells Keep wound moist and clean to speed healing Promote epithelialization, granulation tissue formation, angiogenesis, wound contraction

From Evans RB. An update on wound care. *Hand Clin.* 1991;7:418.

a "three-color concept" to describe wound status. Wounds are described as red, yellow, black, or a combination of two or three colors. The clinical application of this classification system is described by Cuzzel[148-150] in several articles. The following color descriptions for evaluation and treatment are summaries of her articles. Clinical decision making as it relates to therapeutic management by debridement, cleansing, disinfecting, and dressing is reviewed in a brief synopsis as it relates to wound color[1,6,149,151] (Table 18-1).

The Red Wound

The red wound is uninfected, healing according to a predictable schedule, and characterized by definite borders, granulation tissue, and apparent revascularization (Fig. 18-2). The fibroblast, myofibroblast, endothelial, and epithelial cells are active in this wound, orchestrating the events of epithelialization, angiogenesis, and collagen synthesis. Skindonor sites or surgical wounds healing by secondary intention, as in the case of an open Dupuytren's release, are examples of red wounds often seen in the hand clinic. Superficial wounds and acute partial or second-degree burns are classified as red wounds if they are uniformly pink in appearance.

Tissue oxygenation determines the color of the wound. A chronic red wound has pale pink to beefy red granulation tissue and usually is in the late stages of repair. Red wounds closing by secondary intention fill with granulation tissue from the edge of the wound to the center, closing by contraction and epithelialization, or they may be closed by grafting at the appropriate time.

Cellular activity in the clean red wound must be protected and facilitated by the appropriate therapy. Therapeutic goals

are to protect the local wound environment, maintain humidity, protect the wound fluids from desiccation, and protect the newly forming granulation tissue and epithelial cells. These wounds should be cleansed with lactated Ringer's solution or for home care with a nondetergent, mild pump soap such as Ivory or Dove. The soap should be applied to the periwound area only and rinsed with running water. Antiseptics should not be used on the red wound. Topical treatment may include an antibiotic ointment if the patient is at high risk for developing infection. The newly forming cells should be protected from noxious mechanical forces (tapes, dry dressings, wet-to-dry dressings, whirlpool agitation, and wound scrubbing). Occlusive or semiocclusive dressings, which are described in a later section, may be used to protect the local wound environment and wound humidity.

The Yellow Wound

The yellow wound may range in color from a creamy ivory to a canary yellow. Colonization with *Pseudomonas* gives the wound a yellow-green appearance and a distinctive odor. The yellow wound is draining, purulent, and characterized by slough that is liquid or semiliquid in texture; it contains pus, yellow fibrous debris, or viscous surface exudate (Fig. 18-3). The exudate may promote bacterial growth. Cellular activity is dominated by the macrophage, which is stimulated by the presence of bacteria and inflammation. The macrophage functions to clear the tissue of debris and to remove pathogenic organisms; thus, it is critical to bactericidal control and phagocytosis.[23]

Epithelialization and wound contraction, activity controlled by the epithelial cells and myofibroblasts, may be occurring at the pink wound margins but, in general, are

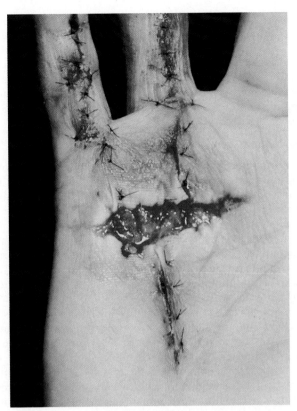

Figure 18-2 A red wound in a Dupuytren's fasciectomy 3 days after surgery. The wound in the palm is beefy red, without infection, with epithelial, endothelial myofibroblast, and fibroblast cellular activity taking place. Note that the digital wounds are already epithelized.

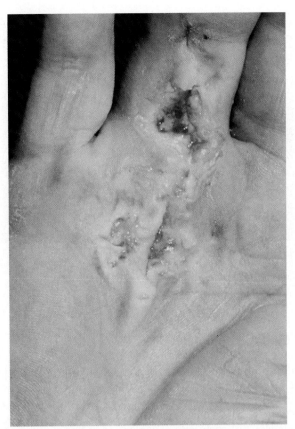

Figure 18-3 A yellow wound infected with *Pseudomonas* in a postsurgical Dupuytren's fasciectomy closed by primary intention with subsequent dehiscence. Although some of the green color is from skin pencil, the wound is yellow-green with a distinctive odor. Cellular activity is dominated by the macrophage, which is stimulated by bacteria and inflammation. (From Evans RB: An update on wound management. *Hand Clin.* 1991;7:419-432.)

delayed until infection or excessive inflammation are under control.

The goal of treatment in the case of the yellow wound is to facilitate cellular activity so that it can evolve into a red wound. Continual cleansing, removal of nonviable tissue, and absorption of excess drainage are important to decrease the workload of the macrophage.[17] These wounds may be aggressively washed with soap and water, irrigated with a water pick[152] or syringe, or treated with sterile whirlpools to separate surface debris and necrotic tissue. Topical antiseptics are cytotoxic and depress leukocyte function, thus depleting the body's natural defense mechanism and are thus to be avoided.[138,139,142,153,154] If bacterial proliferation requires control, an antibiotic such as Silvadene or Bactroban, and not a topical antiseptic, should be used in the wound.[135,155] Wet-to-dry dressings should be placed over only the wound because their application to the periwound area may cause skin maceration. Wet-to-dry dressings should be used with care because their removal may disturb new cells that are forming at the edge of the wound in addition to necrotic tissue. Dressings that absorb excess exudate while maintaining a moist environment, such as semipermeable foams, hydrocolloids, or hydrogels, may be used in the noninfected wound.[142]

The Black Wound

The black wound ranges in color from dark brown to gray-black; it is covered with eschar or thick necrotic tissue (Fig. 18-4). Cellular activity represents several stages of

wound repair that may be occurring simultaneously. The macrophage is working to clear the area of bacteria and debris and to signal fibroblasts to the area. The fibroblast and endothelial cells are beginning to synthesize collagen and new vessels as the debris is removed. This cellular activity is facilitated by the removal of the eschar surgically, mechanically, or enzymatically, in an effort to decrease the workload of the macrophage and to allow for unimpeded cellular migration. Eschar impedes cellular migration and proliferation by acting as a mechanical block and provides a medium in which bacteria can proliferate.

Debridement is the therapeutic goal for the black wound. Meticulous and timely debridement decreases the risk of infection and hastens healing by facilitating normal cellular response. These wounds may be debrided surgically, mechanically, or with proteolytic enzymes[135,142,148] such as Travase or Elase. Before mechanical debridement, the tissue may be softened as it is cleansed with scrubs or whirlpool to loosen dead tissue from the viable wound bed.

Topical antibiotics may soften eschar and decrease bacterial count. These wounds should be dressed to protect the wound environment, soften eschar, and facilitate autolysis. Synthetic dressings may facilitate autolysis by protecting wound fluids that contain the white cells responsible for phagocytosis.

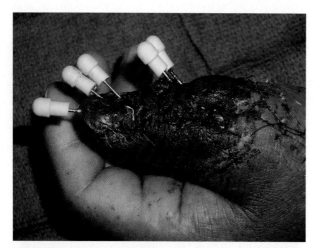

Figure 18-4 A black wound with evident necrosis of the distal thumb following replantation. (Photo courtesy of Dr. Miguel Pirela-Cruz, El Paso, Texas.)

Wound Management

Understanding the normal cellular activity of wound repair and regeneration is critical to accurate wound assessment, which in turn determines successful wound treatment. The key issue in wound management is understanding the physiologic effect of such treatment steps as debridement, cleansing, disinfection, dressing, or the use of modalities or motion on the natural response of wound healing. These treatments all contribute, either positively or negatively, to that cellular response.

The therapist can contribute to the wound-healing process by using management techniques that protect wound fluids, help prevent or control infection, minimize adverse mechanical influences, and control the collagen maturation process. Physical agents may facilitate cellular movement associated with increased blood flow, epithelialization, and macrophage or fibroblast activity and may have a role in the stimulation of growth factors. The deleterious effects of desiccation, mechanical trauma, and some topical treatments have been studied in terms of their inhibition of normal cellular function, and the results should alter some currently popular, but unscientific, wound management techniques.[147,151,156-160]

Protecting Wound Fluids

The positive role of humidity in wound resurfacing, first reported more than four decades ago,[161-163] has been recognized as one of the most important factors in wound healing by several researchers.[17,56,114,126-130,133,164-168] The maintenance of a moist wound environment in the noninfected wound facilitates both biochemical and cellular activity.[4,23,37,132,133,139,142,169-173] Wound fluids contain certain growth factors that interact with the host tissue, promote cellular activity, and contribute to wound metabolism.[4,10,16,21,23,27,131,170,174,175] The tissue fluids that accumulate in a wound create a favorable environment for angiogenesis and granulation tissue formation on which epithelialization can occur.[3,9,16,22,142,163,170,176]

An accelerated rate of healing in moist wounds is supported by histologic evaluation of full-thickness wounds in porcine skin.[3] Neutrophils and macrophages decreased in number more rapidly under moist conditions, and the proliferative phase cells (fibroblasts and endothelial cells) increased more rapidly. More rapid progression to the remodeling phase and advanced angiogenesis were noted in moist compared with dry wounds.[3]

Dessication

In an unprotected wound, evaporation occurs within hours of tissue disruption, allowing wound fluids to escape the wound bed.[142] An open wound exposed to air for 2 to 3 hours becomes necrotic to a depth of 0.2 to 0.3 mm.[163] The desiccated dermis or scab impedes epithelial cell migration and acts as a mechanical barrier, creating a dell or depression in the wound as the epidermal cells are required to migrate from the wound margins deep beneath the dried tissue.[162] This process is minimized in a wound that is occluded and not allowed to dessicate.[128]

Occlusion refers to the ability of a wound dressing to allow the transfer of water vapor and gases from a wound surface to the atmosphere.[17] The concept of sequestering wound fluids in the noninfected open wound for the purpose of enhancing cellular activity or facilitating autolytic debridement with occlusive or semiocclusive dressings has led to the development of many environmental dressings.[56,129,132,142,164-166,168,169,176-179]

These microenvironmental dressings may be categorized as films, foams, hydrocolloids, hydrogels, and calcium alginates.[17,142,165,166,169,172,173,177,180-184] Although there are substantial differences in these dressings, they are similar in that they maintain wound humidity (are impermeable to water but not always water vapor), may permit exchange of gases, reduce pain, reduce mechanical trauma associated with dressing removal, and absorb exudate in some cases.[142] The properties and indications for the dressings are summarized in Table 18-2), and several excellent review articles are recommended for more detailed study.[17,58,114,133,142,169,176,182,184,185]

Human skin has measurable transcutaneous electrical potential differences that are decreased with wounding.[176,186,187] Dehydration of wound tissue may decrease the lateral electrical gradient thought to control epidermal cell migration.[142,188,189] Exposed wounds tend to be more inflamed and necrotic than occluded wounds.[17] In later stages, the dermis of exposed wounds is more fibroblastic, fibrotic, and scarred.[17]

Preventing and Controlling Infection

The therapist can contribute to infection control by using the appropriate therapeutic techniques to maintain a clean wound bed free of necrotic tissue or excess drainage, by protecting the wound from its external environment with the proper dressings, and by instructing the patient concerning home wound care.

Cleansing

Cleanly incised and sutured wounds may be washed with a mild soap and running water as early as 24 hours after surgery.[190] The red wound may be rinsed with lactated

Table 18-2 Properties, Indications, and Precautions for Microenvironmental Dressings*

	Semipermeable Film	Semipermeable Foam	Semipermeable Hydrogel	Hydrocolloid
Indications	Clean, minimally exudative wound; red wound, sutured wounds, donor graft sites (split-thickness grafts), superficial burns, IV site dressing, superficial ulcers	Yellow wound, moderate to high exudate, skin ulcers, odiferous cancers, venous ulcers when combined with stockings or pressure dressings	Donor sites, superficial operation sites, chronic damage to epithelium, yellow exudating wounds; may apply over topical antimicrobials	Yellow wounds, friction blisters, postoperative dermabrasions, decubitus ulcers, venous stasis ulcers, cutaneous ulcers
Characteristics	Semiocclusive, occlusive, nonabsorbent, transparent, thin, adhesive, resistant to shear, low friction, does not control temperature, permeable to O_2 gas and water, impermeable to water and bacteria	Hydrophilic properties on wound side, hydrophobic on other side; limited absorbent capacity; permeable to water vapor and gas; polyurethane foams with a heat- and pressure-modified wound contact surface	Three-dimensional hydrophilic polymers that interact with aqueous solutions, swell and maintain water in their structure; insoluble in water; conform to wound surface; permeable to water vapor and gas, impermeable to water; tape required for fixation	Combine benefits of occlusion and absorbency; absorbs moderate to high exudate; expands into wound as exudate is absorbed to provide wound support; vision occluded; atraumatic removal; outer layer impermeable to gas, water, bacteria
Function	Mimics skin performance protects from pathogens, decreases pain, maintains wound humidity, enhances healing by protecting wound fluids; protects from pressure, shear, friction	Maintains wound humidity absorbs excess exudate, maintains warmth, decrease pain, cushions wound while averting "strikethrough"	Maintains wound humidity; facilitates autolytic débridement; absorbs excess exudate; allows evaporation without compromising humidity; removes toxic components from wound; maintains warmth; decreases pain	Absorbs exudate to form a gel that swells; applies firm pressure to the floor of a deep ulcer; autolytic debridement maintains wound humidity; maintains warmth; removes toxic compounds; decreases wound site
Precautions	Only for uninfected, red wounds; apply to dry periwound area; frame wound by 2 in; break-in seal allows microbes to enter wound from dressing margins	Visual monitoring occluded; low adherence, must tape	Permeable to bacteria; for moderate exudate; dehydrates easily; nonadhesive	Vision occluded; do not use on hairy surfaces

*Disclaimer/contraindications: All environmental dressings must be used in accordance with product information, which provides guidelines for indications, application, and contraindications. Some contraindications are wounds ulcerated into the muscle, tendon, bone; third-degree burns edge-to-edge eschar; wounds associated with osteomyelitis and active vasculitis, ischemic ulcers, and infected wounds. These products are all-inclusive and are not necessarily endorsed by the author or publisher but are provided as a source for further study.

Ringer's solution, which is more biologically compatible with the wound environment than saline. Some wound therapists currently believe that the pH of saline is too acidic for wound care. Saline, however, continues to serve as a common choice for wound cleansing as it does not cause harm to normal tissue and adequately cleanses most wounds.[191]

The red wound should not be scrubbed because this mechanical trauma could disrupt newly forming epithelium and vessels.[192] The yellow and black wound may be scrubbed with a mild soap and water. Dove or Ivory soap are recommended for home care,[193] or Pluronic F-68 or Poloxamer 188, nontoxic surfactants, can be used when more vigorous cleansing is needed.[139,151] A high-porosity sponge (90 ppi) may be used for mechanical scrubs because it is minimally abrasive and thus inflicts less tissue damage.[139] The object of wound cleansing is to separate soil, particle, and debris from the wound but not to create cellular destruction. Hydraulic irrigation with a water pick or whirlpool are indicated only for yellow and black wounds to loosen debris from the wound bed.[155,172] Pressures between 4 and 15 psi are recommended for wound cleansing.[191]

Cleansing solutions such as Hibiclens, hexachlorophene, and povidone-iodine (Betadine) may be used on intact skin before surgery on the periwound area, but if applied to the wound itself, they are cytotoxic and invite infection by destroying macrophages.[118,138,151,158,194]

Several authors have studied the adverse effects of povidone-iodine.[118,139,151,194] Aronoff and coworkers[195] has demonstrated that long-term povidone-iodine topical application may result in systemic absorption with resulting negative effects. Wound epithelialization and early tensile strength are affected negatively by 1% povidone-iodine solution. Researchers have reported that this solution must be diluted to 0.001% concentration to be nontoxic to human fibroblasts.[196] At this strength, the solution is still bactericidal to *Staphylococcus aureus*. However, Rodeheaver[151] has demonstrated that cleansing with povidone-iodine offers no advantage over cleansing with saline solution. He found the same level of viable bacteria in wounds contaminated with *S. aureus* when treated with either saline or povidone-iodine. Both hexachlorophene and povidone-iodine scrubs have been found to instantaneously lyse white blood cells that are critical to wound defense,[151] and povidone-iodine damages red blood cells, resulting in significant hemolysis.[197] Feedar and Kloth[142] urge that povidone-iodine solution in whirlpools and on gauze dressings be reconsidered, and other authors[139,151,198] recommend cessation of this practice altogether.

Although we all have observed wound healing in the presence of these cleansing agents, it may be that the wounds we have treated could have responded more quickly, decreasing time, discomfort, and expense, had we more carefully protected the wound fluids and cellular environment.

Disinfecting

Many wound specialists have condemned the practice of decontaminating a wound after cleansing with topical antiseptics. The often-quoted adage that "the only solution that should be placed in a wound is one that can safely be poured in the physician's eye" is supported by most wound therapists.[156] Rodeheaver and colleagues[155] has demonstrated that all antiseptic agents are cytotoxic, and their only mechanism of action is to destroy cell walls. Almost four decades ago he reviewed commonly used antiseptics and found iodine, chlorhexidine, peroxide, boric acid, alcohols, hexachlorophene, formaldehyde, hypochlorite, acetic acid, silver nitrate, merthiolate, gentian violet, permanganate, and aluminum salts to be cytotoxic.[155]

Hydrogen peroxide (H_2O_2), which has little bactericidal action, is perhaps misused as often as povidone-iodine. Hydrogen peroxide is appropriately used on a crusted wound, or to cleanse periwound skin, but should not be used after crust separation, on new granulation tissue, or on closed wounds.[142]

Researchers have suggested that topical antibiotics are the only antimicrobial agents that are nontoxic and beneficial to wound cellular activity.[155] Mupiricin (Bactroban) is a broad-spectrum antimicrobial recommended for its bactericidal capacity, which is greater than that of other topical antimicrobials. Neosporin ointment has a wide spectrum of bactericidal activity, including against most gram-positive and gram-negative bacteria found in both human and porcine skin.[142] Zinc bacitracin, which is one of the three antibacterial components of Neosporin, was found to increase epidermal healing by 25% compared with controls.[142] Contaminated blister wounds treated with the triple antibiotic in Neosporin (neomycin, polymyxin B, and bacitracin) ointment demonstrated lower bacterial counts and faster healing than with similar wounds treated with only protection or antiseptics.[199] One percent silver sulfadiazine (Silvadene) cream acts on a wide range of gram-negative and gram-positive bacteria as well as fungi. It has been used to prevent infection in burn wounds[200] and to salvage some or all parts of questionable flaps.[135] Silvadene treatment has been reported to reduce bacterial counts in wounds contaminated with less than 10^5 bacteria in 100% of the cases tested.[151] Silvadene also has been found to speed epithelialization in experimental animal studies.[151]

With each dressing change, the wound should be cleansed thoroughly of these ointments, and surface coagulum should be gently removed so that the fresh application of the topical antibiotic can be in contact with the wound bed.[138,201] By using only antibiotic ointments and avoiding the use of cytotoxic antiseptics, bacterial count is controlled and macrophage function, so critical to wound defense, is protected. These ointments may speed epithelialization by keeping the wound moist, thereby preventing crust formation and desiccation, which serve as mechanical barriers to cell migration.

Debridement

Necrotic tissue promotes bacterial growth and, by mechanical impedance, interferes with epithelial cell migration.[139] Removal of this necrotic tissue by meticulous debridement may be the most critical aspect of care to prevent infection in the acute wound and in the management of the contaminated or chronic wound.[139,202]

Debridement can be accomplished mechanically, enzymatically, or biologically through the normal phagocytic activity of white blood cells (autolysis).[142] Mechanical debridement by the surgeon is a critical component of both primary and chronic care. The therapist can remove small areas of black or gray eschar or debris from combination yellow and black wounds with fine forceps and sharp scissors. The necrotic debris should be separated from the wound edges, working toward the center, to facilitate the process of wound contraction. The yellow wound can be gently debrided with a small bone curette, but care must be taken not to fracture new capillaries at the wound edges. Before mechanical debridement, the wound may be cleansed and softened in a clear-water whirlpool. A scab may serve as a biologic dressing and left in place on a superficial wound, but if drainage occurs from beneath the scab, it must be debrided.[135]

Enzymatic debridement with topical fibrinolysin enzymes such as Travase or Elase may be used to hasten separation of eschars, scabs, or fibrinous coagulum.[135,142] Collagenase debridement products Biozyme C and Santyl may hydrolyze undenatured collagen or facilitate debridement of difficult necrotic tissue.[142] Feedar and Kloth[142] categorize these topical enzymes as selective, that is, working on only necrotic tissue, and their claim is supported by others who have demonstrated that these enzymes spare viable tissue.[203,204] Although these proteolytic enzymes may depress leukocyte phagocytosis, they do not significantly interfere with wound healing.[154] Hydrocolloid, alginate, or hydrogel dressings can be used to achieve natural autolytic cleansing.[184]

Autolytic, or biologic, debridement is considered the most selective because it relies on the body's natural defense system.[142] The noted importance of this natural phagocytic activity has led to the concept of sequestering wound fluids to facilitate macrophage debridement and has led to the development of synthetic dressings that enhance autolytic debridement.[142,184]

Selective debridement by careful mechanical, proteolytic, or autolytic means facilitates positive cellular response and is indicated for the yellow or black wound. Nonselective debridement, or that which indiscriminately removes both viable and nonviable tissue from the wound, may disturb new epithelial cells and granulation tissue and should be used with discretion. Nonselective methods includes wet-to-dry, wet-to-wet, and dry-to-dry dressings, whirlpool therapy, vigorous scrubs, Dakin's solution, or hydrogen peroxide solutions.[142]

Dressings

The act of covering a wound is an attempt to reproduce the barrier function of epithelium.[17] The primary dressing, or that which is placed in direct contact with the wound, provides a barrier to the external environment and functions to prevent infection. Nonadherent, nonabsorbent contact layers,

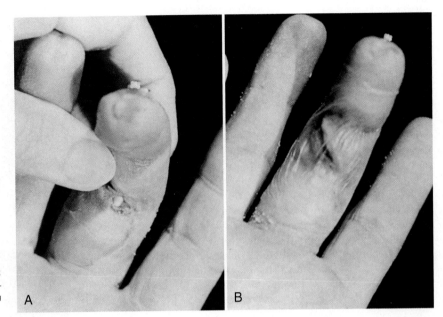

Figure 18-5 A, Exposed repaired flexor tendon 3 weeks after surgery. **B,** A Tegaderm dressing sequestered wound fluids and protected the exposed tendon until the wound was revised.

such as Adaptic, Xeroform, Aquaphor, or Transite, may help prevent desiccation and adhesion of the secondary dressing to the wound. These nonadherent contact layers are used postsurgically before the wound is sealed or epithelialized or can be used on a clean, red wound. The red wound can be protected from its environment with nonabsorbent film dressings such as Tegaderm, Opsite, or Bioclusive (see Table 18-1). These dressings are impermeable to water and provide all the benefits of moist wound healing previously described. Tegaderm has been used successfully to protect the humidity of exposed tendon in the digit. This film allows complete motion, adheres with an airtight seal to the periwound area, and prevents tendon desiccation until the wound is closed by secondary intention or surgical means (Fig. 18-5). These dressings provide a physiologic solution to a difficult problem, but they are not appropriate for infected wounds.

When excess drainage or infection is present, dressing changes should be performed as often as demanded by the accumulation of debris and fluid and the overload of absorbent materials.[17] The absorption of exudate into a dressing reduces the work requirement of the macrophage for phagocytosis and autolytic debridement and also removes a potential substrate for microbial growth.[17] The accumulation of wound fluid to the point of flooding causes maceration and bacterial overgrowth. Therefore, an absorbent dressing should imbibe exudate, but not allow fluid accumulation to the level of the most superficial dressing layer ("strikethrough").[17] If "strikethrough" does occur, a channel is created that will allow microorganisms to enter the wound from the external environment.[17] The absorbent dressing should match the requirement of the wound. The acute, noninfected wound exudes maximally at 24 hours after surgery and may have as its secondary layer sterile absorbent woven or nonwoven gauze products that usually are made of cotton or rayon.[17]

Yellow, noninfected, exudating wounds may be dressed with some of the newer microenvironmental dressings that function to absorb fluid without "strikethrough," encourage autolytic debridement, and maintain body temperature[17,116,166,176] (see Table 18-2). Hydrocolloid and hydrogel dressings are those that combine the benefits of occlusion and absorption and are most often used for chronic yellow wounds.[17,173,177,183] Alginates absorb exudate, facilitate moist wound healing, and can be used to obtain hemostasis in an oozing wound.[166,172,181] Excess exudate also may be absorbed with hydrophilic products.[79] Yellow wounds should be irrigated of the yellow-brown gelatinous mass that remains on the wound after dressing removal when hydrocolloids are used.[17] The yellow wound also may be dressed with a wide-meshed 4 × 4 dressing changed every 4 to 6 hours to absorb purulent drainage, or with a wet dressing saturated with saline or topical medicants. If topical medicants are used, they should not be allowed to dry out because drying increases the concentration of the medication, possibly rendering it cytotoxic.[135]

Open wounds with dead space should be lightly packed with a fine-mesh strip gauze (e.g., Nu Gauze) to keep the superficial portions of the wound open while the deeper layers contract. Tight packing should be avoided because it could retard drainage and create tissue ischemia. A fine-mesh (44/36) gauze prevents epithelial growth into the weave.[135] Despite the negative consequences to healing tissue, the use of wet-to-dry dressings perseveres due to its simplicity and long tradition.[191]

In a systematic review comparing dressings used for surgical wounds healing by secondary intention, insufficient data limited a correlation between dressing choice and wound healing.[205] Limited evidence was found, however, to support the use of foam rather than gauze in terms of pain, patient satisfaction, and decreased nursing time.[205]

Minimizing Mechanical Influences

Mechanical influences that affect healing include wound edema, hematoma, tension at the wound site or incision line, foreign bodies, crust or necrotic tissue, iatrogenic manipulation, and overly aggressive debridement.

Edema

Swelling is a normal occurrence in the inflammatory stage of wound healing, but its control decreases the inflammatory response, which in turn decreases fibrosis.[16] The edematous wound environment contributes to sustaining and perpetuating a chronic inflammatory state associated with excessive scarring.[142] Gross edema in the periwound area decreases vascularization by altering hydrostatic capillary pressure; decreased oxygen and nutrient supply subsequently decrease the proliferation of granulation tissue.[36,124,125] Therapeutic management of edema includes elevation techniques, controlled motion when possible, and application of a bulky dressing during the inflammatory stage. Single self-adherent Coban wraps control edema in digital wounds. The application of stress to injured tissues with manual exercise should be applied judiciously in all phases of wound healing. Exercise that is painful or increases swelling should be avoided.

Hematoma

Hematoma formation compromises the repair process. The space-occupying blood coagulum decreases perfusion capability, may cause graft separation or wound dehiscence, and increases the workload of the phagocytic cells.[206] The increased inflammatory response associated with hematoma increases fibrosis and scar. Hematoma also serves as a perfect culture medium for bacteria and increases the risk for infection.

Correct surgical management with proper hemostasis before closure, adequate approximation of tissue defects, and drains where deemed necessary may prevent hematoma. The postoperative bulky dressing should be used for 24 to 48 hours with most surgical wounds about the hand or wrist and continued with each dressing change for as long as the first 5 to 7 days after surgery for surgeries in the vascular forearm, such as tumor excision or release of the median or radial nerves at this level.

Large-mesh grafts, such as those that provide coverage for the dorsum of the hand, can be dressed with 4 × 4 wide-mesh gauze dressings, wet with saline, to provide a continuous wicking action for exudate and to reduce fluid viscosity. These dressings serve to protect the graft from hematoma and excess accumulation of exudate, which should cause graft separation. These dressings must be kept wet, because allowing them to dry out causes adherence and disturbs the graft tissue during removal. This regimen is carried out in a hospital environment with 24-hour elevation.[207]

Dressings that function to maintain the configuration of a wound or to ensure graft contact to the wound, such as a bolus, should be made of cotton instead of synthetic materials, which compress and lose their shape.[208]

Wound Site Tension

Wound site tension may reduce the rate of repair, compromise tensile strength, and increase the final width of the scar.[15,209,210] Excessive tension at the wound site may cause necrosis by jeopardizing local blood supply.[176,211] Sutures that are tied too tightly may need to be released; tension on an incision line may be relieved with wound tapes, pressure dressings, or orthoses that limit motion and stress.[155,156,212]

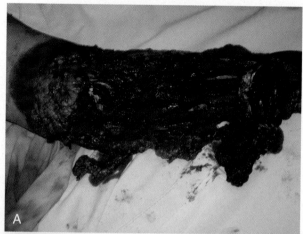
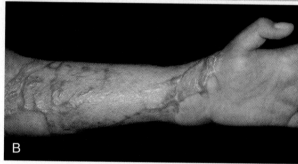

Figure 18-6 **A,** The distal left, nondominant upper extremity of a 16 year-old female after motor vehicle accident involving an 18-wheeler. **B,** Final outcome following negative-pressure wound therapy. (Photos courtesy of Dr. Miguel Pirela-Cruz, El Paso, Texas.)

Negative-Pressure Wound Therapy

Negative-pressure wound therapy is a technique for preventing hematoma formation or serum collection postoperatively as an alternative to protecting skin grafting with bolstered dressings.[213,214] The technique, termed *vacuum-assisted closure* (VAC), uses negative pressure to eliminate fluid collections, to increase oxygen tension, and to decrease contamination. Negative-pressure wound therapy is postulated to increase perfusion, nutrient delivery, and rate of granulation and decrease bacterial levels in wound tissue.[215] It was approved by the FDA in 1995 and has gained popularity due to cost savings in dressings, decreased length of stay, and decreased need for nursing care.[216]

The treatment consists of insertion of sterile sponge into the wound bed connected to the negative-pressure device by a suction hose. Pump settings are adjustable based on specific wound characteristics.[216] For acute wounds, the device is operated at a negative pressure of 125 mm Hg with a 5-minute on, 2-minute off cycle.[213,216] Following mesh skin graft, a continuous pressure setting of 50 to 75 mm Hg is recommended.[216] A nonadhesive layer is placed between the graft and the sponge, with VAC treatment commencing after 5 days.[216] Negative-pressure wound therapy has been used successfully in multitraumatic upper extremity injuries requiring extensive reconstruction and skin-grafting procedures (Fig. 18-6).

Complications with VAC use are reported as primarily technical and include pressure from evacuation tubing on surrounding tissues, maceration of skin caused by occlusive dressing, growth of granulation tissue into the foam dressing, and pain.[216] Precautions for use include active bleeding, the use of anticoagulants, and difficult hemostasis of the wound.[216] It is contraindicated for patients with untreated osteomyelitis and for wounds that are malignant, necrotic, or demonstrate eschar formation.[216] In the postoperative phase, the wound site, VAC parameters, and fluid collection are all closely monitored.[216]

VAC has been used in the treatment of degloving injuries,[217] for the coverage of radial forearm free-flap donor-site complications,[206] and for closure of chronic wounds.[218] Recently, three systematic reviews have been completed to assess recommendations and outcomes for clinical use of VAC. The first review, completed by the Agency for Healthcare Research and Quality, found the literature to be insufficient to support conclusions for effectiveness in completeness of healing, time for healing, or readiness for surgical closure.[219] A second systematic review of VAC for partial-thickness burns reported significant differences in burns at day 3 and 5 that decreased by day 14.[220] No complications were found in the studies under review; however, absence of clinically relevant outcomes such as wound-healing parameters of rate, total time, area, and proportion were identified.[220] The third review included articles that compared topical negative pressure with moistened gauze and other wound care products, such as hydrocolloids, gels, and alginates.[221] The authors found no valid or reliable evidence that topical negative pressure facilitates chronic wound healing, and no difference in effect was found in comparison to alternative dressing choices.[221]

Physical Agents

Physical agents offer the therapist additional options in wound management. The use of physical agents and their effect on cellular function is yet another expanding frontier in the area of wound manipulation, but a detailed discussion is beyond the scope of this chapter. Several sources are suggested for further study on the application of exogenously applied electrical stimulation,[8,25,53,56,184,188,222-224] the effects of ultrasound (US) on the various connective tissues,[56,225-232] and the use of heat and cold as an adjunct to wound treatment.[233-235]

Definitive research is lacking for clinical application of these modalities.[8] A number of review articles offer perspective to the clinician.[53,56,224,229,233]

A few important studies are mentioned to emphasize the point that with all applied modalities, as with other wound management techniques, the therapist should understand the physiologic response of the tissues to the treatment applied.

Electric Stimulation

Therapeutic doses of electric current have been shown to augment healing in chronic wounds in human subjects and induced wounds in animal models.[188] Studies of cell cultures have shown that electric fields can influence migrating, proliferative, and functional capacity of cells involved in the healing process, and that growth factors may be stimulated by electric current.[188] One clinical study has demonstrated the beneficial effect of pulsed electric stimulation on the healing of stage II, III, and IV chronic dermal ulcers, with

treatment times that do not exceed 60 minutes per day, 5 to 7 days per week,[188] a period substantially less than the 20 to 42 hours of stimulation per week recommended in earlier studies.[236] In vitro electric stimulation has been shown to stimulate local growth factor activity, affecting human dermal fibroblasts and leading to greater collagen synthesis.[222]

Isolated epidermal cells, cell clusters, and cell sheets have demonstrated galvanotaxis (electrotaxis) in migrating toward the cathode in in vitro studies.[186,187] Macrophages have been shown to migrate toward the anode,[237] whereas neutrophils have been observed to migrate toward both the anode and cathode.[238]

Researchers have demonstrated that dermal fibroblasts in culture, stimulated with pulsed current at 100 pulses per second (pps) and 100 V, increased the expression of receptors for transforming growth factor-β that were six times greater than those of control fibroblasts.[222] A negative effect has been demonstrated on tendon healing. The effect of pulsed electromagnetic fields (PEMF) stimulation on early flexor tendon healing in a chicken model (using a similar stimulus to that used clinically) caused a decrease in tensile strength and an increase in peritendinous adhesions.[239]

Pulsed Magnetic Field

An in vivo rat model was employed to study the effects of pulsed magnetic field (PMF) on repaired Achilles tendons.[240] Following surgery, two 30-minute sessions of PMF were applied at differing levels.[240] At 3 weeks, a 69% increase in tensile strength was noted compared with controls. The researchers in this study identified PMF as contributory to the speed and efficiency of the cellular response.[240]

Ultrasound

The effect of low-intensity US on the healing strength of 24 repaired rabbit Achilles tendons was studied.[241] The tendons were excised after nine treatments and compared with non-US-treated tendons. The US group demonstrated a significant increase in tensile strength, tensile stress, and energy absorption capacity. These findings suggest that high-intensity US is not necessary to augment the healing strength of tendons, but that low-intensity US may enhance the healing process of surgically repaired Achilles tendons.[241] Rat models have also been used to study the response of Achilles tendons to ultrasound with comparable results. Increased tensile and mechanical breaking strength[242] and increased density and orientation of collagen fibrils[243] have been noted in response to therapeutic US.

A study that describes the influence of US administered at different postoperative intervals on several aspects of healing in the surgically repaired zone II flexor tendon in 76 white leghorn chickens has indicated that use during the early stages of wound healing increases range of motion, decreases scar formation, and shows no adverse effect on strength.[244]

The effect of US on the healing human tendon has not yet been established, and US is not yet ready for clinical application. However, experimental studies suggest that positive effects are found with sonication limited to the very earliest stages of healing, and negative results when sonication is continued for several weeks.[241] Clinical guidelines in regard to timing, duration, and intensity of application have not yet been established, but these parameters evidently must be matched to specific cellular activity to maximize the effectiveness of this modality.

The effect of US on bone repair has been investigated recently. It has been demonstrated that low-intensity US can accelerate the healing of fresh fractures.[227,232] Some preliminary evidence suggests its usefulness in treatment of delayed healing and nonunions as well.[227,228] A single case study credits low-intensity US with union of an ununited hook of the hamate fracture.[226]

Nussbaum[229] provides an interesting review of studies on US of clinical interest to the hand clinician.

Scar Management

Scar management should be addressed from the first wounding day. Judicious planning of surgical procedures, full-thickness skin grafting where necessary, and infection control are immediate concerns.[33] Control of the variables that could lead to infection, an exaggerated inflammatory state, or a dehydrated wound, help minimize fibrosis and hypertrophic scarring.[17]

Adhesion control in the case of the deeper tissues is discussed in other chapters on rehabilitation of the tendon, ligament, and joint. The negative biochemical and biomechanical changes in immobilized connective tissue studied both experimentally and clinically have been defined in many articles and are not reiterated here, except to point out that some controlled motion for these deeper tissues should be applied where possible with respect to the tensile strength of the repair to maintain tissue homeostasis and to promote a more organized deposition of collagen at the wound site.[245] Motion in the inflammatory stage biochemically stimulates cellular response.[42,54,245] Early passive motion has been correlated to an increased fibronectin (FN) concentration in the adult canine tendon; by 7 days after repair, controlled motion flexor tendons had FN concentrations two times that of immobilized tendons.[42] Fibroblast chemotaxis and adherence to the substrate in the days after injury and repair appear to be directly related to FN concentration.[47] Motion during the reparative stages biomechanically affects tissue glide for tendon and ligament and nutrient transport for cartilage. Tissue engineering promises to alter the management of healing connective tissue in the future,[51] but at this writing, none of these new experimental techniques have been as effective as the application of controlled load to healing tendon and ligament.[54]

Techniques for the management of cutaneous scars—pressure garments, elastomeres, silicone gel sheeting, and the use of paper tape—are well known to the hand therapist.[34,123,167,171,210,212,246,247]

Hypertrophic scars are found most commonly in areas of high tension and movement as with the flexor surfaces of the extremities.[210] Applying tension to suture lines with aggressive orthotic positioning and exercise can contribute to hypertrophic scarring on these surfaces and functional limitation. An example of commonly misapplied force by the hand therapist occurs with postoperative Dupuytren's contractures. These cases, along with others, fare better by eliminating tension via orthotic fabrication and careful exercise technique.

Topical silicone gel sheeting (SGS) is used to prevent, control, and reduce hypertrophic scar formation.[210] Clinically, it decreases scar redness and elevation of the scar area, and patients seem to have fewer complaints about itching and painful sensations.[248]

The mechanism of action of the SGS is unknown.[210,248] Pressure exerted by the SGS applied to the scar with paper tape is negligible (<3 mm Hg).[249] Temperature and differences in oxygen transmission have been excluded. The gel is occlusive, with a water vapor loss rate lower than that of skin (4.5 vs. 8.5 $g/m^2/hr$).[123] However, other polyurethane films do not have the same effect on hypertrophic scar. Researchers postulate that because the scar surface does not become wet or macerated with prolonged wear, the SGS may promote hydration of the scar, but changes in scar water content have not been directly measured. Researchers also postulate that the reduction in water vapor loss may decrease capillary activity, thereby reducing collagen deposition and scar hypertrophy.[250] There is no histologic or scanning electron microscopic evidence of silicone absorption, but a chemical effect has not been excluded. Several clinical studies have demonstrated the clinical benefits of SGS in minimizing hypertrophic scarring in surgical scars and keloid scars with at least 12 hours of treatment daily over periods of up to 6 months.[251]

SGS also has been found to prevent development of these scars and is effective as a wound dressing. In a controlled analysis of fresh surgical incisions, SGS was found to significantly inhibit the formation of hypertrophic scar when used at least 12 hours daily for 2 months.[248] They have been used with postoperative punch grafting to prevent cobblestoning and graft dislocation, to provide sterile atmosphere for the grafts,[252] and as a method of treating painful fingertip injuries in children.[246]

Paper tape applied longitudinally along an incision line as soon as epithelialization takes place prevents wound site tension and clinically appears to minimize scarring. This technique has been studied,[167,171,212] with one researcher finding that it is even more effective than SGS.[167] Reiffel applied paper tape longitudinally along susceptible wounds and found that hypertrophic scarring was prevented.[212] He hypothesized that the tape worked by preventing longitudinal stretching of the incision line. He also proposed that SGS was effective in scar management because it prevents tension at the incision line, not because of compression forces.[212]

Summary

The wound-healing process is subject to manipulation and facilitation by the clinician. The importance of a physiologic approach to the management of both the simple and complex wound may prove to speed the processes of epithelialization and contraction and help control collagen deposition. The importance of careful attention to this aspect of our discipline cannot be overemphasized.

REFERENCES

The complete reference list is available online at www.expertconsult.com.

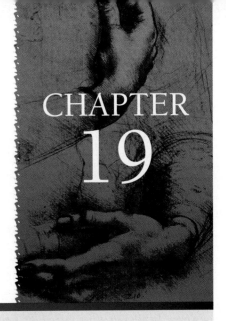

CHAPTER 19

Common Infections of the Hand

JOHN S. TARAS, MD, SIDNEY M. JACOBY, MD, AND
PAMELA J. STEELMAN, CRNP, PT, CHT

CRITICAL POINTS

Acute Paronychia

- Indication: Infection involving the nail fold, most common overall hand infection (usually *Staphylococcus aureus*).
- Diagnostic Pearls: Of all the fingertip areas, the hyponychium is most resistant to infection. Carefully evaluate for infection residing in the nearby nail plate or distal pulp.
- Pitfalls: Misdiagnosis, delayed diagnosis, failure to identify underlying osteomyelitis.
- Surgical Pearls: Incise eponychial fold with nail blade faced away from matrix to avoid nail bed injury.
- Healing timelines and progression of therapy: Daily soaks in dilute povidone-iodine (Betadine) solution; 7- to 10-day course of oral antibiotics, early digit range of motion (ROM).

Felon

- Indication: Closed space infection manifested by a tense distal pulp with or without fluctuance.
- Pitfalls: Misdiagnosis, incomplete decompression of all involved septa, iatrogenic digital nerve or vessel injury, creation of unstable pulp.
- Surgical Pearls: Incision is dictated by the point of maximal tenderness and location of any fluctuance. Digital nerves and vessels at risk, avoid incisions that cross the flexion creases.
- Healing timelines and progression of therapy: Gauze wick for 48 to 72 hours, IV antibiotics for inpatients, Betadine soaks at least three times per day, early digit ROM.

Pyogenic Flexor Tenosynovitis

- Indication: Based on the four classic findings of Kanavel
  1. Fusiform swelling of the digit
  2. Semiflexed posture of the digit
  3. Pain with passive extension of the digit
  4. Tenderness along the flexor tendon sheath
- Pearls: Pain with palpation along flexor tendon sheath and with passive stretch are the most reliable clinical findings; early tenosynovitis may be treated with antibiotics, elevation, and frequent evaluation.
- Surgical Pearls: Early decompression is warranted if symptoms fail to resolve; operative management with sheath irrigation is effective. Irrigate until the effluent within the sheath is clear.
- Healing timelines and progression of therapy: IV antibiotics, repeat debridement if symptoms do not improve, soaks in Betadine solution, pain management to allow early digit ROM.

Fascial Space Infections

- Indications: Dorsal subcutaneous, dorsal subaponeurotic, hypothenar, thenar, and midpalmar space infections. Most are usually the result of penetrating trauma to the hand.
- Diagnostic Pearls: Deep space infections characterized by wide abduction of the digits, difficulty with motion, loss of palmar concavity, semi-flexed positioning and pain with passive stretch.
- Surgical Pearls: Separate dorsal and volar incisions should be utilized. Particular care should be taken to avoid the superficial palmar arch, digital neurovasculature, and deep palmar arch.

233

- Pitfalls: Delay in diagnosis, inadequate decompression, iatrogenic injury to digital neurovascular structures.
- Healing timelines and progression of therapy: IV antibiotics, repeat debridement if symptoms do not improve, soaks in Betadine solution, pain management to allow early digit ROM.

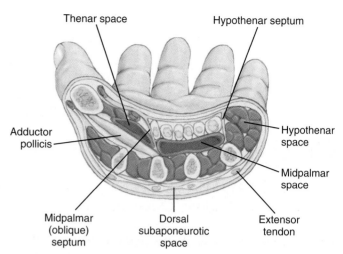

Figure 19-1 Cross-sectional anatomy of hand showing thenar, midpalmar, hypothenar, interdigital (web), and dorsal subaponeurotic spaces. (From Wright PE II: Hand infections. In: Canale ST, ed. *Campbell's Operative Orthopaedics*, 11th ed, Philadelphia, Mosby, 2008, p. 4349.)

Since the discovery of penicillin in 1944 and the pioneering work of Dr. Allen Kanavel, the noted Chicago general surgeon who treated hand infections in the preantibiotic era (early 20th century), the incidence of hand infections has declined and the ability to recognize and treat these maladies has improved. Despite the advances of modern medical care, however, hand and wrist infections remain among the most disabling ailments affecting the upper extremity.[1,2] Hand infections vary from routine problems treated with oral antibiotics, immobilization, and limited incision and drainage to catastrophic surgical emergencies resulting in significant deformity, pain, and loss of function.

A hand infection can predispose the individual to a lifetime of disability, which is why patients often require prolonged hospitalization and rehabilitation. In most cases, a hand infection begins with a minor penetrating trauma or small open wound.[2-7]

Its character and progression are determined by several factors, including its specific location within the specialized tissues, the host environment, the virulence of the particular organism, and, importantly, the administration of timely, appropriate care.[8] A key to minimizing the incidence and severity of hand infections is the prompt administration of treatment for even the most minor injuries. The purpose of this review chapter is to provide a systematic approach to the diagnosis, examination, evaluation, and treatment of both common and uncommon hand infections.

General Considerations

Injuries that break the skin barrier almost always create a wound contaminated by bacteria. Whether the microorganisms multiply and establish an infection is determined by both their virulence and the host's immune response.[6] Poor arterial blood supply, venous congestion,[7] the presence of necrotic or damaged tissue,[6,9] and the presence of foreign bodies are all local factors that increase the likelihood of infection. A patient's resistance can be compromised by certain systemic conditions, the most common of which is diabetes mellitus, which affects 5% to 7% of the adult population of the United States.[9-12] Other patient conditions include AIDS,[13] Raynaud's disease, agranulocytosis, severe chronic illness, immunosuppressive therapy, malnutrition, alcoholism, chronic steroid use, and drug abuse.

Although almost any type of microorganism can cause a hand infection, most cases involve *Staphylococcus aureus* (50% to 80%)[14] and β-hemolytic streptococci (15%).[4,15] The next most common pathogens are *Aerobacter aerogenes* (10%), *Enterococcus* (10%), and *Escherichia coli* (5%).[4] Infections resulting from penetrating trauma usually involve a single species, but those associated with bites and IV drug use are polymicrobic in more than 50% of cases.[15-17] Initial antibiotic therapy traditionally has been empirical, depending on the results of the Gram stain and the most likely organism. The emergence of community-acquired methicillin-resistant *Staphylococcus aureus* (MRSA) has recently become a particularly relevant topic. Multiple studies have shown that the overall prevalence of MRSA ranges anywhere from 34% to 61% in the general population. With an increasing incidence of MRSA, health care providers should consider the use of initial antibiotic therapy targeted against MRSA with the aim of more quickly targeting the causative organism.[18,19] Furthermore, the addition of antibiotics effective against gram-negative organisms has been recommended for high-risk situations, such as infections in IV drug abusers and contaminated outdoor or farm-related injuries. Tables 19-1 and 19-2 summarize the most commonly used antibiotics, antifungals, and antiviral agents used today.

Anatomy

A thorough understanding of the hand's specialized anatomy is crucial in determining the ease of penetration, localization, and spread of infection. An appreciation for the intricate anatomy of the hand also allows for precise surgical exploration and drainage without injuring vital structures or extending the infection to uninvolved tissues.[20] The skin, subcutaneous tissue, tendon sheaths, and joint spaces are some of the specialized structures in the hand, and their anatomy is addressed elsewhere in this text. The fascial spaces and lymphatics are other important components of the hand's anatomy and merit a brief review at this time.

The hand contains five fascial spaces in which pus can accumulate: (1) dorsal subcutaneous, (2) dorsal subaponeurotic, (3) hypothenar, (4) thenar, and (5) midpalmar[20] (Fig. 19-1). Other spaces that provide an optimal environment for the rapid growth of microorganisms include the flexor tendon sheaths and the joint spaces, which contain synovial fluid and are lined with a specialized layer of synovial tissue. Infections within the synovial spaces are among the most devastating of all hand disorders.

The lymphatics of the hand can be classified into two types according to their origin and location. The superficial lymphatics arise in the skin and course through the subcutaneous tissue, and the deep lymphatics arise in deeper tissue and follow the blood vessels.[10] The lymph vessels in the fingers follow the digital arteries and are most abundant on the volar surface. From this point, the channels flow dorsally in the interdigital spaces along the medial and lateral borders of the hand[21] and then travel proximally up the dorsal surface.[10] This anatomic pathway explains how a primary infection in the palmar surface can initially present with dorsal swelling.[10,20,22,23]

Diagnosis

The routine evaluation of a patient with a suggested hand infection consists of a thorough medical history,[11] physical examination, and both standard radiographic and specialized imaging studies as needed. Identification of organisms with culture and antibiotic sensitivity studies aids in the diagnosis of more serious infections and in choosing direct antimicrobial therapy. Surgical procedures, including drainage of abscesses and debridement of necrotic tissues, may be required based on the identification and virulence of the isolated organism(s).

The history usually discloses a trivial injury in which the patient either delayed seeking care or where inappropriate care was initially delivered. If so, it is important to determine the environment in which the injury occurred because it may help to identify the type of organism responsible for the infection. The time course of symptoms is also important, as some infections can be treated with immobilization, antibiotics, and observation, but others may require early surgical drainage and debridement. Significant medical conditions should also be noted because some, including gout, pseudogout, foreign bodies, silicone synovitis, rheumatoid arthritis, and nonspecific tenosynovitis, among others, can easily be confused with infections. Finally, a complete list of medications, particularly antibiotics, should be ascertained.

Erythema, heat, swelling, and a restriction of motion are nonspecific signs of inflammation that are often present in an established infection. Important clues about the location of the infection can be obtained by determining the site of maximum tenderness in relation to the compartments of the hand. Inspection of proximal regions can reveal lymphangitic spread. Areas of fluctuance and spontaneous drainage of purulent material make the diagnosis of a suppurative infection more likely. Radiographs should be reviewed for foreign bodies, osteomyelitis, and fractures. Air density in the soft tissues may indicate gas gangrene, a rapidly progressive and destructive infection caused by clostridial or other anaerobic gas-producing microorganisms. Ancillary laboratory studies, including peripheral white blood count, erythrocyte sedimentation rate, and C-reactive protein titer, are also helpful in confirming the presence of infection and following the body's response to treatment. Additional imaging studies including MRI and ultrasound can be helpful in localizing

deep fluid collections, and indium-labeled radionuclide imaging may be helpful in diagnosing osteomyelitis.

Drainage from wounds should be evaluated with a Gram stain and culture before antibiotics are administered. Initial cultures should always test for both aerobic and anaerobic microorganisms. Special culture media may be required when the presence of certain pathogens such as fungi, atypical mycobacteria, and viruses is suggested.[15]

Although the concept of quantitative bacteriology dates back to World War I, a definitive technique for wound assessment was developed only in recent years.[24] It has been determined that approximately 10^5 bacteria per gram of tissue are required to sustain a clinical infection; however, tissue is rendered more susceptible to bacterial invasion by certain mechanisms such as crushing, shredding, chemical injury, and the presence of penetrating foreign bodies.[14] Patients with more severe infections should be evaluated with a complete blood count and a blood glucose test to screen for diabetes.[11]

Classification

Depending on the tissues involved, four types of hand infections are possible: (1) superficial spreading (cellulitis and lymphangitis), (2) subcutaneous abscess, (3) synovial sheath, and (4) fascial space. Patients usually have one type of infection, but in rare cases, some combination of the these possibilities may exist.[3,20,22] It is vitally important to distinguish an acute spreading infection involving the skin, subcutaneous tissue, or lymphatics from a localized abscess or closed-space infection because the treatment approach for these two entities differs.[5,6]

Principles of Management

Prompt, appropriate care is critical in the management of hand infections. Few significant infections develop after a severe open injury because early wound care is usually administered. Most cases that culminate in bad outcomes usually involve an ostensibly trivial injury that was either neglected or treated inadequately.

Primary care of open hand wounds begins with the application of basic principles espoused by Hippocrates centuries ago and include gentle irrigation to remove debris and foreign bodies, debridement of devitalized tissue, and the application of a dressing to protect against secondary contamination.[5] After an infection has established itself in a hand wound, the anatomic boundaries of the infected area should be defined because the type of infection determines the therapeutic plan. Treatment may include supportive measures, antimicrobial therapy, wound care, surgical drainage, or physical therapy to regain motion and prevent contractures.[8,25,26]

Wound management is critical to resolving infection and allowing for therapeutic intervention to be introduced in a safe and timely manner. Table 19-3 summarizes the authors' preferred wound strategy. Superficial wound infections can often be managed at home with careful patient teaching. The wound can be cleansed daily with soap and running water. A sterile nonstick dressing such as Vaseline gauze can be

Table 19-3 Preferred Strategy for Wound Management

Wound Type	Clean	Infected
Superficial open	Daily self wound care Cleanse with soap and running water Apply nonstick topical dressing (moisture barrier) Clean gauze wrap Self ROM program	Establish empirical antibiotic treatment Daily self or supervised wound care program Cleanse with soap and water or sterile saline Apply sterile nonstick topical dressing Clean gauze wrap Self or supervised ROM program
Chronic nonhealing Superficial open	Apply papain/urea ointment (Panafil) to clean wound Treat as above	Apply papain/urea ointment (Panafil) to clean wound Treat as above
Deep open	Supervised dressing change every day or every 2nd day Cleansing with soap and running water or sterile whirlpool Pack wound with dry, sterile plain or iodoform packing Top with nonstick topical dressing Clean gauze wrap Splint immobilization for comfort Supervised or self ROM program	Establish empirical antibiotic therapy Supervised dressing change every day or every 2nd day Cleansing with soap and running water or sterile whirlpool Pack wound with dry, sterile plain or iodoform packing Top with sterile nonstick topical dressing Sterile gauze wrap Splint immobilization for comfort Supervised ROM program
Chronic nonhealing Deep open	Apply papain/urea ointment (Panafil) to clean wound Treat as above	Apply papain/urea ointment (Panafil) to clean wound Treat as above
Closed infection		Establish empirical antibiotic therapy Splint immobilization for comfort Supervised edema control Supervised ROM program

*Enzymatic debriding-healing ointment, Healthpoint, Ltd. (Fort Worth, Texas).
ROM, range of motion.

applied directly to the wound to act as a moisture barrier. The dressing is finished with a clean gauze wrap. Gauze dressings should be applied in a manner that addresses wound drainage while allowing maximum joint mobility. Deep wounds or wounds with tracts may require sterile whirlpool or supervised therapist cleansing on a daily or every other day schedule, depending on the degree of drainage and inflammation. After cleansing, deeper wounds can be packed with sterile plain or iodoform packing strips and then dressed in the same manner as a superficial wound. In cases of chronic, nonhealing wounds, topical enzymatic debriders such as papain/urea ointment (Panafil) (Healthpoint, Ltd., Fort Worth, Texas) can be applied directly to the wound just prior to application of the moisture barrier. Application of topical antibiotic preparations is not recommended. When wounds are fully healed, application of a dye and fragrance-free moisturizer followed by a moisture barrier aids in restoring the scar area to a healthy state.

Immobilization should be avoided whenever possible as the sequelae of hand infection can lead to fibrosis and contracture. Instead, the component problems of infection, including wounds, edema, inflammation, pain, scarring, and limitation of motion, should be addressed with specific therapeutic interventions designed to address the target tissue. When an infection is accompanied by acute inflammation, a short course of immobilization may be indicated to control pain, prevent the spread of infection through tissue planes, and prevent undesirable joint postures which would lead to contracture and limit hand function. Orthotic immobilization should include only those joints and structures necessary to control inflammation, spread of infection, and contracture formation. Elevation of the affected limb allows early resolution of swelling and an expedient progression of specific rehabilitation protocols. Moist heat can increase local circulation and antibiotic delivery and is especially useful in the treatment of superficial spreading infections. Heat also promotes the ease of joint movement. A program of ROM exercise should be introduced as early in the course of hand infection as is safe given the specifics of the infection. Adjacent joints should be mobilized in all cases, even when specific immobilization is indicated.

When the acute inflammation has subsided, the patient should be progressed to active and passive ROM exercises in all joints to tolerance. Early ROM along with elevation aids edema control, which is critical to controlling pain and preventing fibrosis and contracture. Retrograde massage is to be avoided in the presence of an active infection because it may cause the infection to spread proximally.

The use of antibiotics depends on the clinical situation. Minor infections often resolve with supportive measures alone. Oral antibiotics are effective in the management of superficial infections, and IV antibiotics play a critical role in the treatment of severe infections. The choice of drug is based on the culture results, but initial therapy is directed against the most likely pathogens. A first-generation cephalosporin is generally prescribed because it is effective against most staphylococci and streptococci. Patients who are immunocompromised or have devitalized wounds are more prone to severe infections and should receive broader antibiotic coverage, preferably by the IV route. The detailed aspects of antimicrobial therapy are beyond the scope of this discussion, and the interested reader is referred to specialized texts on the subject.[9,11,27,28] Tetanus prophylaxis is essential in all wounds with soil, animal, oral, or fecal contamination. The patient with a tetanus-prone wound who has never been immunized should be administered 0.5 mL of absorbed tetanus toxoid along with 250 to 500 units of tetanus immune globulin intramuscularly at different injection sites with different syringes. Penicillin also may be considered.[4]

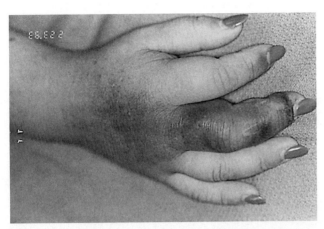

Figure 19-2 Cellulitis. Swelling and redness are present over the dorsum of the middle finger. Note the extension over the back of the hand.

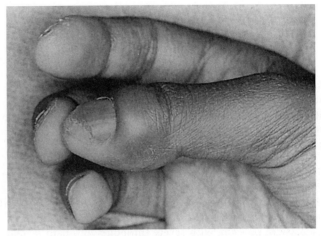

Figure 19-3 This acute paronychia involving the proximal nail fold requires incision and drainage.

Types of Infections

Superficial Spreading Infections

Cellulitis

Cellulitis is a superficial infection of the skin and subcutaneous layer that is characterized by the absence of pus or localized abscess (Fig. 19-2). An area on the dorsum of the finger or hand is usually involved, and the responsible organism is usually streptococcal. Typically, there is a history of a scratch, minor cut, or puncture. The affected area is warm, erythematous, and tender. Treatment involves supportive measures, including elevation, orthotic fabrication, warm compresses, and administration of antibiotics with activity against *Streptococcus*. If the patient has systemic symptoms or a compromised immune system, hospitalization and IV antibiotics may be necessary. After the acute inflammation is controlled, ROM exercises should be initiated to further assist in edema control and prevent joint stiffness.

Lymphangitis

Lymphangitis is much less common than cellulitis but is one of the most serious and rapidly progressing types of hand infections. It often develops from a trivial injury that has been neglected. It can also result from direct inoculation of an extremely virulent organism, usually β-hemolytic *Streptococcus*. The organism spreads quickly through the lymphatics and may produce a generalized infection within a few hours.[6] Red streaking develops from the site of inoculation proximally up the hand and forearm, along the pathways of the lymphatic channels. If untreated, an abscess may form about the elbow or in the axilla near the lymph nodes. Prompt recognition and hospitalization are essential. Treatment includes parenteral antibiotics with activity against *Streptococcus*. In addition, immobilization, elevation, and warm moist compresses are useful therapeutic adjuncts. Unlike closed-space infections, surgical drainage is reserved for cases in which there is definite evidence of localized pus and abscess formation or tissue necrosis.[5]

Subcutaneous Abscesses

Paronychias

A paronychia, otherwise known as a "runaround" infection, is a bacterial infection of the soft tissue fold around the fingernail (eponychium). It is one of the most common hand infections and often begins as a cellulitis of the skin surrounding the nail plate and progresses to pus formation. Acute pyogenic paronychias usually are caused by a hangnail or poor nail hygiene, and the most common isolated organism is *Staphylococcus aureus*. In late cases, the abscess may extend to all three borders of the nail fold (run-around abscess) or spread beneath the nail plate (Fig. 19-3).[4] The treatment of early paronychias consists of warm soaks and antibiotics. However, surgical drainage is necessary after an abscess has formed. If pus has accumulated beneath the nail, partial or even complete nail plate removal may be necessary to achieve adequate drainage.

Chronic paronychias differ from the acute form in that the offending organism usually includes *Candida albicans* along with the pyogenic bacteria (Fig. 19-4). Individuals with occu-

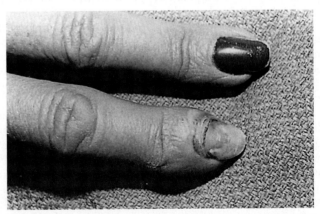

Figure 19-4 Chronic paronychia caused by a combination of bacterial and fungal microorganisms.

pational exposure to moisture appear to be more prone to the chronic variety.[29] The treatment of this condition, which has been less successful than that for acute paronychias, involves partial or complete nail plate removal. Often, long periods of topical antimicrobial agents are needed. Keyser and Eaton[30] have recommended eponychial marsupialization, which requires removing an elliptical segment of skin in the proximal nail fold and permitting adequate drainage from the infected proximal nail bed.

Felons

The distal digital pulp is divided into many tiny separate compartments that are essentially specialized fibrous septa that extend from the skin to the bone. Because of the fixed septa, infection or swelling of the pulp produces a marked increase in pressure with severe throbbing and pain. A felon is a deep infection of the finger pad that involves these small, discrete compartments. There is usually a history of a puncture wound or other penetrating injury. Pus formed in a closed space under pressure causes intense pain, throbbing, marked tenderness, redness, and tense swelling over the fingertip pad. Treatment consists of surgical drainage. The incision may be made directly over the point of the abscess or through its midlateral aspect. After drainage, the wound may be kept open with a loose pack that can be removed for finger soaks.[14,27,29]

Subepidermal Abscesses

Subcutaneous abscesses are localized collections of pus at the subcuticular level. They can occur in the palm or on the volar pads of the fingers between the flexor creases (Fig. 19-5A, B). Like felons, they are usually caused by *S. aureus*. The abscess usually points toward the skin, and it resolves rapidly with simple incision and drainage. If left untreated, it may track deep and invade the flexor sheath or deep compartment of the palm.[11]

Flexor Sheath Infections

Infection within the flexor sheath, or purulent flexor tenosynovitis, is one of the most destructive and devastating of all hand infections. They usually develop after a puncture wound over the flexor crease at the level of the interphalangeal or metacarpophalangeal joint, where the skin is separated from the flexor sheath by only a thin layer of subcutaneous tissue (Fig. 19-6A). This condition also can result from direct extension of a pulp-space infection. Hematogenous spread has occurred in rare cases. *Staphylococcus* or *Streptococcus* is usually responsible, but other organisms such as mycobacteria and *Neisseria gonorrhoeae* can also be causative agents.

The flexor tendon sheath is a closed space rich in synovial fluid and therefore provides an excellent milieu for bacterial growth. After inoculation, the infection spreads rapidly within the confines of the sheath. Even if this infection is identified and treated early, it may still result in permanent adhesions and scarring and severely limit flexor tendon gliding and motion.[1] Sufficient pressure may build to result in tendon necrosis, destruction of the flexor sheath, and extension of pus into the subcutaneous space.

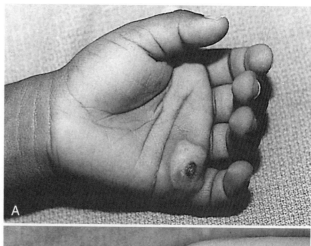
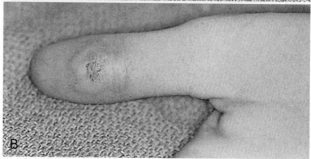

Figure 19-5 Subepidermal abscess of the distal palm **(A)** and volar pad of the thumb **(B)**.

Flexor tenosynovitis can be recognized by the four cardinal signs of Kanavel:[22] (1) flexed posture of the digit, (2) uniform swelling of the digit, (3) tenderness over the length of the involved tendon sheath, and (4) severe pain on attempted hyperextension of the digit (Fig. 19-7).

Infection of the flexor sheath represents a true hand surgery emergency. Prompt recognition is critical to avoiding rapid progression of the infection and destruction of the flexor tendon and sheath. Treatment involves emergent surgical decompression and drainage with irrigation catheters within the flexor sheath (Fig. 19-6B). Patients are hospitalized, and parenteral antibiotics are administered.

In rare cases when the symptoms and infection are recognized early (i.e., within 24 hours), a brief trial of parenteral antibiotics, immobilization, and elevation may be attempted, and resolution might be achieved without surgery. However, if the signs of infection do not resolve rapidly, surgical treatment is required.[4,11]

Fascial-Space Infections

As previously mentioned, pus can accumulate in five fascial spaces: (1) the dorsal subcutaneous, (2) dorsal subaponeurotic, (3) hypothenar, (4) thenar, and (5) midpalmar. Accurate diagnosis and treatment relies on knowing the boundaries of these spaces and the most common routes of extension. Fascial space infections must be differentiated from the two other serious purulent hand infections, those of the flexor sheath and lymphangitis.

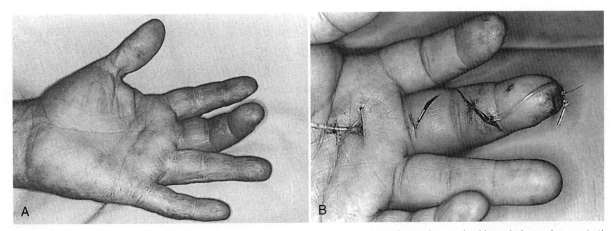

Figure 19-6 Flexor sheath infection. **A,** The hand is shown 24 hours after a puncture wound over the proximal interphalangeal crease in the middle finger. **B,** Treatment involved open irrigation and drainage of the flexor sheath in the finger and palm.

Treatment consists of surgical drainage, which is best done in the operating room under general anesthesia and tourniquet control. Incisions are made to provide adequate drainage, with care taken to avoid extending the infection to adjacent uninfected spaces. Standard sterile technique and precautions are used to prevent secondary contamination by more virulent microorganisms.[3,20,31]

Common Sources of Infection

Human Bites

Depending on the status of an individual's oral hygiene, human saliva may contain as many as 42 species of bacteria and up to 10^8 organisms per milliliter.[23,32,33] The bacteria commonly isolated from human bite wounds include streptococci, staphylococci and other micrococci, spirochetes, *Clostridium, Bacteroides, Fusobacterium, Neisseria,* and other gram-negative species. More rarely, this route has transmitted *Actinomyces, Treponema pallidum,* hepatitis B virus, and *Mycobacterium tuberculosis.*[8,14,28,29,32] Hand wounds contaminated by human saliva are caused by biting, fist-to-mouth contact, nail biting, and accidental penetration by a toothpick or dental instrument.[23] Wounds that are caused by fist-to-mouth contact have the highest incidence of complications and usually occur over the dorsal aspect of the third, fourth, or fifth metacarpophalangeal joint. This area is especially susceptible to infection because the skin over the knuckle is pliant and provides only a thin barrier to the ligaments, synovial space, and articular cartilage over the metacarpal head.[28]

Human bites to the hand usually occur during "evening scuffles," as a clenched fist strikes the mouth of another individual. For a variety of reasons, including inebriation, the patient is often too embarrassed to seek treatment until several days after the incident (Fig. 19-8A, B). Such a delay often necessitates aggressive management to prevent a progressive and severe infection. The wound must be vigorously cleansed and debrided (Fig. 19-8C) and the patient administered broad-spectrum IV antibiotics. Wound care, whirlpool therapy, and ROM exercises must be initiated early to prevent severe tissue fibrosis and contractures. The wound is left open to heal by secondary intention.

Animal Bites

Dogs are responsible for 90% of animal bite wounds, with cats being a distant second (5%).[34] The incidence of infection associated with cat bites, however, is nearly three times greater than that associated with dog bites. This kind of injury may result in a rapidly progressive cellulitis or lymphangitis, especially if treatment is not obtained.[35] *Pasteurella* species, especially *Pasteurella canis* in dog bites and *Pasteurella multocida* subspecies in cat bites, are the characteristic species isolated from these wounds.[17,35] The laboratory should be notified in advance of the possibility of *Pasteurella* species to optimize identification (Fig. 19-9), as cultures often show a polymicrobial infection. Treatment involves cleansing the wound and debridement of any devitalized or necrotic tissue. The wound is left open, and the patient given either combination therapy with penicillin and a first-generation cephalosporin or clindamycin and a fluoroquinolone for *P. multocida* infection.[8,17,34,35]

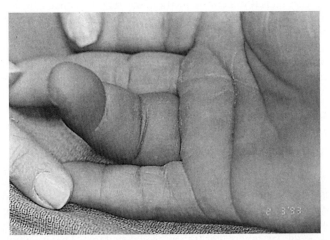

Figure 19-7 The cardinal signs of Kanavel (flexed posture of the digit, uniform swelling, tenderness over the flexor sheath, and pain on hyperextension) indicate the presence of a purulent flexor sheath infection.

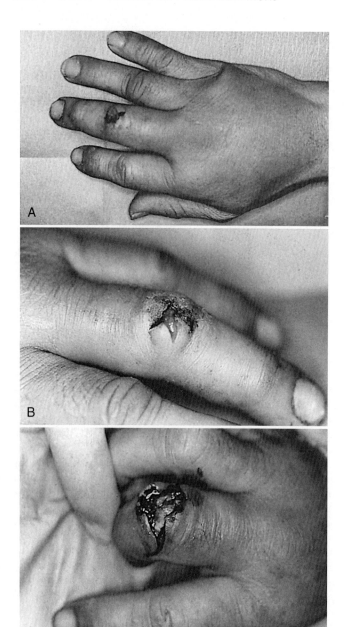

Figure 19-8 A, Appearance of a human bite wound in a bar patron 2 days after a brawl. **B,** There is pus and necrosis of the extensor tendon and surrounding tissues. **C,** Treatment involved surgical irrigation and debridement. Note the extensive involvement of the articular cartilage of the proximal interphalangeal joint.

Intravenous Drug Abuse

IV drug abusers commonly develop abscesses over the dorsum of the hand or forearm at the sites of attempted venous access (Fig. 19-10A, B). Such infections are caused by a combination of locally introduced exogenous pathogens, as well as chemical necrosis from the extravasation of injected materials. Management of hand infections in the IV drug abuser is complicated because the patient is often extremely unreliable and usually seeks treatment only when the infection has reached an advanced stage. Treatment is also more difficult because the individual may be further debilitated by

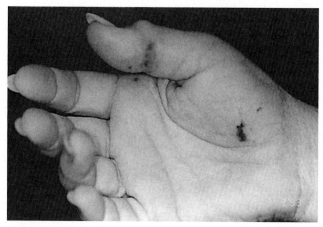

Figure 19-9 Multiple puncture wounds from cat bites, with secondary cellulitis. *Pasteurella multocida* was cultured from the wound drainage.

an altered immune response secondary to malnutrition, chronic infection such as from HIV[36,37] or some other pathogen, or possibly a combination of these factors

Subcutaneous abscesses are incised, drained, and allowed to close secondarily. Infections of the flexor sheath, joint space, and fascial space should be identified and surgically decompressed through appropriate incisions. Broad-spectrum antibiotics should be instituted immediately and the antimicrobial therapy modified when the culture results are obtained. Because of their poor compliance, these patients should be hospitalized until their acute infection has resolved.

Certain drug-abusing individuals may become so desperate for intravascular access for their drug, they may use their radial or ulnar artery as a dangerous alternative site for drug injection. In these patients, the major problem becomes chemical vasculitis rather than infection. Distal necrosis of the digit or hand with dry gangrene and ischemic pain may result.[38] Supportive measures used to treat this problem consist of antibiotics and local wound care. Necrosis in the region supplied by the artery and amputation typically follows.

Mycobacteria

Mycobacterial infections in the hand may be caused by any one of several species, including *Mycobacterium tuberculosis, Mycobacterium marinum, Mycobacterium avium, and Mycobacterium intracellulare.* They most often present as indolent processes that affect the skin, flexor tendon sheaths, carpal canal, extensor tendons, and synovium on the dorsum of the wrist. Infections caused by *M. tuberculosis* have a clinical presentation similar to that of rheumatoid arthritis (Fig. 19-11A, B). Many times there is a delay between the onset of symptoms and diagnosis (often months), and some patients have no history of pulmonary involvement.[39,40]

Of the atypical mycobacteria, *M. marinum* is the species most often responsible for hand infections.[41,42] This organism is a common contaminant of warm water environments, and exposure typically occurs when the patient suffers a skin abrasion or puncture wound while at the beach, lake, river, or pool, or when working with a fish tank. The infection presents as either a chronic skin ulceration or a localized tenosynovitis along the digital flexor sheath, carpal tunnel,

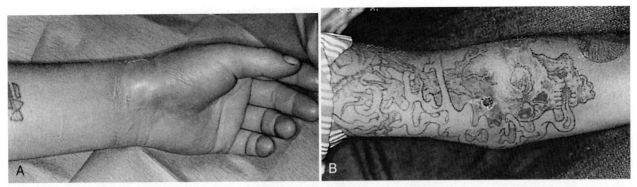

Figure 19-10 Infection secondary to IV drug abuse. **A,** Subcutaneous abscess over the volar radial wrist in a young female drug addict. Note the scars indicating sites of past infection and surgical debridement. **B,** Appearance of a subcutaneous abscess in the antecubital fossa after surgical drainage. The infection had developed after IV injection of cocaine. Multiple tattoos may mask needle marks, or "tracks."

or extensor tendons over the dorsum of the wrist (Fig. 19-12A, B).[16,43] *M. marinum* must be cultured on special media at 30° to 32°C; therefore, it is critical to instruct the microbiology lab to test for this organism. Deep infections are treated by surgical synovectomy and prolonged antituberculous medication.

Viruses

Herpetic whitlow is a superficial infection that manifests as clear vesicles on or near the finger pad. It is often seen in children and medical and dental personnel (Fig. 19-13A). There may or may not be a history of herpes simplex infection elsewhere in the body. It may be accompanied by axillary and epitrochlear adenopathy. The diagnosis can be made on the basis of the clinical appearance and confirmed using the fluorescent antibody test. If recognized early and left to run its 2- to 4-week course, this infection is self-limited. IV antibiotics and acyclovir may be utilized to limit the duration of the outbreak.[42] Incision and drainage should be avoided because it prolongs recovery and may lead to bacterial superinfection (Fig. 19-13B).[7,29,42,44]

Pyogenic Granuloma

A pyogenic granuloma is a growth of granulation tissue above the skin caused by a chronic low-grade infection or foreign body. Continuously moist local environments and bandages

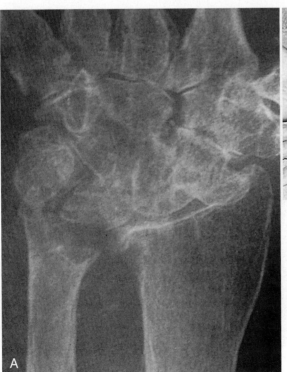

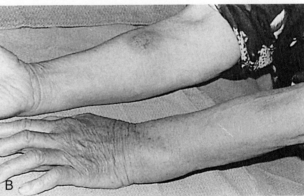

Figure 19-11 This woman from Southeast Asia presented with isolated wrist pain that was thought to be secondary to inflammatory arthritis. **A,** Radiographs demonstrated bony destruction. **B,** The soft tissue over the wrist was swollen, and the purified protein derivative (PPD) skin test on the opposite forearm was positive. Surgical specimens revealed acid-fast bacilli, and cultures were positive for *Mycobacterium tuberculosis*.

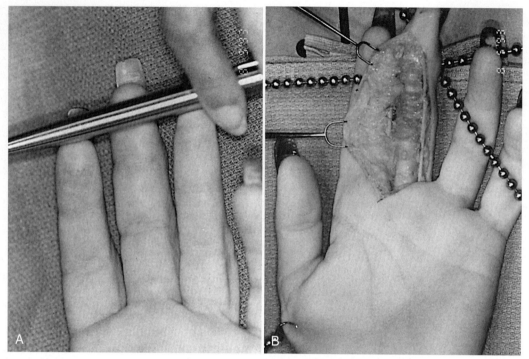

Figure 19-12 A, Chronic *Mycobacterium marinum* infection involving the flexor sheath of the middle finger. **B,** Surgical exposure of the flexor sheath demonstrated extensive tenosynovitis.

favor their development. These infections are common and appear as red friable growths that bleed readily with little provocation (Fig. 19-14A to C). Simple curettage and cauterization with silver nitrate may be performed in the office and is usually curative. Operative excision may be necessary for larger lesions.[4,8]

Summary

The critical step in the treatment of hand infections is a high clinical suspicion that directs the appropriate utilization of laboratory and imaging modalities culminating in an accurate diagnosis. Treating physicians must provide emergent care

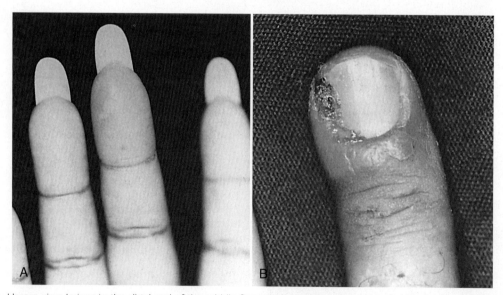

Figure 19-13 A, Herpes virus lesions in the distal pad of the middle finger in a respiratory therapist. **B,** Herpes virus vesicles around the nail fold with a secondary bacterial infection that developed after incision and drainage.

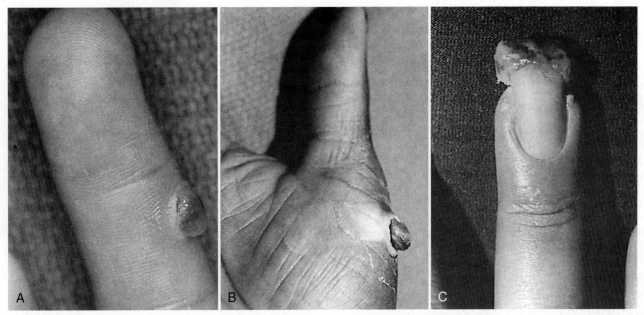

Figure 19-14 Pyogenic granuloma. **A** and **B,** Typical appearance of the lesion. **C,** This large lesion of the distal tip of the ring finger developed after the patient sustained a puncture wound.

for all open hand wounds, including irrigation and debridement, targeted antibiotic therapy, a short period of immobilization, and finally the judicious use of hand rehabilitation modalities, which may include moist heat, gentle ROM exercises, and edema control. The severity and progression of hand infections are determined in part by host factors, but also by the virulence of the organism. It is therefore imperative that the treating physician consider both the immune status of the individual as well as the characteristics of the organism. Common pathogens and sources of transmission must be recognized and treated expeditiously. If neglected, infections involving the hand may result in permanent disability of the upper extremity.

Appropriate treatment of hand infections includes a combination of the judicious use of antibiotics; appropriate therapeutic interventions to promote wound healing, control edema, and prevent contracture; and surgical decompression and debridement as necessary. With this philosophy, hand surgeons and therapists can guide the patient through a difficult clinical situation with the hope of achieving a functional, painless limb.

REFERENCES

The complete reference list is available online at www.expertconsult.com.

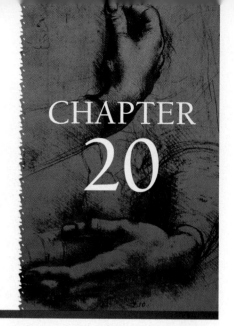

Management of Skin Grafts and Flaps

L. SCOTT LEVIN, MD, FACS

PATIENT ASSESSMENT
MANAGEMENT STRATEGY
SUMMARY

CRITICAL POINTS

- Reconstructive surgery of the upper limb has been advanced by the continual addition and use of new flaps and the increasing use of functional free tissue transfer, with improved microsurgical techniques, postoperative management, and intensive rehabilitation.
- Soft tissue reconstruction options include primary closure, delayed primary closure, healing by secondary intention, skin grafting, local tissue transfer, free tissue transfer, or any combination of these techniques.
- An algorithmic approach to reconstruction of the upper extremity for the evaluation and treatment of upper extremity wounds and defects is based on the extent and severity of the wounds, the functional needs of the patient, and the availability of required tissue elements. This algorithmic approach facilitates localized healing and optimizes each individual patient's functional rehabilitation and overall recovery.

Reconstructive surgery of the upper extremity has developed significantly over the last four decades. Microsurgical techniques, a variety of new flaps, and the increasing use of functional free tissue transfer have greatly enhanced the armamentarium of reconstructive surgical concepts and procedures.[1] At the same time, the continuing sophistication of postoperative wound management has created an optimal environment for wound healing, rehabilitation, and overall recovery. Reconstructive surgery has evolved from the practice of simply providing soft tissue coverage for traumatic defects, to a complex algorithmic process of wound management involving thorough clinical assessment, evaluation of individual functional and social needs of the patient, creation and implementation of a surgical plan, and meticulous

postoperative management. The algorithmic approach offers a reconstructive ladder for the evaluation and treatment of wounds, ranging from acute traumatic injuries to various chronic conditions, including osteomyelitis, nonhealing wounds, and defects following tumor resection.[2] This ladder directs the reconstructive surgeon to the indicated reconstructive surgical approach, based on the extent and severity of the wound, the functional needs of the patient, and the availability of required tissue elements. The initial goal of the reconstructive surgeon is the reconstitution of the soft tissue envelope, providing a well-vascularized, healthy environment to facilitate localized healing. With successful recovery and healing, the reconstructive surgeon can attain the ultimate goal of optimizing rehabilitation based on individual needs, thus maximizing functional restoration, providing patients with the opportunity for rapid social reintegration and the overall improvement of their quality, productive recovery. This chapter discusses an algorithmic approach to reconstruction of the hand and upper extremity, providing examples of excellent reconstructive options for complex surgical problems, ranging from skin grafts, to local tissue flaps, to advanced free tissue transfer. Management strategies for facilitating localized healing and optimizing functional rehabilitation and recovery are outlined.

Patient Assessment

The first step in developing a reconstructive strategy is the assessment of the patient. The surgeon must recognize the clinical reconstructive needs of the patient, based on the severity of a traumatic injury, the extent and complexity of a chronic wound, or a malignant tumor requiring resection. Important considerations include age, significant medical conditions, preinjury functional status, occupation, dominance of the extremity involved, psychosocial considerations, and individual patient motivation and compliance. In patients with acute traumatic injuries of the upper extremity, a thorough clinical evaluation is necessary to first rule out the presence of other significant life-threatening conditions. Once a patient's overall condition is established hemodynamically, the clinician may proceed to further assess the extremities. Evaluation of the hand and upper extremity involves a systematic approach to the extremity as a functional organ.[1] Complete examination includes gross visual inspection, evaluation of limb perfusion, assessment of passive and active motion, and a review of neurologic function. Imaging studies, such as radiographs, ultrasonography, CT, MRI, or angiography are incorporated as indicated, to further establish the extent of soft tissue, bone, and vascular involvement. Once the clinical needs of the patient have been clearly established, an algorithmic surgical management strategy can then be created to optimize the reconstruction, postoperative management, and the overall functional rehabilitation of the patient, based on those individual needs.

Management Strategy

A reconstructive management strategy is created based on the evaluation of an injury or wound and the patient's individual needs. The complexity of the surgical reconstruction is directed by the severity and extent of the wound, the viability of the remaining tissues, and the exposure of underlying vital structures. The first step in surgical wound management is exploration, irrigation, and meticulous debridement. Adequate débridement of all nonviable tissues is required to establish a healthy environment for healing and to decrease the risk of potential infection. Underlying injuries to vital structures must be identified and repaired. Neurovascular injuries need to be repaired either primarily or with the use of conduits if indicated. Fractures must be identified, irrigated, and débrided, and then be stabilized with internal or external fixation. Tendon injuries should be repaired primarily, if possible, or prepared for more extensive future reconstruction as a staged procedure. Following repair of these underlying vital structures, soft tissue coverage becomes the primary consideration. Soft tissue reconstruction options include primary closure, delayed primary closure, healing by secondary intention, skin grafting, local tissue transfer, free tissue transfer, or any combination of these techniques.

Primary Wound Closure

Primary wound closure simply involves reapproximating the wound edges. This is accomplished with the use of sutures, staples, tapes, or skin glue, as a single or multilayered repair. Delayed primary closure suggests a delay in the repair, such as waiting to allow associated edema to resolve enough to facilitate direct skin closing or to allow future reassessment of the soft tissue viability before closure considerations.

Healing by Secondary Intention

Healing by secondary intention refers to leaving a wound open and allowing it to heal spontaneously through contraction and epithelialization. In the hand and upper extremity, healing by secondary intention can be successfully applied to small wounds (with acceptable results) such as fingertip injuries involving less than a 1-cm defect, without exposed underlying bone. Healing of larger hand and upper extremity wounds by secondary intention, however, can result in

significant scar formation and contracture, with subsequent limitations in range of motion (ROM) and function.

Skin Grafts

A skin graft is a harvested segment of epidermis and dermis that has been elevated and separated completely from its blood supply. The first reported transfer of skin was credited to Reverdin in 1870,[3] but skin grafting did not become common until the invention of the dermatome by Padget[4] during World War II. The dermatome simplified the method of elevating a skin graft, providing a reliable instrument for consistently harvesting a graft of a desired size and depth. The dermatome remains the primary tool used today for harvesting skin grafts. With the increased use of skin grafts, it was recognized that their early use for wound coverage could retard the extent of wound contracture, thus limiting deformity and functional disability.[5]

Skin grafts can either be full thickness or split thickness. A full-thickness skin graft is a segment that includes the epidermis and entire dermis. A full-thickness graft resembles normal skin more closely, including texture, color, and potential for hair growth. A full-thickness graft demonstrates the greatest amount of primary contracture, but the least amount of secondary wound contracture. That is, after the harvest of a full-thickness skin graft, it quickly contracts and appears much smaller because of the elasticity of the tissues. However, when that full-thickness graft is applied to a wound defect early, it maintains its size and can completely stop the contracture of the wound. Full-thickness skin grafting does have limitations. There is a slightly greater risk of nonadherence of the graft, and donor site availability must be considered before full-thickness skin harvest. A full-thickness skin graft donor site must be amenable to primary closure, or the created donor defect may require an additional split-thickness skin graft for coverage.

A split-thickness skin graft is a sample of partial thickness that consists of the entire epidermis and a portion of the dermis. Partial-thickness skin grafts can be harvested at varying depths and are classified according to the thickness of dermis included: thin split-thickness grafts, intermediate- or medium-thickness grafts, or thick split-thickness skin grafts. Compared with a full-thickness graft, a split-thickness graft demonstrates less primary contracture following harvest, but greater secondary contracture of the grafted wound. A thin split-thickness skin graft produces the least primary contracture because of the decreased elastic tissues, but it produces the greatest secondary wound contracture. A thick split-thickness graft can decrease the rate of wound contracture, but it does not retard it completely as a full-thickness graft can.

A split-thickness skin graft can be either meshed or unmeshed. Split-thickness grafts are typically meshed at ratios of 1:1 to 3:1, with the ratio selected depending on the size of the defect needed to be grafted and the skin available for grafting. Meshing of the harvested skin graft facilitates expansion of the graft for coverage of more extensive wound defects. A split-thickness graft also may be left unmeshed and used to cover a wound as a sheet graft. A sheet graft avoids the meshed-pattern scarring associated with meshed skin grafts, thus resulting in a better cosmetic appearance.

Skin grafts may be secured to the margins of the wound with sutures, staples, tape, or skin glue. At this point, the wound dressing and the postoperative management take precedence. The postoperative wound care can greatly influence the survival of the transferred skin graft. Various potential postoperative complications can lead to the demise of a skin graft. The best method for avoiding graft failure is prevention by meticulous postoperative management. The number one reason for failure of a skin graft is hematoma. A hematoma can form beneath the graft, preventing adherence and promoting graft loss. Prevention includes meticulous perioperative hemostasis and appropriate postoperative dressings. Dressings over a skin graft must provide lubrication to prevent desiccation, appropriate compression to eliminate the potential space between the skin graft and the wound bed, and local immobilization to prevent shearing of the graft. An appropriate dressing promotes imbibition, inosculation, adherence, and success of the skin graft. A lubricating (petrolatum) gauze such as Adaptic, Xeroform, or Xeroflo initially is placed directly over the skin graft, followed by layered moist cotton balls, cotton sheets, or gauze, saturated in a solution such as Bunnell's, or mineral oil. Bunnell's solution, consisting of benzalkonium chloride, acetic acid, and glycerin, is the lubricating liquid we prefer. A convex wound may only require a simple dressing under which compression can occur naturally because of the projection of the convex surface of the wound. A concave wound often requires a tie-over dressing, also called a *bolster* or *stent*, to compress the skin graft against the surface of the wound defect. This is accomplished with the use of sutures, staples, or a circumferential dressing, to secure the bolster dressing over the skin graft, facilitating graft adherence and healing. Recently the wound vac has been used to stabilize grafts and promote healing.

Graft survival also is enhanced by strict local immobilization. This is achieved by immobilizing the appropriate associated joint(s) with an orthosis, at the level of the digits, wrist, or elbow, to maintain a constant protective position and decrease the risk of shearing of the graft.

Postoperative Follow-up and Management

The dressing over an upper extremity skin graft typically is removed in 4 to 7 days, and the wound is reevaluated. By this time, the skin graft should be adherent to the wound bed, but meticulous wound care is still required to protect the reconstruction. It remains important to maintain a moist/lubricated environment to prevent the persistent risk of desiccation of the skin graft and to facilitate complete healing. This is accomplished with either continued wet-to-wet dressing changes or the application of a lubricating agent such as an antibacterial ointment (e.g., bacitracin). Once complete, epithelialization of the skin graft is recognized, the use of the lubricating ointments and dressings can be discontinued and a simple moisturizing cream started. The continued serial application of a moisturizing cream, such as Eucerin or the equivalent, in combination with gentle massage, can facilitate progressive contoured scar maturation with flattening of the grafted surface and improve the overall cosmetic results. Once adherence of the skin graft is recognized, and as long as there are no significant underlying injuries, rehabilitation of the upper extremity can be initiated and rapidly advanced.

Neurovascular, tendon, and bone injuries influence the rehabilitation plan, the timing of which is directed by the individual extent of their involvement.

Management of the Skin Graft Donor Site

We prefer to simply cover the harvested split-thickness skin graft donor site with an OpSite (Smith and Nephew) transparent, adherent dressing, and allow spontaneous reepithelialization of the donor bed. Reepithelialization of the graft donor site typically occurs in approximately 1 week. If fluid collects beneath the dressing, it is simply drained with a needle and the dressing patched with an additional OpSite, or the entire dressing is changed. Following complete reepithelialization of the donor site, dressings are discontinued and the healing bed can be treated for dryness as needed, using a moisturizing lotion such as Eucerin or an equivalent.

Local Tissue Transfer

Earlier in this chapter, we noted that skin grafts are not appropriate for all wounds. For traumatic defects of the upper extremity involving soft tissue loss, with associated exposure of underlying vital structures, such as blood vessels, nerves, tendons devoid of paratenon, bones devoid of periosteum, or wounds with insufficient vascularity to support a skin graft, a more complex reconstructive approach must be used. The surgeon's initial consideration in this situation is the next step in the algorithmic approach to reconstruction of the upper extremity, that is, use of a local tissue flap. Local tissue transfer refers to the dissection, elevation, and transfer of skin, combined with a varied amount of underlying tissue, potentially including subcutaneous tissue, fascia, muscle, nerve, tendon, or bone. The composition of the tissue harvested and used is determined by the type and extent of tissue loss. During the elevation of a local tissue flap, the local blood supply supporting the flap is preserved. This undivided portion of the flap containing the vascularity required for flap survival, is labeled the pedicle. A local tissue flap can close a local tissue defect, establishing a well-vascularized, healthy environment to potentiate healing of the associated underlying injuries. Local tissue flaps are labeled according to the layers of tissue used, the pattern of the blood supply, and the type of mobilization required.

Skin Flaps

Using a local skin flap for reconstruction of an upper extremity defect refers to rotating adjacent skin and subcutaneous tissue into a wound to supply coverage and closure. A skin flap design is based on the local vascular anatomy of the skin. A random pattern flap is a local skin flap that has no specific arteriovenous system.[6] An axial pattern flap is a single-pedicle skin flap with an anatomically established arteriovenous system along its longitudinal axis.[6] An island flap is an axial pattern flap in which the skin bridge has been separated, leaving only the vascular pedicle intact at the base.[7] Skin flaps are also classified by mobilization techniques, rotational versus advancement. Rotation flaps rotate around a fixed point to reach a wound defect (Fig. 20-1). An advancement flap advances from the donor site to the recipient wound bed in a straight line, without any rotation (Fig. 20-2). Numerous accounts of local flaps are well described in the literature;

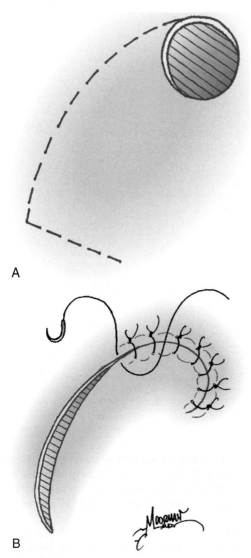

Figure 20-1 Rotation flap. The flap is designed to rotate around a fixed point to reach a wound defect.

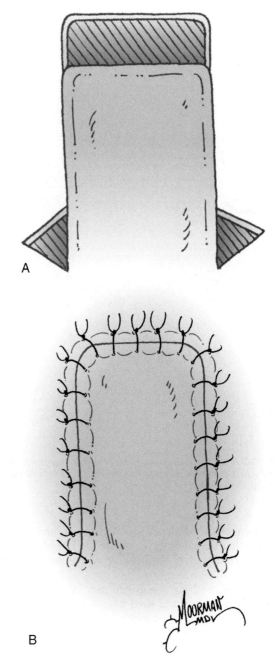

Figure 20-2 Advancement flap. The flap is designed to advance from the donor site to the recipient wound bed in a straight line, without any rotation.

local flaps are traditionally valuable and versatile options in the reconstruction of many upper extremity defects at all levels: the fingers, hands, forearm, and upper arm.

Digital Reconstruction

Our fingers are the tools we use to reach out and engage our environment. Whether at work or at play, our fingers are always in front of us and subsequently are injured often. Fingertip injuries involving a surface area of less than 1 cm, without exposure of bone or vital structures, can simply be allowed to close by secondary intention. Moist dressings can be applied until the wound has reepithelialized. In fingertip injuries involving a surface area defect greater than 1 cm, or digital defects with exposed underlying vital structures, a reconstructive procedure is indicated. The reconstructive goal is to provide wound closure and restore functional sensibility to the finger. As noted before, many well-described local skin flap procedures are illustrated in the reconstructive literature. The selection of a particular surgical procedure is individualized to the patient, based primarily on the size and the location of the wound defect.

V-Y Advancement Flap. The volar V-Y[8,9] or lateral V-Y[10,11] advancement flaps are skin flaps indicated for small fingertip injuries. These flaps offer a reconstructive dimension of 1 to 1.5 cm. Following appropriate debridement of the injured tissues, the volar V-Y flap is created by making a triangular skin incision(s) just below the defect. The subcutaneous tissue is preserved, and the fibrous septa from the pulp to the periosteum is released. The dissected V-shaped flap is then advanced distally to cover the defect, and subsequently closed in a Y-pattern with surgical sutures (Fig. 20-3). The flap is covered with a nonadherent lubricating gauze and protected with a bulky dressing. Sutures are typically removed in 2 weeks, and early motion is initiated.

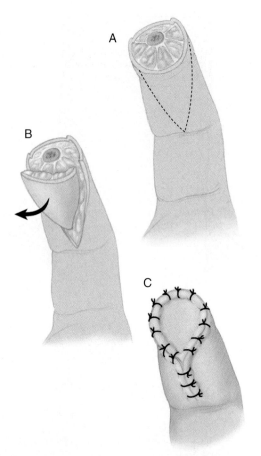

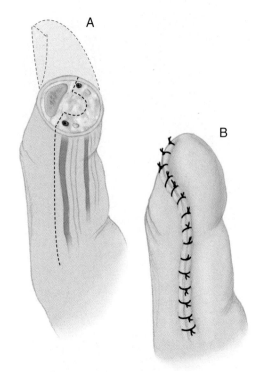

Figure 20-4 Moberg flap. **A,** Distal thumb amputation with planned midlateral incisions. The neurovascular bundles are preserved and advanced with the volar flap. **B,** Advancement of the volar flap and suture closure.

Figure 20-3 V-Y advancement flap. **A,** Fingertip injury with planned V-shaped volar incision. **B,** Elevation of volar flap. **C,** Distal advancement of volar flap and closure in a Y-pattern.

Volar Advancement Moberg Flap. Defects of the pulp of the thumb or other digital defects that are too large for coverage with a V-Y advancement flap may be closed using a Moberg flap.[12]

Moberg's volar advancement flap may be advanced a distance of 1.5 to 2.0 cm and used to cover a traumatic defect involving the entire volar surface of the thumb or another digit. The Moberg flap is created by making midlateral incisions below the fingertip defect. The neurovascular bundles are preserved, and the volar flap is then advanced to cover the defect (Fig. 20-4). This is a reliable, sensate flap that restores sensibility to the pulp. The flap is dressed with a nonadherent lubricating gauze, followed by the application of a protective dressing and orthosis.

Cross-Finger Flaps. A conventional cross-finger flap uses an elevated skin flap from the dorsal aspect of one finger to cover an open volar or tip wound with exposed tendon or bone of an adjacent finger.[13] The donor site is then covered with a skin graft (Fig. 20-5). A reverse cross-finger flap involves dissecting an additional adipofascial flap beneath the skin flap, which is then used to cover a dorsal wound defect of an adjacent finger.[14] The skin flap is then reinset over the donor defect and a skin graft is placed over the transferred adipofascial flap. Each of these flaps can cover a digital defect up to 2 cm. The skin grafts are then supported with a bolster

dressing, and the fingers are immobilized with an orthosis or pinned to protect the flaps. The patient returns in 2 to 3 weeks for separation and insetting of the flap. Hand therapy is initiated early to maintain optimal ROM and function.

Digital Island Flaps. Digital island flaps are excellent reconstructive tools for covering either distal or proximal digital defects up to 2.5 cm, overlying exposed joints or tendons (Fig. 20-6). A skin flap is created in a pattern indicated by the local defect and then harvested based on the proper digital artery and vein.[15] The associated proper digital nerve can be included to add sensibility to the reconstructed flap or preserved in its natural anatomic state. The pedicle flap is then transferred distally or proximally to the digital defect and secured with permanent sutures. The donor site is usually reconstructed with a small full-thickness skin graft.

Muscle, Musculocutaneous, and Fasciocutaneous Flaps

Muscle, musculocutaneous, and fasciocutaneous flaps are more complex reconstructive tools available for surgical coverage of local wound defects of the upper extremity. Reconstruction proximal to the fingers typically involves more extensive injuries with larger soft tissue defects requiring more elaborate reconstruction. Vital structures, such as tendons, blood vessels, nerves, and bone are often exposed, requiring appropriate healthy soft tissue coverage to optimize healing. Muscle, musculocutaneous, and fasciocutaneous flaps, either harvested and used as local flaps or as free tissue transfers, can provide sufficient healthy tissue bulk to fill large wound defects. These soft tissue flaps are based on

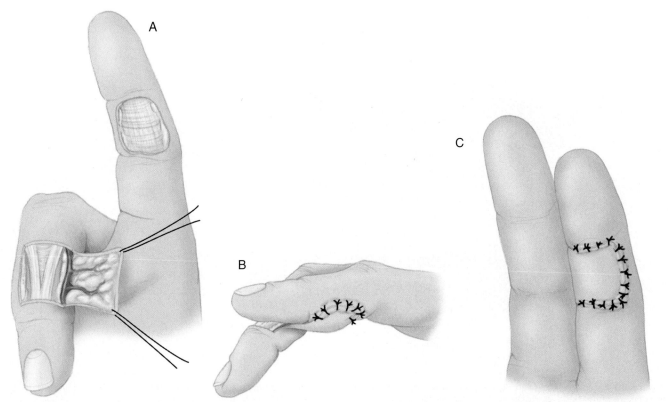

Figure 20-5 Cross-finger flap. **A,** Elevation of dorsal flap from adjacent finger to match defect. **B,** Transfer of the flap to the defect. **C,** Suture closure of the flap. The donor site is covered with a skin graft.

defined vascular anatomy with associated versatility and reliability.[16] The upper extremity offers several excellent choices for local tissue transfers.

Radial Forearm Flap. The radial forearm flap is a fasciocutaneous flap harvested from the volar forearm, based on the radial artery and concomitant veins[17] (Fig. 20-7). This flap offers the reconstructive surgeon an excellent option for

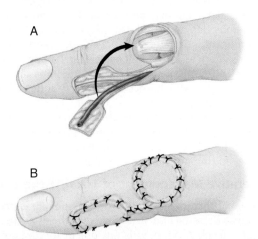

Figure 20-6 Digital island flap. **A,** Dissection and elevation of skin flap based on the proper digital artery and vein, designed to cover the illustrated defect over the dorsal surface of the proximal interphalangeal joint. **B,** Rotation of the island flap to cover the defect and closure of the donor site with a skin graft.

coverage of defects requiring thin, pliable tissue. The radial forearm flap can be raised on its pedicle and rotated locally, either proximally, based on antegrade flow, or distally, based on retrograde flow. This flap also may be harvested as a free flap or combined with a strip of palmaris longus or brachialis for associated tendon reconstruction, a portion of the radius for bony reconstruction,[18] or the lateral antebrachial cutaneous nerve to establish an innervated flap. The disadvantages of this procedure are the sacrifice of a major forearm artery, and the unsightly donor harvest site, which requires a skin graft for coverage.

Posterior Interosseus Flap. The posterior interosseous flap is a fasciocutaneous flap that can be used as a reverse pedicled local tissue transfer based on the posterior interosseous artery, to cover distal defects of the wrist, dorsal hand, and first web space. A reconstructive dimension of 8×15 cm may be elevated and rotated, but any skin island greater then 4 cm wide requires a skin graft for closure of the donor site. This flap is dissected and harvested from the dorsal forearm, rotated distally, and secured into the defect with surgical sutures.

Lateral Arm Flap. The lateral arm flap is an excellent flap for reconstruction of upper extremity soft tissue defects. This flap can be used as a local pedicled flap, based on antegrade or reverse flow, or as a free flap. The lateral arm flap represents an innervated cutaneous flap with a reconstructive dimension of 15×18 cm. It may be harvested as an osteocutaneous flap with a portion of the humerus and may

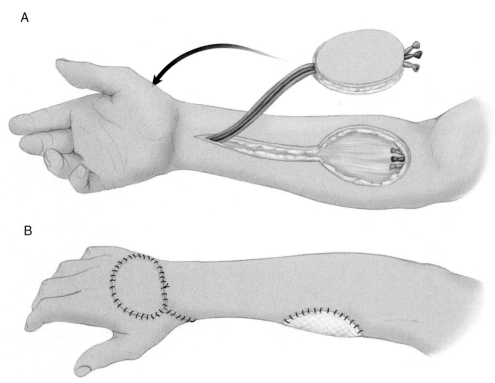

Figure 20-7 Radial forearm flap. **A,** Elevation of the fasciocutaneous flap based on the radial artery and veins, designed to cover a wound defect on the dorsum of the hand. **B,** Rotation of the flap distally and suture closure. Coverage of the donor site with a skin graft.

include a fasciocutaneous forearm extension, or a tendon strip from the triceps, depending on the individual needs for reconstruction.[19] The lateral arm flap may be rotated on its pedicle to cover large defects distally around the elbow. As a free flap, the lateral arm flap may be further used for coverage of defects involving the dorsum of the hand or the first web space.

Groin Flap. The groin flap is an axial pattern flap that provides a reliable surgical option for reconstruction of distal upper extremity injuries. This flap is elevated as a pedicle flap based on the superficial circumflex iliac artery and concomitant veins and then used to cover either hand or forearm defects[6] (Fig. 20-8). The donor defect may close primarily, or it may require a skin graft for coverage. Once the flap is secured to the defect, the upper extremity must be immobilized to eliminate tension on the vascular pedicle. Immobilization of the flap may be achieved with circumferential dressings, tape, or supportive orthoses and carefully maintained as an outpatient. The patient then returns in 2 to 3 weeks for surgical division of the vascular pedicle and final contouring and insetting of the flap. Before division of the flap, gentle ROM of the uninvolved digits should be performed.

Parascapular and Scapular Flaps. The parascapular and scapular flaps are cutaneous flaps based on a branch of the circumflex scapular artery[20] (Fig. 20-9). Each of these flaps has a reconstructive dimension of about 10 × 25 cm. A parascapular or scapular flap can be rotated locally and used as a pedicled flap for coverage of shoulder or proximal,

posterior arm defects. This flap can be harvested and transplanted as free flap for coverage of both forearm and dorsal hand defects.[21] Parascapular and scapular flaps also provide the reconstructive surgeon the opportunity to incorporate additional fascial extensions to provide gliding surfaces for associated tendon repairs, if necessary, or include a portion of scapular bone for reconstruction of segmental forearm defects.

Latissimus Dorsi Flap. The latissimus dorsi flap is an excellent reconstruction option for the coverage of large surface area defects. This flap may be harvested as a muscle or musculocutaneous flap and used as a pedicled tissue transfer to cover significant local defects of the shoulder and upper arm, or as a free flap to cover extensive distal upper extremity wounds. As a free tissue transfer, the latissimus dorsi flap is harvested based on the thoracodorsal artery and concomitant vein[22] and contoured to fit the defect. The thoracodorsal vessels are anastomosed to prepared recipient vessels out of the zone of injury, followed by insetting of the flap to cover the defect. This flap has a large surface area of up to 20 × 35 cm, depending on the size of the individual.

Postoperative Management of Local Tissue Flaps

At the time of the operation, the local tissue flap is protected with a sterile dressing and a supportive orthosis at the appropriate joint level. A window is cut out of the dressing over the created flap to allow direct visualization of the reconstruction. This allows meticulous clinical observation of the local tissue flap vascularity, which is monitored by color and capillary refill. Lack of color or delayed capillary refill may

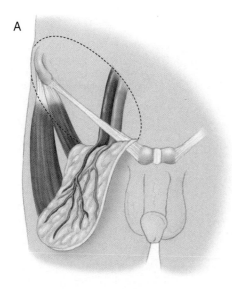

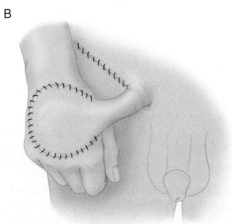

Figure 20-8 Groin flap. **A,** Elevation of the groin flap. **B,** Contouring the flap as a tube for coverage of a complex degloving hand injury.

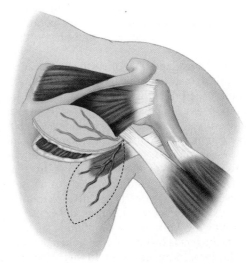

Figure 20-9 Surgical anatomy of the scapular flap.

represent lack of blood flow within the flap, whereas discoloration or rapid capillary refill suggests flap congestion. Each of these clinical findings suggests potential flap failure and the need for continued meticulous clinical monitoring, with a low threshold for surgical reexploration and revision. Postoperatively, the reconstructed upper extremity is elevated on a couple of pillows or a prefabricated foam wedge commercially designed for limb elevation. Elevation is of utmost importance to prevent upper extremity swelling and the associated potential risk of increased flap congestion. Upon discharge home, elevation is continued and orthoses are left intact to maintain support and protection, facilitating complete healing of the local tissue reconstruction.

The patient or a home health care agency monitors operative drains at home, where output is measured and recorded over 24-hour periods. The drains are removed at clinic follow-up when the reported output falls below our set minimum of 30 mL for a 24-hour period. Sutures or staples are removed 2 weeks postoperatively, and an early rehabilitation protocol is instituted to facilitate progressive functional restoration and overall recovery. As noted earlier, the intensity and timing of the postoperative rehabilitation therapy depend on the extent and specific nature of the underlying structural injuries.

Free Tissue Transfer

Reconstruction of an upper extremity wound defect using a local tissue flap is not always feasible. Local tissue transfer may be limited because of the wound location or regional donor site deficiencies. A vascular pedicle may not be long enough to reach a particular defect, or the defect may be too large to cover completely with local tissue. In these instances, the reconstructive surgeon looks to the final rung in the reconstructive ladder, free tissue transfer.

Autologous free tissue transfer refers to the transplant of tissue from one location of the body to another. This is achieved by using an operating microscope and meticulous techniques of microsurgery to perform small-vessel anastomoses between the pedicle of the transferred free tissue flap and the prepared local recipient vessels.

Microsurgery for extremity reconstruction began more than four decades ago with the introduction of the operating microscope for anastomoses of blood vessels, described by Jacobson.[23] The operating microscope was first used to repair injured digital arteries, which began the age of digital replantation in the 1960s.[24,25] In the 1970s, the use of the microscope was expanded to microsurgical composite free tissue transplantation.[26] Composite free tissue transplantation is the harvesting and transfer of a composite (or collection) of tissues, including muscle, fascia, skin and subcutaneous tissue, nerve, tendon, bone, or any combination of these. The vascular inflow and outflow of the harvested free tissue flap is preserved for anastomosis with the local blood supply. Efforts of the modern microsurgeon have expanded from just providing soft tissue bulk for coverage of a wound defect to the ultimate reconstructive goal of full functional restoration.[27]

Free tissue transfer continues to play an increasingly vital role in the reconstruction of upper extremity complex wounds. Free tissue flaps, dissected as muscle, musculocutaneous, or fasciocutaneous flaps, can be harvested out of the zone of injury and transferred to a distant extensive wound, providing healthy tissue for coverage and optimizing the healing potential.

Free tissue transplantation offers many advantages, primarily including early mobilization and rehabilitation. Free flaps also offer the possibility of using composite free tissue transplantation, as a single-stage procedure, even in the acute emergency setting.[28] Free flaps may include a combination of tissues that can be harvested and transferred as a single unit, including vessels, nerves, tendons, muscle, skin, and bone. These flaps can be tailored specifically to fit a particular wound defect, with associated improved cosmesis.

Free muscle flaps can provide potential restoration of specific upper extremity motor function and sensibility.[29] For example, following Volkmann's contracture of the forearm, flexion of the fingers is lost due to the ischemic injury associated with this local traumatic event. In this instance, a gracilis muscle may be harvested with its motor nerve and transferred as an innervated free muscle flap to restore finger flexion. Similarly, an innervated latissimus dorsi free muscle flap may be used to restore elbow flexion in individuals lacking elbow function secondary to traumatic injury or congenital anomaly. A cutaneous sensory nerve also may be preserved with a harvested free fasciocutaneous flap and used to create a neurosensory flap, potentially restoring sensibility to a particular area. In free tissue reconstruction of the upper extremity, the ultimate feat of functional restoration is the replantation of amputated digits or the transfer of entire toes to the hand. In summary, a free flap offers contoured soft tissue coverage, provides a healthy wound environment to facilitate healing, offers functional reconstruction, and allows for early mobilization and rehabilitation to optimize the potential for full recovery.

Numerous excellent free flaps are available for reconstruction of upper extremity wound defects, each individually indicated by the location and extent of the particular wound. Several of these flaps, which can be used for either local tissue transfer or as free flaps for upper extremity reconstruction, were discussed earlier in this chapter, including the radial forearm flap, lateral arm flap, parascapular and scapular flaps, and the latissimus dorsi flap. Other reconstructive options using free tissue transfer are described in the following sections.

Serratus Muscle/Fascial Flap

The serratus flap is harvested as a muscular or fascial flap with or without a skin island, based on the serratus vascular arcade. This flap has a reconstructive dimension of about 10×18 cm, and provides the reconstructive surgeon with another versatile option for repairing upper extremity defects requiring thin pliable tissue or gliding tissues for associated tendon reconstructions. Vascularized ribs may be harvested with this flap, for additional bony reconstruction.

Temporoparietal Fascial Flap

The temporoparietal fascial flap consists of thin, supple fascia, harvested as a free flap, based on the superficial temporal artery and vein[30,31] (Fig. 20-10). This flap has a reconstructive dimension of 8×15 cm and is often used for defects of the dorsal hand, palm, and digits. The temporoparietal

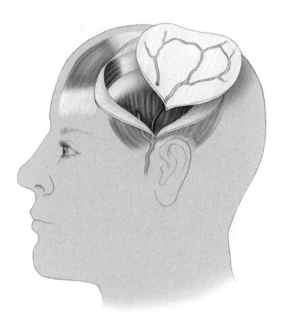

Figure 20-10 Anatomy of the temporoparietal fascial flap.

fascial flap conforms nicely to the contour of a wound surface but requires the addition of a skin graft for completion of the surface coverage. Appropriate dressings are required for maintenance of a moist environment to facilitate skin graft survival and healing.

Gracilis Flap

The gracilis flap can be harvested as a muscle or musculocutaneous flap and transplanted to the upper extremity as a free tissue transfer. This flap is based on the terminal branch of the medial femoral circumflex artery and concomitant veins[32] and can be used to cover defects up to 6×25 cm. The gracilis muscle also can be harvested with a motor branch of the obturator nerve and used as an innervated free muscle flap to restore flexor function to the upper extremity[33] (Fig. 20-11).

Fibular Flap

The fibular flap involves the harvest of bone, with or without a skin paddle or muscle, for reconstruction of segmental defects of the shoulder, humerus, radius, ulna, or wrist, and associated soft tissue loss. This flap is based on the peroneal artery and veins and can include a segment of fibula up to 26 cm.[34] The proximal and distal 6 cm of the fibula are preserved to maintain stability of the extremity. A skin island with a reconstructive dimension of 8×15 cm may be included, based on septal perforators from the peroneal vascular pedicle. The donor site may or may not require a skin graft for closure, depending on the size of the skin paddle harvested.

Postoperative Management of Free Flaps

Following free tissue transfer, the free flap is protected with sterile dressings and a supportive orthosis. When the wound is dressed and the orthosis is molded, great care is taken to avoid any pressure on the vascular pedicle. A window in the

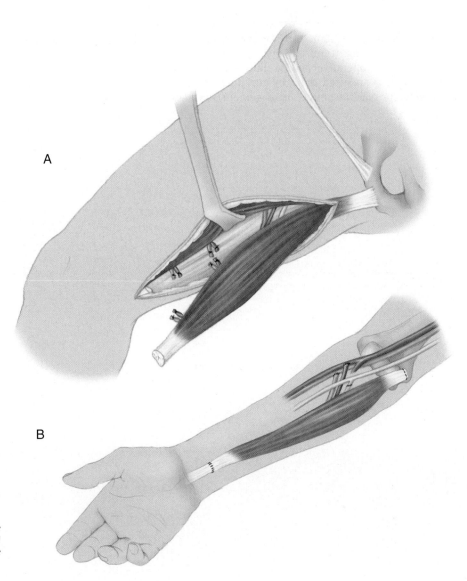

Figure 20-11 A, Elevation of a gracilis muscle flap. **B,** Transfer of the gracilis as an innervated free muscle flap to restore flexor function to the upper extremity.

dressing is created over the reconstruction to allow for meticulous postoperative clinical observation. We prefer to monitor free flaps with the aid of a Cook Doppler flow probe.[23] Once the Cook Doppler probe is secured to the vessel, venous and arterial flow can be heard. Loss of the signal suggests vascular compromise and impending failure of the free flap, unless addressed expeditiously in the operating room. The most reliable method of accurate free flap monitoring remains meticulous clinical observation.

The Cook Doppler probe is typically removed on postoperative day 4. Without complication, our patients are typically discharged the next day—postoperative day 5. At the time of discharge, orthotic immobilization of the upper extremity is maintained for continued support and protection and patients are instructed to continue strict upper extremity elevation. Operative drains are removed from the reconstruction and donor sites when the drain output subsides to a minimum, typically under 30 mL for a 24-hour period. Sutures and staples are left intact for 2 weeks and then removed in the clinic. Depending on the underlying injuries to vital structures, such as tendons or bone, early rehabilitation, including occupational therapy and social reintegration, can now be initiated.

Summary

Reconstructive surgery of the upper extremity has continued to make progressive and significant clinical advances. These impressive advances have been facilitated by the continual addition and use of new flaps and the increasing use of functional free tissue transfer, with improved microsurgical techniques, postoperative management, and intensive rehabilitation. We have successfully incorporated an algorithmic approach to reconstruction of the upper extremity. We have established this reconstructive ladder for the evaluation and treatment of upper extremity wounds and defects, directing the surgeon to the indicated reconstructive surgical options, based on the extent and severity of the wounds, the functional needs of the patient, and the availability of required tissue elements. The reconstructive options, surgical techniques, and postoperative pearls, illustrated and described in this chapter, are used daily in our practice and offered as excellent reconstructive management strategies for facilitating localized healing and optimizing each individual patient's functional rehabilitation and overall recovery.

REFERENCES

The complete reference list is available online at www.expertconsult.com.

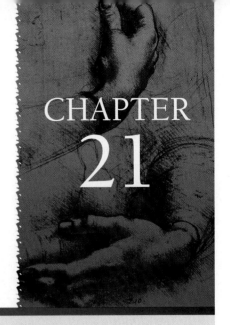

Fingertip Injuries

AARON SHAW, OTR/L, CHT AND LEONID KATOLIK, MD

ANATOMY	HAND THERAPY EVALUATION
SURGICAL CONSIDERATIONS	HAND THERAPY INTERVENTION
AUTHORS' RECOMMENDATION	SUMMARY

CRITICAL POINTS

- Fingertip injuries are common and account for approximately 4% of all emergency department visits.
- Sequelae of fingertip injuries include scar contracture, cold intolerance, hypersensitivity, inadequate pulp volume, and stiffness in adjoining joints and adjacent digits with consequent long-term patient dissatisfaction or frank disability.
- Goals of management include preservation of functional length, durable coverage, preservation of useful sensibility, prevention of symptomatic neuromas, prevention of adjacent joint contractures, short morbidity, and early return to work or recreation.
- All fingertip injuries ultimately require referral to a hand therapy unit for optimization of outcome and minimization of long-term sequelae.

Fingertip injuries are common and account for approximately 4% of all emergency department visits.[1,2] Significant costs are associated with treatment, lost work, and functional disability due to these injuries. Furthermore, long-term sequelae of scar contracture, cold intolerance, inadequate pulp volume, and stiffness in adjoining joints and adjacent digits may lead to chronic patient dissatisfaction or frank disability.

Surgical options for the treatment of fingertip injuries span the spectrum from elegant simplicity to the absolute triumph of technology over reason.[3,4] Treatment decisions should ultimately be based on patient needs. These include preservation of functional length, durable coverage, preservation of useful sensibility, prevention of symptomatic neuromas, prevention of adjacent joint contractures, short morbidity, and early return to work or recreation.

Regardless of medical or surgical intervention, all fingertip injuries ultimately require referral to a hand therapy unit for optimization of outcome and minimization of long-term sequelae.

Anatomy

For simplicity we consider the fingertip as the digital unit distal to the insertion of the flexor digitorum profundus. It consists of the pulp, nail, and underlying phalanx.

The fingertip pulp is a closed space. Vertical fibrous septae anchor the pulp to the periosteum of the underlying phalanx. The pulp contains the distal arborization of cutaneous lymph vessels, as well as the terminal branches of the digital neurovascular system.

The nail unit provides support to the pulp during pincer grasp and tactile functions (Fig. 21-1). It consists of keratinized squamous cells produced by the germinal matrix at the base of the nail bed. The thin epithelium of the sterile matrix provides an adherent layer for firm nail attachment. It is in turn contiguous with the underlying periosteum of the distal phalanx. The eponychium forms the dorsal roof of the base of the nail, and the paronychium is the lateral nail fold. The hyponychium is the junction of the nail bed and the fingertip skin distally.

Surgical Considerations

Fingertip injuries are typically due to a crush or a crush–avulsion type of mechanism. They result in an injury spectrum consisting of disruption of the pulp, injury to the nail unit, and fracture of the underlying bone (Fig. 21-2).

Examination is best performed under loupe magnification, in a hemostatic field, and with the patient made comfortable.

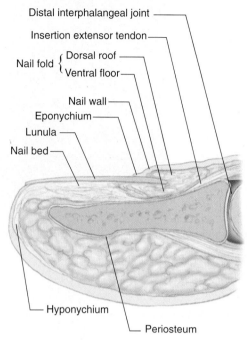

Figure 21-1 The finger nail unit.

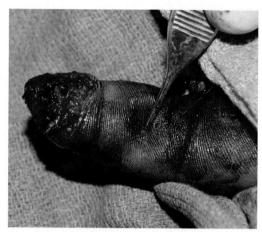

Figure 21-2 Fingertip injury in 32-year-old truck driver with loss of pulp substance, open fracture through distal phalanx, avulsion of fingernail, and laceration of nail bed following blunt injury.

To this end patients are offered a regional anesthetic. It is the authors' preference, for reasons of patient comfort, to administer wrist blockade rather than digital blockade. Multiplanar radiographs of the affected digit are then obtained. A finger cot tourniquet is applied. In the subacute setting, although the wound may initially be hemostatic, examination and debridement will shortly disrupt this. The wound is irrigated with sterile saline solution to clear blood and debris. Detailed and complete assessment is now possible. Once complete,

the fingertip is dressed with nonadherent gauze, surgical sponges, and light compressive dressing. The bulky nature of this dressing generally provides adequate immobilization as well.

Fractures of the distal phalanx with fingertip injuries often involve significant comminution or bone loss. As such, operative intervention for the bony injuries alone is very uncommon.

Recall that the periosteum of the distal phalanx is contiguous with the sterile matrix, and disruption of the nail bed with tuft fractures is generally a certainty. If the overlying nail plate is not avulsed, surgical nail removal and repair of the nail bed is not performed. The overlying nail plate serves as an excellent occlusive dressing to allow for healing of the underlying matrix (Fig. 21-3). If the nail plate is disrupted

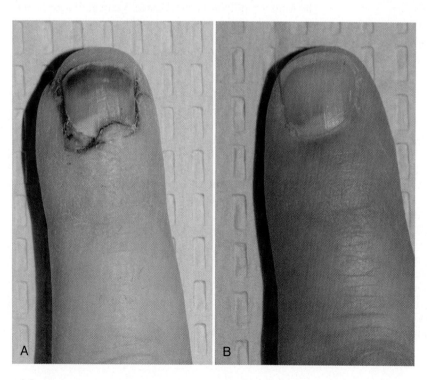

Figure 21-3 Crush injury to fingertip. **A,** Large subungual hematoma but without avulsion of nail from nail fold. This patient was treated with a tip protector orthosis for comfort, mobilization, and edema control. The injured nail fell off at 3 weeks, and at 9 months a new, normal-appearing nail was in its place (**B**).

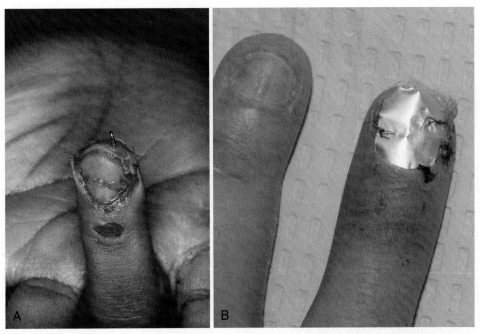

Figure 21-4 A, linear laceration of the nail is approximated with fine gut sutures. **B,** it is commonly our practice to splint the nail folds and protect nail bed repairs with a "foil nail" made of sterile suture packaging. Note inset of the foil into the nail fold, secured proximally and distally with absorbable suture.

or avulsed, it is removed and meticulous nail bed repair is performed with fine absorbable (5-0 gut) sutures. The nail fold is then fixed, using either the native nail plate or a contoured slip of sterile foil from the surgical wrapper (Fig. 21-4).

Linear skin lacerations may be easily repaired with fine absorbable suture. Stellate lacerations are loosely reapproximated. When the laceration involves the proximal or lateral nail folds, care must be taken to restore the anatomy without obliterating the underlying space.

The management of soft tissue loss of the fingertip with exposed bone has engendered tremendous controversy. The patient's work demands and the desire for restoration of appearance guide the choice of treatment. Microsurgical replantation, free tissue transfer, pedicled flap coverage, soft tissue advancement, cross-finger flap coverage, thenar flap coverage, and skin grafting have been described with varying degrees of success.[5-11] However, no single method is universally applicable. Indeed, no method guarantees prevention of

the vexing sequelae of cold intolerance, tip sensitivity, or altered cosmesis.

Revision amputation is the most expeditious approach, but it involves shortening of the digit to the level of the head of the middle phalanx. While allowing for immediate soft tissue coverage, further shortening of an injured digit is not accepted by all patients (Fig. 21-5).

Simple shortening of exposed bone with a rongeur at the time of initial examination followed by dressing changes allowing for healing by wound contraction and granulation allow restoration of satisfactory appearance and sensitivity. It avoids surgical intervention but generally entails a 3- to 4-week period in which meticulous wound care is required two to three times a day. Patients are instructed in dry dressing changes, secured with a lightly compressive wrap (Fig. 21-6). They may incorporate full use of the injured extremity into daily hand hygiene 3 days after the injury, including gentle cleansing of the amputated tip with a mild antibacterial soap.

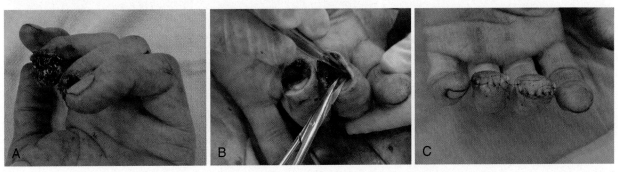

Figure 21-5 Revision amputation. **A,** Patient with multiple digital amputations. **B,** Digits operatively explored, debrided, with neurectomies performed. **C,** Single-stage closure with local tissue.

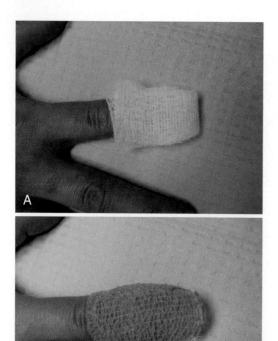

Figure 21-6 A, A single, dry gauze is placed to cover the fingertip without excessive bulk. **B,** This is overwrapped with a light compressive dressing. This may easily be changed daily by the patient.

More recently, the application of topical growth factors with dressing changes[12] has been shown to yield results superior to and less costly than surgical soft tissue reconstruction. It is unclear whether these offer any advantage to less technologically sophisticated wound care.

We have enjoyed great success with this method, but concerns over bone dessication and osteomyelitis lead some to abandon this method except in the smallest of injuries.

Full-thickness skin grafting of pulp and tip defects enjoys limited benefit over simple healing by secondary intention. Although donor site morbidity is minimal, the fingers are immobilized for 7 to 10 days to allow for graft incorporation. A mature graft is relatively anesthetic, and graft contracture may lead to poor cosmesis.

Full-thickness pulp defects, with exposed bone or tendon, are typically not amenable to healing by secondary intention. These injuries have more recently been treated by us through a staged procedure involving the application of an acellular dermal matrix followed by full-thickness skin grafting at an interval of 3 weeks[13] (Fig. 21-7). This technique allows for preservation of length and contour, but carries with it the costs of two procedures and a heavy expense for the acellular matrix template.

Homodigital flaps, such as the V-Y advancement flaps have been in use for decades with little modification of the original technique described independently by Attasoy and Kutler[14,15] (Fig. 21-8). Tissue is advanced based on deep septal perforating vessels. There is no need for prolonged immobilization, and no donor site morbidity results. Clinically, however, the extent that tissue may be advanced distally is limited. Although advancement up to 10 mm is possible, considerable dissection is involved and possibly devitalization of septal perforators.[16]

The adipofascial "turnover" flap[17,18] is a reasonable option for coverage of large full-thickness defects to the dorsum of the fingers. This flap is based on constant dorsal cutaneous perforating vessels arising from the proper digital arteries at the level of the proximal interphalangeal joint. The flap may be extended to offer durable coverage to the entirety of the digit from the proximal interphalangeal (PIP) joint to the fingertip dorsally. A full-thickness skin graft is applied over the flap while the donor site may be closed primarily (Fig. 21-9).

Heterodigital flaps such as thenar flaps and cross-finger flaps further expand the surgical armamentarium for fingertip reconstruction.[19,20] These are random flaps raised either at the base of the thumb or off the doral aspect of an adjoining digit. The injured digit is secured to this flap and sec-

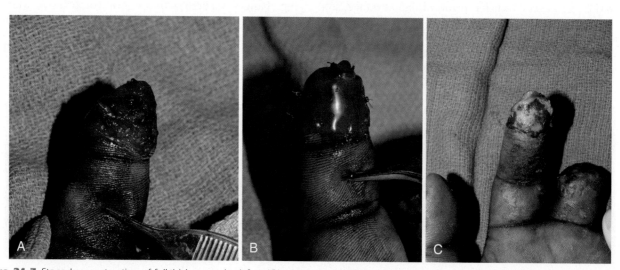

Figure 21-7 Staged reconstruction of full-thickness pulp defect (**A**) with application of acellular dermal matrix (**B**). At 3 weeks the matrix is ingrown and provides a suitable bed for skin grafting (**C**).

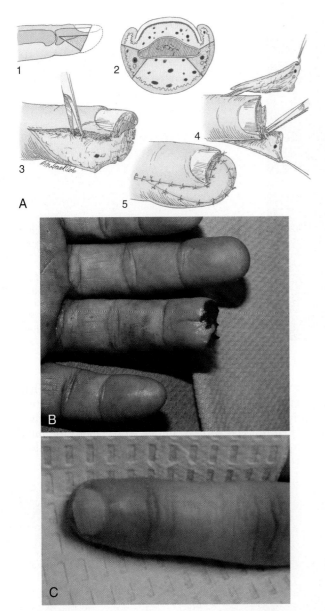

Figure 21-8 A, Artist's rendering of V-Y advancement flap for fingertip coverage (Reprinted with permission from Green D, Hotchkiss R, Pederson W, eds. *Green's Operative Hand Surgery,* 4th ed. Philadelphia: Churchill Livingstone, 1999, p. 1804.) **B,** Clinical case of 32-year-old with transverse amputation through distal phalanx. **C,** Four months following treatment with radial and ulnar V-Y advancement flap.

tioned 14 to 21 days later at a second surgery. The donor site is typically covered with a skin graft (Fig. 21-10). This iatrogenic syndactylization of two digits, often with the PIP joint in midflexion, has an inherent propensity to lead to permanent flexion contracture. Although we have found these complications to be common, several authors assure us that this sequela is rare.[21]

Finger defect coverage using tissue perfused by the metacarpal artery system has become common in the last two decades. In 1990, Quaba and Davison reported a series of finger defects that were covered by island skin flaps from the dorsal hand.[22] These flaps were nourished by the palmar–

dorsal vascular connection in the hand at the level of the metacarpophalangeal (MCP) joint, just distal to the extensor tendon juncturae. Even in the extended fashion, however, these flaps generally reach only far enough to allow coverage of the nail bed.

Impressive advances in tip reconstruction have come from Asia where an extreme primacy is placed on digital tip preservation. Lim and colleagues described a spiral flap for digital tip defects.[9] The flap is designed in a spiral shape and then extended to the fingertip in much the same way one would extend a spring with traction. The resultant proximal donor defect is covered with a skin graft. Amazingly, this group reports normal range of motion (ROM), normal sensation, and no cold intolerance. In an application of free tissue transfer expertise on an extremely small scale, Lee and coworkers published an enormous series of fingertip defects that were reconstructed with pulp from the second toe.[4] In addition to the microvascular anastomoses, these flaps are neurotized by digital nerve coaptation. Of the 854 flaps described, only 3 were outright failures, and there was a minimal revision rate. The authors report that static two-point discrimination averaged 8 mm. This two-point discrimination does not appear to be markedly better than that seen with healing by secondary intent. Operative time, cost, and the availablility of an experienced microsurgical team preclude the recommendation of this option by us.

Authors' Recommendations

We treat fingertip injuries with distal soft tissue loss by meticulous dressing changes, to allow for wound contraction and healing by secondary intention. When bone is exposed, the treating physician must consider the importance of preserving functional length. Often the exposed bone may be rongeured to a level to allow for soft tissue closure.

For transverse amputations through the distal phalanx, homodigital advancement allows for restoration of contour and the provision of durable soft tissue coverage. Full-thickness soft tissue loss to the dorsum of the fingertip has been treated by us with dorsal metacarpal artery flaps. More recently, we have largely abandoned this technique in favor of the adipofascial turnover flap. Although we previously treated full-thickness injuries to the volar aspect of the fingertip with heterodigital flaps, we have now abandoned this technique in favor of staged reconstruction using acellular dermal matrix if pulp is avulsed to bone, or with dressing changes, almost without regard for wound size. In our experience, defects greater than 1 cm[23] are still very easily and very satisfactorily treated in this fashion.

All injuries are followed weekly in the office for 3 weeks and then on a monthly basis for 3 months. Formal evaluation and treatment by a therapist is begun at the first visit.

Hand Therapy Evaluation

Hand therapy assessment should include a detailed history of the injury and any surgical intervention. Injuries to other digits or other portions of the involved limb should be noted. Past medical history should take particular note of diseases

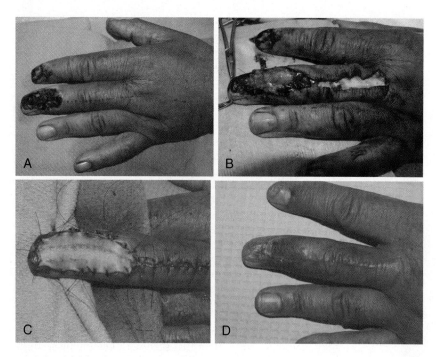

Figure 21-9 Adipofascial turnover flap. **A,** Left hand of a 52-year-old craftsman following auger injury. **B,** Adipofascial flap harvested from proximal finger and rotated distally based on perforating vessels at level of proximal interphalangeal joint. Coverage is obtained to the level of the fingertip. **C,** Full-thickness skin graft applied. **D,** Three months after surgery. Patient was self-employed and returned to work 10 days after surgery following removal of operative dressings. He continued with Coban wrap while at work.

that may interfere with healing, such as diabetes mellitis, peripheral vascular disease, chronic liver disease, alcoholism, poor nutrition, and chronic corticosteroid use. Pain, wound status, edema, and ROM should be formally assessed in the acute injury.

Precautions must be communicated between the referring physician and therapist to allow appropriate protection to the injured limb during rehabilitation. Furthermore, therapy may often proceed without undue worry about the innately grotesque appearance of some wounds. The following

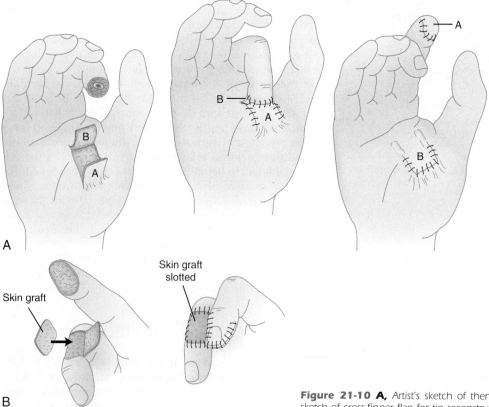

Figure 21-10 A, Artist's sketch of thenar flap for tip reconstruction. **B,** Artist's sketch of cross-finger flap for tip reconstruction.

assessment should be performed within the limits of the precautions prescribed by the treating surgeon. Active (AROM) and passive range-of-motion (PROM) measurements of the injured and adjacent joints should be performed following the standard established by the American Society of Hand Therapists (ASHT).[24] Finger ROM is assessed by placing the stationary and mobile arms of the goniometer on the dorsum of the joint being measured. When measuring ROM in an edematous finger, changing from a dorsal to lateral goniometer placement provides a more accurate assessment of motion. The lateral goniometer placement provides consistent and reproducible measurements as the edema changes.

ROM, and therefore functional hand use, is initially limited by pain and guarding as well as possible postoperative precautions. Some tip injuries, including fractures and tendon lacerations, may have ROM precautions for several weeks. Flexion of the PIP and distal interphalangeal (DIP) joints with sutures located at the nail bed or dorsum of the finger may be uncomfortable for the patient and limit motion. Edema may limit the glide of tendons and the extensor mechanism, making achieving full ROM of both injured and uninjured joints more difficult.[25] Although the DIP joint tends to demonstrate the greatest stiffness in a fingertip injury, patients referred for hand therapy may also demonstrate stiffness of the MCP and PIP joints. Many patients spend the days following acute injury in an extension orthosis, which may include the metacarpal (MP), PIP, and DIP joints. This immobilization period, in addition to the acute inflammatory process, contributes to joint stiffness. Intrinsic muscle tightness and scarring of the extensor mechanism and the lateral bands also becomes more apparent in the finger that has been immobilized for several weeks. A differential diagnosis to determine the structures causing the loss of ROM is necessary. A functional assessment should be completed to determine the patient's ability to perform functional tasks and the amount of compensation needed to be independent with these activities. A clear understanding of the premorbid work and home activities is essential to rehabilitation. Demonstrating hand use in activities of daily living (ADL), instrumental activities of daily living (IADL), and work simulation tasks is ideal, although task performance not demonstrated in the clinic should be acquired through interview and pre-evaluation questionnaires, such as the Disability of the Arm, Shoulder, and Hand (DASH) Questionnaire.[2]

Gripping and turning door knobs, gripping cones and dowels, and using feeding and writing utensils demonstrate motion in addition to the level of hypersensitivity at the fingertip. Functional activities such as holding tool handles, picking up coins and keys, and fastening buttons should be used during the assessment. These tasks determine the patient's ability to manipulate everyday objects and may reveal spontaneous adaptations of normal movement patterns that improve function.

Some patients with fingertip injuries protect the entire hand, and others are able to quickly demonstrate modified function by keeping the injured finger in an extended position and using uninjured fingers to compensate. The patient with a thumb tip injury usually demonstrates difficulty with pinching tasks, whereas those with isolated index or middle

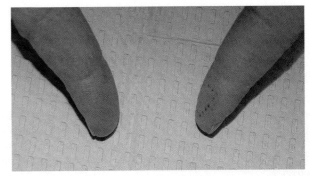

Figure 21-11 Trophic fingertip following pulp avulsion treated by split-thickness skin grafting. Patient has been bypassing fingertip for 12 months.

fingertip injuries may be able to compensate by using the uninjured adjacent finger for pinch activities.

In the case of multiple tip injuries or concomitant hand injuries, the entire hand may not be able to engage in functional tasks due to pain or injury precautions (i.e., tendon, nerve repairs). Any adaptive movement patterns and devices used should be noted because adaptations initially help but often need to be "unlearned" later to return to normal hand function. Continued finger avoidance leads to a trophic fingertip appearance and potential pain with use in spite of expert soft tissue reconstruction and timely therapy (Fig. 21-11). Assessment of typing tolerance may be necessary given the increasing frequency of computer use for work and electronic communication. Having a spare keyboard and mouse in the clinic is a simple way to enable patients to demonstrate their tolerance of keying, which can be measured by words per minute or number of keystrokes with the injured finger. Fingertip hypersensitivity can be more of a barrier than ROM and strength in the person who works with computers.

Soft Tissue

Acute injuries often present with a wound that may vary from a clean sutured partial tip amputation to a draining wound from an untidy crush that was contaminated with debris. Documenting wound size, depth, color, and odor is a standard procedure that can be repeated through consecutive treatment sessions to track progress.

If the nail was amputated in the injury or removed as part of the surgical intervention, a foil nail may be sutured in place to maintain the integrity of the nail matrix while the nail regrows (see Fig. 21-4). The foil nail needs to be protected until it falls off, usually within 2 to 3 weeks. The integrity of an injured but intact nail should be noted; erythema or drainage surrounding the nail bed may indicate infection.

Circumferential measurements of the finger at the proximal, middle, and distal phalanx are appropriate for assessing edema in the tip injury with or without wound. Volumetric measurements have been found to be an objective and accurate measure of edema, although this technique is not used with open wounds or percutaneous pins due to risk of contamination.

If percutaneous pins have been placed, assessing the pin sites for signs of infection, including drainage and redness around the pin, is mandatory. Early recognition allows for the initiation of an appropriate suppressive antibiotic regimen or simple pin removal.

Dysesthesia

Once the soft tissues are stable, hypersensitivity of the tip should be assessed. The density of nerve endings at the fingertip often results in innocuous stimuli causing intense pain. A hypersensitive tip leads to a nonfunctional finger regardless of how well a fracture or wound has recovered.

Barber[23] has developed an organized approach to evaluating and treating hypersensitivity. The assessment involves the three sensory modalities of textures, contact particles, and vibration. The patient orders each of the modalities from least to most irritating. A variety of textures fixed to 10 dowels are rubbed, tapped, and rolled over the sensitive area by the patient. In the next ranking the patient attempts to submerge the hand in tubs of contact particles ranging from soft cotton balls to sharp blocks and again ranks the tubs from least to most irritating. A hand-held vibrator with speed variations measured in cycles per second (cps) is applied to the finger with the patient ranking the tolerance according to duration of application, cps, and whether the stimulus was intermittent or sustained. This ranking forms the basis for treatment of the hypersensitive finger.

Hand Therapy Intervention

Wound Care

The initial intervention for the acutely injured fingertip should address protecting the healing tissue through orthotic fabrication and instruction in activity modification and precautions. For most tuft fractures, nail bed injuries, and soft tissue wounds a DIP static extension orthosis is molded. Some distal phalanx fractures include the terminal extensor tendon and are treated with extension orthoses or percutaneous pinning through the DIP joint. A tip protector orthosis (Fig. 21-12) should be fabricated to protect the pin or to maintain the DIP in full extension if it is not pinned.

Bandaging open wounds with a nonstick dressing under dry finger gauze helps prevent the wound from drying while the gauze absorbs excess drainage. The patient and family need to be instructed in changing the dressings as appropriate, which may be several times a day for a wound with excess drainage, or once a day if there is minimal drainage. Dressings that become saturated with fluid compromise healing and lead to skin maceration (Fig. 21-13). This maceration indicates the bandage needs to be changed more often and the orthosis may need to be molded with perforated thermoplastic to encourage ventilation. If dried blood and fluid stick the dressing to the wound, it can be soaked in warm soapy water to loosen and limit the chance of removing healthy healing tissue when changing.

For fingers with a percutaneous pin and a bandage stuck to the skin it is better to sponge warm soapy water over the bandage instead of soaking. Soaking a finger with a percuta-

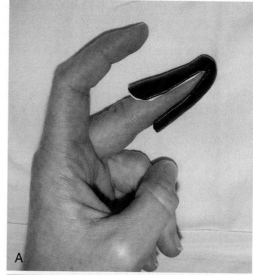

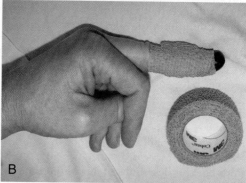

Figure 21-12 Thermoplastic tip protector orthosis (**A**) with Coban overwrap (**B**).

neous pin is contraindicated due to the risk of contamination at the pin site. Percutaneous pins should be cleaned daily with a solution of 50% sterile water and 50% hydrogen peroxide and a cotton swab. Protecting the finger with a percutaneous pin with a simple clam shell DIP extension orthosis helps prevent contamination and accidental bumping of the pin (see Fig. 21-12). The patient and family must demonstrate proper wound and dressing care prior to leaving the clinic. A finger gauze applicator can be purchased at a medical supply store or can be made with scrap thermoplastic material and given to the patient to take home. Fingers that have been fully sutured without any open wound areas can simply be covered with finger gauze for comfort until the sutures are removed.

The patient should be made aware of the signs and symptoms of infection, including fever and chills, swelling, drainage, induration, and erythema. A marked increase in pain, however, is perhaps the most sensitive clinical indicator of infection, even in the absence of marked qualitative change of the soft tissues. Pin tract infections are often marked by pin loosening in addition to local signs such as drainage at the pin site. When recognized early, oral antibiotics are often enough to treat the infection or to suppress infection until the pins may be removed.

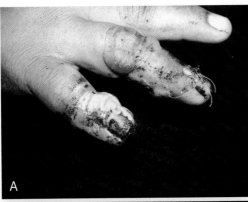

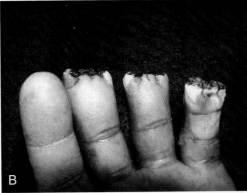

Figure 21-13 *A macerated wound.*

Hypergranulation, also referred to as "proud flesh," is a common phenomenon in the face of even minor trauma to the fingertip or nail unit (Fig. 21-14).

Desensitization

Hypersensitivity of the fingertip is a common and debilitating result of a fingertip injury and should be addressed as soon as wounds have closed. The goal of the therapy is to decrease the uncomfortable and painful response to touch at the

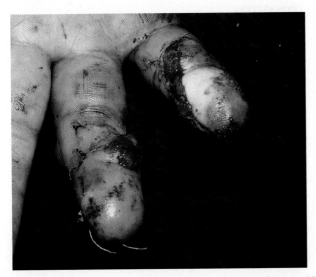

Figure 21-14 *"Proud flesh" at wound margins. This is easily treated by the topical application of silver nitrate.*

fingertip, known as *desensitization*, and increase the tolerance for using the finger during functional tasks. Various modalities of fingertip desensitization following injury may be employed.[26] The sensory modalities of textures, contact particles, and vibration, which were ranked in the assessment phase are now applied with increasingly irritating intensity and frequency. Home exercise performance of the desensitization techniques are done three to four times a day for 10-minute sessions. The patient uses each of the modalities to produce an irritating but tolerable stimuli to the fingertip, and once a modality becomes tolerable, the next in the series is used. This continues until all the modalities are tolerated. This process can take several weeks to several months to reduce the hypersensitivity.

Fluidotherapy can also help with desensitization as it uses fine contact particles in a dry-air-driven whirlpool.[27] With the machine set to produce heat it can also aide in loosening stiff joints through performing AROM during the treatment. In addition to these techniques, the patient who uses power tools such as drills and hand saws should gradually reintroduce these tools as the tolerance for vibration improves.

Desensitization is a gradual process, and until it fully resolves the hypersensitivity can be compensated for by wearing gloves during tool use or wrapping the finger with a self-adherent elasticized bandage such as Coban (3M Coban Self-Adherent Wraps, 3M Company, St. Paul, Minn.) during tasks that cause the most discomfort. A commercially available silicone or gel-lined finger sleeve can be used to cushion the finger against textures and vibration while also having the effect of softening scars.[28,29] The challenge for the patient and therapist is weaning from these protective coverings and getting the finger to tolerate normal activity and contact. The therapist should use activity simulation as well as hand gripping and pinching exercises to increase strength and tolerance for touch and pressure. Gripping and pinching a soft sponge or piece of foam may be done initially then progress to putty gripping, pinching, and raking as hypersensitivity decreases.

Mobilization

Loss of motion of the PIP and DIP joints of the injured finger is common in a tip injury, although all the fingers may manifest stiffness that needs to be addressed in therapy. Stiff fingers should be treated with exercise, stretching, and, if necessary, orthotic positioning.

In a finger injured distal to the DIP joint, the MCP and PIP joints should be mobilized immediately to prevent joint stiffness. AROM and PROM of the PIP can be performed in isolation with blocking exercises or in combination with MP ROM. The patient should be instructed in stretching techniques for home exercise to address a stiff joint, but joint mobilization in addition to stretching techniques can be used in the clinic. Home stretches of the stiff joint should be performed several times a day to improve and then maintain motion.

Heat modalities including fluidotherapy and paraffin wax application can be used to prepare the finger for stretching. Holding the finger in a flexed position with Coban while dipping in paraffin wax (Fig. 21-15) provides a passive stretch with the additional comfort of the heated wax.

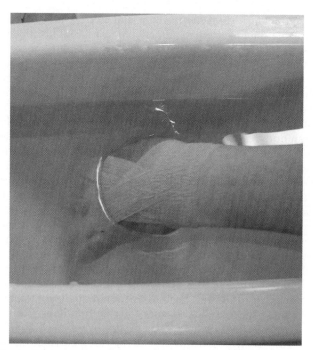

Figure 21-15 *Simultaneous application of a Coban wrap coupled with paraffin bath for static progressive stretch.*

Caution should be taken when first attempting this because even a healed fingertip may be too sensitive to tolerate the heat of the wax. Paraffin should not be used on any hand that has an open wound, a foil nail, or percutaneous pin in place.

The fingertip is often unable to tolerate manual manipulation initially, so DIP joint tightness should be addressed with AROM exercises in the form of blocking and gripping exercises. Functional gripping and prehension tasks with tools used in daily activities, such as hairbrush handles and writing and eating utensils, should be used to encourage DIP joint motion. If the patient's motion prevents gripping small handles, the handles can be built up using foam, Coban, or tape. Using Coban or tape allows for graded reduction in handle size as the patient demonstrates greater ROM.

Buddy-taping can address not only stiffness of the MCP and PIP joints, but also help the patient break the habit of overprotecting the injured finger (Fig. 21-16). Some PIP and MCP joint stiffness is caused or exacerbated by holding the finger in a fully extended protected position to avoid contact. Buddy-taping attaches an injured finger to an adjacent finger while gripping exercises and functional tasks are performed. The stiff finger is provided with AROM through the attached uninjured finger during motion. Using the buddy-tape while exercising with a weight well, cones, or Baltimore Therapeutic Equipment (BTE) is beneficial. Patients returning to heavy manual tasks such as carpentry can use buddy-taping while practicing using power drills, hammers, and screwdrivers again and may be able to wear the buddy-strap when transitioning to full work duties. Because of the length discrepancy of the fingers, buddy-taping is not as effective in addressing stiffness of the DIP joint.

If ROM stretching and exercise fail to return joint ROM, the patient may benefit from static-progressive orthoses. This

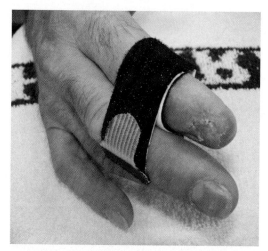

Figure 21-16 *Buddy-straps.*

orthotic approach is applied only to joints that have losses in both AROM and PROM that have not responded to the interventions listed earlier. Static progressive orthoses provide a low-load, long-duration stretch that produces permanent changes in tissue length.[30] The orthosis can be fabricated to apply a flexion or extension force to the MCP or PIP joint without stretching the DIP joint (Fig. 21-17) if it is at risk for forming an extension lag, such as after terminal tendon injury. A static progressive flexion orthosis should be avoided with the terminal extensor tendon injury until it demonstrates limited improvement after several weeks of AROM, PROM, and exercise. There is a significant risk for developing an extensor lag when a flexion orthosis is used after a terminal tendon injury, and gaining flexion at the expense of active extension must be avoided. If the MCP, PIP, and DIP joints are stiff from injury and immobilization, a composite finger flexion orthosis can be fabricated to apply a stretch to all the joints and surrounding tissue (Fig. 21-18). If tolerated, the orthosis should be worn during sleep so the finger can be used functionally during the day.

Summary

The fingertip makes up less than 0.25% of total body surface area. Injuries to this small unit, however, can be quite

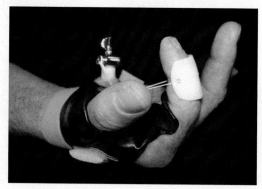

Figure 21-17 *Static progressive orthosis for proximal interphalangeal joint flexion.*

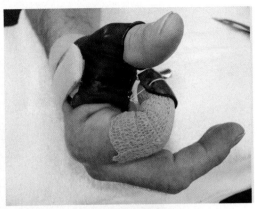

Figure 21-18 Composite flexion orthosis.

debilitating, affecting function of the adjoining digits and the entire hand. Surgical intervention seeks to restore a stable and durable soft tissue envelope. Issues such as stiffness and hypersensitivity are not predictably obviated with surgical intervention alone.

Therapy seeks to maximize gains made through surgical intervention. It involves the patient in their own care, and maximizes functional outcomes while minimizing long-term deficits.

REFERENCES

The complete reference list is available online at www.expertconsult.com.

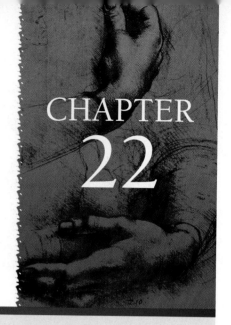

Dupuytren's Disease: Surgical Management

LARRY HURST, MD

CRITICAL POINTS: INDICATIONS AND TIMING OF OPERATIVE TREATMENT

Indications

- Metacarpophalangeal (MCP) contracture 30 degrees or more.
- Proximal Interphalangeal (PIP) contracture 20 to 30 degrees or more with progression.
- Functional disability. Interferes with activities of daily living (ADL) or leisure activity (e.g., golf, piano).
- Acceptable comorbidities for planned surgery and anesthesia.

Preoperative Evaluation

- Thorough history and physical examination.
- Consider the condition of the hand tissues, the rate and extent of the contracture, and the patient's capacity to participate in a hand therapy program.
- Consider the severity in context of the whole patient (Is this a simple procedure under local anesthesia or a recurrent case needing a skin graft and 3 hours of general anesthesia?).
- Be blunt about potential complications, but place the statistical likelihood in practical terms. "It is more dangerous to drive home from work on the highway in the rain than to have a Dupuytren's surgery."

Pearls

- Understand that the normal fascial anatomy is the precursor. Anatomy defines the pathologic cords, which follow predictable patterns.

- Surgery can release the contracture, but surgery can never cure Dupuytren's disease.
- The aim of surgery is release: Dupuytren's tissue cannot be totally excised.
- Make digital incisions after palmar release.
- Expect recurrence, but in older nondiathesis patients recurrence may not interfere with function.
- Dissection is proximal to distal.
- While protecting underlying neurovascular structures, transect the cord at the level of the superficial arch.
- Complete excision does not reduce recurrence.

Technical Points

For MCP Joint Contracture

- Preserving transverse fibers of palmar aponeurosis is optional. The neurovascular bundles are under these fibers.
- Partial fasciectomy and segmental fasciectomy are both effective. There is no evidence that more extensive surgery reduces recurrence.
- Release the tourniquet and avoid hematoma.
- Install a drain if needed within patient's dressing.

For PIP Joint Contracture

- Excise fascia in the proximal digit using zigzag plasty.
- Remember that slight oblique incisions may become longitudinal as contracture is straightened.
- Or use dermofasciectomy and excise skin, fat, and fascia.

- Identify the neurovascular bundles (likely to be displaced).
- Dissect and preserve neurovascular bundles by blunt and sharp dissection in the distal palm first.
- Close zigzag incisions or do Z plasties or V-Y advancements or replace with full-thickness graft.
- Gentle traction on nerve proximally with nerve hook can help identify nerve location distally.

Fixed Joint Contracture Despite Fasciectomy

- Less than 30 degrees of persistent contracture is acceptable.
- More than 30 degrees of contracture, consider PIP joint release.
- Check flap capillary refill and hemostasis at tourniquet deflation.
- Digital vascular tolerance of corrected PIP position should be checked at time of tourniquet deflation.

Pitfalls

- *Nerve division:* The neurovascular bundles can be displaced proximally, superficially, and centrally. Dupuytren's disease doesn't adhere to nerve but repeatedly needing to trace the nerve is tedious, especially in surgery.
- *Artery division:* Critical ischemia may occur if both digital arteries are damaged or if severe PIP contracture is forced to stay in extension (i.e., pinned).
- The surgery is often more difficult, recovery longer, and recurrence more common than the surgeon imagines or the patient understands.

Postoperative Care

- The amount of rehabilitation required varies greatly.
- Spot the patient whose hand is becoming stiff and intervene with therapy and a night extension orthosis.

Functional Use

- The patient is advised not to work or do sports requiring gripping for 3 to 6 weeks. Functional recovery and return to work and sports also varies greatly.

Description and Presentation

Dupuytren's disease is a benign fibromatosis of the palmar and digital fascia of the hand. It develops in the palmar ligaments, with the histologic and surgical pathoanatomic changes occurring primarily in the longitudinal ligaments. The transverse ligaments, such as the intermetacarpal ligaments, can have biochemical changes consistent with Dupuytren's disease but usually develop clinical contractures. Dupuytren's disease starts with a palpable mass in the palm, usually at the level of the distal palmar crease. This mass, the Dupuytren's nodule, may be transient and mildly painful. As the nodule enlarges, it forms pathologic cords that extend distally and proximally. As the cords thicken and shorten, they cause flexion contractures of the joints. The fourth and fifth digits are the most commonly involved, but the thumb, first web, index, and long fingers can also be involved. The

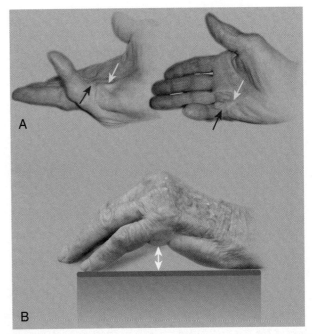

Figure 22-1 A, Palmar and sagittal views of a hand with Dupuytren's disease of the palm and fifth finger. Note, nodules (*red arrows*) and cord (*yellow arrows*). **B,** A positive tabletop test—the palm and fingers cannot be simultaneously placed on the flat surface of the tabletop (*dark gray line*). The distance marked by the double-headed *white arrow* should be zero in the normal hand with a negative tabletop test.

disease on the radial side of the hand is more common in diabetic patients.[1]

The diagnostic workup for Dupuytren's disease includes a careful patient history and physical examination. The severity of the disease can vary considerably. The prognosis for successful treatment and subsequent recurrence clearly relates to contracture quantity and severity. Those patients with a Dupuytren's diathesis (i.e., a more aggressive course of the disease) predictably have multiple surgeries and significant impairment of hand function during their lives. The diathesis group is defined by patient history. The diathesis subgroup, originally defined by Hueston,[2] is composed of whites with a positive family history, bilateral disease, ectopic lesions such as plantar fibromatosis, male gender, and age of onset younger than 50.[3]

The physical exam in Dupuytren's disease reveals palpable nodules and cords with a positive tabletop test[4] (Fig. 22-1). The fixed joint contractures should be recorded with a digital goniometer. Most contractures are static, and the position of one joint does not affect the measurable flexion contracture in the other joints of the same digit. However, dynamic flexion contractures also occur in Dupuytren's disease. For example, a central cord that crosses both the MCP and the PIP joints may produce different degrees of flexion contracture or loss of extension depending on the position of each joint. If the MCP joint is held in neutral extension, then the PIP contracture will be maximized. If the MCP joint is flexed, then the recordable PIP contracture will be significantly reduced (Fig. 22-2). Understanding this potential variability is important when assessing contracture progression, comparing preoperative and postoperative physical findings, or when collecting data to compare one procedure with another.

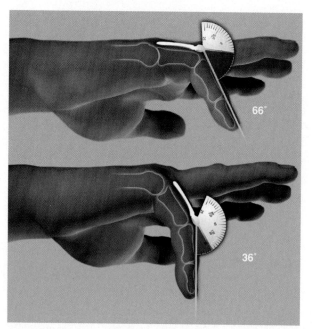

Figure 22-2 Dynamic flexion contracture often seen in Dupuytren's disease when a central cord crosses both the MCP and PIP joints. When the MCP joint is kept at neutral (0 degrees of extension and flexion), the PIP flexion contracture measures 66 degrees (*top image*) but when the MCP is flexed, the PIP contracture is only 36 degrees in this example (*bottom image*).

Nodules, cords, and digital contracture findings are pathognomonic of Dupuytren's disease. Dupuytren's disease is a rare tumorous condition for which an accurate diagnosis can be made without a tissue biopsy. Radiographs and other special diagnostic procedures such as MRI are not needed to diagnose Dupuytren's disease. The rare exception might be the patient with associated osteoarthritis or rheumatoid arthritis for whom arthritic joint change should be delineated by radiography. The arthritic joint changes may be a secondary cause of joint contracture. A second exception might be the use of MRI in the evaluation of the solid knuckle pad or isolated palmar wrist nodule over the palmaris longus insertion into the palmar fascia. In the absence of other signs of Dupuytren's disease, the clinical diagnosis can be uncertain.

Historical Review

Elliot and Tubiana meticulously documented the history of Dupuytren's from the earliest descriptions written in the 12th and 13th centuries to modern times.[5-8] The earliest references are from Orkney and Iceland of miracle cures of Dupuytren's disease. These cures probably represented a traumatic rupture of the Dupuytren's cords. Dupuytren's disease was next described by Swiss physician Felix Plater of Basel in 1614. He thought the disorder was from tendon injury and subsequent digital contracture. The first accurate description of Dupuytren's disease was written by the Englishman John Hunter in 1777. Hunter, the father of English surgery, correctly identified the palmar fascia as the source of Dupuytren's contracture. Interestingly, Dupuytren was born

this same year. Hunter's student Henry Cline proposed fasciotomy. In 1822, Ashley Cooper published the use of a pointed bistoury—a long, narrow surgical knife for closed fasciotomy. In 1831, Dupuytren performed his first open fasciotomy through a transverse incision. He attributed Dupuytren's disease to a traumatic origin and verified the palmar aponeurosis as the source of the contractures. Dupuytren's teachings and procedure were documented in the prolific French medical writings of the time. As a result, palmar fibromatosis became known as Dupuytren's disease even though Cooper's closed fasciotomy remained the surgical treatment of choice. Introduction of general anesthesia in 1842 by Long and Morton and Lister's antiseptic technique in 1865 resulted in the increased use of surgery for the treatment of Dupuytren's disease. The first half of the 20th century brought numerous reports of various surgical incisions and types of fasciotomies and fasciectomies. In the second half of the 20th century and the beginning of the 21st century, surgeon scientists and collaborations between clinicians and basic scientists have exponentially expanded our knowledge of Dupuytren's disease. This knowledge explosion is beyond anything Dupuytren could have conceived in the 1830s; however, this vast expansion of understanding has only begun to expand our therapeutic options. In his textbook, Tubiana documented Hueston's 1992 remark, "I have a dream that one day Dupuytren's disease will be treated without surgery."[9] Hopefully in the near future, the investigational procedure closed enzymatic fasciotomy[10] will be an approved therapy that will, in a small way, fulfill Hueston's dream.

Basic Science

The basic science investigations concerning Dupuytren's disease have undergone an information explosion during the last three decades. A basic understanding of Dupuytren's disease starts with a satellite view of the global epidemiology of this disorder. At the population level, one of the most enduring studies is the Norwegian study,[11] which showed a 9% incidence in males and a 3% incidence in females. This study also showed a clear relationship between the incidence of Dupuytren's disease and aging. In late years, the male/female ratio starts to equalize, but as a global population, the overall gender ratios vary from 2 : 1 up to 10 : 1. Bayat and McGrouther[12] have stated that Dupuytren's disease is the most common heritable connective tissue disease in whites. Tubiana and colleagues estimated the global prevalence at 3% to 6%.[7]

As the focus narrows to a subpopulation view, the pathogenesis of Dupuytren's disease is next characterized in terms of race and genetics, geographic emigration, associated diseases that may increase individual susceptibility, and the potential effects of occupation and trauma on the incidence of the disease.[7,11,13] It is clear that Dupuytren's disease is a disease of Celtic peoples. Where the Vikings, and later the northern Europeans, emigrated, the prevalence of Dupuytren's disease increased. The disease is fairly common in Japan but otherwise rare in Asia and extremely rare in blacks. Dupuytren's is a genetic disorder inherited through an autosomal dominant pattern with a variable penetrance.[14-16]

Dupuytren's disease is associated with diabetes, alcoholism, epilepsy, smoking, AIDS, and vascular disorders. These associations do not imply cause and effect, and not all studies verify these relationships. However, it does appear that subpopulations with certain diseases like diabetes are more frequently afflicted with Dupuytren's disease. Presumably, these patients' comorbidities cause changes at the tissue/molecular level that make their fibroblasts susceptible to the triggers that initiated the dedifferentiation of fibroblasts to myofibroblasts and the beginning of the imbalance in the collagen turnover that leads to nodules, cords, and contractures. Although Dupuytren himself suggested an association between this fibromatosis and heavy use of the hand such as occurred in his coachman's hand from using the whip, this concept has not held up to closer scrutiny. It is now clear that workers whose jobs require heavy manual labor are probably not more susceptible to Dupuytren's disease than those with more sedentary occupations. McFarlane felt that trauma can initiate Dupuytren's disease but not cause it. The asymptomatic nodule that sustains a laceration may rapidly develop a Dupuytren's cord, but heavy use in a normal hand does not cause a Dupuytren's nodule to form. Similarly, a laceration of a normal hand does not cause a nodule or cord in an individual who is not genetically predisposed to Dupuytren's disease. Clearly, one's job does not cause Dupuytren's disease; however, a single injury can initiate clinically evident Dupuytren's in a patient who carries the wrong genes. Dupuytren's disease inheritance follows an autosomal dominant pattern with variable penetrance.

After a subpopulation analysis, the scientific focus narrows to the individual patient and the clinical surgeon treating the patient. The mainstay of treatment remains surgery with frequent recommendations for fasciectomy. The basis for this surgical treatment is a thorough understanding of the anatomy and pathoanatomy of Dupuytren's disease, as described in later sections. The understanding of Dupuytren's disease expands further as excised fascial specimens are brought to the clinical and basic scientists who change our level of observation from the individual to the microscopic and molecular levels.

In the last four decades the histologic, biochemistry, and growth factors associated with Dupuytren's disease have been intensely studied (Fig. 22-3).[14,15,17-27] One of the earliest histologic studies of Dupuytren's disease was Meyerdig's 1940 light microscopic study of Dupuytren's disease and Luck's 1959 classification of it into proliferative, involutional, and residual stages.[28,29] In the 1970s, Gabiani and Majno identified the nodular myofibroblasts and their role in producing the contracture. Soon after, Chiu and McFarlane correlated the cellular findings with Luck's clinical stages of disease.[30] In the next decade, the components of the myofibroblasts' contractile system, including myosin, actin, and ATPase, were identified.[31-34] The density of myofibroblasts was correlated to recurrence, and dermal dendrocytes were identified in Dupuytren's fascia. Next, the microcirculation of Dupuytren's tissue was investigated. Kischer and Speer showed pericyte thickening and speculated on the potential for low O_2 tension.[35] The perivascular smooth muscle cells were shown to turn into myofibroblasts. The observation of low O_2 appears to correlate with epidemiologic studies showing an increased incidence of Dupuytren's with

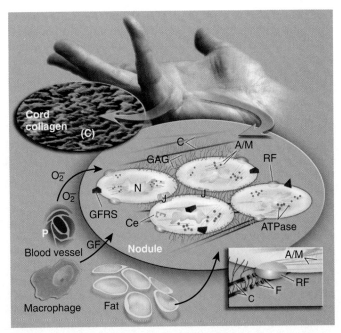

Figure 22-3 Diagrammatic representation of the cellular, molecular, and collagen components of Dupuytren's disease. A/M, actin and myosin filaments; ATPase, adenosine triphosphatase; C, collagen with triple helix; Ce, centrioles; GAG, glycosaminoglycans; GF, growth factors; GFRS, growth factor receptor site for tumor growth factor beta, epidermal growth factor beta, PDGF, platelet-derived growth factor; J, gap junctions; N, indented nucleus; O_2^- oxygen free radical; P, pericyte; RF, α_5, β_1-receptor/fibronexus attachment site.

disorders associated with poor peripheral circulation such as aging, smoking, and diabetes.

The study and understanding of the biochemistry of Dupuytren's disease has also advanced rapidly in the last three decades. The early work of Gelberman and Brickley-Parson found increases in GAGs, type III collagen, and reducible crosslinks in Dupuytren's disease.[21,36] Oxygen free radicals were shown to stimulate the proliferation of myofibroblasts.[37] The connection between the myofibroblasts and the collagen triple helix was elucidated by the important work of Tomasek, Shultz, and Rayan that showed fibronectin strands connecting myofibroblasts to the collagen matrix.[38,39] This made it possible to imagine how the actin/myosin ATPase-driven mechanism in the cytoplasm of the myofibroblasts could pull on the collagen via the fibronexus, shorten the collagen triple helix, and allow subsequent collagen turnover to secure the matrix in a shortened condition. Biochemical studies on Dupuytren's tissue have also shown that prostaglandins are increased in Dupuytren's tissue and can stimulate myofibroblast contraction. Interestingly, prostaglandin abnormalities are also seen in chronic alcoholism, and epidemiology studies show connections between Dupuytren's disease and alcoholism.

In the last two decades, the role of growth factors and cytokines in the mechanism of Dupuytren's disease has also been investigated. Interleuken-1 and growth factors such as tumor growth factor beta (TGF-β), epidermal growth factor beta (EGF-β), platelet-derived growth factor (PDGF), and

EGF have all been implicated in Dupuytren's disease as molecular signals with the potential to stimulate fibroblast transformation to myofibroblasts, collagen production, increased type III collagen production, fibronectin, splicing, and platelet activation.

Given these numerous investigations, it would appear that the sequence of events leading from a normal hand to a symptomatic Dupuytren's contracture would be known in minute details. Alioto, Badalamente, Hurst, Rayan[14,15,17] and others have tried to delineate the concepts from numerous investigations into a "Krebs cycle" that explains Dupuytren's disease. In a recent review, Al-Qattan summarized the basic science knowledge of Dupuytren's disease and proposed a complex algorithm of the multiple factors involved in the pathogenesis of this disease.[40] However, the network diagram of the major genes expressed in a Dupuytren's nodule tissue, which was recently published in Rehman and collaborators' publication, clearly shows that we have only scratched the surface of the true and complete picture of the pathogenesis of this disease.[16] A complete understanding of the signals, pathways, and overall pathogenesis of Dupuytren's disease should lead to numerous new therapeutic options, but for now only hopes precede the new therapeutic alternatives.

Pertinent Anatomy

The skin on the dorsum of the hand is loosely attached but the palmar skin is firmly attached to the skeleton by retention ligaments. These important ligaments keep the skin in place during grasp and pinch. The fascial retention ligaments are part of the normal connective tissue of the hand, and it forms a fibrous continuum that can be divided into the digital fascia, the palmar digital junctional fascia, and the palmar fascia (Fig. 22-4). Normal connective tissue structures are called fascia, ligaments, or bands. Excellent descriptions of the normal anatomy have been provided by Bojsen-Moller, Gosset, Kaplan, Landsmeer, McGrouther, Milford, Rayan, Stack, and White.[22,41-47,54]

The digital fascia is composed of the lateral digital sheath; superficial fibrofatty palmar and dorsal fascia; Cleland's ligaments, which are located dorsal to the neurovascular bundle; and Grayson's ligaments, which are located volar to the bundle. All these ligaments serve as retention ligaments for the digital skin. Except for Cleland's ligaments, all of these structures can become pathologic components of Dupuytren's cords. In the normal state, the fibrofatty palmar and dorsal fascia is scant with tiny, thin, individual fascial fibers, but in the pathologic state, this tissue thickens, coalesces, and becomes a well-defined part of pathologic anatomic structures such as a central cord.

The fascial structures at the palmar digital junction include the spiral band, the natatory ligaments, and the vertical fibers of Legueu and Juvara. In the digit, these structures connect to the proximal portion of Grayson's ligament and the lateral digital sheath. In the palm they connect to the pretendinous band and the superficial transverse ligaments.

The palmar fascial structures include pretendinous bands, superficial transverse bands, and vertical septa. In the sagittal plane, pretendinous bands are the most superficial structures and include thin vertical fibers attached to the skin. The

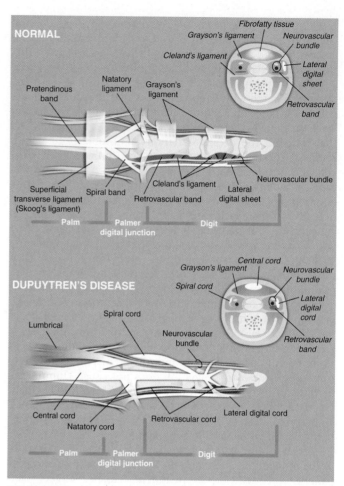

Figure 22-4 Normal fascial anatomy (*top*) and pathoanatomy of the common cords (*bottom*) of the distal palm, palmar digital junctional area, and the digit.

superficial transverse bands are perpendicular and dorsal to the pretendinous band, and the vertical septa are the deepest structures. The vertical septa run dorsally adjacent to the metacarpal necks and attach to the sagittal bands of the extensor hood at the MCP joint level. The vertical bands make a fibrous channel enclosing the flexor tendons and metacarpal and isolate the neurovascular bundle and the lumbrical in separate channels as well. The vertical bands (septa) attach to five structures, septa of Legueu and Juvara, volar plate, deep intermetacarpal ligament, sagittal bands, and loosely to the A-1 pulley. There is no significant connection between the pretendinous band and the A-1 pulley. There is usually an easily dissectible plane between the cord and the A-1 pulley portion of the flexor sheath.

As McFarlane pointed out,[48] these normal fascial structures are the building blocks of the pathologic cords of Dupuytren's disease. The commonly seen cords of Dupuytren's disease are the pretendinous, central, spiral, natatory, abductor digiti minimi, lateral retrovascular, commissural, and radial thumb. Understanding the pathoanatomy of these predictable cords is critical to the safe and effective surgical treatment of Dupuytren's contractures. Cords can act alone or in combination to produce finger contractures.

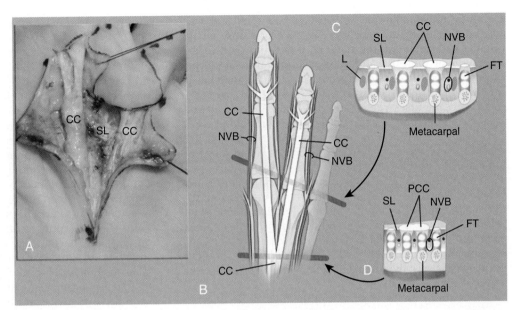

Figure 22-5 Dupuytren's disease—central cord. CC, central cord; FT, flexor tendon; L, lumbrical; NVB, neurovascular bundle; PCC, proximal central cord; SL, Skoog's ligaments.

Pathoanatomy

Knowledge of the anatomic transformation of the normal fascial bands to pathologic cords that, either alone or in combination, alter the normal hand function is essential to the surgical treatment of Dupuytren's disease (see Fig. 22-4). It is critical to understand which components of the palmar and digital fascia are contracted, the involvement of the neurovascular bundle, and how to use the correct surgical maneuvers to safely remove the pathological cords. The works of Barton, Hall-Findlay, Landsmeer, McFarlane, McGrouther, Stack, Tubiana, and White[7,9,44,45,47-54] provide important detailed references concerning the pathoanatomy of these complex cords.

The pathologic central cord (Fig. 22-5) originates from the pretendinous band and palmar superficial fibrofatty fascia. The central cord's first layer is composed of thin vertical bands, which go to the skin, and a middle layer, which constitutes most of the cord, and a deep layer connecting dorsal structures via vertical fibers. The cord inserts into the skin over the proximal phalanx. More distally this cord attaches to the tendon sheath just distal to the PIP joint, periosteum at the base of the middle phalanx, and the lateral digital sheath. This cord is a common cause of combined MCP and PIP joint contractures and the primary cause of dynamic contractures in which measurements vary secondary to finger position. Generally, the cord splits twice just distal to the PIP joint level. On each side of the digit the divided cord surrounds the neurovascular bundle, with part going to the base of the volar middle phalanx and part to Grayson's ligaments and the lateral sheath. Therefore, the divided cord surrounds both the radial and ulnar neurovascular bundles with pathologic cord tissue. Because of this attachment distal to the PIP joint, the central cord frequently results in a PIP joint contracture. When Grayson's ligaments are involved with a central cord, the neurovascular bundle can be pulled toward the midline of the digit at the distal insertion site of the central cord.[48]

The pathologic spiral cord (Fig. 22-6) originates from five separate fascial structures: the pretendinous band, the spiral band of Gosset, the lateral digital sheath, the vertical band, and Grayson's ligament. All these fascial structures coalesce, thicken, and contract to form this cord. Thus, the only part of the palmar digital junction's web coalescence not involved with the spiral band is the natatory ligament. The other components of the web coalescence—the vertical septa band of Legueu and Juvara, the spiral band, and the lateral sheath—are all part of the spiral cord. In the normal hand, for example, the common digital nerve between the ring and little fingers (see Fig. 22-4) divides at the level of the MCP joint, and the radial digital nerve of the little finger passes over the radial fifth spiral band and continues distally to its midlateral position between Grayson's and Cleland's ligaments. In the pathologic state, the spiral cord pulls the radial digital neurovascular bundle proximally, centrally, and superficially as the spiral cord thickens and shortens. Anatomically it is the *neurovascular bundle that actually spirals* as it goes over the spiral cord and then goes dorsally and twists radial to its

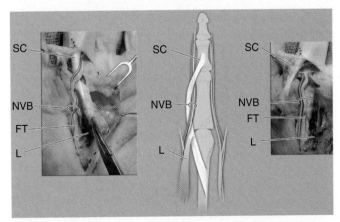

Figure 22-6 Dupuytren's disease—spiral cord. FT, flexor tendon; L: lumbrical; NVB, neurovascular bundle; SC, spiral cord,

anatomic midlateral position between Grayson's and Cleland's ligaments in the digit (see Fig. 22-6). Because of this peculiar pathoanatomy, the spiral cord puts the neurovascular bundle at more risk for surgical injury than any other Dupuytren's cord. As the surgeon cuts through the skin at the level of first digital flexion crease in the presence of a spiral cord, the first structure encountered can be the neurovascular bundle and not the fascia of the cord. Spiral cords can cause severe PIP joint contracture. The severity of this contracture is the most reliable method of diagnosing the presence of a spiral cord. However, in my experience, perfectly accurate preoperative prediction of a spiral cord is not possible. Therefore, dissection of the neurovascular bundle in the palm and assessing the bundle's location is important before extending the incision and cord dissection from the palm into the palmar digital junction region. Only when the position of neurovascular structures is identified should a more aggressive palm–digital junction fascial dissection be undertaken.

The anatomy on the ulnar side of the little finger is different from the normal interdigital web anatomy. There is no natatory ligament; however, the tendon of the abductor digiti minimi can be the origin of a pathologic Dupuytren's cord called the abductor digiti minimi cord (Fig. 22-7). In patients with a fifth finger contracture, approximately one quarter will have an abductor digiti minimi cord. This cord usually originates from the musculotendinous junction area of this intrinsic abductor muscle. This cord can act like a spiral cord and draw the neurovasculature toward the middle line of the proximal phalanx. In addition to the ulnar digital nerve spiraling around the abductor digiti cord in a proximal ulnar, radial, and distal ulnar path, the dorsal ulnar sensory nerve also lies in close proximity to this cord (see Fig. 22-7). The dorsal sensory ulnar nerve supplies a significant area of sensibility to the lateral side of the fifth digit. Like the spiraling fifth ulnar digital neurovascular bundle, the dorsal ulnar sensory nerve can also be easily damaged during dissection of this cord, and therefore, its proximity must be appreciated and its location identified if possible.

The lateral cord (see Fig. 22-4) results from contracture of the lateral digital sheath. This sheath is formed proximally

from the coalescence of the natatory ligament and the spiral band. The ulnar side of the small finger does not have this fascial arrangement; however, the abductor digiti minimi tendon acts as a lateral cord. The lateral cord generally inserts into the dermis of the finger and does not result in severe PIP joint contracture. In the small finger, however, it can attach to the middle phalanx via Grayson's ligaments and cause a PIP joint contracture. It can also cause distal interphalangeal joint contracture because of distal extension of the cord beyond the PIP joint. It does not cause displacement of the neurovascular bundle. The retrovascular cord arises from digital fascia dorsal to the neurovascular bundle and it is separate from the transverse Cleland's ligaments. The retrovascular cord runs in a longitudinal direction. On its own it does not cause contracture of the PIP joint, but in combination with the lateral cord can result in a hyperextension contracture of the distal interphalangeal joint.

The commissural cord results from contracture of first web natatory ligaments, which are identified in the first web as the distal commissural ligament and the proximal commissural ligaments. Surgery is indicated when the contracted first web interferes with thumb function during pinch and grip. Minor commissural cords usually occur in older patients and can be surgically approached with a first web Z-plasty. In younger patients with aggressive disease, skin grafting is often needed. Prior to fasciectomy of the cord, the vulnerable radial digital neurovascular bundle of the index and both the radial and ulnar digital neurovascular bundles of the thumb must be identified and protected. Commissural cords can occur in combination with the radial cord of the thumb. The radial thumb cord rarely causes contracture of the thumb MCP or IP joints but when contractures interfere with function, a fasciectomy may be needed.[9,55]

Cord combinations are not uncommon and can result in continued contracture after individual cord release. The most common cord combination is a central cord/lateral cord combination. This combination contracts both the MCP and PIP joints, and the neurovascular bundle may be drawn centrally. Another common cord combination is the central cord/spiral cord combination. Initially separate, this combination can become a solid sheet encasing the neurovascular bundle. The central cord/natatory cord combination or the spiral cord/natatory cord combination can cause simultaneous MCP contractures in two adjacent fingers (Fig. 22-8). These Y-shaped cords provide a special opportunity when performing a closed enzymatic fasciotomy because a single injection at the apex of the Y can simultaneously correct contractures in two adjacent digits.

Indications for Treatment

In appropriate patients, the amount of contracture improvement and functional correction is predictable and useful, but the durability of the correction varies. The indications for surgical treatment are an MCP contracture of 30 degrees or greater or a PIP contracture of 20 degrees or greater with documented progression. An MCP or PIP contracture of this degree produces a positive tabletop test and begins to cause functional complaints such as difficulty putting the hand in tight places, such as pockets. If contractures are allowed to

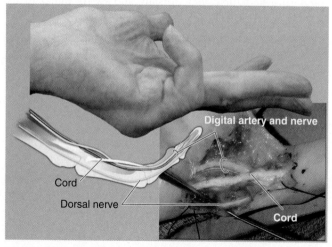

Figure 22-7 Dupuytren's disease—abductor digiti minimi cord; note similar nerve relationships as seen in the spiral cord.

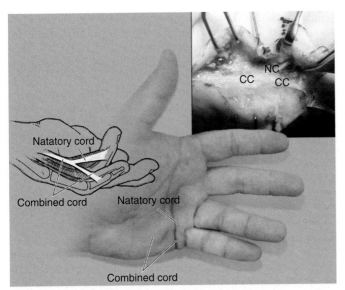

Figure 22-8 Dupuytren's disease—combination cord involving central cord (CC) and natatory cord (NC).

get significantly more severe, then surgery is more difficult to perform, and the outcome, especially in the PIP joint, is less predictable. However, for a patient with a nonprogressing 20-degree PIP contracture who has been followed at appropriate intervals and does not have functional complaints, surgical treatment is not mandatory. With appropriate education, patients with a nonprogressing contracture in a functional hand can decide for themselves when to return for further evaluation or surgical treatment. However, for those patients who present with more than the minimally indicated contracture, then surgery should be recommended because contractures tend to worsen over time. The contracture then interferes more with hand function and surgical treatment is more complex. When recommending surgical treatment, the risks of surgery, potential benefits, limitations of treatment, and alternatives including observation should be discussed frankly with the patient in terms they can understand.

Thousands of patients with Dupuytren's disease are helped each year by surgery, but each patient must be evaluated individually and advised in the context of his or her own complaints, goals, and examination. The patient's ADLs level, the anticipated type and duration of anesthesia, medical evaluation, preoperative labs, electrocardiograph, and American Society of Anesthesia (ASA) level must all be assessed before a final operative decision is made. If the presenting complaint is a Dupuytren's nodule and a minor cord that has not caused a significant contracture, then reassurance, education, and observation are indicated. The associated problems of young age, advanced age, alcoholism, recurrent disease, severe osteoarthritis, rheumatoid arthritis, previous complex regional pain syndrome, and Dupuytren's diathesis must all be part of the patient's evaluation before recommending surgery for Dupuytren's disease. The likelihood of recurrent disease or recurrent disease severe enough to necessitate repeat surgery must be reviewed with each patient. It is my opinion that recurrent disease and disease in areas previously not affected is high (20–80%), but recurrence mandating

repeat surgery for those whose first surgery was after age 50 is not as frequent but still possible. As is true for all musculoskeletal surgery, educating the patient about realistic expectations is extremely important when recommending surgical treatment of Dupuytren's disease.

Types of Surgery

The operative choices include open fasciectomies,[42,51,56-61] closed fasciotomy,[16] needle fasciotomy,[49,62,63] and enzymatic fasciotomy (experimental).[10,64-68] There is no perfect surgical solution for Dupuytren's disease. Surgery does not cure Dupuytren's disease; its goal, instead, is to release the joint contractures and improve hand function. Surgery cannot eliminate the disease.

As stressed by McGrouther,[53] each surgical procedure must manage first the skin, second the fascia, and finally any residual joint contracture after release or excision of the fascia.

Numerous surgical skin incisions have been described for Dupuytren's surgery. Essentially all fall into four groups (Fig. 22-9). All incisions must follow basic hand surgery principles. First, no incision should cross a flexion crease at right angles at the time of wound closure. Second, thin, potentially avascular, skin flaps should be avoided. Disease-free

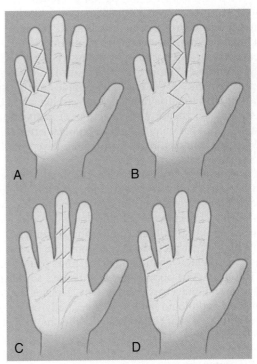

Figure 22-9 Four basic skin incision patterns for Dupuytren's fasciectomies: **A,** The zigzag plasty incision with its linear extension proximal to the palmar flexion crease. In the finger there can be one oblique incision between flexion creases (e.g., fifth finger) or two oblique incisions between flexion creases (e.g., fourth finger). **B,** The Littler–Brunner incision with small transverse extensions. Watson uses these for V-Y plasty closures, Bedeschi leaves them open in the honeycomb technique. **C,** The longitudinal incision, which is closed by Z-plasties (oblique incision lines). **D,** The transverse incisions of McCash's open-palm technique.

subcutaneous tissue should be left on the flaps whenever possible. If the Dupuytren's tissue is intimately attached to the skin, especially in recurrent tissue, then skin excision with subsequent grafting is indicated. Third, the dissection is started proximally and proceeds distally. It is appropriate to make an incision in the palm, partially release the cord, identify the neurovascular locations, then incise the skin of the palmar digital junction, and finally incise the digital skin. A partial cord release in the palm starts to correct the contracture and makes the proper distal incisional design easier. Occasionally, in the palmer digital junction area the neurovascular bundle must be dissected from both a proximal and a distal direction to ensure its identification and proper mobilization away from the pathologic tissue being excised.

The fascial contracture management in Dupuytren's disease can be done with open limited segmental fasciectomy, open limited fasciectomy, open radical fasciectomy, open fasciectomy with skin grafting (dermofasciectomy), open fasciectomy without complete skin closure (McCash's technique), open or closed fasciotomy, needle fasciotomy, or by an enzymatic fasciotomy.

Open limited fasciectomy is the most popular surgery for Dupuytren's disease today.[2,53,57,58] The advantage of this procedure is excellent exposure of the pathologic cord and normal structures such as the neurovascular bundles. This procedure allows correction of the contracture and removal of the bulk of the longitudinal pathologic cords. The uninvolved fascia is left in place unless excision is needed for exposure. I prefer to incise and partially remove the superficial intermetacarpal ligaments of Skoog in order to expose and protect the neurovascular bundles. At the level of the palmar digital junction where the common digital arteries and nerves divide, the location of these structures should be carefully identified. The proximal extent of the fasciectomy is the proximal end of the cord and nodules or to a specific landmark such as the superficial palmar vascular arch. During the dissection, exposure and resection of pathologic cord hemostasis should be obtained with a bipolar cautery. Cautery should be used carefully in order to avoid inadvertent damage to the digital vessels.

The open radical fasciectomy has become less popular in the last 50 years. In this procedure, not only the longitudinal pathologic cords causing contracture are excised but all normal-appearing fascia as well. Presumably, this became popular when anesthesia and antiseptic technique became available and longer procedures were possible. In the 1950s, McIndoe and Beare[69] championed the total palmar fasciectomy. The aggressive approach was intended to release the contracture and prevent recurrence by excising fascia that did not look pathologic but could potentially be the source of recurrent disease. Unfortunately, the more extensive surgery and larger skin flaps caused more surgical morbidity and did not reduce recurrence rates significantly, especially in the PIP joints.[51,53]

The dermofasciectomy is a different approach to surgical management of Dupuytren's disease. This procedure was advocated by John Hueston.[57] More recently, McGrouther[53] has emphasized the utility of this surgical approach. In this procedure, the fascia that causes the contracture is excised with the overlying skin. Then a skin graft is used to cover the entire volar surface of the proximal digit or parts of the palm (or both). The advantage of dermofasciectomy, as McGrouther reports, is that the skin graft acts as a "fire break" of new tissue between the residual fascial tissues. Skin grafting does reduce the chance of recurrence but does not guarantee zero recurrence. Dermofasciectomy in young patients with recurrent aggressive Dupuytren's disease with skin involvement or skin shortage is advocated by many Dupuytren's surgeons.[53,55,57,70,71]

In older patients with inadequate skin because of chronic severe contractures, transverse incisions, originally described by McCash,[59] can be used to expose and excise the Dupuytren's cords. The transverse portion of incisions can be left open and skin grafts avoided. The transverse elliptical skin deficits will heal with a linear transverse scar over 6 to 8 weeks. During this time the patient can do hand soaks and range of motion (ROM) exercises with the hand therapist. Unlike patients with skin grafts that require a period of immobilization, patients with open incisions can start vigorous ROM exercises immediately, which is important in older patients who may have mildly arthritic joints that can become stiff so easily.

Closed and open fasciotomy in which the pathologic cords are cut but not removed have been used for years. Ashley-Cooper described closed fasciotomy in 1822, and Dupuytren did an open fasciotomy for his original procedure.[5,6] In current practice, most surgeons have abandoned the closed fasciotomy, especially in the palmar–digital junction area and digit because of the potential for nerve injury. Open fasciotomy is still used in selected cases where significant functional improvement can sometimes be achieved by a single cut of the central cord in conjunction with a gentle closed manipulation.

An intermediate approach that falls between the limited fasciectomy and open fasciotomy is Moerman's segmental open fasciectomy.[61] He performs a segmental excision of a portion of the longitudinal cord through a series of short curved incisions. Like the open fasciotomy, this has the advantage of limited surgical dissection secondary scarring (Fig. 22-10).

Two additional closed fasciotomies are closed needle fasciotomy and the enzymatic fasciotomy. The closed needle fasciotomy was started in the 1970s by a group of French rheumatologists.[49,62,63] Percutaneous needle fasciotomy is performed with a 25-gauge needle mounted on a syringe. Some surgeons use small amounts of local anesthesia, but others don't. The needle is used blindly to pierce the skin and cut the cord with repeated needle insertions into the cord at multiple levels. As the cord is cut, the finger is passively extended to complete the rupture of the cord. No formal hand therapy is used. Proponents of needle fasciotomy note that patients can use their hand optimally within a week. The complications associated with this technique are tendon rupture (0.05%), digital nerve injury, and a 58% recurrence rate at 3 years.[72] In a recent comparison study between needle fasciotomy and limited fasciectomy, Van Rijssen showed an extension deficit improved 63% (38 degrees reduction in the contracture) in the needle group compared to 79% in the fasciectomy group.[63] MCP joint contracture responded better than PIP joint contracture. His group concluded that percutaneous needle fasciotomy was not suitable for severe contractures.

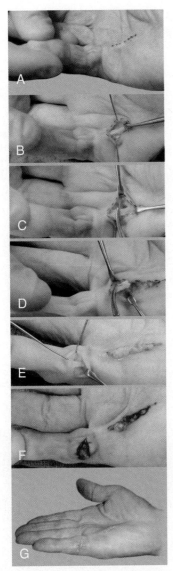

Figure 22-10 Dupuytren's fasciectomy—segmental fasciectomy (steps A–G). **A,** Palmar incision. **B,** Central cord in palm. **C,** Central cord in clamp. **D,** Central cord transected proximally. **E,** Central cord exposed over proximal phalanx area. **F,** Two segments of central cord removed. **G,** Hand flat postoperatively with full correction of contracture.

The closed enzymatic fasciotomy is an investigational procedure.[10,64-68] This procedure has undergone intensive study (Table 22-1). The clostridial collagenase under investigation is derived from *Clostridium histolyticum* and consists of multiple collagenase subtypes that are not immunologically cross-reactive, have different specificities, and act synergistically. Furthermore, the mixed collagenase has well-described collagenolytic properties. The collagenase is injected into the cord, where it disrupts the collagen bonds. This enzymatic activity weakens the cord. The following day the contracted joint is passively extended, usually without anesthesia, and cord rupture occurs. Further details are described later in the author's preferred methods section. Collagenase is an orphan drug. For a new drug application to be submitted to the FDA, the enzymatic fasciotomy has been rigorously studied with double-blind, placebo-controlled phase I, II, and III studies.

More than 2600 injections in more than 1000 patients have now been given worldwide.[24]

Recent phase III studies have been very encouraging. Preliminary data from the double-blind phases of the CORD I and CORD II (Collagenase Option for Reducing Dupuytren's) trials were recently released (Table 22-2).[73] A statistically significant difference was observed for the primary end point correction to 0 to 5 degrees of normal (0 degrees of extension) after the last injection—between collagenase and placebo in CORD I (64% vs. 6.8%, respectively; $P < .001$) and CORD II (44.4% vs. 4.8%, respectively; $P < .001$). The most commonly reported adverse events were pain, swelling, bruising, and pruritus at the injection site. No systemic allergic reactions were reported. Overall, seven serious adverse events possibly related to collagenase were reported from more than 1000 treated patients, including three confirmed tendon ruptures (two in the CORD studies and one in a pharmacokinetic study); one pulley ligament injury; one complex regional pain syndrome; one deep vein thrombosis; and one tendinitis. These results confirm those from earlier studies and support clostridial collagenase as a potential treatment alternative for patients with Dupuytren's contracture.

The primary treatment of Dupuytren's nodules remains observational. Palmar nodules are usually mildly tender, but the tenderness usually resolves even if the nodule remains. Ketchum has recommended treating symptomatic nodules with triamcinolone. After an average of 3.2 injections, he showed 97% regression of the nodules but 50% experienced recurrence.[74] Further study is needed to demonstrate clear disruption of the progression of the contracture by these injections.

The surgical excision of a Dupuytren's nodule is reserved for two special situations. First, the nodule superficial to a trigger finger that requires surgical release should be excised during trigger finger release. Second, the nodule that produces unrelenting pain, especially any night pain, should also be excised. In the first situation, if a nodule is incised while approaching the flexor sheath and not removed, it may progress rapidly and quickly produce a Dupuytren's cord and contracture. Therefore, the nodules and surrounding fascia should be removed during trigger finger surgery. In the second situation, the extremely rare possibility of fibrosarcoma in a young patient must be considered and an excisional biopsy of the nodule performed.[7,14]

The primary treatment for ectopic knuckle pads is also observational. Occasionally, a single knuckle pad can be the presenting sign of Dupuytren's disease, and the diagnosis may not be certain. Then surgical excision may be indicated. Surgical treatment may also be indicated when the knuckle pads are persistently painful, excessively large, or interfere with activities such as wearing a ring. If surgical treatment is considered, recurrence must also be considered. The fibrous mass representing the pad can be approached through a longitudinal, straight, or curvilinear dorsal incision (Fig. 22-11). The dissection should be started proximally where the pad is adhering to the extensor tendon. There is no interval between the extensor tendon and the pad, so the dissection must be done sharply with iris scissor or scalpel. Great care must be taken to preserve the extensor hood and prevent a postsurgical boutonniere deformity.

Table 22-1 Collagenase Studies*

	Population and Treatment	Results
In vitro Studies		
Rat-tail tendon model[75]	Tail tendon was exposed and injected with purified clostridial collagenase (150 or 300 units) or sterile distilled water	Clear evidence of collagen lysis with fibril and bundle discontinuity after 24 hours No extravasation to adjacent tissues No neurovascular damage noted
Biomechanical study[40]	20 Dupuytren's cords were surgically removed from patients and randomly assigned to treatment with collagenase (150 units, 300 units, or 600 units) or control buffer	300 units of collagenase was the minimum effective dose sufficient to cause cord rupture by the normal extensor forces of the index, long, ring, and small fingers Collagen lysis increased with incremental doses of collagenase
Phase 2 Studies		
Open-label, dose-escalation, phase 2, pilot study[31]	6 patients received single injections of 300, 600, 1200, 2400, 4800, or 9600 units of collagenase; 29 patients received single injections of 10,000 units (0.58 mg) of collagenase	No clinical benefit observed until 9600 units collagenase was given 88% of MP joints and 44% of PIP joints treated with 10,000 units of collagenase achieved 0–5 degrees of normal
Single-center, randomized, placebo-controlled, double-blind study with open-label extension (Study 101)[32]	49 patients received single injections of 10,000 units (0.58 mg) of collagenase or placebo 36 MP joints 13 PIP joints	More collagenase-treated cords than placebo-treated cords achieved 0–5 degrees of normal ■ 78% vs 11%, respectively, for MP joints and 71% vs 0%, respectively, for PIP joints after 1st injection
	Up to 3 injections per joint (5 total) were permitted in the open-label phase	
Randomized, double-blind, placebo-controlled, dose-response study with an open-label extension (Study 202)[32]	80 patients received single injections of 2500 (0.145 mg), 5000 (0.29 mg), or 10,000 (0.58 mg) units of collagenase or placebo 55 MP joints 25 PIP joints	10,000 units (0.58 mg) of collagenase is the minimum dose that results in clinical benefit 78% of joints receiving 10,000 units of collagenase, 45% of joints receiving 5000 units, and 50% of joints receiving 2500 units achieved 0–5 degrees of normal No response to placebo observed
	Up to 3 injections per joint (5 total) were permitted in the open-label phase	
Safety[31,32]	Minor, transient AEs such as injection site tenderness, hand ecchymosis, and edema were reported, but all resolved within 6 to 7 weeks of the injection Collagenase injection did not induce an adverse systemic immune reaction, even after repeated administration	
Completed Phase 3 Studies		
Randomized, double-blind, placebo-controlled study (Study 303)[33]	35 patients with Dupuytren's contracture were randomized in a 2:1 ratio to receive up to 3 injections of collagenase 10,000 units (0.58 mg) or placebo 21 MP joint contractures 14 PIP joint contractures	91% of joints receiving collagenase and 0% of joints receiving placebo for a primary joint achieved 0–5 degrees of normal ($P < .001$)
Open-label extension of Study 303 (Study 404)[33]	19 patients (35 joints) from Study 303 who did not achieve 0–5 degrees of normal, or who had other involved joints of the same or contralateral hand, continued treatment (maximum: 3 injections per joint, 5 total)	89.5% of joints achieved 0–5 degrees of normal in at least 1 treated joint
Safety and recurrence[33]	All AEs were graded as mild to moderate with most resolving within 1 to 3 weeks Most frequently reported AEs: injection-site pain, hand ecchymosis, and edema During long-term follow-up, joints treated in studies 303 and 404, 4 PIP joints and 1 MP joint, had recurrence	

AEs, adverse events; MP, metacarpal; PIP, proximal interphalangeal.
*A series of preclinical and clinical trials investigating the efficacy of collagenase for the treatment of joint contractures caused by Dupuytren's cords.

Author's Preferred Treatment Method

When it is approved* by the Food and Drug Administration, collagenase will be my first-line treatment for

_____
*In 2010 the FDA approved collegenase for treatment of Dupuytren's contractures.

Dupuytren's contractures. My research experience in the double-blind, placebo-controlled studies has convinced me that collagenase is safe and efficacious. The indications for injection and manipulation are similar to current surgical indications. Treatment is dictated when the MCP contracture equals 30 degrees or greater or when a progressing PIP contracture is 20 degrees or greater. Contractures of this degree or greater usually cause a positive tabletop test and interfere with hand function. A final

Table 22-2 Collagenase Phase III Trial Results*

	CORD I		CORD II	
	Collagenase†	Placebo	Collagenase	Placebo
Evaluable joints, n	203	103	45	21
Joints achieving 0–5 degrees of normal, % (n/N)	64 (130/203)	6.8 (7/103)	44.4 (20/45)	4.8 (1/21)
Improvement, % (baseline/after last injection)	79.3 (50.2°/12.2°)	8.6 (19.1°/45.7°)	70.5 (53.2°/16.7°)	13.6 (50.0°/44.3°)
Joints achieving ≥50% reduction in contracture from baseline, % (n/N)	84.7 (172/203)	11.7 (12/103)	77.8 (35/45)	14.3 (3/21)

*Four additional phase 3 studies, **C**ollagenase **O**ption for **R**educing **D**upuytren's (CORD) I and CORD II, and JOINT I and JOINT II, are ongoing. The primary end point of the studies is normalization of the joint to within 0–5 degrees of normal after up to 3 injections of study treatment. Upon completion of the double-blind phases of the CORD studies, patients who initially received placebo or who had other affected joints were eligible for enrollment in open-label extension phases, during which all patients are receiving collagenase treatment.
†All differences between collagenase and placebo are statistically significant ($P < 0.001$).

indication is a web contracture that interferes with grasp or pinch.

Collagenase injections are given with sterile technique using a 27-gauge needle and an insulin syringe (Fig. 22-12). Prior to injection, the cord is placed under tension while the proximal end, the distal end, and area where the cord is maximally separated from the flexor tendon are determined by observation and palpation. At the level of the affected joint, the needle is inserted into the cord at a point where the cord is maximally separated from the underlying flexor tendons. A collagenase dose of 0.58 mg in 0.25 mL is used for cords causing an MCP contracture. A dose of 0.58 mg in 0.20 mL is used for cords causing a PIP contracture. The 0.58-mg dose is divided into thirds. One third of the dose is placed in three close but separate spots in the cord (see Fig. 22-12). This can be done by inserting the needle in the cord once and moving the needle tip to place one third of the dose in three slightly different locations in the cord, or alternatively the needle can be inserted three separate times. The dose must be injected into the cord and not through it. The hand is then placed in a bulky dressing, finger motion is limited, and the hand is elevated until bedtime. At bedtime, the patient removes the dressing. The next day the patient returns for manipulation of the finger. Sensation and tendon function is checked. In the research protocols, anesthesia has generally not been used, but local lidocaine block has been used occasionally. Before manipulating the finger, the flexor tendon is protected by flexing the wrist. The affected joint is then passively extended. If the MCP joint is being manipulated into extension, then the PIP joint is kept flexed. If the PIP joint is being manipulated, then the MCP joint is kept flexed as much as possible. Frequently, passive extension of the previously injected cord results in a palpable or sometimes audible snapping of the injected Dupuytren's cord. Immediately after rupturing the cord, the patient is asked to flex and extend the finger to demonstrate tendon integrity. When the cord does not snap, it often still stretches over the course of several weeks. All patients are started on passive stretching exercises. Frequently, over the next week, the cord that has not snapped completely continues to stretch, thereby reducing the Dupuytren's flexion contracture. All patients wear an orthosis in extension at night for 3 months. In the research protocols, patients who do not correct their contracture to 5 or less degrees were offered a second and third injection at 30-day intervals. The excellent results obtained with this treatment are detailed in Tables 22-1 and 22-2. At this point more than 2600 joints in more than 1000 patients have been injected. The adverse events (complications) with this treatment have been minimal and mild except for three flexor tendon ruptures, which all occurred while injecting cords at the PIP joint of the little finger (Table 22-3). Protocol modifications have so far decreased this complication. The modifications of the manipulation technique have included not injecting the area immediately adjacent to the little finger PIP joint flexion crease and being extra cautious about inserting the needle too deeply during injections. Again, the collagenase must go into the cord, not through it. For cords

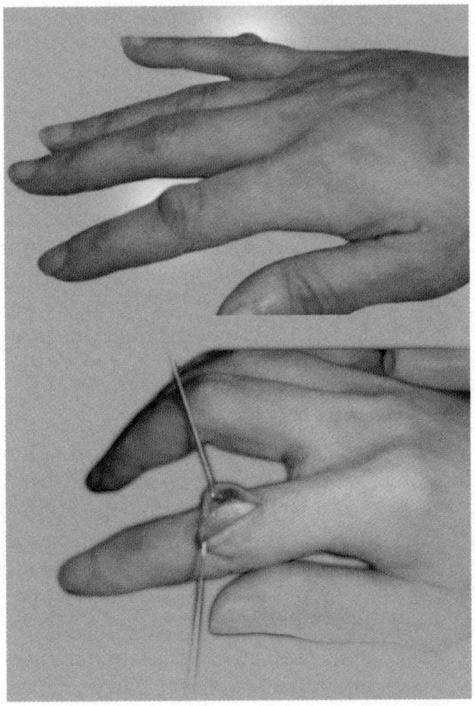

Figure 22-11 Dupuytren's disease—knuckle pads. Preoperative view of large painful knuckle pads on the index and little fingers *(top)*. Excised index finger knuckle pad within intact extensor hood *(bottom)*.

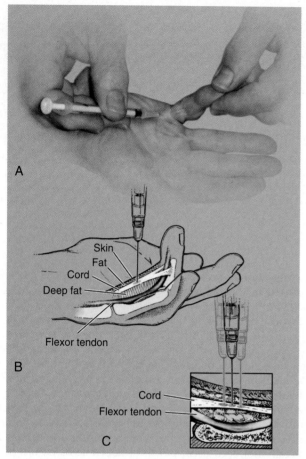

Figure 22-12 Dupuytren's enzymatic fasciectomy. **A,** 0.58 mg in 0.25 mL injected into central cord. **B,** Collagenase (*green*) diffuses in cord. **C,** One third of the 0.58-mg dose placed in three separate areas in the cord.

Table 22-3 Adverse Events Associated with Collagenase Treatment

CORD I	CORD II
Arthralgia	Lymphadenopathy
n = 8 (3.9%)	*n* = 11 (12.4%)
6/8 on 1st injection	Paraesthesia
2/8 3rd injection	*n* = 4 (8.9%)
Lymphadenopathy	
n = 20 (9.8%)	
Most on 1st injection	
Lymph node pain	
n = 21 (10.3%)	
Paraesthesia	
n = 3 (1.5%)	
Hypoesthesia	
n = 3 (1.5%)	
Tendon ruptures	
2 (5th finger PIP) occurred before the revised injection technique	
One in CORD I and one in PK study	
1 (5th finger PIP)	
CORD I	
To date, more than 2600 injections have been given in more than 1000 patients, with an occurrence rate of 0.2%	

CORD, **C**ollagenase **O**ption for **R**educing **D**upuytren's; PIP, proximal interphalangeal; PK, pharmacokinetics.

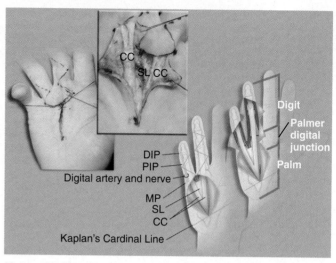

Figure 22-13 Dupuytren's zigzag limited fasciectomy technique. CC, central cord; DIP, distal interphalangeal joint; MCP, metacarpophalangeal joint; SL, Skoog's ligaments.

contracting the fifth finger PIP joint, the needle should be brought into the cord in a horizontal plane, not a vertical one, if possible. In addition, the bevel of the needle is about 1.25 mm, and the needle should not be inserted more than 2 to 3 mm into the skin near the fifth finger PIP joint. The recurrence of any joint contracture in these studies has been approximately 10% for MCP joints and 20% for PIP joints at 5-year follow-up.

My current treatment for Dupuytren's contracture in my clinical practice is a limited partial fasciectomy done through a zigzag (Brunner type) skin incision. This surgical technique has been previously described in detail in *Blair's Techniques in Hand Surgery*.[58] This surgical approach is straightforward (Fig. 22-13). All incisions and dissections should be done with loupe magnification. In this surgical approach, the incision starts proximally at the level of the superficial vascular arch and then extends as a straight longitudinal incision to the distal palmar crease. From this point distally the incision continues in a zigzag manner into the involved digit(s). The palmar digital junction area is incised cautiously after checking the location of digital neurovascular bundles through the initial longitudinal palmer incision and first limb of the zigzag incision. The final design and incisions in the finger are done after partial release of the cords in the palm. After partial correction and extension of the digit, the proper obliquity of the limbs of the zigzag design can be better appreciated. If there are coexisting cords in the little and ring fingers, for example, then the longitudinal palmar portion of the incision can be placed between the two cords. The palmar–digital junctional area is exposed by using a distally based web flap (see Fig. 22-13). After making the palmar portion of the incision, the fasciectomy is started proximally at the point where the cords coalesce. Each digit's cord is dissected separately from this proximal point distally. The fasciectomy is initiated by cutting the cord transversely at the level of the superficial arch while protecting these underlying vascular structures. The superficial intermetacarpal ligaments are incised to allow easy visibility of the neurovascular bundle in the distal half of the palm. Next, the vertical septae are cut. These initial releases in the palm frequently allow considerable correction of the contracture. The dissection is then continued carefully through the palmar–digital area. In the digit there can be one or two limbs of the zigzag incision between the first and second transverse digital creases (see Fig. 22-13). Varying the limb design allows the surgeon to keep the skin flaps as thick as possible, thus avoiding a flap that is too thin or excessively soft at its base. The pathoanatomy of the cord guides the dissection, especially in the palmar–digital area and digit.

The fascial excision is done to release the contracture and remove the nodules and any large palpable portions of the cord. I do not attempt to remove all the pathologic fascia. If there is greater than a 30-degree residual PIP contracture after fascial excision, then I consider a PIP volar release and gentle manipulation.

I agree with McGrouther that all Dupuytren's surgery should be done under tourniquet. but the tourniquet should be deflated before wound closure and bleeding carefully controlled with a bipolar cautery. If there is any residual bleeding, the transverse portions of the incision should be left open or a small drain should be used. In the ambulatory surgery setting, the drain is left under the dressing and removed the following day in the office.

In older patients with significant contractures causing considerable functional complaints but who also have significant co-morbidities, I substitute a limited segmental fasciectomy or open fasciotomy for the partial fasciectomy described earlier. In young patients with recurrent disease, I use a dermofasciectomy with skin grafts from the medial arm or groin. In older arthritic patients with associated skin problems, I try to avoid skin grafting and use the open palm McCash technique, which allows for immediate active ROM exercises.

Surgery for recurrent disease also requires special consideration. First, the patient must have an obtainable goal in mind. Full correction of the contracture is unlikely. Second, the dissection is more difficult and takes longer. Third, a careful preoperative exam is needed to identify previously damaged nerves and vessels. Fourth, the incidence of neurovascular injury is higher during repeat fasciectomy because the normal anatomy is always distorted. Fifth, the recovery and postoperative therapy is more intense. Finally, ancillary procedures such as PIP joint release, PIP fusion, or arthroplasty or amputation may be needed.

Complications

Managing patients' expectations before and after surgery is extremely important. The patient must understand that Dupuytren's surgery usually improves function but cannot cure this disease. Except in young patients, I think it is safe to advise that recurrence is common, but the need for repeat surgery for those older than 50 is fairly uncommon. In a litigious society, an emphatic but balanced discussion of all potential complications **must** be done preoperatively.

The complication rate from Dupuytren's surgery has been reported as high as 17%. In my experience, however, complications that cause permanent harm that leaves the patient functionally worse off than before surgery are rare.

Potential complications include failure to correct the contracture, loss of flexion, digital nerve laceration (1.5%),[7] arterial laceration, skin flap loss, digit loss, tendon sheath or flexor tendon damage, hematoma, infection, complex reflex sympathetic dystrophy (RSD; otherwise known as complex regional pain syndrome), and recurrence or extension of disease and contractures. The first step in managing these complications is prevention and managing the patient's expectations before surgery. MCP contractures are almost always corrected to neutral or very close. With PIP contractures, the surgeon should anticipate that complete correction is unlikely and that some loss of correction will occur over time. If there is a PIP contracture greater than 30 degrees at the end of cord excision, then a volar release of the PIP joint should be done as an adjunct to the fasciectomy. Flexion loss is not easily corrected and should be avoided by early hand therapy and by limiting the surgical dissection as much as possible, especially in patients with co-morbidities such as osteoarthritis. Any digital nerve lacerations that occur during surgery should be repaired immediately. To ensure that these repair opportunities are not missed, the neurovascular bundles should be scrutinized before wound closure. A significant number of patients experience numbness immediately after surgery. The majority of these are secondary to neuropraxia caused by digital nerve retraction. In these patients, protective sensation is almost always intact. Lacerated digital arteries should also be repaired before closure if they are recognized. Before wound closure, the tourniquet should be deflated, homeostasis should be cautiously achieved with a bipolar cautery, and digital capillary refill assessed. Putting warm saline-soaked sponges on the palmer and digital wounds at the time of tourniquet deflation facilitates capillary refill by quickly ending vasospasm. If a digit fails to "pink up," then the fingers should be put in a more flexed position and more warm soaks should be reapplied with or without lidocaine bathing of the neurovascular bundle. If the digit is still not profusing after an appropriate time, the arteries should be explored for a missed laceration. Skin flap loss should again be prevented by assessing flap viability at the end of the procedure. As needed, small avascular parts of a flap can be removed, transverse parts of the incision left open, or skin grafts performed. The potential for digit loss in severe contractures, especially of the fifth PIP joint, must be explained to the patient preoperatively and the possibility of amputation discussed. If a digit becomes ischemic after surgery, amputation at the appropriate level should be done. A small opening of the tendon sheath can usually be left as long as the A2 and A4 pulleys are intact. Other tendon injuries should be repaired or reconstructed as needed. Any significant hematoma should be drained in an operating room environment, but wound evaluation with the tourniquet deflated, open palm technique, and the use of drains should minimize this complication. Complex RSD should be considered in any patient with unrelenting pain that is out of proportion with the surgery performed. Whenever complex RSD is considered, pain center consultation, hand therapy, and appropriate medications must be started promptly. Recurrence and extension of the disease must be explained to the patient as regular occurrences in Dupuytren's disease. When contractures reoccur that are severe enough to interfere with function, repeat surgery may have to be considered, but with repeat surgery, the risks are greater and cure is still not achievable. Some patients can be helped in these recurrent cases by PIP fusion with shortening, PIP joint replacement with shortening, or by amputation. Finally, it should be understood that some patients have contractures that represent very real functional problems that cannot be safely helped by further surgical treatment.

Postoperative Management and Hand Therapy

Essentially, all Dupuytren's surgery is now done in an ambulatory or day surgery setting. At the conclusion of the surgical procedure, the hand and fingers should be placed in an orthosis in extension with a comfortable bulky dressing or a combined dressing and orthosis. Ice packs against the dressing are also recommended during the first 48 hours. Patients are sent home in a sling but should be advised to take the upper extremity out of the sling at home and keep the hand elevated above the heart for the first 48 hours. Elevation should be continued until the dependent position is *not* accompanied by throbbing, swelling, or paresthesias. The patient should do gentle active motion within the constraints of the bulky dressing. The patient is told that this motion will cause discomfort but will not be harmful. Between 1 and 5 days, the bulky dressing is removed. The wound and neurovascular status is checked. If a drain was used, the first visit is done on postoperative day 1. At this visit the drain is removed. Next, a new small dressing is applied. The patient is then sent to the hand therapist, who starts ROM exercises and makes a removable nighttime extension orthosis. If an open palm technique has been used, soaks and dressing changes are also started. The night orthosis is used for 3 to 4 months. With PIP contractures, the orthosis may require frequent modification. At the next postoperative visit 10 to 14 days after the surgery, the skin sutures are removed. Routine bathing and incisional area massaging is begun at this visit. After this visit, patients are seen at monthly intervals until their result has stabilized. Therapy visits are recommended one, two, or three times weekly, depending on the patient's needs. Patients must understand that the therapist is a teacher and that doing their "homework" (i.e., exercises and using their orthosis) is their responsibility and that exercises must be done several times a day in order to optimize the outcome. Additional therapy modalities may be needed

if the PIP joint has been released, if a flare reaction occurs, or if there is any sign of RSD. A "flare reaction" is a complication that occurs in patients who otherwise show good progress during the first few weeks after surgery and then experience a flare of edema, redness, increased pain, and stiffness. It usually occurs during the third or fourth week after surgery. The therapist should contact the surgeon whenever the patient's progress is abnormal. The reader is referred to Chapter 23 for a detailed discussion of the postoperative management of Dupuytren's contracture.

Results of Treatment

If patients are followed long enough, recurrence after surgery to some degree probably reaches 100%, as stressed by McGrouther.[53] Further development of visually evident disease in areas not previously involved (i.e., disease extension) is also common. Surgical recurrence rates vary from 8% to 54%.[55,71] The exact surgical procedure does not affect the recurrence rate significantly except for dermatofasciectomy, for which recurrence rates are somewhat lower.[70] The longer patients are followed, the higher the recurrence rate. PIP joint contractures reoccur more often than MCP joint contractures. Recurrence after collagenase injection is approximately 10% for MCP joints and 20% for PIP joints at 5 years. The recurrence rate for percutaneous needle fasciectomy at 3 years has been reported at 58%.[72]

Summary

This chapter reviews the history, basic science, and anatomy that are important background information for those surgeons diagnosing and treating Dupuytren's disease. Further, the chapter reviews the indications for treatment and all currently available treatment options. The author's preferred surgical method of partial fasciectomy is described in detail along with a review of potential complications and postoperative management. Finally, the chapter has reviewed collagenase which has recently been approved by the FDA for the treatment of Dupuytren's disease.

REFERENCES

The complete reference list is available online at www.expertconsult.com.

Therapeutic Management of Dupuytren's Contracture

ROSLYN B. EVANS, OTR/L, CHT

CRITICAL POINTS: KEYS TO SUCCESSFUL POSTOPERATIVE MANAGEMENT FOR DUPUYTREN'S CONTRACTURE

- Proper preoperative evaluation of associated problems (carpal tunnel syndrome [CTS], triggers, abductor band)
- Early referral to therapy; proper wound care, and edema management
- *No-tension orthosis* for the first 3 postoperative weeks
- Gentle exercise technique to protect against wound and neurovascular tension
- No suture removal before 2.5 weeks after surgery; 24-hour paper tape for an additional 3 to 4 weeks
- Early identification of problems related to infection, sympathetic flare, or CTS
- Progression to static or dynamic extension orthosis at 3 weeks after surgery
- Attention to stretch for the intrinsic muscles, oblique retinacular ligament (ORL), and facilitation of the flexor digitorum profundus (FDP) tendon
- No repetitive gripping exercise or forceful passive motion
- Extension orthosis at night for 4 to 6 months

The purpose of this chapter is to examine postoperative rehabilitation techniques following surgical intervention for Dupuytren's contracture (DC), with particular focus on improved functional outcomes and diminished postoperative complications. The reader who is interested in a more comprehensive review of the subject can follow links in the bibliography for more in-depth study. This chapter will emphasize the author's preferred techniques.

Clinical experience teaches that some complications following Dupuytren's fasciectomy may be attributed in part to aggressive management of the tissues by the therapist or patient with exercise and orthotic use; late referral to therapy, short-term follow-up, or undiagnosed pre-existing CTS or triggering digits. The rational, clinical research, and experience for this observation are defined in a previous paper and in the online appendix.[1]

Description

Dupuytren's disease (DD) is a proliferative and progressive fibroplasia affecting the palmar fascia that can lead to flexion contracture in the metacarpophalangeal (MCP) and the proximal interphalangeal (PIP) joints, causing functional disability. The pathologic findings vary with the stage of the disease, progressing from early cellular nodules to dense fibrous cords.[2-6]

This disease has been studied extensively since being described by Dupuytren in 1834[7] in terms of anatomy,[8] etiology,[3,9-11] genetics,[12-16] pathophysiology,[17-20] associated ailments,[21,22] demographics,[10,22,23] surgical technique,[24-31] and functional outcomes.[32-34]

Nonoperative treatment for DC including enzymatic fasciotomy, skeletal traction and use of progressive mechanical tension orthoses, radiation, dimethyl sulfoxide, vitamin E, allopurinol, ultrasound therapy, steroid injection, interferon, and orthotic use have been studied and are summarized elsewhere.[35] Most conservative interventions demonstrate only limited short-term improvement, but some of the newer procedures, including collagenase injection (enzymatic fasciotomy) with manipulation,[36] and needle fasciotomy,[37] have demonstrated promising results and gained popularity due to limited complication rate and quicker recovery. Long-term results for these interventions are not yet available.

Although DC is now better understood, with much new research on biochemical and cellular aspects, the true cause of the disease continues to be unknown,[6,20,22,38-40] and little data is available about the response of these cells to various agonists such as mechanical stress.[19,41,42]

Although techniques for surgical intervention and nonoperative treatment for DC are well described and reviewed in the literature,[6,31,35] reference to postoperative therapy is, for the most part, inadequate and anecdotal, without much evidence other than clinical observation.[32,43-47] Au-Yong and associates recently surveyed 141 hand surgeons regarding practice patterns for surgical and postoperative decision making in the treatment of DC. Questions regarding practice patterns and results of their survey addressed clinical decision making with regard to surgery, but revealed little information regarding postoperative management other than referral to therapy and time in orthoses with no details given on orthoses design with reference to joint angles or to actual therapeutic regimens.[46]

Literature review produces few studies to support therapeutic interventions and conflicting support about the benefit,[48] or lack of benefit for these interventions.[34] As of this writing, no matches were found for evidence-based medicine or randomized controlled studies for physical agents or exercise protocols following surgical intervention for DC.[49] Postoperative orthotic use as a therapeutic intervention also has little definition. Clinical experience and literature review show that postoperative orthotic use among hand surgeons and therapists varies significantly from relaxed extension, aggressive extension, tension relieved, to no tension.[1,29,38,43-45,50-54] The antitension regimen for orthotic use and exercise described by the author is the only study that attempts to objectively correlate the effect of postoperative mechanical stress to complications of inflammation, sympathetic flare, hypertrophic scar, and functional range of motion (ROM).[1] Currently, a multicenter, randomized, controlled trial is underway to determine the effectiveness of postoperative orthotic positions and duration of use.[47]

The Value of Preoperative Therapy

There is a limited role for therapy post-operatively in DC. A single presurgery visit with the therapist is valuable for the patient because the therapist can support the surgeon's interview by reiterating the postoperative sequelae, time frames for rehabilitation, and the need for prolonged night orthotic use, a well as help define *realistic* expectations for outcomes. Such a visit also benefits the physician because the therapist can assist with documentation of preoperative ROM; sensibility for each digital nerve; function of the flexor digitorum profundus (FDP), oblique retinacular ligament (ORL); degree of intrinsic tightness; documentation of abductor digit minimi band;[55] screen for carpal tunnel syndrome (CTS) and triggering digits; and document the patient's functional self-assessment with standardized outcome measures.[56,57] Early troubleshooting, especially with a screen for CTS, digital triggers, and the presence of an abductor band, can help prevent postoperative complications.

Several investigators have had success with preoperative continuous traction techniques to improve joint extension,

but these devices have not gained popularity among surgeons, do have some complications, and the patient still requires fasciectomy.[58-61] The author has a small series of patients ($n = 9$) (referred by Paul Dell, MD, Shands Teaching Hospital, Gainesville, Florida) that have been treated preoperatively for 3 weeks with serial finger casting[62] (Fig. 23-1, online) to improve proximal interphalangeal (PIP) joint extension by applying a low load continuously[63] to connective tissues about the joint and to the Dupuytren's fascia. The distal interphalangeal joint (DIP) is left free to stretch the ORL and to activate the FDP. This requires two serial cast changes per week, with exercise each session to work the PIP joint into extension, and to focus on activating the FDP and stretch for the ORL. On average, about 25 to 40 degrees of PIP extension are gained before surgical release with serial casting, and improvements are noted for FDP function and stretch to the ORL, but the study is ongoing. It has not been established if this technique shortens rehabilitation time or improves final results, but the referring physician feels that the serial casting simplifies the release and may help to improve final results. As these patients are usually in the age group for Medicare insurance, the issue about limited visits is a concern to therapists in free-standing rehabilitation units, so presurgical treatment should be kept to a minimum.

Postoperative Management: Author's Preferred Technique

Postoperative complications, including infection, flap necrosis, white finger, nerve damage, sympathetic flare, hypertrophic scar, scar contracture from a poorly designed incision, joint stiffness, recurrence, and disease extension, have been well documented.[22,32,46,64-71] We can anticipate that patients with more than two involved digits, radial disease, PIP flexion contracture greater than 45 to 60 degrees,[71] and a ruddy type complexion (a clinical observation) can be expected to produce more postoperative complications. Rehabilitation protocols, as they relate to postoperative complications, have received limited attention in the literature, but may be a significant variable.[1]

The goals of postoperative management are to foster uneventful wound healing by protecting wound fluids, preventing infection, minimizing adverse mechanical influences, and controlling the collagen maturation process.[72-74] Basic wound-healing principles should be respected to regain joint motion and soft tissue extensibility without contributing to inflammation. Stressful exercise can compromise corner flaps and skin grafts, encourage the development of hypertrophic scar, and may contribute to sympathetic flare from aggressive stretch to the neurovascular bundles.[74]

It is not uncommon for therapy protocols to include aggressive use of extension orthoses in early wound-healing phases and aggressive manual therapy, which, experience teaches, contributes to inflammation and postoperative complications noted earlier. A better approach is for the therapist to think in terms of tissue nutrition instead of ROM. Tension to the neurovascular bundles and cutaneous repair should be avoided. The rationale for this "no-tension" technique is that applied tension to digital vessel and nerve may contribute to local hypoxia and inflammation.[1] Tissue anoxia may

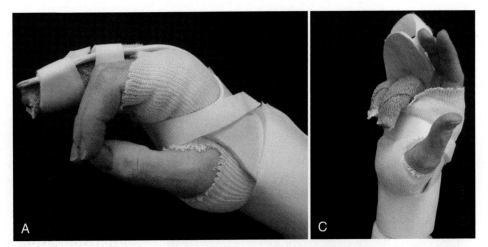

Figure 23-2 A, Dorsal static protective orthosis utilized immediately postoperatively for the no-tension applied (NTA) protocol following Dupuytren's fasciectomy. This dorsal orthotic design allows for flexion, but not MCP joint extension, in a controlled range preventing neurovascular and wound tension the first 2.5 weeks after surgery. **C,** The patient exercises within the orthosis, strapping the interphalangeal joints to the dorsal hood between exercise sessions.

contribute to free-radical release and adverse cellular response,[75–78] as well as hypertrophic scar formation in the lines of tension.[72,79–82]

Postoperative Care—Weeks One and Two

In the author's clinical setting, patients are treated 24 hours after surgery. Patients are always treated while they are supine the first postoperative visit to prevent a vasovagal episode and to decrease anxiety. Initial wound care includes drain removal (if present), wound cleansing with sterile water, cool compresses to reduce edema, and sterile dressing changes. Wounds are treated with mupirocin (Bactroban) topical antibiotic and contact layers (Adaptic if the skin is macerated, Xeroform if it is not). Digital wounds are dressed with ⅝-inch tube gauze with enough dressing (2 × 2-inch sterile gauze pads) to absorb any bleeding, and then a single layer of 2-inch self-adherent wrap (Coban) to control edema for the digital wounds. Dressing to maintain humidity speeds epithelialization, prevents dressing adherence, and avoids painful dressing changes. The benefits and science for moist wound healing are reviewed elsewhere.[74] The patient is fitted with a dorsal blocking type orthosis with the wrist positioned at neutral, MCP joints at 35 to 45 degrees of flexion, and the interphalangeal (IP) joints in relaxed extension (Fig. 23-2A). The thumb is positioned in mild abduction if the first web was operated. Only the operated digits are included (Fig. 23-2B, online).

Patients are instructed verbally as well as given written notations concerning hand elevation and sleeping techniques and the need to keep the dressing dry and to avoid exercise the first few days, both for the operated hand and for their usual total body exercise regimen. Shoulder management includes proper positioning for elevation and sleeping that prevent shoulder impingement positions, and exercises that keep the shoulder joint capsule extensible. The upper trapezius and levator scapulae muscles may develop trigger points from improper positions of elevation, posturing, and disuse associated with postoperative sequelae. Cervical stretches for bilateral upper trapezius and the levator scapulae, and myofascial massage for both, address these symptoms.

Patients usually return to the clinic again in 48 hours for wound care and to begin gentle exercise. Wound care advances to a *mild* (Dove or Ivory pump) soap and water wash[83] at the sink supervised by the therapist, with the predescribed dressing application. Patients are instructed to exercise with *gentle* composite digital flexion, within the confines of the orthosis, and to avoid stress to the corner flaps of the incisions (Fig. 23-2C). Exercise to end range of digital extension and flexion are avoided. Many patients, especially the retired male who is used to an aggressive approach in business and sports, tend to overwork and to edit the therapist's instructions. These patients need a firm approach and written instruction with clear definition.

Postoperative Care—Week Two to Three

Week two to three includes exercise advancement to increased angles of flexion and extension with respect to wound healing. The IP joints are best worked by the therapist with gentle manual, axial traction to prevent cartilage abutment. Aggressive passive exercise only compromises the wound and increases joint inflammation, so it should be avoided. If wound healing is progressing satisfactorily, digital orthoses including the proximal phalanx (P1), middle phalanx (P2), and distal phalanx (P3) applied to the volar aspect of the digit can be applied four or five times per day with 1-inch Transpore tape (Fig. 23-3). The tape applies light extension forces to the PIP joints. Functional electrical stimulation (FES) can be utilized as a type of muscular reeducation and to facilitate flexor and extensor tendon glide. FES to improve digital extension should be applied both with the MCP joints manually blocked in flexion to transmit forces to the PIP level by week three, and for composite extension. Wound care progresses to lighter dressings, continued single-layer Coban wraps, and suture removal when the wound edges demonstrate adequate tensile strength. Early suture removal with wound dehiscence results in wider and often hypertrophic scar.[1,74] A frequent scenario for wound complication is suture removal at 10 days or less after surgery by the nurse or physician assistant before the surgeon sees the patient, with resulting wound dehiscence. Suture removal at 16 to 17 days, or even longer if the patient is diabetic and the corner flaps are

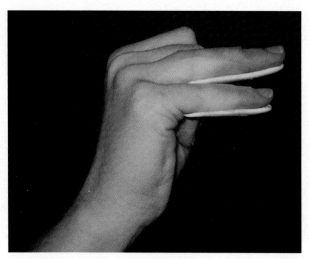

Figure 23-3 If wound healing is progressing satisfactorily, digital orthoses including the proximal phalanx (P1), middle phalanx (P2), and distal phalanx (P3) are applied to the volar aspect of the digit four or five times per day with 1-inch Transpore tape, applying light extension forces for 10 to 15 minutes per session.

repetitions per exercise). The patient is instructed in intrinsic stretch, isolated DIP motions with the PIP joints at 0 degrees to facilitate ORL stretch. A dynamic extension orthotic can be utilized (applied week 2–4) for the more difficult cases where MCP and PIP joint extension are not satisfactory and when the application of multiple digital static orthotics are difficult for the patient to apply independently (Fig. 23-4B). Digital orthotics can be placed inside the traction loops intermittently to provide a composite extension stretch. Therapy aides such as putty and hand grippers are not utilized because they increase pressure in the carpal tunnel and at the A1 pulley region,[87,88] and, if overdone, cause flexor tendon inflammation.[94] Again, overly aggressive exercise should be cautioned against.

Postoperative Care—Weeks Four to Six

By week four the wounds are epithelialized, edema should be under control, and motion should, for the most part, be reestablished. Therapy can be discontinued or decreased to one or two times per week unless the patient has not progressed satisfactorily. Exercise progression continues with a

not stable, helps to prevent the formation of painful or hypertrophic scar. Attention to basic wound-healing principles minimizes complications.[74]

Scar management progresses to 24-hour paper taping once sutures are removed to *minimize skin tension*. One-inch Micropore paper surgical tape placed longitudinally along incision lines, or lines of tension, especially where the incision crosses a joint, minimizes scar/skin tension and thus the development of hypertrophic scar.[84,85] Patients are instructed to change the paper tape when they shower. The scar should be massaged prior to showering with gentle transverse motions, and then following showering the scar and volar tissues are cleansed of any oils with isopropyl alcohol. For the paper tape to adhere, the skin must be free of oil and completely dry. Silicone gel sheeting is applied to the scar at night if the scar is hypersensitive or hypertrophic. The silicone is worn inside the night extension orthosis. Molded elastomer can be used in combination with a night orthosis for larger palmar areas, however, paper tape is less expensive and actually gets equal or better results than the more expensive gels or elastomers.[84,85]

The antitension orthosis continues until week three, and then daytime use is discontinued. The dorsal orthosis is remolded to a volar hand-based extension device with straps placed strategically over the MCP and PIP joints to maintain or improve joint extension and is worn at night (Fig. 23-4A). If carpal tunnel symptoms are exhibited, the orthosis should include the wrist at 2 degrees flexion and 3 degrees ulnar deviation.[86] The patient should be cautioned about repetitive composite fisting, which elevates pressures at the A1 pulley[87,88] and in the carpal tunnel.[89–92] Controlled stress to the tendon and ligament systems progresses with gradual increase in composite extension as the neurovascular bundles begin to accommodate increased tension. Isolated flexor tendon gliding,[93] including hook, and full fist are recommended at least five times per day for short intervals (15–20

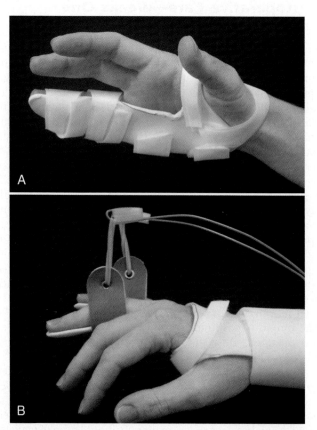

Figure 23-4 A, The dorsal orthosis is remolded to a volar hand-based extension orthosis with straps placed strategically over the metacarpophalangeal (MCP) and proximal interphalangeal (PIP) joints to maintain or improve joint extension by week three. The splint is worn at night, and the digital extension orthoses are worn for short intermittent periods during the day. **B,** Dynamic extension orthoses can be used during the day (applied weeks 2–4) for the more difficult cases when MCP and PIP joint extension are not satisfactory and when the application of multiple-digit static orthoses are difficult for the patient to apply independently.

light strengthening program. This should include isometric strengthening with a 2-inch dowel instead of exercises such as putty squeezing, which bring the fingers into the palm and if utilized repetitively, as mentioned earlier, increase pressure in the carpal tunnel and A1 pulley region. Exercise with the home program should continue to include stretch to the intrinsic muscles and ORL; FDP gliding relative to the FDS; strengthening and facilitation of the zone III and IV extensor tendon gliding; and overall strengthening for the wrist extensors and rotator cuff musculature for return to sports or heavier activity. Gloves with a gel pad in the palmar region decrease pressure for sports activity that requires grip. Composite digital extension orthoses are best continued for 3 to 6 months, with intermittent use of a daytime digital extension orthosis or dynamic extension orthosis as deemed necessary.[52,95,96] Patients benefit from brief periodic visits to the therapist to ensure compliance with long-term orthotic use. In the author's clinic, quick courtesy rechecks are done at no charge and serve to emphasize the need for prolonged orthotic use and as intervention if joint extension is lost due to noncompliance.

Needle Fasciotomy

Patients referred following needle fasciotomy[37] for Dupuytren's bands typically do not require much intervention. The same principles should apply for a gradual increase in extension orthotic use without an aggressive approach for either exercise or the orthosis, and the use of padded gloves for activities, such as racket sports, golf, or gardening, that apply stress to the palmar aspect of the hand. In the author's experience, these patients expect to see the therapist for only one or two visits and plan to return to normal activities immediately.

Intervention for Complication

The therapist should intervene quickly for complications related to infection, inflammation, edema, or sympathetic flare by sending the patient to the physician for assessment and medication change,[97–99] and by altering therapeutic protocols to address the specific problem. Sympathetic flare related to the development of carpal tunnel symptoms that were either missed preoperatively or develop postoperatively[100] may require carpal tunnel release (CTR).[66] In the author's experience, patients followed immediately postoperatively following CTR or trigger release associated with Dupuytren's surgery, or as an intervention for postoperative complications, progress well with careful management of the involved tissues.

Inflammatory problems can be addressed with changes in exercise patterns, orthotic positions, and the use of high-voltage galvanic stimulation and cold applications. Edema can be addressed with Isotoner gloves, Coban wraps, fluid-flushing exercises, and elevation.[101] Painful or hypertrophic scar can be treated with ultrasound or iontophoresis with dexamethasone sodium phosphate, paper taping and silicone, desensitization, and massage. Physical agents used as therapeutic interventions for edema, pain, and inflammation are reviewed elsewhere in this text,[102] but as mentioned previously, no evidence exists other than clinical experience to support these interventions with DC.

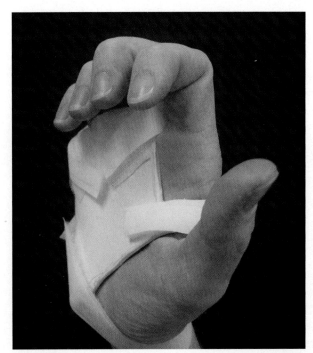

Figure 23-5 Trigger orthosis: A volar hand-based static orthosis that immobilizes the metacarpophalangeal joints at 0 degrees reduces pressure at the A1 pulley level, which helps to reduce inflammation and edema in the flexor system. This position also promotes differential flexor tendon gliding as well as synovial diffusion for these tendons and has demonstrated good results for conservative management of triggering digits.[88]

Triggering digits can be addressed by altering forces at the A1 pulley[88] with a hand-based MCP extension orthosis or use of a profundus orthosis only (P2, P3 dorsal orthotic) during the daytime and by limiting repetitive gripping (Fig. 23-5).

Difficult PIP flexion contractures can be treated with serial casting (see Fig. 23-1) for several weeks,[62] or intermittent digital orthotic use taped precisely over the PIP joint with 1-inch Transpore tape (see Fig. 23-3). Dynamic digital-based orthosis are recommended by some authors, but tend to migrate and are difficult to fit for the small finger. If PIP joint flexion or intrinsic stretch is an issue, a volar wrist control with lumbrical block (MCPs at 0 degrees) can be applied with flexion vectors for the PIP to stretch the intrinsics and to improve PIP joint flexion (Fig. 23-6). Composite flexion issues are often more related to intrinsic tightness than limitations with joints or the extensor system. Improving excursion of the intrinsic muscles facilitates composite digital flexion.

A home exercise program is critical to maintaining motion gained in surgery and therapy. Patients need to be required to reproduce exercises without cue as well as proper orthotic application. Typically, most patients do not exercise with precise exercise position, repetition, or force application, and most become lax once they are discharged from formal therapy. Written exercise programs, questioning in therapy, and quick rechecks after discharge help to ensure compliance with home programs.

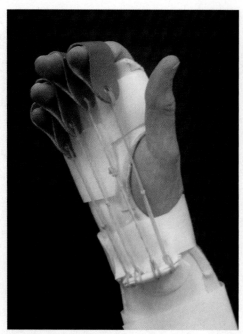

Figure 23-6 A volar wrist control with a lumbrical block (metacarpophalangeal joints at 0 degrees) can be used with dynamic traction applied to the proximal interphalangeal (PIP) joints if PIP joint flexion or intrinsic tightness is an issue.

Rationale and Clinical Experience for the No-Tension Technique

The effect of mechanical stress on Dupuytren's palmar fascia and cellularity,[11,19,30,42,103–105] occlusion of capillary endothelium,[78,106] tissue anoxia and oxygen free radicals,[75–77,106–109] and growth factor release has been studied.[11,17,110–113] In an attempt to understand the pathogenesis of this condition, studies have defined the role of the myofibroblast in force transmission to the extracellular collagen and matrix in DD.[19,114,115] Research into therapeutic regimens have examined the effect of continuous stress on the collagen fibers of Dupuytren's tissue applied prior to surgery, with results indicating that preoperative stress on these tissues can trigger the release of enzymes that weaken collagen.[58,116–119]

These studies, which address the biochemical and biomechanical response of these tissues to mechanical agonists, may raise questions regarding some popular rehabilitation techniques that apply tension to vessel, nerve, and incision lines with orthotic use and exercise techniques that often apply stress beyond the physiologic limits of accommodation in this operated tissue. Tissue nutrition in the early postoperative phase following Dupuytren's fasciectomy has not received enough attention by therapists, and mechanical stress applied by the therapist or patient may be a critical variable in the complication rate and outcomes that has been overlooked.

The author and associates hypothesized in a previous study[1] that orthotic use on the operated digits under tension following fasciectomy may contribute to negative alterations in neurovascular function, altered tissue nutrition, and facilitate hypertrophy of scar in lines of tension; and that stressful exercise technique that contributes to edema or inflamma-

tion may also contribute to localized hypoxia. This theory finds some support in basic science studies that look at cellular response to mechanical stress and tissue anoxia.*

Clinical Experience: Materials

The authors first reported clinical experience is defined elsewhere in a review of 268 patients treated exclusively by the author over a 17-year period, comparing the results of patients treated with *tension applied* to the operated digits immediately after Dupuytren's fasciectomy versus those treated with the *antitension technique* described earlier (Table 23-1, online). The patients were operated on by 49 surgeons, with no controls on surgical technique.

The first group *tension applied* (TA), n = 103, consisted of 76 male and 27 female patients with a mean age of 67.15 (±8.91) and average number of operated digits 1.96 (±0.71). These cases were evaluated retrospectively from 1983 to 1993, and prospectively from 1993 to 1999. The primary author treated the cases from 1983 to 1993 with an extension orthosis immediately postoperatively as standard accepted protocol. Cases included in this group from 1993 to 1999 were those sent to the primary author at 2 weeks or greater postoperatively wearing physician-applied orthoses. A limited number (n = 13) were seen as follow-up after being treated first at other therapy units.

The second group was the *no tension applied* group (NTA), n =165, which consisted of 128 male and 37 female patients with a mean age of 69.33 (±6.78) and an average number of operated digits 1.6 (±0.7). These patients were all studied prospectively from 1993 to 1999, and treated with the no-tension protocol following the clinical observation by the primary investigator that following Dupuytren's fasciectomy a number of patients treated with tension applied developed flare.

Treatment Protocols: Methods

Patients in the TA cohort received an orthosis with tension applied to the operated palmar and digital regions with efforts to obtain extension immediately postoperatively from 20 to 0 degrees at the MCP and to neutral PIP joint extension (Fig. 23-7). Extension orthoses were worn intermittently during the day (with self-exercise sessions prescribed four to six times per day), and during the night. Exercise efforts were

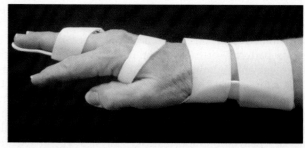

Figure 23-7 Volar static extension orthosis utilized immediately postoperatively for group I (TA) patients. This orthosis applied extension forces to both the metacarpophalangeal and proximal interphalangeal joints as a hand-based extension orthosis or with the wrist included.

*See Appendix online for more in-depth review.

directed to regaining digital extension immediately postoperatively according to standard postoperative protocol. No attempt was made to apply aggressive tension for the sake of this study, and the technique of applying tension was not utilized by the primary author after 1993.

NTA cases received orthoses with no wound tension to the operated palmar or digital regions by blocking the last 40 to 45 degrees of MCP extension with a static dorsal blocking orthosis that supports the wrist at 0 degrees of extension, MCP joints at 40 to 45 degrees of flexion, and PIP joints in neutral position allowing controlled flexion but no digital extension beyond these parameters (see Fig. 23-2A, B [online], C). The dorsal blocking orthosis was prescribed for 24-hour wearing time, with the patients advised to work with gentle active flexion exercise within the orthosis every 2 hours. Careful attention to gentle exercise technique and no repetitive forces prevented wound tension from being applied to these tissues with exercise. At 7 to 10 days after surgery the operated digits were fitted with volar digital extension orthoses (see Fig. 23-3) to improve PIP extension (to be worn intermittently during the day and at night), and by 2.5 weeks to 3 weeks after surgery the blocking orthosis was discontinued during the daytime and replaced by a static volar MCP and PIP extension orthosis (see Fig. 23-4A) at night, usually hand-based.

Both groups were treated with flexion exercise for each digital joint, including both composite motion and individual joint blocking exercise. Distal joint motion was encouraged to stretch the often tight ORL and to encourage tendon gliding for the FDP tendon.

Clinical Experience: Data Analysis

Each case was analyzed with respect to age, sex, surgeon, number of digits operated, therapy technique (orthotic attitude and exercise), days from start of therapy to discharge, number of therapy visits required for rehabilitation, MCP and PIP ROM, degree of flare, and degree of scarring. No attempt was made to match the effects of diathesis, osteoarthritis, or surgical technique. All comparisons were made based on the TA versus NTA rehabilitation technique.

All recordings of physical characteristics were made by the principal investigator. Flare was graded using the criteria defined in Table 23-2. Flare complications for each patient

Table 23-2 Grading System Used to Evaluate Flare

Grade	Description	Treatment Required
Grade 0	No inflammation beyond normal wound healing	Edema control
Grade 1	Inflammation limited to operated fingers, with redness, stiffness, edema lasting beyond 2–3 weeks	Edema control, high-voltage stimulation, cold, anti-inflammatories
Grade 2	Sympathetic symptoms extending beyond operated digits	TENS, stellate blocks, gabapentin (Neurontin), steroids, stress loading

TENS, transcutaneous electrical nerve stimulation.
Printed, with permission, from Evans RB, Dell PC, Fiolkowski P. A clinical report of the effect of mechanical stress on functional results after fasciectomy for Dupuytren's contracture. *J Hand Ther.* 2002;15:333.

Table 23-3 Grading System Used to Evaluate Scarring

Grade	Description	Treatment Required
Grade 0	Soft, pliable, nonpainful flat scar	Light massage, longitudinal paper tape at 2 weeks
Grade 1	Thick, widened scar with no joint limitation, tender, hypersensitive	Silicone gel sheets ultrasound, orthosis use, massage
Grade 2	Hypertrophic, inflexible scar with joint limitation, hyperemic, itching, pain	Silicone gel sheets ultrasound, iontophoresis, orthosis use, serial casts, massage

Printed, with permission, from Evans RB, Dell PC, Fiolkowski P. A clinical report of the effect of mechanical stress on functional results after fasciectomy for Dupuytren's contracture. *J Hand Ther.* 2002;15:335.

were assigned a number (0, 1, 2) based on symptoms and required treatment. Similarly, the scar was graded and was assigned a number (0, 1, 2) by using the criteria defined in Table 23-3.

For comparison of ROM, individual t-tests with a Bonferroni correction were used to compare the ROM at the PIP and MCP joint for each of the four fingers. The independent variable was tension, or the lack thereof, with the dependent measure being ROM, in degrees. A separate 3×2 analysis of variance (ANOVA) was run using tension, age, and the number of days between surgery and start of treatment as the independent variables, whereas days to discontinuation of treatment and number of visits were the dependent variables. Duncan's post-hoc test was used to test the individual effects of independent variables, should any differences be indicated by the test results. Chi-square tests were used to examine relationships between the application of tension and the development of scar and flare. Chi-square tests were also used to examine the association of gender with these developments. Significance was set a priori at 0.05.

Clinical Experience: Results

The results of the ANOVA using age, gender, and tension as independent variables indicated that neither gender nor age demonstrated an effect on the time spent in rehabilitation. Also, there was no interaction among the variables of age, gender, and treatment on the number of visits required or the days until discharge. The only significant difference in these measures was seen when comparing TA and NTA. In order to achieve similar results, the TA cohort required 20 therapy visits compared with 13 for NTA ($p < 0.01$) (Fig. 23-8, online). Similarly, TA patients were in therapy for an average of 67.73 (±47.21) days, but NTA patients were in therapy for only 36.49 (±22.83) days from the initial visit until discharge ($p < 0.01$) (see Fig. 23-8, online). Average time between surgery and therapy for the TA group was 5 days, NTA group 2 days.

Final ROM in flexion for both the MCP and PIP joints was significantly improved in the NTA group compared with the TA group only at the PIP level in the long, ring, and small digits, and these differences were 4.03, 3.83, and 4.04 degrees, respectively ($p < 0.05$) (Fig. 23-9, online). Similarly, the two treatments resulted in a significant difference in the extensor deficit at the PIP joint level only. These differences were 5.39, 6.91, and 6.32 degrees in the long, ring, and small digits, respectively ($p < 0.05$) (Fig. 23-10, online).

Analysis of the subjective grading for flare and scar revealed differences between the groups. There was a significant difference between the two groups with regard to flare development ($p < 0.01$) (Table 23-4, online) and degree of scar complication ($p < 0.01$) in favor of the NTA (Table 23-5, online).

Positioning of the MCP joints in flexion for the first 2.5 weeks of wound healing to relieve tension did not result in any loss of ROM in digital extension, but it did result in fewer therapy visits, less time to discharge (therefore, less expense for treatment was incurred), and decreased complications of flare and scar. Final ROM was clinically similar for both groups; however, the TA group required more therapy to reach similar measurements obtained in the NTA group.

Discussion

Patients in the NTA group had fewer scar complications, developed less flare response, and required less therapy. The final ROM at time of discharge was statistically significant in favor of the no-tension protocol, but for practical purposes (differences of 4–9 degrees per digit) was not clinically significant. *No motion was lost to extension with this protocol.*

Clinical experience shows that among hand surgeons and therapists orthosis use after Dupuytren's fasciectomy varies from relaxed extension, aggressive extension, tension relieved, to no orthotic. Clinical experience teaches that large variations in force application exist from therapist to therapist and with patient self-exercise as well. Many patients tend to overexercise with repetition and stress that creates local inflammation. Therapy "aides" such as exercise putty, hand grippers, and sponge balls, often used postoperatively for these cases, elevate pressures at the A1 pulley region[87] and within the carpal tunnel[89–92] and can contribute to problems of carpal tunnel symptoms and triggering of the unoperated digits.[83,94] Delaying PIP joint extension orthotic use by 7 to 10 days does not result in loss of motion gained from surgical release, nor does delaying MCP joint extension orthotic application by 2.5 to 3 weeks following MCP joint release.

The no-tension technique described in this study may decrease adverse tissue response and complication rate because it may facilitate improved tissue nutrition, decrease inflammation, and decrease incision line tension. The rationale for this theory finds support in studies on tissue anoxia, inflammation, and mechanical stress. The studies validating these concepts are reviewed in an appendix available in the online version of this text.

Continued Study

The antitension technique[1] continues to be supported by the author's clinical experience over the past 8 years and suggests that applied mechanical tension may be an important

variable in complication rates following this surgery. An updated chart review of 119 cases (149 digits) treated by this author from January 1, 2002, until June 30, 2008, with similar demographics and from a wide referral base treated with the no-tension technique continues to support this technique, with average therapy visits 12, average days in therapy 35.2, average time between surgery and therapy 1.9. Final ROM in flexion mirrored the original research, with average MCP flexion 85 degrees; PIP flexion 91.5 degrees; DIP flexion 50.5 degrees; and extension deficit index 9 degrees, long 5.1 degrees, ring 6.2 degrees, small 8.5 degrees. Results regarding complications for scar and flare were similar to the original study; eight patients had complications associated with postoperative digital nerve neuropraxia, postoperative triggering digits and the development of CTS, or inflammation related to overexercising. No patient developed a significant sympathetic flare. All patients received treatment for scar with paper tape, silicone, ultrasound, and massage, but only five patients in this review were documented as having more than the expected postoperative scar tenderness and complications.

Summary

Although the initial study was limited by methodologic flaws[120,121] relating to the soft methods of evaluating flare and scar, the data support the conclusion that patients treated with no tension, and therapeutic exercise with low load and repetition during the early phase of wound healing have better outcomes than those treated with tension applied. Furthermore, no motion of the MCP or PIP joints or composite joint flexion is lost to extension with the no-tension rehabilitation technique.

In summary, many complications can be avoided by proper preoperative evaluation and education, a no-tension technique of orthotic application and exercise, proper management by a therapist who has perspective regarding tissue nutrition instead of aggressive efforts to force ROM, and early recognition and treatment of flare or inflammation. The no-tension technique has proven to be more effective in terms of reduced complications, improved motion, decreased flare and scarring rate, fewer needed therapy visits, and decreased expense to the patient.

REFERENCES

The complete reference list is available online at www.expertconsult.com.

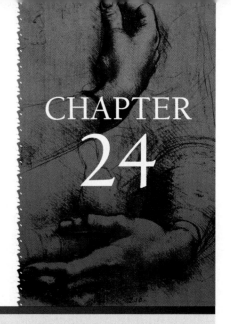

Soft Tissue Tumors of the Forearm and Hand

STEPHANIE SWEET, MD, LEO KROONEN, MD, AND
LAWRENCE WEISS, MD

CRITICAL POINTS

- Perform a biopsy and culture all tumors treated operatively.
- Rheumatologic workup should be considered with suggestive synovitis pattern (i.e., atraumatic ulnar wrist swelling in young patient).
- Nonhealing wound or chronic infection can mimic a soft tissue tumor.
- Consider checking the adjacent joint for satellite lesions when resecting a giant-cell tumor of the tendon sheath.
- Pyogenic granuloma has a relationship with inflammatory bowel disease and pregnancy.
- Atypical mycobacterial infection mimics soft tissue masses and must be specifically cultured.
- Ultrasound is particularly useful when there is a suggestion of a foreign body which is not confirmed by plain radiographs.

Masses of the forearm, wrist, and hand are one of the most common presenting conditions seen in an upper extremity surgeon's office. The vast number of masses that occur within the soft tissues of the forearm and hand are benign. However, the treating surgeon must be familiar with a large differential diagnosis. Tumors may originate from any of the elements of soft tissue in the upper extremity, including synovium, fat, skin, lymphatics, nerves, blood vessels, or bone. A high index of suspicion for such masses is necessary so that an

appropriate workup and treatment plan can be formulated when indicated. The goal of this chapter is to familiarize the reader with the more common types of hand and forearm masses and to present a logical approach to rendering appropriate diagnosis and treatment.

Assessment of Masses in the Upper Extremity

A detailed history and physical examination are the essential starting points when a patient presents with an upper extremity mass. If a classic history can be obtained for a common tumor, then physical examination alone can confirm the diagnosis. This might obviate the need for a biopsy. It is important to ask when the mass was first noticed. Was there any history of trauma? Has the mass changed in size, shape, color, or consistency? Is the mass growing? If so, how fast? It is also important to identify any "red flags" that might be more suggestive of malignancy. Has the patient had any constitutional symptoms, such as fever, weight gain, weight loss, fatigue, night sweats, or pain awakening from sleep? Past medical history is important, as many common conditions seen in the hand surgeon's office manifest with a soft tissue mass. Examples of these conditions include rheumatoid arthritis, Dupuytren's contracture, gout, and infection. Moreover, since metastatic disease can manifest in the hand, history of any prior malignancies should also be sought. Obtaining a good family history might lead one to the diagnosis of a hereditary condition such as neurofibromatosis.

Physical examination should include the entire upper extremity. The size, shape, and consistency of the lesion should be noted. Location of the lesion, any skin induration or discoloration, and neurovascular involvement are important. Plain radiographs are recommended in all cases beyond the most straightforward diagnoses. Even though these masses are present in the soft tissues, radiographs can often reveal mass effect on the underlying bone or calcifications within the soft tissues. If there is any concern at all for malignancy, more advanced imaging should be obtained. Although computed tomography (CT) and bone scan both can have a role, magnetic resonance imaging (MRI) has become the test of choice for delineating the anatomy of the lesion. The additional use of gadolinium may enhance the image, which is particularly valuable for a malignancy workup. More recently, Cheng and colleagues[1] reported their experience with ultrasound in the diagnosis of soft tissue tumors of the hand and forearm. They found ultrasound to be reliable in determining whether a lesion was cystic or solid, and where the lesion was located relative to other structures.

Principles of Biopsy

Once an appropriate radiographic workup has been completed and a limited differential diagnosis has been compiled, a biopsy is often indicated. Though certain common diagnoses, such as ganglion cysts, are obvious, most solid tumors seen by the hand surgeon warrant biopsy or excision (or both). Certain red flags, such as rapidly increasing size or recurrence after initial biopsy, are suggestive of malignancy and are of concern. This type of information helps determine the type of biopsy to be performed.

The techniques used to perform a biopsy of a lesion vary from needle biopsies that can be performed in the clinic setting, to open surgical biopsies that must be done in the operating suite. Small, clearly benign lesions can be addressed with an excisional biopsy, in which the entire tumor is removed. However, if there is any question about the diagnosis and whether it is malignant, an incisional biopsy is indicated. An incisional biopsy is performed by surgically removing only a portion of the lesion, with the intention of coming back to address the remainder of the tumor once a diagnosis has been established. Most orthopedic oncologists recommend that incisional biopsies be performed only by surgeons who are comfortable doing the definitive resection.[2]

When performing a biopsy, certain principles should be applied. First and foremost, longitudinal skin incisions are always preferred if there is any chance that the lesions could be malignant. Second, in contrast to standard surgical techniques, the surgical dissection when performing the biopsy should attempt to stay within a single compartment instead of proceeding within an internervous plane. Last, it is prudent to culture all biopsy specimens, as indolent infection can often be confused with neoplasm.[2]

Masses in the upper extremity can be separated into tumor-mimicking lesions, benign tumors, and malignant tumors. Box 24-1 lists the most common soft tissue masses of the upper extremity. The remainder of the chapter focuses

---

Box 24-1   Most Common Soft Tissue Masses of the Upper Extremity

Tumor-mimicking lesions
    Rheumatoid nodules
    Gout
    Pseudogout
    Ganglion cysts
Benign neoplasms
    Giant-cell tumor of the tendon sheath (fibrous xanthoma)
    Lipoma
    Vascular tumors
        Hemangioma
        Congenital arteriovenous malformation
        Lymphangioma
        Aneurysm
        Glomus tumor
        Pyogenic granuloma
Inclusion cyst
Nerve tumors
    Neurilemmoma (benign schwannoma)
    Neurofibroma
Fibromatosis
    Calcifying aponeurotic fibroma
    Dupuytren's contracture
    Garrod's nodes
Epithelial tumors
    Skin warts
    Dermatofibroma (cutaneous fibrous histiocytoma)
    Keratoacanthoma
    Bowen's disease
    Sweat gland tumors
    Malignant neoplasm
Malignant skin tumors
    Basal cell carcinoma
    Squamous cell carcinoma
    Malignant melanoma
Soft sarcomas
    Epithelioid sarcoma
    Synovial sarcoma
    Malignant fibrous histiocytoma
    Rhabdomyosarcoma
    Leiomyosarcoma
    Lymphangiosarcoma
    Kaposi's sarcoma
    Malignant peripheral nerve sheath tumors
Metastatic disease

---

on the defining characteristics of each of these individual tumors.

Tumor-Mimicking Lesions

Non-neoplastic conditions can mimic tumors. Rheumatoid arthritis (RA) and gout can both manifest as a solitary soft tissue mass. Rheumatoid arthritis has several characteristics that can confuse the unsuspecting surgeon. Isolated soft tissue swelling associated with synovitis, particularly in the prestyoid recess of the wrist in a young female, can be a cardinal presenting sign of RA. Rheumatoid nodules can also present as a solitary finding, though this is rare. These nodules result from rheumatoid factor and immunoglobulin G (IgG), causing small vessel arteritis, which results in tissue necrosis and subsequent granulation tissue. Despite surgical excision, these nodules typically recur, unless medical intervention with disease-modifying agents is implemented. They may be seen in advanced rheumatoid disease.[3]

Gout and pseudogout are two other common diseases that can manifest with soft tissue lesions. Gout occurs as the result of a disorder in the metabolism of purines associated with DNA synthesis. Pseudogout is the result of accumulation of calcium pyrophosphate crystals within the joints and soft tissues. Pseudogout is classically seen on the ulnar side of the wrist. When calcifications are noted on plain radiographs in the location of the triangular fibrocartilage complex (TFCC), pseudogout should be prominent on the list of differential diagnoses. As with RA, gout and pseudogout can manifest for the first time with isolated swelling and synovitis that could be indicative of neoplasm. With longstanding disease, patients can develop tophi, which are accumulations of the monosodium urate crystals (gout) (Fig. 24-1) or calcium pyrophosphate crystals (pseudogout) within the soft tissues. In most cases, a thorough history reveals the previous diagnosis of gout/pseudogout, allowing the current diagnosis to become obvious. It is important to diagnose this prior to biopsy, as surgical treatment of a tophus may be unnecessary and may result in clinical flareup of the gouty condition. In the rare case of a tophus that begins to break through the skin, a debulking procedure may be entertained, and in the most severe cases amputation may be required.[4]

Ganglion cysts are discussed in detail as they are the most common soft tissue masses of the hand and wrist. Other conditions that manifest as soft tissue masses include Dupuytren's contracture, tendon sheath fibroma, and localized calcium deposits, such as those that form secondary to a hematoma. Unusual entities such as atypical mycobacterial infection may be seen in immunocompromised hosts. Herpetic whitlow is also seen in the hand and manifests with a classic vesicular appearance that should not be drained because it spreads the lesion (Fig. 24-2). Foreign body reaction can develop in an occult scenario, sometimes months or years later. Skin lesions are also included in this chapter as they are common.

Ganglion Cysts

According to Galen, the word *ganglion* means "anything gathered into a ball." Ganglion cysts are widely acknowledged as the most common soft tissue mass in the upper extremity, comprising approximately 15% to 60% of all soft tissue masses in the upper extremity.[5,6] They are synovial cysts that arise from the synovial lining of either a joint or a tendon sheath. It has been suggested that these masses are actually herniations of the synovial lining that fluctuate in

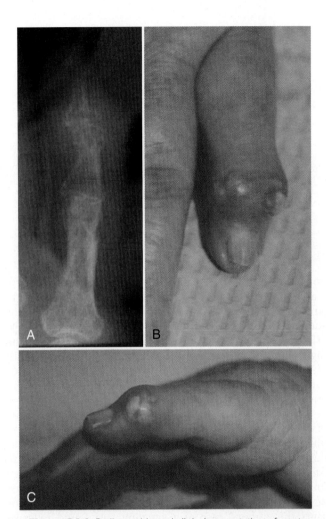

Figure 24-1 *Radiographic and clinical presentation of gout.*

size as a result of a one-way valve that forms at the joint of origin.[7]

As with most benign soft tissue masses, the clinical presentation of a ganglion is as a painless mass. However, when it becomes large enough to exert a mass effect on surrounding structures such as the terminal branch of the posterior interosseous nerve at the level of the wrist capsule, pain can be present. Patients often report some pain with full flexion or extension of the wrist and weight bearing, as with doing pushups. Patients classically report a mass that may wax and wane in size, or spontaneously decompress. There is often no history of trauma, although they are often seen in the young female population with ligamentous laxity, particularly of the scapholunate ligament. Ganglion cysts should not be confused with a carpometacarpal boss or with extensor tenosynovitis.

Diagnosis of a ganglion is usually straightforward. The patient presents with a mass that is typically nontender, but is either cosmetically or functionally bothersome. It is sometimes correlated with antecedent trauma or repetitive microtrauma, but often there is no clear cause. On physical examination, it is a well-circumscribed lesion with smooth borders and is sometimes multilobuled. Because these lesions are filled with a gelatinous fluid, if large enough, transillumination is diagnostic (Fig. 24-3).

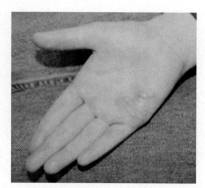

Figure 24-2 Herpetic whitlow.

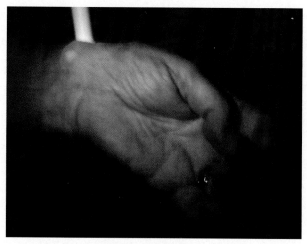

Figure 24-3 Transillumination of a ganglion cyst.

Ganglion cysts are most often found in characteristic locations. The dorsal wrist ganglion most often arises from the scapholunate interval (Fig. 24-4). On the volar surface of the wrist, the radioscaphoid joint, scaphotrapeziotrapezoid joint, and the flexor carpi radialis tendon are the most common origins (Fig. 24-5). An Allen's test is important when evaluating volar carpal ganglions, as the radial artery is usually intimately associated with the ganglion. A volar ganglion should not be confused with a pseudoaneurysm of the radial artery. It is important to recognize that the surface location of these masses does not always correspond with their joint of origin, such that a mass that appears on the middle or ulnar side of the dorsum of the wrist may still originate from the scapholunate interval when one traces it down to its origin. Ganglia may be found in Guyon's canal and may cause intrinsic dysfunction in the hand secondary to compression of the motor branch of the ulnar nerve. Figure 24-6 represents the authors' case of a ganglion cyst found to cause intrinsic paralysis in an avid drummer. Recovery was complete after excision of the ganglion.

Two other common examples of a ganglion are the retinacular cyst and the mucous cyst. A retinacular cyst is a ganglion that originates from a tendon sheath, most often on the flexor tendon sheath. Classically, these appear at the volar side of the proximal interphalangeal (PIP) or metacarpophalangeal (MCP) joint and arise from the A2 or A1 pulleys (Fig. 24-7). Triggering may be seen in association with these cysts, although it is not common. Mucous cysts

form in association with degenerative osteoarthritis at the distal interphalangeal (DIP) joint. They typically form at the dorsal base of the distal phalanx and are associated with an underlying osteophyte and a nail deformity[8] (Fig. 24-8).

Another rare variant of the ganglion is the intraosseous ganglion.[9,10] These variants are often found incidentally on radiographs, most commonly within the scaphoid and lunate. In these cases, it is difficult to determine if the intraosseous ganglion is the cause of wrist pain. Nuclear bone scan imaging can be used to detect metabolic activity associated with these entities to determine whether the cyst is the cause of the patient's pain. If the surgeon believes that the intraosseous cyst is the cause of the patient's pain, these lesions can be successfully treated with curettage and bone grafting. The authors believe that arthroscopy in this setting is a useful adjunctive tool, especially for assessing the scapholunate ligament in association with a radial-sided intraosseous lunate cyst.

Treatment of ganglion cysts varies. Nonoperative care may include aspiration of the cyst with or without injection of a corticosteroid. Aspiration of these cysts usually reveals a straw-colored thick, mucinous fluid, which confirms the diagnosis. The recurrence rate of dorsal wrist ganglion cysts after aspiration is 60% with a single aspiration, though

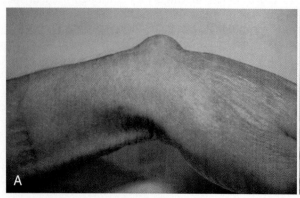

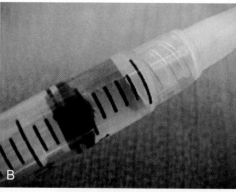

Figure 24-4 Appearance of dorsal carpal ganglion (**A**) and resultant aspirate (**B**).

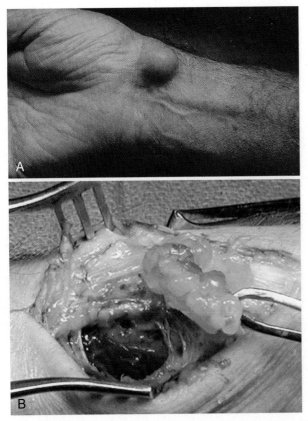

Figure 24-5 Volar carpal ganglion (**A**) and subsequent excision (**B**).

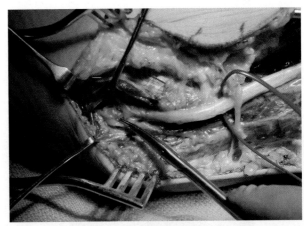

Figure 24-6 Ulnar tunnel level ganglion cyst causing ulnar motor paralysis.

repeated aspirations have achieved up to 85% cure rates.[11] In 1963, Bruner[12] anecdotally reported cure rates in 14 of 15 retinacular cysts. Aspiration is not recommended in volar wrist ganglia because of their proximity to the radial artery. Our preferred technique is surgical excision if the ganglion is large or symptomatic. When excising a ganglion, a portion of the joint capsule is also excised in order to decrease the chance of recurrence. The surgical excision of a dorsal wrist ganglion can be performed with either an open or arthroscopic technique. The arthroscopic technique has the theoretical advantage of causing less postoperative pain and allowing for smaller incisions.[13-15] Arthroscopic resection is most suitable if the ganglion arises from the scapholunate interval so it can

be decompressed when the 3–4 radiocarpal arthroscopic portal is established surgically. The recurrence rate with either open or arthroscopic technique is similar, at between 2% and 10%. When surgical excision of the mucous cyst is undertaken, it is imperative that the underlying osteophyte also be removed to limit recurrence. For retinacular cyst excision, a small noncritical window of flexor sheath is usually excised.

Surgical treatment of ganglion cysts, though routine, is not without complications. Watson and colleagues[16] reported a case of scaphoid rotary subluxation after ganglion excision, presumably caused by overzealous intercarpal ligament resection. Dorsal sensory branches of the radial nerve are at risk during the dissection of a dorsal wrist ganglion. Mucous cysts, when they occur, are often associated with attenuation of the skin overlying the cyst. In severe cases, this attenuation of skin may require skin grafting or a rotation flap.

Ganglion cysts in the pediatric population warrant special consideration. Although much less common than in young adults, their natural history appears to be different. In 1989, Rosson and Walker[17] reported on a series of 29 ganglion cysts in patients younger than 15 years old, and saw 20 of 29 resolve without any treatment within 2 years. In a similar study, Wang and Hutchinson[18] followed 14 children under the age of 10, and found that 11 of 14 cysts spontaneously

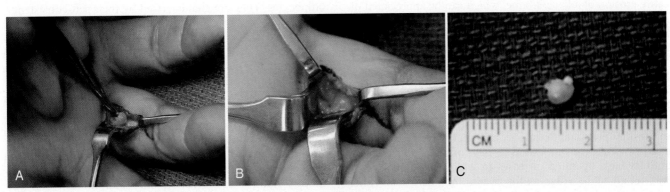

Figure 24-7 Retinacular cyst with subsequent excision from flexor tendon sheath.

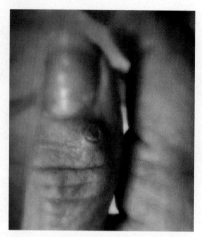

Figure 24-8 Mucous cyst near the proximal nail fold.

resolved within 2 years. For this reason, observation is recommended initially for ganglion cysts in children.[17-20]

Giant-Cell Tumors of the Tendon Sheath

Giant-cell tumors of the tendon sheath (GCTTS) are the next most common soft tissue tumors of the upper extremity, after ganglions. These benign tumors are known by a number of different names, including fibrous xanthoma, localized nodular tenosynovitis, and benign synovioma.[4] They are commonly classified into nodular and diffuse varieties, with the diffuse type being closely related to pigmented villonodular synovitis (PVNS). There is a slight female predominance (3 to 2), and they most commonly occur in the fifth and sixth decades of life.[21]

Clinically, they manifest as a painless soft tissue mass, oftentimes having been present for many years. They can be found on either the dorsal or volar side of the hand or digit. Most commonly they are found on the volar aspect of the digit, at the level of the proximal phalanx (Fig. 24-9). As with ganglion cysts, they can uncommonly cause a local mass effect, compressing neurovascular structures to cause numbness or sensitivity distal to the lesion. Ward and coworkers[22] reported one case of GCTTS manifesting as acute carpal tunnel syndrome. Similarly, longstanding tumors can cause erosion of adjacent bone, which can be appreciated on plain radiographs. Histologic examination reveals that these lesions are very similar to PVNS. Foam cells with small nuclei and lipid-laden granules within the cytoplasm are characteristic. These cells are accompanied by brown deposits of hemosiderin.[23]

Treatment for GCTTS is surgical excision (Fig. 24-10). Meticulous technique is imperative in order to completely excise the mass. Identification of the neurovascular bundles in the digit proximal to the lesion is imperative prior to excision. For this reason, extensile incisions are utilized. The authors have operated on cases in which the digital nerve was found to be volar to the lesion and the artery either midsubstance or dorsal. Recurrence rates for these tumors is

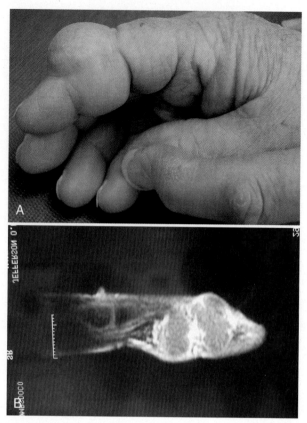

Figure 24-9 Clinical and MRI appearance of giant-cell tumor of the tendon sheath.

high—up to 50%[4]—but can be diminished with good technique. Gholve and colleagues[24] examined the treatment of a pediatric population with GCTTS treated with surgical excision, and at 2-year follow-up there were no episodes of recurrence. They attributed their success to "meticulous dissection and excision" under loupe magnification. Surgical dissection may require evaluation of joint involvement, as GCTTS may extend intra-articularly and require arthrotomy for complete excision.

Lipomas

Lipomas are common soft tissue tumors composed of mature adipocytes. They are characterized by their soft consistency; however, in the hand they can take on a number of varied appearances. They are typically painless and often are not noticed until they reach a significant size. These tumors can arise from any place in which there is adipose tissue. Some hypothesize that they can be related to prior blunt trauma.[25] They vary in size from quite large in the arm, to smaller lesions within the hand and finger. In the hand, they can be found in intramuscular locations within the intrinsic muscles.[26,27] Babins and Lubahn[28] and Vekris and associates[29] reported palmar lipomas that caused compression of the median nerve, producing symptoms of carpal tunnel syndrome. Azuma and collaborators[30] and Ersozlu and colleagues[31] reported the cases of a subcutaneous lipoma of the

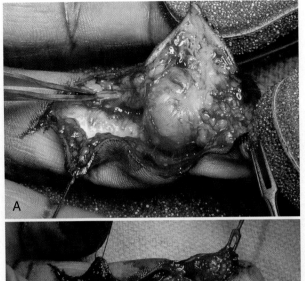

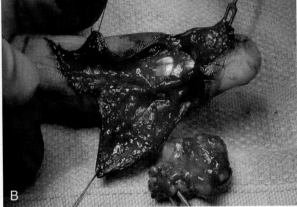

Figure 24-10 Surgical resection of giant-cell tumor of the tendon sheath.

index that manifested as a bulging of the entire fingertip. The deep palmar space is the most common location to find a lipoma within the hand.

Radiographically, MRI can be of assistance in making the diagnosis of lipoma. MRI demonstrates a soft tissue lesion that shares the same signal as surrounding subcutaneous fat on all sequences. Histologically, these lesions show the same mature adipocytes that are seen in surrounding fat. However, they also often demonstrate a thin capsule. Atypical lipomas present with intermediate level of MRI signal intensity, which may require biopsy for evaluation.

If the diagnosis has been confirmed with MRI, one can safely observe these lesions with little concern for malignant degeneration. Marginal excision is adequate for symptomatic masses, and recurrence rates are low.

Vascular Tumors

Vascular tumors in the upper extremity can be either congenital or acquired. Hemangioma, congenital arteriovenous malformations (AVMs), and lymphangioma represent congenital failure of differentiation. Aneurysms, glomus tumors, and pyogenic granulomas are all acquired. In general, the clinical presentation of vascular tumors is a blue or purplish red lesion. They can be painful or painless and may or may not be pulsatile.

Hemangiomas are abnormal collections of blood vessels that often occur in the hand as a soft tissue mass. They may also present within the skin (strawberry nevus, port wine stain, etc.), within muscles, or within bone as an intraosseous hemangioma. It is unclear whether they represent a true neoplasm or a hamartoma. These lesions take on a characteristic life cycle, with rapid growth in the first year, followed by growth proportional with the patient. Finally, they involute in up to 70% of cases by age 7 years.[32] These lesions are more common in females, with a ratio of 3 to 1. They are a disease of young patients. Because the vast majority involute on their own, their presence in the elderly is very rare. Treatment of hemangiomas initially consists of observation and education of the patient about the natural history of the process. For lesions that persist, surgical treatment can be entertained. Surgical management consists of ligation of both feeder vessels and excision of the hemangioma. In a rare complication of hemangiomas, known as Kasaback–Merritt syndrome,[33] platelets are absorbed within the hemangioma, leading to a consumptive coagulopathy that can be quickly fatal. Treatment is aimed at addressing the underlying coagulopathy.

Arteriovenous malformations are another variety of vascular tumor that results from an error in development of the vascular tree during embryogenesis. Clinically, they often share the appearance of a hemangioma. It is important, however, to differentiate these lesions from hemangiomas, because AVMs do not spontaneously involute. They are commonly separated into slow-flow lesions, which come from the venous or lymphatic side of the circulatory system, and fast-flow lesions, which are arterial in nature. Lesions may also demonstrate mixed characteristics.[34] Patients with AVMs typically present with complaints of either deformity associated with the lesion or a sense of pain or "heaviness" of the hand.[4] Plain films sometimes reveal calcifications, or phleboliths, within the soft tissues. Ultrasound is useful for determining the type of flow within the lesion, though MRI is the imaging modality of choice. Angiography is used primarily for preoperative planning. Initial treatment of AVMs should start with nonoperative treatment, such as compression gloves, elevation, calcium channel blockers and α-adrenergic agonists, and pain medications. Surgical excision of vascular malformations is reserved for painful lesions in which nonoperative modalities have failed. In these cases, selective embolization can be used in high-flow lesions to limit bleeding during surgery, though the risk of ischemia to the remainder of the extremity is present.

Lymphangiomas originate from the lymphatic system, but are otherwise similar in nature to hemangiomas. They are present at birth, and enlarge with time until they become symptomatic. Surgical resection is the treatment of choice as nonoperative treatment will fail.

Glomus tumors are painful lesions most commonly found in the subungual region of the fingertip. The glomus body is a normal structure within the body that is responsible for thermoregulation. These tumors are characterized by a classic triad of cold hypersensitivity, paroxysmal pain, and pinpoint pain.[35] MRI demonstrates a classic hyperintense signal, which is enhanced further with gadolinium contrast (Fig. 24-11). They can occasionally erode into the underlying bone. The treatment of choice is surgical excision, first removing the

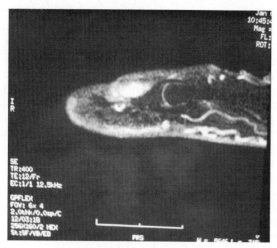

Figure 24-11 Glomus tumor.

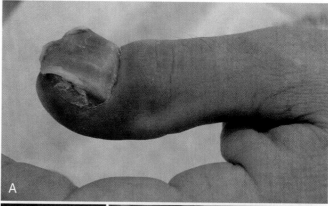

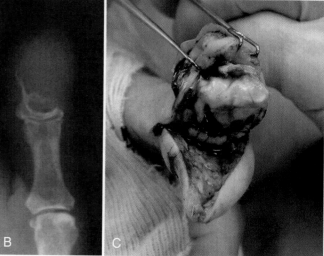

Figure 24-13 A, Epidermal inclusion cyst causing clinical deformity. **B,** Distal phalangeal erosion is noted on radiographs. **C,** White, pearly appearance is noted upon resection.

nail plate, and then repairing the nail bed after excision. Maxwell and coworkers[36] noted that up to one quarter of patients have multiple lesions, and that wounds should be thoroughly explored at the time of surgery for additional tumors. He also noted that if symptoms persist for more than 3 months after initial excision, the wound should be reexplored to look for additional lesions.

Pyogenic granuloma is another lesion characterized by abundant capillary proliferation. In contrast to the other vascular lesions, most believe that this lesion is secondary to trauma, with a subsequent superimposed infectious component. Clinically, these lesions appear as beefy red, friable masses that bleed (Fig. 24-12). These lesions do not tend to resolve spontaneously. Treatments with electrocautery, silver nitrate, and lasers have all been attempted with some success. The mainstay of treatment remains careful excision including a small cuff of normal tissue along with primary closure of the wound.

Inclusion Cysts

Inclusion cysts are common in the hand. They are thought to be the result of penetrating trauma. The traumatic event causes epithelial skin components to become lodged within the subcutaneous layer. Another theory is that embryonic cells that have been dormant are stimulated by trauma.[37] The cells then proliferate in the subcutaneous layer and produce keratin, thus forming a tumor. Because this process can take many years to occur, the history of a definite traumatic event cannot always be elicited.

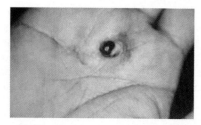

Figure 24-12 Pyogenic granuloma.

These cysts are commonly found in manual laborers who subject their hands to light trauma more frequently. Usually, they are found on the volar surface of either the palm or the digits. Although they are most often solitary lesions, multiple lesions in the same hand have been reported.[3] In addition to the subcutaneous tissues, these cysts can also be found within the flexor tendons or bony elements.[38]

The treatment for symptomatic inclusion cysts is surgical excision. These masses usually have a discrete wall filled with a foul-smelling, cheesy material. Histologically, the cell wall is composed of epithelial cells, and the cheesy material is composed of keratin. Excision should have the goal of removing the entire wall of the cyst, in addition to the cyst's contents. Some recommend that an ellipse of skin be taken around the cyst to ensure complete excision. Goebel and associates[3] emphasized the importance of everting the skin edges when closing the wound to decrease the chance of recurrence. When these lesions are found within a bone, the bone should be curetted back to a bleeding cancellous bed. In extreme cases bone erosion may be so severe as to require en bloc resection with reconstruction. Figure 24-13 demonstrates the authors' case in which most of the distal phalanx was eroded by inclusion cyst. Reconstruction was performed with iliac crest bone grafting and nail plate preservation,

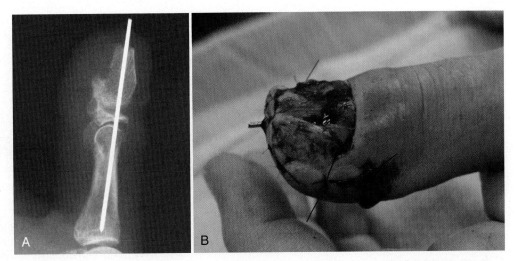

Figure 24-14 Reconstructive efforts for epidermal inclusion cyst. Use of iliac crest graft allowed for substitution of missing distal phlalanx. The nail matrix was able to be preserved for later nail growth.

achieving an excellent functional and cosmetic result (Figs. 24-14 and 24-15).

Nerve Tumors

Neurilemmoma (or schwannoma) and neurofibroma are the two most common nerve tumors. These are rare tumors, representing less than 1% of tumors of the hand. Both of these tumors originate from the Schwann cell, the cell responsible for production of the myelin sheath around a nerve. However, whereas the neurilemmoma only involves the myelin sheath portion of the nerve, the neurofibroma also involves the underlying nerve fibers.[4]

Neurilemmomas are the more common of the nerve tumors and represent 1% to 10% of all soft tissue tumors. They occur in the third to fifth decades of life and have equal incidence in men and women. As such, it is usually possible to excise them without damaging the underlying nerve fibers. A microscope is often required to perform the resection. Neurilemmomas are benign, well-encapsulated tumors of the Schwann cell. Clinically, they are usually slow-growing,

painless tumors. They do not usually produce any neurologic symptoms. However, given their proximity to the nerve, a Tinel's test over the mass may produce paresthesias. They are characterized histologically by two different characteristic patterns referred to as Antoni-A and Antoni-B cells. The Antoni-A cells are spindle-shaped cells that are packed densely together and often line up in a "picket-fence" pattern. This configuration is referred to as a Verrocay body. The Antoni-B cells are arranged in a much looser pattern and usually have smaller nuclei. These two patterns of cells alternate in the classic neurilemmoma. These lesions only very rarely demonstrate malignant transformation.[39-41]

Neurofibromas, although also originating from the Schwann cell, additionally involve the underlying nerve. Ninety percent of patients have a solitary tumor. The other 10% have multiple neurofibromas—a condition referred to as von Recklinghausen's disease, or neurofibromatosis. Neurofibromatosis is also characterized by café au lait spots and other orthopedic manifestations such as scoliosis. Because these tumors often involve nerve fibers, they are more likely to manifest with neurologic symptoms such as paresthesias. Malignant transformation can be seen in about

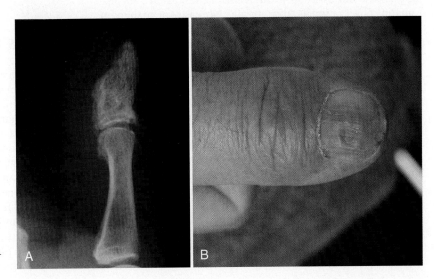

Figure 24-15 Final result after reconstruction of epidermal inclusion cyst.

5% of patients with neurofibromatosis. The surgical management of a neurofibroma is much more difficult than for neurilemmomas as it is difficult to avoid damaging the underlying nerve. Although the histology of neurofibroma can be similar to neurilemmoma, it is distinct in that it often demonstrates nerve fibers going through the lesion.[39] In addition, lymphocytes, mast cells, and xanthoma cells are often appreciated.

Other masses, such as ganglion cysts, lipomas, and hemangiomas, can also occur in close proximity to a nerve and cause symptoms and radiographic findings similar to those for nerve tumors. In addition, repetitive trauma to a digit can lead to fibrous enlargement of a nerve, such as in bowler's thumb, a radial digital nerve neuritis.

Fibromatosis

Fibromas can form in several different structures within the upper extremity. Dupuytren's contracture, Garrod's nodes, and calcifying aponeurotic fibroma are a few examples. Fibromatosis can occur in any age range, though certain diseases are more common in certain age ranges. For example, Dupuytren's contractures are usually found in the sixth and seventh decades of life, whereas calcifying aponeurotic fibroma is typically found in children. These processes are all characterized by proliferation of fibroblasts with abundant, dense collagen formation.

Calcifying aponeurotic fibroma can manifest in an identical fashion to that of GCTTS. This lesion was first reported in 1953.[42] It is a rare lesion that was originally believed to only occur in children in their first two decades of life. As such, it was initially termed *calcifying juvenile aponeurotic fibroma*. However, since then, cases have also been reported in the adult population. The lesions are about twice as likely to occur in men, and they usually originate in the palmar fascia. They can be distinguished from the more common GCTTS by MRI. On MRI imaging they demonstrate a less distinct margin, heterogenous enhancement, and often calcifications.[43] The surgical treatment is excision in order to confirm the diagnosis. However, the recurrence rate for these lesions is about 50%, so if the recurrent lesions are asymptomatic, observation is appropriate. No cases of malignant transformation have been documented.[44]

Dupuytren's contracture was first described in the early 1800s and remains a common disease in the hand surgeon's practice. It can often manifest as an isolated nodule, usually in the ulnar side of the palm. As the disease progresses, it often leads to joint contractures of the MCP and PIP joints. The condition itself is usually painless. Dupuytren's contracture has a strong male predilection of about 10 to 1. It is far more common in people of Scandinavian or Celtic heritage. However, it has also been reported in some Asian populations and in some case reports in African-Americans.[45,46] The myofibroblast is the cell responsible for producing the contractile collagen. Patients who have "Dupuytren's diathesis" of associated knuckle pads, plantar fibromatosis (Ledderhose's disease), and Peyronie's disease (fibromatosis involving the penis) are thought to have more aggressive disease and are more likely to experience recurrence after surgical excision.

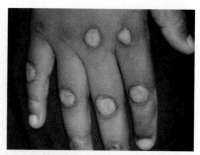

Figure 24-16 Garrod's nodes (knuckle pads).

The procedure of choice is a fasciectomy, excising the diseased fascia. Collagenase injection and needle aponeurotomy have both shown early success as alternative treatments to fasciectomy. Because these contractures are often longstanding, the releasing of the contractures often leads to deficits in skin coverage that require skin grafting. The open-palm technique is still utilized in severe cases involving multiple digits and often completely heals in about 4 to 6 weeks. This technique also allows for drainage of hematoma and early motion. Postoperative nighttime and intermittent hand-based extension orthosis use is an essential component of Dupuytren's disease treatment. Additionally, it is the authors' opinion that the careful use of a small amount of steroid given in the wound after closure has dramatically diminished pain, swelling, and postoperative Dupuytren's flare reaction.

Knuckle pads (Garrod's nodes) is fibromatosis of the dorsum of the hand in the area of the PIP joints (Fig. 24-16). They occur in about 20% to 40% of patients with Dupuytren's. However, they rarely have any functional effect on the patient, so the need for surgical excision is rare. They are, however, more common in patients who have evidence of fibromatosis in other areas of the body and therefore represent a poorer prognosis. In the pediatric population, these may develop as a result of habitual biting and may be resistant to treatment without behavior modification. (See Chapters 22 and 23 for a detailed discussion of the surgery and rehabilitation for Dupuytren's contracture.)

Tumors of the Epithelium

The epithelium of the skin is the most superficial layer covering the human body. Dermatologists manage these tumors most frequently. However, several of these tumors can manifest in the hand and upper extremity. These tumors, though small, are sometimes premalignant lesions. It is, therefore, important for the hand surgeon to be familiar with them so prompt diagnosis and treatment can be rendered. The more common skin tumors include verruca vulgaris and verruca plana, dermatofibroma, keratoacanthoma, Bowen's disease, sweat gland tumors, and the skin carcinomas (squamous cell carcinoma and basal cell carcinoma).

Skin warts come in two different varieties: verruca vulgaris and verruca plana. They are both the result of a viral infection with the human papillomavirus. Verruca vulgaris, the common wart, is characterized by a raised, rough surface. Verruca plana, the flat wart, is flush with the surrounding skin and can commonly be found on sun-exposed areas, such as the dorsum of the hand. The clinical course of these warts is self-limited, with complete resolution usually occurring without any treatment after 1 to 2 years. If these lesions persist, or occur in a location that causes discomfort or cosmetic concerns, treatment should be considered. Initial treatment consists of a topical salicylate, which is then covered with an occlusive dressing. Cryotherapy is also used commonly in the primary care and dermatology clinic setting, especially for genital and facial warts, though it can also be considered in warts on the hand.[47] Surgical excision can lead to the formation of satellite lesions due to viral spread, so treatment with the other methods is preferred.

Another common epithelial lesion is the dermatofibroma, also known as cutaneous fibrous histiocytoma. This lesion appears as a firm nodule within the skin that is often pigmented with yellow, brown, or reddish purple. Though it has a particular predilection to the lower extremity, it may occur in the hand. It is common in young to middle-aged adults and has a slight female predominance. The histologic characteristics of dermatofibroma include an increased number of fibrocytes within the dermis, accompanied by other inflammatory cells (lymphocytes, macrophages, eosinophils, neutrophils, or plasma cells).[48] The surrounding tissues are usually hyperplastic. Excisional biopsy is indicated with these lesions, as they can be easily confused with malignancies such as malignant fibrous histiocytoma or even malignant melanoma.

Keratoacanthoma is another epithelial tumor that can be difficult to differentiate from malignancy. This lesion may be confused with squamous cell carcinoma. Keratoacanthomas arise from the pilosebaceous units and hair follicles of the skin. They are typically quick-growing and manifest as a hyperkeratotic, dome-shaped lesion that is often red or brown in color.[49] They often demonstrate a central keratin plug.[50] Clinically, they look remarkably like a squamous cell carcinoma. However, they are not usually well fixed to the underlying tissues. Also, they often resolve on their own, which distinguishes them from squamous cell carcinoma. The treatment for these lesions is again excisional biopsy to confirm the diagnosis and verify that no malignancy is present. Although the two entities are distinct, keratoacanthoma is believed by some to be a precursor lesion to squamous cell carcinoma.

Bowen's disease is a squamous cell carcinoma that is limited to the epidermis. Because it is limited to the epidermal layer, it does not metastasize. However, 3% to 11% of these lesions develop into invasive squamous cell carcinoma.[50] Two thirds of these lesions are solitary.[51] Various factors such as exposure to arsenic and sunlight are thought to have a role in development of these tumors. Human papillomavirus has also been implicated.[51] Clinically, they manifest as scaly plaques. The treatment for Bowen's disease is surgical excision of the lesion and its surrounding dysplastic tissues or cauterization.

Sweat gland tumors, though arising in the epithelium, are more often clinically confused with giant-cell tumors and hemangiomas. These tumors can take on any number of forms from benign to malignant. The benign form goes by

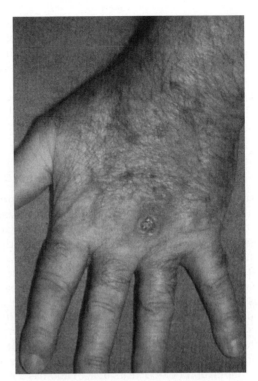

Figure 24-17 Squamous cell carcinoma.

several names, including eccrine spiroadenoma, dermal cylindroma, eccrine poroma, and hidroacanthoma. These benign masses can be treated with simple excisional biopsy. It is important that they be examined by the pathologist because their malignant counterparts can also appear benign. Aggressive benign varieties of these tumors are called aggressive digital papillary adenoma and should be treated with appropriate surgical margins for aggressive lesions.[52]

Malignant epithelial tumors include basal cell carcinoma, squamous cell carcinoma, and malignant melanoma.[53] Each of these seem to have a direct link to sunlight exposure. Basal cell carcinoma is the least common of the three in the hand and upper extremity. It has a classic pearly raised edge along its border. Treatment is usually under the direction of a dermatologist, and the use of Mohs' microsurgery has revolutionized the treatment of these lesions.

Squamous cell carcinoma is the most common skin malignancy in the upper extremity. These lesions have the potential to be fatal. They can vary in size from very small lesions that appear quite benign to larger lesions with significant areas of necrosis. Squamous cell lesions are most common in fair-skinned individuals with a history of significant sun exposure. Australia, with its proximity to the equator and large population of fair-skinned people, has the highest rate of skin cancer in the world.[50] Clinically, these lesions can be quite heterogenous in their appearance. Often they are scaly or crusted, sometimes with ulceration (Fig. 24-17). At this time, Mohs' surgery is the procedure of choice for treating these lesions, and it provides the lowest recurrence rate.[54,55] In larger, more involved cases, and those cases involving the nail bed, amputation is recommended. Metastatic diseases most commonly involve the lymph nodes, so sentinel node biopsy can be valuable.

Malignant melanoma is the final malignant tumor of the skin. It originates from melanocytes within the epidermis. The prognosis of these lesions is directly related to the depth of the lesion. Again, Mohs' surgery is the treatment of choice for accurately and completely excising these tumors. However, melanoma involving the nail bed is a poor prognostic sign and often requires amputation through the interphalangeal joint proximal to the lesion.[56]

Soft Tissue Sarcomas

Soft tissue sarcomas are rare malignant tumors that originate from cells of mesenchymal origin, including muscle and connective tissues. These are rare tumors, but they are malignant and possess the ability to metastasize. Aggressive early treatment offers the best prognosis, so clinicians should actively look for these lesions when a patient presents with a soft tissue mass. In general, these tumors are named based on their tissue of origin with similarity to the benign tumors mentioned earlier. A few notable exceptions are epithelioid sarcoma and synovial sarcoma, which we discuss first.

Epithelioid sarcoma is the most common soft tissue sarcoma of the hand. The lesion typically occurs in the younger population (10–35 years of age) and has a predilection for the volar surface of the digits. They are more common in males. They usually do not appear aggressive, but their clinical behavior is very aggressive. Steinberg and colleagues[57] presented their experience with 18 patients carrying a diagnosis of epithelioid sarcoma and found that those treated with marginal excision had significant recurrence and mortality rates. As such, the treatment of choice is wide resection or amputation. In addition, they have often metastasized to the lymph nodes by the time of diagnosis, so sentinel node biopsy is recommended.

Synovial sarcoma, despite its name, does not take its origin from the synovial linings of joints. They are commonly found in regions of the body that are near the joints, and histologically they share some of the characteristics of synovial cells. They do often take their origin from bursae and tendon sheaths. These tumors can be found in the upper extremity, though they rarely involve the digits. Similar to epithelioid sarcomas, they present as seemingly benign soft tissue masses and often demonstrate distal metastasis at the time of diagnosis. They are treated in the same manner as epithelioid sarcoma, with wide surgical excision or amputation.[39]

Malignant fibrous histiocytoma is the malignant analogue to calcifying aponeurotic fibroma. These lesions are more common in the elderly population, though they have been reported in a patient as young as 3 years old.[58] These tumors arise from the connective tissues and muscle of the forearm. They are treated with wide local excision or amputation, with adjuvant chemotherapy or radiation therapy.

Malignant soft tissue tumors of muscle origin include rhabdomyosarcoma and leiomyosarcoma. Rhabdomyosarcoma originates from skeletal muscle cells, whereas the origin of leiomyosarcoma is from smooth muscle cells such as those found in the sweat glands and hair follicles. Rhabdomyosarcomas can be classified into embryonal, alveolar, and pleomorphic variants based on its histologic appearance. Although the embryonal variant is the most common

throughout the body, the alveolar subtype is most common in the hand. These tumors are found in the pediatric age group. Leiomyosarcoma in the hand represents only about 1% of all leiomyosarcomas, but they are important for the hand surgeon to consider because their clinical presentation is very benign. The treatment for both rhabdomyosarcoma and leiomyosarcoma is wide surgical excision with adjuvant radiation or chemotherapy (or both).[39]

Lymphangiosarcoma and Kaposi's sarcoma are both malignancies of lymphatic tissue origin. Lymphangiosarcoma is seen after mastectomy for breast cancer in association with the chronic lymphedema that develops. Kaposi's sarcoma is seen most commonly in patients with AIDS. It manifests as painless pigmented nodules that can progress to ulcers. Treatment typically consists of surgical biopsy to confirm diagnosis, followed by treatment with chemotherapy or radiation therapy. The prognosis of lymphangiosarcoma without metastatic spread is very good. However, the prognosis of Kaposi's sarcoma in patients with AIDS is dismal, with only 20% survival at 2 years.[59]

Malignant tumors taking origin from nerves are termed malignant peripheral nerve sheath tumors. These tumors are found in patients in their fourth to six decades of life. Upper extremity lesions represent about 20% of all malignant peripheral nerve sheath tumors. Multiple neurofibromas (von Recklinghausen's disease) are at increased risk. Wide excision is the treatment of choice, though when they are intimately involved with the adjacent nerve, chemotherapy can be used. Radiation therapy is not usually beneficial. The overall survival rate for these tumors is about 20% at 3 years.[60]

A number of other soft tissue sarcomas have been reported in the upper extremity, but are very rare. These include clear-cell sarcoma (malignant melanoma of soft parts), fibrosarcoma, and alveolar soft-part sarcoma. The basic approach to all of these soft tissue sarcomas is the same. Having a high index of suspicion even in benign-appearing soft tissue tumors is paramount. Surgical biopsy provides a tissue diagnosis. Further treatment decisions can then be made in close consultation with both orthopedic and medical oncologists.[61,62]

Metastatic Disease

Although metastatic disease is the most common malignancy in bone, it is relatively rare in soft tissues. It may manifest as a destructive distal lesion in the fingertip (Fig. 24-18). Metastatic disease in the hand represents only 0.1% of all metastases of bone, and the number in soft tissues is even less. Bush reported three cases in his series.[5] One of them was a forearm lesion initially mistaken for an infection. It was an adenocarcinoma of unknown primary origin. The other two cases were metastatic squamous cell carcinoma and metastatic adenocarcinoma of the stomach. A high index of suspicion for metastasis is necessary in an elderly patient who has a chronic "nail bed infection" that will not heal. Treatment of soft tissue metastatic disease is aimed at palliative relief. Reconstructive surgery is not usually performed except in a structurally weight-bearing bone.

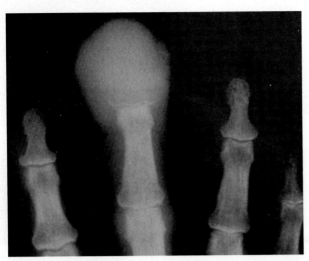

Figure 24-18 Metastatic lesion to distal phalanx.

The Role of the Therapist

The close relationship of the therapist with the patient allows for significant insight into the patient's concerns and fears when being treated for a tumor of the upper extremity. The therapist can be a true patient advocate by conveying such fears to the surgeon and by reassuring the patient in clear-cut cases. In addition, the hand therapist plays a critical role in the appropriate setting of functional goals after oncologic surgery, in which cases can range from simple ganglion excision to complex reconstructive surgery and amputations. Especially in dealing with the patient with a malignant upper extremity tumor, a multidisciplinary team approach is essential to optimal patient care. Close consultation of the hand surgeon with oncologists, psychologists, social workers, and hand therapists can provide maximum benefit for the patient.

Summary

Soft tissue masses of the upper limb present frequently to both the hand surgeon and therapist. Recognizing the hallmark features of these lesions is required to ultimately allow for successful treatment. Management may range from observation to radical treatment. The correct diagnosis and treatment are of paramount importance in the patient's outcome

REFERENCES

The complete reference list is available online at www.expertconsult.com.

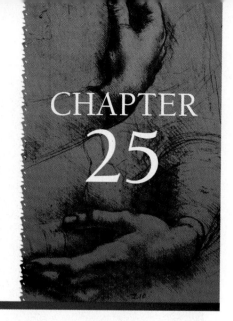

Management of Burns of the Upper Extremity

ROGER L. SIMPSON, MD, FACS

ACUTE PERIOD
RECONSTRUCTIVE PERIOD
SUMMARY

CRITICAL POINTS

- Thermal burns to the upper extremity constitute a major injury and source of disability, despite the disproportionately small body surface area involved.
- The depth of burn injury predicts the course of treatment and the degree of functional recovery. Correct assessment is essential.
- Early excision and grafting of deep burns is preferred.
- Burn contraction and surface contour determine therapy planning and plateaus.
- The quality of the burn scar, its response to therapy, and the expected functional outcome suggest the timing and extent of the burn scar reconstruction.

Every year in the United States, approximately 700,000 people receive treatment for a burn injury, of whom 40,000 require hospitalization.[1,2] Of those burned patients admitted to the hospital, nearly 80% have a burn injury involving the upper extremity.[3,4] Flame burns are the predominant cause of burn injury in adults admitted to the hospital. Scald burns from hot liquids are the most common cause of burn injury in children; 45% of children sustaining burns are younger than 5 years. Work-related injuries account for 25% of all burn-related hospital admissions.[3]

Burns of the hand and upper extremity result in permanent functional and esthetic deformities. The extent of the deformity is directly related to the severity of the initial injury. Thermal burns to the hand constitute a major injury, despite the disproportionately small body surface area involved. Proper evaluation, assessment of burn depth, and coordinated management of the burned upper extremity can improve the level of functional return and shorten the period of time before a return to productivity and work.[5,6]

Acute Period

Knowledge of the cause of the burn as well as the length of time of exposure play a significant role in assessing the depth of the injury, the recovery time, the plan for treatment, and the anticipated level of functional recovery. A burn wound heals by reepithelialization if the depth of injury is confined to the dermis or epidermis. The concentration of uninjured hair follicles, neural elements, and sweat glands at the depth of the unburned dermis determines the rate of reepithelialization. The greater the remaining concentration of these uninjured adnexal elements in the dermis, the faster the burn wound will heal and the better the quality of the resultant burn scar. Complete loss of the dermis, as occurs in full-thickness burns, requires skin resurfacing. The quality of a healed burn scar heavily influences the degree of functional return. Correct assessment of the depth of injury is the first step in managing the upper extremity burn.

Burn care involves a team management approach. A total patient care plan must be established within the first 24 hours. The physicians are responsible for resuscitation and the management plan. The nursing staff coordinates and implements dressing change protocols and family interaction. Their constant patient contact allows the nurses to provide physicians with the information necessary to make appropriate decisions regarding pain management and times of dressing change, therapy, and rest. Occupational and physical therapists coordinate a plan for orthosis use and exercise and interact with staff. Nutritionists plan the appropriate calorie and protein content and coordinate with nurses and physicians regarding ongoing procedures. The social service department plays a significant role in establishing benefits for the patient and answering insurance coverage and job-related questions. Many others play a role in total patient care. Management strategies are formulated in twice-weekly multidisciplinary conferences. The patient and family are immediately aware of the treatment planned as well as the changing goals for optimum functional improvement. Strict attention to upper extremity function during total

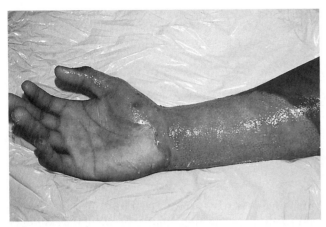

Figure 25-1 Superficial second-degree burn depth that is expected to heal within 10 days with minimal scarring.

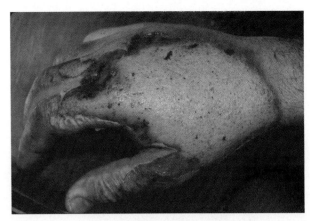

Figure 25-2 Deep second-degree burn with moderate-thickness eschar.

patient care is a responsibility of all involved in the treatment of the burn patient.

Assessment

The initial extent of the total burn injury is assessed using the "rule of nines."[7,8] The total body surface area burned is estimated using this easily reproducible protocol. This information predicts the overall severity of the burn injury and estimates early patient fluid resuscitation. The upper extremity constitutes 9% of the total body surface area; the hand by itself represents 3%.[3,9] The depth of burn injury as well as the total surface area and location involved predict the course of treatment and the functional recovery. This assessment also provides early valuable information to the patient and family concerning time of recovery.

A first-degree burn is confined to the epithelial layer of skin, producing erythema and mild discomfort. The injured area is red, and blisters are usually not seen on examination. Full function remains, reduced, however, by the acute pain. Symptoms of pain and swelling are of short duration. Topical application of a moisturizer to the exposed surface of the burned area reduces the pain. Reepithelialization begins within 48 hours. No restrictive scar results.

By definition, second-degree burn injury penetrates into the dermis (Fig. 25-1). These levels of injury are classified into superficial second-degree and deep second-degree burn. The superficial second-degree injury involves the upper level of the dermis and is expected to reepithelialize within 10 to 14 days with topical wound care.[10] The appearance of the burn is characterized by blisters, intact or ruptured, a thin eschar, and severe pain. The periphery shows an erythema as the level of burn injury becomes progressively more superficial.

The deep second-degree injury extends to the depth of the dermis, injuring a greater concentration of the adnexal hair follicles and sweat glands. This diminishes the ability for reepithelialization and results in delayed healing—taking between 14 and 21 days to completion. The appearance of this injury, in contrast to the superficial second-degree burn, shows the absence of blisters and sometimes a moderate-thickness eschar (Fig. 25-2). Immediate pain is less intense because the superficial nerve endings are injured by the burn at this depth. The quality of the resultant burn scar healing after these depth injuries can be poor, increasing the risk of later hypertrophy and secondary scar contracture.

The specific location of injury also helps guide the management plan. Areas of thin skin, flexion and extension creases, and fine joints of the fingers are severely affected by the persistent inflammation of slowly healing wounds and the resultant restricting scars. When poor-quality healing or hypertrophic scar is anticipated, early resurfacing with better quality skin must be considered.

Full-thickness burn injury, or third-degree burn, destroys the entire dermis, and with it the potential for reepithelialization and healing. The presence of a thick inelastic eschar defines the depth of injury (Fig. 25-3). Initially, the burn surface is not painful. Skin graft resurfacing is indicated because no spontaneous epithelialization is possible. Early grafting reduces the morbidity of anticipated contracture and subsequent reduction of function. The small joints of the

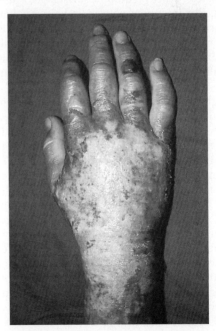

Figure 25-3 Third-degree burn with full-thickness loss of tissue.

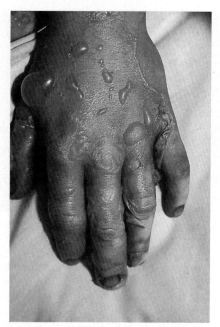

Figure 25-4 Mixed deep and superficial second-degree burns. The depth of the burn is related in part to the thickness of the skin.

hand are extremely sensitive to any degree of skin restriction.

A fourth-degree burn results from prolonged thermal contact and involves the soft tissue and underlying tendon, joint, and bones.[4] The injured tissue at this depth is charred. Prolonged hot immersion, extended flame contact, and electrical burn injury may show this depth of tissue destruction. Extensive reconstructive procedures and, more often, amputation result.

Burn depth in the hand is often mixed (Fig. 25-4). Superficial areas of injury heal spontaneously by epithelialization, whereas others require resurfacing to prevent functional loss. The treatment plan must be individualized after careful burn assessment. The management goal is to resurface all burns that are not expected to reepithelialize within 14 to 21 days with suitable quality grafts.[11] Burns that will reepithelialize sooner are carefully assessed for improvement daily.

Although the depth of burn is important, additional information concerning the injury permits the treatment team to plan more precisely. The source of the thermal injury is extremely important. A scald injury traditionally produces a burn more homogeneous in depth and appearance. Knowledge of the temperature of the scalding liquid and the length of the contact time helps to better define the depth of injury. Water at 158°F causes full-thickness injury in a child within 1 second.[7] Lower temperatures also produce equal-depth burn if the contact time is prolonged. Liquid with fat or grease added retains greater heat, producing a deeper burn in less time (Table 25-1). Fire burns in open air at approximately 500°F. Contact with burning substances or ignition of clothing produces a full-thickness burn injury almost immediately.

The thickness of the skin in the involved area also plays a very significant role. The thickness of the dermis in the

Table 25-1 Time Needed for Hot Water Immersion to Produce Third-Degree Burns

Temperature (°F)	Time
158°	1 sec
150°	2 sec
140°	10 sec
130°	30 sec
127°	1 min
120°	10 min

injured area determines the speed with which the skin can reepithelialize. The depth of injury relative to the skin thickness also predicts the quality of the healing process. The skin of the dorsum of the finger, the dorsum of the hand, the volar wrist, and the inner arm represents relatively thin dermal areas. A deep second-degree burn at any of these levels is associated with delayed epithelialization and a poor quality restricting burn scar. Scar breakdown, fibrosis, and injury in proximity to joints compromises function because of associated joint contracture and restricted motion. The same source and contact time of the burn injury applied to the palm, however, may be associated with a more rapid epithelialization with no functional long-term restriction owing to the rich concentration of adnexal elements in the dermis of palmar skin. The quality of the skin at the level of injury is another important factor in determining the outcome.

The severity of the burn is determined by the combination of the temperature of the source, time of contact, thickness of the skin, and area of the burn injury. This information, as well as the early appearance on examination, permit decision making for either continuation of conservative management or an early plan for excision and grafting of the wound. The goal of burn management is maximum restoration of function with stable soft tissue coverage in the earliest possible time.[12,13]

The management of each burn must be individualized. Patient compliance, understanding the type of work the patient performs, and overall burn size are important factors in the management plan. The experience of the surgeon and therapist in evaluating the progressing clinical picture in light of the expected outcome is an extremely important part of the treatment protocol.

Acute Management

Admission to a burn treatment facility is indicated for second-degree burns in excess of 10% to 15% of body surface and for third-degree injuries as small as 3%. Patients requiring resuscitation or those having smaller areas of burn requiring specialized care meet the criteria for hospital admission as well.[2] A large number of minor burn injuries are also treated on an outpatient basis in major centers or physicians' offices. Initial management involves evaluation of the burn wound severity and the selection of a treatment plan. The burn surface is cleaned and all foreign debris is removed. Broken blister epithelium is débrided. When blisters are intact, the treating physician is faced with a decision to either débride the blisters or leave them intact until the

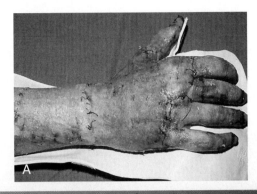

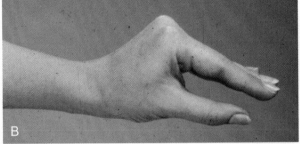

Figure 25-5 A, Universal orthosis used to protect ligaments and fine joint capsules. **B,** MCP joints at 90 degrees and IP joints in full extension.

next dressing change.[14,15] As a matter of protocol, when the blisters are covered by thin epithelium, they are débrided along with the exudate. Blisters in the palm are usually covered by a thicker epithelium. These blisters are incised, the fluid is removed, and the epithelium is used for resurfacing the wound as a biological dressing. This provides effective wound coverage, diminishes pain, and permits epithelialization below. For wounds without epithelial coverage, an impregnated gauze dressing or skin substitute may be used as temporary coverage with dressing changes at 24 to 48 hours.

A more extensive burn injury requiring fluid resuscitation produces local and often generalized edema. An orthosis should be applied immediately to maintain joint position of the wrist in extension and the metacarpophalangeal (MCP) joint at 90 degrees of flexion to protect ligament tension. The interphalangeal (IP) joints are positioned in full extension (Fig. 25-5).[12,13] This extended position decreases tension on IP joint capsules, ligaments, and the overlying burned skin. The extended position also provides protection, when indicated, from exposure of the extensor tendon through the severely injured thin skin covering the proximal interphalangeal (PIP) or distal interphalangeal (DIP) joint.

Fibrosis and persistent small-joint inflammation is a cause of postburn stiffness and joint deformity. The longer the burn wound remains open, the longer inflammation around the fine joints continues. This inflammation is the source of progressive scar formation and restriction of motion. Intensive hand therapy during the acute period is scheduled at least twice daily, with the nursing staff continuing exercises between dressing changes. Pain, high levels of sedation, and significant swelling may preclude full active or passive joint motion. Continuous passive motion (CPM)

devices can be employed in an attempt to maintain overall range until the patient can participate in active exercises.[5] Compliance, however, is often altered by pain, and goals are all too often not completely met during the acute period.

Most patients with burns of the upper extremity have additional areas of burn injury. Forty-five percent of nonfatal burns involve the upper extremity.[2] The burn patient is assessed for the extent of the total burn injury. Fluid resuscitation and airway patency are first ensured. When the patient's emergent condition is stabilized, management of the upper extremity becomes a definitive part of the overall burn care. Evaluation of the hand and upper extremity begins with an appreciation for the presence of compartment swelling. Observation of the extremity with dressings removed is essential. Circumferential burns of the hand, fingers, and extremity increase venous pressure and begin acting as a tourniquet. Combined with an increase in soft tissue swelling, compartment pressure may increase above 30 mm Hg, causing tissue necrosis. An initial clinical diagnosis may be sufficient when the pattern of burn involvement is extensive and deep.[16] Burn injury, however, may show progressive swelling with slowly increasing pressure and less acute signs of compartment syndrome. Clinical signs of severe distal swelling despite elevation, progressive loss of sensibility, intrinsic negative posturing of the hand, and constant unrelenting pain suggest increased compartment pressures.

Anticipation of increasing pressure suggests the need for compartment measurements performed with a baseline value obtained for comparison over the first 24 hours. Increased pressure values or the expectation of a compartment syndrome as edema continues indicate the need for an emergency escharotomy (Fig. 25-6).[17] Complete decompression of all compartments involved in the burn injury is then indicated. The axial escharotomy incisions of the fingers and the upper extremity result in immediate reduction of pressure. Individualized compartment releases in the hand, including the intrinsic muscles, may be necessary to achieve pressure reduction.[18] Escharotomy is, however, not a guarantee of tissue survival. The origin of the burn and length of exposure may be too extensive for soft tissue survival of the distal digits (Fig. 25-7). Clinical observation of progressive distal swelling, intracompartment measurements, and pulse oximetry have been used to evaluate these conditions.[19]

The thin dorsal skin of the hand and fingers is often involved in deep burns of the extremities based on initial protective motions such as firm fist making. Immediate management of all burns includes surface lavage of all debris and débridement of nonviable epithelium and blisters. Topical silver sulfidiazine antibacterial cream is applied with soft bulky nonconstricting gauze dressings, contoured to the burned areas of the extremity. Custom-fitted orthoses are fabricated at the bedside to maintain individual functional positions and to protect the small joints.

Management of second-degree burns of the extremity is guided by burn depth and area of involvement. Conservative management with dressing changes, whirlpool, and active and passive range of motion (ROM) exercises provided by a therapist is appropriate for burns that are expected to heal satisfactorily in a defined period of time. Early excision and grafting are advocated for those injuries for which no healing, or poor-quality healing is anticipated.

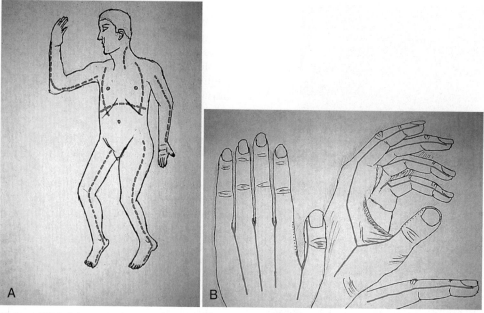

Figure 25-6 Schematic diagram of escharotomy procedures for immediate compartment decompression.

Several authors have advocated delayed excision of deep second-degree and even third-degree burns of the hand, allowing additional time to see if epithelialization will occur.[20] In a selected group of patients with deep second-degree burns, Salisbury and Wright showed that intensive therapy produced functional results similar to those achieved in hands in which the burns were excised and grafted early in their course.[11] Patient compliance is essential in these circumstances. In my experience, deep second-degree burns of the hand and fingers that are not expected to epithelialize within 14 days are excised early and immediately skin-grafted. This has resulted in a predictable return to function and less long-term stiffness.

Direct tangential excision or fascial excision is indicated for burns that will not heal by reepithelialization.[21,22] Early excision is preferred as soon as possible after the decision to excise is reached and the patient is stable for anesthesia. Tangential excision under tourniquet control removes all

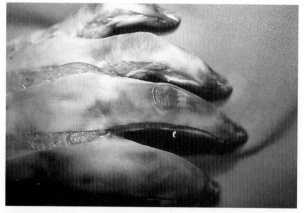

Figure 25-7 Escharotomy had been indicated, but tissue injury resulted in necrosis of the fine soft tissue distally.

injured tissue, leaving only viable dermis and a well-vascularized bed for a skin graft (Fig. 25-8). If the burn injury involves the entire dermis and includes thrombosis of the subdermal vessels, the plane of excision must be deeper at the fascial level. In the hand, all attempts are made to excise above the neurovascular plane of the dorsum. Excision involves surgical judgment to ensure complete resection of nonviable burn tissue. This plane is characterized by white, soft, pliable tissue. Once complete excision is achieved, the tourniquet is deflated and the wound is observed for dermal or subcutaneous bleeding. Questionable areas are reexcised until all nonviable tissue is removed. Hemostasis is obtained, temporary pressure dressings are applied, and the hand and extremity are elevated as preparations are made for skin graft harvest.

Once hemostasis is complete, the skin graft is applied to the bed. Sheet grafts, piecrusted for drainage, generally measuring approximately 0.012 inches in thickness for the average adult, are preferred for the hand and fingers. Resurfacing a child's hand requires thinner grafts. Meshed grafts in ratios of 1:1.5, 1:2, or 1:3 may be used to minimize the use of available remaining noninjured skin (see Fig. 25-8). Conservation of donor skin is critical when the patient has sustained injuries over more than 50% of the body's surface. The interstices of these meshed grafts heal by epithelialization over scar and are subject to somewhat greater contraction than the sheet graft. If the wound is initially thought unsuitable for graft coverage, application of a topical skin substitute or frequent dressing changes are preferable to immediate grafting. Delayed secondary grafting is preferable to incurring a significant risk of graft loss on a less than optimal recipient bed.

The graft is applied to the bed with the hand in the functional position of gentle flexion of the fingers and wrist extension.[23] The graft is secured with sutures, staples, or fibrin glue (or a combination).[24-26] An interface dressing is

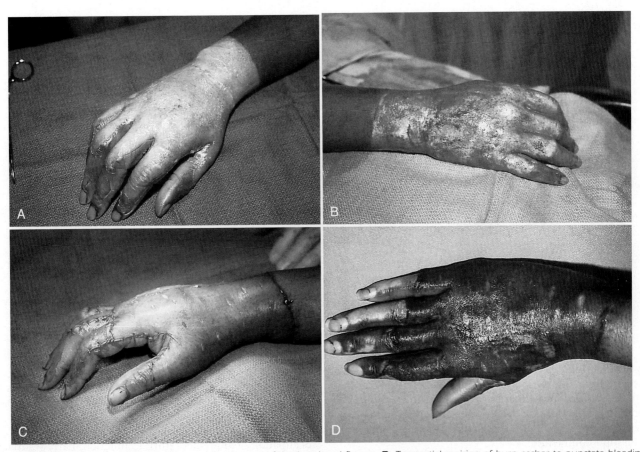

Figure 25-8 A, Deep second-degree burns on the dorsum of the hand and fingers. **B,** Tangential excision of burn eschar to punctate bleeding in dermis. **C,** Application of split-thickness skin graft. **D,** Supple graft at 3 months with expected hyperpigmentation.

used, followed by a bulky soft dressing and an immobilizing orthosis. Vacuum-assisted closure (VAC) is a technique of wound management that seals the wound with a foam dressing and applies *negative pressure* to the wound bed by tubing threaded through the dressing. The vacuum pressure can be applied continuously to the skin-grafted site. Use of the VAC dressing supports the graft, prevents shear forces, and is associated with a lower need for secondary grafting.[27,28] Initially, graft observation and assessment are performed at 24 to 48 hours after the acute excision, depending on the confidence in the hemostasis obtained. If no fluid collections are noted, the next dressing change can be at postoperative day 3 to 5. Hand therapy begins at 4 to 5 days after grafting, when graft adherence is secure.[29] Exercises consist of active and gentle passive ROM. Orthoses are designed with an emphasis on wrist extension and MCP joint flexion. Dynamic orthoses may be used when the graft is stable and active ROM is slow to return because of stiffness or lack of compliance. Pain management is an essential part of the therapy plan. (See Chapter 26 for an in-depth discussion of therapy for the burned hand).

Burns of the palm often require a more conservative management plan (Fig. 25-9). The specialized skin of the palm and volar aspect of the fingers has a thick epidermis and a dermis rich in adnexal elements. Burn depth based on palmar skin thickness and a protective flexion response to injury

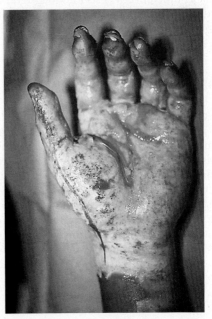

Figure 25-9 Palmar burns are managed conservatively until the burn's depth is fully demarcated.

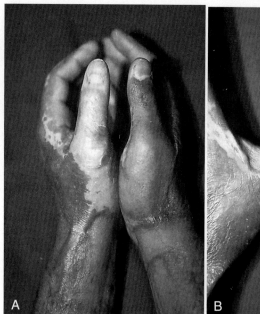
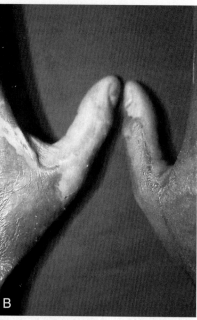

Figure 25-10 A, Significant functional difference between the grafted right hand and the left hand after second-degree burn. Note the parchment-like epithelium, hypertrophic scarring, and the loss of pigmentation on the left. **B,** Note the poor-quality scar and the contracting webs associated with secondary healing on the left compared with skin grafting resurfacing on the right.

may permit high-quality reepithelialization in a shorter than expected time. More conservative treatment is suggested until the depth of the palmar burn is fully defined. When the palmar burn is full-thickness, resurfacing is indicated to prevent the functional loss brought about by late palmar and digital joint contracture.

Advocates for resurfacing of the palm with either full-thickness or split-thickness skin have based their decisions on long-term wound hypertrophy, recurrence of contractures, and development of burn syndactyly.[30] A split-thickness graft offers the best alternative in the acute burn wound. Graft take is often better because of the shorter time to revascularization and the ability to resurface larger areas. No appreciable difference was seen in long-term contracture results in deep palmar burns. Full-thickness grafting can be reserved for later reconstructive procedures when graft take presents less of a risk for loss.[31]

Reconstructive Period

Once the acute burn wound has healed completely, attention is given to a program of improved motion, stretch, and positioning during scar maturation. Hand therapy includes frequent visits for active and passive motion. Serial orthosis use maintains position; a dynamic orthosis is often used for constant and progressive stretch between exercise periods. Massage, silicone sheeting, and conformer application are part of the management plan during the maturing phase of approximately 12 months. The therapist's role is to bring all joints of the extremity to their maximum function and aid in soft tissue softening and desensitization. The therapist and treating physician must also identify when functional improvement reaches a plateau.

The quality of the burn scar influences the ease of return of hand and extremity motion. A poor-quality thick scar is associated with stiffness that is more pronounced after sleep

or inactivity. Improvement in scar quality as softening occurs over the first 6 to 12 months updates the prognosis for improved or full-joint function. Strict attention to anticipated time of healing of the initial burn wound, scar fibrosis and thickening, proximity of the injury to fine joints, age, and occupation help predict return to function. Early resurfacing of a deep burn injury with a better-quality skin produces a better long-term result. The following case study outcome defines the practical meaning of quality results in burns of the hand.

A 19-year-old man was admitted to the burn center when he sustained burns to the dorsal aspect of both hands and fingers while working on a car engine. The entire dorsal aspect of both hands and fingers were noted to have deep second-degree burns with extensions onto the thenar eminence and distal wrist. Left and right hands were similar in involvement. The palmar surfaces were not burned. There was no suggestion of compartment syndrome or increased pressure. A decision was made to excise the deep burns early with immediate skin graft resurfacing, beginning with the right hand and following 48 hours later with the left.

All fingers and the dorsum of the right hand and wrist underwent an uncomplicated excision and graft procedure. Graft take was complete. Just before scheduling the left hand for a similar procedure, the treating physician made a decision to allow more time for reepithelialization rather than grafting the left hand. The management plan was changed. The left hand had completely epithelialized by the 20th postburn day. The patient showed excellent compliance in therapy and achieved full flexion of all digits of both hands. He returned to his work as an auto mechanic approximately 4 months after his injury.

At 6 months, during routine follow-up examination, this patient provided a superb insight into the quality of burn healing (Fig. 25-10). He noted that the right hand showed no stiffness on awakening, and he had a full ROM of all digits. He was comfortable and had no pain in making a fist. The

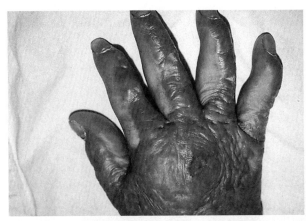

Figure 25-11 Extensive fibrosis and hypertrophic scarring has resulted from prolonged secondary healing of this second-degree burn. The resultant stiffness will be permanent.

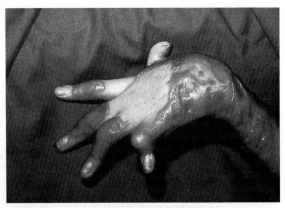

Figure 25-12 Burn scar deformities on concave surfaces of the flexor portions of the wrist and digits result in decreased forces opposing contracture.

stability of the hand grafts was excellent, and he described no wound breakdown since the graft had been applied. He had no trouble going about his work, even sustaining frequent superficial injuries against the engine block. The left hand, however, was extremely stiff in the morning, taking up to 20 minutes for him to overcome the stiffness in the small joints and obtain full flexion. The left hand had a constant general aching, and wound breakdown in response to minor trauma was frequent. The appearance of the left hand showed parchment-like burn scar and web syndactyly as opposed to the smooth, well-pigmented graft on the right hand.

The patient was not about to undergo a secondary procedure unless absolutely necessary for unstable scarring or web restriction. The patient achieved full coverage of the burn wound of both hands and, with therapy, achieved full active and passive ROM. The difference in quality of the function of the healed burn wounds is clearly appreciated in this patient interview. Appreciation of expected wound quality is an important part of decision making during the acute period. The notion that if the wound becomes hypertrophic or unstable then one can always return for resurfacing is not valid. The fibrosis, soft tissue shortening, and tendon imbalance that occur cannot be improved satisfactorily after long-standing stiffness and decreased motion (Fig. 25-11). Early aggressive wound management based on a thorough knowledge of wound healing decreases many of the problems seen in the reconstructive period.

Basic principles in planning burn scar reconstruction involve a serious appreciation of forces of contraction.[32] Understanding how the contracture developed increases the possibility that a reconstructive procedure will be successful, avoiding an early recurrence and its associated functional restriction. These principles assume that the burn scar is well healed and fully mature and that all therapy has reached the maximum level of improvement.

Montandon and colleagues write that a scar or skin graft continues to contract until it meets an opposite and opposing force.[33-35] Scar and graft contraction progresses over the first 3 months of maturation. The surface over which a contracting burn scar lies also influences the contraction process. Scar over concave surfaces meets less resistance than that over convex surfaces, allowing greater migration of the scar and webbing. Examples of this include axillary contractures,

distal migration of the dorsal finger webs, and flexion contractures on the antecubital surface of the elbow (Fig. 25-12). The quality of the scar, its response to therapy, and the expected functional result based on the contour of the area in question help determine the timing and extent of the burn scar reconstruction.

A burn scar is always synonymous with a skin deficit. In planning a reconstructive procedure, the deficit of soft tissue after scar release is always larger than expected. A diagram of the original burn-injury surface helps to anticipate the reconstruction defect. A generous overcorrection with skin graft alone does not ensure a successful reconstruction because the forces of contraction are governed by the surface characteristics of the area. Adding more skin grafts to the release of a severe axillary contracture does not guarantee that restriction of the arm abduction will not recur. External orthosis application and the early return of abduction motion adds resistance to the contractile forces. The graft will simply continue to contract until it meets the precise opposing force, also determined by surface characteristics.

Palmar Contractures

The resting posture of the hand normally maintains the fingers and wrist in slight flexion. Moderate to deep burn injury across the volar wrist, the palm, and the palmar surface of the digits can easily produce a flexion contracture if the details of proper treatment are neglected (Fig. 25-13). Palmar burns that heal by epithelialization or even those that require skin graft coverage have a common tendency to contract, producing flexion deformities. ROM and stretch exercises as well as sequential orthosis use during the period of scar maturation counter the forces of contraction and result in well-balanced motion. Failure to satisfactorily improve this flexion deformity as the burn scar matures prompts consideration for early scar contracture release, skin graft or flap application, and renewed hand therapy to restore ROM.

Flexion contraction that progresses despite extension orthosis use results in secondary joint contractures as the burn scar matures and contracts. Progressive pain with orthosis use and the inability to obtain full extension of the digits reduce the amount of passive stretch that can be tolerated. The contracture becomes permanent and reduces

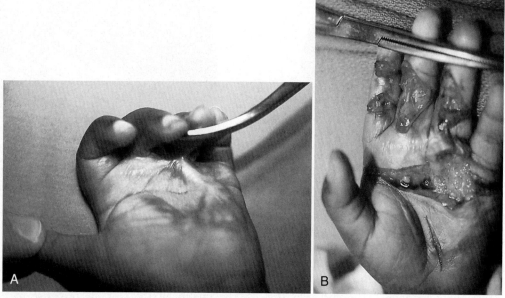

Figure 25-13 A, Palmar contractures result in significant soft tissue deficit. Burn contractures in the palm almost always necessitate the addition of skin. **B,** Note the significant tissue deficit resulting from simple release of burn scar contractures.

motion and function. Surgical reconstruction is indicated before further joint contraction is appreciated. Radiographic examination is obtained prior to reconstruction to verify the alignment of the joint surfaces. Kurtzman and Stern classified PIP joint contractures based on their degree of skin deficit and joint narrowing.[36,37] More severe and long-standing flexion contractures may require volar joint release in addition to resurfacing of the volar skin deficit. Arthrodesis must be considered in those fingers in which secondary joint destruction precludes full extension, despite adequate soft tissue release.

Complete soft tissue release perpendicular to the direction of maximum contracture is indicated. A transverse incision from midaxial to midaxial point is necessary to release all tissue tension.[38] Passive stretch of the contracted joint after soft tissue release defines existing tension. Complete excision of contracted scar is usually not indicated because residual hypertrophic burn scar will mature and soften when the tension forces are released. Resurfacing of the deficit is often achieved using full-thickness skin graft.[39] When contracture release involves exposure of tendon, a local flap, if available, is the procedure of choice.[40-43] Soft bulky dressings and extension orthotic positioning continue during the postgrafting period. Once adequate release of a contracture in children was established, longitudinal growth did not necessarily produce a recurrence of the contracture. Active extension exercises increase the resistive forces against the graft contraction, diminishing the rate of recurrence.

Dorsal Hand Burns

Maturing dorsal hand burns are characterized by restricted motion and pain. Rehabilitation begins in the acute period with early motion and excision of the burn for deep second-degree or full-thickness burns. The relatively thin dorsal skin of the hand and digits contracts when thermally injured, making digital flexion difficult and producing extension deformities. Achieving maximum flexion at the MCP joints increases resistive force over the dorsum of the hand and is the best prevention against extension contractures. Active ROM, passive stretch into flexion, and dynamic flexion orthotic positioning all attempt to achieve a flexion posture of the fingers during wound healing and maturation.[5] This progressive flexion increases the force over the dorsum of the hand and is strong enough to prevent contractures. Failure to achieve progressive improvements in flexion results in hyperextension deformities of the MCP joints and secondary flexion deformities at the PIP joints (Fig. 25-14). This deformity occurs more easily in the ring and small fingers because of the higher degree of metacarpal flexion in these fingers at the carpal–hamate articulation.[44,45] As these metacarpals are pulled into increasing extension, the resistance against continued MCP hyperextension continues to decrease. If uncorrected, the outcome produces fixed MCP joint hyperextension and PIP flexion deformities. This pattern differs from the stable second and third carpal metacarpal (CMC) joints—the fixed unit of the hand. Similar hyperextension deformities at these joints are seen only in the most severe burn contractures.

The ability to overcome hyperextension stiffness across the dorsum of the hand and fingers demands persistence, compliance with therapy, and tolerance of pain. Some patients, despite analgesia and encouragement, cannot or will not achieve sufficiently improved digital flexion at the MCP level necessary to overcome the increasing forces of contraction. As the dorsal graft or reepithelializing burn scar continues to contract until it meets an equal and opposing resistive force, the MCP joint extension contraction steadily increases toward fixed deformity contracture (Fig. 25-15). The fourth and fifth metacarpals descend progressively into palmar flexion, creating a more concave dorsal surface at the MCP joint level. Resistance to graft contraction is therefore further reduced. This accentuated hyperextension is more prominent on the ring and small fingers. If this cycle is not broken, fixed MCP joint hyperextension results, followed by secondary flexion deformities at the PIP joints. The PIP joint deformity

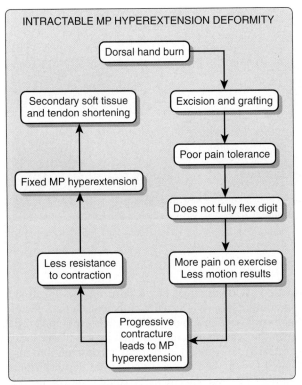

INTRACTABLE MP HYPEREXTENSION DEFORMITY

Dorsal hand burn

Secondary soft tissue and tendon shortening

Fixed MP hyperextension

Less resistance to contraction

Excision and grafting

Poor pain tolerance

Does not fully flex digit

More pain on exercise
Less motion results

Progressive contracture leads to MP hyperextension

Figure 25-14 Metacarpophalangeal hyperextension deformities may be prevented by early initiation of hand therapy. Range of motion and passive stretch exercises diminish contractions before secondary soft tissue shortening.

in these cases originates from MCP joint hyperextension and not from direct injury to the central slip over the PIP joint. Because these PIP joint flexion changes are secondary, this deformity is termed *pseudo*boutonnière deformity, as opposed to a true boutonnière deformity resulting from primary deep tendon injury at the PIP joint level.[44]

Reconstruction of MCP joint extension contractures begins as hand therapy reaches a plateau. The dorsal soft tissue contracture is released transversely, including the MCP joint capsules when indicated, and the deficit covered with a split-thickness skin graft.[46] Postoperative orthosis

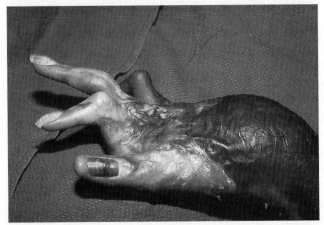

Figure 25-15 Intractable hyperextension deformities at the metacarpophalangeal joints with secondary proximal interphalangeal flexion deformities.

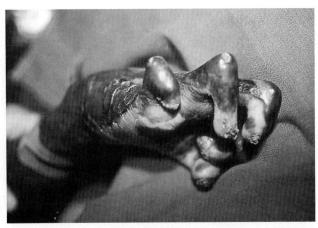

Figure 25-16 True boutonnière deformities following burn injury are the result of exposure or attenuation of the central slip and capsule over the proximal interphalangeal joint.

application following the graft application and the use of dynamic flexion orthoses after the graft has taken (5–7 days) help maximize improvement of the contracture deformity. However, these results depend on the overall suppleness of the released MCP joint and the continued ability to overcome capsular and soft tissue contraction.

Long-standing extension contractures over the dorsum of the hand, if unresolved, produce fixed hyperextension MCP joint deformities (Fig. 25-16). Simple release of the overlying contracted skin may not reduce the entire soft tissue tension present at the capsule level and surrounding the extensor tendons. Forced passive stretch of the MCP joint may achieve the desired degree of flexion. K-wire pin fixation can hold the MCP joint at near 90 degrees if the surgeon anticipates significant residual tension as may remain in the longitudinal contraction of the extensor tendons over the dorsum. This unresolved extrinsic extensor tightness favors recurrence of the hyperextension deformity, frequently within weeks of the contracture release. In this instance, a relative discrepancy persists between skeletal length and available soft tissue.

Fixed MCP joint extension contractures caused by soft tissue shortening following burn injury can only be resolved by lengthening the foreshortened composite soft tissue or shortening the skeleton length, returning this soft tissue to skeletal ratio to 1:1. Available techniques for these intractable deforming contractures include metacarpal shortening, MCP joint replacement, arthrodesis (skeletal length shortening), and extensor tendon lengthening with dorsal flap reconstruction (composite soft tissue elongation). An advanced technique using a tissue expander placed *below* the extensor tendons stretches these tendons as well as the overlying soft tissue and skin graft, creating a composite soft tissue stretch, returning the skeletal/soft tissue length ratio to normal. Slow, progressive inflation of the expander is not associated with an increased risk of morbidity and complication, even in burn-scarred soft tissue. On removal of the expander, release of the dorsal MCP joint capsule permits passive flexion to 90 degrees with no restriction from the now stretched extensor tendon. A dynamic orthosis protocol permits the extensor tendon to rebalance itself against normal MCP joint flexion exerted by the patient. The strength of this unrestricted digital flexion is now sufficient to bring about a lasting

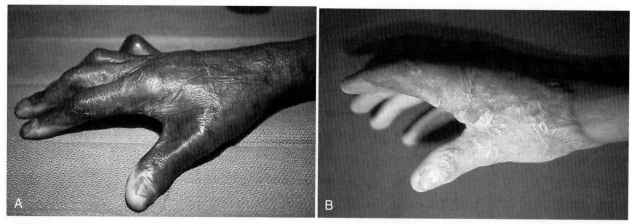

Figure 25-17 A, Mild to moderate postburn contracture of the first dorsal thumb index web space. **B,** Progressive loss of thumb abduction is appreciated with more severe contracture.

resolution to the extension contracture. The overlying skin and soft tissue remain stable and do not recontract once the force of flexion is unrestricted.[47]

Deep burns occurring over the PIP joints may produce secondary extension contractures or may result in true boutonnière deformities, depending on the depth of involvement (see Fig. 25-16). The dorsal skin is extremely thin, and exposure or injury to the underlying extensor tendon is not uncommon in patients sustaining deep flame burn injuries. Extension orthosis use protects the tendon from exposure in the acute period depending on the original depth of injury. Early graft resurfacing provides quality tissue if the underlying tendon was not injured.

Injury to the central slip of the extensor tendon overlying the PIP joint progressively results in a true boutonnière deformity. If the quality of the overlying skin remains poor, arthrodesis of the PIP joint into an optimum position of function shortens the skeleton length relative to the available, often unstable, soft tissue. Multiple procedures for soft tissue reconstruction of a postburn boutonnière deformity have been described.[48-50] When the overlying skin quality is good, results of tendon reconstruction are fair at best. Stiffness and tendon imbalance persist. Late complications are related to overlying poor-quality skin breakdown and unresolved joint stiffness. Arthrodesis of the PIP joint is a reproducible procedure that improves function of the hand and, by shortening, establishes decreased soft tissue tension and stable wound coverage.

Thumb Index Web Contractures

Contracture of the first web space of the hand results in reduction of thumb abduction and opposition (Fig. 25-17).[51] Once contraction progresses, static and dynamic orthoses become less effective because their force is dissipated by the radial deviation of the MCP joint of the thumb. Secondary contracture and stiffness of the first dorsal interosseous muscle fascia and the metacarpal trapezial joint can result in a more severe restriction of function.[52,53]

The classification of the thumb index web contracture can be based on the severity of injury.[54] A simple web-band contracture, often resulting from a palmar burn, restricts only

abduction. With minimal or no burn on the dorsal skin, a lengthening Z-plasty is usually sufficient. When dorsal *and* palmar surfaces show burn scarring, the anticipated deficit exceeds the soft tissue gain provided by a Z-plasty local flap (Fig. 25-18). A three-dimensional reconstruction may be indicated to lengthen the scar and regain depth of the web. A double Z/V-Y advancement is suitable coverage for the moderate contracture deficit. A tighter web contracture is characterized by a greater skin deficit, exceeding the lengthening possibility with local flap tissue alone. Release of the contracture and resurfacing with full- or split-thickness skin

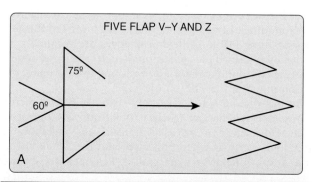

FIVE FLAP V–Y AND Z

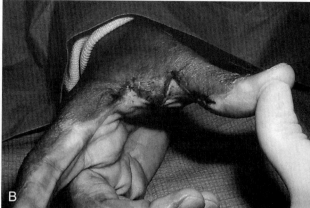

Figure 25-18 A, Design of interdigitating flaps to lengthen the scar contracture and deepen the web space. These flaps are most successful in contractures showing little skin deficit. **B,** Restoration of web contour and depth.

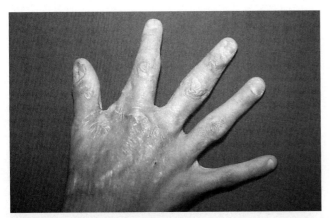

Figure 25-19 Burn scar syndactyly showing distal migration of the dorsal burn scar, distorting the web spaces.

grafts permits maximum functional return in those cases.[55-61]

Very severe contractures involve contraction of the first dorsal interosseous muscle and fascia and even the joint capsule of the metacarpal trapezial joint. The thumb is slowly pulled into the plane of the palm with severe restriction in all directions of motion. The release of the skin deficit contractures, muscle fascia, and, if needed, the CMC joint capsule, permits the return of the thumb to a functional position. Flap coverage is then necessary (radial forearm, free flap, groin, random) to reliably resurface the large defect and possible basal joint exposure.[62,63]

Maintenance of joint position after contracture releases ensures good graft or flap contact to the underlying bed. The immobilization of the area is maintained for 5 to 10 days until complete graft take or flap stability permits motion without risk of shear. Positioning of the thumb index web space has been described using pin fixation or an external fixator in the more severe cases.

Burn Syndactyly

Burn syndactyly is anticipated on any concave web surface where scar or graft has been pulled distally by contraction (Fig. 25-19). This distal migration continues until the scar has reached its maximum tension against resistance. Acute burn injuries of the dorsal hand and fingers often produce burn syndactyly in the web spaces as scar contraction matures. In deep dermal burns that are allowed to reepithelialize over time, burn syndactyly reconstruction is expected as part of the reconstructive plan at some point in the future. In deep hand burns that are excised and grafted, injury extending into the web and dorsally onto the digits ensures web syndactyly during the healing and maturing period. The details of early skin grafting should include the application of deep darts from the dorsal to volar aspect of the web in an attempt to break the anticipated straight-line contraction of the graft interface with healthy soft tissue. Application of a dart elongates the graft surface. This technique may not be sufficient to counterbalance the distal pull of the contracting graft that advances the soft dorsal skin distally toward the digit, creating a prominent dorsal hood.

Pressure garments with conformers inserted into the web create extrinsic pressure in an attempt to restrict the distally

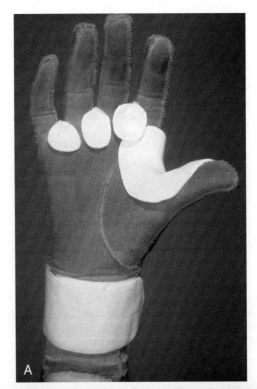

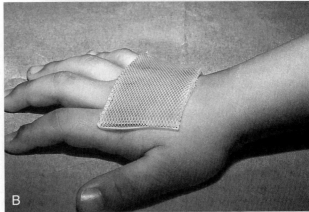

Figure 25-20 A, Compression gloves or gauntlets provide pressure on the dorsal hand burns. Web space conformers (beneath the glove) or silicone **(B)** sheeting also plays a role in softening contracting and hypertrophic scars.

migrating contraction (Fig. 25-20). This pressure is maintained until the wound is mature. Any residual burn syndactyly can be reconstructed at that time.[64] A neglected burn, allowed to heal mostly by secondary intention, may produce a tight web between digits with severe functional restriction.

Many techniques of reconstruction have been described, varying according to the location and extent of the skin deficit. A simple midline split with placement of the skin graft simply re-creates the original contraction pattern; recurrences are therefore common. Local flap rotations may be sufficient for the minimal syndactyly web. The basic principle of skin deficit must not be underestimated. The use of a dorsal flap physically separating portions of the skin graft usually re-creates the dorsal web slope and offers significant protection against recurrence (Fig. 25-21A). The composite

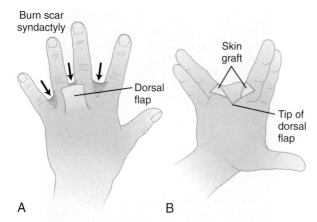

Figure 25-21 A, Burn scar syndactyly using reliable dorsal flap. **B,** Mandatory skin deficit requires full-thickness skin grafts.

tissues in the dorsal flap show minimal contraction. Placing the skin graft against the lateral and medial aspect of the digits, separated by the dorsal flap, protects the finger from future distal scar migration and recurrent contraction. Pressure garments and conformers are continued until complete scar maturation is complete (approximately 12 months).

Distal Finger Burn Contractures

Burn scar contracture over the middle and distal phalanges often results in extension contractures of the DIP joint and deformities about the nail and eponychial area.[65] Once the contracture is present, active exercise and passive stretch are not completely successful in restoring full flexion. Pain is often a symptom of the sensitive DIP joint being pulled into hyperextension. Release of the contracture centered over the DIP area is preferred with either graft or flap coverage.[66,67] The deformity of the eponychial fold from longitudinal contraction causes proximal migration of the nail fold (Fig. 25-22). Restoring the curvature of the nail cuticle from extrinsic contracture requires release across the DIP area, perpendicular to the line of contraction. Improvement of motion and a restored nail fold often result. Direct burn injury may, however, result in destruction of the nail matrix,

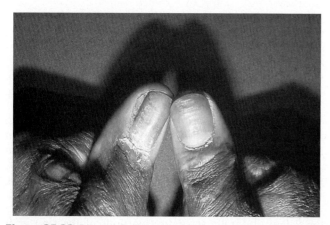

Figure 25-22 Release of proximal nail fold contracture at the interphalangeal joint level. Addition of full-thickness skin graft decreases tension and restores paronychial contour.

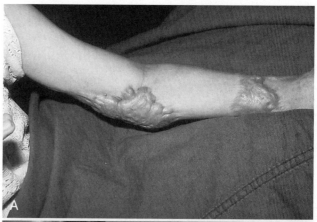

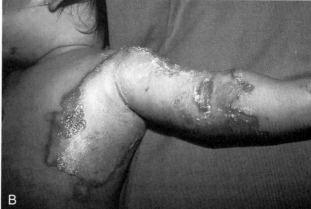

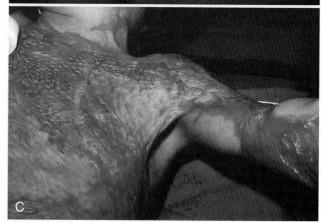

Figure 25-23 A, Extra-articular contracture of the elbow precluding full extension. Fibrosis of soft tissue and joint capsule is appreciated. **B,** Axillary burn scar can create a contracture on the concave surface, resulting in functional restriction to motion. **C,** Longstanding contracture with hypertrophy.

which cannot be restored by simple resolution of the contracture. Techniques at postburn reconstruction of the entire nail and nail matrix have produced fair results.[68,69]

Elbow and Axillary Contractures

Kurtzman and Stern classified elbow flexion contractures into extra-articular and intra-articular contractures.[36] The extra-articular contractures involve the skin, possibly tendon structures, and the underlying joint capsule (Fig. 25-23).

Scar contraction at the level of the capsule is not fully appreciated until all of the overlying structures are first released. The complete antecubital release is approached by a horizontal midaxial-to-midaxial incision.[70] With maximum elbow extension achieved and a stable soft tissue base present, a split-thickness skin graft can be applied. Extension positioning is maintained with an orthosis until full graft take is appreciated. Passive stretch and use of a dynamic orthosis can apply even greater force to improve extension after the graft is stable.[71] If the elbow joint is exposed during the course of deep multilevel contracture release, local or regional composite flap reconstruction is required.[72] Release to within 30 degrees of full extension permits most activities of daily living.[36]

Heterotopic ossification occurs in less than 2% of all burns of the upper extremity.[36,73] X-ray examination before contracture release will document its presence. Resection after maturation of the bone formation is possible with difficulty. Indications for surgery include failure of improvement of elbow motion, inability to reach the mouth or perineum, and a total ROM of less than 50 degrees. Injury to articular cartilage or nerve compression about the elbow is not uncommon. Surgical correction usually at about 18 months postinjury has resulted in an improved ROM and absence of recurrence.[74]

Contractures of the anterior axillary or posterior axillary fold result in restricted abduction, flexion, and extension of the shoulder. Restriction and progressive loss of motion, refractory to therapy, indicate early release.[75] In some cases the central portion of the axilla is spared from burn injury and contraction. The concave surfaces of the anterior and posterior folds allow progressive contraction because full abduction is often limited by pain. Release of the contracted axillary fold perpendicular to its axis and use of split-thickness skin grafting extending into the axilla and beyond the folds allow for early active abduction and stretch, once the graft is secure. Release often must be carried on to the lateral chest wall to include the pectoralis fascia if that portion participates in the contracture.

When the soft tissue of the axilla is also contracted, successful long-term release is difficult. Resurfacing the axilla after complete release requires an abduction orthosis until active stretch is possible. The large surface area of graft in this case is associated with recurring contracture on both the anterior and posterior surfaces. Secondary release once the skin graft is mature and abduction has been maximized is not uncommon. Lateral chest wall flaps or distant muscle flaps may reduce the rate of recurrent contracture significantly in the more severe cases.[76]

Tissue Expansion

The use of tissue expansion in burn reconstruction can replace the deficient soft tissue with donor skin and

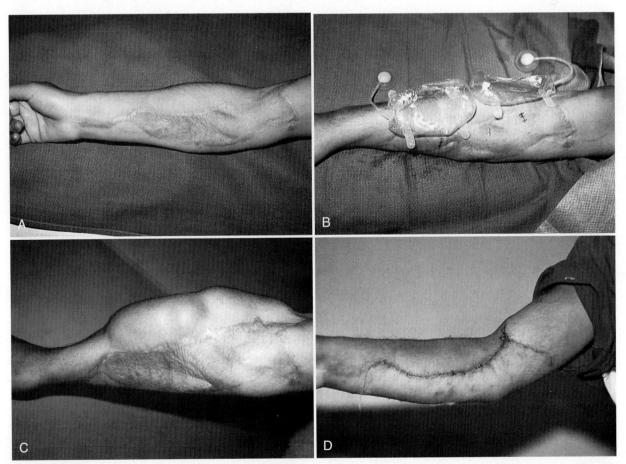

Figure 25-24 Tissue expansion for unsightly or unstable scarring **(A).** Multiple expander insertion **(B)** and progressive expansion **(C).** Subsequent resection of burn scar and advancement of healthy composite flaps **(D).**

subcutaneous tissue of similar color, thickness, and texture.[47] Resection of unstable or unsightly scars is possible by advancement of the expanded, better-quality, sensate skin. An attempt is always made to hide the resultant scars in concealed sites when possible (Fig. 25-24). Longitudinal defects lend themselves better to expansion reconstruction than do wide horizontally oriented burn scars on the upper extremity. The broad lateral-based flaps have a more reliable base circulation. Excessive tension in the expanded flap after advancement necessitates a staged reconstruction of the burn scar. It is prudent not to resect the entire scar until the expanded flap is completely advanced and its tension assessed.[77]

Summary

Management of the burned upper extremity begins with attention to detail during the acute phase. Appreciation of burn depth, potential for contraction, and loss of function indicate an aggressive approach of burn excision and resurfacing. Therapy plays a significant role in preventing early burn deformity and in maximizing functional return following closure and resurfacing of the burn wound. Once this management has reached a maximum improvement, a decision concerning additional reconstructive procedures must be weighed against the potential benefit of functional gain. Burn scar is synonymous with *skin deficit,* and the concave and convex surface contours play a significant role in planning the reconstructive procedure. Attention to these details prevents secondary contracture where possible. Maximum functional return of the upper extremity with quality skin coverage is the goal for each thermally injured patient.

REFERENCES

The complete reference list is available online at www.expertconsult.com.

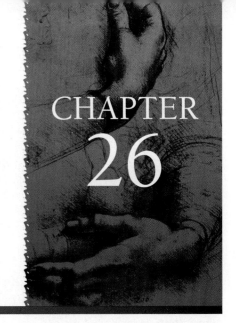

Therapist's Management of the Burned Hand

PATRICIA A. TUFARO, OTR/L AND
SALVADOR L. BONDOC, OTD, OTR/L, CHT

HYPERTROPHIC SCARS AND SCAR CONTRACTION
PHASES OF BURN RECOVERY
THERAPEUTIC MANAGEMENT OF COMMON
    DEFORMITIES OF THE BURNED HAND
RETURN TO WORK AND SCHOOL
FUNCTIONAL OUTCOMES
SUMMARY

CRITICAL POINTS

- When treating the burned hand, therapists spend a
  great deal of time in limiting, reducing, or preventing
  the negative effects of hypertrophic scarring and scar
  contraction on hand structures and function.
- The positioning program for the burned hand is
  designed to minimize edema, prevent tissue
  destruction, and preserve soft tissues in an elongated
  state to facilitate functional recovery.
- Hypertrophic scars appear red, raised, and rigid to
  touch. Gentle pressure on the scar during palpation
  causes transient blanching.
- Keloid scars are distinguished from hypertrophic scars in
  that they have an irregular shape (often bulbous or
  pendulous), extend beyond the boundary of the
  wound, and encroach on the surrounding skin.

The hand accounts for only 3% of the total body surface area
(TBSA).[1-3] Despite this small percentage, an injury to the
hand can cause lifelong deformity and disability. Musculoskeletal impairment and loss of the normal appearance can
influence the patient's self-image, occupation, and lifestyle.
Skilled therapeutic intervention is imperative in order to
preserve motion and joint integrity, prevent scarring, restore
cosmesis, and ultimately optimize function of the hand.

Hand burns are the leading cause of impairment following
a burn injury.[4] They are typically seen as an isolated injury;
however, the hands are rarely unaffected in larger burns.[4]
The American Burn Association classifies a hand burn as a
major injury requiring treatment at a burn center.[5] Although
a burn to the hand is typically not life-threatening, it can,
however, be devastating. Loss of hand use results in an
impairment rating of 95% for the involved extremity and a
57% loss of the whole person's function.[6] Early wound
closure and rehabilitation can facilitate restoration of hand
function. This chapter describes the role of the therapist
during each phase of healing, emphasizing scar assessment,
prevention, and management.

Hypertrophic Scars and Scar Contraction

Loss of hand function following burns may be attributed to
a variety of factors including loss of sensation due to damage
to sensory nerves and nerve endings as well as the loss of
motion due to contractures. Contractures may be functionally defined as shortening of soft tissues, including skin,
muscle, tendon, ligament, and fascia, which restricts the
ability to perform full range of motion (ROM) of a joint. In
the burned hand, contracture formation may be a primary or
secondary outcome of scar formation and contraction.
Primary contractures following a burn are mainly due to the
formation of hypertrophic scars and excessive contraction of
scars (Fig. 26-1).

During typical wound healing, spatial reduction of the
wounded area commences once a matrix of collagen and
proteoglycans known as cicatrix is formed. Within 1 week
after injury, the cicatrix covers the wound and actively contracts to form scar. Scar conversion is an active process, but
may extend further into *scar contraction*, in which the scar
shortens, gathers, and pulls the surrounding unscarred tissue.
Scar contractures are dense, adherent to underlying tissues,
relatively immobile, and painful with pinpoint pressure.
Many physicians and therapists do not distinguish between
scar *contraction* and scar *contracture*. As a point of clarification, scar contraction is a process in which scar contracture
is the ultimate outcome.

Scar contractures tend to occur more in areas where skin
is loose or more pliable. Typically, a scar continues to contract until it meets an equal or opposing force. Skin immediately surrounding scar contractures tends to be less pliable

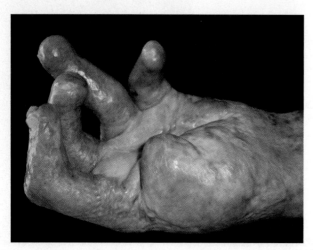

Figure 26-1 An example of excessive scar and contractures limiting hand motion. Note swan-neck deformity on ring finger and proximal interphalangeal joint flexion contractures (perhaps boutonnière deformities) on other digits.

as it gets pulled taut by the scar and therefore could result in movement limitations in joints and soft tissues. Over time, the taut surrounding skin loses its extensibility even if it is uninjured.[7] A simple "pinch" test could give the therapist an idea of the extent of the scar contracture's centripetal pull. The pinch test assesses the degree of tautness and extensibility of the surrounding skin and compares it with the contralateral side or comparable skin on an unburned body part (Fig. 26-2). Decrease in skin pliability reduces joint movement, accessory joint play, and, in certain cases, tendon glide. For example, scar contracture on the dorsum of the hand tends to pull the metacarpophalangeal (MCP) joint in hyperextension. Attempts to actively complete a fist position may be difficult since the scar adds resistance and drag against typical MCP joint arthrokinematics. In addition, adhesion of the scar to the extensor digitorum communis may limit distal excursion of its tendon and cause the tendon to be passively insufficient before optimal MCP joint flexion is reached.

Postburn scars become hypertrophic due to excessive proliferation of dermal tissue during the healing process.[8] Scar formation is marked by deposition of bundles of disorganized collagen and production of fibrous tissue matrices, creating

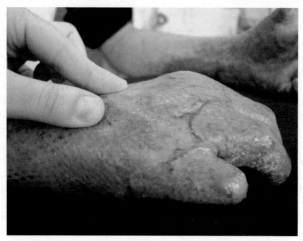

Figure 26-2 The pinch test to assess scar extensibility.

a meshwork on the site where skin and adjacent tissues were disrupted. Over time, collagen cross-linking increases and subsequent reorganization of fibers occurs in response to mechanical stress on the skin and underlying soft tissues. The collagen fibers that were once bundled and disorganized like hay in a haystack become flatter and more parallel to follow the same orientation as the skin surface. This process of collagen reorganization is evident within 3 to 5 weeks after injury.[9] However, in hypertrophic scars, this process of collagen reorganization is significantly protracted and is further complicated by persistent fibroplasia and local chronic inflammatory reaction.[9]

Through visual inspection, one may find that hypertrophic scars appear red, raised, and rigid to touch. Gentle pressure on the scar during palpation causes transient blanching. As the scar matures, it becomes flatter, paler, and more pliable. With consistent scar management, the process of scar maturation is expected to last at least 6 months following the burn. Certain populations, especially those with higher melanin pigmentation (skin of color), may experience a greater challenge with scar maturation, including keloid scar formation. Keloid scars are distinguished from hypertrophic scars in that they have an irregular shape, are often bulbous or pendulous, extend beyond the boundary of the wound, and encroach on the surrounding skin. Beyond familial tendencies, keloids are proposed to be different histologically, biochemically, and immunologically; however, these differences are not necessarily accepted universally.[10,11] Clinical observations and anecdotal evidence suggest that keloids often do not appear to respond as readily as hypertrophic scars to the traditional treatment of pressure application.

The extent of hypertrophic scarring and scar contraction in burns is related to various factors, including the size and depth of the injury.[12] In a classic study by Deitch and colleagues,[13] which investigated the factors predictive of the development of scar hypertrophy, the most predominant factor appeared to be the time needed to obtain complete closure of the wound. If the burns healed between 14 and 21 days, 33% of the sites became hypertrophic, and if the healing took longer than 21 days, 78% of the sites became hypertrophic. In a related study conducted by Smith and coworkers,[14] increases in both the percentage of third-degree burn and in the number of weeks after injury were associated with an increase in serum anticollagen antibody level. Smith proposed that such an increase in the anticollagen antibody may have lead to an increase in collagen accumulation at the burn site.[14]

Another important predictor in the formation of hypertrophic scars is the anatomic location of the burn. Richards and associates[15] postulated that skin tension may be a factor in scar formation and contraction due to the directional variance in skin movement between the volar and dorsal skin surfaces. Myer and McGrouther[16] found that skin that typically receives multidirectional tension during various limb movements is more likely to develop hypertrophic scar due to overstimulation of collagen-producing fibroblasts. The mechanism proposed by Myer and McGrouther[16] may partly explain why hypertrophic scars develop more often in the hand and larger areas such as the axilla due to the greater degrees of freedom and multidirectional skin tension afforded during joint movements of the hand and shoulder.

Another predictor of scar-induced contracture is the timing and the type of surgical intervention. Sheriden and colleagues[17,18] demonstrated that early eschar excision and sheet grafting in 90% of patients with deep thermal burns had function consistent with independent performance of activities of daily living. A full-thickness skin graft (FTSG) can almost completely inhibit wound contraction, whereas the amount of wound contraction seen with a split-thickness skin graft (STSG) is inversely proportional to the thickness of the graft.[19]

In rehabilitating the burned hand, therapists must spend a great deal of time to limit, reduce, or prevent the negative effects of hypertrophic scarring and scar contraction on hand structures and function. The processes of scar hypertrophy and contraction essentially begin almost as soon as the wound begins healing and are most "active" for the first 4 to 6 months after the injury. However, as time goes by along the continuum of burn recovery, therapists may also need to focus on addressing secondary contractures. Secondary contractures may arise due to substantial reduction in mobility and tension in the soft tissues, which over time decrease their elasticity. Contractures are consistently considered as anticipated sequelae of any traumatic or postsurgical injury of the upper extremity due to immobilization. In the burned hand, immobilization may be a necessity earlier in the recovery process for safety reasons such as in postgrafting procedures. However, in the latter stages of recovery, secondary contractures may evolve due to primary contractures caused by hypertrophic scarring and scar contraction.

Once scar maturation activity abates, the scar is said to be mature. The period of scar maturation for children is 12 to 24 months; for adults this period is 6 to 24 months. While the scar is active, especially early on, hypertrophy and contraction can be minimized or corrected by therapeutic interventions such as ROM exercises, pressure application, and orthotic intervention. Scar maturation can also bring about development of flexible deformity or worse, the formation of fixed deformities. Once the scar maturation is complete, scar management may no longer respond to nonsurgical interventions.

Another motivating factor to the therapist's management of hypetrophic scars is cosmetic appearance of the hand. Next to facial and genital disfigurement, the cosmetic appearance of the burned and scarred hand is deemed to be most concerning to a patient's body image and self-esteem.[20]

Phases of Burn Recovery

The therapist's role in management of the burned hand is discussed in four phases of burn recovery: (1) the emergent phase, (2) the acute phase, (3) the skin-grafting phase, and (4) the rehabilitation phase. Depending on the particular burn injury and treatment approach, a hand that has sustained a burn can be in more than one stage of recovery at any given time or, because of early grafting, may even "skip" the acute phase.

Emergent Phase

The emergent phase of burn recovery is generally considered to be the first 24 to 72 hours after injury. In a survey on

therapeutic interventions conducted by Whitehead and Serghiou,[21] 91% of those surveyed reported that initial evaluations are performed within the first 24 to 48 hours after acute admission. At this time, the therapist's goals are to examine the patient and develop treatment goals and a plan of care. This should include minimizing edema, obtaining optimal positioning of the hand, initiating motion, and maximizing function. Early and timely intervention by the therapist is necessary to help minimize the deforming effects of both the injury and the natural sequelae of healing, as well as to maximize functional recovery.

Acute Initial Evaluation

The medical record is reviewed and the following information should be collected: age, TBSA, cause of burn, procedures (intubation, escharotomy, fasciotomy), social history, and previous medical history.[22,23] Additional components of the initial evaluation include: burn wound assessment (e.g., depth, color, texture, moisture, location, joints involved), edema (description of and location), pain (via a visual analog scale), cognition, ROM (active and passive), sensation (particularly light touch), muscle performance, gross and fine motor coordination (e.g., hand dominance, opposition, diadochokinesia, i.e., rapid execution of opposite movements such as quick repetitions of pronation and supination), and activities of daily living (ADLs) or play.[22,23] In order to prevent infection, ROM measurements are performed over the patient's dressings. Special tests are often not performed at this stage due to dressings covering the hand and upper extremity.

Edema

In response to the injury and also to fluid resuscitation, the extremity becomes edematous (Fig. 26-3). Fluid translocates to the extravascular space of both burned and unburned tissue in patients who have sustained greater than 25% TBSA burn injuries. For many years, this fluid shift was thought to be caused by an increase in capillary permeability. However, research has shown that although increased capillary permeability is contributory to edema formation, burn-induced

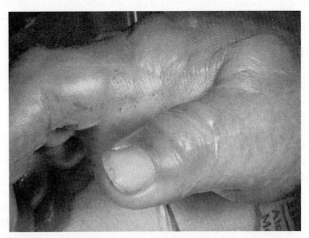

Figure 26-3 A child with deep partial-thickness and full-thickness hand burns on day of admission to hospital. Note how the edema is contributing to flattening of the palmar arches, metacarpophalangeal joint extension, and interphalangeal joint flexion.

edema in the emergent phase is caused primarily by interstitial components generating a strong negative tissue pressure.[24,25] Deep partial-thickness and full-thickness burns produce more prolonged and severe edema than do superficial partial-thickness burns,[26] but the typical full-thickness injury gives less edema and exudation than does a partial-thickness injury.[27,28] Edema develops from 8 to 12 hours after the burn injury, peaks up to 36 hours after the injury, begins to resolve after 1 or 2 days, and usually is completely gone by 7 to 10 days after the injury.[24]

Edema may cause several problems, such as ischemia and fibrosis, particularly in conjunction with inelastic burn tissue. Compromised blood flow to the intrinsics can lead to intrinsic tightness. Edema places the hand in a deforming position restricting motion and interfering with performance of ADLs and other functional activities. The protein-rich components of unresolved edema 42 to 72 hours after the burn injury may become organized around joint capsules, ligaments, and other soft tissue structures and form a scar tissue matrix, leading to contracture and loss of motion.[29–31] Chronic edema may result from damage to or destruction of dorsal veins or lymphatic vessels.

Escharotomy of the Hand

As previously described in Chapter 25, burn eschar (destroyed, nonviable tissue) is inelastic. Therefore, when the injury is circumferential, such inelasticity in conjunction with the development of hard, immobile edema produces a tourniquet effect. Intervention is necessary to prevent fibrosis and ischemic necrosis of the intrinsic muscles of the hand,[32] nerve damage,[33] and gangrene of the digits.[34] If circulation is compromised, a surgeon must perform an escharotomy. A fasciotomy may be necessary if the circulation is not restored by an escharotomy (Fig. 26-4).

ROM exercises (active and passive) are permitted in extremities that have undergone an escharotomy. In the case of a fasciotomy it is especially important that the wound is viewed prior to performing ROM to ensure the viability and gliding of the tendons. In some cases, ROM may need to be performed when the dressings are down to ensure gliding of the tendons in the case of exposure. Typically, patients are cleared for full ROM; however, in the case of a fasciotomy ROM may be limited due to the nature of the exposed structures.

Positioning

Proper positioning is one of the keys to the successful rehabilitation of a burn patient.[29] A burn patient's positioning program is designed to minimize edema, prevent tissue destruction, and maintain soft tissues in an elongated state to facilitate functional recovery.[29] Ninety-five percent of surveyed burn centers in 2006 reported that positioning begins within 24 hours of admission as opposed to 54% in 1994.[21] Ideally, the upper extremity is positioned at or above heart level with the elbow in extension, forearm is either supinated or in neutral, wrist in neutral, and hand in an intrinsic plus position.[29,31,35–37] In the case of a palmar burn, the digits are positioned in, with interphalangeal (IP) joints in extension, and the first webspace in a slight stretch.[28] With circumferential hand burns, hand positioning may alternate every 12 hours to account for both a palmar and dorsal burn. A foam

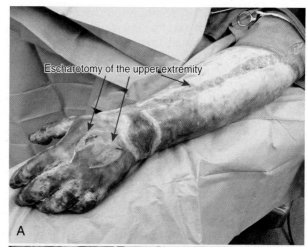

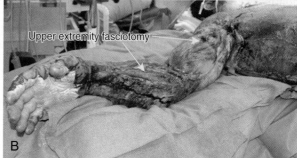

Figure 26-4 A, Escharotomies of the forearm and dorsum of the hand. **B,** Fasciotomies of the forearm and upper arm.

wedge is an effective and inexpensive positioning device (Fig. 26-5). It is easy to apply and keep in place, is well accepted by patients and staff, and was found not to cause any adverse reactions such as pain or sensory problems.[38] Other upper extremity elevation devices include commercial arm troughs, pillows, blankets, bedside table, and surgical netting (Fig. 26-6).

Complications can arise from incorrect positioning of the upper extremity. Elevation beyond heart level may result in decreased arterial supply to the hand.[38] Excessive weight-

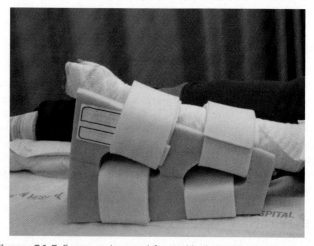

Figure 26-5 Foam wedge used for positioning and edema management that is widely accepted by patients and hospital staff.

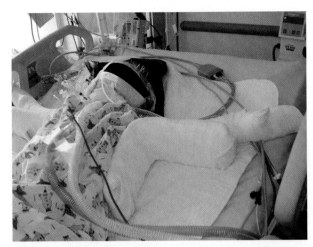

Figure 26-6 Example of an abduction arm trough from orthotic material for positioning of the upper extremity.

bearing stress to the olecranon of the elbow, especially with a flexed elbow, should be avoided since this may lead to pressure on the ulnar nerve. Helm[39] has cautioned therapists to regard neurologic considerations when positioning the burn patient. Helm cited Wadsworth and Williams,[40] who demonstrated how the prolonged position of the elbow in acute flexion or forearm pronation may cause compression on the ulnar nerve. This may result in motor weakness of the intrinsic muscles and impaired sensation in the ulnar-nerve distribution in the hand. In addition to proper elevation of the hand to help control edema, exercise and orthotic intervention may also be beneficial in helping control edema and minimizing the adverse effects of edema.

Orthotic Intervention

During the emergent phase, a static orthosis is often used to counteract the deforming position of edema, support the hand, and maintain joint alignment.[41–46] Edema, pain, and tight eschar immediately after a burn are the leading reasons why a person may demonstrate impaired ROM.[41–45] The hand is commonly positioned in an orthosis following a burn.[47] Whitehead and Serghiou[21] found that 61% of surveyed burn centers in 2006 initiated orthotic intervention within 24 hours of admission as opposed to 54% of responding centers in 1994. Burn depth, ROM limitations, as well as level of arousal (intubated vs. nonintubated) should be taken into account when considering orthotic intervention. The duration of wear time has not been adequately studied and is facility-dependent. Malick[47] suggests removing orthoses every 2 hours for cleaning to prevent patient contamination. If the patient is alert, many facilities recommend the orthosis only be worn when asleep.[48] In the case of the intubated patient, orthoses are often worn at all times except during burn care and therapy.

To counteract the position of deforming forces and to protect the structures of the hand, an orthosis that positions the hand in wrist slight or neutral extension, MCP joint flexion, IP joint extension, and the thumb away from the palm is recommended. This position is commonly referred to as the "protected," or "safe," position of the hand. Placing the wrist in slight extension facilitates MCP joint flexion by

action of the extrinsic forearm muscles—the *tenodesis effect.* Boswick[49] described the basic burned hand orthosis as one that positions the wrist in 30 degrees or more of extension, contributing to MCP joint flexion. When the MCP joints are flexed, the flexor tendons are on slack, which, along with the pull of the intrinsic hand musculature, facilitates the positioning of the IP joints in extension. The position of the IP joints in extension prevents adaptive shortening of the volar plate and collateral ligaments and the development of IP joint flexion contractures.

However, as Richard and colleagues[50] discovered in a review of the literature, a set of universal, standard dimensions for what exactly constitutes the "basic" burn orthosis, and even what its name is, does not exist. They found more than 40 different descriptions of how to position dorsal hand burns as well as a variety of names for such an orthosis. Although most practitioners agreed that the wrist should be in slight extension and all agreed that the MCP joints should be flexed, a wide range of specific joint angles have been cited. Surprisingly, almost one fourth listed that the proximal interphalangeal (PIP) joints should be flexed, and an assortment of combinations of positions for the thumb were reported.

We recommend that the wrist be positioned in 15 to 20 degrees of extension, the MCP joints flexed 60 to 70 degrees, the IP joints extended fully, and the thumb positioned midway between radial and palmar abduction, with the thumb MCP joint flexed 10 degrees and the IP joint fully extended. In addition to maintaining thumb opposition and abduction, the orthosis must maintain the thenar webspace and properly support the MCP joint of the thumb, which the 10 degrees of thumb MCP joint flexion aids. Failure to properly support the thumb MCP joint could result in a swan-neck deformity.

The burned hand orthosis described previously is not applied to hands when only the palm is burned or to hands that have sustained other specific burns such as those of just the thenar webspace. When applying an orthosis to a palmar hand burn, the wrist should be positioned in neutral or slight extension, the fingers in full extension and abduction, and the thumb in radial abduction and extension. This is typically called a "pan" orthosis (Fig. 26-7). As healing progresses, the orthosis should be molded to maintain the palmar arches. Burns involving only the thenar webspace are positioned in radial abduction, but care must be taken to support the thumb MCP joint. This is typically called a "C-bar" orthosis.

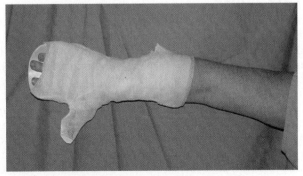

Figure 26-7 Example of a static pan orthosis.

Prefabricated hand orthoses can be applied initially if a therapist is not immediately available to construct custom orthoses. However, such orthoses, when commercially made, may need to have their forearm troughs widened before initial application so that they can accommodate both edema and bulky bandages.[43]

In the case of an alert adult patient, hand orthoses are usually applied with strapping for easy application. Pediatric hand orthoses and those of an intubated patient are secured with an elastic gauze bandage such as Dermacea. The elastic gauze prevents poor positioning of the orthosis in patients who wear them for longer durations and is more challenging for a child to remove. If orthotic intervention is not chosen at this time, a small roll of gauze can be placed or wrapped in an intubated patient's hand to help maintain the thenar webspace and the palmar arch. All hand burns are not always routinely positioned in orthoses. Whether to use an orthosis during the emergent phase is determined by the experienced therapist (in accordance with physician orders) based on the depth and extent of the wound and on the ability of the patient to cooperate with exercise, positioning, and ADLs. The therapist should evaluate the patient daily to determine the need for orthotic intervention and to ensure the correct fit.

Although orthotic intervention is commonplace in burn rehabilitation, decisions regarding initiation of an orthosis, duration of wear, and design vary significantly among burn centers. Further research is necessary to determine best practice within each phase of recovery.[51]

Motion

Initiation of ROM, specifically active range of motion (AROM), is vital to preserving function and preventing deformity.[51-54] The purpose of active motion during the emergent phase is to preserve ROM, tendon gliding, and muscle function. Active motion, in conjunction with elevation, is also effective in the early management of edema. Simple wiggling of the digits is not as effective as focused efforts on full active motion. The muscle contraction must be forceful enough to serve as a pumping mechanism to help venous blood and lymph return.[55] Whitehead and Serghiou[21] found that 96% of surveyed burn centers initiated AROM within 24 hours of admission. If tendon involvement is suggested, precautions should be taken. See the following section on Acute Phase for considerations on the management of exposed and ruptured tendons.

Acute Phase

The acute phase generally extends from the emergent phase until *wound closure*. Wound closure is defined here as either the surgical closure of the burn wound, which in the hand usually is accomplished by the application of skin graft(s), or as closure of the burn wound by secondary-intention healing so that any remaining partial-thickness wounds are approximately less than the size of a postage stamp. The reader should note that according to the description and delineation of phases of healing in this chapter, an acute phase technically may not exist for some hand burns. As a result of advances in surgical techniques, some hand burns may be grafted 1 to 2 days after the burn

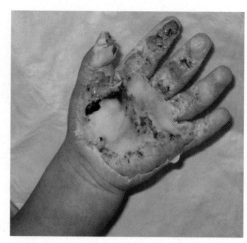

Figure 26-8 *Contact palmar hand burn. Inelastic eschar may compromise active range of motion of the newly burned hand.*

injury. This is particularly true of small TBSA burns of known depth.

The goals of the therapist during the acute phase are to increase or preserve ROM, preserve tendon gliding, maintain muscle activity, inhibit contraction, and promote function. Clark[56] reported that collagen synthesis may begin as early as 3 days after injury and remain rapid for up to 6 months. After 6 months, this process slows and continues for 1 to 2 years after the injury. Therefore early intervention is imperative for orientation of the collagen fibers that are being deposited so that deformity caused by scar formation is minimized or prevented.

Motion

The therapist should continue with the AROM exercises previously described. During the acute phase, the therapist should be aware that full AROM can be compromised by fibrous (not pitting) edema, inelastic eschar (Fig. 26-8), or tension from newly deposited collagen. The scar band from newly deposited collagen can appear in the open wound as well as in the closed wound, particularly when there is a protracted acute phase. To help judge whether more active motion should be expected from the patient when he or she appears to be at maximum range, gently press the band (e.g., the thenar web in radial abduction) to test the tension. If it is as taut as a stretched rubber band and blanching occurs, the patient is indeed at maximum range. If not, the patient should be encouraged to achieve more motion. This same method can be used during the rehabilitation phase with a scar in a closed wound. ROM, especially in children, may be more accurately assessed while the patient is under anesthesia before surgical procedures or during a dressing change.

If the patient has limited AROM, passive or active assistive stretching can be performed to increase ROM. Other exercises that are typically incorporated into a hand treatment or home exercise program are tendon glides, opposition, blocking exercises at the digits, and contract–relax exercises. When exercising the burned hand, the therapist should support the joint proximal to the joint being stretched. Pain should be considered to determine the intensity of the exercises.[52] To avoid unnecessary pain, support should be provided where eschar is present rather than on granulation tissue. Gentle passive range of motion (PROM) may be the only type of ROM that the therapist is able to administer to young children because they are often not able to cooperate with an AROM exercise program.

Care should be taken while performing PROM. Scar tissue ultimately responds well when passive force is applied in a steady, controlled manner, over a period of time.[52] Overly aggressive passive ranging constantly reinjures the fragile new tissue, resulting in an increase of collagen deposition and consequently more scarring.[57]

Active motion, with emphasis on isotonic contraction, should be encouraged. The patient should be carefully instructed about his or her exercise program and then observed to be sure that the exercises are performed correctly. At this time, spontaneous use of the hand and upper extremity should be strongly encouraged. Functional activities should be incorporated into the treatment plan.

The use of virtual reality (VR) and video gaming has become an increasingly popular treatment intervention. Virtual reality and video gaming are often utilized during painful or anxiety-provoking interventions such as dressing changes and therapy. These interventions offer an escape and often distract patients, allowing them to tolerate more aggressive debridement and ROM and encouraging them to actively move more freely within the game.[58]

Exposed and Ruptured Tendons

Upon initial wound assessment and as the eschar is debrided, the therapist should look carefully for tendon exposure (Fig. 26-9). Tendon exposure can also appear in the recently healed wound. If tendon involvement is suggested because of the depth of the injury, the therapist should proceed with the same precautions that would be used if tendon involvement were confirmed. Two of the most common sites for tendon exposure are the dorsum of the hand, where the skin is thin, and the extensor tendon over the PIP joint. In a review of 50 patients with hand burns, Hunt and Sato[59] found that the more distal the tendon exposure, the less the functional deficit noted, and the worst functional outcomes were from damage to the extensor tendon over the PIP joint. Loss of the central slip of the extensor tendon to the PIP joint can result in a boutonnière deformity (see Fig 26-1).

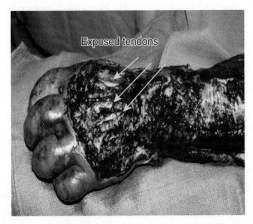

Exposed tendons

Figure 26-9 Examine for exposed extensor tendons in the wound bed.

After tendon exposure has been noted, close monitoring and care by the surgeon, nurse, and therapist is critical to preserve as much tendon integrity and function as possible. Saffle and Schnebly[60] stated that exposed tendons rapidly become desiccated and dissolve as a result of the action of surrounding leukocytes and bacteria. To prevent desiccation, the exposed tendon must be kept covered with a protective dressing that will keep it from drying, which will also assist with healing.

Exercise and Orthotic Intervention of the Exposed Tendon: Before Grafting. Choice of the specific orthotic intervention and exercise program depends on the extent and location of the exposure, the apparent integrity of the tendon and surrounding tissue and structures, and the willingness or ability of the patient to comply with the plan of care. These conditions and factors must be assessed daily. Exercises are performed under the supervision of a therapist who has received physician orders.

Some therapists and physicians opt for more aggressive ROM regimens if the tendon appears healthy and the exposure is small. For example, when the extensor digitorum communis (EDC) is exposed over the MCP joint of the index finger, the wrist is positioned in 15 to 30 degrees of extension, the involved MCP joint in 30 to 40 degrees of flexion (to prevent tightening of the collateral ligaments), and the IP joints in full extension.[61] When ROM exercises are being performed at the IP joint, the MCP joint and the wrist should be positioned in extension to put the tendon at maximum slack. Conservatively, gentle passive extension of the PIP and distal interphalangeal (DIP) joints and active flexion of the PIP and DIP joints can also be performed. When the central slip of the extensor tendon over the PIP joint is exposed, the PIP joint must be maintained in extension.[62] However, *gentle, isolated* ROM exercises in the available ROM at the DIP joint can be performed. The previously stated advisory should be kept in mind. Exercises are performed to help preserve joint ROM and to ensure tendon gliding and may help maintain oblique and transverse retinacular ligament length.[63]

A finger orthosis, typically called a finger gutter, has been found to be effective for immobilization of exposed tendons of the PIP joint while still allowing MCP joint flexion.[64] Gutter orthoses may be applied before, and worn under, traditional hand burn orthoses, although some adjustment may be necessary to accommodate them. Use of ⅙-inch thermoplastic material in the construction of finger orthoses limits the amount of space they occupy; limiting each orthosis to cover just the volar aspect of the digit reduces bulk and minimizes the finger abduction that can result from using multiple finger-based orthoses. Finger abduction should be avoided because it may cause malalignment and may limit MCP flexion due to tension on collateral ligaments. In addition, the finger orthosis should cover only the proximal and middle phalanges so that active flexion and extension of the MCP and DIP joints can be accomplished. Gutter orthoses may be secured with Coban.

Pullium[65] advised the use of a full volar orthosis if damage appears to extend beyond the extensor hood. A more restrictive exercise program is also indicated in such cases. When an exposed tendon is present, ADL tasks should be monitored to prevent accidental rupture. In the case of a dry or ruptured tendon, ROM is avoided at the joint to prevent further damage.

Orthotic Intervention

Generally, a hand that is healing without complications does not have to be positioned in an orthosis unless there is a limitation in active motion of the MCP or IP joints of 20 degrees or greater in extension, or MCP or IP joint flexion is less than 70 degrees. If active MCP or IP joint extension is limited by 20 degrees or greater, the therapist can initiate serial extension orthotic fabrication. If MCP joint flexion is less than 70 degrees, the therapist should position the hand as close to the previously described position of 15 to 20 degrees of wrist extension, 60 to 70 degrees of MCP joint flexion, full extension of the IP joints, and the thumb positioned midway between radial and palmar abduction with the thumb MCP joint flexed 10 degrees and the IP joint fully extended.[29,41–44,50,66,67] The orthosis can be adjusted as MCP joint flexion increases. When a limitation in motion does exist, the therapist should evaluate and make any necessary changes to other components of the therapy program, such as exercise and participation in ADLs, which might help increase ROM.

In addition to evaluating the wound, the therapist must evaluate the fit of the orthosis and check to see if it is being applied correctly. If an orthosis is applied incorrectly and not secured adequately, it can slip forward, contributing to the deforming forces of thumb adduction, MCP joint hyperextension, IP joint flexion, and breakdown from pressure at the carpometacarpal joint. Changes in bulk of the bandages also affect the fit of the orthosis.

As the patient's ROM and level of arousal improves, the use of the orthosis during the day can be decreased. If the patient is unwilling or unable to cooperate, the orthosis should be worn continuously and removed only for dressing changes, self-care activities, and therapy. The orthosis should be worn during all hours of sleep. It is not unusual for a patient to lose significant range because the orthosis was not applied during the night.

The therapist should be careful not to overly immobilize the patient. This can result in joint stiffness, contractures, and soft tissue adhesions. Children can tolerate immobilization longer than adults because of the elasticity of their joints and soft tissue, but they still need to be monitored.[53,54] In addition to immobilization caused by orthotic intervention, the therapist should note whether the patient is causing the increased joint stiffness by self-immobilization or muscle guarding, which typically results from pain.

Skin-Grafting Phase

Once it is determined that a patient requires skin grafting (see Chapter 25) and surgery is scheduled, it is crucial to obtain full ROM prior to grafting because the patient will need to be immobilized for approximately 2 to 5 days after surgery (Fig. 26-10). However, in some cases of early excision and grafting, some edema is still present or reports of pain may limit full ROM at the time of grafting. For most hand burns, an orthosis that positions the hand in the previously discussed antideformity position (wrist extension, MCP joint flexion, IP joint extension, and the thumb midway

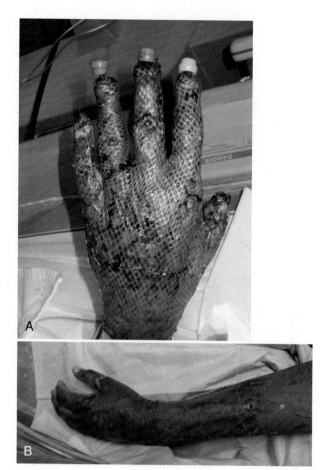

Figure 26-10 Skin grafts. **A,** Mesh split thickness with digital pinning. **B,** Sheet split thickness.

between radial and palmar abduction) should be applied by the therapist in the operating room immediately after grafting. This orthosis is worn for approximately 5 days. Adjacent nongrafted areas may be mobilized. As previously discussed in the case of a palmar burn, the wrist and digits are positioned in extension and thumb in radial abduction and extension.

Protocols for when to initiate motion and how much motion is permitted following grafting vary from facility to facility. Some prefer immobilization of the hand for up to 5 days, whereas others may initiate some or full motion much earlier.[68] Specific reintroduction of motion depends on the appearance of the graft and on the ability of the patient to cooperate. Motion should not be performed on hands when grafts appear wet or discolored, or when bleeding is excessive. Assuming graft integrity and patient cooperation, gentle AROM in isolated ranges can be performed on the second postoperative day. By the third or fourth day, gentle full AROM may be permitted. Also by the fourth day, the orthosis may be removed during the day and worn at night only. In the case of a FTSG, ROM is typically initiated between 5 and 7 days after surgery, depending on how well the graft takes to the palm (Fig. 26-11).

Cultured Epithelial Autograft

Cultured epithelial autografts (CEA) are more fragile than traditional STSGs, often lacking long-term durability.[69,70]

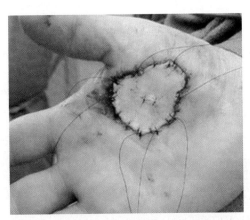

Figure 26-11 In the case of a full-thickness skin graft, range of motion is typically initiated between 5 to 7 days postoperatively, depending on how well the graft takes to the palm.

Ensuring graft adherence and survivability of CEA frequently requires adjustments in the therapy program. Resumption of motion often is delayed until 7 to 10 days postoperatively or longer after CEA application rather than the typical 4- to 5-day immobilization period common with standard STSGs. The implementation of orthoses or pressure garments also may be delayed or limited because of their potential stress and shearing forces.

Dermal Analogs

As previously described in Chapter 25, Integra is an artificial skin comprising two layers, both of which are essentially temporary. One significant benefit of Integra is that scar formation is minimal.[71] One of its shortcomings, however, is that the final dermis does not contain hair follicles and sweat glands; however, Burk,[72] a pioneer in the development of artificial skin, reported that sensory function returns to the same level and on the same time course as it does following normal split-thickness autografting.

Initiation of ROM and removal of orthoses following Integra placement depend on the surgeon's preferences. Integra Life Sciences Corporation states that the site of placement should be immobilized for 5 days, with ROM beginning on the fifth day.[73] No other therapeutic guidelines are outlined. Some facilities only allow partial ROM until final coverage, but others progress to full ROM prior to final coverage. It is important that the therapist views the Integra prior to and during the initiation and progression of ROM. If the ROM program is too aggressive, it causes the Integra to tear or lift off of the wound bed.

Rehabilitation Phase

The rehabilitation phase generally extends from the time of graft adherence or wound closure until scar maturation. The primary goals of therapy at this time are to protect the new spontaneously healed wound or the fragile graft, preserve joint mobility, increase strength and function, and inhibit the development of scar contraction and hypertrophy.

Evaluation

In addition to the typical hand therapy clinical examination, evaluation of the burned hand during the rehabilitation phase should include evaluation of the scar. If the patient has suffered anoxia or an electrical injury, assessment of other burn-related aspects, such as muscle tone and cognition, should be included. Several dexterity measures are available; however, there has been minimal testing within the burn population. Anecdotally, evidence has suggested the use of objective measures such as the Jebsen's Hand Function Test, Minnesota Rate of Manipulation Test, Purdue Peg Board, and Grooved Peg Board test.[74] More functional-based nontimed assessments, such as the Manual Ability Measure, are emerging, which incorporate a self-rating by the patient and clinician. Upper-extremity-specific outcome measures that are self-reports and not clinician-driven include the Michigan Hand Outcomes Questionnaire (MHQ) and the Disability of Arm, Shoulder, and Hand Questionnaire (DASH). Both measures assess beyond the impairment level. In the case of a pediatric patient, developmental assessments or screenings should be administered, particularly those that assess fine motor skills.

Scar Evaluation

Scar is evaluated to provide both an objective and a subjective description, to assess the need for and efficacy of treatment, and to estimate maturation. Several methods and tools for evaluating scar have been presented:

1. Oximeter to measure transcutaneous oxygen tension as an index of maturity[75]
2. Laser Doppler flowmeter to measure microcirculation in grafts and healed wounds to assess such variables as likelihood of hypertrophic scar formation and scar maturity[27,76,77]
3. Tonometer to measure scar pliability, firmness, and tension (data that can be used to quantify the course of cicatrization and evaluate the effectiveness of therapy)[78-81]
4. Elastometer to measure elastic properties of scar to objectively document scar response to treatment or scar maturity[82]
5. Quasistatic extensometer to measure extensibility of hypertrophic scar[83]
6. Dermal torque meter to measure viscoelastic properties of scar and grafts to assess various components of pliability[84]
7. Ultrasound (US) to measure scar thickness to monitor the progress of hypertrophic scar[79,80,85]
8. Objective measurements from positive molds of the scar[86]
9. Shear velocity device to measure propagation of an auditory shear wave through the skin surface to assess biomechanical alterations (e.g., stiffness) of scar[87]
10. Scales with visual and other components[88-93]

Although all of these tools are useful in measuring aspects of scar and the scarring process, no instrument or method has been accepted or used universally.[51] Many are costly, time-consuming, and impractical within the clinic setting.[93]

In 1990, the Vancouver Scar Scale (VSS) was developed by the Occupational Therapy Department at Vancouver General Hospital, Vancouver, British Columbia, Canada (Fig. 26-12). This instrument is currently the most widely utilized scar assessment tool among burn therapists.[89] The VSS rates four characteristics of burn scar: pigmentation, vascularity,

Name: _____

Date of evaluation: _____ / ___ / _____

Burn   ▨ ▨ ▨   ___ / ___ / ___

Donor   ▧ ▧ ▧   ___ / ___ / ___

Skin graft   ▦ ▦ ▦   ___ / ___ / ___

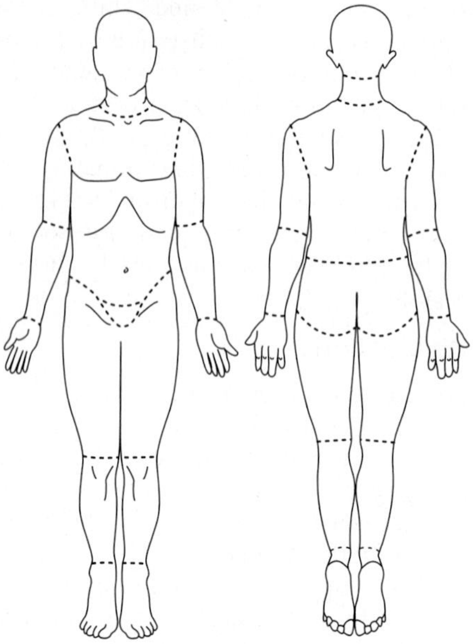

AREA	PIGMENT	VASCULARITY	PLIABILITY	HEIGHT	SCORE
Head					
Neck					
Ant. trunk					
Post. trunk					
R. buttock					
L. buttock					
R.U. arm					
L.U. arm					
R.L. arm					
L.L. arm					
R. hand					
L. hand					
R. thigh					
L. thigh					
R. leg					
L. leg					
R. foot					
L. foot					
TOTAL					

Signature _____   Date _____

A

Vancouver burn scar grading system

PIGMENTATION - This is assessed by applying pressure with a piece of clear plastic (i.e., UVEX) to blanch the scar. This eliminates the influence of vascularity, so that a more accurate assessment of pigmentation can be made. The blanched scar is compared to a nearby blanched area of the person's unburned skin. A variation from the normal skin color indicates a pigment change. Scale ratings are as follows:

0 = normal *(minimal variation)*
1 = hypopigmentation
2 = hyperpigmentation
3 = mixed pigmentation

VASCULARITY - This is assessed by observing the color of the scar at rest. In addition, the scar is blanched with the clear plastic and the rate and amount of blood return are observed. The more intense the color return, the higher the rating. Scars which are congested and refill slowly or cannot be completely blanched are grouped in the purple category.

0 = Normal   *color and rate of its return, closely resembles that of normal skin*

1 = pink
2 = red
3 = purple

PLIABILITY - To assess, the scar is positioned to minimize its tension, afterwhich it is manually palpated between thumb and index finger to assess how easily it distorts under this pressure.

0 = normal   resembles pliability of normal skin
1 = supple   flexible with minimal resistance
2 = yielding can be distorted under pressure without moving as a single unit, but offers moderate resistance
3 = firm   inflexible; car moves as single unit
4 = banding   rope-like tissue that blanches with extension of the scar, full range of movement
5 = contracture permanent shortening of scar producing limited range of movement

HEIGHT - The height of the scar is visually estimated to be the maximum vertical elevation of the scar above the normal skin. A millimeter scale is included on the form to facilitate this assessment.

Scale in mm

0 = normal *flat, flush with normal skin*

1 = >0 to 1 mm *(more than one quarter of the area being rated is raised more than 0, but less than 1 mm)*

2 = >1 to 2 mm *(more than one quarter of the area being rated is raised more than 1 mm, but less than 2 mm)*

3 = >2 to 4 mm *(more than one quarter of the area being rated is raised more than 2 mm, but less than 4 mm)*

4 = >4 mm *(more than one quarter of the area being rated is raised >4 mm)*

Figure 26-12 A, Vancouver Scar Scale (VSS).

Temple Burn Center
Temple University Health System

Date of evaluation: _____ / _____ / _____

Burn ▨   _____ / _____ / _____

Donor ▧   _____ / _____ / _____

Skin graft ▦   _____ / _____ / _____

Left   Right

Left   Right

Areas of scar banding/contractures denoted xxxxxxxx

AREA	PIGMENT	VASCULARITY	PLIABILITY	HEIGHT	SCORE
R. dorsal hand					
L. dorsal hand					
R. volar hand					
L. volar hand					

_____   _____
Signature   Date

Vancouver burn scar grading system

PIGMENTATION - This is assessed by applying pressure with a piece of clear plastic (i.e., UVEX) to blanch the scar. This eliminates the influence of vascularity, so that a more accurate assessment of pigmentation can be made. The blanched scar is compared to a nearby blanched area of the person's unburned skin. A variation from the normal skin color indicates a pigment change. Scale ratings are as follows:

0 = normal *(minimal variation)*
1 = hypopigmentation
2 = hyperpigmentation
3 = mixed pigmentation

VASCULARITY - This is assessed by observing the color of the scar at rest. In addition, the scar is blanched with the clear plastic and the rate and amount of blood return are observed. The more intense the color return, the higher the rating. Scars which are congested and refill slowly or cannot be completely blanched are grouped in the purple category.

0 = Normal   *color and rate of its return, closely resembles that of normal skin*

1 = pink
2 = red
3 = purple

PLIABILITY - To assess, the scar is positioned to minimize its tension, afterwhich it is manually palpated between thumb and index finger to assess how easily it distorts under this pressure.

0 = normal   resembles pliability of normal skin
1 = supple   flexible with minimal resistance
2 = yielding can be distorted under pressure without moving as a single unit, but offers moderate resistance
3 = firm   inflexible; car moves as single unit
4 = banding   rope-like tissue that blanches with extension of the scar, full range of movement
5 = contracture permanent shortening of scar producing limited range of movement

HEIGHT - The height of the scar is visually estimated to be the maximum vertical elevation of the scar above the normal skin. A millimeter scale is included on the form to facilitate this assessment.

Scale in mm

0 = normal *flat, flush with normal skin*

1 = >0 to 1 mm *(more than one quarter of the area being rated is raised more than 0, but less than 1 mm)*

2 = >1 to 2 mm *(more than one quarter of the area being rated is raised more than 1 mm, but less than 2 mm)*

3 = >2 to 4 mm *(more than one quarter of the area being rated is raised more than 2 mm, but less than 4 mm)*

4 = >4 mm *(more than one quarter of the area being rated is raised >4 mm)*

B

Figure 26-12, cont'd B, VSS, the occupational therapy department at Temple University Hospital, Philadelphia.

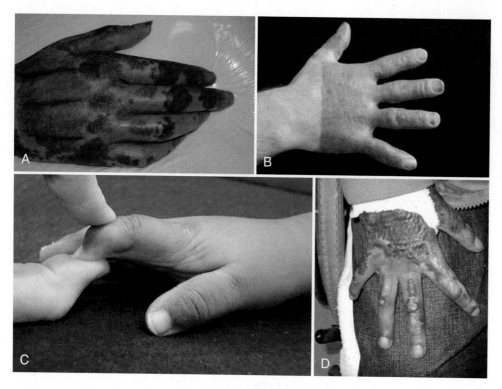

Figure 26-13 The Vancouver Scar Scale rates four characteristics of burn scar: pigmentation **(A)**, vascularity **(B)**, pliability **(C)**, and scar height **(D).**

pliability, and scar height[89] (Fig. 26-13). The originators of the VSS believe such characteristics relate to the healing and maturation of wounds, cosmetic appearance, and function of the healed skin.[89] Several authors and clinicians have made or proposed modifications to the VSS, including Nedelec and coworkers,[91] whose proposed changes relate to improving the scale's construct validity. Forbes-Duchart and associates[93] modified the scale to include two color scales for Caucasians and Aboriginal clients and to adopt the Plexiglas tool developed by Baryza and Baryza.[92] At the conclusion of their study, they further suggest omitting the pigment section and reclassifying the color scales as "light," "medium," and "dark." It is recommended that the VSS be performed following autografting and at every reevaluation thereafter.

Although not objective, photographs are helpful in cataloging change in a scar. They should be taken in a standardized fashion (i.e., distance from subject, angle, lens) at regular intervals and can be used with a visual assessment scale).[85] Because donor sites occasionally develop hypertrophic scar, the therapist should evaluate the donor site or sites in addition to evaluating healed burned and grafted sites.

Currently no published studies have evaluated the relationship between a patient's subjective scar evaluations and that of the therapist's objective measurement. Nor are there any studies that relate these two findings to function and return to life roles.

Edema

The continued presence of edema during the rehabilitation phase can be addressed by several means. If some wounds still remain open, edema management may be initiated to the digits via self-adherent wraps such as 3M Coban or

Co-Wrap.[94-96] However, care must be taken to protect fragile new tissue or recently adherent grafts, and circulation should be monitored during the period they are worn. If reduction in edema is a treatment goal, objective measurements (circumferential measurements at joint or phalanx) should be taken before and after intervention to determine and monitor the intervention's effectiveness. Once the hand is completely healed, wrapping the entire hand can be initiated, or commercially available interim compression gloves, such as an Isotoner Therapeutic Glove, can be utilized.[95] Due to the fragile nature of newly healed tissue and grafts, it is recommended that compression initially remain on for only a few hours.

Scar Massage

Massage has been reported to be effective in increasing and preserving mobility (by freeing restrictive fibrous bands) and in increasing circulation.[97] However, in one study of 15 pediatric patients who received 10 minutes daily of massage over a 3-month period,[98] no differences were found in the vascularity, pliability, and height of the scars, as measured by a modified VSS, although there were reports of decreased itching in some patients. Massage may be helpful in alleviating the commonly reported itching sensation that is partly caused by excessively dry and cracked skin resulting from damage to the sweat glands[99] and from increased evaporative water loss from scar tissue.[100] Massage appears to have other therapeutic benefits as well. Field and colleagues[101] compared burn patients who received massage therapy with a control group who did not. The group who received massage therapy had reduced itching, pain, anxiety, depressed mood, and showed long-term improvements on these measures from the first to the last day of the 5-week study.

In a pilot study conducted by Morien and coworkers[102] eight pediatric burn survivors received massage over a grafted area once a day for 3 to 5 days. Each massage session lasted 20 to 25 minutes. Therapeutic massage on scar tissue consisted of 5 minutes of lengthening using long light strokes (effleurage); 5 minutes of stretching and rolling strokes, which consisted of lifting and rolling the tissue between hands, fingers, or thumbs (petrissage); and, depending on the pain tolerance of the child, 2 to 5 minutes of small cross-fiber movements (friction) to loosen the scar tissue from the underlying tissue. The last 5 minutes of the massage session consisted of general lengthening and rolling. Overall the massage was found to increase ROM in children with burn scars; however, no change in mood was noted. The authors account for this by the fact that the study was conducted during a burn camp, so the kids were excited about the week ahead.[102]

Only gentle massage should be performed on newly spontaneously healed or recently adherent grafts because the skin is fragile and friction can result in skin breakdown and blister formation. New or fragile skin may appear translucent and wet, be sensitive to touch, or appear as though it will break open with slight pressure. As the skin becomes thicker and stronger, greater pressure can be exerted by massaging in a rotary motion along the scar. Creams that are not water-based, such as BIOTONE dual-purpose massage creme, are recommended because they are good lubricants and are not rapidly absorbed into the skin. One should not massage over small open areas because this could result in delayed wound healing at those sites. The skin should be massaged at least twice a day and up to six times a day for 5 to 10 minutes.[67,96] After the massage, the excess cream should be removed and pressure garments reapplied. An electrical or battery-operated massager may be utilized and may be helpful for carryover of the home exercise program. Heat attachments may be used; however, skin checks should be performed regularly[67] (Fig. 26-14).

Motion

When evaluating ROM in the recently healed burned hand, the therapist should look at the total ROM across several joints and evaluate individual joint motion. A patient with a dorsal hand burn may have full passive flexion of the MCP and PIP joints individually yet still be unable to make a full fist actively. Contracting scar, leading to loss of skin mobility, also can cause loss of active motion in an adjacent, unburned area. For example, the patient with a burn to the dorsum of the hand may be able to actively make a fist with the wrist extended but, because of scar contraction, may not be able to do so with the wrist at neutral or in slight flexion.

The exercise program, performed a minimum of three times a day, should consist of exercises to achieve full active and passive wrist motion and full total active motion (TAM) and total passive motion (TPM) of the digits in flexion and extension. Isolated tendon gliding exercises for the flexor digitorum profundus and flexor digitorum superficialis, as well as intrinsic muscle exercises, should be included. PROM should be performed if there is individual joint or tendon tightness. Joint ROM can be facilitated by mild traction.[103] Webspaces should be stretched both actively and passively.[103] The thumb should be exercised in all planes of motion. It is particularly important to maintain thumb opposition and to maintain the thumb webspace in both radial and palmar abduction. Spontaneous use of the hand should be strongly encouraged to help the patient overcome the fear of potential skin breakdown or pain with use.

Strength and Coordination

Resistive exercises and activities that challenge finger dexterity should be increased in pace with the patient's tolerance (Fig. 26-15). Cronan and colleagues[104] reported that because muscle tissue is one of the most mutable tissues in the body; a burn injury can affect the musculoskeletal system as well as the skin. In a study of burn patients returning to work, Cronan and colleagues[104] demonstrated that those patients given isokinetic exercise in addition to isometric and isotonic exercises were found to produce a better test outcome than those receiving isometric and isotonic exercise training only. Citing other work[105] that shows that slow-twitch and fast-twitch muscle fibers are present in an equal ratio, Cronan and colleagues[104] stated that therapy must involve training of both types of fibers. They explained that fatigue results from improper training of slow-twitch fibers and that joint pain after increased activity or inability to perform certain work loads for extended periods may be caused by improper training of fast-twitch fibers. Training involved the use of isokinetic exercise equipment. Cronan and colleagues[104] stated that light submaximal contraction selectively recruits slow-twitch fibers, moderate submaximal contraction adds fast-twitch fibers, and maximal contraction leads to an "all-or-none" recruitment of both fiber types.

The unburned hand also may need to be included in the therapy program. In a study of hand function after major burns, Covey and coworkers[104] found that the unburned hand also can show impairments in strength, TAM, and coordination at the time of hospital discharge. By 3 months after discharge, all study participants had normal TAM, and most had achieved normal grip strength and coordination; however, some required as long as 12 months after discharge to regain normal strength and coordination.

In addition to weakness that can occur as the result of any hospitalization, many metabolic disorders, including altered

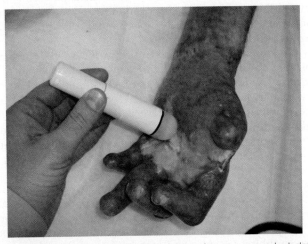

Figure 26-14 An electrical or battery-operated massager may be helpful for carryover of the home exercise and desensitization program.

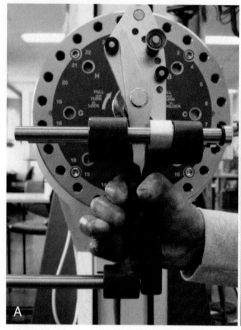
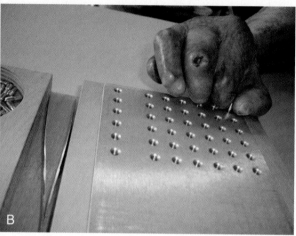

Figure 26-15 Resistive exercises **(A)** and activities that challenge finger dexterity **(B)** should be increased in pace with the patient's tolerance.

protein kinetics with muscle weakness, result from burn injury. Investigators[106] compared muscle dysfunction in burn-injured rats in the absence of apparent immobilization with muscle dysfunction after immobilization alone. Their findings suggest that muscle dysfunction after immobilization alone occurs primarily as the result of loss of muscle mass, whereas muscle dysfunction after burn injury on days 1 to 7 is a result of a decline in specific tension, and at day 14 is the result of a decline in specific tension and muscle mass. Research on rats with 40% TBSA scald burns showed that although the muscles directly beneath the burned skin were not damaged by the burn, they demonstrated dramatic apoptotic (cell death initiated by the cell itself) changes.[107] Apoptosis also was confirmed at muscle sites distant from the injury. These changes peaked at postburn days 3 and 7, indicating to the investigators the need for early and continuous intervention.

Pressure

Use of compression therapy dates back to the 16th century. Rayer utilized pressure in the treatment of keloids in 1835 and Unna in 1881 for burned scars.[108] Its use gained popularity in the 1970s when alterations in burn scar tissue were noted with the use of vascular support garments and orthoses.[109,110] Since that time burn therapists have generally accepted and utilized pressure garments (PG) as the first line of defense against scarring, despite the lack of evidence supporting its clinical effectiveness.

A large body of dermatologic, histologic, clinical, and anecdotal or case study evidence supports the effectiveness of PGs; however, the working mechanism has not been fully proven.[111] Studies[112,113] on tissue gases in normal dermis and in hypertrophic scars have found that pressure of approximately 25 mm Hg is believed to decrease the blood flow to rapidly metabolizing collagenous tissue. The authors of these studies noted that hypoxia does not appear to result in cell death but does indirectly affect the metabolic pathway (e.g., collagen formation) of scar growth or maturation. Another viewpoint is that pressure only causes dehydration of the scar (by indirectly affecting mast cells) and that the temporary diminished size of the scar noted after application of pressure is caused by the close approximation of collagen cross-linking.[114,115]

In 2009, Anzarut and associates[116] performed the first meta-analysis of the effectiveness of PG therapy for the prevention of scarring after a burn injury. The review included 316 patients from six randomized controlled trials. After reviewing scar assessments, they were unable to find a difference between scars that received PG and those that did not; however, there was a trend toward decreased scar height. Although the findings of this study do not fully support the use of PGs, the investigators conclude that the review had several limitations due to small number of studies. Despite lack of objective data, the therapist can take advantage of the positive effects seen clinically.

PG compliance varies and can be as low as 40% in some instances. A majority of the problems are physical, such as sweating, overheating, itching, pain, and difficulty performing various movements. A lack of communication between the therapist and patient and a patient's perceived lack of information may also lead to noncompliance.[117,118] Patients often complain about the quality of the garments, noting rapid wear and tear and the high cost to replace.[117,118]

Initiation of Pressure. Pressure is applied when a graft is adherent or wounds are almost closed (open wounds are smaller than a quarter). The purpose of pressure at this time is not just to inhibit scar contraction and hypertrophy but also to inhibit vascular and lymphatic pooling and to avert hypersensitive, fragile skin.[119]

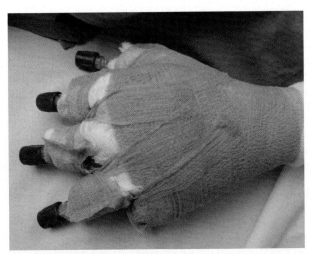

Figure 26-16 A Coban glove is used for edema management and as an early form of pressure.

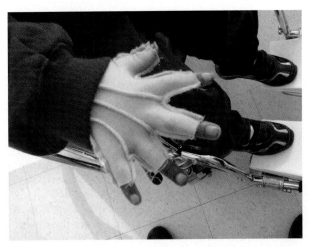

Figure 26-17 Example of an initial, noncustom pressure glove.

Interim Pressure Bandages and Gloves. Interim pressure bandages or gloves may be used until the patient can tolerate commercially custom-made gloves. The choice of type of interim pressure bandage or glove depends on how much pressure the patient can tolerate, which typically increases over time. A progression of interim pressure bandages and gloves commonly is used until the patient receives commercially custom-made gloves. The therapist should postpone application of interim pressure bandages or gloves if the skin appears too fragile.

Early forms of pressure include self-adherent elastic wraps such as Coban or commercially made compression or edema gloves such as an Isotoner Therapeutic Glove. Several companies make self-adherent elastic wraps. They are available in several colors and widths and can be easily applied to a digit, hand, or over a dressing. A Coban glove may be a better option for a child who is noncompliant with an interim glove (Fig. 26-16). The Cincinnati Shriners Burns Institute guidelines[96] are as follows:

1. Wrap each finger, beginning at the nail bed and wrapping in a spiral fashion proximally to the webspace.
2. The fingertip should be left exposed so that capillary refill can be monitored.
3. Then wrap the hand in a spiral fashion, starting at the knuckles and ending 1 inch past the wrist. When wrapping, the self-adherent wrap should be stretched up to 25% of its elasticity.
4. A small layer of moisturizer can be applied over the wrap to eliminate any tackiness.[67,96]
5. The glove should be removed daily for skin inspection and washing.

Several of the custom PG companies also manufacture interim gloves. They are typically softer and provide less pressure than the custom gloves. Sizes for adult interim gloves typically range from extra small to large. To fit a pediatric glove, a therapist must measure the circumference of the hand at the distal palmar crease (Fig. 26-17). Any of these pressure bandages and gloves can be worn over small open wounds. A light, nonadherent dressing should be placed over the open area prior to application of pressure.

Commercially Made Custom-Fitted Pressure Gloves. Commercially made custom-fitted gloves can be ordered from several companies, such as Barton-Carey Medical Products (Jellico, Tennessee); Bio-Concepts, Inc. (Phoenix, Arizona); Torbot Group, Inc. (Toledo, Ohio); Gottfried Medical, Inc. (Toledo, Ohio); Empathy Inc.; and Medical Z Inc. (San Antonio, Texas). Depending on the company, several types of materials, colors, adaptations, and individual custom designs are available. The therapist should select according to the requirements of the individual patient, and these may change over time depending on factors such as stage of scar maturation, the need for inserts, and the patient's daily activity regimen.

Glove Materials and Options. A therapist may select from several materials. Depending on the manufacturer, gloves may be constructed from one of several different materials (or from a combination of two or more), with each material having its own properties of smoothness and stretch. Gloves may be made from softer material for patients who have more fragile skin or who cannot tolerate regular material. For durability, gloves for children should be made from regular material, unless the child is younger than 1 year of age. Then a softer material may be considered, particularly if the skin is fragile over the MCP joints and amputation sites.

Gloves can be ordered with zippers, Velcro closures, or without either.[30,96] These closures can be placed almost anywhere on the dorsal, volar, or ulnar aspect of the glove. There are pros and cons with the use of closures. If skin tear is a concern, zippers are ordered in the first set of gloves to decrease friction on new, fragile skin. Patients and family members may also prefer zippers because they make it easier to put on or take off gloves, especially in the case of a child. If the therapist anticipates that the patient will need an insert, the glove should include a zipper to ensure proper placement of the insert and to provide ease of application.

The addition of a zipper or Velcro closures should be carefully considered as it decreases or disrupts pressure across the burn scar. The closures take the place of elastic material, are nonmobile, and can ripple, thereby causing disruption of pressure on and around their location. This may be particularly true in a pediatric glove where the zipper may make up a proportionally large part of the glove. In some cases the zipper leaves may leave an indentation on the skin and cause breakdown. If an insert is not anticipated and a skin tear is not a concern, the glove should be ordered without a zipper or Velcro closure.

Other modifications to the glove include slanted inserts at the webspaces. It is standard to request a glove with inserts if a client has self-healed skin or grafted areas surrounding the webspaces. On request, the glove manufacturer may also sew a dart almost anywhere in a glove to help provide pull in a particular direction. For example, a dart sewn in the area of the thenar eminence may help pull the thumb into opposition. In addition, when gloves have open fingertips, it is easier to ensure that the glove webspaces are flush with the webspaces of the hand than when the tips are closed. It also allows for improved dexterity. However, if the scar extends to the DIP and beyond, the fingertips should be enclosed. Additional glove options include extending the length of the glove past the wrist to include to the forearm or ordering a gauntlet if the digits are not involved.[30,96]

Grip Enhancements. Often the PG fabric makes it difficult to perform ADLs, work, and play due to a lack of friction and sensation at the palmar surface of the gloved hand.[120-122] Recent addition of grip enhancements to the palmar surface of the glove have increased dexterity. O'Brien and colleagues[121] developed the New York-Presbyterian Dexterity Glove (NYPDG) in conjunction with Torbot Group, Inc. (Toledo, Ohio). They added Silon to the volar surface of the digits and MCPs (Fig. 26-18). Medical Z, Inc. (San Antonio, Texas), also offers grip enhancements on their gloves. Dewey and coworkers[120] performed a case series analysis of five different silicone and rubber grip enhancements developed and manufactured by Medical Z, Inc. The enhancements included rectangular rubber tabs, honeycomb pattern silicone, wave-like pattern silicone, line pattern silicone beads, and line pattern silicone beads embedded into the fabric. The researchers concluded that the wavy silicone pattern embedded into the fabric provide the best combination of grip and durability.[120] The following companies currently manufacture gloves with grip enhancements: Barton-Carey Medical Products, Inc. (Jellico, Tennessee); Bioconcepts, Inc. (Phoenix, Arizona); Gottfried Medical, Inc. (Toledo, Ohio); Medical Z, Inc. (San Antonio, Texas); and Torbot, Inc. (Toledo, Ohio).[120]

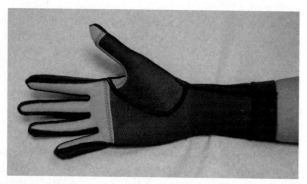

Figure 26-18 New York-Presbyterian Dexterity Glove (NYPDG) with grip enhancements to the palmar surface of the glove for increased dexterity.

Wear and Care of Gloves. Commercially made custom-fitted pressure gloves are worn 23 hours per day until scar maturation, at which time the scar is no longer active (i.e., hypertrophying and contracting) and permanent removal of the glove will not lead to relapse.[123-125] While the scar is active, the glove is removed only for bathing. The glove and added inserts can inhibit full AROM and at times may need to also be removed for exercise. Because of a developing child's need to use his or her hand for both sensory and motor input, a child's glove may need to be removed for specified periods throughout the day. Two sets of gloves are recommended due to the continuous wearing schedule, so that one can be worn while the other is being laundered.

The burn glove should fit snugly but not too tightly. A glove is too loose if the material can be pinched up from the skin. Custom-made pressure garments can lose their elasticity (and therefore their pressure) due to the frequent, rapid, and complex movements of the hand. Although seeming to fit adequately, new sets may be necessary approximately every 2 to 3 months to ensure that adequate pressure is being provided.

Many factors contribute to the breakdown of elasticity. Some of these factors are normal wear and tear ("normal" can vary widely according to occupation or daily activity), the use of petroleum-based lotions and ointments, and laundering. Some glove manufacturers recommend washing your glove in the delicate cycle; however, this has been observed to lead to quicker wear and tear. It is recommended that gloves be hand-washed with a mild soap and warm water and laid out to dry. Avoid "ringing out" of the glove as this further stretches the material. Even without daily wear and tear, gloves may need to be adjusted or new measurements taken to accommodate for edema and weight changes, contractures, or normal growth in a child.

Dynamics of Pressure and the Use of Inserts. The amount of pressure the gloves are designed to apply varies according to the individual manufacturer. In addition, some manufacturers design gloves to provide a uniform pressure, whereas other manufacturers design gloves to apply a gradient pressure (i.e., pressure that decreases distally to proximally). Although the gloves are designed to apply a specific amount of pressure over a specific body part, the actual pressure being applied may be below what is considered therapeutic or vary depending on the position of the hand.[126] In addition, despite the fact that pressure garments are custom-made and appear to fit well, there still may be problems with hard, thickening, or contracting scar. If this is so, pressure in those areas may be insufficient.

To be effective, pressure must be conforming. The palm of the hand is a concave surface. The best-made custom-fitted glove always bridges across this area while fitting snugly over convex areas. When a glove is applied to a hand with a burn on the palmar surface, an insert must be used to achieve adequate pressure. Many materials can be used as inserts. Some examples are Rolyan Silicone Elastomer, Rolyan 50/50 Mix Elastomer Putty, Rolyan Polycushion, OTOFORM-K/c Elastomer, Rolyan Prosthetic Foam, or Rolyan Ezemix Elastomer Putty. When Rolyan Polycushion or any sponge with an adhesive side is used as an insert, the paper backing

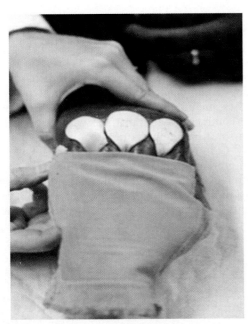

Figure 26-19 Webspacers may be fabricated to apply conforming pressure in the webspaces.

is removed from the adhesive side and a stockinette or similar fabric is placed on the adhesive side. The sponge side is placed against the patient's skin. The glove manufacturer can sew a pocket in the palmar, dorsal, or other specified part of the glove to secure an insert. However, a pocket may interfere with the conformity of the insert to the surface of the skin, and therefore care should be taken in this regard.

Most hand burns involve the dorsal rather than the palmar surface. Although the dorsum is a convex surface, inserts still may be necessary. Interdigital webspaces are concave surfaces that can hypertrophy even when a glove is worn. These areas are a problem not only because they are concave but because there is essentially little opposing force for the webspaces. One can compensate for this by using a dynamic webspacer or by adding conforming pressure with the use of inserts (Fig. 26-19). Webspacers can be constructed from many materials. Some examples are Rolyan Polycushion, Neo-Plush Sheet, $\frac{1}{16}$-inch Aquaplast, Beta-pile, Otoform-K/c Elastomer, and Rolyan Silicone Elastomer and Oleeva FOAM.

When a custom-made glove is used, pressure is usually greater over harder surfaces of the body than over softer ones. Therefore, inserts may be needed over softer surfaces. Where inserts are used, the skin must be checked routinely for maceration or breakdown. Inserts, especially more rigid or bulky ones, also can limit motion or function. For these reasons, even though constant pressure is preferred, it may be possible to use inserts only part of the day. Softer or less restricting inserts can be used during the day and more rigid inserts used at night.

Inserts can also be fabricated specifically to be worn in an orthosis. Ideally, the insert is fabricated on a perforated material, and then the patient's hand is placed over the insert as it is setting. The insert conforms and somewhat seeps into

the perforations and is therefore less likely to slide. Orthoses also can be made of $\frac{1}{16}$-inch Aquaplast. Both types of orthoses can be adjusted or reconstructed regularly as scar or ROM changes. Because this type of pressure inhibits hand use, these types of orthoses may be desirable for only a brief period or may be used solely at night, while a glove and an insert are worn during the day. The orthosis is attached with an elastic gauze wrap or with Coban. A sponge or gauze roll insert over the dorsum of the hand can be wrapped in to inhibit curling of the fingers and provide excellent conforming pressure and traction.

Silicone Gel Sheets. Silocone gel sheets (SGS), which are soft, semiocclusive, and flexible sheets, have been utilized in the United States with increasing popularity since the 1980s.[127] Some brands have a tacky or adhesive surface that helps the sheet to better stay in place. SGS are indicated in a scar that remains raised and with decreased pliability despite PGs. The scar may or may not affect ROM. It is contraindicated in patients with open wounds and known allergies to silicone. The addition of an SGS increases pressure against the scar and adds to the risk for breakdown if worn for 24 hours upon initiation. Therefore, it is recommended that patients begin with 4 hours the first day and gradually increase the wearing time over the next 5 days. If a patient complains of a rash or increased itchiness, the SGS should be removed and therapist notified as the patient may be having an allergic reaction. In this case silicone-free Silon and Silipos products can be tried. The SGS should be washed daily with warm water and a mild soap and laid out to dry. If an SGS is indicated over a joint, patients may often only wear it at times of rest even if they could benefit from longer use. If the joint is frequently flexing and extending it may cause the silicone to roll up under the pressure garments.

Controlled studies report topical SGS to be effective in both the prevention and the treatment of hypertrophic scars and of keloids, and in increasing ROM that has been limited by burn scar contracture.[80,127-138] In a study that included subjective assessments and objective measurements, Ahn and coworkers[134,135] showed that SGS placed on hypertrophic scar for a minimum of just 12 hours daily and worn for a duration of only 2 months were effective in increasing scar elasticity and in flattening established hypertrophic burn scars. They were also effective in preventatively limiting large-scar volume of surgical scars. Although SGS were effective in studies in inhibiting the development of hypertrophy of all surgical scars, not all established hypertrophic scars responded to treatment by SGS.[80,135] They were beneficial in treating longstanding hypertrophic scars, some as old as 3 years.[134] Wessling and colleagues,[133] in a controlled investigation involving patients with limited ROM resulting from bilateral elbow burn scar contractures, demonstrated that SGS and exercise achieved greater gains in AROM than did the use of exercise alone; they also found that these gains were not the result of a placebo effect.

The Cochrane Collaboration reviewed the use of SGS in the prevention and treatment of hypertrophic scarring and keloid scars.[8] They reviewed 15 trials, involving 615 patients. From this literature they concluded that evidence for the effects of SGS are obscured by the poor quality of the research.

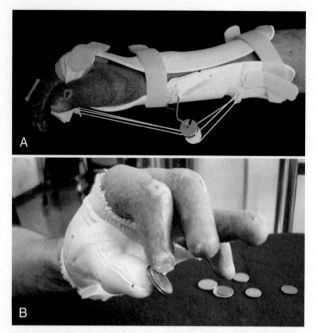

Figure 26-20 A, Static progressive orthosis to increase metacarpophalangeal joint flexion. **B,** Static orthosis to increase prehensile function.

There appeared to be few abnormal scars in people at high risk associated with use of SGS; however, they report that these findings are highly susceptible to bias.

There are many SGS options. The therapist needs to consider the flexibility of the insert, application site, the width, and if an adhesive backing is required.[96] Oleeva Fabric works well over the dorsal hand because of its fabric backing. It decreases friction and allows the glove to slide over the insert more easily. Topigel and Oleeva Clear are also two types of thinner, adhesive SGS that can be utilized over the dorsum of the hand and dorsal or volar wrist.

Orthotic Fabrication

Orthotic fabrication is used initially during the rehabilitation phase to preserve ROM by opposing the force of contracting scar, usually during periods of patient inactivity. Traction also is used to correct scar contractures. Static and static progressive orthoses are typically used, but in some cases dynamic orthoses may be helpful[30] (Fig. 26-20).

Recently, Bio Med Sciences, Inc., developed an orthosis material called Silon-LTS that combines both thermoplast and silicone. This material works well in areas, such as the palm and webspaces, in which it is typically difficult to apply steady, even pressure. When wearing an orthosis made of this material, it is recommended that the patient remove the glove in order to get the scar management effects of the top, conforming silicone layer.

A great resource for burn orthoses is *An Atlas and Compendium of Burn Splints.*[139] The editors compiled a single comprehensive resource of burn orthoses. Sections 4 through 9 are dedicated to the upper extremity. Materials needed, fabrication instructions, advantages, disadvantages, indications, precautions, and supporting references are listed with each orthosis.

Casting

Casting to provide positioning or serial casting to correct scar contractures or to increase ROM can be used at almost any time throughout the acute and rehabilitation phases. Casting may delay or eliminate the need for surgical correction of contractures, including finger deformities, MCP joint hyperextension contractures, thumb–index webspace contractures, and other soft tissue contractures, that may occur after burn injuries.[140] Casting theory is based on Brand's work of using plaster to promote elongation of tissue and collagen realignment through application of continuous force in a desired corrective position.[141] Serial casting also can result in flatter, softer, and more supple tissue.[142] In addition, casts can provide protection for wounds or exposed tendons. Casts have advantages over orthotic fabrication in that they cannot be removed by the patient and they do not slip,[143] and, depending on the specific cast, they can provide a higher degree of conformity. They are particularly useful when traditional methods of therapy have been ineffective[142] or when multiple joints are involved.

Casts may be applied over dressings or inserts. They can be circular, univalve, or bivalve, and made of either plaster or synthetic material. 3M Soft Cast and Delta-Cast Soft are synthetic casts that appear particularly suited for children because they are light, semirigid, and easy to apply. Both can be removed via scissors or unraveling by a therapist or parent. Such removal may be less frightening to the child than removal by a cast saw. Specialist plaster bandages also may be removed without a cast saw by soaking the cast in warm water and unrolling it.

With the goal of increasing finger flexion of all involved joints, Harris and associates[144] serial casted 15 grafted, burned hands that had limited ROM. Most of the casts were removed and reapplied in 1 day, and most of the second casts were worn for more than 1 day but for fewer than 6 days. A mean increase in total ROM of 51.1% was achieved. The greatest increase in motion was found at the MCP joint, and the greatest gains were obtained with the second cast.

Rivers[142] recommends casting as a way to increase motion in the burned hand when the hand is stiff in both flexion and extension. In such cases, serial casting is performed alternating flexion with extension casts. Casts may be particularly effective in maintaining MCP joint flexion in toddlers while allowing active flexion of the digits,[145] and serial casting may be effective in correcting scar contractures even in the small digits of children.

The choice of specific casting procedure varies according to the individual patient's status and needs. The therapist should consider the type of cast material used and ensure that the water temperature is cool and that the cast-application environment is well ventilated and has a moderate temperature and humidity. Patients with uncontrolled edema, circulatory problems, or neuropathies are not good candidates for casting. If a cast is to be applied over a wound, the wound must be clean and free of infection. Any necessary topical agents and nonadherent dressings are placed on the wound prior to casting. In some cases, it may be beneficial to measure the size of the open wound before casting and following removal. The use of nonbulky dressings reduces the potential for cast migration and resultant skin shear. If an insert is being used, it is secured in an area requiring particular conforming pressure; it should be placed over intact skin only. An insert should not be initiated the day of casting. It is important to ensure that a patient is tolerating the insert well prior to casting to eliminate the possibility of an allergic reaction. Next, a stockinette, terrycloth liner, or cast padding is then donned. Cast padding such as Rolyan Padding or Polycushion should be applied over bony prominences and can be utilized along the line of cut. A strip of felt can also be taped to protect the patient from the vibration of the cast saw during cast removal.[11] If the goal of casting is to increase ROM, the tissue usually is placed on maximum or near-maximum stretch. However, serial casting that is executed with low increments in ROM and with low force applied over burn scar reduces the risks of edema, skin breakdown, tissue rupture, and increased scar formation. If the cast padding is too bulky or if the cast is applied too loosely, the maximum benefits of casting may not be achieved. However, if the cast is applied too tightly, the excessive pressure can result in skin breakdown, vascular compromise, and peripheral neuropathies. The practitioner also should be alert to wrinkles in the padding, which can cause skin breakdown because of the increased skin fragility in burn patients. The hand position is checked and adjusted as necessary. The desired position is held until the cast is dry or hard, but care should be taken to avoid indentations from the therapist's fingers.[133] Depending on the specific patient, the cast is changed between twice per day[142] and a week.[133] On average a cast is left on for 2 to 4 days.

Another method of casting utilizes Delta-Cast conformable (polyester cast) tape. Two to four layers of cast material are placed in a parallel fashion over the area of concern (e.g., just proximal to dorsal PIPs to midforearm to promote MCP flexion). The roll is then wrapped in a spiral fashion up and down the length of cast (e.g., PIPs to two thirds up forearm). One of the advantages of the Delta-Cast material is that it can later be removed and used as an orthosis. It also sets quickly, can be washed in the dishwasher, dried with a hair dryer, and worn during swimming. The gains achieved through casting must always be maintained through orthotic fabrication, pressure, exercise, and other indicated treatments.

Physical Agents

Besides the physical agents already discussed, many other methods may be beneficial in scar management of the burned hand. More studies and documentation concerning the use and effectiveness of many of these modalities with the burned hand are needed.

Paraffin. The use of paraffin in treating burn scar contractures has been described by Head and Helm,[146] who state that paraffin, when combined with sustained stretch, can increase collagen extensibility, make the skin more pliable, decrease joint discomfort, and increase joint ROM. The paraffin is mixed with mineral oil (12 pounds of paraffin to 1 quart of mineral oil), and the temperature is lowered to 115°F.[147] Patients with limited finger flexion can be flexion wrapped with a self-adherent tape such as Coban or they should make a tight fist around a cone or cylinder before dipping the hand into the paraffin. Often patients cannot tolerate the heat of the paraffin bath, in which case the paraffin should be painted on with a paintbrush or piece of gauze.[148] After the paraffin has been applied, the hand is covered with plastic wrap, and the position of finger flexion is maintained with an elastic wrap.

Gross and Stafford[147] described a modified method for paraffin application. Pieces of coarse mesh gauze are dipped in paraffin and applied on the scar area. A layer of plastic wrap and a towel are then applied. With the wax in place, gentle long stretch and active exercises are performed.

Paraffin should not be used on patients with fragile skin or decreased sensation. Many burn patients appear to have increased sensitivity to heat or may be fearful of hot liquids.

Continuous Passive Motion. Therapists may use continuous passive motion (CPM) machines in the treatment of hand burns to help maintain or restore ROM.[149-151] The machines can be applied over dressings. CPM machines do not replace the therapist; they are an adjunct to therapy. In addition, hand CPMs do not take all of the finger joints through the full ROM. Studies on the use of CPM with patients with hand burns that required excision and grafting found no difference between CPM and non-CPM groups in the degree of and length of time to regain TAM and TPM, in the rate of edema reduction, in reported pain, and in loss of graft attributable to motion.[149,150] The authors of one study[149] concluded that those who would most benefit from CPM included patients with extensive burns covering multiple joint areas; patients who have decreased cognitive function and who require passive motion over a protracted period; and patients who demonstrate little active motion because of pain, edema, and anxiety.

Functional Electrical Stimulation. A pilot study reported by Apfel and colleagues[152] investigated the use of functional electrical stimulation (FES) with three patients with three severely burned hands that had not responded to traditional ROM and exercise techniques. The FES was applied to the flexor digitorum superficialis in hands with an intrinsic-plus imbalance. Objective measurement showed late improvement in hand function after the use of FES. However, FES appears to be used rarely in burn care.

Ultrasound. Ultrasound (US) has been used in the treatment of scars to increase ROM, reduce pain, and decrease scar formation.[151] In 1954, Bierman[153] reported increases in ROM and reduction of pain after US treatments of scars. Except for one patient who had sustained a burn 2 months before initiation of US treatments, the age of the scars was not specified. However, in 1993, Ward and coworkers[154] reported no difference in ROM or in perceived pain between a control group that received placebo US followed by passive stretching and an experimental group that received US followed by passive stretching. As pointed out by Nussbaum,[155] this study also omits detail, such as time from initial injury and breakdown of results for different burn sites, that might be relevant to a discussion of the study's findings. In 1970, Wright and Haase[156] examined biopsies and photographs of keloids of six individuals before and after a period of 24 US treatments and found no difference between treated and untreated scars. Because all of their specimens revealed a great deal of hyalinized connective tissue, Wright and Haase[156] concluded that

US was unsuccessful in the treatment of keloids in the later stages, when a great deal of hyalinized tissue had developed, and that the favorable reports of US in the literature represented keloids or hypertrophic scars that had been treated in the fibroblastic or fibrous stage.

The aforementioned US studies state or imply that the pain being treated by US was scar pain, and the results of the studies were conflicting. Despite such incongruities in the effectiveness of US in treating scar pain, Head[63,146] pointed out that US is useful in the treatment of painful joints in burn patients.

Iontophoresis. In two separate case studies when used with exercises and manual treatment, iontophoresis with iodine (Iodex) and with methyl salicylate ointment (because of its sclerolytic effect), can be an effective agent for reducing post-traumatic scar adhesions.[157,158] We have used saline with 0.9% to 3.0% concentration as a means of hydrating the tough and adherent burn scars before mobilization with encouraging results. When applying iontophoresis to a scar, we recommend lower intensities and longer delivery time because tissue resistance and permeability of scars is greater than in unburned skin. To maximize tissue diffusion, the buffered pad should be left on the patient's skin for a few hours. We find this method to be safe since the fluid composition of the human body is primarily made up of saline. However, we have yet to demonstrate the efficacy of our methods through empirical means (Fig. 26-21).

One agent, tranilast, appears to be the only known medication in the literature that has been examined extensively in the treatment of scars. Tranilast, an antiallergenic agent, has been shown to inhibit collagen synthesis in the treatment of keloid and hypertrophic scars when delivered via iontophoresis.[159,160] This agent appears to be widely used in Japan where it was developed; however, we are not aware of any comparable studies conducted in the United States.

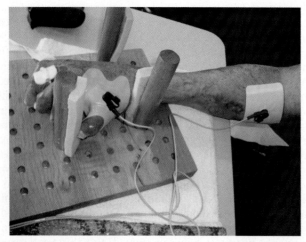

Figure 26-21 Iontophoresis with iodine (Iodex) and with methyl salicylate ointment may be an effective agent for reducing post-traumatic scar adhesions.

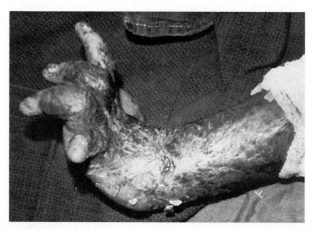

Figure 26-22 Extreme example of deformity that can result from scarring and other deforming forces in the deeply burned hand.

Therapeutic Management of Common Deformities of the Burned Hand

Scarring and Contracture Deformities in the Hand

As noted previously, scar hypertrophy and contraction are major forces during the healing of the thermally injured hand that can contribute to decreased function, deformity, and disability. Besides the obvious effect scar hypertrophy and contraction can have on the appearance of the hand, without intervention they can have a devastating effect on the structures and function of the hand (Fig. 26-22).

The location of the scar contracture is of greater relevance than its size when it comes to the effect on function. A 1-cm scar contracture on the dorsal surface of the PIP joint can produce far more devastating effects than the same sized scar on the palm. In a retrospective review of 659 adult patients with hand burns who were treated over a 10-year period, 90% of hands with injuries not involving the extensor mechanism, any joint capsule, or bone eventually regained normal function.[18] In a parallel study with children, Sheriden and colleagues found that only 20% of children with hand burns involving the underlying tendons and bones resulted in normal hand function, although 70% were able to perform basic ADLs.[17] Scar size and its effect on function is also relative to its proportion to the body. For instance, a 1-cm scar on the palm of an adult may cause little loss of motion. That same 1-cm contracture in a small child's hand may cause a more significant loss of motion.

In a retrospective study of 985 patients with burns, nearly 1 out of 4 demonstrated a hand contracture.[161] From this subset group of 226 patients, an average of 10 joint contractures was found per patient, for a total of 2320 hand joint contractures. This number is not surprising, given the proximity of the joints of the hand and how they functionally interrelate during prehensile movements. Given the complexity of the hand and the extent of the functional effect of postburn contractures, therapists should get a sense of the gravity and complexity of the rehabilitative process.

Boutonnière and Pseudoboutonnière Deformity

Boutonnière deformity of the finger is a common problem in the burned hand (see Chapter 25 for pathophysiology). Given the complexity of the development of a boutonnière deformity, there is no simple solution to management. With nonoperative or preoperative rehabilitative management, patients with boutonnière or pseudoboutonnière deformity could benefit from a finger gutter orthosis that maintains the PIP joint in extension but allows some degree of DIP flexion. The extension at the PIP helps preserve the length of the volar plate, whereas the allowance for active DIP flexion facilitates dorsal displacement of the lateral bands by passive tension. In addition to maintenance of the PIP in extension, finger abduction and adduction exercises could promote proximal migration of the extensor mechanism with concomitant dorsal displacement of the lateral bands. To minimize PIP and DIP stiffness due to collateral ligament tightness or oblique retinacular ligament shortening, patients must be instructed to perform ROM exercises with the next proximal joint (i.e., MCP and PIP joints, respectively) in neutral extension.

When the central slip of the extensor tendon to the PIP joint has ruptured, the PIP joint is immobilized in extension for 6 weeks and active flexion exercises of the DIP joint are performed. DIP joint flexion with the PIP joint held in extension requires lengthening of the oblique retinacular ligaments and helps to prevent the DIP joint hyperextension component of the boutonnière deformity. After 4 weeks, the orthosis may be removed for AROM exercises to the PIP joint. PIP joint flexion should be done with care to avoid stressing the healing central slip and the development of an extension lag at the PIP joint. Flexion can be performed in a limited arc at first, and the ratio of exercises can be done in favor of PIP joint extension over flexion. By the sixth week, the orthosis is worn only at night, and PROM may be initiated as long as there is no significant extensor lag. Use of the orthosis may be discontinued after 8 weeks if no significant extensor lag is present.

Multiple surgical techniques are suggested in the literature,[162-164] but with little consensus from the literature, there appear to be two general prevailing principles in the surgical repair of postburn boutonnière deformities: (1) maintenance of the lateral bands dorsal to the PIP axis of rotation with the ability to extend the PIP and DIP simultaneously, and (2) restoration of the continuity of the central slip in the extensor mechanism (see Chapter 25 for further discussion).

Proximal Interphalangeal Joint Contractures

Contractures at the PIP joint after a burn may develop in various ways. One such pathomechanical sequence is PIP contractures due to boutonnière deformity, pseudoboutonnière deformity, or scar banding of the palmar surface of the finger. Other potential means of PIP joint contracture development include inadequate positioning that renders the PIP joints in partial flexion and prolonged dorsal hand edema in which extra fluid deposit produces tautness on the dorsal skin, flattening of the hand, and compression of the extensor tendons.

Rehabilitative management of the PIP joint contractures requires a multidimensional approach. Stern and MacMillan

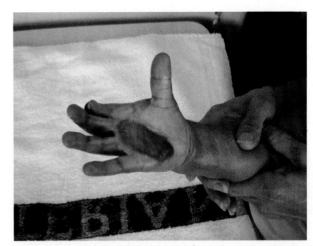

Figure 26-23 Example of a type I proximal interphalangeal joint contracture due to scar contraction.

proposed a three-level classification of PIP joint contractures after a burn.[165] Type I refers to PIP joint contractures that are due to scar alone (Fig. 26-23). Type II refers to PIP joint contractures due to involvement of articular structures, including the collateral ligaments and the volar plate. Type III occurs when the stiffness is most remarkable or the joint has arthrodesed. By highlighting various types of contractures, Stern and MacMillan have also presented different mechanisms in which PIP joint contractures may evolve.[165] Thus, it is necessary to determine the exact pathomechanics of the contracture for treatment to be most effective. To illustrate, if the PIP joint contracture is due to scar banding (type I), it is logical to manage the scar and the contracture together. A "two-bird-with-one-stone" solution is the use of a finger gutter orthosis that extends to the DIP joint distally and MCP joint proximally. Not only is the orthosis more mechanically advantageous than a three-point orthosis as it spreads the force application and lengthens the moment arm of the corrective forces, the broad surface area creates a wide pressure application over the volar PIP joint scar. Although an infrequent occurrence in hand burns, singular PIP joint contractures may also be treated with dynamic or static progressive orthoses with a hand-based dorsal outrigger device. Whether the therapist opts for a static or dynamic/static progressive orthosis, the aim of orthotic fabrication must be to provide low-load passive stretching of the PIP joint volar structures (Fig. 26-24).

Other interventions for PIP joint contractures include joint mobilization with sustained distraction through end ranges and serial casting for contractures that do not respond to conventional orthoses and traditional thermal agents. In 15 patients (total of 34 joints), Bennett and colleagues[140] demonstrated that with unresponsive burn contractures, an average of 54% gain in joint ROM can be achieved through systematic application of serial casting.

Flattening of the Hand

The various configurations of carpals and metacarpals along with strong ligamentous support create three important arches of the hand: (1) the very stable proximal transverse arch; (2) the very mobile distal transverse arch; and (3) the variable longitudinal arch. All three arches are a necessary

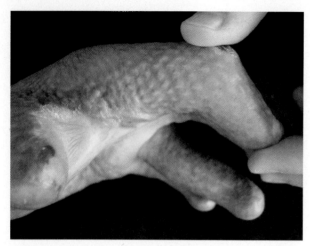

Figure 26-24 The aim of orthotic fabrication must be to provide low-load passive stretching of the proximal interphalangeal volar structures.

foundation to the various prehensile and grip patterns of the hand. In addition, the longitudinal arch has varying degrees of mobility and stability. The ulnar column, which is formed by the fourth and fifth metacarpals and the triquetrohamate articulation, offers carpometacarpal mobility necessary for power grip, and cylindrical and spherical grasps. Meanwhile, the radial column, which is formed by the second and third metacarpals and the lunocapitate and scaphocapitotrapezoid articulations, offers proximal stability for more prehensile precision patterns, such as tip and tripod pinch. Flattening of the hand can disrupt the anatomechanical configuration necessary for efficient and coordinated hand function.

As suggested earlier, flattening of the hand may be a direct outcome of dorsal hand edema. In our observation, scar contractures from dorsal hand and wrist burns are by far more common factors in producing flattening of the hand. In very few cases, postsurgical complications of partial-thickness grafts with excessive pulling of the dorsal skin may contribute to flattening of the hand.

Flattening of the hand may be treated with function-based activities that encourage use of the hand in various configurations. It may be necessary to add extra inserts within the compressive glove to the dorsum of the hand to increase the pressure on the scar. As a proactive measure during the early stages of recovery, therapists must continually evaluate the effect of the resting hand or pan orthosis on the arches of the hand. Preservation of the arches of the hand is just as important as maintaining the required joint angles of the wrist and digits. An effective orthosis is one that does both.

The opposite of flattening is cupping of the hand, in which the distal transverse arch of the palm becomes exaggerated or less mobile. This phenomenon is typically seen in patients with palmar burns and heavy scar bands. With hand use mainly consisting of frequent pressure contact on the palm such as during in-hand manipulation tasks or gross grip, many scars mature faster and become more pliable. Although cupping of the hand can be disabling, the extent of its effect on functional is comparably less than in persons whose burned hand has flattened.

Webspace Contractures and Syndactyly

Contractures in the webspaces of the fingers or the thumb are commonly observed in deep partial- or full-thickness burns that are located in the hand dorsally or circumferentially[30] (Fig. 26-25). Two ways in which contractures at the webspaces typically form are syndactylism and scar banding. Syndactyly forms when scar or grafted skin advances over the webspace, creating a "hooding" over what normally is a down-sloping webspace between the fingers or between finger and thumb.[166] Webspace contractures may occur on palmar, dorsal, or both surfaces and frequently require reconstructive surgery (see Chapter 25 for further discussion). On the other hand, scar bands develop across or along the lines of tension on the skin or on the borders of grafts.[30] When either scar band or hood forms in the webspaces, abduction and opposition of the fingers (especially the ulnar rays) become limited. Consequently, patients have functional limitations in tasks that require spherical grasp, such as grabbing an apple and any other movements that requires cupping of the hand. In addition, scar bands over or across the webspace or hooding over the webspace may create "pockets" that pose additional functional challenges, especially for hand hygiene.

Since syndactylism and webspace contractures are mainly driven by scarring, specific considerations must be taken when it comes to the use of pressure gloves. Pressure inserts that are custom-made to individual webspaces have been demonstrated to be effective in reducing scar advancement, increasing digital ROM, and even restoring the anatomic slope and dorsal slant of the webspace.[167,168]

One highly disabling complication of scar banding is when it involves the thumb. Salisbury estimates that the thumb accounts for 50% of hand function. Practically, most prehensile movements requisite to normal ADLs involve the thumb.[169]

Compressive garments and pressure inserts to manage scar banding of the thumb may not be sufficient. As previously discussed in the pathogenesis of hypertrophic scars,

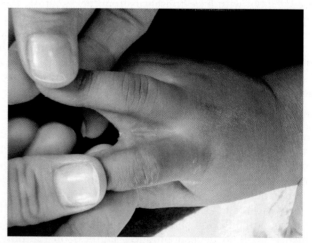

Figure 26-25 Contractures in the webspaces of the fingers are commonly observed in deep partial- or full-thickness burns that are located in the hand dorsally or circumferentially. (Howell JW. Management of the burned hand. In: Richard RL, Staley MJ, eds. *Burn Care and Rehabilitation Principles and Practice*. Philadelphia: FA Davis; 1994:531–575.)

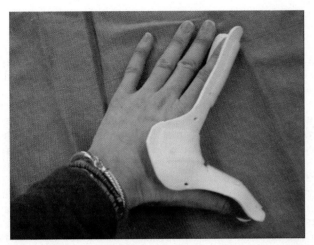

Figure 26-26 The C-bar or radial/palmar abduction orthosis to provide prolonged and progressive pressure over the scar of the thumb webspace.

multidirectional tension that is produced on the healing skin during thumb movements is proposed as the primary stimulus for scar band development. Thus, the thumb web needs a more rigid implement, such as an L-bar or radial/palmar abduction orthosis (Fig. 26-26) to provide prolonged and progressive pressure over the scar, stretch over the contracture, and limitation of multidirectional tension on the skin of the thumb web. A thin moldable insert such as Otoform K/c Elastomer may be placed underneath the orthosis to give added pressure over the scar band. If functionality is preferred, a wide C-bar orthosis that offers MCP and IP mobility of the thumb and composite flexion of the index finger may be provided during times when the patient is more active; alternating the C-bar with the L-bar orthosis during resting times can promote more prolonged pressure on the scar.

Small-Finger Deformity

Of the four fingers, excluding the thumb, the fifth is the most mobile. As a result, the fifth finger is most vulnerable to the formation of burn boutonnière.[170] At times, the deformity may include torque malrotation and abduction of the fifth finger at the MCP joint due to scar bands. Unlike other digits of the hand, the origin of fifth digit boutonnière and associated deformation is typically nontraumatic, meaning there is no exposure, disruption, or rupture of the central slip at the PIP joint. If early attention is not given to the positioning of the fifth digit, severe scar contracture extending to the extensor mechanism and articular structures may ensue. To prevent MCP joint hyperextension and subsequent PIP joint flexion especially in the early stages of rehabilitation, we use separate strapping or a thermoplastic bar in the resting hand or pan orthosis for the fifth finger.

Other than its hypermobility, one additional explanation for the fifth finger's tendency to deform is that people often do not fully include the fourth and fifth fingers in ADLs; instead they mainly use two-point, three-point, or lateral prehension to accomplish many tasks. This may be especially true of individuals who have sustained a burn to the hand

because many of the deforming forces tend to flatten the palmar arches and extend or hyperextend the MCP joint; they therefore position the fifth finger in a manner such that the disinclination to use it and the difficulty to include it when performing ADLs is greater. It is therefore important to encourage and prompt patients to maximize volar surface contact on objects with the fifth finger during certain manipulation tasks such as holding a bottle or turning a doorknob.

Return to Work and School

Work

Return to work, whether to the same or a different job, should be considered early in the course of treatment. Ideally, this goal requires a collaborative effort among the patient and his or her family, employer, medical professionals, workers' compensation personnel, and insurer. When possible, referral to a work program is preferable for vocational assessment, work hardening, and work adaptation. Zeller and coworkers[171] reported that 91% of burn patients returned to work after completing a work-hardening program versus 60% of patients with other diagnoses. The high success rate was attributed to early referral to the program and to the focus on rehabilitation in the burn center.

Helm and associates,[172] in a study of time elapsed until return to work in patients with hand burns, examined the variables of (1) percentage of TBSA burned, (2) which hand was burned (dominant vs. nondominant), (3) whether grafting was required, (4) patient age, and (5) occupational category. The best indicator of time elapsed until return to work was percentage of TBSA burned. The second-highest predictor was found to be distributed equally between the categories of those patients requiring grafting and those patients with both hands burned.

In a continuation of the previous study, including additional variables and patients with and without hand burns, Helm and Walker[173] again found that percentage of TBSA burned was the best predictor of time elapsed until return to work. Although patients with hand burns had smaller TBSA burns than the general burn population, they required a significantly longer time until they returned to work.

In a study of return to work of patients who had been employed before the burn injury, Saffle and colleagues[174] found that the length of hospitalization, number of surgeries, TBSA and full-thickness burn size, and patients' subjective assessment of their functional ability (including hand function), as well as their subjective assessment of scarring and appearance, correlated with time off from work. Also more likely to return to work than expected were patients who were covered by health insurance, whereas patients covered by Medicaid and those involved in injury-related lawsuits were less likely to return to work. The authors of the study noted that objectively assessed functional status may not be the only or primary indicator affecting return to work, rather an individual's attitude and ability regarding return to work may be profoundly affected by personal, psychological, legal, and societal influences. Other investigators who studied the influence of various factors that might affect return to work in persons who had sustained severe burns (not specifically hand burns) found that burn severity and other acute factors (e.g., receiving grafts) were not the strongest factors predicting whether an individual returned to work; rather, the strongest positive predictors were being employed before the injury, receiving workers' compensation, not blaming oneself, and being white.[175]

Back-to-work status after a burn injury depends on the preinjury employment status, the extent of the burn injury, the resulting physical limitations, and the patient's motivation for returning to work. With transitional modified or light-duty job placement, environmental considerations, and job adaptations, most patients can successfully return to work. A detailed determination of the job requirements and description of the work environment are required before allowing the patient to return to work. No open wounds should be present, and skin fragility must be taken into account when considering job demands. Light-duty transitional jobs with environmental restrictions may need to be negotiated as a step toward reintegrating the patient back into work.

School

Although school reentry programs and anecdotal information on return to school have been described, actual studies are sparse. Just as with return to work, return to school should be considered early in the course of treatment. Some hospitals have school programs or tutors, and some school districts provide a teacher to help the child continue school work during hospitalization. Tutors are provided as necessary when the child is an outpatient. Successful return to school is the result of a cooperative effort between the child and his or her family, medical professionals, school professionals, and classmates.

School reentry programs that involve visits to the school by medical professionals or the use of videos or puppet programs have the goal of facilitating the child's physical, social, and emotional return to school. School guidance counselors can assist in coordinating such programs with the parent and member of the burn center (often the play therapist or community outreach coordinator). Information is provided to the child's classmates about his or her appearance and scars, what happened to the child, and the purpose of pressure garments and orthoses. The inappropriateness of teasing, the noncommunicability of scars, and fears are discussed. Highlighted is the fact that, although the child may not look the same, he or she is still the same on the inside and can still participate in and accomplish most, if not all, activities, or soon will be able to. The information presented to classmates is graded according to age. Specific instructions concerning orthoses, pressure garments, any wounds and dressings, skin care and sun precautions, and itching are provided to teachers, the school nurse, and other school personnel. The presence of bandaged open wounds does not preclude a student from returning to school. Contact with and coordination of services with a school occupational or physical therapist is indicated in some cases. The student may be restricted from recess or physical education activities, at least initially, because of skin fragility. Just as with return to work, sun and heat precautions should be taken.

Functional Outcomes

Evaluation of the effectiveness of burn treatment protocols is encouraging. The assessments of functional return of the thermally injured hand have shown promising results. As to be expected, individuals who have sustained the deepest burns requiring grafts appear to demonstrate the greatest dysfunction in ROM, grip strength, and coordination. One year or more may be required for normal function to return.

A prospective longitudinal study by Roberts and coworkers[176] investigated the relationship of strength recovery to living skills in the burn-injured child. All subjects had functional ROM. At 6 weeks after hospital discharge, all subjects tested normal for tip-to-tip pinch strength. At 6 months, 75% of the children achieved normative values for grip, lateral pinch, and tripod pinch strength. Subjects in the 14- to 19-year-old age group reached norms at 6 weeks after hospital discharge, and those in the 9- to 11-year-old age group reached norms at 6 months. The investigators speculated that this difference in recovery rate was secondary to the older age group having higher expected responsibilities and greater capabilities in skilled performance. However, because of the limited number of subjects, the investigators could not determine from the study whether limitations in hand prehension hindered independent performance of age-appropriate ADLs.

An investigation of physical and psychological rehabilitation outcomes of pediatric patients who had sustained 80% or more TBSA, 70% or more full-thickness injuries, found that 80% were independent in basic ADL skills and that 86% of children ages 10 years and older were independent in advanced ADL skills.[126] Patients with amputated fingers were significantly more dependent in ADL skills than those without amputations. However, finger amputation alone was not the best predictor of functional independence. One or more finger amputations had to be paired with a major burn, one or more amputations of either limb, joint fusion, or brain anoxia. Encouragingly, psychosocial adjustment was normal.

Research has been performed to assess sensibility of grafted skin. Investigators, particularly in the past, have not always agreed. Several variables may contribute to the presence of sensory deficits and final sensory outcome. Such variables include the depth of injury, the type (or depth) of excision, the type of graft used, and age (but probably only if the individual is a young child). It also has been suggested that larger grafts or flaps may limit the number of axons available for reinnervation.[176] Another explanation given for the diminished sensation is that increased scar formation impedes axon regeneration in skin grafts, and it may take up to 1 or 2 years to achieve final sensory return.[178]

The skin's function, both to help regulate body temperature by sweating and to act as a water barrier to inhibit evaporative water loss, may be altered in the spontaneously healed or grafted burn wound. STSGs do not contain sweat glands,[179] although sweat glands may be present in the interstices of meshed grafts.[99] The loss of sweating may contribute to heat intolerance, especially in larger BSA burns.[99] One report of poorly recognized sequelae of thermal hand injuries showed that those patients who had skin-grafted hands had more complaints of heat intolerance and altered perspiration than those whose hands were not grafted.[180] In the study by

Apfel and colleagues[181] of enzymatically debrided and grafted partial-thickness hand burns, no sweating was seen initially in the grafted areas. However, by the second half of the year, more sweating was noted than in areas next to the graft. Apfel and colleagues[181] stated that the presence of sweating was because of the preservation of the original dermal sweat glands and indicated one of the benefits of enzymatic (vs. surgical) excision and early autografting of the hand with deep dermal burns. A study by Cadwallader and Helm[99] showed a decrease in the number of functioning sweat glands in hypertrophic scar tissue. However, interestingly, an increase in the activity of sweat glands was noted in burned areas as compared with control, unburned areas.

Studies of evaporative water loss from healed burn wounds revealed that grafted wounds had significantly lower rates of water loss than did normal skin.[100,182] Partial-thickness wounds that healed with hypertrophic scarring had higher rates of evaporative water loss than did partial-thickness wounds that healed without hypertrophic scarring and grafted wounds with and without hypertrophic scarring.[100] Such water loss results in extreme dryness of the skin and perhaps is another cause of patients' common complaints of itching.[100]

Psychology

A burn injury is sudden and can be quite frightening and overwhelming. Often, its psychological effects are not felt until after discharge from the hospital. Patients and their families must be instructed early and encouraged regularly about the extensive time involved and the commitment to often unforgiving treatment regimens required for good results. Goals regarding function should be set high and should be set in conjunction with the patient. If the therapist expects less, the patient also will expect less.

Many patients and their family members benefit from one-to-one counseling and support groups following a burn injury. Burn facilities frequently offer monthly parent and burn survivor support groups. Online support groups and chat rooms can also be found. The Phoenix Society (2153 Wealthy Street SE, #215, East Grand Rapids, MI 49506, 800-888-BURN), a nonprofit burn support organization, offers many programs such as school reentry, peer support, annual World Burn Congress, online resource center, and scholarships for burn survivor students.

Summary

Rehabilitation of the burned hand begins immediately following injury. Early therapy by a skilled clinician is essential to maximizing the functional outcome and cosmesis of the hand. Therapists must have a good understanding of the anatomy and kinesiology of the hand and phases of wound healing, specifically scar maturation, in order to adequately treat a burn injury. Further research is necessary to identify best practices for the treatment of burned hands.

REFERENCES

The complete reference list is available online at www.expertconsult.com.

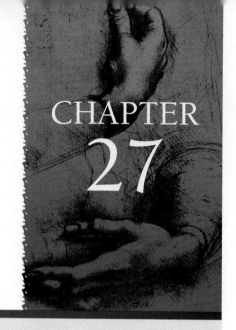

Acute Care and Rehabilitation of the Hand After Cold Injury

DOUGLAS M. SAMMER, MD

CRITICAL POINTS

- Frostbite is a severe, freezing-temperature, cold-induced injury.
- Tissue injury occurs by two mechanisms: cellular injury due to ice crystal formation, and progressive tissue ischemia.
- Frostbite primarily affects three groups: (1) the military, (2) the homeless, alcoholic or drug-addicted, and those with psychiatric illness, and (3) cold-weather sports enthusiasts.
- The traditional grading of frostbite injury by "degrees" of severity does not correlate well with outcomes.
- The risk of bony amputation correlates with the proximal extent of injury.
- Rapid rewarming is the cornerstone of management in the emergency department, but thawing and refreezing in the field should be avoided at all costs.
- Treatments aimed at blocking the arachidonic acid cascade likely reduces tissue injury.
- Rehabilitation goals include edema control, wound care, and preservation of motion.

Introduction and Definitions

Cold-induced injuries can be divided into major and minor categories. Major cold injuries include frostbite and immersion foot (also known as trench foot). Minor cold injuries include pernio (or chilblains) and frostnip. Cold-induced injuries can also be categorized by the temperature at which they occur. Frostbite and frostnip both occur at freezing ambient temperatures, whereas pernio (chilblains) and immersion foot occur at above-freezing temperatures.

Frostbite is defined as the freezing of tissues with accompanying ice crystal formation leading to tissue injury and death. It is a severe injury that can result in tissue loss and permanent disability. Frostnip, on the other hand, is not as clearly defined in the literature. Clinical signs of frostnip include numbness, pallor, and paresthesias that resolve immediately on warming. Although this has not been clearly demonstrated, ice crystals may temporarily form in frostnip.[1] Unlike frostbite, frostnip does not result in permanent tissue injury. Pernio (chilblains) is a mild cold-induced injury that occurs with prolonged and repetitive exposure to above-freezing cold temperatures. Clinical findings include a patch of erythematous, edematous, and pruritic skin. Pathologic studies reveal vascular and perieccrine inflammation.[2] The condition is usually self-limiting and resolves in a matter of weeks.[3] If pernio occurs in the same anatomic location season after season, a chronic form (which may include skin ulceration) can develop. Immersion foot (trench foot) is the result of prolonged exposure to above-freezing cold temperatures and moisture. Initially the foot is blanched or mottled, and the patient experiences an anesthetic effect described as "walking on air."[4] Clinical findings include poor pulses and sluggish capillary refill due to vasoconstriction. After rewarming, the extremity becomes hyperemic with bounding pulses. However, capillary refill remains poor and petechiae are seen, indicating damaged microcirculation. Blisters and desquamation follow. After healing, it can take months or years for cold sensitivity, hyperhydrosis, paresthesias, and pain to resolve.

Frostnip and pernio are mild self-limiting injuries that rarely require the services of a surgeon or hand therapist. Immersion foot occurs almost exclusively in the lower extremity and is not the focus of this chapter. Of the previously mentioned cold-induced injuries, frostbite is most likely to result in a significant injury to the hand.

History

Frostbite injuries have been well documented throughout history because they frequently occurred during large military campaigns. For example, historical records suggest that thousands of soldiers died from frostbite and other cold-induced injuries when Hannibal and his troops crossed the Alps in 218 BCE. The first large medical report of frostbite was made in the early 19th century by Baron Larrey, the surgeon-in-chief for Napoleon during the winter campaign in Russia. He also introduced "snow friction massage," a treatment method that was used until the 1950s. Frostbite injuries continued to plague military campaigns into the 20th century. During World Wars I and II and the Korean War, there were an estimated 1 million cases of frostbite.[1] Frostbite injuries were particularly common among high-altitude bombers who were exposed to below-freezing temperatures.[5] Frostbite management took a great stride forward in the 1950s and 1960s when Merryman and Mills introduced the concept of rapid rewarming, a treatment modality that remains the basis of management today.[6-9]

Epidemiology

Frostbite most often occurs in adults aged 30 to 50 years, and it predominantly affects males (10:1). As would be expected, it is more common in colder climates. In Finland, for example, the yearly incidence is 2.5 cases per 100,000. In Antarctica, the incidence is much higher at 65.6 cases per 1000. Unfortunately, there are no large population studies in the United States, but it is fair to assume that frostbite occurs more commonly in the northern parts of the country.

Three population groups tend to be affected by frostbite: (1) the military, (2) the homeless, drug-dependent, or those with psychiatric illnesses, and (3) cold-weather sports enthusiasts. Throughout history, frostbite has been considered a military disease. However, a recent 19-year study of cold-weather injuries by the U.S. Army revealed that the yearly incidence has been decreasing rapidly, likely due to increased awareness and efforts aimed at prevention.[10] Alcohol and drug use, homelessness, and psychiatric illness are also strongly associated with frostbite injuries. A 12-year retrospective epidemiologic study performed in the northern prairies of Saskatchewan showed an association with alcohol consumption in 46% of cases, and psychiatric illness in 17% of cases.[11] Another study from Montreal noted that alcohol was involved in 62% of cases, psychiatric illness in 19%, other drugs in 15%, and homelessness in 8%.[12] Some authorities suggest that in the urban setting, psychiatric illness plays a role in as many as 65% of cases. Finally, cold-weather sports enthusiasts such as mountain climbers, snow-mobile riders, skiers, and sky-divers commonly suffer frostbite injuries. A recent survey of 637 experienced mountaineers showed an incidence of 366 frostbite injuries per 1000.[13]

Pathophysiology

Type of Cold Exposure

Tissue freezing occurs more rapidly as the ambient temperature falls further below the freezing point (of water). In addition, the duration of cold exposure and the conduction properties of the substance to which the body is exposed are crucial factors. For example, because metal is a more efficient conductor of heat than is wood, a cold metallic object pressed against the skin induces frostbite more rapidly than a piece of wood can at the same temperature. Like wood, air is a relatively poor conductor of heat. However, as the wind-speed rises, heat loss through convection increases, creating the basis for the wind chill index.[14] For example, at 20°F with a brisk 35-mph wind the risk of frostbite is equivalent to that at 0°F with no wind. Other variables like skin moisture[15] or insulating clothing also affect the speed at which frostbite occurs.

Physiologic Factors

Physiologic factors also play an important role in the pathogenesis of frostbite. Normal cutaneous circulation is approximately 200 mL/min, but can vary dramatically. When a person is exerting physical effort, cutaneous circulation can rise to 8000 mL/min. On the other hand, an immobile person in a cold environment might have cutaneous circulation as low as 20 mL/min.[1] Increased cutaneous circulation results in loss of body heat but an increase in skin temperature. Conversely, a slowing of cutaneous circulation results in a drop in skin temperature, with preservation of body heat. As the ambient temperature drops, cutaneous vasoconstriction occurs. This allows the body to preserve heat, but also results in a decrease in skin temperature, making it more susceptible to frostbite. As the ambient temperature continues to decrease, another phenomenon called cutaneous intermittent vasodilation (CIVD) occurs.[16] During CIVD, blood vessels in the skin periodically dilate for a short period of time, increasing blood flow and warming the skin without a significant loss of body heat. CIVD has a protective effect for the skin and helps to prevent tissue freezing during cold exposure. The CIVD response varies from person to person and may account for differences in individual susceptibility to frostbite. Other physiologic factors contribute to frostbite, including impaired local circulation from smoking, diabetes, peripheral vascular occlusive disease, or vasoconstrictive medications.[17] Exertion and physiologic stress also alter cutaneous circulation and can affect susceptibility to frostbite.

Mechanisms of Injury

Tissue injury occurs by two mechanisms in frostbite: direct cellular damage and progressive tissue ischemia.[17,18] Direct cellular damage occurs with the formation of extra- and intracellular ice crystals. Extracellular ice crystals form first as tissue temperature drops. These crystals create an osmotic gradient that draws water out of the cell and into the extracellular tissue. This results in high electrolyte concentrations within the cell, which trigger programmed cell death

Table 27-1 Traditional Classification of Frostbite

Degree	Findings
1st	Numb white plaque, surrounding edema, or erythema
2nd	Blisters, filled with clear or milky fluid
3rd	Hemorrhagic blisters (reticular dermal damage), eschar formation
4th	Frankly necrotic tissue, into subcutaneous tissue, muscle, or bone

Data from McCauley R, Killyon G, Smith D, et al. Frostbite. In: Auerbach P, ed. *Wilderness Medicine*, 5th ed. Philadelphia: Elsevier; 2007.

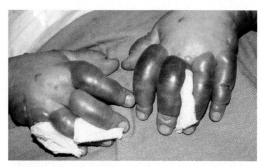

Figure 27-1 Second- and third-degree frostbite. Note the large bullae, some of which contain hemorrhagic fluid.

(apoptosis).[17] As temperatures continue to decline, ice crystals form within the cell, resulting in expansion and mechanical destruction.[19]

The second mechanism of tissue injury, progressive tissue ischemia, is more complex. Cold-induced vasoconstriction and direct endothelial injury initiate a cascade of fibrin deposition, platelet aggregation, and the release of local and systemic mediators.[17] Thrombosis occurs, resulting in further ischemia and propagation of the cycle. Prostaglandin F2-alpha and thromboxane A2 are important mediators of this process. They are found in high concentrations in frostbite blister fluid,[20] and drugs that block their effects have been shown to reduce tissue damage in animal studies.[21]

Clinical Presentation

Classification

Frostbite has traditionally been divided into four degrees of increasing severity (Table 27-1). First-degree frostbite is a numb white plaque with surrounding erythema. Second-degree frostbite involves clear blister formation. In third-degree injury, hemorrhagic blisters form and eschar may develop, an indication that the reticular dermis is involved (Figs. 27-1 and 27-2). Fourth-degree frostbite presents as frank tissue necrosis, with involvement of subcutaneous tissue, muscle, or bone.[1] Unfortunately, this traditional classification system does not correlate well with final outcomes.[17] Because of this a number of other classifications have been devised.

The Cauchy classification system (Table 27-2) defines four grades of increasing severity, based on physical examination immediately after rapid rewarming and again on injury day 2. It also incorporates the results of a

technetium-99 bone scan on injury day 2.[22] The advantage of the Cauchy system is that it attempts to provide prognostic information for each grade. Cauchy also demonstrated that in the hand, the risk of amputation correlates with the proximal extent of the injury.[22] If the distal phalanx alone is affected, there is only a 1% chance of amputation. If the injury extends into the middle phalanx, the risk increases to 31%. Proximal phalangeal extension results in a 67% chance of amputation at some level, and metacarpal or carpal extension means almost certain amputation.

One of the most important features of frostbite is the prolonged demarcation period. On average it takes 3 weeks for frostbitten tissue to fully demarcate, although it is not unusual for it to take many months. Often remarkable improvement takes place over time, and tissue that initially appeared necrotic or severely injured can survive. This characteristic of frostbite injuries is the basis for delaying surgical débridement as long as possible.[17]

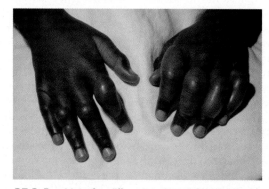

Figure 27-2 Frostbite of a different patient demonstrating sparing of the fingertips, due to clenched fist position at time of exposure.

Table 27-2 Cauchy Classification

Grade	Initial Exam	Exam Day 2	Bone Scan Day 2	Prognosis
1	No lesion	No blisters	N/A	No amputation
2	Lesion distal phalanx	Clear blisters	Hypofixation of radiotracer	Soft tissue loss
3	Lesion middle or proximal phalanx	Hemorrhagic blisters	Absence of radiotracer	Bone amputation
4	Lesion on metacarpal/carpal	Hemorrhagic blisters (carpal)	Absence of radiotracer (carpal)	Bone amputation, possible systemic symptoms

Data from Cauchy E, Chetaille E, Marchand V, Marsigny B. Retrospective study of 70 cases of severe frostbite lesions: a proposed new classification scheme. *Wilderness Environ Med.* 2001;12:248-255.

Imaging

The utility of imaging studies in frostbite injury is controversial. Plain radiographs should always be obtained, not for diagnostic purposes, but to provide a baseline for future comparison. A number of other imaging modalities have been advocated, with the goal of identifying tissue demarcation levels earlier in the course of treatment. Radioisotope scans including [131]I (iodine-131), [133]Xe (xenon-133), and [99]Tc (technetium-99) have been used.[23-25] Angiography, MRI, and magnetic resonance angiography (MRA) have also been studied.[17,26-28] Although some of these imaging techniques may become useful in the future, it currently appears that none is completely accurate until 2 to 3 weeks after frostbite injury.[1,17] By then, physical examination can usually determine demarcation levels reliably.

Treatment

Prethaw Treatment

Initial management in the field should include removal of any wet clothing, followed by padding of the hand and application of an orthosis. No attempt should be made to rewarm the hand in the field or during transport to the hospital. Thawing followed by refreezing causes a more severe injury than freezing alone.[17] Rubbing the skin, or "snow friction massage," should also be avoided. Frostbitten skin is fragile and susceptible to shear injury. Once in the emergency department, hypothermia should be treated before any attempt at rewarming of the hand. Once hypothermia has been addressed, rapid rewarming should be performed.

Rapid Rewarming

Rapid rewarming was developed and studied by Merryman and Mills in Alaska during the 1950s and 1960s.[6-9] Studies that have since been performed comparing slow rewarming with rapid rewarming (with or without adjunctive therapies) demonstrate better results with rapid rewarming.[29-31] Rapid rewarming involves immersion of the hand in circulating warm water with a dilute antimicrobial agent. The temperature should be carefully maintained at 40–42°C (104–108°F). Higher temperatures can result in thermal injury to the skin, and lower temperatures are less effective. Rapid rewarming takes 20 to 30 minutes in most cases and should be performed until the skin is pliable.[19,32]

Post-Thaw Treatment

After rapid rewarming, treatment is largely nonoperative. Surgical débridement should be delayed for at least 3 weeks and should not be considered until tissue has clearly demarcated. Early surgery should be reserved for surgical infections or escharotomy. There are case reports of early soft tissue débridement and coverage of ischemic bone with vascularized soft tissue transfers.[33] Although this approach may be useful in some situations, it has not yet become the standard of care. Figures 27-3 through 27-8 demonstrate the

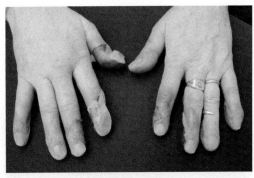

Figure 27-3 Another patient. Dorsal view within days of injury. Note that most of the bullae contain nonhemorrhagic fluid.

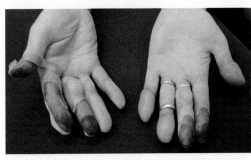

Figure 27-4 Palmar view within days of injury. Note the deeper injury at the fingertips.

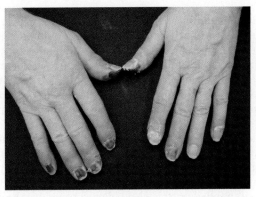

Figure 27-5 Dorsal view 3 weeks after injury. Note that most areas have healed, with the exception of the fingertips.

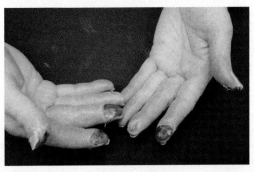

Figure 27-6 Palmar view 3 weeks after injury. Note eschar formation at fingertips, consistent with deeper dermal injury.

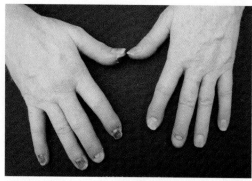

Figure 27-7 Dorsal view at 3 months after injury. Note complete healing of skin, with persistent discoloration of nail beds. Also note loss of nail plate on bilateral long fingers.

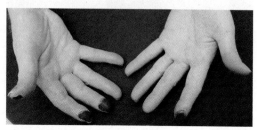

Figure 27-8 Palmar view at 3 months after injury. Note well-demarcated eschar at fingertips. Patient went on to heal completely over the next 2 months without surgical débridement or skin grafting.

demarcation and healing of a frostbite injury over time. Although this injury initially appeared quite severe, the patient went on to heal completely without surgery.

Standard nonoperative management after rapid rewarming includes (1) ibuprofen, (2) penicillin, (3) tetanus prophylaxis, (4) débridement of clear blisters, (5) topical aloe vera, and (6) elevation of the hand. Ibuprofen (400 mg PO q12h) is used to block the arachidonic acid cascade. Clear blisters are gently débrided at the bedside or in a whirlpool in order to remove thromboxane and prostaglandins from the wound surface. Hemorrhagic blisters should be left intact to prevent exposure and desiccation of the deep dermis. Topical aloe vera (applied q6h) is also believed to reduce thromboxane levels.[1,17]

A number of other modalities, including hyperbaric oxygen, dextran, heparin, and thrombolytics, have been used.[18,34-38] Some evidence from animal studies indicates that these adjuncts might prove useful, but as of yet there are no compelling human studies.

Rehabilitation

The hand therapist plays a crucial role in the treatment of frostbite, both in terms of acute wound management, and in the maintenance of mobility. Early in the postinjury period edema formation occurs. If untreated, it causes a number of problems. It results in a relative decrease in tissue oxygen tension and can potentially worsen the severity of the injury. It also reduces the natural antistreptococcal properties of the

skin. Finally, it severely limits active and passive motion. Orthotic use and elevation, as well as periodic active finger flexion and extension, are appropriate edema control measures. Compressive wraps or garments should be avoided in the early postinjury period to reduce the risk of compressive ischemia or shear injury.

Daily whirlpool and hydrotherapy should be instituted. Whirlpool fluid should be warmed to about 40°C (104°F) and should contain a dilute antimicrobial agent. Whirlpool/hydrotherapy sessions should focus on two goals: débridement and maintenance of motion. Whirlpool and gentle pulse lavage can be used to assist with débridement of broken blisters and loose necrotic tissue. This is also an ideal time to work on passive and active range of motion. These sessions have the added benefit of improving circulation. It is important to note that the dependent position of the hand during the whirlpool treatment can contribute to an increase in edema. For this reason limiting the duration of the whirlpool treatment to 5 minutes at a time is recommended.[39]

Postinjury orthosis use should focus on prevention of contractures, and protocols similar to those used in burn patients are appropriate. The hand and wrist should be fixed in a comfortable position of function. Tight Velcro straps should be avoided. Initially the orthosis may be held in place with lightly applied gauze wrap. As edema resolves, the orthosis will need to be adjusted and Velcro straps may be applied to allow a more secure fit.

The patient should be instructed in active and passive motion out of the orthosis. In areas where the degree of tissue injury is unclear, it is important to limit stress to the injured tissue through very gentle exercise. Light functional activities may begin as soon as wound healing permits. An assessment of the patient's ability to perform activities of daily living is called for with provision of assistive equipment or adaptive techniques as needed. The extent to which the injury affects the individual's ability to work and fulfill his or her roles and responsibilities in relation to family and home is addressed and adaptations are suggested. Finally, the hand therapist may be asked to assist with scar management and desensitization after the wounds have healed.

Summary

Frostbite is a severe cold-induced injury that occurs at below-freezing temperatures. It primarily affects three types of patients: (1) those in the military, (2) the homeless, drug-addicted, or mentally ill, and (3) cold-weather sports enthusiasts. Tissue injury occurs by two mechanisms: direct cellular injury by ice crystals, and progressive tissue ischemia mediated by the arachidonic acid cascade. The initial management of frostbite involves transfer of the patient to a treatment center where rapid rewarming can be performed. Post-thaw treatment includes ibuprofen, penicillin, tetanus prophylaxis, débridement of clear blisters, topical aloe vera, and elevation of the hand. Surgical débridement should be delayed until tissue has clearly demarcated. This may take weeks or months, and tissue that initially appears severely injured often survives. The hand therapist should be involved early on in the care of the patient. Orthotic use, elevation, and range of motion should be initiated at the time of injury. Compressive dressings should be avoided. Whirlpool and hydrotherapy can be helpful for débridement and assist during range of motion exercises. Postinjury orthotic use should focus on prevention of contractures, with care taken to avoid tissue compression. Finally, the therapist plays an important role in scar management and desensitization after the wounds are healed.

REFERENCES

The complete reference list is available online at www.expertconsult.com.

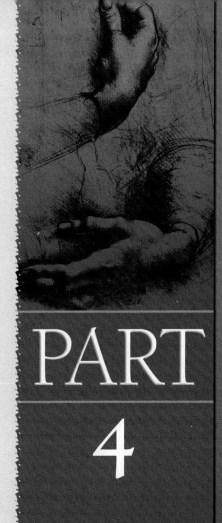

PART

4

Hand Fractures and Joint Injuries

Fractures: General Principles of Surgical Management

EON K. SHIN, MD

PATIENT EXAMINATION
CLASSIFICATION OF FRACTURES
CHOICES FOR FRACTURE FIXATION

FRACTURE HEALING
COMPLICATIONS
SUMMARY

CRITICAL POINTS

Fracture Fixation

- Unstable fractures require surgical stabilization.
- Kirschner wires provide adequate stability with minimal soft tissue exposure. Pin tract infections can be treated with oral antibiotics or early pin removal.
- Plate–screw fixation generally provides rigid stabilization and allows for early mobilization. However, hardware removal with soft tissue releases may be necessary when used to treat phalangeal or metacarpal fractures.
- Intramedullary fixation is being used to treat metacarpal injuries, some distal radius fractures, and midshaft humerus fractures.
- External fixation is useful for severely comminuted or open fractures.

Fracture Healing

- The *inflammation phase* is characterized by bleeding from the fracture site and hematoma formation.
- The *repair phase* occurs when gentle range-of-motion exercises can generally be instituted. Radiographs depict callus formation at the fracture site.
- The *remodeling phase* continues long after the fracture has clinically healed.

The care of hand and upper extremity fractures continues to challenge surgeons and therapists alike. A detailed understanding of the surgical and rehabilitative management of upper extremity injuries is critical, given how frequently upper limb fractures are encountered. Fractures of the metacarpals and phalanges, for example, are among the most common injuries seen in the upper extremity.[1] Unfortunately, metacarpal and phalangeal fractures are often neglected by referring physicians or regarded as trivial injuries,[2] leading to less than optimal outcomes. Swanson himself once stated, "Hand fractures can be complicated by deformity from no treatment, stiffness from overtreatment, and both deformity and stiffness from poor treatment."[3]

The goals of fracture care for the upper extremity are straightforward, but sometimes difficult to achieve. These include

- Stabilization of fractures for bony healing
- Elimination of angular or rotational deformities
- Restoration of the articular anatomy
- Care of associated soft tissue injuries
- Rapid mobilization

Patient Examination

History and Physical Examination

A thorough history, physical examination, and radiographic assessment should be performed for each patient presenting with an upper extremity fracture. Before delving into the historical details of the specific injury, it is important to determine the injured individual's occupation and hand dominance. When taking the history, determining the mechanism of injury is critical to understanding the patterns of skeletal and soft tissue damage. For work-related trauma involving heavy machinery, for example, it is essential to obtain a detailed description of the devices involved. Such details may include the distance between rollers in a metal-working machine, the degree of contamination of moving metal parts, and so forth. These details offer clues to the

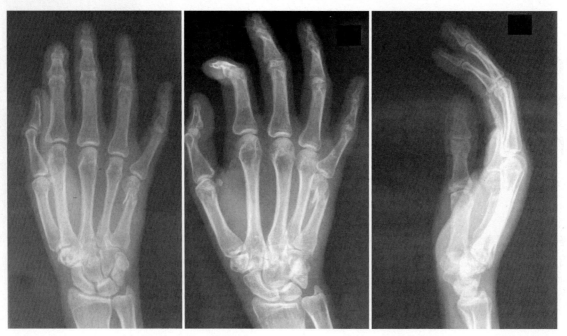

Figure 28-2 Anteroposterior, oblique, and lateral views of the hand for evaluation of a small finger metacarpal neck fracture with comminution.

practitioner about the extent of soft tissue involvement, which often dictates final outcomes following fracture fixation (Fig. 28-1, online).

The patient should also be questioned about any initial deformities that may have resulted from the traumatic injury, such as finger dislocations that were reduced, open bleeding wounds that were sutured closed, or any symptoms of motor or sensory disturbance. Such clues can help to focus the clinical examination and develop an appropriate treatment plan. Patients with open wounds should be asked about their tetanus vaccination status and the use of prophylactic antibiotics, if any. The time of injury is also significant for patients who present with an open fracture or dysvascular limb.

General questions encompass the medical and surgical background of the patient, the use of routine medications, and an allergy history. The habitual use of tobacco products has been shown to delay bony healing,[4,5] therefore information about tobacco use should also be solicited in an initial examination.

The physical examination should involve inspection of the entire limb. Clothing should be moved or removed to permit appropriate visual and manual inspection of the proximal articulations even for simple hand or distal forearm injuries. The presence of ecchymosis, deformity, and tenderness is usually sufficient to confirm the diagnosis of fracture. However, palpation of the entire extremity should be performed to rule out other areas of injury or possible associated soft tissue damage. When evaluating fractures of the metacarpals or phalanges, the examiner must determine the alignment of the digits both on initial examination and, if indicated, after fracture reduction. Alignment is determined clinically by viewing the relationship of the fingernails to one another with the digits in full extension. The nail plates should be almost parallel in this position. Conversely, the alignment of the fingers can be assessed by asking the patient to flex the digits. In this position, the finger tips should point toward the scaphoid tuberosity. When in doubt, the alignment of the fingers in the injured hand can be compared with that on the contralateral side for patients who might demonstrate normal anatomic variability.

The integrity of the flexor and extensor tendons of the injured limb should be individually determined and documented. Both closed and open skeletal trauma may also be associated with injury to the nerves and vessels. Testing distal to the area of injury is usually sufficient to document the limb's neurovascular status. Sensibility should be documented by response to light touch and also to two-point discrimination. Circulation can be determined by visual inspection and timed capillary refill of the digits.

Radiographic Evaluation

Comprehensive radiographic studies should be obtained. The tubular skeleton of the hand requires three radiographic views (anteroposterior, lateral, and oblique) to accurately assess the position and integrity of these small skeletal units (Fig. 28-2). Fractures involving a single digit must have at least anteroposterior and true lateral views of the individual digit. Failure to obtain a true lateral view of the affected finger can result in misdiagnosis or misinterpretation of injury severity. The Brewerton view is a special radiographic aspect that can assess collateral ligament avulsion fractures of the metacarpal head and is obtained with the metacarpophalangeal (MCP) joint flexed 65 degrees and the dorsum of the fingers lying flat on the radiographic plate with the tube angled 15 degrees in an ulnar-to-radial direction.[6]

With fractures of the forearm and humerus, it is advised to obtain radiographs of the joints proximal and distal to the site of injury to avoid misdiagnosis. Radial neck fractures about the elbow, for example, can lead to distal radioulnar

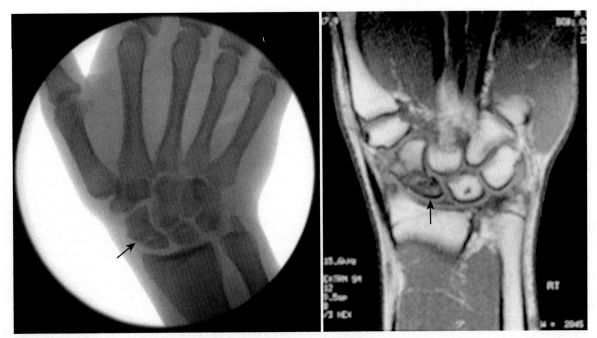

Figure 28-4 *Proximal pole scaphoid fracture (arrow). With MRI, decreased vascularity to the proximal portion of the scaphoid is visualized (arrow).*

joint disruption and possible interosseous membrane injury (Essex–Lopresti fracture).

Computed tomography (CT) may be necessary to characterize fractures involving the articular surfaces or those with significant comminution. The latest generation of CT scanners can produce precise bony detail and incredibly realistic three-dimensional images (Fig. 28-3, online). Magnetic resonance imaging (MRI) can also serve as an adjunct to plain radiographs but is typically reserved to document soft tissue injury or avascularity (Fig. 28-4). Occasionally, MRI studies are useful in diagnosing an occult fracture, such as a scaphoid injury, which may not appear initially on radiographs. Finally, radionuclide imaging such as bone scans can help to identify areas of occult injury. However, its use is typically limited for acute fracture care as the findings from a bone scan are largely nonspecific. High-quality plain radiographs are generally sufficient to treat and care for most fractures of the upper extremity.

Classification of Fractures

The mechanism of hand and upper limb injuries varies considerably. Most occur from falls onto outstretched extremities or from direct impact. In general, fracture patterns emerge based on the nature and direction of the traumatic force. Although the Orthopaedic Trauma Association (OTA) has developed a formal classification system of most upper limb fractures, descriptive terms are typically employed to document the fracture pattern as visualized on plain radiographs (Table 28-1).

Location Within Bone

Fractures are usually defined according to the location in the affected bone. When this involves a long bone such as a radius, metacarpal, or phalanx, the fracture can be described as being diaphyseal (within the midportion of the bone shaft), metaphyseal (within the area of the bony flare close to the articular surface), or articular when it engages the end of the bone and enters the joint (Fig. 28-5). Articular fractures can be further subclassified as condylar, T-condylar, or Y-condylar. Articular fractures can also involve the rim of the joint surface, which suggests an avulsion of a portion of the capsule, collateral ligament, or tendon (Fig. 28-6).

Displacement

The degree of fracture displacement is typically measured in millimeters for upper limb injuries or as a percentage of the fractured bone's diaphyseal width. Although significant fracture displacement may be better tolerated in a larger bone like the humerus, a critical eye should be used to evaluate displacement of intra-articular fractures. Articular

Table 28-1   Fracture Classifications

Criteria	Examples/Comments
Location within bone	Diaphyseal
	Metaphyseal
	Articular
Displacement	Measured in millimeters
	Measured as diaphyseal percentage
Pattern	Transverse
	Oblique
	Spiral
	Longitudinal
	Stellate
	Simple
	Comminuted
Open vs. closed	Subclassified by soft tissue injury

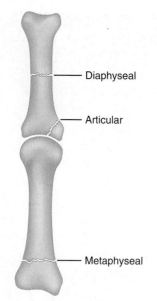

Figure 28-5 Fractures may be classified according to their location in the bone: diaphyseal, metaphyseal, and articular.

incongruity for intra-articular fractures may lead to decreased ability to remodel as the joint stepoff exceeds the thickness of the cartilage ends. In distal radius fractures, for example, Knirk and Jupiter[7] found that articular incongruity predisposed patients to the development of degenerative joint disease in the radiocarpal joint. In their study of young patients, the absence of joint stepoff following treatment for an intra-articular distal radius fracture led to arthrosis in only 11% of patients. Stepoffs of 2 mm or greater, however, led to degenerative joint disease in 91% of patients.

Catalano and colleagues[8] also found a strong association between intra-articular stepoff and degenerative joint disease but found that all patients presented with good or excellent outcomes an average of 7 years following surgery regardless of the initial deformity. Goldfarb and coworkers[9] followed up on this study by evaluating the same cohort of patients an average of 15 years after surgery. The authors found that patients continued to function at high levels, that strength and range-of-motion (ROM) measurements were unchanged, and that the joint space was reduced an additional 67% in those patients with radiocarpal arthrosis. No correlation was noted between the presence or degree of arthrosis and upper

extremity function as measured by the Disabilities of the Arm, Shoulder, and Hand (DASH) questionnaire or other objective criteria.

Though intra-articular stepoff in upper extremity fractures may not be as significant as previously believed, less than 2 mm of displacement is recommended and minimal incongruity is desirable[10] by most current standards.

Pattern

Fractures can be described by the angle of the fracture line through the bone. Common configurations include transverse, oblique, or spiral patterns as seen on plain radiographs (Fig. 28-7). Less common patterns include longitudinal fractures, which span the length of the bone from proximal to distal, or stellate injuries, which usually represent significantly comminuted fractures radiating from some central point (Fig. 28-8). Fractures are described as simple if the injury produces two major fracture fragments, or comminuted if multiple fragments are visualized on radiographs.

Deformity (Rotation or Angulation)

Rotational deformities are difficult to assess on plain radiographs. Metacarpal or phalangeal fractures are best assessed clinically by asking the patient to simultaneously flex all of the digits.[11] If significant overlap of the digits is noted with composite digital flexion, then corrective open reduction should be considered. Angular deformities can be assessed with plain radiographs. Significant angulation between fracture fragments may lead to malunion and should be corrected with closed or open reduction. Metacarpal neck fractures can accept varying degrees of angular deformity, particularly as one moves from the radial to the ulnar side of the hand due to increasing mobility at the proximal carpometacarpal articulations.

However, angulation of other upper limb bones tends to be less well tolerated. Treatment of distal radius fractures, for example, has evolved since Abraham Colles provided the first description to the English-speaking community in 1814.[12] In his initial report, Colles noted that these fractures tended to do well despite considerable angular deformity. This assertion was later supported by Cassebaum in 1950.[13] Finally in 1988, McQueen and Caspers[14] demonstrated a clear correlation between malunion of the distal radius and poor functional outcomes. Since then, we have witnessed a growing

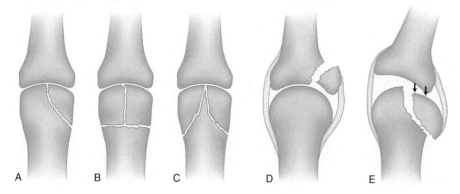

A   B   C   D   E

Figure 28-6 Articular fractures are further subclassified as (**A**) condylar, (**B**) T-condylar, (**C**) Y-condylar, (**D**) articular avulsion, or (**E**) articular depression.

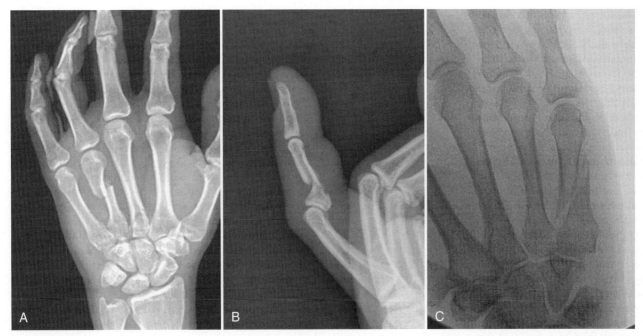

Figure 28-7 Fractures can be described according to the angle of the fracture line through the bone: **A,** transverse fracture of the ring finger metacarpal; **B,** oblique fracture of the index finger middle phalanx, and **C,** spiral fracture of the small finger metacarpal.

body of literature devoted exclusively to surgical techniques for correcting angular deformities of distal radius fractures.

Guidelines for optimal positioning of the distal end of the radius have evolved such that most orthopaedic and hand surgeons strive for radial inclination greater than 15 degrees; radial tilt between 15 degrees of dorsal angulation to 20 degrees of volar angulation; radial length with less than 5 mm of shortening at the distal radioulnar joint; and less

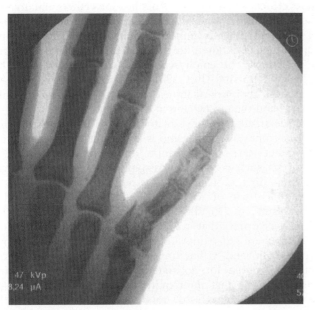

Figure 28-8 Stellate intra-articular fractures of the proximal and middle phalanges of the small finger secondary to gunshot wounds.

than 2 mm of intra-articular stepoff between fracture fragments[15] (Table 28-2, online).

Open Versus Closed Injuries

Open fractures require special consideration for treatment. All open fracture wounds should be considered contaminated because of communication between the fracture site and the outside environment. Until about 150 years ago, an open fracture was virtually synonymous with death and generally necessitated an immediate amputation of the injured limb.[16]

Open hand and upper extremity injuries have traditionally been classified using the Gustilo and Anderson classification system[17,18] (Table 28-3, online). The basic objectives in the management of open fractures include prevention of infection, bony union, and restoration of limb function. Antibiotics have been shown to reduce significantly the risk of postoperative infection. Patzakis and associates[19] found that infection rates decreased sixfold from 13.9% to 2.3% with the administration of appropriate antibiotics as compared with placebo. Antibiotics should be administered in the emergency department once an open fracture has been identified. This typically includes the use of IV cefazolin (Ancef) and possibly an aminoglycoside for type III injuries. Ampicillin or penicillin should be added to the antibiotic regimen when conditions favor development of anaerobic infections, such as clostridial myonecrosis (gas gangrene), as occurs in farm accidents and vascular injuries.[20] The tetanus toxoid status of the patient must be ascertained and the appropriate tetanus booster or immunization given as needed.

Though wound cultures have been emphasized in traditional teachings, their utility has recently been controversial because they often fail to identify the causative organism.[21,22] In one prospective, randomized, double-blind trial, only 3 (18%) of the 17 infections that developed in a series of 171 open fracture wounds were caused by an organism identified by the initial cultures.[23] Thus, initial cultures are generally no longer recommended.

Despite the effectiveness of antibiotics in preventing infection, no principle is more important in the care of an open fracture than aggressive irrigation and debridement. Penetration of antibiotics into necrotic tissue is still under investigation.[24,25] The wound should be thoroughly debrided to remove devitalized tissues and gross debris. Oftentimes, it is necessary to have patients with open injuries return to the operating room for revision debridements to ensure that all devitalized soft tissues are removed and to decrease the risk of possible deep infections. Traditionally, closure of open fractures after initial debridement has been delayed to minimize the risk of complications.[26] However, recent studies comparing primary with delayed closure have not demonstrated an increased rate of complications.[27-31] The optimal time for wound closure continues to remain controversial.

Bony stabilization should be achieved as soon as possible to prevent further soft tissue injury. This can require the use of external fixators, which span the defect but avoid the placement of foreign materials (e.g., titanium plates and screws) within an open and contaminated wound.[32,33] External fixation is also technically expedient and is associated with minimal blood loss. Later conversion to open fixation with plates and screws or intramedullary nailing can be undertaken once the soft tissue envelope has been reestablished. With minimal contamination or wound conversion from "dirty" to "clean," open fixation may be used initially to provide bony stabilization.

Although the Gustilo and Anderson classification has withstood the test of time in general orthopedic practice for predicting rates of infection and nonunion, its applicability is more limited for evaluating open hand injuries. Gustilo and Anderson's original study examined 673 open fractures in long bones, which included the tibia and fibula, femur, radius and ulna, and humerus.[17] Unfortunately, no provision was made for the classification and treatment of open carpal, metacarpal, or phalangeal fractures.

The Swanson–Szabo–Anderson classification of open hand injuries subdivides hand fractures into two categories. Type I injuries feature clean wounds without significant contamination or delay in treatment and no systemic illnesses. Type II injuries feature (1) grossly contaminated wounds, (2) a delay in treatment greater than 24 hours, or (3) significant systemic illness (e.g., diabetes, rheumatoid arthritis). The rate of infection from a type I injury was noted to be 1.4%. The rate of infection with a type II infection was 14%. Neither primary internal fixation nor immediate wound closure was associated with an increased risk of infection in type I injuries. Primary internal fixation was not associated with increased risk of infection in type II injuries.[34]

It is obvious that the rate of complications increase as open fractures increase in their severity. Avascular necrosis and blood supply loss due to comminuted fragments need to be carefully considered. In addition, open fractures carry a higher risk of delayed union or nonunion with resultant fixation failure. The soft tissue envelope certainly must be con-

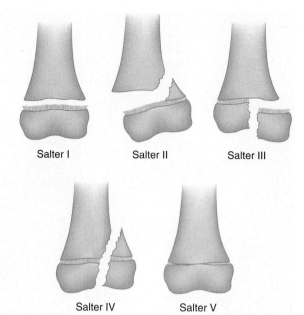

Figure 28-9 *Salter–Harris classification of physeal fractures.*

sidered as a casualty of such complicated fractures, as adhesions binding soft tissue planes to fracture sites are common. Thus, the attentive repair of essential soft tissue gliding structures and their early mobilization through proper therapy are cornerstones for postoperative success.[35-37]

Pediatric Fractures

Fractures in children can be described in a manner similar to those in adults in terms of location within the shaft of the bone and whether a fragment of bone has been avulsed from the articular region. However, pediatric fractures become more critical when they cross ossification centers and involve the epiphysis or physeal growth plate. Accurate reduction of such fractures is important, although the remodeling capabilities in children far exceed those in adults. Fractures that do cross the epiphyseal lines have been classified by Salter and Harris[38] (Fig. 28-9). According to Hastings and Simmons,[39] epiphyseal injuries occur 34% more commonly in the hand than elsewhere in the skeleton.

Understanding the anatomy of the metaphysis–physis–epiphysis relationship is important in understanding the Salter–Harris classification. Injuries that damage the epiphysis, such as Salter–Harris types III, IV, and V fractures, are more likely to result in growth abnormalities or growth cessation. Lack of accurate reduction of these injuries may result in articular incongruity in addition to the angular deformity that may result if Salter–Harris type I and II injuries are not reduced. Accordingly, some Salter–Harris type III, IV, and V fractures require open reduction and internal fixation for accurate reconstitution of the joint surface. Those that do require operative intervention are more likely to be referred to the hand therapist for early protected motion and may be more of a rehabilitation challenge.[40-42]

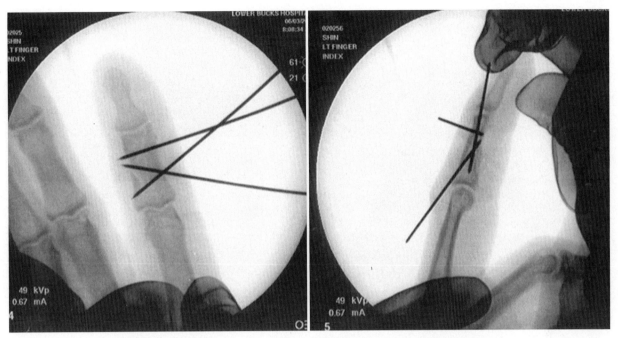

Figure 28-10 Percutaneous pinning of a comminuted middle phalanx fracture.

Choices for Fracture Fixation

Fracture stability is judged both radiographically and clinically. Cast or orthosis immobilization is an appropriate treatment for nondisplaced fractures and stable displaced fractures that have been reduced. It may also be appropriate for low-demand patients who cannot tolerate surgery for medical reasons.

Certain fracture patterns cannot be adequately reduced or maintained in a reduced position, including comminuted fractures; fractures with bone loss; intra-articular fractures; and oblique, spiral, or transverse fractures with malrotation, angulation, or shortening. Stability can be determined clinically by manually assessing whether a fracture reduction can be maintained or, instead, immediately redisplaces after reduction. Malrotation is assessed by having the patient actively flex the fingers while the examiner looks for digital overlap or spreading. Open fractures and fractures with associated injuries to adjacent structures result from high-energy trauma and tend to be unstable. In these situations, the hand surgeon must rely on an armamentarium of techniques to obtain stable bony fixation.

Kirschner Wires

Because of the limited bone stock available in the hand and upper extremity, preoperative planning and implant selection are of critical importance. There are certainly advantages and disadvantages to using different techniques or implants for bony stabilization. Kirschner wires (or K-wires) require minimal soft tissue and bony exposure (Fig. 28-10). If wire placement is initially unacceptable when visualized under fluoroscopy, it is generally a simple matter to reinsert the wire or make reduction adjustments as needed. K-wire

fixation can also be augmented with the use of a wire loop or tension band construct, which can provide greater compression of the fracture site. However, a greater exposure of the fracture site is required.[43-45] Although K-wires are often appropriate for fixation of certain distal forearm and many hand injuries, the surgeon should be prepared for conversion to open fixation techniques using plates and screws. The fixation provided by K-wires is relatively weak fixation,[46,47] and pin tract infections can develop that may necessitate premature removal.

Multiple Screws

With oblique or spiral fractures of the hand that can be reduced through closed means, multiple screws can be placed in a percutaneous fashion to avoid periosteal stripping and blood supply disruption. Screw fixation performed in this manner permits rigid compression of the fracture site and only requires exposure sufficient for drill placement.[48] Headless screws are typically used to stabilize scaphoid fractures and feature screw ends with differing pitch to confer compression across the fracture site. The ends of the screw are buried beneath the articular surfaces of the bone to allow early motion.

Open Reduction and Internal Fixation

Open fixation with plates and screws provides the greatest rigidity for fracture repair, thereby permitting early ROM[49] (Fig. 28-11). However, open techniques require greater exposure of the fracture site, with potential compromise of the soft tissue structures and the blood supply. Open reduction and fixation of proximal phalangeal fractures, for example, often requires an extensor tendon splitting

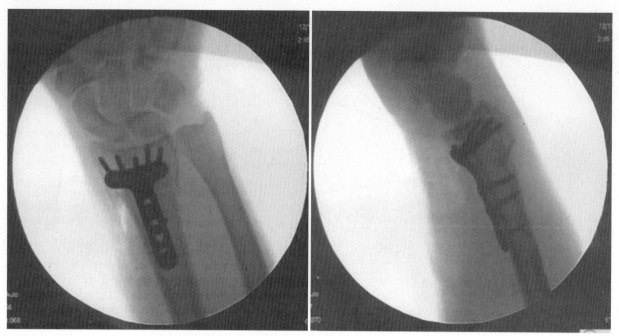

Figure 28-11 Open fixation of a distal radius extra-articular fracture.

approach. Therefore, the potential for adhesion formation and stiffness following open fixation is significant. Plates can also be bulky and may require hardware removal once the fracture has healed. Finally, tenolysis may be necessary should the patient develop significant stiffness.[50]

One study examining outcomes following metacarpal and phalangeal open fixation found that major complications, including stiffness, nonunion, infection, and plate prominence, were encountered in 36% of fractures.[51] However, in injuries involving the distal radius, forearm, and upper limb, open fixation is usually preferred because the soft tissue envelope is more forgiving of the additional bulk a plate confers. Both surgeon and therapist must take a collaborative approach in maximizing postoperative mobility while respecting the stability of fixation. If stable internal fixation is achieved, an orthosis is initially used for comfort, and active mobilization is started within 2 weeks following surgery.

Intramedullary Fixation

The popularity of intramedullary fixation has been fueled, in part, by the successful management of lower extremity long bone fractures. Intramedullary nailing is now an accepted treatment for humerus fractures and certain forearm fractures. Intramedullary devices increase fracture stability of the affected bone, allow load transfer across the fracture site, minimize soft tissue problems by minimizing scarring and adhesions, and maintain the vascular blood supply to promote fracture healing. However, reaming the humeral canal has been associated with a number of complications, namely injury to the neurovascular structures,[52-54] insertion site morbidity at the shoulder,[55] and iatrogenic fracture and comminution.[53]

Intramedullary implants have recently been described for use in distal radius fractures. These devices are indicated for metaphyseal distal radius fractures with minimal articular involvement.[56,57] The long-term results from use of these implants are still uncertain. For transverse midshaft metacarpal fractures, K-wires can also be used to provide intramedullary fixation using percutaneous techniques.

External Fixation

Occasionally, the hand surgeon is faced with a situation in which direct fixation cannot be achieved using wires, screws, or plates. With significant open fractures of the upper limb or intra-articular fractures that defy internal fixation, external fixators may prove useful for temporary distraction of the fracture site and even definitive management. External fixators provide ligamentotaxis that can help to maintain fracture reduction, thereby preventing collapse. In addition, they function by neutralizing compressive, torsional, and bending forces across a fracture site.

For unstable fracture–dislocations involving the proximal interphalangeal (PIP) joint, for example, various K-wire configurations can be applied for dynamic distraction/external fixation.[58] Such devices permit immediate mobilization of the affected digit while maintaining concentric reduction of the PIP articulation (Fig. 28-12). A disadvantage of external fixation is the lengthy period of treatment, which may lead to pin tract infections and loosening. The hand therapist is a frequent observer of the external fixator and is usually the first to alert the surgeon when such problems arise. Treatment generally entails the use of appropriate antibiotics and possibly pin removal to prevent or treat osteomyelitis.

Fracture Healing

Following fracture fixation or stabilization, the process of fracture healing and repair goes through a series of phases that can be clinically judged by both physical and

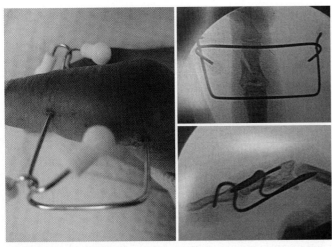

Figure 28-12 Dynamic distraction external fixator applied for treatment of a proximal interphalangeal joint fracture–dislocation. (Courtesy of Stephanie Sweet, MD.)

radiographic examinations. These phases include (1) development of hematoma and traumatic inflammation, (2) organization, (3) union by callus, and (4) remodeling of callus and bony union.[59] An assessment of fracture healing can help the physician and therapist decide when to increase activity levels.

Inflammation Stage

During the inflammation stage, bleeding from the fracture site and surrounding soft tissues creates a hematoma, which provides a source of hematopoietic cells capable of secreting growth factors. Vasodilatation of vessels and hyperemia in the soft tissues surrounding the fracture take place. Clinically, this stage is marked by significant localized pain and swelling. Subsequently, fibroblasts, mesenchymal cells, and osteoprogenitor cells are present at the fracture site, and fracture hematoma is gradually replaced by granulation tissue around the fracture ends.

Repair Stage

The repair stage occurs within 2 weeks from the time of injury. If the bone ends are not in continuity, bridging (soft) callus develops and is replaced later by woven bone (hard callus). With closed treatment and cast or orthosis immobilization, periosteal bridging callus is seen on plain radiographs, which represents the "rubbery" mass seen at the fracture interface. With rigidly fixed fractures (e.g., compression plating), primary bone healing occurs in the absence of visible callus. Callus-free healing requires absolute stability of the construct and exact reduction of the fracture fragments. In fractures treated by external fixation, the presence of callus depends on the rigidity of the fixator construct. In less rigidly fixed fractures, bridging soft callus is seen on early radiographs. In more rigidly fixed injuries, primary bone healing occurs as seen with compression plating. Pain levels generally decrease markedly by this point as the bone ends become stabilized.

From this point forward, associated swelling, pain, and tenderness generally diminish rapidly as the callus matures. It is the resolution of much of the edema and tenderness that signals that one can begin to add significant forces across the fracture and be confident that displacement of the fracture is unlikely. Generally, by the fourth to sixth week in most fractures in adults (and the third to fourth week in most fractures in the hand and forearm in children), forces of active and active-assisted ROM can be increased. However, this always depends on the full assessment of the fracture and considerations of the initial stability, type of reduction used, general health and reliability of the patient, and radiographic appearance.

Remodeling Stage

The remodeling stage begins during the middle of the repair phase and continues long after the fracture has clinically healed. Remodeling allows the bone to assume its normal configuration and shape based on the stresses to which it is exposed. Throughout the process, woven bone formed during the repair phase is replaced with lamellar bone. Fracture healing and remodeling is complete when the marrow space is repopulated.

Fracture healing may be influenced by a variety of biologic and mechanical factors. The most important biologic factor in fracture healing is blood supply. Nicotine from smoking has been shown to increase the time to fracture healing, increase the risk of nonunion, and decrease the strength of the fracture callus.[4,5] Patients with systemic diseases (e.g., diabetes mellitus) may also experience delays in healing due to poor limb vascularity.[60] These considerations should be taken carefully into account by the treating surgeon and therapist. Stable compression loading of fractures, such as can be accomplished with internal fixation, can improve fracture healing and functional recovery. Such stability can allow early guarded motion to improve limb movement and adjacent joint flexibility.

Complications

Malunion

Malunion is a relatively common bony complication of fracture treatment and describes a nonanatomic positioning of the bone. Angulation of metacarpal fractures, for example, can disrupt the intrinsic balance of the hand and result in prominence of the metacarpal heads in the palm with pain on gripping. Malrotation may cause the digits to "scissor" and interfere with simple activities of daily living (Fig. 28-13). Dorsal angulation of the distal radius—which is most frequently seen following improper casting techniques—may cause chronic pain and increase the likelihood of developing degenerative joint disease. Proximal forearm fractures that are malunited may interfere with elbow motion or forearm rotation.

A malunion generally requires an osteotomy procedure to realign the limb's bony elements. A variety of techniques have been described to correct malunions of the phalanges,[61,62] the carpal structures,[63,64] and especially the distal

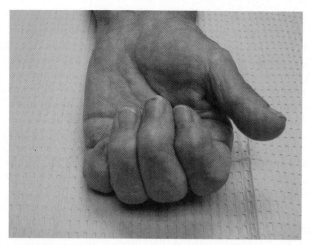

Figure 28-13 Malunion of the small finger metacarpal, resulting in digit overlap. Note the incidental presence of Heberden's nodes affecting the index, middle, and ring fingers.

radius[65-69] (Fig. 28-14, online). The common goals of these procedures are to correct deformity, to improve the limb's mobility, and to eliminate the pain that sometimes accompanies malunion.

Nonunion

Failure of opposed fracture ends to unite by bone is considered nonunion. Basic requirements for fracture healing include mechanical stability, an adequate blood supply, and bone-to-bone contact (Table 28-4, online). Though nonunion is relatively uncommon in the hand, it can occur with extensive soft tissue injury, bone loss, and open fractures with contamination and infection. Grossly contaminated wounds require meticulous management and appropriate antibiotics depending on the injury setting (e.g., barnyard contamination, brackish water, bite wounds), local wound care with debridement as necessary, and possible delayed closure. Infections may result in motion and instability at the fracture site as implants loosen in infected bone.

It has been demonstrated that nonsteroidal anti-inflammatory drugs (NSAIDs) negatively affected the healing of experimentally induced fractures in several animal studies.[70-72] Clinical studies have also documented delayed union or nonunion in human subjects taking NSAIDs.[73] Although a growing body of literature exists implicating NSAIDs as a factor in delayed fracture healing, no true consensus exists. Even for those who believe the negative effects exist, the biochemical mechanism of action still remains obscure.

Nonunions are surgically managed with bone graft and rigid fixation. Areas with poor vascularity, such as proximal pole scaphoid fractures, may require a vascularized bone graft using microsurgical techniques to increase the likelihood of healing.[74,75] Left untreated, scaphoid nonunions can progress to carpal collapse and a predictable pattern of radiocarpal arthrosis.[76]

Stiffness

Joint contractures may result if patients receive an improperly placed orthosis or if the orthosis is in place for too long.

In treating finger or hand injuries, it is important to keep the hand fixed in a "position of safety"—the MCP joints flexed to 70 degrees or more and the IP joints maintained in full extension. Following surgery, loss of motion may be secondary to tendon adherence, especially at the level of the PIP joint. If limitations with motion persist beyond 3 to 6 months, it is reasonable to consider a tenolysis procedure in a motivated patient whose hand has not responded to therapy measures. Schneider[77] recommended removal of hardware, if present, and aggressive soft tissue releases with possible palmar–dorsal capsulectomies. Local anesthesia may be beneficial for obtaining direct patient input during the procedure.

Stiffness can also occur secondary to heterotopic bone formation, which can be seen following burns, trauma, repair of distal biceps tendon rupture, or operative treatment of forearm fractures (Fig. 28-15, online). Many options have been recommended for treatment of heterotopic bone formation with variable results.[1,53,78,79] These surgeries generally incorporate excision of the heterotopic bone with possible soft tissue or synthetic material interposition. Adjuvant treatment with radiation therapy or NSAIDs has also been recommended after excision.[70,80]

Osteoarthritis

Finally, post-traumatic osteoarthritis may result from a failure to restore articular congruity of affected joints. Though post-traumatic arthrosis is easily determined using plain radiographs, the degree of functional impairment must be assessed clinically to decide if surgical intervention is needed. In healed distal radius fractures with significant degenerative joint disease, limited or total wrist fusions may be beneficial to alleviate pain[81] (Fig. 28-16, online). Alternatively, prosthetic replacements are a consideration. For example, displaced fractures of the radial head that fail operative fixation may be treated with radial head excision and interposition with soft tissue or a vitallium implant. Some fractures, such as injuries about the MCP or PIP joints, may require primary silicone implant arthroplasty for load sharing,[82] though such applications are not common.

Summary

Management of upper extremity fractures requires careful handling by both the hand surgeon and therapist for optimal patient outcomes. It requires an understanding of the anatomy and the physiologic processes associated with fracture repair. Though fractures do require appropriate stabilization to prevent the development of malunion or nonunion complications, mobilization must take place as expediently as possible to prevent soft tissue adhesions and contractures. In the end, limb mobility and functional capacity define how well fracture care has been performed.

REFERENCES

The complete reference list is available online at www.expertconsult.com.

Hand Fracture Fixation and Healing: Skeletal Stability and Digital Mobility

CHAPTER 29

MAUREEN A. HARDY, PT, MS, CHT AND ALAN E. FREELAND, MD*,†

"The most common complication of hand fractures is not malunion or infection. Rather, it is joint contractures and tendon adhesions."[1]
BARATZ AND DIVELBISS, 1997

CRITICAL POINTS

- Fracture reduction
- Fracture stability
- Soft tissue mobility
- Zone of injury (ZOI)
- Minimally invasive surgery (MIS)
- Clinical physiological correlation of tissue healing
- Clinical progression based on fracture healing and soft tissue response

Hand fractures do not occur in isolation. Every hand fracture has a proportionate closed or open injury to and response within its adjacent embedding soft tissues, creating a "zone of injury" (ZOI)[2,3](Fig. 29-1A). Immediately after fracture, a central hematoma occurs within the space between the fragments and expands about the fracture. Interstitial edema accumulates within the impacted soft tissues and deposits fibrin as part of the acute inflammatory response to injury. The peripheral margins of the edematous response define the ZOI (Fig. 29-1B–D).

Initial local signs of hand fractures include primary bone deformity, secondary joint deformities, motion and instabil-

ity at the fracture site, pain, tenderness, swelling, ecchymosis, and heat. Without treatment, all of the tissues encompassed within the ZOI tend to become progressively bound into a single amalgam (one wound/one scar) by the fibrin, fibronectin, and mucopolysaccharides ("tissue glue") contained in the extracellular matrix (ECM)[2,4] (Fig. 29-2). Joints adjacent to the fracture are often affected and can develop permanent intrinsic or extrinsic (or both) adhesions, stiffness, and deformity. Pseudoclaw deformities may develop (Fig. 29-3). Tendons tend to adhere to adjacent structures, sometimes impairing gliding. Progressive stiffness, atrophy, dysfunction, and pain may result ("fracture disease").[5]

The essence of hand fracture management is restoration of anatomic osseous integrity and stability throughout fracture healing; together with simultaneous preservation of the normal length and elasticity of the ligaments and joint capsules; and facilitation of early independent joint motion, tendon gliding, and functional recovery of the hand and digits.[1,6-12] Gentle, progressive, controlled, passive range-of-motion (PROM) and unresisted active range-of-motion (AROM) exercises should be initiated as soon as the fracture is reduced and stable. Early motion stimulates parallel interstitial collagen fiber alignment, which enhances scar elasticity and prevents or disrupts early adhesions in the interstitial spaces between disparate tissues during concurrent fracture healing and joint and tendon rehabilitation. The more severe the injury, the more extensive and proliferative the fibroblastic response; and thus, the more compelling early motion becomes. The duration and intensity of exercises are gradually advanced in accordance with the stability of the fracture, the response of the soft tissues, and the patient's pain tolerance. The resting hand and digits should be positioned and protected in the functional (intrinsic plus) "safe"

*This work is dedicated to our mentors, William Burkhalter, MD, Wyndell Merritt, MD, and Evelyn Mackin, PT, for sharing their knowledge and lending their support and encouragement through the years. We would also like to acknowledge and thank Alvra Jenkins for guiding and supporting each stage of manuscript development and Virginia Keith for her always superb editorial assistance. Any errors are our own.

†Disclosure: Dr. Freeland receives departmental and institutional support from AO North America and royalties from Elsevier Publishing Company. No funding was received for this article.

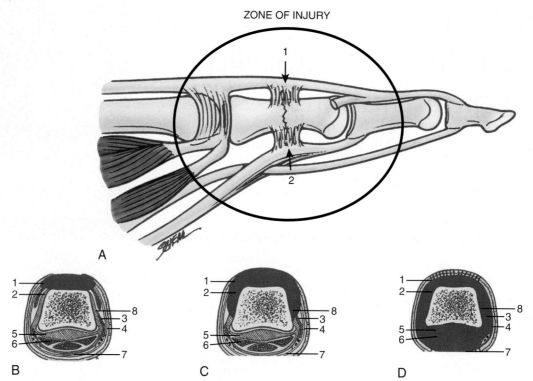

Figure 29-1 Every fracture results in a zone of injury (ZOI) proportional to the extent of trauma. **A,** The ZOI can encompass both extensor and flexor tendons with potential restrictive adhesions. (A, 1 Adhesions from extensor mechanism to proximal phalanx following digital fracture; A, 2 Adhesions from flexor tendon to proximal phalanx following digital fracture.) **B,** A localized edematous response (*dark area*) on the dorsum of the proximal phalanx involves the central extensor mechanism; **C,** a more edematous response spreads the ZOI to include the lateral bands; and **D,** a marked traumatic response radiates the ZOI circumferentially around the digit, incorporating all soft tissues. (1, Extensor tendon mechanism; 2, collateral ligament; 3, digital artery; 4, digital nerve; 5, volar plate; 6, FDS at proximal phalanx level; 7, flexor tendon sheath; 8, transverse retinacular ligament.)

posture between exercise sessions to prevent joint contractures and central slip attenuation.[9-15]

Fracture and soft tissue healing are processes, not events that occur over time. Bone healing and scar formation undergo three discrete yet artificial and overlapping stages of progression: the acute or inflammatory phase, the reparative or proliferative phase, and the remodeling or maturation phase.[2,9,11,12,16-18] Knowledge of the molecular and cellular interactions throughout the stages of bone healing and scar formation, the timing of events, and how these processes simultaneously interrelate within and adjacent to the common environment of the ZOI allows the physician and therapist to correlate incremental clinical functional rehabilitation with cellular and molecular events and tissue recovery. The physician, therapist, and patient must work together as a committed team to achieve the best outcome possible.

Fracture Disease

Immobility leads to so-called fracture disease.[5] Fracture disease begins with uncorrected deformities of bone and joints, acute pain, and persistent edema. Without intervention, fracture disease evolves to include stiffness, tendon adhesion, capsular and ligamentous contracture or attenuation, central slip attenuation, infiltrative scar formation, and pseudoclawing. Additional edema may occur due to limb dependency, tight dressings, and pressure points over bone or joint prominences. Consequently, fracture disease may spread beyond the ZOI and become complicated by local or regional chronic complex regional pain (CCRP, reflex sympathetic dystrophy [RSD]). Joint deformities may become progressively fixed as early as 3 to 6 weeks after injury, and CCRP (RSD) may develop. Pain may become chronic, disproportionate to expectations, and unresponsive to ordinary treatment. Algodynia and hypersensitivity may occur. If undeterred, trophic changes gradually develop, including extensive fibrosis, brawny skin induration, shiny skin, digital tapering, loss of rugal pattern, hair loss, nail growth changes, temperature and sweating abnormalities, and local or regional osteopenia. Fracture disease and CCRP become progressively recalcitrant to treatment over time. Therefore, early intervention with fracture stabilization and digital exercises is essential.

Fracture Management

Ensuring anatomic fracture position and stability are the primary initial goals of hand fracture management.[1,6-8] Hand fractures that are undisplaced and inherently stable do not require reduction, but do need some protection against deforming forces and additional impact during early healing. A small cohort of hand fractures have inherent stability following manipulative reduction. They also require the use of a protective static or functional orthosis for 3 to 4 weeks. The remaining hand fractures require closed or open reduction and either temporary or permanent implant fixation to restore their anatomic integrity and stability as fracture healing and rehabilitation progress.

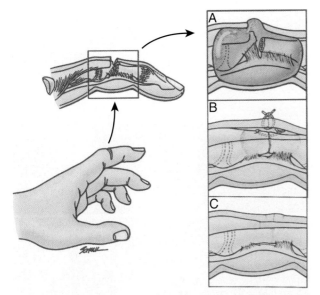

Figure 29-2 One wound/one scar concept. **A,** Initially, all tissues within the zone of injury are encompassed in the common inflammatory soup. **B,** As healing ensues, fibrin (soft tissue response) and callus (bone response) form across tissue planes, potentially welding both stationary and moving structures together. **C,** A healed, but poorly remodeled response with restrictive adhesions can occur in the absence of therapeutic stress (controlled motion programs). (Reprinted, with permission, from Hardy M. The biology of scar formation. *Phys Ther.* 1989;69(12):1014-1024.)

Early fracture reduction and stability control pain, restore fracture surface apposition and the normal proportionate relationships between bone and adjacent soft tissues, promote bone healing, and provide a platform both for any necessary soft tissue repairs and for timely rehabilitation. Function follows form.[1,6-8] Stability prevents "false motion" at the fracture site and allows revascularization and healing of repaired tissues to proceed without disruption. Fracture fixation should be as "atraumatic" as possible to prevent or limit additional bone devascularization, soft tissue damage, and

fibroplasia. Subperiosteal dissection, flexor tendon sheath injury, and extensor tendon injury over the proximal finger phalanges in particular, stimulate additional fibroplasia.

Initial Treatment

Definitive fracture treatment may be delayed for up to 5 to 7 days in closed, low-energy hand fractures having two fragments with little alteration of outcome. Open fractures require urgent attention to débride, cleanse, and catalogue the wound; reduce the fracture; provide at least provisional fracture stabilization; and prevent infection.[1,6-8] Simple (two-part) fractures with clean, limited skin lacerations may be safely and definitively stabilized and the skin repaired primarily. Soiled and complex wounds should initially be left open and then ideally reassessed within 48 hours. Additional cleansing and debridement performed at that time should render most wounds clean and suitable for definitive bone, tendon, and nerve and skin repair.[19,20] If not, the cleansing, debridement, and wound assessment may be repeated at 24- to 48-hour intervals until the wound is rendered clean. The least invasive method of internal fixation should usually be selected from equally applicable methods.[1,6-8]

Reduction

Although limb length, appearance, and function were probably somewhat impaired, primitive humans and animals in the wild have successfully healed markedly displaced, untreated fractures (Fig. 29-4, online). Early indirect fracture healing evolved in an environment where mobility favored survival. The need to secure nourishment and avoid predators resulted in motion about the fracture site that often stimulated callus formation. Over time it became evident that fractured bones held in anatomic reduction healed with better outcomes. The oldest record of fracture reduction is found in Egyptian hieroglyphics (2450 BCE) depicting orthoses made from papyrus that were used to reduce and support distal forearm fractures[21] (Fig. 29-5, online).

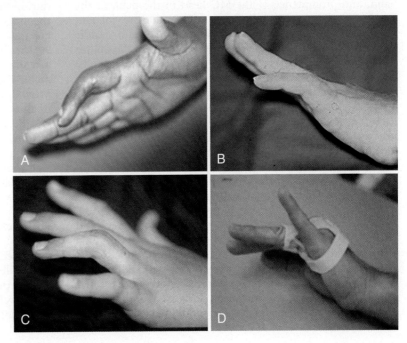

Figure 29-3 Pseudoclaw finger secondary to fracture with extensor and flexor tendon adhesions, contracted proximal interphalangeal joint, and compensatory metacarpal (MCP) joint hyperextension as seen in **A,** index digit, **B,** small digit, **C,** ring digit, and correction with MCP joint blocking orthosis (**D**).

Shortening, angulation, and rotation are the principal elements of deformity and may be seen individually or in combination.[1,6-8] Alterations of bone anatomy may affect functional outcome commensurate with their severity. Reduction restores the fracture fragments to their prefracture anatomy. Although a perfect reduction is of course ideal, the hand and digits have a remarkable capacity for functional adaptation to and tolerance of small and, sometimes, greater fracture deformity.[22]

Anatomic Parameters and Functional Correlations

Recent reports have illuminated the correlation between deformity and functional loss and may help the physician to decide whether to accept or correct a residual deformity. Hand dominance, occupation, or special individual needs may play a role. Observation of and discussion with the patient and the timing of presentation may also be critical in the decision-making process. The risk of postoperative digital stiffness may outweigh the benefit of lesser gains in anatomic fracture restoration in instances of small deformities, particularly in late-presenting inveterate fractures that have the early formation of a soft or hard callus that prevents closed manipulative fracture reduction.[22]

Metacarpal Fractures

Metacarpal (MC) shaft fractures tend to angulate dorsally, owing to the unbalanced pull of the interosseous muscles and extrinsic finger flexors on the distal fragment (Fig. 29-6). Intrinsic muscle shortening and altered muscle tension dynamics lead to increasing grip weakness after 30 degrees of dorsal MC angulation.[23-27] There may also be loss of knuckle contour, pseudoclaw deformity, and a palpable or even visible MC angular deformity on the dorsum of the hand, and prominence of the MC head in the palm of the hand. The ring and small finger MCs are more tolerant of dorsal angulation than those of the index and middle fingers due to their increased carpometacarpal flexibility. Satisfactory results have been reported with as much as 70 degrees of dorsal angulation of subcapital MC (boxer's) fractures.[28,29]

Approximately 7 degrees of extensor lag may develop for each 2 mm of residual finger MC shortening after fracture healing.[30] The intermetacarpal ligaments usually prevent greater than 3 to 4 mm of shortening of finger MC fractures.[31] Internal MCs (third and fourth) have more restraint than border MCs (second and fifth) since the distal fragment is anchored by intermetacarpal ligaments on both sides of the MC head. The intrinsic hand muscles contribute 40% to 90% of grip strength.[26,27] As great as 8% loss of grip power may result from every 2 mm of MC shortening. Based on this information, finger MCs may tolerate as much as 3 to 4 mm of shortening, and occasionally more, with only minimally noticeable clinical deformity and functional loss. In individual instances, surgeons may choose to accept 3 to 4 mm or perhaps more shortening as an alterna-

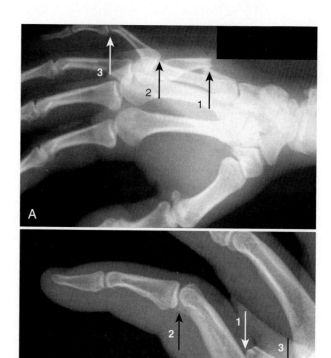

Figure 29-6 A, Fifth metacarpal fracture with apex dorsal angulation (*arrow 1*), compensatory metacarpophalangeal joint hyperextension (*arrow 2*), and slight proximal interphalangeal (PIP) joint flexion (*arrow 3*). **B,** Proximal phalanx fracture with apex volar angulation (*arrow 1*), compensatory PIP joint flexion (*arrow 2*), and slight metacarpophalangeal joint hyperextension (*arrow 3*). *Note:* Both uncorrected deformities constitute pseudoclaw fingers.

tive to the risks of scarring and stiffness from surgical intervention.[22]

Lateral MC angulation of 5 to 10 degrees may be tolerated, provided that no significant finger impingement occurs during motion.[8] MC angulation may be best observed with the fingers straight, whereas impingement becomes more apparent as the fingers progressively flex.

The intermetacarpal ligaments between the MC heads provide some rotational stability to the distal fracture fragment. The internal MCs have more restraint than border MCs. Rotational deformity greater than 5 degrees may result in finger impingement, or "scissoring" (overlap).[32,33] Seitz and Froimson reported that 10 degrees of MC malrotation resulted in 2 cm of overlap at the fingertips.[34] Rotational deformity of the fingers may be apparent with full digital extension, but becomes progressively more pronounced as the collateral ligaments tighten with finger flexion.

Phalangeal Fractures

Displaced fractures of the proximal phalangeal shaft characteristically display an apex palmar angulation (see Fig. 29-6). The intrinsic muscles flex the proximal fragment, whereas the attachment of the central slip to the dorsal proximal border of the middle phalanx extends the distal fragment.

The axis of rotation of proximal phalangeal fractures lies on the fibro-osseous border of the flexor tendon sheath.[35] The distance of the moment arm from the rotational axis of the fracture site to the extensor tendons is greater than that between the axis and the flexor tendons, further contributing to apex palmar angulation. Coonrad and Pohlman reported limitation of finger flexion with palmar angulation of greater than 25 degrees in extra-articular phalangeal fractures at the base of the fingers and advocated correction of greater deformities.[36] More recently, Agee reported shortening of the dorsal gliding surface of the proximal phalanx relative to the length of the extensor mechanism if volar proximal phalangeal angulation exceeds 8 to 15 degrees.[35] As palmar angulation incrementally shortens the fractured proximal phalanx, the extensor mechanism may have as much as 2 to 6 mm of reserve, owing to its viscoelastic adaptive properties, before the sagittal bands tighten to produce a progressive extensor lag at the proximal interphalangeal (PIP) joint of an average of 12 degrees for every millimeter of bone–tendon discrepancy.[37] Skeletal alignment sufficient to prevent or minimize extensor incompetence at the PIP joint and to restore the floor of the flexor tendon sheath is critical in the effort to restore both extensor and flexor tendon gliding and function.[35-37] A persistent palmar angular deformity of the proximal phalanx may lead to permanent attenuation of the central slip, extensor lag, and pseudoclawing of the finger that may persist despite later correction of the osseous deformity.[12,14,15] Apex palmar deformity of middle phalangeal fractures manifests similar problems with skeletal shortening, extensor lag of the distal interphalangeal joint, and alteration of flexor tendon gliding and dynamics.

Stability

Although functional recovery (motion) is the ultimate overall goal of hand fracture management, stability is the ultimate purpose of reducing fracture fragments. Fractures that do not displace spontaneously or with unresisted exercises are considered stable.[8] Inherently stable fractures safely tolerate incremental tendon gliding and joint motion, maximizing their functional recovery. Reduced fractures that displace spontaneously or with unresisted motion cannot maintain their alignment. These fractures require some form of additional support or fixation to ensure that correct anatomy is maintained during fracture union. Fracture fixation methods vary from external to internal support. Miniscrews, miniplates, tension band wiring systems, and "90-90" wiring provide secure fixation and allow healing to occur by direct bone formation. Less secure, "flexible" fixation methods, such as Kirschner wires (K-wires) and external minifixators, internally fix fractures. "Flexible" fixation allows nondisruptive micromotion at the fracture site, thus supporting and stimulating indirect bone healing. Flexible fixation permits sufficient exercising to prevent tendon adhesions and joint contracture in most instances. Exercises must initially be restricted in their arc and intensity to prevent loss of reduction, wire migration, or skin and soft tissue irritation. Balancing the need to maintain fracture stability with the safe introduction of motion is based on scientific predictability and yet is the art and craft of hand fracture management.

Fracture configuration, impaction, periosteal disruption, muscle forces, and external forces may influence stability. Transverse and short oblique fractures have a stable conformation, whereas long oblique and comminuted fractures and those with bone loss have unstable patterns. Periosteal disruption correlates with the severity of the injury and the amount of fracture displacement. An intact or restored periosteum or bone impaction can support fracture alignment. Unbalanced muscle or external forces can cause fracture displacement or collapse. The "safe" hand position neutralizes the effects of muscle forces at the fracture site and thus, enhances fracture stability.

Fracture Stabilization

Nonoperative Management

Stable Undisplaced or Minimally Displaced Fractures

A majority of closed extra-articular hand fractures are simple (two-fragment), undisplaced or minimally displaced, and stable, and therefore may be safely and effectively treated by minimal protective orthoses and early motion.[38-41] This is especially true of impacted transverse or short oblique fractures at the base of the proximal phalanx and subcapital MC fractures with no rotational malalignment.[28,29] Indirect (secondary, enchondral, "biological," "physiologic," or undisturbed) bone healing occurs.

Displaced Fractures That Are Stable After Closed Reduction

Closed displaced transverse or short oblique simple extra-articular hand fractures may often be successfully reduced by closed manipulation (closed reduction, CR) and heal indirectly, or biologically.[41-46] Fractures with simple angulation are typically more easily reduced. The cortices on the angulated side of the fracture act as a hinge to implement reduction. The periosteum may be sufficiently intact to contribute to stability following reduction. Distal proximal phalanx fractures may have tenuous stability owing to their diminished cross-sectional area and the leverage of muscle forces at the fracture site. Successfully reduced fractures may require static immobilization for 3 weeks. External orthoses that protect the fracture and allow early ROM are optimal (Fig. 29-7).

Internal Fixation

Indications

The physician must weigh the risks to benefits of nonoperative versus operative correction and stabilization for each fracture and deformity. Internal fixation is reserved for unstable fractures, irreducible fractures, lost closed reductions, comminuted fractures, fractures with bone loss, multiple hand fractures, hand fractures accompanied by ipsilateral extremity injuries, open fractures, and pathologic fractures.[1,6-8] Secure stabilization may be advantageous for polytraumatized patients with a lower extremity long bone fracture to facilitate patient treatment, transfers, and the use of crutches or a walker for ambulation. Hall has reported the

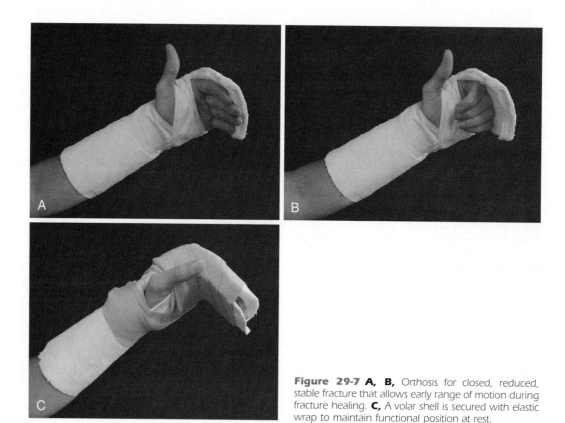

Figure 29-7 A, B, Orthosis for closed, reduced, stable fracture that allows early range of motion during fracture healing. **C,** A volar shell is secured with elastic wrap to maintain functional position at rest.

advantages of using secure fixation in noncompliant patients.[47] Maintenance of anatomic fracture position, wound access, early edema management, and the ability to initiate early and intensive exercises are relative benefits of secure internal fixation.

When surgery is necessary, the physician must also choose among approaches and implants. Fracture implants do not necessarily have to be the strongest available, but rather should be adequate in strength to reliably hold the fracture through the early stages of fracture callus formation and maturation.[48]

Minimally Invasive Surgery

Hand surgeons have long known the perils of indiscriminate open reduction and internal fixation and have been among the first to encourage minimally invasive surgery (MIS). MIS with closed reduction and internal fixation (CRIF) preserves periosteal integrity and circulation at the fracture site, minimizes expansion of the ZOI, allows for biological (undisturbed) fracture healing, and reduces the risk of additional adherent scar formation.[48,49] CRIF is advocated for unstable simple closed hand fractures whenever possible. CRIF aligns the fracture fragments; avoids periosteal dissection, bone exposure, and disturbance of the blood supply; minimizes implant-to-bone contact; allows physiologic interfragmentary stress and strain; stimulates callus formation; and allows graduated exercise.

Transverse or short oblique phalangeal and MC fractures may be stabilized with single or multiple intramedullary wires.[50-55] Locking pins or subcortical buttressing of the wires at one or both ends of the fragments adds stability at the fracture site. Oblique closed diaphyseal phalangeal fractures may be stabilized with percutaneous transfixation wires.[50,51] Percutaneous wires may be inserted transversely through an intact adjacent MC into one or both fragments of a closed simple unstable MC fracture to provide fixation.[56] Complex pilon fractures at the PIP joint can be reduced and the joint structure remodeled with the MIS percutaneous application of a transverse wire through the middle phalanx. The wire is dynamically attached to a moving component on an orthosis. Traction reduces the fracture length, while the intact and stretched periosteal sleeve compresses the fracture fragments (Fig. 29-8).

Open Reduction and Internal Fixation

Stable, or rigid, fixation is achieved at the price of a second planned wound to address the initial fracture injury.[8,11,12] Sharp, low-energy, neutrally placed incisions are less traumatic than random, high-energy, blunt impact, but they nevertheless create additional fibroplasia. The greater potential for soft tissue scarring with open reduction methods may be partially offset by the opportunity for earlier and more intensive exercise.

Most hand fractures are approached with a dorsal incision. Surgeons should try to avoid violation of the peritenon between the skin and tendon and between the tendon and bone as much as possible. Incising the skin and MC periosteum to one side of the extensor tendon and placing

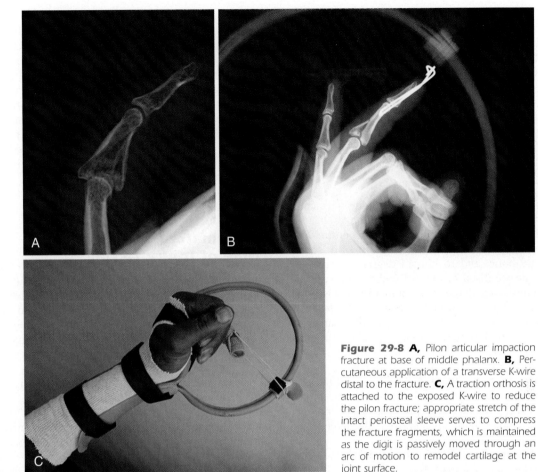

Figure 29-8 A, Pilon articular impaction fracture at base of middle phalanx. **B,** Percutaneous application of a transverse K-wire distal to the fracture. **C,** A traction orthosis is attached to the exposed K-wire to reduce the pilon fracture; appropriate stretch of the intact periosteal sleeve serves to compress the fracture fragments, which is maintained as the digit is passively moved through an arc of motion to remodel cartilage at the joint surface.

retractors between the periosteum and the bone helps to accomplish this goal.[8] Neutrally placed midlateral incisions and lateral band retraction or excision may facilitate phalangeal exposure for selected proximal phalangeal fractures, minimizing the risks of tendon attrition, scarring, and intrinsic tightness that may occur with lateral band incision and repair over an implant.[57] Open fractures may often be approached by extending the laceration or wound.[58] It may be prudent to secure the fracture with the most stable available implants that resources and the fracture configuration and operative exposure will allow.

Two or more miniscrews may be used to secure and often compress an oblique diaphyseal fracture.[1,6-8,59-68] Miniscrews may be thought of as small straight K-wires with a head and threads. The screw head buttresses the adjacent cortex while the threads grip the opposite cortex and enhance stability by compressing the fracture. The miniscrews protect each other from shear, rotational, and bending forces during rehabilitation and have the additional advantage of remaining in place for the duration of fracture healing. Miniscrew fixation supports primary bone healing. Miniscrews are usually removed only if they become symptomatic.

Although the dissection required for plate application, particularly in closed fractures, is technically demanding and may devascularize adjacent bone, delay bone healing, and generate additional fibroplasia, miniplates that compress the fracture provide excellent stability at the fracture site throughout healing.[6-8,64-73] In open fractures, especially those with complex wounds, comminution, or bone loss, priority must often be given to anatomic fracture restoration and healing.[58,74-79] Secure miniplate fixation provides for earlier and more intensive exercises than does flexible fixation and may at least partially offset the disadvantages of operatively generated fibroplasia.[8,11,12] "To operate on a fracture and fail to take advantage of the opportunity for early motion exposes the patient to the worst of both worlds: the injury is compounded and the potential gain is squandered."[73]

Miniplates positioned dorsally under the extensor tendons or dorsal apparatus may restrict the extremes of digital motion by their physical presence, especially as their edges approach adjacent joints. This is especially true of miniplates applied on the proximal phalanx adjacent to the PIP joint.

Straight miniplates are customarily applied to mid-diaphyseal fractures. Mini condylar plates have a fixed angle blade or locking peg that may assist in fracture reduction and may be applied either dorsally or laterally for juxta-articular fractures.[80,81] Primary or delayed primary bone grafting may be performed at the time of plate application in most patients.[75-79,82] Puckett and colleagues reported that microplates that allow closure of the periosteum have improved results in phalangeal fracture plating compared with larger miniplates that prevent periosteal closure.[83] Fracture stabilization, bone grafting when necessary, wound closure or coverage, and the initiation of rehabilitation within 3 to 5 days of injury may provide the best opportunity for optimal functional recovery of open or operated hand fractures.[8,20,58]

Pathophysiology

Regeneration is the restoration of damaged tissue with cells of the same kind. Although some species such as lizards (e.g., salamanders) and starfish can regenerate entire lost limbs, humans have retained this potential in only select tissues, liver, and bone, and to limited degrees. Peripheral nerves may regenerate distal to the cell bodies, and superficial skin lacerations regenerate true epidermis. Most soft tissue injuries heal instead through a process of *repair*, in which fibrous scar tissue forms to weld the damaged cells. Scar, then, is the biological "glue" that allows tissues to heal that have lost their regeneration potential. Bone heals by either primary or secondary regeneration. If the fragments are too distant from each other or insufficiently stable, regeneration cannot occur.[16,17] Conversely, small degrees of nondisruptive cyclic compression at the fracture site stimulates secondary bone regeneration and, later, bone remodeling.

Bone regeneration and soft tissue repair depend on complex processes—mechanoreception and cell signaling—to recruit migration of progenitor cells to the wound and to modulate proliferation and differentiation of these multipotential mesenchymal cells into cells capable of forming bone or scar tissue. This newly formed tissue must mature, strengthen, and reform its configuration to duplicate or approximate the original architecture and tissue function.

Bone must eventually heal with new bone by either passing through a temporary fibrocartilagenous phase prior to ossification (indirect healing) or through direct osteonal regeneration across the fracture site (direct healing). Both types of fracture healing ultimately lead to the regeneration of strong mature lamellar bone.

Indirect Bone Healing

Indirect fracture healing has also been called secondary healing, healing by enchondral ossification, or biological (undisturbed) bone healing.[16,18,48] Indirect bone healing evokes an evolutionary design wherein the requisite cellular response is matched to the wound environment to ensure that the repair process leads to bone formation. A fusiform external callus surrounds the periphery of the fracture site and cascades through the entire spectrum of connective tissue from hematoma to granulation tissue, fibrous tissue, hyaline cartilage, woven bone, and, ultimately, lamellar bone to weld the fracture fragments and ultimately allow cancellous and medullary healing. Five factors are necessary for indirect bone regeneration: (1) a fracture hematoma as a source of signaling molecules, (2) a vibrant, diversified cell population to ensure healing progression and nutrition, (3) an adequate blood supply, (4) an evolving scaffold for cellular differentiation, and (5) a mechanical environment of relative stability that minimizes interfragmentary strain.[84,85] This programmed sequence of tissue differentiation allows the most robust cells—fibroblasts and chondroblasts—to endure through an environment of compromised circulation, oxygen depletion, and instability until the metabolic and mechanical conditions are conducive to successful osteoblastic bone replacement. Finally, fragile woven bone is stress-remodeled into strong lamellar bone. Cyclic reciprocal micromotion (compression–distraction) facilitates this process.[86]

Inflammatory (Acute) Phase (Time of Injury to Day 5)

The bones of the hand have a rich periosteal, intramedullary, and metaphyseal blood supply. No cell lies more than 300 μm from a blood vessel.[87] Histamine-mediated vasodilation occurs during the first several minutes following fracture. Whole blood pours into and expands the space about the fracture fragments and torn soft tissues, creating a liquid hematoma (Fig. 29-9A, online). Local compression, secondary vasoconstriction, platelets, and the clotting cascade lead to the formation of a gelatinous blood clot. There are no functioning blood vessels in the fracture clot.[88]

The hematoma and injured periosteum have important and complementary roles in the cellular events necessary for normal fracture healing. Consequently, early evacuation of the hematoma or excision or stripping of the damaged periosteum retards indirect healing.[89-91] The blood clot contains growth factors, cytokines, and other complex peptides that stimulate neoangiogenesis and attract white blood cells, macrophages, and multipotential mesenchymal cells to the fracture area.[92-94] Within 24 hours after fracture, endothelial cells that line intramedullary capillaries enlarge and migrate into the damaged area, initiating neoangiogenesis. Cells, nutrients, and cell-signaling peptides diffuse into the periphery of the blood clot from local soft tissues and new capillaries. White blood cells secrete lysozymes that dissolve the blood clot. Macrophages and osteoclasts phagocytize the clot and necrotic debris. Macrophages and platelets generate many of the additional complex cell-signaling peptides that modulate mesenchymal cell differentiation and tissue development. Mesenchymal cells recruited from the damaged periosteum, adjacent muscle, and regenerating blood supply differentiate into fibroblasts in the initially acidic and hypoxic environment and invade the periphery of the blood clot.[95] The periosteum is the principal source of multipotent mesenchymal cells. Granulation tissue (fibroblasts and white blood cells) form the early pliable fusiform external fracture callus on the periphery of the blood clot and between the fragments.

Reparative (Proliferative) Phase (Day 5 to Day 21)

Healing by natural means (indirect or secondary repair) involves a gradual substitution of tissues that protects the fracture while bone is regenerated. Tissue oxygenation gradually improves and acidity proportionally decreases as neoangiogenesis progresses, facilitating centripetal healing of the external fusiform fibrous fracture callus from its periphery toward the center of the fracture. Mesenchymal cells now differentiate into chondrocytes rather than fibroblasts, until the fibrous callus is replaced by nonmineralized hyaline cartilaginous scaffolding that encompasses the fracture site (Fig. 29-9B, online). If the bone gap is not bridged by cartilaginous callus within 2 to 3 weeks after injury, the initial callus response may fail.[16]

As stability increases, tissue oxygenation continues to improve and the ECM becomes alkaline. At 10 to 21 days after injury, the cartilage matrix begins to undergo progressive centripetal enchondral ECM calcification.[96] Bone morphogenic protein 7 (BMP-7), also known as osteogenic protein 1 (OP-1), modulates new mesenchymal precursor cells to become osteoblasts. The new osteoblasts invade the cartilaginous callus to form immature trabecular "woven bone" across the fracture site. Cartilage cells undergo apoptosis and are removed by chondroclasts. From the second to the sixth week after injury, intermittent axial compression can increase corticomedullary blood flow and stimulate chondrogenesis and, later, osteogenesis throughout the callus.[84,97,98] Conversely, excessive shearing motion during this time can impede neoangiogenesis and delay or prevent fracture healing by damaging new arterioles and capillaries. Throughout this process, the external fracture callus progressively solidifies and becomes stronger. The periosteal, intracortical, cancellous, and intramedullary blood flow normalizes. Intramedullary healing proceeds. Interfragmentary motion (IFM) progressively decreases and finally ceases at approximately 4 to 6 weeks after injury. At this point the fracture is clinically stable, even though radiolucent portions of the fracture may be seen on radiograph.

Remodeling (Maturation) Phase (Day 21 to 18 Months)

The reparative phase of healing extends into the remodeling phase. The initially accreted immature woven bone is randomly aligned and weaker than normal lamellar bone. The ideal goal of fracture healing is to regain the original form and function of the healed bone (Fig. 29-9C). Progressive remodeling of primary immature trabecular bone along the lines of axial stress forms compact lamellar bone (Wolff's law) and reestablishes the Haversian canals.[99] During this process, osteoclasts remove the weaker woven bone from the tension sides of trabeculae, and osteoblasts accrete linear layers of mature new bone on the compression sides parallel to the stress forces. Osteoclastic metabolism (bone resorption) is initially 50 times greater than osteoblastic activity (bone accretion). This initial imbalance creates temporary local bone porosity that facilitates neovascularization into the Haversian canals. Bone remodeling and metabolic equilibration takes approximately 5 months to complete in the tubular bones of the hand.[100] These forces direct the orientation of newly formed bone to provide better mechanical advantage and duplicate the original shape and strength of normal bone. Each region of each bone responds to a particular amount of intermittent strain, creating an "optimal strain environment"

for remodeling.[101,102] Static loading has little influence on bone architecture. A distinctive "dose/response" curve is generated by daily short, intermittent stimulation exposure with strain magnitudes within the physiologic safe range for the bone. Fracture remodeling is optimally influenced by a regimen of dynamic, diverse activities that do not exceed the strain tolerance level of the bone.[103-105] Remodeling does not always occur simultaneously in all areas of the fracture.[106] The injured bone regains approximately 80% of its original strength within 3 months after fracture, although 18 to 24 months is often required to regain normal tensile strength.

Remodeling allows some correction of angular deformities along the lines of linear stress in younger children, and occasionally in adolescents and adults, but does not correct rotational deformities. The ability of bone remodeling to correct angular deformities by remodeling diminishes with age.

Direct (Primary) Bone Healing

Primary (contact) bone healing begins when the gap between fragments is eliminated and the reduced fragments are compressed and held with secure fixation.[17,107-109] In primary healing, one or more compression implants (miniscrews, miniplate, tension band, or 90/90 wiring) anatomically and physiologically replace the external enchondral fusiform callus. Union occurs by the direct formation of bone across the cortex and intramedullary canal at the fracture site. Compression prevents motion at the fracture site, yet allows load transmission that stimulates healing and remodeling. The implants initially bear the entire load of forces across the fracture site. The forces proportionately shift to the bone as healing proceeds so that little load is borne by the implants at the culmination of fracture healing. Although periosteal excision or stripping can initially inhibit fracture healing, secure fixation can be maintained throughout fracture healing. Tensile strength at the fracture site becomes comparable to that of undisturbed fracture healing at approximately 12 weeks of healing.

Even with good reduction and compression, not all interfragmentary areas are in perfect contact. Contact areas and small gaps of less than 1 to 2 mm coexist at the interface of the fracture fragments. Osteoblasts are recruited from the periosteum into the small gaps and begin to synthesize osteoid between the fracture edges. New woven bone forms. This process called *gap healing* is somewhat comparable to road crews filling in potholes prior to resurfacing.

Basic multicellular units (BMUs) begin to form in the cortical bone adjacent to both sides of the fracture within 48 hours after surgery. BMUs are composed of osteoclasts, osteoblasts, and small nutrient vessels (Fig. 29-10, online). Macrophage-derived osteoclasts tunnel toward the fracture, phagocytizing necrotic bone, hematoma, and debris, and form a "cutting cone" as they migrate toward the fracture (Fig. 29-11, online). Mesenchymal cells differentiate into osteoblasts and line the trailing surface of the cutting cone and are supported by central regenerating small blood vessels that supply nutrients and remove soluble waste material. The osteoblasts accrete immature and lamellar bone as they travel toward the fracture in the wake of the osteoclasts. BMUs are active at a low level in adult bone, maintaining a balance between bone resorption and deposition. After fracture, local BMUs experience a 20- to 30-fold increase in activation.[110] New osteons, the basic building units of bone, are formed across the fracture site within 5 to 6 weeks after stabilization.

Reparative (Proliferative) Phase (Time of Surgery to Day 21)

The acute phase is converted into the repair phase by open reduction, internal fixation, and compression at the fracture site. Axial cutting cones from the major cortical fragments tunnel toward one another. At approximately 7 days after fracture fixation, new bone formation from both contact and gap healing is advancing across the defect. The ongoing BMU activity of osteoclastic resorption with osteoblastic bone formation becomes the major Haversian remodeling factor. BMU remodeling is not in balance, however, as osteoclastic (resorption) activity is 50 times greater than osteoblastic (formation) action. This initial imbalance allows for greater porosity in the bone, facilitating ingrowth of new blood vessels into the Haversian canals.

Remodeling (Maturation— Day 21 to 18 Months)

By 5 to 6 weeks, lamellar bone has replaced all of the immature bone.[111] Primary and secondary callus strengths in similar fractures become equivalent after 6 weeks.[84] The return of well-ordered lamellar bone that resembles the pre-injury bony architecture requires 12 or more weeks. Despite the appearance of mature vascularized lamellar bone in the fracture area, much of the bone lacks axis organization relative to stress. Normal cancellous bone is structured with its axes perpendicular to the forces of muscle tension.[112] Healing fractures attain stiffness with early bone formation to resist strain or tissue deformation and refracture. Repetitive loading of skeletal tissue results in adaptation of bone configuration by changing its structure, density, and orientation through BMU activity.

Even at 12 weeks, the lamellation throughout the defect remains in a distinctly different plane than surrounding non-injured bone. As immature bone is removed, new mature bone is laid down perpendicular to the load. Although stiffness is achieved early in fracture healing, normal lamellar realignment and bone strength requires greater than 3 months to achieve.[113]

Healing fractures attain stiffness with early bone formation to resist strain or tissue deformation (refracture). Stiffness does not mean strength. Repetitive loading of skeletal tissue results in adaptation of bone configuration by changing its structure, density, and orientation through BMU activity. As immature bone is removed, new mature bone is laid down perpendicular to the load. Stiffness is achieved early in fracture healing, whereas normal bone strength requires many months to regain lamellar alignment. Stiffness determines when the healed fracture is ready to handle normal physiologic forces; strength determines when high-work forces and sports can be resumed.[114]

Interstitial Scar Formation

Inflammatory (Acute) Phase (Time of Injury to Day 5)

Edema (excessive interstitial fluid) rapidly accumulates in the affected soft tissues and tissue planes as a result of local injury, relative acidity, increased hypoxia, and capillary permeability.[2,9-12,115] The extent of the edema defines the ZOI (see Fig. 29-1). The soft tissue disruption may be confined to the surrounding periosteum and subcutaneous tissue in low-energy, closed two-fragment fractures. High-energy crush or blast injuries initiate a substantially greater ZOI than closed fractures and may cause bone comminution and complex wounds.

Edema fluid, which contains fibrin, polymorphonucleocytes, lymphocytes, monocytes, and macrophages, invests or permeates tissue planes in both injured and uninjured soft tissues within the ZOI adjacent to the fracture.[2,9-12,115] Fibroblasts may be seen in the ZOI as early as 48 hours after fracture. Fibroblasts enlarge, duplicate, and begin to synthesize and extrude fibrin at 3 to 5 days after injury. Mucopolysaccharides, fibronectin, and fibrin permeate the ECM within the ZOI. Fibronectin attaches to tissue surface cells and also acts as a latticework to guide fibrin migration. Fibrin strength is negligible until 3 to 5 days after injury.

Reparative (Proliferative) Phase (Day 5 to Day 21)

Over time, fibrin evolves into scar tissue.[2,10-12,115] Mucopolysaccharides within the ECM gradually solidify to form a fibrin and fibronectin-reinforced "tissue glue" that can cause permanent tissue adhesions and joint contractures. At this phase, the entire wound and all injured structures are bathed by the same "inflammatory soup." Without treatment, the tissues immersed in the inflammatory soup within the ZOI tend to congeal into a single inelastic amalgam of randomly oriented fibrous tissue and ECM adjacent to the regenerating bone, creating the concept of "one wound/one scar."[2]

The ratio of collagen fibers to ground substance varies, providing different tissue flexibility and strength characteristics in diverse tissues. Low oxygen tension and an acidic (lactic and pyruvic acid) environment favor the evolution of fibroplasia. Extracellular fibrin follows randomly arranged fibronectin channels to align randomly in the ECM (Fig. 29-12, online). Fibronectin and fibrin attach to the surface cells of adjacent soft tissues and may form adhesions that contract over time. Soft tissue injury associated with fractures further compounds fibroplasia and confounds treatment.

Digital motion facilitates edema resorption, stimulates fibrin and early collagen fibers to align parallel to the lines of axial stress, inhibits the attachment of fibronectin and fibrin to adjacent soft tissues, promotes collagen elasticity, and may shear early adhesions with minimal additional trauma. Proliferative fibroplasia spikes on the seventh day after injury, continues for 2 weeks, and then gradually diminishes over the next 3 months. Opportunities for regaining normal tissue integrity and motion are gained or lost during this period of high tissue turnover.

Soft tissues heal by an inferior connective scar tissue "patching process," termed *repair*, that occurs between reapproximated lacerated or torn tissues with adhesions that join the adjacent tissues. The lacerated or lost tissue is not regenerated, but rather replaced with collagen (scar) tissue spawned from biologically abundant fibroblasts. Approximated soft tissue lacerations heal by primary intention, that is, direct fibroblastic scar formation. Skin or tendon edges must be sufficiently apposed and stable while healing to prevent disruption. Small incremental degrees of nondisruptive to-and-fro motion stimulate physiologic (parallel) fibrin alignment, viscoelasticity, strengthening, and maturation of the collagenous bond during healing, while preventing interstitial tissue adhesions to adjacent structures.

Wound defects heal by secondary intention. Granulation tissue (white blood cells and fibrin) replaces the initial hematoma clot with randomly oriented fibrin molecules that form on the periphery of the wound and progress toward the center of the wound as wound contracture simultaneously occurs (centripetal healing). Larger wound defects may require skin grafting or flap coverage.

Remodeling (Maturation) Phase (Day 21 to 6 Months)

Although collagen metabolism remains elevated in the wound relative to noninjured tissue, a balance between synthesis and degradation is gradually regained. Wound strength initially depends on relatively weak intramolecular collagen bonding that occurs within each collagen fiber. Insoluble disulfide bonding (intermolecular bonds) between collagen molecules begins to occur at 21 days and substantially accelerates and increases the tensile strength of scar tissue. Digital motion continues to align collagen molecules in parallel along the lines of stress and prevents tendon adhesions and joint contracture while allowing repaired structures to remodel and strengthen. Collagenase degrades random fibers, and collagen is remodeled along the lines of tension. Cells that are no longer needed are removed after apoptosis. Although metabolically elevated, collagen synthesis and lysis come into balance in normal wound healing. The sinusoidal pattern of parallel realigned collagen fibers allows the reestablishment of normal soft tissue viscoelasticity, expansion and contraction, and tensile strength. Scar tissue becomes more pliable as the excessive blood vessels recede, changing the wound color from red to pink to pale.

Malpositioned statically held ligaments, capsule, or an attenuated central slip dorsal to the PIP joint begin to remodel in inelastic contracted or attenuated resting positions.[11-15] Adhesions may also form. Secondary pseudoclawing of the fingers can occur and become fixed. Proper hand positioning and early exercises implement physiologic remodeling, tendon gliding, and joint motion.

Rehabilitation

Functional recovery is the fundamental goal of hand fracture rehabilitation.[10-12] The physician must inform the therapist of the date and extent of injury; the date(s) of CR, CRIF, or open reduction and internal fixation (ORIF); the method and reliability of fixation; and any anticipated deformities or projected problems. Together, the physician and therapist must formulate a plan and timeline for rehabilitation. They must inform, educate, encourage, and monitor the patient until treatment goals are achieved and the patient has reached a point of maximum medical improvement (MMI).

Acute (Inflammatory) Phase (Time of Injury or Operation to Day 5)

Rehabilitation begins with a well-padded protective orthosis supporting a stable reduced fracture and, properly positioned, the resting hand. Swollen digits tend to assume a dysfunctional posture with MCP joint extension, PIP joint flexion, and thumb web space narrowing. The resting hand should be positioned in the "safe" (rehabilitation ready) position with the MCP joint in 50 to 70 degrees of flexion and the PIP joints in full extension.[13] Metacarpophalangeal joint flexion prevents MCP joint extension contracture by maintaining the collateral ligaments in their lengthened position. MCP joint flexion also creates a distal glide of the extensor hood over P1, providing additional soft tissue support for digital fractures. PIP joint extension allays extensor lag, central slip attenuation, and flexion contracture. The thumb is palmar-abducted, and the first web space is maintained to facilitate pinch and grasp. Bone and joint prominences should be protected by adequate soft padding or orthotic relief to avoid pressure points. A few degrees of digital motion within the dressing is permissible.

The RICE regimen of **rest–ice–compression–elevation** can be carried out at home immediately following injury, CR, CRIF, or ORIF.[11,12] The RICE regime initially moderates edema and the other acute inflammatory responses of injury and, later, facilitates their dissipation. Compression must be judiciously applied and carefully monitored. Continuous, writhing unremitting pain signifies a pressure point or tight dressing and must be relieved as soon as recognized. Complaints should be addressed swiftly.

Repair (Proliferative or Fibroblastic) Phase (Day 5 to Day 21)

The initial orthosis and any surgical dressings are ideally gently removed within 3 to 7 days following injury or operation. Incisions and wounds can be inspected, evaluated, cleaned, and redressed. Radiographs may be taken to confirm the fracture and implant positions.

Proper orthotic use, hand elevation, and the recovery of motion are the most important elements of functional recovery.[10-15,103-105,116-118] Orthoses must be light in weight and comfortable. Strength and endurance are relatively easily regained once the fracture has achieved inherent stability and joints have recovered mobility during the healing process.

Prefabricated or custom-made fracture-specific, protective static or dynamic orthoses can be applied for MC or phalangeal fractures. The orthosis supports and protects the fracture and the adjacent soft tissues and joints. The hand is positioned in the safe rehabilitation-ready position. The wrist is positioned in 15 to 20 degrees of flexion in instances of

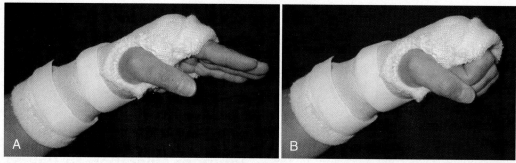

Figure 29-13 A, Proximal phalanx fracture orthosis that positions the metacarpopalangeal joint in flexion, draws the extensor mechanism distally to further compress the fracture, and places the extrinsic extensor tendons on stretch to facilitate proximal interphalangeal joint extension. **B,** Full digital flexion is also encouraged.

phalangeal fractures to allow the extrinsic extensor tendons to assist the intrinsic muscles in extending the PIP finger joints (Fig. 29-13).[10] Conversely, the wrist is extended 15 to 20 degrees in patients with MC fractures to facilitate digital flexion. An attachment may be added to the orthosis to hold the PIP joints fully extended between therapy sessions and at night. The attachment is removed to allow early controlled exercise sessions. Proper positioning of the resting hand and early exercise augment joint recovery, tendon gliding, and collagen remodeling while limiting the opportunities for tissue adhesions, joint and thumb web space contracture, central slip attenuation, and PIP joint lag. Joints may be released from orthotic protection once full active motion is recovered (serial orthotic reduction).[44] Serial orthotic reduction, allowing controlled graduated wrist motion proximally and digital motion distally as the fracture heals, decreases morbidity. Protective orthoses are worn until pain, swelling, and tenderness abate and until joints adjacent to the fracture have recovered full or maximum active motion.

Hand elevation and early digital motion minimize the accumulation of additional edema and enhance edema resorption, decreasing the hydrostatic resistance to tendon, ligament, and capsular excursion. As local signs recede and fracture stiffness and strength improves, exercises may be proportionately increased in intensity and duration. Progress is guided by soft tissue response, fracture stability, and the patient's pain tolerance; stopping short of generating additional inflammatory or fibroblastic response.

Although some evidence suggests that exercises may be delayed as long as 21 days after injury for low-energy, minimally displaced, closed simple MC or phalangeal diaphyseal injuries, the preponderance of evidence indicates better results and less morbidity with very early initiated rehabilitation, especially in high-energy closed crush injuries, open fractures, and fractures requiring ORIF.[103-105,119] Adhesion and contractures have either not occurred or are in an early stage of formation when they can more easily be modified or overcome. Fracture stability limits pain and allows more rapid implementation of exercises. Careful Coban digital wrapping and retrograde massage may diffuse edema and assist the recovery of motion in finger fractures treated with stable fixation.[120]

The rehabilitation of proximal phalangeal fractures correlates very closely with that of zone II flexor tendon injuries, and the rehabilitation of MC fractures corresponds similarly to that of extensor tendon lacerations in zones V and VI.[10-15,103-105,114-118,121,122] Duran and Houser reported that the recovery of 4 to 5 mm of flexor tendon excursion during the 4 weeks following flexor tendon repair in zone II reliably prevented the formation of permanent adhesions between bone and tendon and correlated with good to excellent final digital motion in 90% of patients with zone II flexor tendon lacerations.[123] Less than the recovery of 4 to 5 mm of flexor tendon exclusion during the 4 weeks following surgery predicted fair or poor results. Extrapolation of these findings to proximal phalangeal fractures and allowance for 4 to 5 mm of both adjacent flexor and extensor tendon excursion would require a 40 to 50 degrees partial arc of PIP joint and total active finger motion (TAM). A recent report suggests that only 1 to 2 mm of tendon excursion may be necessary to prevent tendon adhesions.[124]

Early controlled, soft tissue, and pain-modulated digital motion and tendon-gliding exercises are therefore given priority during the reparative stage of healing. PROM exercises primarily move and stretch early formative scar tissue distal to their points of fixation. AROM exercises are necessary to mobilize scar tissue proximally from their points of fixation. Combined PROM and AROM exercises helps to ensure parallel alignment and ultimately remodeling, elasticity, and motion of interstitial collagen and scar tissue.

In fractures treated with flexible fixation (Kirschner and cerclage wires or external fixation), rehabilitation should be limited to tendon-gliding exercises and short-arc PROM and AROM exercises for approximately 21 days after surgery. These limitations help to avoid wire loosening and migration as well as fracture displacement[10-15,103-105,114-118,121,122] (Fig. 29-14). These exercises alternately focus on gradually regaining full extension and approximately 60 to 70 degrees of flexion of the PIP and MCP joints.

PIP joint extensor lag with central slip and dorsal capsular attenuation and volar plate adhesions commonly complicates proximal phalangeal fractures. A dorsal incision over the proximal phalanx or PIP joint may further confound the outcome due to the exposure of the extensor apparatus to additional fibroplasia. A pseudoclaw deformity may occur and become fixed over time. Resting the PIP joint in full extension and early focus on terminal active PIP joint extension and differential gliding exercises of the central slip and lateral bands may prevent PIP joint lag or deformity.

Composite progressive full-arc digital exercises are delayed in fractures treated with coaptive fixation until inherent

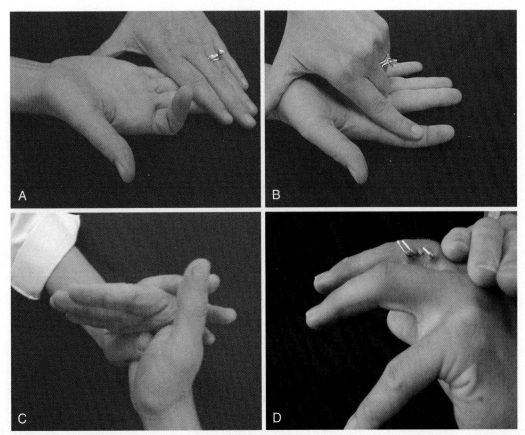

Figure 29-14 Tendon-gliding exercises to maintain mobility for: **A,** flexor digitorum superficialis, **B,** flexor digitorum profundis, and **C,** central slip. **D,** Patient with percutaneous K-wires performing central slip-gliding exercise.

stability is ensured and K-wires or external minifixators have been removed at approximately 21 to 28 days after fixation. Inherently stable fractures and fractures treated with stable fixation (miniscrews, miniplates, or tension band or 90–90 wires) may progress as tolerated with all soft tissue–moderated exercises from the outset of treatment. Composite full-arc digital exercises allow the common muscle to the ulnar three profundus tendons to activate cohesively, simultaneously, and with more force and control than do isolated digital exercises. Fingers work best that work together. Although isolated digital exercises play an important role in recovery, composite full-arc digital exercises also help to prevent stiffness in fingers adjacent to the fracture site (quadriga).

An orthosis with a wrist-lock allows protected, active, progressive reciprocal-wrist extension, finger and wrist flexion, and finger extension. These exercises may be initiated within the first week after injury or operation for patients with secure fracture fixation and after 3 to 4 weeks for patients with flexible fixation. PIP joint extensors are weak and have a poor moment arm. Simultaneous wrist flexion and finger extension allows the extrinsic finger extensors to assist the intrinsic PIP joint extensors to recover the critical position and active function of full PIP extension. It is important to maintain the PIP joint in full extension at rest until full active extension is recovered or until maximum improvement. Although supportive use of orthoses and controlled progressive exercises to recover motion may inhibit intrinsic

muscle recovery, they tend to decrease morbidity and implement return to work and athletics.[125]

Once incisions and wounds are cleaned, closed, and dry, massage softens, desensitizes, and mobilizes scar tissue. Any number of creams, including white petrolatum, cocoa butter, and those containing aloe or vitamin E, may be used as a vehicle for massage. Adherent topical silicone sheeting may also soften scar tissue and be used as a method of scar management. Scar management and desensitization may be beneficial for up to 6 months from the time of injury or ORIF.

Patients are instructed and checked out for daily home programs (DHP) of rehabilitation. Written instructions and diagrams are provided whenever possible. Outpatient progress can be checked concurrently at the time of physician follow-up. Reinforcement can be provided and advancements integrated. As long as the patient is progressing satisfactorily, the DHP can continue under periodic outpatient supervision. If the patient fails to progress or loses ground, additional more intensive outpatient therapy and supervision can be scheduled.[126] This strategy combines excellence in care with cost-effectiveness.

Remodeling (Maturation) Phase (Day 21 to 6 Months)

At 4 weeks after injury, fracture callus is usually sufficiently developed, and pain, swelling, and tenderness are adequately

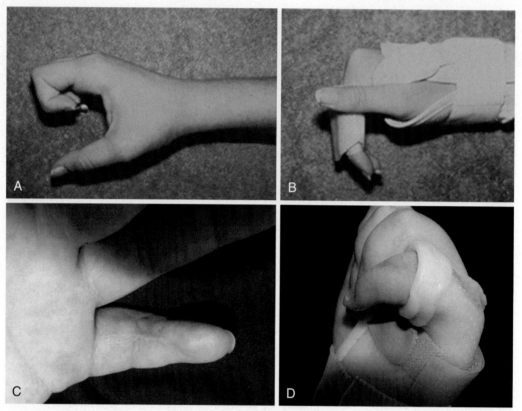

Figure 29-15 A, Metacarpal (MC) fractures can result in limited MCP joint flexion. **B,** Circumferential orthotic blocking of the proximal interphalangeal (PIP) joints concentrates extrinsic flexor action at the MCP joint (note wrist orthosis to prevent compensatory wrist flexion with effort). **C,** Proximal pha-langeal fractures can result in loss of terminal PIP joint extension initially, followed by loss of PIP joint flexion. **D,** A short circumferential blocking orthosis of the MCP joint, allows extrinsic extensor and flexor tendon power to be directed more distally to the PIP joint.

improved or resolved, such that temporary K-wire fixation may be removed. At the same time, patients are weaned from their orthotics as soon as fracture stability, functional recovery, healing, pain, and tenderness allow. Once calcified fracture callus bridges the fracture fragments on radiographic examination, the fracture is "locked," and adequate fracture healing and stability are ensured. This ordinarily occurs within 4 to 6 weeks after injury. Callus strength is then sufficient to support intensified exercises, including strengthening and conditioning, passive stretching, electrical muscle stimulation, and exercises with static joint blocking with minimal risk of fracture displacement.[10-12,127]

Patients with MC fractures, dorsal edema, secondary MCP joint extension, and inhibition of the intrinsic MCP joint flexors tend to develop extensor tendon and capsular adhesions to the fracture callus or MCP joint, limiting MCP joint flexion and leading to a pseudoclaw deformity. An incision overlying the MC or MCP joint may further compound the problem. Use of a static orthosis of the interphalangeal joints in full extension and active MCP joint flexion exercises translate the full force of finger flexion to the MCP joints and across the MCP–extensor tendon interface to overcome dorsal adhesions and reestablish extensor tendon excursion and MCP joint flexion (Fig. 29-15A, B). PIP joint extension contractures are less common than flexion contractures, but do occur. MCP joint blocking orthoses allow simultaneous forceful PIP joint flexion of all of the fingers and may facilitate improvement (Fig. 29-15C, D).

Stretching creates tension at the sites of interstitial adhesions. Tension, applied to healing soft tissues during remodeling, stimulates strengthening in tissues. Collagen turnover, through synthesis and degradation, remains higher in the healing tissue than in normal noninjured tissue. Fibroblasts and the collagen fibers they produce, line up in parallel with lines of tension.[128] As collagenase cleaves and removes the initial randomly oriented fibers, the fibroblasts synthesize new collagen in line with the tension. The resorption of weak fiber alignment, and replacement with parallel fiber alignment, directs the healing tissue to regain its preinjury form and function. The normal mechanical factors of tension, compression, and stretch, when reintroduced appropriately during healing, cause an increase in tensile strength through the mechanically induced change in tissue architecture. In addition to passive stretching and blocking exercises, low-load, long duration or cyclical dynamic orthoses designed to overcome tendon and joint adhesions may also be safely applied once calcified bridging fracture callus is radiographically apparent. Dynamic orthoses may be used in conjunction with passive stretching exercises and blocking exercises or may be reserved for patients whose fractures fail to respond to exercise therapy. Dynamic orthoses should be worn for 6-hour intervals at least once a day for maximum effectiveness. Serial casting may be applied for more severe, long-standing, or recalcitrant deformities. Serial casts can be worn for 6 days prior to being replaced.[129] It is important to stretch and mobilize developing scar tissue in both the proximal and distal directions from points of fixation in order to achieve maximum elasticity and functional improvement. Continued AROM exercises facilitate stretching and blocking exercises and the use of dynamic orthoses and serial casting in achieving this goal.

Heat effectively implements stretching. When collagen tissue temperature exceeds 40°C, there is a 25% increase in potential elongation[130,131] Lentell and coworkers found that the use of heat applied during stretching produced twice the gains in half the time as occurred with heat or stretch used alone.[132] Superficial heat with paraffin wax, hot packs, and fluidotherapy are excellent methods for heat delivery because the temperature rise and depth of heat penetration are adequate for the small volume of the hand.

Outcomes and Complications

Outcomes and complications are irrevocably linked. Complications are the obverse of excellent and good results. There currently is no universally accepted criterion for classification of results following hand fracture healing. Variances in inclusion criteria, fixation, follow-up interval, and evaluation make comparison and meta-analysis of results difficult. Nevertheless, implications may be drawn from available data.

Digital motion correlates highly with functional recovery after fracture union. Total active range of motion (TAM) of the injured digit serves as an indicator of functional recovery. The formula for functional determination is TAM = AF (active flexion) of the MCP, PIP, and DIP joints minus extension deficits of all three. Thus, any joint contracture or extensor lag is subtracted from the sum of the joint flexion of the MCP, PIP, and DIP. Hyperextension, if present, is recorded as 0 degrees and is noted.

The criteria applied to recovery of digital motion following flexor tendon repair has been applied to hand fracture evaluation.[51,58,133] Eighty-five percent to 100% of total active finger motion (TAM) (220–260 degrees in the finger and 120–140 degrees in the thumb) is an excellent result. Seventy percent to 85% of TAM (180–220 degrees in the fingers and 95–120 degrees in the thumb) is a good result. Fifty percent to 70% of TAM (130–180 degrees in the fingers and 70–95 degrees in the thumb) is a fair result. Anything less than 50% TAM is a poor result. Another commonly applied alternative and more stringent classification for finger recovery considers more than 210 degrees a good result, 180 to 210 degrees a fair result, and less than 180 degrees a poor result.[59,65-68,74,76] An excellent result using these criteria should also have greater than 100 degrees of PIP joint finger flexion and less than 15 degrees PIP joint extensor lag or contracture.[42,134] A good result should include greater than 80 degrees of PIP joint finger flexion and less than 35 degrees of PIP joint extensor lag or contracture. Any result with less than 80 degrees of PIP joint finger flexion or more than 35 degrees of PIP joint extensor lag should be considered a poor result. The inclusion of fractures having modest loss of motion in either the good or excellent category attests to both the frequency of residual digital stiffness and the capacity of the hand to accommodate to these residuals.

Some researchers consider only those patients with healed fractures, no functional deformity, and recovery of full TAM as having excellent results; however, this criterion has not been expressed in previous reports. Motion in comparable fractures are often improved at 6 months or more of follow-up as compared with those limited to 6 weeks of follow-up, emphasizing the importance of extended follow-up in evaluating functional recovery in patients that have not recovered full TAM.[42]

Stiffness is the most common complication of hand fractures.[135-137] Among the digits, thumb fractures have the best prognosis. MC fractures tend to have better results than comparable fractures of the proximal phalanx. Initial soft tissue and fracture severity correlate very highly with functional outcome[58,66-69,75,77,119,138] (Fig. 29-16, online). Simple skin lacerations alone usually do not adversely affect the results in hand fractures. Age over 50 years and systemic diseases can impair or delay fracture healing.

Inherently stable undisplaced or minimally displaced simple phalangeal and MC fractures and those that are stable after reduction, or stabilized with flexible fixation, have approximately 90% or greater good or excellent results.[39,41,50,51] Percutaneous or open pin or screw fixation provides comparable results of approximately 90% good or excellent results in unstable oblique proximal phalangeal and MC fractures.[39,50,51,59-62] Morbidity may often be substantially decreased by allowing early motion.[10-12,103-105] Continuous static immobilization of joints adjacent to the fracture should not exceed 21 to 28 days.

As many as 15% of patients with simple hand fractures treated with percutaneous K-wire fixation may experience skin irritation; digital nerve injury; pin tract infection; wire loosening, migration, or bending; joint penetration; tendon impalement or attrition; or fracture settling or collapse.[139,140] Permanent functional impairment is rare in simple fractures. Permanent adhesions or persistent infection rarely occur if the wires are removed within 4 weeks after insertion.

The magnitude of some injuries precludes good or excellent results despite the best efforts of treatment and rehabilitation.[58,66-68,75,77,120,138] Intra-articular, comminuted, and multiple hand fractures; fractures with skin or bone loss; and fractures requiring miniplate fixation have fewer good or excellent and more fair or poor results than low-energy, closed, simple isolated extra-articular fractures treated nonoperatively or with MIS.[39-45,51-54,59-63] Extensor, flexor, or combined tendon injuries further adversely affect treatment and results. Fractures with complete tendon laceration are likely to lose more motion than those with partial lacerations. Contamination and delay in wound or fracture care may also have a deleterious effect. Patients with more than one of these risk factors and those with segmental tendon injuries are in even greater peril.

Secure fixation and early motion favorably affect outcomes even in many patients with one or more risk factors for stiffness.[66-68] An aligned, pain-free digit with adequate sensation and circulation may often be integrated into useful hand function, despite substantial stiffness, and is preferable to ablation. Flexor hinge function at the MCP joint may allow a stiff finger to participate in limited pinching and gripping activities, handling of objects, tool or machine use, and two-handed undertakings.

Nonunion is rare in simple hand fractures.[38,39] The nonunion rate may slightly escalate in comminuted fractures and fractures with inadequate stability or fixation, bone loss, or with more severely complex wounds.[77,119] Inadequate K-wire fixation of comminuted fractures has been commonly associated with MC and phalangeal nonunions.[141] Delayed or nonunion can cause loss of fixation or miniplate fatigue breakage.[75]

Although one study reported a 13% incidence of malunion of proximal phalangeal fractures and another reported 10% in hand fractures, the overall incidence of functionally impaired hands owing to malunion is probably below 5%.[119,138] Malunion rates are influenced by fracture severity, delay in seeking or obtaining treatment, and technical errors of fixation.

Infections have been reported in from 2% to 10% of hand fractures.[75,77,119,138] Open fractures, especially in soiled or mutilated hands, are much more likely to acquire infection than closed fractures or those treated with elective surgery. Osteomyelitis is rare, but does occur.

As many as 30% of patients, especially manual workers and patients with dominant-hand injuries, may have various degrees of difficulty returning to work.[66,67] As many as 15% may have to modify work or change jobs to sustain gainful employment.[59]

CCRP (RSD) may occur and is probably underreported. CCRP–RSD introduces a second wave of inflammation and fibroplasia of varying intensity and severity. CCRP–RSD can be followed by stiffness, atrophy, cold intolerance, algodynia, and hypersensitivity to touch and percussion. CCRP–RSD confounds and prolongs fracture treatment and can further compromise outcome. Early recognition and vigorous treatment is the key to successful treatment.

Summary

Successful management of hand fractures simultaneously requires interfragmentary stability for fracture healing and soft tissue mobility to recover tendon gliding and joint motion and to promote interstitial scar tissue remodeling in both closed and open hand fractures in order to achieve optimal results. Understanding these coincident requirements of bone, soft tissue, and scar tissue facilitates optimal progressive healing and functional recovery. This is the art as well as the science of hand fracture treatment and rehabilitation.

Adequate fracture reduction and stability should ideally be restored with the first 5 to 7 days following injury. Fracture reduction and stability minimize the risks of malunion, delayed union, nonunion, and secondary infection and lay the groundwork for controlled graduated soft tissue response-modulated exercises to recover tendon gliding and joint motion during the reparative (proliferative) phase of healing before adhesions, joint contractures, or extensor lag can become established. Patients with flexible fixation of their fractures must be restricted to short-arc, tendon-gliding and differential sublimus and profundus exercise for approximately 21 days following fracture and surgery to prevent loss of reduction and yet achieve the requisite few millimeters of tendon gliding that avoids interstitial adhesions. Patients with secure fixation may be advanced within their soft tissue tolerance throughout the healing phases. The recovery of an arc of TAM that includes full PIP joint extension and at least 40 to 50 degrees of flexion is crucial during the reparative stage and must be accomplished gradually, judiciously, and with finesse rather than force.

K-wires and external minifixators are removed from simple fractures between 3 and 4 weeks after insertion. Miniscrews, miniplates, and tension band or 90–90 wires remain attached for the duration of fracture healing and are only removed for cause.

The resting hand should be maintained in the position of function with the MCP joints flexed and the PIP joints straight until fracture healing is signaled by a resolution of local signs, radiographically evident interfragmentary callus, and recovery of full or maximum active PIP joint extension.

After visible interfragmentary callus is verified, usually between 4 and 6 weeks after fracture and surgery, the recovery of motion may be pursued more vigorously, and progressive blocking, strengthening, conditioning, passive stretching, and work-hardening exercises may be initiated. Dynamic traction or serial casting may be commenced for more recalcitrant joint stiffness that fails to respond to exercises. Work simulation and return to work and recreational activities constitute the final stages of therapy.

Treatment outcomes and complications are most highly correlated with initial fracture severity. Stiffness remains the most frequent, and often the most serious, complication of hand fractures, especially those of the proximal phalanx. Anatomic position and stability of the fracture and early digital motion to restore joint function and tendon gliding are paramount to achieving successful results. Hand surgeons have long recognized the risks of fibroplasia and scar generation and the penalty of digital stiffness resulting from open surgical treatment of closed hand fractures, particularly in fractures adjacent to the flexor tendon sheaths ("no person's land"), and have admonished against injudicious open surgical procedures.[4-6,17-19,46,80,114] Minimally invasive surgery is an important adjunct to treating closed, and occasionally open, simple unstable fractures. The risk of increased fibroplasia accompanying open operative fixation may be offset, at least to some extent, by secure fracture stability that allows early and more intensive exercise than either nonoperative treatment or K-wire fixation.

As clinicians we strive to develop fracture management strategies that balance the need to protect fracture stability for skeletal union against the need for movement required for soft tissue integrity. The goal of fracture healing then is to maintain the stable position of the fracture while allowing progressive recovery of motion. Ultimately our goal is to train the fibroblasts and osteoblasts to work well together.

An understanding of the process of fracture healing and how it relates to the methods of fracture fixation empowers us in our clinical decisions. Better decision making in initial fracture management, technical advances in implant design, improved surgical design with respect for gliding structures, and early controlled mobilization contribute to reducing the incidence and severity of complications with hand fractures.

REFERENCES

The complete reference list is available online at www.expertconsult.com.

Extra-articular Hand Fractures, Part I: Surgeon's Management— A Practical Approach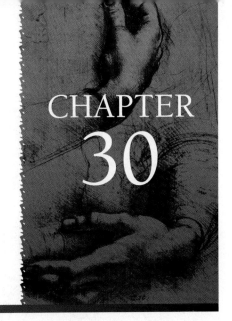

MARK R. BELSKY, MD AND MATTHEW LEIBMAN, MD

METACARPAL SHAFT FRACTURES
PHALANGEAL SHAFT FRACTURES
COMPLICATIONS OF METACARPAL AND
   PHALANGEAL FRACTURES
SUMMARY

CRITICAL POINTS

- Early return to motion is key to achieving the best outcome.
- Rigid internal fixation methods make early return to motion possible.
- The choice of treatment is determined by the specific circumstances of the fracture, balancing the benefit of anatomic reduction with minimal soft tissue injury and patient expectation.
- Methods of fixation range from simple casting, closed reduction and internal fixation (CRIF) with percutaneous Kirschner wires (K-wires), to open reduction and internal fixation (ORIF) with screws and sometimes plates, and for mutilating injury combining ORIF and external fixation.
- Failure to obtain a satisfactory closed reduction is an indication for ORIF.
- Collaboration between the surgeon and therapist is essential to achieving the optimal outcome of hand fracture management.

The metacarpals and phalanges extend from the carpus and project the carpal arch as they shape the palm and digits (Fig. 30-1). As the hand interacts with the environment, skeletal trauma may result. Fracture renders the hand effete with disruption of the stable aligned skeleton. Much of the remarkable function is lost.[1] A practical approach to fractures of the shaft of the metacarpals and the phalanges follows, including multiple methods of treatment. It is important to consider many factors in determining the ideal treatment for a given patient with a specific fracture. To achieve the best outcome,

contemporary teaching supports an early return to motion made possible by rigid internal fixation methods. The enthusiasm for this surgical philosophy is tempered by the inherent soft tissue injury caused by surgical dissection. For certain fractures closed reduction and pinning gives a more predictable favorable result with less risk. Our choice of treatment is determined by the specific circumstances of the fracture balancing the benefit of anatomic reduction with minimal soft tissue injury and patient expectation.

A careful and comprehensive hand examination is performed prior to treatment. An inspection of the hand is made noting the precise location of swelling, ecchymosis, abrasions, lacerations, and deformities. Gentle palpation of the bony and joint surfaces is done noting the areas of maximum tenderness. Acute injuries are tender. It is important to evaluate adjacent joints and bones in order to avoid missing concurrent injury.

Rotational deformity is best assessed with finger flexion. If the injury is too painful, sometimes the nail plate orientation suggests the rotational deformity, but this is not as precise as asking the patient to flex the digits.

Metacarpal Shaft Fractures

The digital metacarpals reside in the hand and are surrounded by the interosseous and abductor digiti minimi muscle bellies. Extrinsic extensor tendons glide smoothly over the dorsal surface of these bones separated by thin fascial planes. Fractures of the metacarpal shaft often disrupt the continuity of this soft tissue "envelope." The care of bony fractures includes treating the injured surrounding soft tissues. The surgical treatment can result in adhesions, which limit motion.

Fractures from the neck to the middle third of the metacarpal shaft typically occur after a punch or when the hand is struck by a hard object. The dorsal apex of the fracture causes a visible, palpable, and tender deformity. If this patient is not seen until the day after injury, the surrounding swelling may obscure the deformity.

Angular deformities due to neck and shaft fractures often are undertreated either due to misinterpretation of the literature or patient preference.[2] There is a distinction between

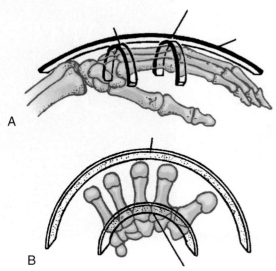

Figure 30-1 These figures demonstrate the arched design of the hand. **A,** The metacarpals project out from the "roman" arched carpus. **B,** The metacarpal heads and the carpal bones represent the "golden arches" of the hand.

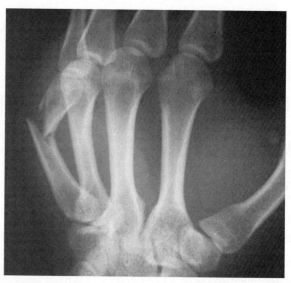

Figure 30-2 A distal shaft fracture of the left small finger metacarpal with 45 degrees of angulation. Closed reduction and internal fixation affords a simple method of treatment.

impacted head and neck fractures, for which up to 40 degrees of angulation may be acceptable, and angulated distal shaft fractures, which are usually not acceptable with more than 20 degrees of deformity.[2] A residual unsightly dorsal bump can interfere with excursion of the overlying extensor tendons and weaken grip strength.[3] With the metacarpal head flexed into the palm, in addition to its prominence interfering with palmar grasp, the patient experiences loss of extension and appears to have an "extensor lag."

Our preference is to reduce all angulated metacarpal shaft fractures of 20 degrees or more or if the deformity is unacceptable to the patient. If the apex is a palpable deformity, it will remain palpable unless reduced. In true impacted neck fractures in which the head is rotated down, up to 40 degrees can be accepted with little if any loss of function.[2]

If the patient punched another in the mouth, "teeth marks" may be seen in the dorsal skin over the metacarpal head. This injury is treated as a human bite wound. A wound extending to the fracture constitutes an open contaminated fracture. This injury is treated with extensive débridement (excision) of all contaminated layers of the wound and IV antibiotics. Following reduction, fixation may be necessary to stabilize the fracture. The decision to use fixation devices such as a K-wire or plate in an open fracture is a judgment call. One choice is to postpone definitive fracture fixation until the wound is satisfactorily healing and no longer contaminated. However, an unstable fracture in an infected or severely contaminated wound is the worst combination, and in this instance the fracture may be pinned with a longitudinal K-wire.

If the wound is untidy and the preference is not to approach the fracture through the metacarpal head, the pin may be placed in an antegrade fashion. Jorge Orbay developed a technique and a device to place an intramedullary pin antegrade from the base of the metacarpal through the shaft and into the metacarpal head.[4,5] This method offers limited advantages for an uncomplicated closed shaft fracture and

often requires removal of a buried bent pin at the base of the metacarpal, which may require a return to the operating room.

Closed Reduction of Metacarpal Neck and Shaft Fractures

Most of these fractures can be reduced by simple methods, especially if the patient is treated within 7 days of injury. A well-fitting cast application is an acceptable method of treatment. The challenge is to maintain the reduction, keep the patient's hand comfortable, maintain the metacarpophalangeal (MCP) joint in at least 60 degrees of flexion, and still allow adequate radiographic imaging to assess the position of the fracture and identify any loss of reduction.

Technique

The sedated patient is in the supine position with involved arm comfortably abducted on an arm table. A tourniquet is applied to the upper arm but usually not inflated for this procedure. The upper extremity is prepared and draped in the usual sterile fashion. Satisfactory anesthesia is achieved with either wrist or axillary block.

We prefer to use wrist block anesthesia. For the small finger MC (Fig. 30-2) a combination of an ulnar nerve and dorsal sensory ulnar nerve block gives complete anesthesia. For the ring finger MC, we add the median and superficial radial nerve blocks at the wrist. Once anesthesia is achieved, a closed reduction is performed. For most MC neck transverse or short oblique shaft fractures, reduction is performed as follows.

Apply longitudinal traction to the involved digit, then flex the MCP joint. Dorsally directed pressure is applied by the digit through the MP head. Pushing up on the MC head should straighten out the angular deformity. This reduces the dorsal apex of the fracture to its normal gentle curve. Any rotational deformity is reduced at this time. The reduction

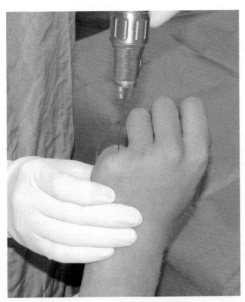

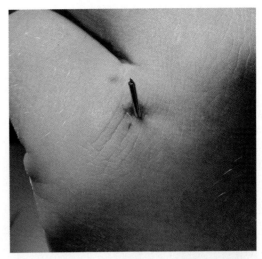

Figure 30-4 *Note the skin tension that is proximal (to the right) of the wire. The distal skin (to the left) needs to be incised to release the tension. The direction of the tension is from distal to proximal, and the skin will migrate in that direction after release.*

Figure 30-3 *A power drill is used to place a longitudinal Kirschner wire down through the extensor and metacarpal head on its way down the shaft to the subchondral bone of the metacarpal.*

can be held by pushing up on the flexed proximal interphalangeal (PIP) joint with the surgeon's thumb and down on the apex of the fracture with the index and middle fingers. A C-arm image intensifier and a power drill are used to maintain the reduction with a longitudinal K-wire. This is the CRIF technique.[6]

Satisfactory reduction is verified with the C-arm. Exposure of the surgeon and patient's hands to the x-ray beam is minimized. The spread of the substantive x-ray exposure is about 15 inches wide.[7,8] Staying 3 feet away from the beam decreases radiation to 25%. The maximum exposure is on the side facing the image intensifier where maximum scatter occurs.

Using a power drill (Fig. 30-3), a 0.054-inch diameter K-wire is drilled through the metacarpal head and down the shaft. There is a tendency to be too volar and ulnar with the initial K-wire. The intent is to deliver the wire to the base (subchondral bone) of the MC but not cross the carpometacarpal (CMC) joint. Once the position of the fracture and K-wire are verified, the K-wire is cut off 3 mm outside the skin.

The resultant position of the MCP joint is at least 60 degrees of flexion. The flexed position maintains the length of the MCP joint's collateral ligaments avoiding an extension contracture. Skin tension must be assessed and released around the protruding wire (Fig. 30-4). The tight skin reflects the direction of the tension. Incise the loose skin (Fig. 30-5) in line with the tension to release it. This prevents an infection around the pin site. Satisfactory reduction of the fracture and position of the K-wire are verified with the C-arm in both the anteroposterior and lateral planes (Fig. 30-6).

The pin site is covered with Xeroform gauze. A short arm cast is applied for 3 weeks, immobilizing the involved and adjacent digits. In compliant patients, the cast can be shortened at 1 week to allow some passive PIP motion. The cast and pin are removed at 3 weeks. Using a heavy needle holder, spin the wire then apply longitudinal traction as the wire is extracted.

Most MC shaft fractures treated this way are healed enough to remove the K-wire by 3 weeks, that is, if the fracture is not tender despite the radiograph not reflecting healing. In this instance, the fracture is healed enough to allow the return of motion for the next 3 weeks. It is a little difficult to get all the MCP joint extension immediately after wire removal. The patient is encouraged to perform active assisted range-of-motion (ROM) exercises. Buddy taping to the adjacent finger facilitates the motion for the first few weeks after cast removal. Some patients require a removable molded ulnar gutter orthosis during the transition for the first week out of the cast. Six weeks after CRIF, more resistive exercises and weight-bearing activities can progress as tolerated.

CRIF technique can be applied to transverse and short oblique fractures for all the MCs. When satisfactory closed reduction cannot be achieved, as in cases with a long obliquity, segmental fragments, or soft tissue interposition, ORIF is preferred.

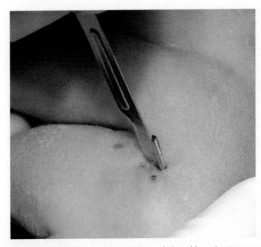

Figure 30-5 *The distal skin is incised, and the skin migrates proximally (to the right) and releases the tension.*

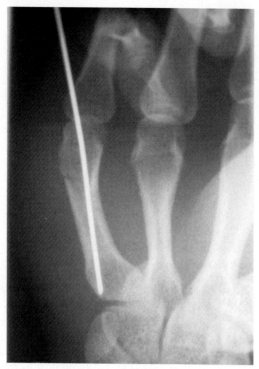

Figure 30-6 *The fracture is satisfactorily reduced and the K-wire placed on this oblique view. The posteroanterior and lateral views are omitted.*

Open Reduction with Internal Fixation

Certain MC shaft fractures are preferably treated with ORIF.[9-12] The *long oblique fractures* of the MC shaft are amenable to ORIF with interfragmentary self-tapping screw fixation. Torque forces create spiraling fractures down the MC shaft and disrupt the attached interosseous muscles. These adjacent muscles can interpose in the fracture and prevent a satisfactory closed reduction. Also these attached muscles contribute to shortening of the unstable fracture.

The goal of ORIF is to accurately restore the anatomy with enough stable fixation that the motion can begin before frac-

ture healing. If stability cannot be achieved, then motion must be delayed until healing takes place.

MC shaft fractures are best approached through a longitudinal dorsal incision set between the MCs.[11,12] The patient is positioned, prepared, and draped as with CRIF but axillary (or supraclavicular) block is preferred. The arm is exsanguinated and a tourniquet applied at the upper arm, set 100 mm Hg above systolic pressure, not to exceed 300 mm Hg.

A longitudinal skin incision is made between the extensor tendons. The extrinsic extensor tendons are gently retracted. A longitudinal incision along the bony cortex is made, sharply dissecting the periosteum and muscle attachments off the fracture to expose just enough of the fracture. In an effort to preserve the bone's blood supply and promote healing, all soft tissue attachments to fracture fragments are preserved. Longitudinal traction is applied and the fracture reduced. Derotation and restoration of length are addressed.

It is especially gratifying to spend the time to reduce the fracture anatomically. As little as 1 mm of missed rotational deformity may cause an unsightly rotatory deformity of the digit. The average circumference of a MC is less than 3.6 cm. Each millimeter of rotational misalignment represents at least 10 degrees of rotational deformity. Usually, more than 5 degrees is unacceptable clinically and will interfere with function.

Once reduced, a fracture clamp is placed and then a K-wire is provisionally fixed perpendicular to the fracture. Imaging verifies satisfactory reduction. The provisional K-wire is placed to indicate where the interfragmentary screws will go. Nondisplaced fissures in the bone are carefully identified, and placement of a screw in a fissure is avoided. The screws are placed perpendicular to the plane of the fracture as much as possible and well spaced along the fracture. The holes are drilled, on the near cortex overdrilled, so compression can be applied across the fracture. It is preferable to direct the screw from the smaller to the larger fragment. Placing a screw within one screw head diameter of the fracture line, an adjacent screw, or near the apex of the fracture fragment is avoided (Fig. 30-7). Countersinking the interfragmentary screws prevents irritation of the overlying tendons and

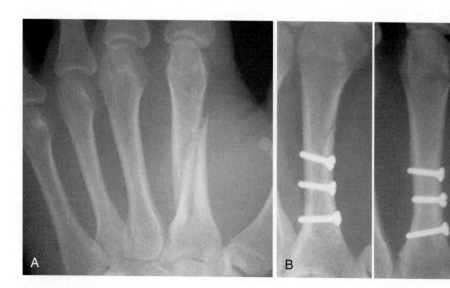

Figure 30-7 A, *This long oblique index metacarpal shaft fracture was treated with open reduction and internal fixation (**B**) and secured with three interfragmentary screws. The patient was able to start immediate range-of-motion exercises a few days after surgery.*

improves fixation of the diaphyseal fracture.[11,12] This is particularly important for fixation of the phalangeal shaft fractures (see section on Phalangeal Shaft Fractures). The size of the screw is in the range of 1.3 to 1.5 mm in diameter but is determined by the anatomy of the particular patient.

Once reduction and fixation are completed, the soft tissues are restored anatomically. If possible, repair the fascial edges of the muscle attachments. It is best to have as many intact soft tissue layers as possible between the fracture and the skin. The hand is placed through a passive ROM using the tenodesis effect to verify that the digits are well aligned and that the natural cascade of the digits is restored.

With the incisions closed, the tourniquet is released. Gentle compression is applied to the hand during the hyperemic phase and restoration of the circulation verified. The hand is placed in a supportive orthosis with a circumferential gently compressive dressing. The MCP joints are flexed at least 60 degrees, and the wrist extended to 30 to 45 degrees. Usually 4 to 7 days following surgery, the dressing is removed and gentle active ROM exercises are begun in a protected environment (Fig. 30-8). A cooperative patient, or with the supervision and guidance of a certified hand therapist, begins a series of exercises to get the tissues gliding, the joints moving, and to ensure MP joint flexion. Emphasis is placed on and successful recovery indicated by the achievement of MCP joint flexion and PIP extension. Intrinsic tightness is to be avoided or minimized by starting appropriate intrinsic stretching exercises early when tolerated.

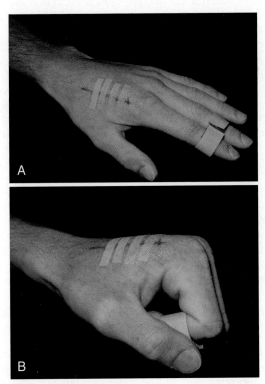

Figure 30-8 A and **B,** Photos of the left hand for the same patient seen in Figure 30-7, 10 days after surgery demonstrating active range of motion facilitated with buddy taping with Velcro. Note the longitudinal incision for exposure of the index metacarpal shaft fracture.

Transverse, Short Oblique, and Multiple Metacarpal Shaft Fractures

Certain MC shaft fractures are best treated with plate fixation to provide more stable fixation and earlier postoperative rehabilitation. Transverse, short oblique, and comminuted fractures, especially those associated with a more severe soft tissue injury, are considered for plate fixation. An open fracture involving bone, muscle, and skin is considered a combined injury because it involves more than one system. When the combined injury is more extensive, such as in a log splitter crush injury of the hand that causes comminuted MP shaft fractures, plate fixation is particularly helpful. This allows an earlier return to motion and function, preventing the inherent scarring, adhesions, and fibrosis of the otherwise immobile injured soft tissues.

A variety of commercially available modular hand systems can be used for plating MC fractures. Plates held with 2.0 mm diameter screws provide enough stability to allow early ROM with these fractures. Some of the modular handsets have added locking plate technology. If the screw is locked to the plate, the construct is even more stable, especially in metaphyseal fractures with poor bone quality and comminution.

Application of the plates does require more dissection, but only just enough to apply the plate after fracture reduction[11,12] (Fig. 30-9). Plate length allows for at least two screws (four cortices) on either side of the fracture. If there is comminution, as occurs with a butterfly fragment, complementary interfragmentary fixation contributes to further stability. Closure of the soft tissues to cover the plate facilitates tendon excursion of the adjacent intrinsic and extrinsic tendons. The postoperative care is the same as for patients with ORIF as described earlier.

The previously discussed methods can be used to treat most MC shaft fractures. However, a few cases always occur for which these methods must be supplanted with others. When a major loss of bone or soft tissue has occurred, external fixation may be necessary temporarily before later reconstruction with bone grafts and soft tissue flaps. In some cases cerclage wiring serves as a supplementary fixation. These extensive injuries are beyond the scope of this discussion.

Phalangeal Shaft Fractures

Swanson suggested that the outcome following a proximal phalangeal fracture often suffers either from neglect or overtreatment, or worse still, from poor treatment. Unfortunately, this most common of hand fractures lends itself to all three. Although radiography is necessary to image the fracture, it is the intimate relationship of the fracture to the delicate soft tissue envelope that determines the outcome. Finding the right balance between fracture reduction and surgical assault through the tissues to treat the fracture is the critical judgment.

Closed proximal phalangeal shaft fractures are classified as transverse and short oblique, long oblique, and comminuted. For most transverse and short oblique fractures that result from low-velocity injury at the neck, midshaft, and base of shaft, CRIF is a simpler, less invasive, and reproducible

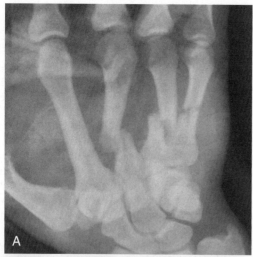

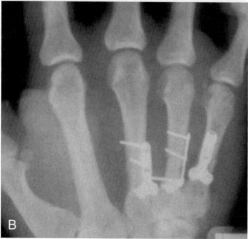

Figure 30-9 A, *Severe crush injury with associated metacarpal shaft fractures of the middle, ring, and small metacarpals. The patient's hand was crushed in a log splitter.* **B,** *Open reduction and internal fixation.*

method.[12,13] The oblique and comminuted fractures are more amenable to CRIF, ORIF, or external fixation, and sometimes a combination of methods.[11-13]

Closed Reduction and Internal Fixation of Phalangeal Shaft Fractures

The common proximal phalangeal (P1) shaft fracture at the base or midshaft is ideally suited for CRIF[12,13] (Fig. 30-10). The approach to such a fracture is similar to CRIF for an MC fracture. These fractures are inherently unstable after reduction and require additional fixation.

Under adequate wrist block anesthesia, the hand is prepared and draped in sterile fashion. Closed reduction is achieved with longitudinal traction in the line of the digit and then flexing the MCP joint. The apex of the base and midshaft of P1 and P2 fractures is inherently volar. This collapse pattern is predictable based on the mechanism of injury, the imbalanced pull of the extrinsic flexors flexing the PIP, and the intrinsic flexors flexing the MP and extending the PIP. If treated within 5 to 7 days of injury, most of the fractures are reducible by closed means. Any angular or rotatory

deformity is addressed by applying force to reduce it appropriately.

Reduction is verified with the C-arm. It is critical to remember that a satisfactory closed reduction must be achieved at this point to be able to proceed with CRIF. A 0.045-inch K-wire is drilled through the metacarpal head, across the flexed MP joint, and down the shaft of the proximal phalanx. The K-wire should stop at the subchondral bone in the head of the proximal phalanx (see Fig. 30-10D).

The pin is cut 3 mm outside the skin and skin tension is released. A circumferential cast incorporating the involved and adjacent digits is used for 3 weeks. The cast is applied with the MCP joint and adjacent MCP joints flexed, but the interphalangeal joints are allowed to extend to a comfortable position (intrinsic plus position, also called the position of comfort or protection).

At 3 weeks the cast is removed and the pin is pulled. The fracture is usually not tender at this time. To pull the pin, a heavy needle holder is used and the K-wire is gently twisted until it is loose. It is then pulled and twisted at the same time.

The patient is started on ROM exercises. Initially the patient is unable to fully extend the MP joint. Over the next week with active assisted range-of-motion (AAROM) exercises, the motion is restored. At 6 weeks after surgery, the patient can proceed to strengthen the hand with resistive exercises as tolerated.

Long oblique fractures of the proximal phalanx are treated by either transverse parallel K-wires with CRIF methods or with ORIF with interfragmentary screws. Each method has its own advantages and disadvantages. Our preference is to avoid incisions through the extensor tendons that surround P1. When a satisfactory closed reduction cannot be achieved or when early motion is critical, ORIF with screws is preferable.

After reduction is completed for oblique P1 and P2 fractures, CRIF begins with application of a fracture clamp through the skin to hold the reduced fracture. The clamp is placed in the middle of the fracture. Two 0.035-inch K-wires are drilled transversely and parallel across the digit. Beginning at either end of the fracture, the clamp is removed to place a third K-wire, in the middle (Fig. 30-11). For the index and small fingers, we prefer the K-wires to protrude from the skin on the border (radial side of the index and ulnar side of the small). For the central digits the pins are either buried or cut shorter to avoid irritation of the adjacent digit's skin and a solid short arm cast is applied.

After 3 weeks the cast is removed. Since the pins do not cross a joint (see Fig. 30-11C), AAROM can begin. The patient usually wears a molded resting orthosis when not exercising. The K-wires are removed at 4 weeks. The patient then progresses with specific exercises to regain full motion.

Open Reduction and Internal Fixation of Phalangeal Shaft Fractures

If ORIF of a P1 shaft fracture is required, incisions can be made either midaxial or dorsal.[11,12] The midaxial approach allows for retraction of the extensor, whereas the dorsal approach requires incision and repair of the extensor. If it is incised, repair and handling of the delicate soft tissues is a major factor in determining the resulting motion.

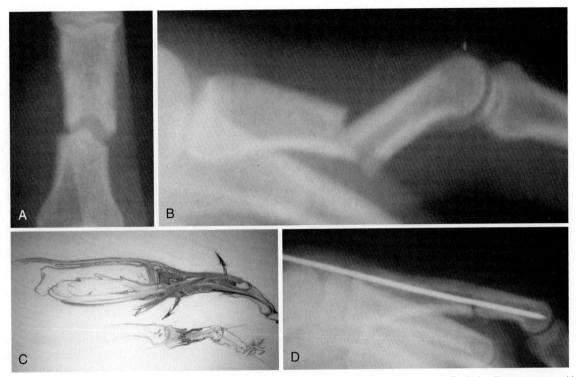

Figure 30-10 A and **B,** Midshaft proximal phalangeal (P1) shaft fracture as a result of a low-velocity injury. Typical collapse pattern with apex volar is noted. **C,** The forces that caused this displacement are indicated in this classic drawing by Littler. The MCP joint is flexed by the intrinsics and the proximal interphalangeal joint is flexed by the flexor superficialis. **D,** Once reduced and fixed with percutaneous internal fixation with a 0.045-inch K-wire, the fracture is well reduced and stable enough to spend the next 3 weeks in a cast. The pin is removed at 3 weeks and motion started.

The approach to placing the interfragmentary screws for a long oblique fracture of P1 or P2 is similar. The skin is incised, the extensor retracted or, if necessary, incised, and the reduction performed with longitudinal traction. Any malrotation is reduced, and then provisional fixation applied. Nondisplaced fracture lines that look like little fissures should be cautiously looked for. Placement of the screw within one screw head diameter of one of these fissures is avoided. With meticulous technique, holes are drilled and depth measured. Self-tapping screws are placed in and coun-

tersunk. It is important to make sure the screws don't protrude on the opposite cortex. The hole on the near cortex can be overdrilled to the diameter of the screw thread, which allows compression of the fragments. Usually 1.3- to 1.5-mm diameter screws of appropriate length are satisfactory for phalangeal fractures[11,12] (Fig. 30-12).

Some fractures are amenable to more than one approach. There is always some healthy tension between advocates for CRIF and advocates for ORIF for fractures such as shown in Figure 30-13.

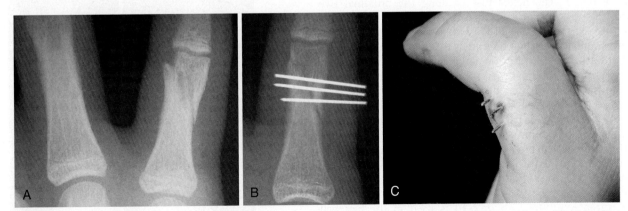

Figure 30-11 A, Short oblique fracture of the proximal phalanx of the small finger is amenable to closed reduction and internal fixation with transversely oriented K-wires. **B,** Longitudinal traction reduces the fractures. A fracture clamp is applied before three 0.035-inch K-wires are drilled from the ulnar border (from the smaller fragment to the larger fragment) of the small finger. **C,** Once placed, the wires are cut off outside the skin along the border of the digit (in this case the ulnar side of the small finger).

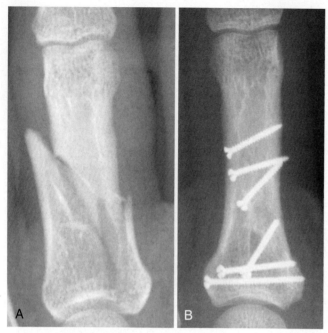

Figure 30-12 A, A comminuted fracture of the proximal phalanx treated with open reduction and internal fixation with interfragmentary screws (**B**). More screws of a smaller size were used for this particular fracture.

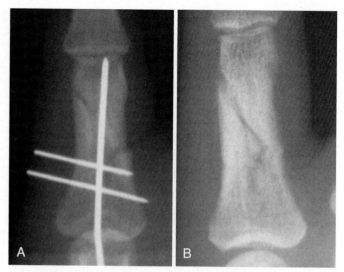

Figure 30-13 A, Similar comminuted P1 fracture treated with closed reduction and internal fixation. **B,** Note healed fracture with pins out.

Distal Phalangeal Shaft Fractures

Fractures of the distal phalanx (P3) usually result from crush injuries of the nail bed. Care for these fractures includes caring for the nail bed—both the germinal and sterile matrices. The nail bed resides on the cortex of the distal phalanx. If the midshaft fracture of P3 is displaced, the nail bed is likely torn. Crush injury of the nail bed with a large hematoma often includes fracture of P3. If unstable, it is better to pin the fracture.

For the tuft fracture, pinning is unnecessary. Fractures near the base and midshaft are more likely to displace. Due to the differential insertions of the extensor and flexor tendons, an imbalance deformity may result after midshaft fracture. The extensor inserts at the very base of the dorsal surface of P3. The flexor inserts along the proximal two thirds of the volar cortex, which usually results in a flexion deformity at the fracture of P3 with a dorsal apex.

An angulated P3 shaft fracture is treated with a power drill and a C-arm. If necessary, the nail plate is removed to expose the fracture and the nail bed injury. This permits reduction of the fracture and meticulous closure of the nail bed. A 0.035- or 0.045-inch K-wire is placed through the tip of P3 (Fig. 30-14). It can be used to manipulate the distal fragment and achieve reduction under direct vision through the rent in the nail bed. The pin is then driven proximally. Depending on the level of the fracture, the pin is driven either into the base of P3 or across the distal interphalangeal joint into the midshaft of P2.

Resorbable suture (5-0 or 6-0) is used in the nail bed repair. Contrary to other literature, it is not necessary or even preferable to replace the nail plate in the sulcus unless the tear of the nail bed extends into the germinal matrix. Most

shaft fractures of P3 involve nail bed injuries through the sterile matrix. For these cases we place a single layer of Xeroform gauze on the nail bed and make no effort to place it into the sulcus under the eponychium. If the tear extends into the germinal matrix, the Xeroform is sutured into the sulcus with chromic suture to prevent a synechia (adhesion between the roof and floor of the germinal matrix). Replacement of the nail plate does not always prevent a split nail. The biggest problem with replacement of the nail is that it may adhere to the sterile matrix. If this occurs then the patient suffers as the new nail plate grows in, as it creates "the world's largest hang nail" which may require excision

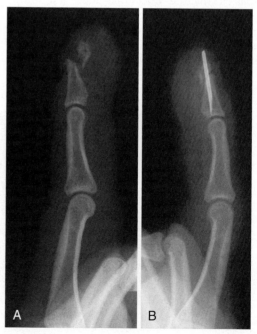

Figure 30-14 A, Distal shaft fracture of P3 treated with pin fixation after open reduction and nail bed repair (**B**).

under anesthesia a month after injury. This painful scenario can be avoided by just leaving the single layer of Xeroform in place on the nail bed, which dries and adheres to the nail bed until it can be easily peeled off painlessly by the patient.

The K-wire in P3 remains in place for 4 weeks before removal. The pins are removed as previously described. However, if the pin is only to the base of P3, one can wait until there is radiographic evidence of healing. By 6 weeks the pin may loosen due to bone resorption around the pin and slides out easily.

Complications of Metacarpal and Phalangeal Fractures

Loss of MCP joint flexion due to the contracted MCP joint collateral ligaments is common and results from the MCP joint being immobilized in extension. If not responsive to therapy, capsulotomy may be necessary. After the neglected MC shaft fracture, the unsightly dorsal apex creates an extensor lag due to the malposition of the metacarpal head and from extensor adhesions. Osteotomy is necessary for the nascent or fully healed malunion to be realigned.[14] With rigid plate fixation, early motion can begin within a week of surgery. If for any reason the plate must be removed, we wait until healing is verified after 6 months with a CT scan.

Pin site infection is extremely rare if skin tension is released and a solid cast is applied at the time of the surgery. CRIF with K-wires does not pretend to be rigid fixation. The pins are just internal "orthoses" and must be supported with a solid cast for the first 3 weeks. If the pin site infection is deeper than the skin, the pin is removed. If there is any drainage or cellulitis, the pin is removed, the wound débrided, and IV antibiotics started. The resulting deformity is treated at a later date once the tissues have healed and the infection resolved.

Intrinsic tightness after hand injury is common and often overlooked. Bunnell's test is used to assess intrinsic tightness.[15] "Knuckle roll back" exercises (Fig. 30-15) are an excellent method of stretching the intrinsics. The patient extends the MCP joints and flexes the interphalangeal joints. With the other hand the patient grasps a finger passively, flexing the interphalangeal joints while extending the MCP joint. If intrinsic tightness remains severe, the contracted intrinsic component is excised under local anesthesia through a dorsal approach.[16]

Adhesions of the adjacent extensor or flexor tendon to the phalangeal fracture may occur. If needed, tenolysis is postponed to at least 4 to 6 months after surgery so the screws or plates can be removed at the same time. Tenolysis is performed under local anesthesia so the patient can actively participate. Intrinsic release may be helpful at the same time.

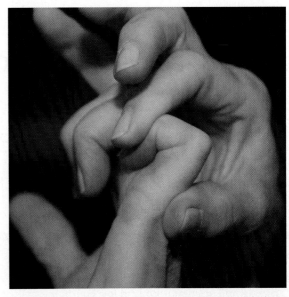

Figure 30-15 Knuckle roll-back exercise. The patient actively extends the metacarpophalangeal (MCP) joints while flexing the interphalangeal (IP) joints. The patient uses the other hand passively to extend the small finger MCP joint further while maintaining the flexion of the IP joints, one finger at a time. This stretches the intrinsics while gaining motion of all the joints in the digit.

A volar spike of the fracture can impale the flexor sheath even with CRIF. A flexor tenolysis is performed through a midaxial approach.

Malunion of a phalangeal fracture may cause rotatory and/or angular deformity.[11,14] Reconstruction of a P1 malunion is complex. Osteotomy of the phalanx or at the MC level is described in Jupiter and Ring[11] and Freeland and Lindley,[14] but is beyond the scope of this discussion.

Summary

Most displaced phalangeal and MC shaft fractures are simple to reduce. The methods of fixation range from simple casting, CRIF with percutaneous K-wires, to ORIF with screws and sometimes plates, and for mutilating injury a combination of ORIF and external fixation. Failure to obtain a satisfactory closed reduction is an indication for ORIF. The surgeon must approach the hand fracture with all these modes of treatment available. The least invasive, most effective treatment is chosen for a particular fracture in a particular patient.

REFERENCES

The complete reference list is available online at www.expertconsult.com.

Extra-articular Hand Fractures, Part II: Therapist's Management

LYNNE M. FEEHAN, BScPT, MSc(PT), PhD, CHT*

BACKGROUND
REHABILITATION: GENERAL PRINCIPLES
EARLY MOBILIZATION: FRACTURE-SPECIFIC
  CONSIDERATIONS
SUMMARY

CRITICAL POINTS

Clinical Factors Defining Relative Stability of a Fracture

- Which bone; where in bone
- Nature and number of fracture line(s)
- Initial fracture displacement and alignment
- Type of reduction and fixation
- Postreduction and fixation alignment
- Nature of additional soft tissue injury
- Time since fracture/surgery
- Normal daily functional demands and priorities of the individual

Essential Elements to Gaining This Understanding

- Referral: Complete and detailed fracture information
- Imaging: Pre- and postreduction fixation imaging
- Operating Room Report: Written (or verbal) report from referring surgeon (if applicable)
- Team Work and Communication: Patient and family, physician and surgeon, and therapist

Background

Epidemiology and Fracture Distribution

Second only to forearm fractures in incidence, hand fractures account for up to 20% of fractures in adults and children, with an annual incidence of 36/10,000 people.[1-3] Hand

fractures in both genders occur most commonly in early adolescence, just after the period of most rapid bone growth.[3-8] Across the lifespan, males have twice the risk of sustaining a hand fracture, with most of this risk occurring between the ages of 15 and 40, the most active and productive working years. As with other "fragility" fractures, women older than 65 are at higher risk (1.5:1) for sustaining hand fractures than men.[3,9]

Phalangeal fractures (distal, middle, and proximal) account for more than 50% of hand fractures. However, metacarpals (MCs) are the most common bones fractured, accounting for 35% to 45% of hand fractures, followed by 20% to 25% in the distal phalanx, with the middle and proximal phalanges each accounting for about 15%. Fractures within the fifth (little) ray make up about 40% of hand fractures, with the first (thumb) and fourth (ring) rays each accounting for about 15% to 20%. Extra-articular hand fractures account for 75% to 85% of hand fractures. Work-related hand fractures account for 14% of all hand fractures, with distal phalangeal fractures accounting for up to 60% of extra-articular fractures in a working population, as the fingertip is the most exposed and vulnerable to traumatic occupational injury. In the general population, MC fracture is the most common extra-articular hand fracture.[9-12]

Medical and Surgical Management

Most patients present with simple, closed, extra-articular hand fractures that are managed nonsurgically with closed reduction, followed in some instances by percutaneous transfixing or intramedullary Kirshner wire (K-wire) fixation to help maintain fracture alignment during initial healing.[13-18] The advantage of closed reduction, with or without percutaneous pin fixation, is that additional surgical trauma can be avoided. It is generally recommended that closed, extra-articular hand fractures be "immobilized" in a cast or a rigid thermoplastic orthosis for at least 3 to 4 weeks for additional external protection of the healing fracture.[13-18] Commonly, the cast or orthosis immobilizes the regional hand and wrist joints in the position of function (10–15 degrees of wrist extension, 70 degrees of metacarpophalangeal [MCP] joint flexion, full interphalangeal [IP] joint extension, thumb

*Special thanks to my friends and colleagues for their assistance with this chapter; Judy Colditz (USA) and Sarah Ewald (Switzerland) for providing images of orthoses, Maureen Hardy (USA) for her review, and Susan Harris (Canada) for editing.

palmar abduction with web space maintenance), with the flexion creases of noninvolved joints remaining clear for movement.[19,20]

Although some extra-articular hand fractures can be reduced in a closed manner, others may remain structurally fragile or significantly malaligned following attempts at closed reduction. In addition, some hand fractures manifest as more complex clinical injuries, involving significant bone loss or comminution, articular disruption, or open injury in conjunction with other regional tendon, nerve, vascular, and skin tissue injuries that also require treatment. In these circumstances, it is usually recommended that an open surgical or direct fracture reduction be done, supplemented by some form of more stable or rigid internal or external fixation to facilitate direct fracture healing and early motion.[13-18]

Open reduction and rigid fracture fixation can be technically difficult in the small, contoured hand bones and often require extensive regional soft tissue and periosteal disruption, creating a more clinically complex injury with increased risk for scarring, stiffness, and the need for secondary surgical interventions.[13,14] Therefore, it is not uncommon for surgeons to opt for less invasive surgical approaches for fracture reduction or less rigid or more flexible forms of fracture fixation that help maintain fracture alignment. These approaches, however, do not necessarily provide significant additional structural strength or stability to the healing fracture. In these instances, it is generally recommended that the regional hand and wrist joints be immobilized for up to 4 weeks to protect the healing fracture.[13-18]

Micromotion and Early Fracture Healing

Animal studies have shown that limited or controlled cyclic (usually compressive) microstrain or micromotion introduced during the initial days of healing clearly influences the initial genetic and molecular expression in the callus.[21,22] This, in turn, affects initial cellular proliferation and differentiation, all of which ultimately influence the morphologic changes and biomechanical strength of the fracture throughout the early stages of healing, leading to improvements in both quality and rate of fracture healing.[23-45] However, these same studies also show that too much micromotion of the fracture negatively influences the quality and rate of early fracture healing. Until recently, it was unclear if early, controlled passive motion of regional joints surrounding a potentially unstable fracture in a non-weight-bearing limb would have a positive or negative effect on quality and rate of early fracture healing. In a study of closed, extra-articular third MC fractures in non-weight-bearing limbs in a rabbit, Feehan and colleagues[46] compared fractures treated with immobilization to those treated with a controlled passive motion protocol combined with gentle local pinch fracture stabilization initiated on the fifth day. These authors found statistically and clinically significant improvements (>25% better) in the biomechanical properties (strength and stiffness) and fracture alignment of the healing fracture at 28 days after fracture, providing support for the concept of early controlled and protected motion in the management of fragile extra-articular hand fractures in humans.

Early Motion: Changing Trends and Clinical Evidence

Not all extra-articular hand fractures are immobilized during the early healing phases, as some are considered strong or stable enough to withstand active regional joint motion; these more stable fractures can be categorized into two clinical scenarios. The first is the fracture that has been managed with a more rigid fixation. This is based on the original principle underlying the Arbeitsgemeinschaft für Osteosynthesefragen/Association for the Study of Internal Fixation (AO/ASIF) fracture fixation philosophy from the 1950s to 1960s. This concept considers that rigid fixation not only provides a "no-motion" healing environment that facilitates direct internal fracture healing and remodeling without formation of an external callus, but also a mechanical construct of sufficient strength to allow early functional active motion of surrounding joints.[47]

In theory, the concept of rigid fracture fixation combined with early motion sounds ideal. However, the actual functional outcomes from case series studies following rigid (usually plate or screw or plate and screw) fixation in the hand have been less than ideal.[13,48-53] This is likely due in part to the intimate and complex regional soft tissue anatomy in the hand, with multilevel, interstitial motion planes that do not tolerate additional restrictive scarring secondary to extensive surgical dissection. However, this is conjecture because clinical evidence to support or refute the use of more rigid fixation alternatives in extra-articular hand fracture management is lacking.[54] Clearly the efficacy and effectiveness of rigid fracture fixation alternatives in extra-articular hand fracture management are areas that need further investigation.

The second scenario for early motion is based on the concept of functional fracture bracing. Generally, this type of bracing is recommended for simple, closed, minimally displaced extra-articular long bone fractures.[55,56] Sarmiento and Latta[57] have been strong advocates for functional fracture bracing of long bones for more than 30 years, and Colditz provides an excellent overview of the history, theory, and role of functional fracture bracing in the management of closed stable upper extremity fractures, including MC and proximal phalanx fractures (see Chapter 127). Latta and coworkers[58] state that fracture bracing is a philosophy rather than merely the use of orthotic devices, predicated on the belief that immobilization of the joints above and below the fracture is not necessary for secondary fracture healing.

The intent of the fracture brace is not to immobilize the fracture fragment, but to provide sufficient fracture alignment and stability when regional joint motion occurs. The functional fracture brace is designed to provide circumferential regional support of the long bone; the brace is adjustable for variations in swelling or girth of the surrounding soft tissues, with joints both proximal and distal to the fracture free to move through an unrestricted arc of active motion. From an evidence-based practice perspective, there is support from several independently conducted, limited-quality, randomized clinical trials showing consistent potential for improved rates of recovery of mobility, strength, and return to work with no significant risks of harm in simple, closed extra-articular finger MC fractures treated with various forms of "flexible" or more "rigid" forms of external regional fracture bracing and early regional joint motion compared with metacarpal fractures treated with regional immobilization.[54,59-67]

During the last decade, a philosophical shift has taken place in the principles of long bone fracture fixation in humans.[68] This shift is moving away from the original AO/ASIF concept of direct (open) anatomic reduction and rigid compressive fracture fixation followed by immediate functional reactivation (absolute or high-stability fixation), to indirect (closed or limited open), near-anatomic reduction combined with minimally invasive, limited contact, flexible fixation methods (relative or low-stability fixation), followed by early protected or controlled mobilization of the affected limb.[69,70] This newer concept, known as biologic, or flexible long bone, fixation, was described by Perren[71] as finding a balance between maintaining the biological integrity of the healing fracture and providing a stable mechanical environment that allows for fracture healing and early controlled functional motion rather than immobilization.

In theory, functional fracture bracing is consistent with the concept of biological or flexible fixation, in which a functional fracture brace is defined also as a noninvasive, external, indirect form of flexible fracture fixation. As is true of many of the more commonly used less or minimally invasive techniques, flexible hand fracture fixation alternatives provide some additional fracture alignment and limited structural stability but not necessarily a rigid or no-motion environment for fracture healing. A number of case series studies have reported results for early active motion, combined with variations of fixation that could be defined as biological or flexible fixation options, including K-wire, cerclage wire, and semirigid external fracture fixation for management of extra-articular MC and phalangeal fractures. Good outcomes with few complications were reported in these series.[72-82] Only one randomized clinical trial compared rigid lag screw fixation with more flexible percutaneous wire fixation. This trial noted no long-term differences in pain, strength, or mobility in oblique and spiral proximal phalangeal fractures for which active motion was initiated 1 week after fracture.[83] Thus, it is difficult to compare the relative efficacy (risk or benefit) of rigid fixation plus early motion with that for flexible fixation plus early motion in the management of extra-articular hand fractures.

As outlined in the literature, the primary concerns with motion surrounding these more flexible K-wires and external fixators is the increased risk for pin track infections and pin migration or loosening associated with regional soft tissue motion around the pins.[84-89] As well, the motion options that might be available with these types of fixation depend on what soft tissues and joints are skewered with these devices, because such skewering certainly limits the amount of possible soft tissue excursion or joint motion. If the fixation crosses over or through a joint, or through or across a muscle or the extensor apparatus, motion of these joints or full excursion of the muscle or extensor mechanism are not an option until the fixator is removed. Given the concern about increased risk for pin-related complications, it is important to stress that early motion around fractures managed with more flexible forms of pin or wire fixation should be intro-

duced gradually, in a controlled fashion, during the initial stages of fracture healing.

Outcomes and Complications

The most common complications after hand fracture are not delayed union or nonunion or other fracture healing complications (e.g., infection), but rather reduced tendon gliding and tethering, resulting in secondary joint lag, stiffness or contracture, and decreased muscle function (strength, endurance, flexibility, coordination) associated with immobilization.[48-53,82,83,90] Single, nondisplaced, closed hand fractures treated with no or closed reduction, no fixation, and limited immobilization are associated with minimal long-term morbidity. In contrast, clinical factors associated with increased risk of secondary fracture complications requiring additional or prolonged treatment include multiple fractures, bone loss, other associated regional soft tissue injury, proximal phalangeal fracture, surgical intervention, plate fixation, and immobilization exceeding 4 weeks.[12,13,49,50,91-93]

Fortunately, most people with uncomplicated, extra-articular hand fractures regain normal or near-normal regional tissue (joint, tendon, muscle, neurovascular) function and the ability to return to normal participation in daily activities without limitation within 12 weeks after fracture.[13,54,60,72,90,94-96] However, as with other fragile, healing soft tissue injuries in the hand, it is better to try to prevent or reduce postfracture regional tissue dysfunction and facilitate a person's return to normal daily functioning as soon as possible during the recovery through early thoughtful and controlled therapeutic interventions.

Rehabilitation: General Principles

Defining Relative Stability or Structural Strength

Traditionally, initiation and progression of rehabilitation and functional reactivation of individuals following extra-articular hand fractures have been based on the concept of clinical stability—the point in time when the fracture is considered structurally strong enough to withstand nonresisted, active motion without fracture displacement.[13,18,85] In many instances during the initial healing phases, extra-articular hand fractures are considered to be clinically unstable. Early postfracture rehabilitation is often limited to providing an immobilization orthosis and some additional supportive education and advice, with active motion and graduated functional reactivation initiated only after a period of immobilization when regional tissue complications are already established.[13,18,85]

The more traditional concept defines the clinically stable fracture as one that can tolerate active motion; a clinically unstable fracture requires immobilization. This chapter presents an alternative view of rehabilitation progression, defining a fracture's current structural strength as falling somewhere along a continuum of relative stability throughout recovery (Fig. 31-1). This alternative view leads to a number of graduated-motion, external protection, and functional reactivation rehabilitation options based on the current

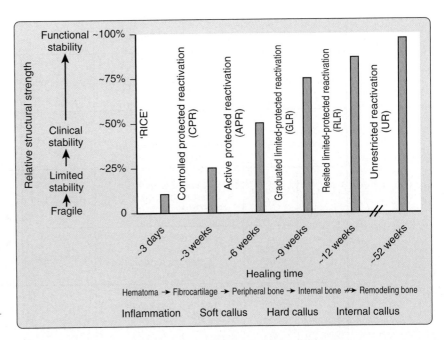

Figure 31-1 Fracture-relative strength and rehabilitation progression.

structural strength or relative stability of a fracture in any individual patient at any given point in time during healing and recovery. Following the same principles used when designing, implementing, and progressing through an individualized rehabilitation plan after any fragile healing soft tissue injury (e.g., a tendon, ligament, or nerve injury), therapy should begin within a few days of the injury. Motion is limited or controlled and protected, with functional reactivation as the goal. The degree of protection is progressively decreased, and the types of physiologic loads and functional activities are increased over the next few weeks until full functional recovery has occurred, usually about 3 months after injury.

Defining the current structural strength or relative stability of a healing fracture at any point in time depends on a number of clinical factors as well as the individual's functional demands and priorities. This involves the same clinical decision-making process as for any other healing, fragile, soft tissue hand injury. In all cases, the structural strength of any healing tissue is relative to the type of stresses or loads the tissues must withstand. As is also true for such tissues, there are no recipes or rules regarding the best type or timing for specific rehabilitation interventions. Each fracture is unique, and the rehabilitation plan must be tailored to each patient's clinical presentation, specific personal needs and priorities, and daily functional demands. Understanding these unique factors and the specific clinical fracture presentation is critical to developing an efficient and effective rehabilitation plan focused on maximizing the quality and rate of functional recovery.

These factors are detailed in the following discussion.

Which Bone and Where in the Bone?

The fracture location and surrounding soft tissue anatomy define the regional static and dynamic forces that may compromise skeletal alignment. Potential deforming forces acting on a fracture in the neck of a fifth finger MC are quite different from those acting on a fracture in the base of a first MC or the shaft of a second proximal phalange. The clinician needs to understand the nature of these forces in order to plan the appropriate resting joint posture. The correct posture helps neutralize these forces and mitigates or counterbalances them when motion is introduced around a fracture (Fig. 31-2). Understanding the regional anatomy offers insights into what other regional soft tissues may have been injured or compromised functionally due to the initial injury and what secondary surgery or fixation (plus subsequent immobilization) may be needed. As mentioned earlier, the most common complications after a hand fracture are secondary soft tissue complications in the regional joints, tendons, and muscles, not complications associated with fracture healing. Understanding what regional soft tissue complications are likely to occur is the first step in planning a rehabilitation program to prevent them.

Number and Nature of Fracture Line(s)

The pattern of bone structural failure helps define how much the fracture has undermined the inherent structural strength of the bone. Intrinsically, the number of fracture lines and their orientation within the bone determine what types of forces are likely to displace the fracture fragments and in which direction. An oblique or spiral fracture in the midshaft of an MC compared with a transverse fracture in the same location is displaced by different types of (compression, traction, bending, rotation) and directions of (axial, anteroposterior [AP], radioulnar [RU]) forces acting on the bone. Oblique and spiral fractures are displaced more easily with axial compression and rotation forces than are transverse fractures, which are more susceptible to AP and RU forces. The nature and number of fracture lines also characterize the type or pattern of fracture fixation that can be used to help maintain and stabilize fracture alignment during healing.

Bone	Region	Regional deforming forces	Pattern of malunion	
Metacarpal (MC)		**Intrinsic muscle:** distal flexes	Apex dorsal	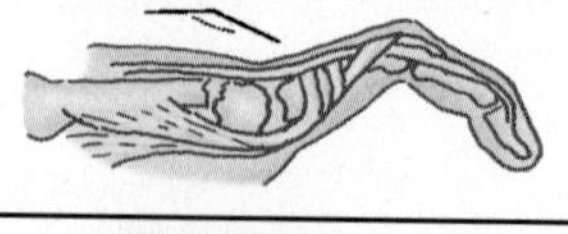
Proximal phalanx (P1)		**Intrinsic muscle:** proximal flexes **Extensor mechanism:** distal extends	Apex volar	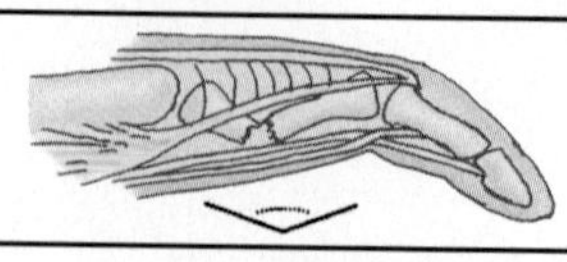
Middle phalanx (P2)	Proximal 1/3	**Central tendon:** proximal extends **FDS:** distal flexes	Apex dorsal	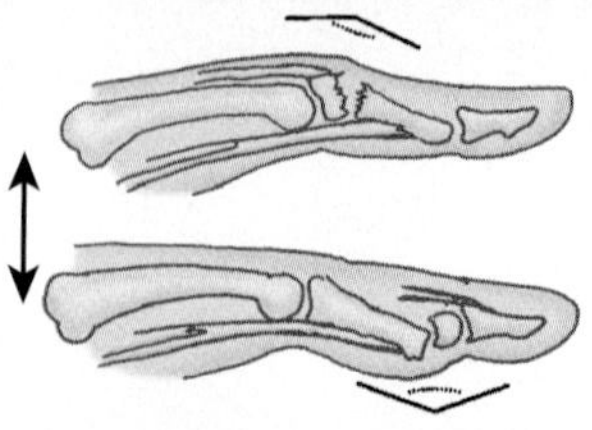
	Distal 1/3	**FDS:** proximal flexes **Extensor tendon:** distal extends	Apex volar	
Distal phalanx (P3)	Shaft	**Extensor tendon:** N/A (nail bed injury) **FDP:** distal flexes	Apex dorsal	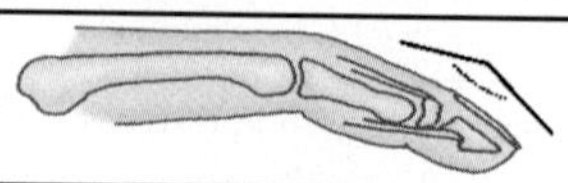
	Tuft	N/A: no tendon insertions	N/A	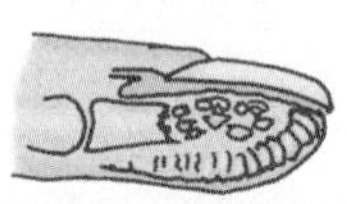
Note: All malunions - functional bone shortening +/− digital rotation or lateral angulation distal to fracture				

Figure 31-2 Regional deforming forces and common patterns of fracture malunion. FDP, flexor digitorum profundis; FDS, flexor digitorum superficialis; MC, metacarpal.

Initial Fracture Displacement and Alignment

The degree of displacement (amount of associated periosteal disruption) and direction or pattern of actual displacement of the bone fragments at the time of injury also determine the inherent structural damage caused by the fracture; the more periosteal disruption and internal structural bony collapse or failure (comminution) at the time of injury, the greater the loss of intrinsic structural strength even after reduction. In addition, the degree and direction of initial bone fracture displacement define the type and direction of forces required to reduce or realign the fracture fragments. Fractures are generally reduced by introducing forces in a pattern opposite to the original pattern of bone failure or injury and are also generally more tolerant of forces and loads associated with physiologic joint motions distal to the fracture introduced opposite to the pattern of bone failure. If a bone failed from a compression/hyperextension injury, then it is reduced with traction and volar displacement and flexion forces acting on the distal fragment. This same fracture is also likely to be more tolerant of joint motions distal to the fracture moving into flexion rather than end-range extension.

Type of Reduction and Fixation

The type of reduction (closed, limited open/minimally invasive, or open) and the kind, pattern, and location of any additional fixation (none, wire, screw or plate, or both) influence the nature of underlying healing (direct or indirect). Additionally, the type of reduction and fixation defines how bone vascularity and regional soft tissues may have been disrupted and may continue to be affected due to ongoing metal impingement or encroachment. The type of fixation also establishes how much and what types of additional structural strength or stability might be expected from the fixation mechanical construct (minimal, flexible, or low-stability fixation vs. absolute, rigid, or high-stability fixation).

Postreduction and Fixation Alignment

Although the ultimate goal of fracture reduction and fixation is to achieve perfect anatomic alignment, this is often not possible, especially if the fracture has been managed with minimal or closed reduction and minimal or more flexible fracture fixation. Often, the quest for perfect alignment and stability (the perfect radiograph) requires more extensive surgical interventions and greater amounts of residual metal left in the bone or hand, both of which have potential negative effects on the underlying healing and the patient's functional recovery.

Fortunately, the hand tissues and the person affected have the capacity to compensate and recover functionality, even with extra-articular fractures that heal with a degree of malunion. However, there are limits to the degree and type of malunion that are tolerated or compensated for. What is tolerable varies markedly based on the bone affected, the site of the malunion, and the patient's needs and priorities for cosmetic and functional recovery. In general, the hand tissues and the patient are better able to compensate for and tolerate volar or dorsal angulation deformities than lateral angulation or rotational deformities that cause the fingertips to move away from the thumb during pinching and gripping activities.

Although the potential risk–benefit ratio of various surgical options is a decision made between the surgeon and patient, therapists need to understand the potential functional implications of different patterns of malunion. This understanding is important not only to ensure that planned therapeutic interventions do not increase the potential for worsening a malunion, especially in situations where the fracture has minimal or no additional fixation, but also to plan specific orthosis use or exercises that will help reduce or prevent complications associated with malunion, in particular any functional bone foreshortening and subsequent loss of active end-range joint motion (or joint lag) in joints distal to the fracture.

Nature of Additional Soft Tissue Injury

The degree of associated soft tissue injury, both from the injury and from any surgical trauma, also needs to be identified as it determines the other regional tissues to be included in the rehabilitation plan. The greater the complexity of associated soft tissue injury, the more complex the rehabilitation plan and the greater the need to ensure that therapy begins early to try to prevent the secondary complications associated with immobilization. Frequently, in the case of multiple tissue trauma injuries, surgeons opt for more extensive surgical interventions and more rigid fracture fixation options in an effort to facilitate earlier rehabilitation. Even when there are no apparent direct soft tissue injuries (such as a tendon or nerve laceration), therapists still need to understand the specific details of how the fracture reduction and fixation were achieved, that is, the technical details of what soft tissues were dissected, retracted, impaled, clamped, and sutured or not sutured; how difficult the reduction and fixation were to achieve; and how confident the surgeon is with the fixation.

It is important to remember that even in conservatively managed, closed-hand fractures, the fracture is just the most obvious injury because it can be seen on the radiograph. Almost all hand fractures are multitissue traumatic injuries and include soft tissue trauma, even if not externally evident. Closed crushing, hitting, torsion-type forces transmitted through the finger or hand with enough force to create underlying bone failure likely cause similar regional neurovascular, muscle, tendon, tendon sheath, or joint capsule–ligament crush, contusion, or tearing-type injuries.

Time Since Fracture or Surgery

The time since fracture or surgery sets the stage for fracture healing, whether the healing is through direct or indirect mechanisms.[85] In general, the longer the time from fracture or surgery, the more structural strength is provided by the underlying bone healing or mineralization process. The majority of extra-articular hand fractures heal through indirect or secondary fracture callus healing, passing through the initial inflammatory phase in the first few days, then through the proliferative fibrocartilage, or soft callus, stage, followed by peripheral bony union or mineralization or hard callus, and then into a final internal bony bridging or mineralization phase. As this progressive mineralization of the fracture callus increases, relative structural strength (stiffness) is regained at the fracture site; this progressive increase in stiffness associated with bone healing or mineralization tends to

define the phases or types of rehabilitation interventions and functional reactivation that can occur following a fracture (see Fig. 31-1 and Table 31-1).[85,97,98]

For fractures that have been managed with more rigid fixation, it is important to remember that these forms of fixation do not provide the same relative structural strength as normal bone, and so are not functionally stable. Rather, they provide the relative structural strength equivalent to a clinically stable fracture or a fracture that is able to tolerate unrestricted active motion of the joints adjacent to the fracture without displacement or additional protection during the initial 3 to 4 weeks after fracture. These fractures still need to be protected during functional use, especially during the first 3 to 4 weeks, and they should not be subjected to progressive resisted motion, composite passive stretching, or unprotected moderate to heavier functional use until there is evidence of internal mineralization across the fracture. In terms of timelines, internal mineralization of the fracture following rigid fixation usually occurs around the same time that internal mineralization begins in fractures healing through indirect or secondary fracture callus healing—sometime around 6 weeks after fracture.[97,98]

Normal Daily Functional Demands and Patient Priorities

Understanding the patient's normal daily functional demands and priorities is crucial to determining the level of protection needed for the fracture during functional use, as well as for defining the priorities and timelines for functional reactivation around the healing fracture. In most instances, a planned and graduated return to normal functional activities, including work, sport, leisure, and personal care activities, can be achieved through the thoughtful design and use of serially reduced or modified external fracture orthoses or braces, as well as a targeted functional reactivation plan consistent with the person's needs and priorities. The advantage of early, protected functional reactivation throughout fracture healing is that the affected hand is less likely to develop losses of hand pinch and grip strength and endurance associated with early postfracture immobilization and prolonged functional disuse.

Gaining This Understanding

The essential components for gaining an understanding of a fracture's relative stability are:
- A complete and detailed report from the referring physician or surgeon
- Access to pre- and postfracture reduction and fixation imaging
- An operating room report (if applicable) or direct communication with the referring surgeon regarding details of the surgery
- Team work and communication among therapist, physician and surgeon, and patient

Without these essential components of information and support, therapists are essentially treating hand fracture patients "in the dark," with limited ability to maximize functional recovery. Fortunately, most hand therapists have established close TEAM (*together everyone accomplishes more*) (see Chapter 29) working relationships with referring physicians and surgeons who are used to providing detailed

Table 31-1 Rehabilitation Progression: Extra-Articular Hand Fractures

Relative Stability: (Structural Strength)	Approximate Timeframes	Acronym	Motion (Joint(s)/Tendon)	External Protection (Fracture)	Reactivation Limitations (Function)
Fragile	~0–3 days	**R** est/Recover **I** mmobilize **C** ompression **E** levation	No joint motion: immobilization	Immobilization orthosis: >2 regional joints (worn at all times)	Rest/recover: Elevation/compression Limited pain-free personal functional use (with cast or orthosis)
Limited Stability	~3 days–3 weeks	**C** ontrolled: stabilized (motion) **P** rotected (fracture) **R** eactivation (function)	Controlled stabilized joint motion ▪ Type ▪ Arc/direction ▪ Number of joints ▪ Frequency	Serial orthosis reduction/modified fracture brace: 1 joint distal + 1 proximal to fracture (off for hand hygiene)	Light pain-free functional activities (with modified fracture brace)
Clinical Stability	~3–6 weeks	**A** ctive (motion) **P** rotected (fracture) **R** eactivation (function)	Full-arc isolated joint motion: active + passive	Fracture brace: no joints (off at rest/night + light activities)	Moderate pain-free functional activities (with fracture brace)
	~6–9 weeks	**G** raduated (motion) **L** imited: protected (fracture) **R** eactivation (function)	Full-arc composite joint motion: active + passive (end-range stretching + orthosis)	Limited fracture brace: no joints (on for selected heavier use)	Heavy pain-free functional activities (with fracture brace)
	~9–12 weeks	**R** esisted (motion) **L** imited—protected (fracture) **R** eactivation (function)	Resisted, full-arc composite joint motion: resisted active (strengthening)	Limited fracture brace: no joints (on for high-risk use)	High-risk (sports, recreation, work) pain-free functional activities (with fracture brace)
Functional Stability	>12 weeks	**U** nrestricted **R** eactivation	Unrestricted joint motion	No protection	No limitations

information and referrals to therapists for other types of fragile healing hand injuries. Additionally, many therapists have improved access to imaging and surgical reports as most are now available in digital form and easily transferred and viewed in the clinic on any computer. As with other acute hand injuries, it is the therapist's responsibility to understand the details of the injury and surgery before beginning intervention and to consult with the physician or surgeon for further details if this information is not available at the time of referral. In addition, therapists and surgeons typically work together to ensure that the patient is the central team member, ensuring that he or she understands the details of the hand fracture and the goals and timelines for recovery, with the therapist and surgeon focusing on monitoring, supporting, and encouraging the patient to achieve the best possible outcome.

Phases of Rehabilitation: Based on Relative Stability

The phases of rehabilitation following an extra-articular hand fracture are essentially the same as those after a healing tendon or nerve repair, beginning with a few days of rest and recovery during the inflammatory stages of healing following the injury, progressing over the next 3 to 4 weeks to limited or controlled motion with a light, functional reactivation program introduced in conjunction with the external protection or support needed. In the weeks that follow, a progressively graduated program of composite active motion, followed by passive stretching, resisted exercise, and functional reactivation, is introduced in conjunction with progressively decreasing or reduced external protection or support for the healing fracture.

Postfracture rehabilitation can be divided into six phases, corresponding to the progress of perceived structural strength or relative stability of the healing fracture (see Fig. 31-1 and Table 31-1). However, the initiation and progression or modification of therapy following any hand fracture varies and must be based on an assessment of the fracture's relative stability at each point in time. These phases of rehabilitation are general guidelines that need to be tailored to each patient.

Phase 1: Fragile Fractures—Rest, Ice, Compression, Elevation (RICE)

During the first 3 to 5 days after injury, an initial hematoma and inflammatory response to the traumatic fracture are seen. During this period, there is no biological or functional advantage to using the hand except for very light and essential self-care. Other than potentially contaminated, open injuries in need of further wound care and monitoring, hand fracture injuries are best left to rest and recover during the first 3 to 5 days after injury. Light, compressive, immobilization dressings or orthoses and hand elevation are effective strategies for minimizing postfracture edema and pain during these initial days. Around 3 to 5 days after fracture, the symptoms of aching pain at rest, at night, and with dependency begin to subside. These are general indications that the degree of fracture immobilization or support can be serially reduced or modified and some early controlled and protected motion and light protected functional reactivation can begin (see Table 31-1).

Phase 2: Limited Stability—Controlled, Protected, Reactivation (CPR)

Around the third to the fifth postinjury day, most fractures have some limited stability and can tolerate controlled joint motion, as well as light functional use, if introduced in conjunction with appropriate support and a protective orthosis. Most fractures are not yet strong enough to withstand unrestricted active joint motion or functional use without this additional protection and are often treated with ongoing immobilization. Fortunately, as with other fragile healing soft tissue injuries, many less forceful controlled-motion options can be considered at this time. A number of modified fracture brace designs can provide protection and support during functional use. These modified braces also stabilize or immobilize at least one joint proximal and distal to the fracture at rest and during functional use, while providing the opportunity to introduce controlled motion in the joints under controlled circumstances (see Table 31-1).

Phase 3: Clinical Stability—Active, Protected, Reactivation (APR)

After 3 to 4 weeks in most fractures with initial limited stability, and within 3 to 5 days in fractures managed with more rigid forms of plate or screw fixation, enough structural strength or clinical stability is usually achieved to withstand unrestricted, full-arc, regional joint motions. However, the fracture has not yet gained enough strength or stability to withstand composite, end-range, passive-stretching, resisted motion for moderate functional activities without ongoing external support or protection. At this point, functional use of the hand for moderate, pain-free activities is facilitated if the immobilization orthosis or modified fracture brace used during the early phases of rehabilitation is serially reduced to a more traditional, functional fracture brace design so that it provides circumferential support around the fracture but does not include either of the joints proximal or distal to the fracture (see Table 31-1).

Phase 4: Graduated, Limited-Protected, Reactivation (GLR)

Around 6 weeks after injury, most extra-articular hand fractures have developed enough structural strength to withstand end-range, composite, active motion and passive end-range stretching exercises or orthosis use, progressive-resisted (light strengthening) exercises, and moderate functional activities without the need for additional fracture support or protection. However, the external support or protection (functional fracture brace) should still be applied when the person uses the hand for heavier strengthening or functional activities (see Table 31-1).

Phase 5: Resisted, Limited-Protected, Reactivation (RLR)

About 9 weeks after injury, most extra-articular hand fractures are strong enough to withstand moderate levels of functional demands for occupational and sports-related activities and heavier resisted therapeutic exercises without

any additional protection or support. However, fractures still need to be protected with external support or functional fracture bracing during higher-risk, high-impact activities until at least 3 months after fracture (see Table 31-1).

Phase 6: Unrestricted Reactivation (UR)

Because no residual hand tissue impairment or dysfunction usually remains 3 months after fracture, the individual should be able to resume normal functional activities without the need for additional support or protection. This is not always the case, however, and the focus at this point is to continue to maximize the recovery of any regional tissue, joint, tendon, and muscle impairment through continued exercises and orthosis use as required. If the patient has yet to return to a typical level of participation in occupational, sports, or other functional activities by 3 months after fracture, further attention should be given to defining specific barriers or limitations to this return and what further modifications or plans are needed to facilitate return to the previous functional level (see Table 31-1).

Therapeutic Options: Motion, External Protection, and Functional Reactivation

Figure 31-3 provides an overview of a number of motion, external protection, and functional reactivation alternatives and progressions that therapists might consider following when treating an extra-articular hand fracture. Although these clinical options may appear complex, they are no different from similar clinical options for other fragile, healing hand injuries.

Motion Options

Traditionally, motion of joints surrounding an extra-articular hand fracture is delayed, occurring after removal of an immobilization cast or orthosis, or earlier when a fracture has been managed with more rigid fixation or when it is considered to be clinically stable. In these instances, the motion usually starts with active, full-arc, composite motion of the affected digit or hand. However, a number of motion parameters can be controlled or limited and introduced earlier, when a fracture has more limited relative stability or progressed to more forceful motion options when a fracture has greater relative stability.

The motion parameters that can be limited or controlled include (see Fig. 31-3):
1. Arc of motion (limited or full)
2. Type of motion (passive, active-assisted, unresisted active, passive end-range, or resisted active)
3. Direction of motion (flexion or extension, or both)
4. Number of joints moving (isolated or composite motion)
5. Frequency of motion (how many, how often)
6. Conditions of motion (with local fracture stabilization, under supervision, in protective orthosis or unlimited)

How and when to progress motion following a hand fracture depend on the fracture tolerance and how well the patient achieves the motion goals introduced to date. There are no specific timelines or rules for progression, other than achieving pain-free motion based on the relative stability of

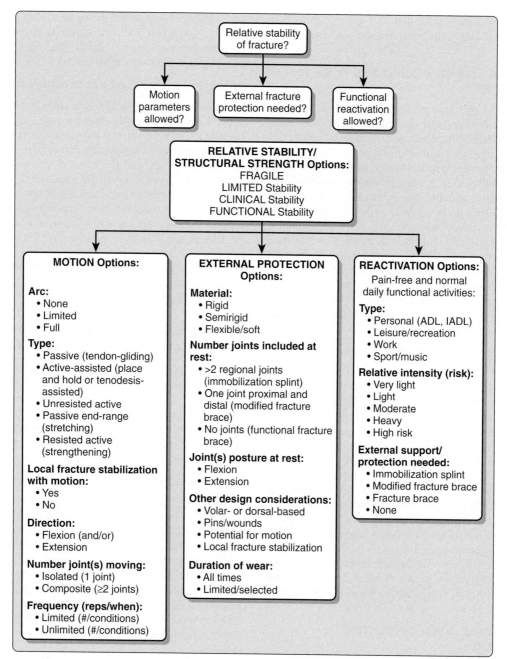

Figure 31-3 Therapeutic options: Motion, external protection, and functional reactivation. ADL, activities of daily living.

the underlying fracture. If a patient can successfully and consistently achieve a pain-free, limited-arc, passive, isolated joint motion, then progression can be considered. If, however, such motion is not possible, it is time to revisit and modify the motion goals to a less strenuous or forceful exercise regimen that can be tolerated. If the fracture tolerates this goal and the patient can successfully and consistently achieve a pain-free full arc of unresisted active motion of the joints distal to the fracture, then it is time to consider progressing to composite full-arc or light-resisted active or gentle end-range passive stretching exercises, with or without additional local fracture stabilization or external fracture protection. Alternatively, if this same patient can achieve full, pain-free,

composite active flexion of the joints adjacent to the fracture, but cannot consistently maintain full active extension of these joints, then daytime extension blocking orthoses or exercises and nighttime full-extension resting orthosis use should be continued.

External Protection Options

During the initial 3 to 4 weeks after fracture, hand fractures are traditionally managed with some form of rigid external cast, orthosis, or brace within which the regional joints in the affected finger, hand, wrist, and forearm are included, effectively immobilizing all joints within the external support. Although these supports provide adequate protection of the fracture during initial healing, they are not function-friendly, nor do they allow for safe introduction of limited or controlled motion. Secondly, these bulky external supports are often removed completely at 3 to 4 weeks to enable introduction of active motion and light functional use. However, at this point, the underlying fracture is still relatively weak, needing protection from other than light functional use, which means that the patient needs to continue to limit participation in many normal daily functional activities.

The external protection parameters that can be modified or adapted throughout recovery are (see Fig. 31-3):

1. Material (rigid, semirigid, soft or flexible)
2. Number of joint(s) included at rest (immobilization orthosis [>2 joints]; modified fracture brace [1 joint ± fracture]; functional fracture brace [no joints, circumferential support only]);
3. Joint(s) posture at rest (flexion, extension)
4. Other design considerations (volar- or dorsal-based; pin and wound access; strapping options for potential for motion, or additional local stabilization)
5. Duration of wear (all times; selected or limited)

As with controlled-motion options, there are no rules or best orthosis designs for any given extra-articular hand fracture. Postfracture orthoses or braces should in most cases be custom-designed and molded to suit the individual patient and fracture. The art of designing and fabricating individualized orthoses or modified fracture braces involves finding a balance between ensuring that the design and material provide adequate support and protection for the healing fracture during functional use, while minimizing the number of joints included in the orthosis or brace at rest, and facilitating the introduction of early and controlled-motion alternatives without the need for orthosis removal. In most cases no one orthosis or brace design is adequate throughout a person's recovery. However, in many cases most custom-designed orthoses can be designed to be serially reduced or modified easily as the relative strength of the fracture increases throughout recovery. Some examples of modified functional fracture brace designs and serial reduction options for different extra-articular hand fractures are presented later in this chapter.

Functional Reactivation Options:

The functional reactivation parameters that can be integrated into a rehabilitation plan are based on the patient's daily functional demands, needs, and priorities and should be identified early in recovery, along with establishing clear goals. Again, the specific functional demands and protection needed throughout recovery differ for any two individuals presenting with very similar fractures. Functional reactivation for a single, male, competitive college football player wanting to return to his sport is different from that for an elderly retired widow who lives independently and walks with a cane. Both should be able to return to some planned and graduated leisure, occupation, or sporting activities with appropriately designed functional fracture support or protection soon after the fracture. Over the weeks immediately following the fracture, both patients should also have an individualized, planned, and graduated increase in the type, intensity, and duration of activities with a gradual reduction

of the required fracture protection needed during functional use (see Fig. 31-3).

Early Mobilization: Fracture-Specific Considerations

Metacarpal Fractures

Regional Deforming Forces: Intrinsic muscle (see Fig. 31-2)
Malunion: Apex dorsal angulation with bone foreshortening ± lateral deviation or rotation of the distal fragment (see Fig. 31-2)
Common Soft Tissue Complications

1. Extensor tendon adherence to underlying callus = active finger composite extensor lag and limited end-range composite flexion (fist)
2. Intrinsic muscle contracture = limited end-range IP flexion with MCP extension (tuck)
3. Dorsal incision scar contracture = limited end-range composite finger flexion (fist)

Early Mobilization Considerations

1. *Orthosis Design:* MCP held in at least 70 degrees of flexion at rest with circumferential and three-point fracture (apex dorsal) stabilization of the fracture. Provision for additional dynamic local stabilization at the fracture when moving into MCP extension/abduction combined with IP flexion (Fig. 31-4)
2. *Extensor Tendon-Gliding Exercises:* Early passive or active stabilized composite finger extension (see Fig. 31-4)
3. *Intrinsic Muscle Exercises:* Early stabilized composite finger extension abduction/adduction progressed to composite IP flexion with MCP extension (finger tuck—intrinsic stretch) (see Fig. 31-4)

Clinical Example

Figure 31-5 shows an example of an orthosis design that could be used for a fifth MP fracture that has limited early stability or has been managed with some form of flexible fixation. The initial volar-based immobilization orthosis can be reduced to free the IP joints or serially reduced to a modified functional fracture brace design including only the MCP and the CMC joints within the orthosis (one joint distal and proximal to the fracture). In addition, the orthosis includes an additional three-point (apex dorsal), counterpressure, semirigid dorsal insert and adjustable strapping to ensure consistent circumferential support of the fracture that accommodates variations in swelling and that is consistent with the concept of circumferential functional fracture bracing.

This same orthosis allows the potential for limited or controlled motion of the MCP joint into extension with additional local stabilization of the fracture with a gentle pinch or local compression to counterbalance the dynamic deforming forces associated with increasing tension in the intrinsic muscles as the finger moves into MCP extension and abduction with IP flexion (see Fig. 31-4). Finally, this same modified fracture brace can be reduced serially by removing the distal component that holds the MCP in flexion, effectively converting this orthosis into a more traditional functional fracture brace design, providing circumferential support for

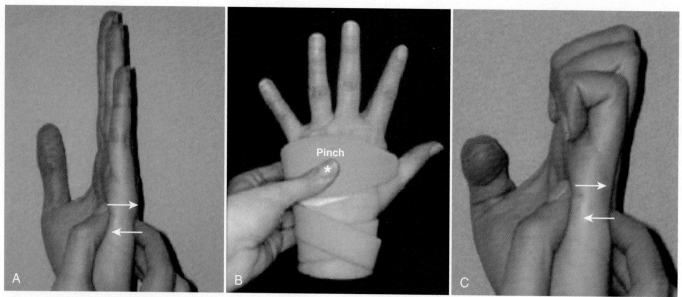

Figure 31-4 Fifth metacarpal key exercises: **A,** Stabilized active composite finger extension (shown with no orthosis). This same exercise can be initiated in the modified fracture brace shown in Figure 31-5. **B,** The exercise is progressed to stabilized active finger abduction with finger composite extension (shown in a modified fracture brace) with × indicating the location of additional local stabilization with a gentle pinch or local compression. **C,** Progressed further to full active, composite proximal interphalangeal and distal interphalangeal flexion with metacarpophalangeal extension (finger tuck).

the fracture without significantly limiting the motion of joints proximal and distal to the fracture. This brace can continue to be worn selectively for the next few weeks during progressive daily functional use and therapeutic exercises. In another example, Figure 31-6 shows a fracture brace that can be used for a first metacarpal fracture with limited early stability.

Proximal Phalangeal (P1) Fractures

Regional Deforming Forces
Intrinsic muscle and extensor mechanism (see Fig. 31-2)
Malunion: Apex volar angulation with bone foreshortening ± lateral deviation or rotation of the distal fragment (see Fig. 31-2)

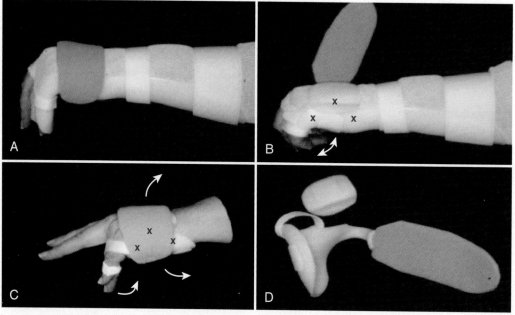

Figure 31-5 Fifth metacarpal (MC) fracture: Modified fracture brace. **A,** A volar-based orthosis that holds the wrist, hand, and fourth and fifth fingers in a position of function with an adjustable dorsal circumferential strap across the MC region. **B,** The dorsal strap is removed to expose a three-point counterpressure, semirigid insert that adds additional fracture support. The orthosis has been serially reduced to allow proximal interphalangeal and distal interphalangeal motion. **C,** Further serial reduction to free the wrist, with a buddy strap distally to control rotation of the finger during motion. **D,** The component parts of the same orthosis shown in C.

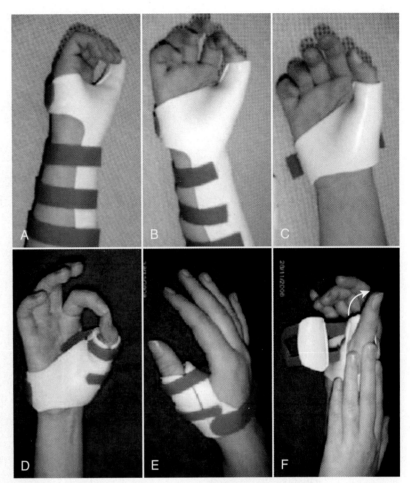

Figure 31-6 Thumb metacarpal fracture orthosis: **A,** Full-thumb spica orthosis (interphalangeal [IP], metacarpophalangeal [MCP], and carpometacarpal joints, and wrist included). **B,** Reduced to free the IP. **C,** Reduced to free the wrist. **D–F,** A simple dorsal window cut out over the proximal phalanx that is held in place with straps during functional use and at rest. These straps and dorsal window can be released to allow stabilized active MCP joint extension exercises, similar to early stabilized MCP joint extension exercises for metacarpal fractures in the second through fifth rays. This same dorsal window cut-out modification also can be done to the longer-thumb spica orthoses shown in A and B.

Common Soft Tissue Complications
1. Extensor mechanism adherence to underlying callus = active PIP extensor lag/flexion contracture and limited end-range composite IP joint flexion (fist and tuck)
2. Flexor digitorum superficialis (FDS) adherence to underlying callus = limited end-range composite finger extension and limited active isolated DIP and composite IP flexion (fist and tuck)

Early Mobilization Considerations
1. *Orthosis Design*: MCP joint held in at least 70 degrees of flexion and PIP held in extension at rest with circumferential and three-point fracture (apex volar) stabilization of the fracture. Provision for additional dynamic local stabilization of the fracture when moving actively into end-range PIP extension or composite PIP and DIP flexion (Fig. 31-7)
2. *Extensor Tendon-Gliding Exercises*: Early passive or active stabilized composite finger PIP and DIP extension (Fig. 31-8)
3. *Flexor Digitorum Profundus (FDP) and Flexor Digitorum Superficialis (FDS) Tendon-Gliding Exercises*: Early passive or active stabilized isolated DIP or composite PIP and DIP flexion, as well as early passive or active stabilized PIP flexion with DIP maintained in extension (see Fig. 31-8)

Clinical Example

Figure 31-7 shows examples of orthosis designs that can be used with a proximal phalangeal fracture with limited early stability or one that has been managed with some form of flexible fixation. These dorsal-based orthoses allow for the potential for limited or controlled motion of the IP joint into flexion. This can occur with or without additional local stabilization or local compression to counterbalance the dynamic deforming forces associated with increasing tension in the intrinsic muscle/extensor apparatus as the finger moves into composite IP flexion or end-range PIP extension. Figure 31-8 shows an example of three early active tendon-gliding exercises for P1 fractures. However, if a proximal phalangeal fracture has limited early stability or has been managed with some form of flexible fixation, initiation of early motion might begin with only one joint (PIP or DIP) or two joints (PIP and DIP) moving passively, through a limited arc (0–50 degrees) of flexion and extension progressed as tolerated to full-arc, active tendon-gliding exercises. This is similar to a passive tendon-gliding exercise done following a flexor tendon repair, ensuring sufficient glide or excursion of the extensor apparatus and the flexor tendon at the level of the fracture to reduce or prevent tendon adhesion.

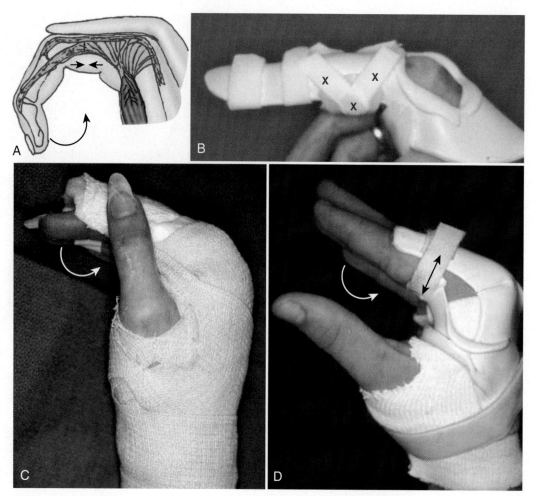

Figure 31-7 Proximal phalangeal (P1) fracture: Modified fracture brace. **A,** Diagram of metacarpophalangeal (MCP) joint blocked in flexion with active composite finger flexion; causing distal excursion of the extensor mechanism creating a volar cortical compression force that stabilizes P1 fractures. Modified, with permission, from Reyes FA, Latta LL. Conservative management of difficult phalangeal fractures. *Clin Orthop Relat Res.* 1987;214:23-30. **B,** A modified P1 brace design including a distal extension of the dorsal orthosis that holds the interphalangeal (IP) joints in extension at rest with straps that can be released to allow IP flexion motion. Also shows a three-point (apex volar), semirigid thermoplastic volar component and strap that provide additional support to the fracture and a dorsal window over the metacarpophalangeal joint that accommodates protruding K-wires (not shown). **C** and **D**, Variations of P1 modified fracture braces made from rigid-cast (**C**) and thermoplastic orthosis materials (**D**). **C** and **D** reprinted, with permission, from Feehan LM. Early controlled mobilization of potentially unstable extra-articular hand fractures. *J Hand Ther.* 2003;16:(2)161-170.

Middle Phalangeal (P2) Fractures

Regional Deforming Forces: Proximal = FDS and central tendon. Distal = FDS and terminal extensor tendon (see Fig. 31-2)

Malunion: Proximal = apex dorsal angulation with bone foreshortening ± lateral deviation or rotation of the distal fragment. Distal = apex volar angulation with bone fore-shortening ± lateral deviation and or rotation of the distal fragment (see Fig. 31-2)

Common Soft Tissue Complications

1. Extensor mechanism adherence to underlying callus = active DIP extensor lag/flexion contracture and limited end-range composite IP flexion (fist and tuck)
2. FDP adherence to underlying callus = limited end-range composite finger extension/flexion contracture and limited active isolated DIP and composite IP flexion (fist and tuck)

Early Mobilization Considerations

1. *Orthosis Design:* PIP and DIP held in extension at rest with circumferential stabilization of the fracture. Provision for additional dynamic local stabilization at the fracture when moving actively into PIP flexion or end-range extension or isolated DIP or composite IP flexion (Figs. 31-9 and 31-10)
2. *FDS Tendon-Gliding Exercises:* Early passive stabilized isolated PIP finger flexion/extension exercise, progressing to active motion (see Fig. 31-10)
3. *Terminal Extensor and Flexor (FDP) Tendon-Gliding Exercises:* Early active stabilized isolated DIP flexion and extension (see Fig. 31-10)

Clinical Example

Figure 31-9 shows examples of orthosis designs that could be used with a middle phalangeal fracture that has limited

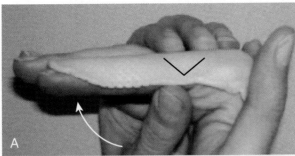
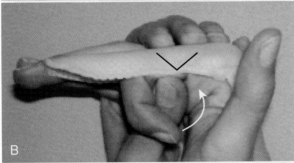
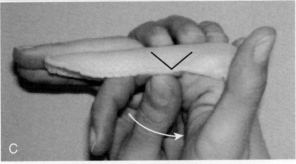

Figure 31-8 Proximal phalangeal (P1) fracture: Stabilized active tendon-gliding exercises. **A,** Extensor mechanism tendon gliding = stabilized/active interphalangeal (IP) extension initiated through a limited arc (–30 to 0 degrees) and progressed to full arc. IPs should rest in extension if there is any lag at the proximal interphalangeal (PIP) or distal interphalangeal (DIP) joint. **B,** Flexor digitorum profundus tendon gliding = stabilized/active composite DIP and PIP flexion, initiated with active DIP flexion or starting with limited-arc composite motion and progressed to full-arc motion. **C,** Flexor digitorum superficialis tendon gliding = active PIP flexion with DIP extension, progressed from limited to full arc of motion. Note: This figure shows only a dorsal orthosis template and local pinch stabilization at the fracture site. The Velcro straps and three-point volar counter-support are removed for better visualization of the exercises.

early stability or has been managed with some form of flexible fixation. Volar-based orthoses do not allow for the potential of motion, so they must be removed if early exercises are to be introduced. Dorsal-based orthoses allow for the "potential" for limited or controlled motion of the IP joint into flexion in the orthosis, with or without additional local pinch stabilization to counterbalance the dynamic deforming forces associated with motion. Figure 31-10 shows two early P2 fracture "stabilized" tendon-gliding exercises (passive PIP flexion and extension and active DIP flexion and extension) that can be introduced one at a time and with a limited arc of motion if the fracture has very limited stability.

Distal Phalangeal (P3) Fractures

Regional Deforming Forces: Proximal shaft (epiphysis in children) FDP. Tuft generally stable (see Fig. 31-2)

Malunion: Shaft = apex dorsal ± nail bed injury (see Fig. 31-2)

Common Soft Tissue Complications
   1. Open wound = wound care
   2. Crush/neurovascular injury = pain or hypersensitivity, avoidance behavior with functional pinch and grip activities.

Early Mobilization Considerations
   1. *Orthosis Design:* Dorsal-based mallet-type DIP extension orthosis ± fingertip dressing. Orthosis removed for wound care or early DIP motion. Discontinue orthosis as pain tolerance allows (usually within the first few days) and use light, flexible dressing materials to facilitate DIP motion.
   2. *DIP Motion:* Early pain-free limited arc, progressed to full arc, DIP flexion and extension. Monitor for DIP extensor lag and manage like a mallet finger injury if lag develops.
   3. *Buddy Strap:* To facilitate use of the injured fingertip with functional use

Summary

Most patients present with simple, closed, extra-articular hand fractures that are managed nonsurgically with closed reduction, followed in some instances by percutaneous wire fixation to help maintain alignment. Other more complex fracture injuries involving significant bone loss or comminution, articular disruption, or an open injury in conjunction with other regional tendon, nerve, vascular, and skin tissue injuries are managed with an open surgical or direct fracture reduction and supplemented by some form of more stable or rigid internal or external fixation. Traditionally, initiation and progression of rehabilitation and functional reactivation following extra-articular hand fractures have been based on the concepts of clinical stability or instability, with many hand fractures considered clinically unstable during the early stages of healing and immobilized for up to 4 weeks, when regional tissue complications are already established.

This chapter presents an alternative view, based on the concept of a fracture's structural strength falling along a continuum of progressively increasing relative strength throughout recovery, defining rehabilitation progression through six phases of recovery, including a phase of limited structural strength or stability in the early phases of healing. This chapter focuses on an overview of the general principles of graduated-motion, external protection, and functional reactivation rehabilitation following extra-articular hand fractures, with specific clinical examples. Early progressive mobilization and reactivation of extra-articular hand fractures follows the same principles used when designing, implementing, and progressing with an individualized rehabilitation plan after any fragile healing soft tissue injury (e.g., tendon, ligament, or nerve injury), for which therapy begins within a few days of the injury with limited or controlled and protected motion and functional reactivation, followed by a

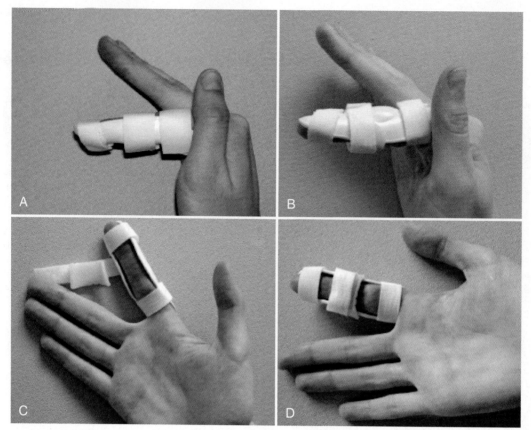

Figure 31-9 Middle phalangeal (P2) fracture: Modified fracture brace. **A,** Volar, finger-based proximal interphalangeal (PIP) and distal interphalangeal (DIP) extension orthosis. **B,** Dorsal, finger-based PIP and DIP extension orthosis (lateral view) with additional volar semirigid thermoplastic orthosis/strap component over P2 providing additional circumferential support of the fracture. **C,** Same dorsal, finger-based PIP and DIP extension orthosis (volar view) with strap released showing volar thermoplastic component**. D,** Same orthosis (volar view) with all straps in place. The dorsal and volar finger-based orthosis can be extended proximally to a hand-based orthosis that holds the metacarpophalangeal joint in flexion for additional fracture support.

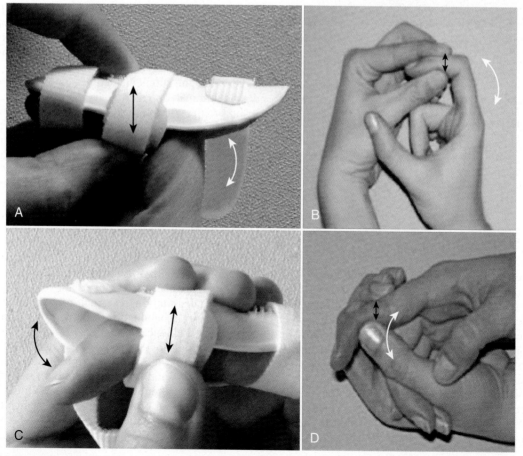

Figure 31-10 Middle phalangeal (P2) fracture: Stabilized tendon-gliding exercises. **A** and **B,** Stabilized, passive proximal interphalangeal flexion and extension (**A,** in orthosis; **B,** out of orthosis). **C** and **D,** Stabilized, active blocked distal interphalangeal flexion and extension. (**C,** in orthosis; **D,** out of orthosis).

progressive decrease in the degree of protection and increase in the types of physiologic loads and functional activities over the next few weeks until full functional recovery has occurred—usually about 3 months after injury.

And as with other fragile healing tissues, there are no recipes or rules for the best type or timing for specific rehabilitation interventions. Each fracture is unique, and the rehabilitation plan must be tailored to each patient's clinical presentation, personal needs and priorities, and daily functional demands. It is the therapist's responsibility to understand these unique factors prior to developing a rehabilitation plan focused on maximizing the quality and rate of functional recovery. Thankfully, most hand therapists have access to fracture imaging and operating room reports. Therapists typically work closely with the referring physician and surgeon to ensure that the patient is the central team member, and they also understand the details of the hand fracture and the goals and timelines for recovery. The therapist and physician or surgeon focus on monitoring, supporting, and encouraging the patient to achieve the best possible outcome.

REFERENCES

The complete reference list is available online at www.expertconsult.com.

Intra-articular Hand Fractures and Joint Injuries: Part I— Surgeon's Management

CHAPTER 32

KEVIN J. LITTLE, MD AND SIDNEY M. JACOBY, MD

CRITICAL POINTS

- The numerous ways and circumstances in which humans can position their hands places the hand and finger joints at risk for injury.
- A thorough knowledge of the articular and ligamentous anatomy is paramount to providing the best treatment for each patient.
- A good working relationship with the therapist providing care is critical in returning patients back to their vocational and recreational activities with the goal of having a painless and functional extremity.

The activities of daily living require that our hands have stability and motion at numerous joints. The vital usefulness of the hand in so many activities thereby renders it susceptible to trauma, and it is therefore the most commonly injured part of the upper extremity.[1] The incidence of injury peaks during youth and young adulthood due to participation in athletics and industrial vocations. The phalanges and metacarpals account for 10% of all fractures referred to hand surgeons. Soft tissue injuries and dislocations are common injuries as well.[2] The treating physician's and therapist's goal is to balance the joint immobilization required for healing with mobilization necessary to prevent stiffness and pain. Swanson stated in his landmark article: "Hand fractures can be complicated by deformity from no treatment, stiffness from overtreatment, and both deformity and stiffness from poor treatment."[3] The precise balance of proper surgical and therapeutic techniques is critical. Based on a thorough diagnostic evaluation and individualized treatment plan created to address the injuries identified, clinicians may maximize patient recovery and satisfaction and speed return to vocational and recreational activities.

Evaluation

After an injury occurs, a thorough history of the injury should be obtained from the patient, including mechanism, finger position during injury, the presence of deformity, previous treatments received, and a subjective sense of stability. The primary goal of the physical exam is to assess the stability of the injured joint. Observation for symmetrical or asymmetrical edema (consistent with unilateral collateral ligament injury), ecchymosis, and deformity is a critical first step. Palpation should be performed in a standard fashion, utilizing the examiner's knowledge of the appropriate anatomy to discern patterns of injury.

A radiographic evaluation should be performed prior to assessing range of motion (ROM) and stability in order to exclude obviously unstable or severe injuries. Posteroanterior (PA) and lateral radiographic views of the affected finger are mandatory, and oblique views may be of additional benefit in judging the extent of articular injuries. Occasionally, further imaging using CT or MRI may be required to completely assess intra-articular pathoanatomy. A two-stage functional assessment of the joint should be performed, using a digital or wrist block if motion is limited by pain[4] (Fig. 32-1). It is important to assess the motion of the joint while the patient voluntarily flexes and extends it. The degree of instability and the angle at which the instability occurs

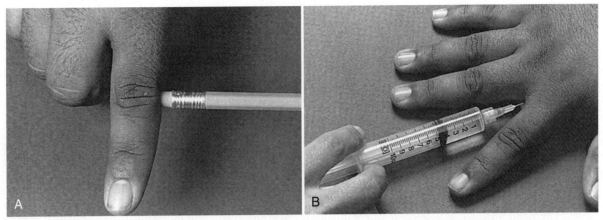

Figure 32-1 *Examination of the injured proximal interphalangeal joint. Specific area(s) of tenderness about each major retaining ligament should be localized* **(A).** *A metacarpal block may be helpful before functional range-of-motion testing in the painful, acutely injured joint* **(B).**

should be noted and used to help determine the specific anatomic site of injury. Loss of active motion but full passive motion can be indicative of tendon injury; for instance, an extensor lag may indicate damage to the extensor tendon. Passive manipulation of the joint in flexion and extension as well as lateral deviation should be performed after active motion is assessed. Crepitus during motion and lateral stability should be assessed at full extension and 30 degrees of flexion to determine if the collateral ligaments are injured. The continuity of the volar plate can be assessed via passive hyperextension and dorsal shear stress applied to the joint. Comparison with uninjured digits can be helpful in discerning whether mild instability patterns are physiologic or due to injury.

Proximal Interphalangeal Joint

The proximal interphalangeal (PIP) joint is essentially a ginglymus, or hinge joint, allowing a 110-degree arc of motion although articular asymmetry allows for 9 degrees of supination with full flexion.[5] Anterior/posterior stability is achieved primarily through articular congruity due to the thicker anterior and posterior lips of the middle phalanx. The bicondylar nature of the proximal phalanx, articulating with the biconcave fossae and intermediate ridge of the middle phalanx, provides additional stability against lateral translation. The radial and ulnar collateral ligaments supply lateral angular stability of the joint. The proper collateral ligaments (PCL) are anatomically confluent with the accessory collateral ligaments (ACL), although they are divided by their respective insertions. Both the PCL and ACL originate eccentrically from the dorsal lateral aspect of the proximal phalanx. The PCL traverses volarly and distally and inserts onto the lateral tubercle on the middle phalanx, which lies on the volar aspect of the middle phalanx. The ACL inserts onto the thick, fibrous portions along the lateral aspect of the volar plate (VP), which forms the floor of the PIP joint. Thus the PCL, which attaches more dorsally, is tight in flexion and loose in extension, and the ACL is tight in extension and loose in flexion.[6] The VP attaches along the entire volar lip of the middle phalanx, with thicker attachments at the

confluence of the collateral ligaments laterally. The thinner, central portion blends with the periosteum of the middle phalanx, allowing for greater range of flexion. Proximally, the VP tapers centrally and forms cordlike check-rein ligaments laterally, which originate off the periosteum of the proximal phalanx, inside the distal aspect of the second annular pulley (A2) and confluent with the first cruciate pulley (C1). These stout ligaments prevent hyperextension of the PIP joint[7] (Fig. 32-2).

Dynamic stability of the PIP is provided by the extensor and flexor tendons that traverse the joint. The central slip of the extensor tendon attaches to the dorsal lip of the middle phalanx, whereas the flexor digitorum superficialis (FDS) tendon divides proximal to the PIP joint and has separate lateral insertions along the middle phalanx confluent with

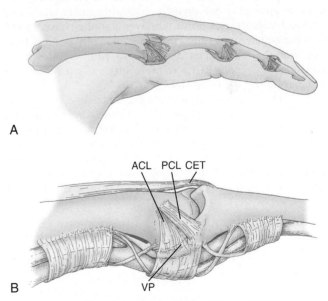

Figure 32-2 A, *Lateral view of metacarpophalangeal (MCP), proximal interphalangeal (PIP), and distal interphalangeal (DIP) joints demonstrating the capsuloligamentous structures.* **B,** *PIP joint. The major retaining ligaments of the PIP joint include the proper and accessory collateral ligaments (PCL and ACL, respectively), the volar plate (VP), and the dorsal capsule with its central extensor tendon (CET). The VP acts as a gliding surface for the flexor tendon.*

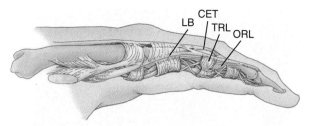

Figure 32-3 Many structures give supplemental stability to the proximal interphalangeal joint. These include the central extensor tendon (CET), the lateral bands (LB), the transverse retinacular ligament (TRL), and Landsmeer's oblique retinacular ligament (ORL).

the A3 pulley. The hand intrinsic muscles combine with the lateral bands of the extensor mechanism to form the conjoined lateral bands, which traverse dorsal to the center of rotation of the PIP joint. The transverse retinacular ligament (TRL) enshrouds the PIP joint and collateral ligaments as it courses from the VP to the conjoined lateral bands, thus preventing dorsal subluxation during extension. The oblique retinacular ligament (ORL) of Landsmeer runs from the flexor tendon sheath proximal to the PIP joint and inserts on the terminal extensor tendon traveling volar to the PIP joint axis of rotation. The course of this ligament effectively couples PIP joint extension with distal interphalangeal (DIP) joint extension and acts as a secondary restraint to PIP hyperextension[7] (Fig. 32-3).

Collateral Ligament Injuries

The wide range of motion of the shoulder and elbow allows for the hands to be placed within a large volume of space. This relative freedom predisposes to hand injury, especially during sports and recreational activities. If enough angular stress is applied to the digits, collateral ligament strain and eventual rupture can occur. Cadaveric studies have shown that the collateral ligament avulses proximally in most injuries, but the VP avulses distally.[7,8] In addition, the radial collateral ligament (RCL) is more often injured than the ulnar collateral ligament (UCL).[9]

Collateral ligament injuries are graded based on the pathoanatomy of the injury (Table 32-1). Grade I injuries involve a strain to the ligament with microfibril rupture, but the ligament remains intact. Pain is elicited by direct palpation of the involved collateral ligament, and angular stress testing reveals less than 20 degrees of passive instability. In this injury pattern, the joint is stable throughout active range of motion (AROM) and passive range of motion (PROM) testing, and can be managed nonoperatively with a brief period of positioning with an orthosis for pain control, followed by AROM within a week of injury. Buddy-taping or strapping the digit adjacent to the injured digit allows for ROM activities and passive protection of the joint.

Grade II injuries involve a complete rupture or tear of the ligament without instability of the joint during AROM. These injuries may be associated with a small avulsion fracture of the base of the middle phalanx. Stress testing that notes passive instability involving greater than 20 degrees of angular deviation is indicative of a grade II tear, as long as frank dislocation is not identified.[8] These injuries require more aggressive treatment with 2 to 4 weeks of gutter splinting; however, early motion can be initiated if angular stress can be avoided via buddy-straps or under the supervision of a therapist.

Grade III injuries imply complete collateral ligament rupture combined with VP or dorsal capsular rupture. Instability during AROM testing as well as with PROM testing occurs in both lateral and either dorsal or volar stress. Dislocation with either spontaneous or manipulative reduction is likely to be noted with these injuries.[10] Nonoperative treatment requires concentric reduction to be obtained and maintained during ROM activities. Blocking orthoses can be used to prevent subluxation and dislocation by preventing motion in ranges where instability is present. If concentric reduction cannot be maintained, operative treatment is necessary.

Dorsal Dislocations

Dislocations of the middle phalanx dorsally on the proximal phalanx represent 85% of dislocations at the PIP joint.[11] These injuries are the result of hyperextension stress applied to the joint with some element of longitudinal compression directly leading to varying degrees of bony injury. In pure PIP dislocations the VP is commonly ruptured distally; however, on rare occasions it can rupture proximally and, along with the check-rein ligaments, become interposed, thereby preventing attempts at closed reduction.[11,12] The dissipation of energy through the PIP joint during hyperextension follows a predictable pattern and is subdivided into three groups, proposed by Eaton and Littler.[4] The initial hyperextension results in rupture or avulsion of the thin central portion of the VP along with longitudinal tears in between the fibers of the ACL and PCL. However, the thick, lateral portions of the VP—the so-called critical corner—remain

Table 32-1 Ligament Injuries Involving the Proximal Interphalangeal Joint

	Grade I	Grade II	Grade III
Pathology	Sprains/diffuse fiber disruption	Complete disruption of one CL	Complete disruption of one CL as well as volar and/or dorsal structures
Functional ROM testing	Active → stable Passive → <20 degrees of angulation	Active → stable Passive → >20 degrees of angulation	Active → unstable Passive → unstable
Treatment	Immobilize, slight flexion 3–10 days, and buddy-taping	Immobilize 3–4 weeks, may begin early protected motion	Closed treatment if stable after reduction versus early open treatment

CL, collateral ligament; ROM, range of motion.

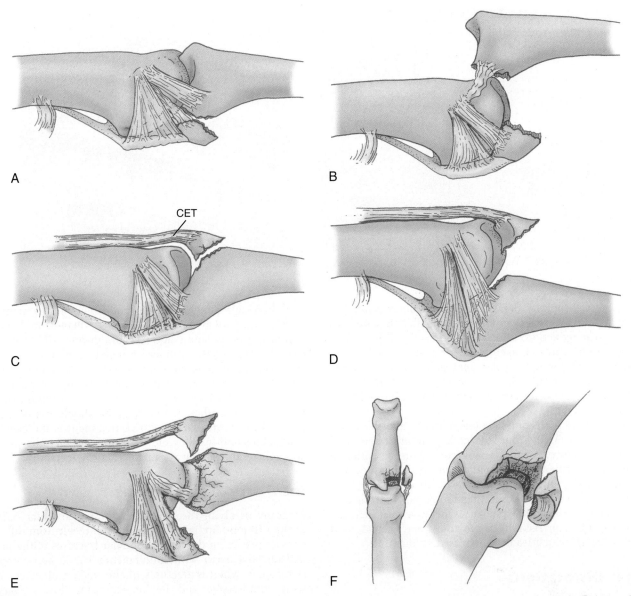

Figure 32-4 A, Avulsion fracture of the volar base of the middle phalanx. The volar plate remains attached to the fracture fragment. **B,** Intra-articular volar fracture with dorsal dislocation. With 40% articular involvement, the middle phalanx displaces dorsally, decreasing tension in the collateral ligament fibers that remain attached to the shaft at the middle phalanx. **C,** Avulsion fracture of the dorsal lip. The central extensor tendon (CET) remains attached to the fracture fragment. **D,** Intra-articular dorsal fracture with volar dislocation. The dorsal support is lost, and the middle phalanx displaces volarly. **E,** Pilon fracture. An axial loading force causes depression of the central articular surface, while the remainder of the articular surface shatters and displaces. **F,** A lateral compression fracture, caused by axial and angulatory forces, produces depression of the lateral articular surface by the proximal phalanx condyle.

intact. The initial injury to the joint can result in locked hyperextension that must be manually reduced. As the energy increases, the critical corners are injured, and the middle phalanx dislocates dorsally, often held colinearly to the proximal phalanx via intact fibers of the PCL, which are split from the ACL, which additionally remains intact. These type II injuries manifest as a pure dorsal dislocation in which the volar lip of the middle phalanx is perched on the condyles of the proximal phalanx and they may be associated with a small avulsion fracture of the base of the middle phalanx. Type III injuries involve simultaneous collateral ligament injury and some degree of lateral instability, but often manifest as dorsal dislocations (Fig. 32-4).

Most dislocations can be treated with closed reduction under digital block followed by an assessment of stability during AROM and PROM. If the joint remains stable up to 25 degrees short of full extension, positioning in an extension block orthosis can be initiated, such as with a figure-of-8 orthosis.[13] These orthoses allow for active flexion of the PIP joint, while preventing subluxation at increasing degrees of extension (Fig. 32-5). Dislocations with small avulsion fractures of the base of the middle phalanx can be treated as though they represent pure dislocations. The splints are eliminated at 3 weeks, and ROM exercises are continued. Reductions that remain unstable or are stable in greater than 25 degrees of flexion, require operative stabilization with

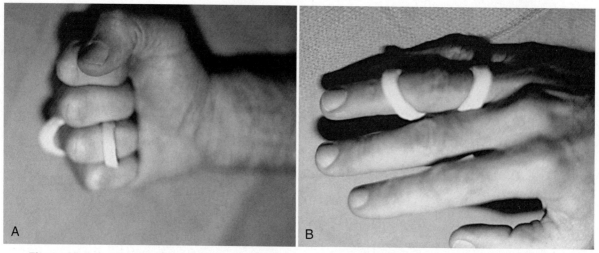

Figure 32-5 A, Figure-of-eight orthosis. **B,** Figure-of-eight orthosis prevents hyperextension while allowing full flexion.

volar plate arthroplasty (VPA),[14] extension block pinning,[15] and dynamic external fixation.[16] Irreducible dislocations require open reduction, which can be accomplished via a limited dorsal approach, using a Freer elevator to reduce the interposed soft tissue. A volar approach requires a larger incision in order to mobilize the flexor tendons around the joint, but does allow for concomitant repair of injured volar structures or VPA.

The most common complications from dorsal dislocations are residual instability due to inadequate treatment and flexion contracture. A mild flexion contracture is common and has been termed a *pseudoboutonnière deformity*; however, it is not a true boutonnière deformity since the DIP joint remains flexible and the central tendon remains attached to the dorsal lip of the middle phalanx. Operative treatment can introduce infection risks from pin tracts and increase soft tissue scarring, which leads to increased stiffness.[17]

Volar Dislocations

In comparison with dorsal dislocations, volar dislocations are rare but more problematic because they frequently involve an avulsion of the central slip at its dorsal attachment.[18] Concomitant unilateral collateral ligament injury can lead to rotatory subluxation of the middle phalanx as it rotates around the intact collateral ligament tether.[19] The difference between these two entities must be elucidated clinically since the treatment algorithm is different. Pure volar dislocations occur with a longitudinal and volar force applied to a semi-flexed PIP joint, whereas rotational torque on the joint can lead to rotatory instability.[19] As the joint dislocates volarly, the dorsal capsule tears, allowing the head of the proximal phalanx to herniate in between the lateral band and central tendon. These two structures can form a "noose" around the condyles of the proximal phalanx, preventing reduction via longitudinal traction, which tightens the noose. Reduction can be performed with wrist extension and metacarpophalangeal (MCP) flexion, to loosen the extrinsic and intrinsic extensors, respectively, followed by middle phalanx flexion and dorsal pressure. If closed reduction is unsuccessful after several attempts, open reduction should be performed.[20]

Following reduction, the central slip should be manually tested to assess if avulsion has occurred. If the central tendon is intact, and no subluxation occurs during AROM testing, early ROM exercises can be initiated to prevent stiffness. However, if central tendon injury occurs, positioning the PIP joint in full extension in a gutter orthosis must be performed for 6 weeks to allow for healing. Active DIP motion should be initiated immediately, and this joint should not be immobilized in the orthosis. Operative treatment is indicated for residual instability following reduction and includes pinning and collateral ligament repair for rotatory instability.[21]

Intra-articular Fractures

Fractures involving the distal and proximal articular surfaces of the PIP joint are fairly common, but result from different stresses placed on the joint. Condylar fractures of the proximal phalanx occur with simultaneous lateral and compressive forces, whereas fractures of the middle phalanx occur with compressive and flexion–extension forces. Varying degrees of longitudinal stress applied to the joint can lead to increasing amounts of comminution in the fractures. Fractures about the PIP joint are prone to develop stiffness; thus the goal of treatment is to maximize the stability of the fractures with minimal soft tissue trauma so that active motion can begin quickly.

Volar shearing fractures commonly occur as dorsal fracture–dislocations of the PIP joint. The extent of injury is graded by the amount of articular surface involved, which is directly related to the inherent stability of the fracture. Fractures involving less than 30% of the articular surface are stable and can be treated with extension block positioning and early mobilization. Fractures involving 30% to 50% of the volar articular surface are variably stable and depend on the extent of collateral ligament injury. Fracture fragments larger than 40% of the articular surface generally encompass most of the PCL, rendering the middle phalanx unstable to closed treatment. Fractures with greater than 50% articular surface injury have little collateral ligament stability and have lost the cup-shaped articular surface that provides intrinsic stability to the joint.[22] Nondisplaced fractures and stable

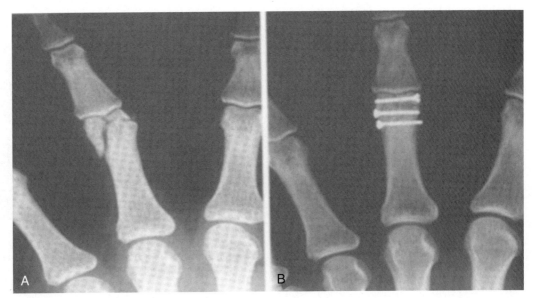

Figure 32-6 Proximal interphalangeal (PIP) fracture treated with open reduction and internal fixation. **A,** PIP fracture with intra-articular extension and angular deformity. **B,** Anatomic reduction with three lag screws.

displaced fracture patterns are treated with a protective orthosis of the PIP joint while allowing for active MCP and DIP motion.[13] Careful, close follow-up is mandatory to ensure that fracture displacement or joint subluxation does not occur during healing. Orthosis use can be discontinued and AROM/PROM initiated once fracture healing is identified, although protected AROM exercises supervised by a therapist can be considered after 2 to 3 weeks with stable patterns. An orthosis should not be used on fractures for longer than 30 days, nor positioned in greater than 30 degrees of flexion, as flexion contractures are likely to develop.[1]

Unstable fracture patterns require open treatment, and in recent years, numerous techniques have been added to the hand surgeon's arsenal. Simple large fracture fragments are ideal for open reduction and internal fixation (ORIF) with lag screws or Kirschner's wires (K-wires) (Fig. 32-6). This can be performed through a volar approach using Brunner's incisions and opening the flexor sheath between the A2 and A4 pulleys. The most important aspect of surgical correction is restoration of the volar lip of the middle phalanx, which provides most of the stability that prevents recurrent dorsal subluxation.[23] However, comminution is frequent and can be underestimated on radiographs. If such comminution is encountered, the fracture fragments can be excised and the fibrocartilaginous VP advanced to fill the defect.[14] This VPA can be attached with suture anchors or through pull-out sutures or narrow-gauge wire placed around the extensor mechanism (Fig. 32-7). This procedure should not be attempted when greater than 50% of articular comminution is present because the significant advancement may lead to flexion contracture and the pliable surface of the VP can allow for dorsal subluxation.

For comminuted fractures involving greater than 50% of the articular surface, a relatively new technique known as hemihamate arthroplasty has been shown to be extremely effective[24] (Fig. 32-8). With this procedure, the dorsal lip of the distal articular surface of the hamate, which closely approximates the biconcave fossae of the proximal aspect of the middle phalanx, is harvested and placed in the defect so as to recreate the volar lip and provide stability against dorsal

subluxation. This procedure can restore most PIP motion, even when reconstruction is delayed; however, lengthy delays can lead to decreased motion, and most patients have at least a small residual flexion contracture due to the extensive soft tissue mobilization required. Persistent dorsal wrist

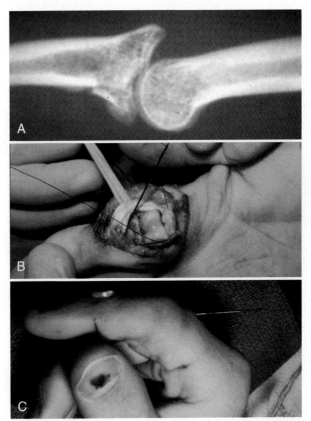

Figure 32-7 Volar plate arthroplasty. **A,** Preoperative lateral radiograph demonstrating impaction fracture of 50% of the volar lip of the proximal interphalangeal joint. **B,** Intraoperative photograph demonstrating proximal "check-rein ligament" release and distal advancement of volar plate. Flexor tendons are retracted by Penrose drain. **C,** Final clinical photograph demonstrating volar plate advancement with pull-out button over dorsal surface of digit at distal interphalangeal joint.

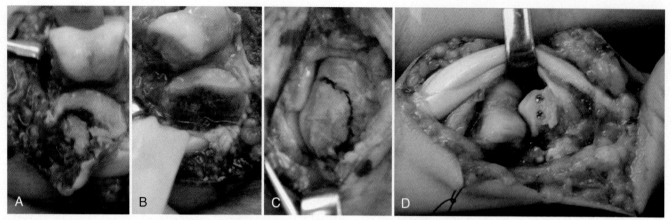

Figure 32-8 Hemihamate arthroplasty. **A,** Intraoperative photograph depicting large central defect with impaction of the base of the middle phalanx. **B,** Intraoperative photograph demonstrating preparation of the middle phalanx following osteotomy and contouring of the impacted fracture in order to accept hamate graft. **C,** Intraoperative photograph demonstrating dorsal view of hamate and outlined portion of bone to be osteotomized and grafted to defect at the base of the middle phalanx. **D,** Final photograph demonstrating screw fixation of hamate graft to the base of the middle phalanx, effectively reconstituting a normal joint surface.

pain and carpometacarpal (CMC) joint instability have not been reported with this procedure.

Another option for large, comminuted volar lip fractures is dynamic external fixation (Fig. 32-9). Numerous methods have been described;[25] however, the underlying principle is the same; fractures are reduced through traction via ligamentotaxis, and the subluxation is reduced and maintained with the appropriate placement of the external fixation pins. These devices allow for AROM to be initiated immediately within the constraints of the system; however, pin tract infections (≤25%) frequently occur.[26] Typically, these do not result in long-term sequelae if treated appropriately with oral antimicrobials. Additionally, closely monitored radiographic follow-up is required to ensure maintenance of the reduction.

Fractures of the dorsal lip of the middle phalanx involve an avulsion injury of the central tendon and must be approximated to prevent late boutonnière deformity. Fracture fragments that are reduced within 2 mm of anatomic alignment with an extension orthosis can be treated with full-time immobilization that allows for DIP motion. Failure to reapproximate the central slip of the extensor tendon can lead to imbalance at the PIP and DIP joints, resulting in a boutonnière deformity (flexion contracture of the PIP joint and fixed hyperextension of the DIP joint). Active flexion can be initiated after fracture healing occurs, generally within 4 weeks of the injury. Simple displaced fractures can be treated with pinning or open reduction. Extension block pinning may be performed; however, it is important to place the pins obliquely

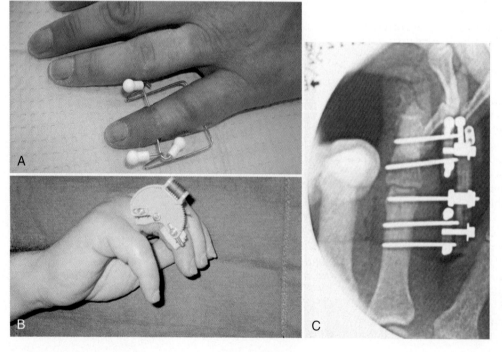

Figure 32-9 Dynamic external fixation. **A,** Clinical photograph depicting dynamic distraction of a proximal interphalangeal (PIP) fracture–dislocation. With the use of K-wires, distraction helps to disimpact fracture fragments via ligamentotaxis. Care must be maintained to keep pin sites clean to prevent infection with this technique. **B,** Clinical photograph demonstrating a compass hinge, a more substantial and supportive form of external fixation. Progressive flexion is achieved via periodic adjustments to the external device. **C,** Radiograph (posteroanterior view) demonstrating a compass hinge applied to a PIP fracture–dislocation. Frequent radiographs are needed in external fixation systems to ensure maintenance of a concentric reduction and early identification of any fracture displacement.

between the central slip and the lateral bands to prevent scarring, thereby limiting PIP and DIP motion.[27]

Dynamic external fixation is additionally the treatment of choice for patients with comminuted, depressed pilon fractures involving the entire articular surface.[16] These fractures are generally not amenable to open treatment with interfragmentary fixation. Dynamic fixation reduces subluxation and can realign the dorsal and volar fragments although longitudinal traction cannot reduce the depressed articular surface. Interfragmentary pins can be placed to reapproximate markedly displaced fragments, and articular remodeling can occur, leading to a stable joint.[1] However, post-traumatic arthritis and loss of motion are common due to the extensive damage sustained in the initial injury. The use of immediate joint arthroplasty or arthrodesis has been reported sporadically in the literature. Arthrodesis is generally not recommended in the ulnar digits, though it is a useful tool for the index PIP joint, as key pinch (the predominant use of the index digit) is performed in PIP flexion and requires absolute stability of the PIP joint.

Longitudinal, angular force can result in fractures of the condyles of the proximal phalanx and are especially common in athletes. Because these fractures do not involve joint subluxation and ROM can be preserved, they are often misdiagnosed as sprains and patients do not seek treatment until late deformity or persistent pain develop. These fractures can be classified into three categories based on severity. Type I fractures are stable, nondisplaced, unicondylar fractures; type II injuries are unstable, displaced unicondylar; and type III are bicondylar or highly comminuted fractures.[28] Nondisplaced unicondylar fractures can be treated with orthotic positioning and close radiographic follow-up, as displacement is common despite adequate treatment. Unstable fractures require stabilization with either percutaneous pinning or ORIF using screws or a minicondylar plate via a midlateral approach. A percutaneous tenaculum clamp can aid in fracture reduction, and provisional fixation allows for anatomic alignment, even in type III injuries. Dynamic external fixation can play a role in markedly comminuted fractures where fixation cannot be achieved with pins or screws. Provided the articular surface remains aligned, outcomes are generally good, and patients may continue to improve postoperative motion for more than 1 year after surgery due to articular remodeling.[29]

Distal Interphalangeal Joint and Thumb Interphalangeal Joint

The anatomy of the DIP and thumb interphalangeal (IP) joints is similar to that of the PIP joint in that it is a ginglymus joint with stout collateral ligaments providing stability. The terminal tendon of the extensor mechanism and the flexor digitorum profundus (FDP) and flexor pollicis longus (FPL) provide additional dynamic support for the joint. Due to the decreased lever arm and the added stability of the terminal tendons, dislocations are not as frequent at the DIP joint; however, because of the thinner soft tissue envelope they more frequently involve skin lacerations. Fractures and fracture–dislocations about the DIP joints are common

during athletic endeavors, but can be misdiagnosed as sprains due to lack of early deformity.

Pure dislocations at the DIP joint are rare and are most often stable after closed reduction. Soft tissue interposition that prevents reduction is unusual, but may be due to entrapment of the flexor tendons, fracture fragments, or aberrant sesamoid bones into the joint.[30] Open reduction must be performed if reduction cannot be achieved under local block. Open dislocations require thorough irrigation and debridement in a sterile setting. Articular congruity must be assessed with radiographs after reduction and AROM and PROM testing are performed. Residual instability can be treated with an extension block orthosis for 2 to 3 weeks, followed by increased AROM. Marked instability can be treated with trans-articular pinning for 4 weeks, followed by slow rehabilitation.

Fractures involving the DIP joint are more common than dislocations, and more often require surgical treatment. Pediatric patients may develop physeal fractures with displacement under the nail sterile matrix. These are termed *Seymour's fractures* and must be treated as open fractures if a subungual hematoma is present.[31] Care must be taken to repair any nail bed injuries.[32] These fractures generally heal in 3 to 4 weeks with the use of a protective orthosis and close radiographic follow-up to ensure the reduction is maintained.

A direct axial load onto a flexed DIP joint commonly results in an avulsion of the terminal extensor tendon at the dorsal lip of the distal phalanx. This avulsion can be purely tendinous or may involve an avulsion of bone ranging from a small fragment to a significant amount of the joint surface. This spectrum of injury is termed a *mallet finger* and can be called a "bony" or "soft tissue" mallet injury[33] (Fig. 32-10). The discontinuity of the terminal tendon places the DIP joint in a flexed posture, and, although full extension is passively attainable, active extension is absent. The overpull at the PIP joint with resultant hyperextension combined with DIP flexion is termed a *swan-neck deformity*. All mallet injuries should be radiographed to evaluate for fractures and joint subluxation. The amount of articular surface involvement predicts stability as fractures with less than 43 degrees of flexion remain congruent, and fractures with greater than 52 degrees always subluxate.[34] Isolated soft tissue mallet fingers can be treated with full-time use of an extension orthosis at 180 degrees extension (Fig. 32-11); hyperextension at the DIP joint can lead to decreased microvascular perfusion at the terminal tendon and may inhibit healing.[35] The orthosis allows for full active PIP motion and is worn for 6 weeks full time, then gradually weaned over 2 weeks. The orthosis should be worn during athletic endeavors for 2 to 3 months after the injury.

The indications for surgical treatment include open injuries, patients with professions that prevent them wearing an orthosis (i.e., health-care workers), large articular fractures (>30% articular surface), fracture displacement of greater than 2 mm, residual extensor lag of greater than 35 degrees, and joint subluxation.[26] Soft tissue mallet injuries can be treated with transarticular pinning for 6 weeks, followed by gradual remobilization. Displaced fragments can be reduced with extension block pinning or ORIF, if large fragments are noted. Surgery at the DIP is not without complications,

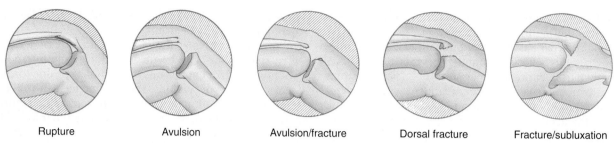

Figure 32-10 Mallet deformity can be produced from extensor tendon rupture, avulsion of terminal extensor tendon, or avulsion of bone with extensor tendon. Dorsal fracture of distal phalanx and fracture–subluxation, although not tendon injuries, can manifest as mallet deformities. (From Management of acute extensor injuries. In: Hunter JM, Schneider LH, Mackin EJ, eds. *Tendon Surgery in the Hand.* St Louis: Mosby; 1987.)

including deep infection, joint incongruity, and persistent nail deformities, which can occur in up to 54% of patients.[26]

Fractures and fracture–dislocations of the palmar base of the DIP joint are rare and commonly involve an avulsion injury of the FDP or FPL tendons. These most commonly result from an extension force applied to a flexed DIP joint and are termed *rugger-jersey injuries*. The patient presents with a swollen DIP joint that he or she is unable to actively flex, although passive flexion is possible. The avulsed fragment can be pulled down the flexor sheath and predictably is caught in one of three locations. Examination for masses or tenderness in the palm and the flexor sheath, combined with radiographs of the entire hand assist in locating the fragment. In type I injuries, a small fragment is brought into the palm due to the avulsion of both the vinculae and held there by the lumbrical muscle attachment to the FDP. In type II injuries, the fragment is held at the level of the PIP joint due to intact vinculae superficialis. In type III injuries, the large fragment is caught in the distal aspect of the A4 pulley and both vinculae are usually intact.[36]

All displaced volar lip fractures should be treated surgically to restore DIP joint flexion. Either a midlateral approach or Brunner's incisions should be carried out to find the avulsed fragment in the flexor sheath. The avulsed fragment can be reapproximated with screw fixation; however, the screws must not penetrate the dorsal cortex more than 10 mm distal to the dorsal lip of the PIP joint to prevent nail deformities due to damage to the germinal matrix. A pull-out suture or wire can also be used and placed through the sterile matrix of the nail bed and tied over a button on the nail plate. Care must be taken to preserve the A2 and A4 pulleys to prevent bowstringing, as well as to minimize trauma to the flexor sheath to prevent adhesion formation during passage of the avulsed fragment. The injury should be rehabilitated like a zone I flexor tendon injury with early active motion to prevent stiffness.

Metacarpophalangeal Joints 2 Through 5

The MCP joint is condyloid in nature, though it has a complex articular geometry that allows for motion in different planes depending on the position of the joint. The base of the proximal phalanx is shallow and concave, and the head of the metacarpal is narrow in extension and wider in flexion. In full extension articular congruity is limited, allowing for motion in radial and ulnar deviation, whereas in full flexion the articular congruity is greater in this plane, thereby limiting motion. This arrangement allows for increased total motion as compared to the IP joints. The collateral ligament complex is similar in nature to that of the IP joints, with a PCL origin that lies dorsal to the axis of rotation and inserts on the base of the phalanx. Thus the ACL is tightest in flexion and works in concert with the greater articular congruity to stabilize the joint at this position. The ACL origin lies volar to the axis of rotation and inserts on the stout VP of the MCP joint, although it is less robust than the PCL and allows for limited radial and ulnar deviation. The VP of the MCP joint has a thick fibrocartilaginous distal insertion throughout the base of the joint and a thin membranous portion proximally.

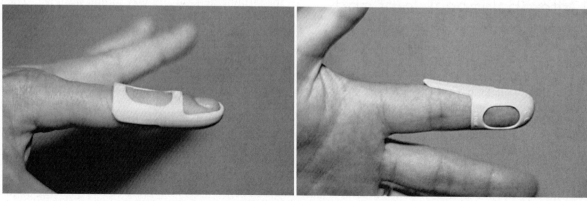

Figure 32-11 Mallet orthosis. (Link America Inc., Hanover, New Jersey.)

This geometry allows for increased hyperextension of the MCP joint, while allowing for full flexion as the thin membranous portion tucks into the volar recess. Dorsally only a thin capsule is present, and the bulk of stability is provided by the extensor mechanism, which is held in place dorsally by the sagittal bands. Extrinsic palmar stability is provided by the flexor tendon sheath with the A1 pulley attaching to the VP.[37]

Collateral ligament injuries are rare and commonly missed during initial presentation. The stability of the collateral ligaments is best assessed in full flexion because the PCL provides more true stability than the ACL when the joint is in a flexed posture. Any passive deviation of greater than 15 degrees without a definitive endpoint is deemed pathologic and indicative of a grade III tear. The rupture or avulsion occurs in nearly equal proportions at either the proximal origin or the distal insertion.[38] Grade I and II injuries should be treated nonoperatively; however, the joint should be immobilized in flexion in an "intrinsic plus" posture to prevent the collateral ligament from healing in a contracted attitude, thereby preventing full joint flexion. MRI can be a useful radiographic correlation to the clinical findings and helps delineate concurrent osteochondral and VP injuries. Grade III injuries can be treated with 12 weeks of continuous buddy-taping, although acute surgical repair is indicated in professional athletes and highly active individuals.[39] Recently, Stener-like lesions (see thumb MCP injuries) have been described in the fingers, where the avulsed collateral ligament gets trapped nonanatomically outside of the sagittal bands.[40] Although this occurred in only 6 of 38 injuries as compared with 25 of 39 thumbs,[41] these lesions will likely fail nonoperative treatment similar to the thumb. If surgical repair is elected, numerous methods have been described. Acute tears can be repaired anatomically with a suture anchor or pull-out sutures, whereas chronic ruptures may necessitate reconstruction with a palmaris longus or plantaris tendon graft. Avulsion fractures with large osteochondral fragments can be repaired with a screw or K-wire.[39]

Pure Dislocations

Although less common than PIP dislocations, MCP joint dislocations commonly occur after a fall onto an outstretched hand with hyperextension of the MCP joints. These injuries may be underreported and underrecognized due to spontaneous relocation. During hyperextension the VP fails proximally as the joint dislocates, perching the proximal phalanx dorsally on the metacarpal head. Both hyperflexion and hyperextension mechanisms have been documented to cause volar MCP dislocations.[42,43] The VP may become interposed into the joint, preventing closed relocation. Additionally, the head of the metacarpal may become entwined in a noose formed by the volar soft tissues between the lumbrical tendon radially, the profundus tendon ulnarly, the superficial transverse metacarpal ligament proximally, and the natatory ligament distally.[44] Additionally, the first dorsal interosseous tendon, juncturae tendinae, and sesamoid bones have all been reported as becoming interposed in the joint, preventing relocation.[30]

Simple dislocations are defined as those that reduce spontaneously or with provocative maneuvers. Many MCP dislo-

cations prove to be complex, or irreducible by closed means, and even simple, reducible dislocations may become irreducible if improper attempts at reduction are performed. Most simple dorsal or volar dislocations may be reduced under local anesthesia by pushing the proximal phalanx volarly or dorsally, respectively, while avoiding longitudinal traction, which may pull the VP into the joint. Following successful relocation, the patient may be treated in a dorsal blocking orthosis at neutral, while allowing full flexion, unless concomitant collateral ligament injury is suggested.

Open treatment is indicated for irreducible or open dislocations. A simple dorsal approach may be chosen for a dorsal dislocation in which a Freer elevator is placed into the joint to remove the offending structure, thereby allowing for successful relocation. This approach also allows for excellent visualization of the joint for osteochondral fractures. Many authors advocate a volar approach, which allows for better visualization of damaged structures. However, the tenting of the metacarpal head under the skin often pushes the neurovascular bundle immediately beneath the skin, placing it at risk during the skin incision.[45] A volar approach additionally allows for inspection of the flexor tendons and incision of the A1 pulley, which relaxes the flexor tendons, thereby allowing quick reduction of the joint. Volar dislocations rarely require open treatment, and a dorsal approach is generally preferred. Prompt remobilization is encouraged following open reduction with an extension block orthosis applied in 30 to 50 degrees of flexion to prevent recurrent instability.

Intra-articular Fractures

Intra-articular injuries to the metacarpal head usually occur as a result of direct trauma to a flexed joint or crush injury. In this position only the skin, extensor tendons, and joint capsule protect the articular surface from damage. Traditional radiographic views often miss metacarpal head fractures, due to the joint overlap seen on the lateral view, so the alternative use of Brewerton's view or the skyline metacarpal[46,47] view is often helpful in delineating fracture patterns. Many of these injuries are open, commonly due to urban pugilism. These must be treated appropriately with surgical irrigation and debridement and antimicrobial therapy to prevent pyarthrosis. Physeal fractures are common at the MCP joint as it is the only joint in the hand with a physis in both the proximal and distal bones of the joint.

Small, nondisplaced fractures can be treated nonsurgically with the MCP joints kept in an "intrinsic plus," or "safe," position. The indications for open treatment are fractures involving greater than 25% of the articular surface or those with more than a 1-mm articular stepoff. Large osteochondral fractures are associated with MCP dislocations and should be treated with ORIF with headless screws. Comminuted metacarpal head fractures are difficult to treat and often require creativity in treatment with K-wires, cerclage wiring, or osteochondral allografting using local bone or toe metacarpal graft.[48] Dynamic and static external fixation may also be used to maintain articular alignment. Some articular remodeling can occur, and often painless ROM is noted in patients with articular incongruity as these joints are non-weight-bearing. Severely comminuted fractures can be treated with immediate arthroplasty with either silicone or pyrolytic carbon implants. Silicone should not be used in the index finger due to excessive pinch stress nor in cases of inadequate soft tissue coverage or excessive bone loss.[1]

Small or nondisplaced ligament avulsion fractures at the lateral or volar base of the proximal phalanx can be treated closed. The indications for open treatment were listed earlier. ORIF can be performed percutaneously with K-wires or open through a volar approach with screws or K-wires. More complex fractures of the base result from an axial load, more often in the index finger, due to the increased stability imparted by its CMC joint. T-Condylar fractures require stabilization with percutaneous K-wires placed either through or around the metacarpal head with the joint in flexion. Unstable fractures can be treated with a dorsal extensor splitting approach and a minicondylar plate. Significant comminution or bone loss is an indication for external fixation.

Carpometacarpal Joints 2 Through 5

Fractures and dislocations at the base of the metacarpals, although rare, are under-recognized injuries that can contribute to significant functional impairment if not adequately treated. The significant stability imparted by the dorsal and volar carpometacarpal (CMC) ligaments as well as the intermetacarpal ligaments can prevent displacement from occurring. Additionally, the extrinsic wrist flexor and extensor tendons attach at the base of these joints and impart additional stability. The second and third metacarpals form the central pillar of the hand, which provides stability to hand function, whereas the fourth and fifth metacarpals are less stable, allowing for increased motion of the ulnar digits in grasping and palmar cupping activities.[49] The articular morphology of the base of the second and third metacarpal provide more intrinsic stability and less motion than the fourth and fifth. The second metacarpal base has radial and ulnar condyles that envelop the trapezoid and additionally articulate with the trapezium and capitate, respectively. The extensor carpi radialis longus (ECRL) inserts on the dorsal radial condyle, and the flexor carpi radialis (FCR) inserts on the volar base of the metacarpal. The base of the third metacarpal is slightly concave and has a dorsal–radial styloid process that helps lock the joint against the capitate and second metacarpal. The extensor carpi radialis brevis (ECRB) additionally inserts along this styloid process. The ECRL and ECRB provide wrist stabilization in extension, where power grip occurs. The second CMC joint allows for 11 degrees of flexion–extension motion, whereas there is only 7 degrees of flexion–extension in the third CMC.[49]

The fourth and fifth metacarpal bases have relatively unstable morphology as they articulate with the hamate, which allows for increased motion at these joints. The trapezoidal base of the fourth metacarpal has no extrinsic muscular attachment and is stabilized by the buttress of the radial and ulnar adjacent metacarpals and stout ligamentous attachments; therefore, isolated fourth metacarpal base instability is rarely, if ever, seen. The base of the fifth metacarpal is convex in its articulation with the hamate, which has an

ulnar slope. This articular morphology allows for increased flexion–extension motion (fourth, 20 degrees; fifth, 28 degrees [with fourth CMC locked], and 44 degrees [unlocked fourth CMC]); as well as pronation and supination (27 degrees, 22 degrees) and radioulnar deviation (7 degrees, 13 degrees).[50] The attachments of the extensor carpi ulnaris (ECU) on the dorsal–ulnar aspect and the flexor carpi ulnaris on the volar base provide extrinsic deformative forces on the base of the fifth.

Injuries to the CMC joints of the hand often can occur as a result of direct trauma, longitudinally directed force (punching), or athletic collisions. The articular and ligamentous stability of the second and third metacarpals does not allow for force dissipation through joint motion, and thus the applied forces tend to lead to fractures at the basilar joint. Simple sprains are common and are diagnosed by physical examination findings with point tenderness at the specific ligament. A brief period of immobilization is usually sufficient treatment for these injuries. Careful scrutiny of radiographs is crucial if injury to the CMC joints is suggested. Standard PA, oblique, and lateral views are mandatory for all suggested injuries in this area, and CT scans can be a useful adjunct for delineating intra-articular pathology. The fifth metacarpal is the most common location for dislocations that can occur dorsally and, less commonly, volarly. Volar dislocations usually result from crush injuries and can injure the motor branch of the ulnar nerve (fourth and fifth) or the deep palmar arch (third metacarpal).[49] Multiple dislocations are indicative of high-energy injuries and, due to their instability despite anatomic reduction, should be treated operatively with percutaneous pinning (Fig. 32-12).

Dorsal avulsion fractures of the ECRL and ECRB insertion can occur along with simultaneous tendon injury. The avulsed fragments can malrotate in situ or be pulled as far

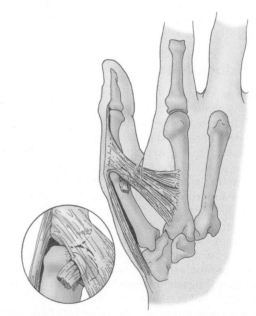

Figure 32-12 Diagram and enlargement of the Stener's lesion. A hyperabduction force results in complete rupture of the ulnar collateral ligament at its distal insertion, with displacement proximally. The adductor aponeurosis blocks the ligament from returning to its insertion site, thus preventing adequate healing.

proximal as the forearm. Additionally, the stout intermetacarpal ligaments cause avulsion fractures, which are more apparent in the second and fifth metacarpals. More commonly found in the fifth metacarpal, this injury is termed a *baby Bennett* or *reverse Bennett* injury when the avulsed fragment is in anatomic location and the metacarpal displaces dorsally and ulnarly due to the unbalanced pull of the ECU tendon.[51,52] In the second metacarpal this has been termed a *ligament-reversed Bennett fracture* because the radial condyle is pulled off and remains attached to the subluxated first metacarpal.[53] Due to the decreased stability afforded by the ulnar metacarpals, fracture–dislocations and displaced avulsion fractures are more commonly noted in these digits.

Minimally displaced fractures that are in anatomic alignment can be treated nonoperatively with a 3-week period of immobilization followed by progressive ROM exercises. Dislocations that are stable after closed reduction can be treated nonoperatively as well, provided close radiographic follow-up is initiated. No consensus over operative indications exists for the treatment of these rare injuries except in cases of multiple dislocations, persistent instability, and failed closed treatment. Nonoperative treatment has been advocated for second and third metacarpal base fractures because their inherent immobility limits the effect of articular incongruity, although extensor tendon ruptures over a bony prominence and persistent pain and weakness have been reported from undertreated injuries. Displaced tendon avulsion injuries should be reduced and fixated with K-wires or screws, and concomitant tendon injuries repaired with suture anchors or pull-out sutures if necessary. Unstable fracture dislocations, predominately seen in the fifth metacarpal, require percutaneous pinning or ORIF if large fragments are present.

Thumb Metacarpophalangeal Joint

The thumb MCP joint, although markedly similar in anatomic appearance to those in the fingers, essentially functions as a hinge, or ginglymus, joint. The wide variation in articular morphology found in this joint makes it the most varied motion of all joints in the body, with anywhere from 6 to 86 degrees in flexion–extension considered normal. The primary function of the thumb MCP joint is to provide stability for grasping and pinching activities, with the joint showing equal stability in all ROMs. Compared with the finger MCP joints, thumb MCP joint stiffness is tolerated much more than instability. Sesamoid bones are nearly always present at this joint and are embedded in the VP. The flexor pollicis brevis (FBP) and abductor pollicis brevis (APB) muscles insert partially on the sesamoids and provide stability against hyperextension forces. The ligamentous anatomy is analogous to that seen in the finger MCP joints, with extrinsic tendons providing additional support.

Dorsal dislocations at the thumb CMC joint often occur following hyperextension injuries and can be simple or complex. The VP avulses proximally in most cases and can become entrapped in the joint, preventing closed reduction. Radiographic evidence of joint space widening or sesamoids in the joint is indicative of complex (irreducible) dislocations in which the metacarpal head buttonholes through the VP

and can be trapped by the FBP and APB. Following reduction, the joint should be radiographed again to ensure articular congruity is achieved. Hyperflexion injuries can cause dorsal capsule tears or extensor pollicis brevis (EPB) tendon ruptures, which are diagnosed on physical exam.[54] Volar thumb dislocations have been reported infrequently in the literature, always associated with entrapment of part or all of the extensor mechanism, which prevents closed reduction. Concomitant ligament injury to the collateral ligaments should be tested following relocation of all dislocations as collateral instability may require further treatment. Following stable reduction, the joint should be immobilized with an opponens orthosis in slight flexion for 3 weeks, followed by gradual remobilization. Persistent instability in extension is rare, and operative fixation of the VP is contraindicated in the acute setting.

Ulnar Collateral Ligament Injuries

A combined radial deviation and hyperextension force applied to the thumb MCP joint often results in damage to the UCL of the thumb. The UCL is injured 10 times as often as the RCL.[55-57] An acute injury often caused during skiing by a fall in which the ski pole is forcibly removed from the hand is termed *skier's thumb*. This term for the acute injury is used interchangeably with *gamekeeper's thumb*; however this second injury is due to repetitive stress and resultant chronic attenuation of the ligament, originally described in Scottish gamekeepers as they euthanized rabbits.[58] Acute injuries most commonly involve a distal avulsion of the PCL. The current of injury may continue through the VP, ACL, and dorsal capsule as well. Excessive radial deviation of the proximal phalanx during the injury may bring the ligament on top of the adductor aponeurosis. This may be palpated as a painful, superficial mass and was termed *Stener's lesion*, after being described by Stener in 1962[41] (see Fig. 32-12). Stener postulated that the ligament could not heal outside the aponeurosis, and the injury would lead to chronic instability if not treated, a finding that was confirmed in multiple subsequent studies.

The treatment of UCL injuries hinges on an accurate diagnosis that differentiates a complete (type III) rupture from an incomplete sprain (types I and II). On examination patients have point tenderness at the avulsed ligament site, and occasionally a Stener's lesion may be palpated. Instability to stress testing is the key to diagnosis, and testing should be performed in full extension and 30 degrees of flexion. The ACL is taut in full extension and a laxity of more than 35 degrees to valgus stress, or more than 15 degrees compared with the contralateral thumb, is indicative of a complete rupture of the ACL. Stress testing in 30 degrees of flexion tests the competence of the PCL, and laxity of more than 30 to 40 degrees to valgus stress, or more than 15 degrees compared with the contralateral thumb, indicates complete rupture. Some authors advocate that the lack of a firm endpoint is highly indicative of a complete rupture as well.[30] Standard PA and lateral radiographs of the thumb MCP joint should be obtained because UCL ruptures show an avulsed fracture fragment in up to 50% of cases.[59] Stress radiographs may be helpful as well, provided the patient tolerates the manipulation (Fig. 32-13). If pain precludes adequate stress

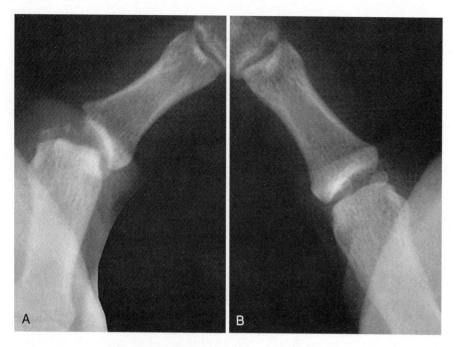

Figure 32-13 Comparative stress radiography of a 32-year-old skier who sustained injury to the left thumb metacarpophalangeal (MCP) joint **(A)** during a fall. Note the amount of displacement and an associated chip fracture. The right thumb MCP joint **(B)** is normal.

testing, an intra-articular local anesthetic can assist in pain control. Additionally, arthrography, ultrasound, or MRI may be used to confirm the diagnosis of complete rupture or the presence of a Stener's lesion.

Grade I and II injuries are treated in a hand-based thumb spica orthosis or cast that allows for IP motion. The orthosis is discontinued after 2 to 4 weeks, depending on painless ROM of the MCP joint, and mobilization is begun. Key pinch exercises and strengthening exercises are then gradually increased for 3 to 4 weeks; however, excessive stress to the UCL with active tip-pinch or grasping is avoided until 8 weeks after treatment. Stability of the MCP joint is preferred over full motion, and aggressive therapy should be avoided. Most surgeons advocate surgical exploration and repair for complete ligament tears since nonoperative treatment can be unpredictable. If a Stener's lesion can be definitively excluded with advanced imaging, nonoperative treatment can be attempted in a thumb spica cast or orthosis for 4 to 6 weeks. This is followed by gradual mobilization that avoids valgus stress across the joint. Minimally displaced avulsion fractures involving less than 30% of that articular surface can be treated in a cast or orthosis as well.

Operative exploration is achieved though a curvilinear dorsal approach, which exposes the ligament tear under the adductor aponeurosis. Midsubstance ruptures can be primarily repaired or sutured to the periosteum. Distal avulsions can be treated with any number of techniques, including suture anchors, pull-out sutures, or fishhook cables (premade pull-out wires). The joint is pinned in slight overcorrection for 4 weeks to prevent stress on the repair, and a cast or orthosis is worn until the pin is pulled. Large avulsion fractures can be repaired with screws or K-wires, with or without joint pinning, for added stability. Protected ROM exercises are begun at 4 to 6 weeks, and return to full activities is allowed at 3 months. Chronic instability for gamekeeper's thumb or delayed presentation should be treated surgically.

Often a substantial portion of the ligament can be found and reattached to the proximal phalanx with suture anchors. If no ligament can be found, reconstruction with palmaris longus or plantaris tendon graft is the preferred treatment. Recently attempts at using bone–ligament–bone constructs for reconstruction have been reported with excellent short-term results.[60]

Radial Collateral Ligament Injuries

Ligament injuries to the radial side of the thumb are less frequent and less disabling than UCL injuries. The RCL is usually torn in forced adduction injuries or rotational stress applied to the MCP joint.[55] The RCL is important for strong key pinch and typing or pushing movements. A Stener's lesion of the RCL has been reported only once in the literature and is rare due to broad anatomy of the abductor aponeurosis, which completely overlies the RCL dorsal to the axis of rotation.[61] Additionally, RCL injuries more commonly involve midsubstance ruptures than distal avulsions. Injuries to the RCL are graded similarly to the UCL, and instability of greater than 30 degrees on stress testing is indicative of a complete tear. The physical exam and radiographs may demonstrate ulnar and volar subluxation of the proximal phalanx due to dorsal capsule injury. Minimally displaced avulsion fractures are treated in a cast similar to the treatment for UCL injuries. Some authors advocate nonoperative treatment for RCL injuries due to the paucity of Stener's lesions preventing healing. However, others suggest that the ulnar pull of the extensor pollicis longus (EPL) tendon and the tendency for volar subluxation in complete ruptures are indications for surgical repair or reconstruction. Surgery is indicated for volar subluxation greater than 3 mm, laxity greater than 30 degrees or 15 degrees compared with the contralateral side, and chronic instability. Surgery is performed similarly to UCL injuries with either primary repair or suture anchor fixation for viable ligaments or reconstruction for attenuated or fibrotic tissue. The rehabilitation is similar to that for UCL injuries; however, key pinch is delayed and the thumb is protected from varus stress until 8 weeks to ensure adequate healing.

Thumb Carpometacarpal Joint

The articular configuration of the trapeziometacarpal joint is unique in the human body. Both the trapezium and metacarpal base have perpendicularly opposed, saddle-shaped articular surfaces, which allow for motion in the flexion–extension, palmar abduction–adduction, and pronation–supination planes. The ligamentous anatomy imparts additional stability to this joint, predominantly through the volar oblique ligament, which runs from the tubercle of the trapezium to the volar beak of the metacarpal. This ligament resists the tendency for dorsal subluxation during CMC flexion and adduction, when key pinch is performed. Additional stability is provided by the dorsoradial, intermetacarpal, and dorsal oblique ligaments. The dorsal oblique ligament provides stability during thumb abduction and opposition as it tightens during pronation and locks the volar beak of the metacarpal into the trapezium via a screw-home mechanism.[62] There is debate whether the volar or dorsal oblique ligament is most important in preventing dorsal dislocation of the CMC joint, but most authors agree that both ligaments must be disrupted for a complete dislocation to occur. The abductor pollicis longus (APL) tendon is the only muscle that inserts at the metacarpal base and can provide stability to the joint; however it is more often considered a deforming force with fractures and dislocations at the CMC joint.

Pure dorsal dislocations of the CMC joint are rare, and commonly occur with an axial load placed on a flexed joint. The dorsal capsule and oblique ligaments tear or are stripped subperiosteally off the metacarpal or trapezium.[62] Although exceedingly rare, anterior or volar dislocations have been reported.[63] Ligament sprains are more difficult to diagnose because less subluxation is seen with incomplete tears. Clinically, patients present with traumatic basilar thumb pain, but subluxation is difficult to elicit due to the inherent stability of the trapeziometacarpal joint. Comparison with the contralateral joint indicates the normal physiologic stability of this joint. Standard radiographic views often miss injuries to this joint unless PA and lateral views of the thumb CMC joint are specified. A "prayer" view, or bilateral stress radiograph taken with the patient forcefully pushing the thumb phalanges together, is a helpful adjunct in diagnosing CMC stability as both thumbs are included on the radiograph. Partial ligament tears can be treated with a thumb spica cast or orthosis for 4 weeks followed by gradual remobilization. Complete dislocations usually can be reduced under local anesthesia and may be treated in a cast with the thumb abducted and slightly extended.

Surgical stabilization is indicated for residually unstable injuries following relocation and is primarily accomplished with percutaneous pinning. However, many authors have reported recurrent instability, likely due to interposed ligament or a chondral fragment that prevents anatomic reduction despite what appeared to be adequate radiographic reduction. Open exploration via Wagner's dorsal approach with capsulorrhaphy and ligament reconstruction with a hemi-FCR tendon is indicated for incongruent reduction or residual instability due to delayed presentation or failed prior treatment.

Intra-articular Fractures

Dorsal subluxation or dislocation of the thumb CMC joint can also occur through a bony avulsion of the volar oblique, or volar beak, ligament. This fracture remains in anatomic location while the metacarpal subluxates dorsally, proximally, and radially and is termed a *Bennett fracture*. This fracture is mechanistically similar to pure dislocations, and the unopposed pull of the APL, EPL and adductor pollicis muscles tends to displace this fracture. Axial compression in less flexion tends to cause a pilon injury to the metacarpal base with three or more fragments noted. These injuries have been termed *Rolando's fractures,* even though the original description by Rolando in 1910 included only Y- and T-shaped intra-articular fragments.[64]

The key to successful treatment is obtaining joint congruity via anatomic reduction.[65] Closed treatment is reserved only for small, nondisplaced Bennett fractures. A percutaneous pin placed across the trapeziometacarpal joint is advocated for fragments that are less than 20% of the articular surface. The fracture is typically reduced with traction, pronation, and abduction while the pin is advanced under fluoroscopic guidance. Fractures that involve greater than 30% of the articular surface or that have greater than 1 to 2 mm of articular stepoff require open reduction via Wagner's dorsal approach. Minifragment screw fixation is preferred for large fragments, and early motion can be initiated if stable fixation is demonstrated intraoperatively. Pins are pulled at 4 weeks, and the thumb is immobilized with an orthosis until healing is demonstrated. Rolando's fractures require operative intervention, although outcomes are poor with any method chosen. Large fracture fragments can be reduced anatomically and held with a minicondylar plate or K-wires.[1] Comminuted fractures are best treated with external fixation or traction mechanisms, although anatomic alignment is rarely obtained.

Future Directions

Arthroscopic small joint surgery represents a technologic advancement that can assist physicans in treating small joint fractures, dislocations, and joint injuries. Specific advantages of small joint arthroscopy include smaller incisions with less dissection and the preservation of the stabilizing dorsal capsule, collateral ligaments, and tendons in the hand. Small joint arthroscopy allows direct visualization and palpation of chondral defects and synovial tissue as well as the assessment of concurrent intercarpal ligament injuries and instability. Arthroscopic assessment of fracture reduction is also superior to fluoroscopy used in standard open cases because of its ability to magnify and brightly illuminate the fracture reduction. Other benefits to a minimally invasive approach to the small bones of the hand are the potential for lower morbidity, expedited recovery, improved motion, and ultimately greater patient satisfaction. With such powerful capabilities, arthroscopically assisted reduction and internal fixation (AARIF) of small joints may one day be considered the gold standard for both diagnosis and treatment of small joint pathology. Future directions include the expansion of AARIF to include PIP joint injuries, as well as controlled studies to compare the efficacy of this technique to other techniques such as closed reduction and percutaneous pinning and ORIF.

Summary

The numerous ways and circumstances in which humans can position their hands places the hand and finger joints at risk for injury. A thorough knowledge of the articular and ligamentous anatomy is paramount to providing the best treatment for each patient. A good working relationship with the therapist providing care is critical in being able to return the patient to vocational and recreational activities with the goal of having a painless and functional extremity.

REFERENCES

The complete reference list is available online at www.expertconsult.com.

Intra-articular Hand Fractures and Joint Injuries: Part II— Therapist's Management

KARA GAFFNEY GALLAGHER, MS, OTR/L, CHT AND
SUSAN M. BLACKMORE, MS, OTR/L, CHT

CRITICAL POINTS

- Most fractures and soft tissue injuries heal on a common timeline, and rehabilitation principles and goals coincide with this period of healing.
- The specifics of each patient's injury, the stability of the involved joint, degree of healing, and expectations for final outcome influence the rehabilitation program, which is developed by the hand therapist in consultation with the hand surgeon.
- The benefits of early motion for intra-articular hand fractures and joint injuries include potentially improved fracture and soft tissue healing and improved mobility of the involved and surrounding joints and tissues.
- The custom fabrication of orthoses by a certified hand therapist used and modified during all phases of rehabilitation is an integral component of the rehabilitation program.
- Activities and exercises incorporated in a therapy program must be carefully selected and monitored to ensure that the desired motion and muscles are activated; poorly selected activities may end up reinforcing compensatory movement instead of the desired movement patterns.

The hand provides one of the most effective ways of interacting with the world around us. Capable of a seemingly endless array of activities, the hand is designed for both strenuous work such as operating a jackhammer as well as detailed fine tasks like embroidery or playing the violin. Congruent articulations, supported by soft tissue complexes, link the 19 bones of the hand. This intricate design allows simultaneous joint stability and mobility plus efficient transmission of muscle force from the forearm to the fingertips. The distal position of the hand on the upper extremity exposes it to external forces that can injure the bones and the soft tissue structures that provide stability and mobility. Injury to the joints of the hand can result in intra-articular fracture of the bones or damage to the supporting joint capsule and ligament systems, causing multiple degrees of instability, dislocation, subluxation, or contracture.

This chapter reviews rehabilitation following intra-articular fractures and joint injuries in the hand. The surgeon's management is covered in Chapter 32.

Intra-articular Hand Fractures

Metacarpal and phalangeal fractures are the most common upper extremity fractures.[1] A study in 1998 showed that of all hand and forearm fractures in the United States, 23% were phalangeal and 18% were metacarpal.[2] Metacarpal and phalangeal fractures are often unnoticed or treated as insignificant injuries.[1,3] Adults and adolescents typically require some form of rehabilitation following a fracture in the hand. To enable the patient to safely and successfully achieve an optimal result, the therapist must understand fracture terminology, management, and healing. This information coupled with a thorough knowledge of soft tissue injury and healing is the cornerstone to treatment. Most fractures and soft tissues heal on a common timeline, and rehabilitation principles and goals coincide with this period of healing. However, the injury patterns of intra-articular fractures and their concomitant soft tissue injuries, as well as the operative techniques for reduction, are more varied. So, the specifics of each patient's intra-articular fracture, associated soft tissue injuries, status of stability, degree of healing, and expectations for final outcome must be discussed with the physician to ensure that an appropriate rehabilitation program is developed.

Several terms are used to describe the initial state of a fracture. "The anatomic restoration of bone integrity, or *reduction*, is crucial to provide the normal anatomic base needed for motion."[4] A *nondisplaced* fracture indicates that the bones are well-aligned with no alteration in normal bone anatomy.[5] The bones in a *displaced* fracture are not well aligned. A displaced fracture must be reduced to its normal anatomic alignment and may require fixation to maintain that normal anatomy.[4] After the anatomy of the bone has been restored, the physician determines if the fracture will maintain its position naturally. A *stable* fracture maintains the reduction and does not displace either spontaneously or with motion.[4] Fractures that displace spontaneously or with motion are *unstable*. Additional management by the physician is needed to resolve the instability and convert it to a stable fracture.[4] Fractures are described as either *intra-articular* or *extra-articular*. Intra-articular fractures occur within the joint articulation at the base or head of the bone. Extra-articular fractures occur outside the joint articulation in the shaft or neck of the bone. Additional information on fracture terminology is provided in Chapter 29.

When the physician is planning surgery, "the need for biomechanical stability must be balanced with the need to preserve biologic integrity and blood supply while minimizing the risk for scarring. The additional stability of the implant must offset the risks of operative dissection."[6] Restoration of anatomy without function does not provide a desired outcome.[6] More recently developed implants for fracture fixation can potentially provide stability and optimize outcomes with minimal soft tissue dissection through the use of small joint arthroscopy and intraoperative imaging.

Choices for fracture stabilization are based on the type of fracture and soft tissue injuries. Fixation methods include (1) immobilization with a cast or orthosis either with or without a closed reduction; (2) closed reduction and external or internal fixation (external fixator, Kirschner wires [K-wires]); or (3) open reduction with coaptive (K-wires, intermedullary pin), stable (screw, tension band), or rigid (lag screw, plate, 90/90 wiring) fixation.[5] A full description of fixation methods for specific injuries is provided in Chapters 30 and 32.

There are excellent resources available that provide a thorough understanding of the fracture-healing process. The reader is referred to the *Journal of Hand Therapy*, 2003, volume 16, issue 2, special edition on hand fracture management for more detailed information.

Fractures heal with new bone, as opposed to scar tissue, which develops to repair soft tissue injuries. Regenerated new bone unites the fracture ends by either primary or secondary healing methods. The type of fracture healing that occurs depends on the method of fixation.

Stable and rigid fixation methods described earlier provide compression across the fracture and prevent any motion across the fracture, which and allows for primary healing.[5] A fracture callus does not form when healing occurs primarily. The advantages of stable and rigid fixation are "precise anatomical reduction, avoidance of peripheral callus with potential tissue adherence, full access to the hand for wound or edema control, immediate initiation of motion to maintain length in capsular joint structures, immediate gliding of tissue interfaces and the allowance for rehabilitation of any concomitant soft tissue injuries."[5] These advantages are only realized if an early motion program begins soon after surgery. It is also important to understand that rigid fixation methods allow for earlier and less protected motion; however, the fracture repair process is not accelerated. So, time must pass before the fracture site can tolerate the stress of resisted activities.

When the fracture is treated with external immobilization, closed reduction and immobilization, closed reduction and external fixation (CREF), closed reduction and internal fixation (CRIF), or open reduction and semirigid internal fixation (ORIF), such as with K-wires, secondary healing occurs. In secondary healing, the bone heals through initially forming a callus followed by remodeling into bone. The new bone that begins to form with secondary healing is weak, non-stress-oriented bone, so integrity of the repair site depends initially on the strength of the implant. At 2 to 3 weeks after the injury a clinical union is present with the development of callus formation.

During the healing period, motion is minimized, but not eliminated across the fracture gap. Micromotion at the fracture site actually stimulates blood flow to enhance fracture healing. The benefits of early motion with fixation types that allow for secondary healing are the preservation of blood supply and soft tissue integrity around the fracture site.

Healing timetables for fractures and associated therapy intervention is listed in Figure 33-1.[5]

Joint Injuries of the Hand

The activities of daily living (ADL) demand that the joints of the hand be both stable and allow for mobility. The hand requires stability to intricately transmit power from the forearm musculature to the fingertips. At the same time, the hand requires mobility to position the digits for countless tasks. The articulations of the joints of the hand are exceptionally designed to provide both characteristics.[7] However, despite this ingenious design, the joints are vulnerable to damaging forces that may injure the supporting joint capsules and ligament complexes.[7] Similar to fracture management, knowledge of joint terminology related to injury, treatment, and healing timelines is critical to helping the patient achieve an optimal recovery.

The complexity of a joint injury ranges from stable dislocation to contracture. *Dislocation* indicates a temporary displacement of bone from its normal position in a joint.[8] Joint injury includes disruption to various structures such as ligaments and supporting joint capsule. Additionally, the dislocation can occur with an associated intra-articular fracture (i.e., *fracture–dislocation*). The direction of the dislocation (e.g., dorsal, volar, lateral) describes the position of the bone

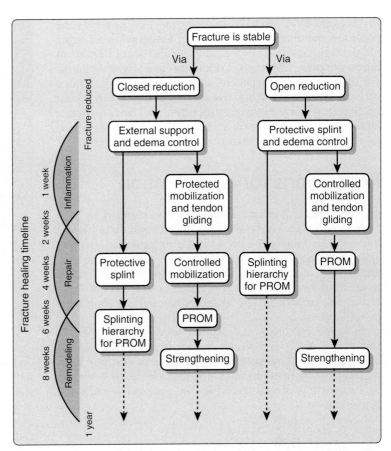

Figure 33-1 Fracture healing timeline and therapy intervention: When the fracture is stabilized, via a closed or open reduction, an external support or protective orthosis (or brace) is needed. The external supports after a closed reduction may include casts, braces, orthoses, or external fixators. Coupled with the external support or protective orthosis during the inflammatory stage is the need to control (i.e., reduce or prevent the formation of) edema. Protected mobilization in the form of gentle active or passive motion (during the external immobilization phase after closed reduction) to the nonimmobilized joints is needed to avoid joint contractures proximal or distal to the fracture site and to glide soft tissue structures. Active motion should be emphasized for controlled mobilization and for tendon gliding. Although positioning in a protective orthosis still is needed during the repair phase, treatments that address passive range of motion (PROM) deficits can be initiated after open reduction; PROM interventions after a closed reduction are delayed until the remodeling stage. Strengthening typically is initiated after closed and open reductions in the remodeling stages. The hierarchical splinting regimen and strengthening is not often continued past the first 6 months, but these interventions may be required (the stippled arrows) for 1 year. (From LaStayo PC, Winters KM, Hardy M. Fracture healing: Bone healing, fracture management, and current concepts related to the hand. *J Hand Ther*. 2003; 16:81–93.)

relative to the injured joint.[8] For instance, a dorsal dislocation of the proximal interphalangeal (PIP) joint indicates that the middle phalanx lies dorsal to the proximal phalanx. An *unstable* dislocated joint indicates a joint that does not maintain stability following anatomic reduction. In a *joint contracture*, the soft tissue around the joint becomes tight in the shortened position, thus limiting range of motion (ROM).[8]

The soft tissue structures affected in a joint injury progress through three phases of healing to produce and remodel scar.[5,9] The inflammation phase occurs from 0 to 5 days; followed by the prolific fibroplasia phase, lasting 5 days to 4 to 6 weeks; and the scar-remodeling phase, which begins approximately 6 weeks after the injury and continuing for years.[5,9] Tendon healing to bone without operative intervention requires 6 to 8 weeks before placing unrestricted tension on the tendon (e.g., soft tissue mallet and central tendon injuries).

Treatment Philosophy

Feehan[10] has developed comprehensive guidelines regarding early controlled motion of potentially unstable extra-articular hand fractures (see Chapter 31). Concepts from this article can be applied to the management of potentially unstable intra-articular fractures. Although evidence-based literature is lacking, clinical studies recommend an early motion program even following potentially unstable injuries.[10,11] The benefits include the potential to improve the quality and rate of fracture healing through the use of intermittent and limited loads, improved connective tissue healing due to physiologic stress applied early on, and improved soft tissue mobility (tendon excursion) around the injury site.[1,12-14] These benefits are negated if the motion contributes to fracture malunion or nonunion or joint instability. On the other hand, prolonged immobilization leads to pain, degenerative changes, arthrofibrosis, and joint stiffness. Immobilization beyond 4 weeks for fractures in the hand generally have long-term detrimental effects.[15]

The timing for introduction of early motion depends on the "structural strength" of the tissue over time. In theory, fibrin gains enough strength by day 3 to 5 to allow for active motion. Edema control measures and rest or immobilization are appropriate for the preceding days. The hand assumes a position of wrist flexion, metacarpophalangeal joint hyperextension, and PIP flexion when edema is not controlled. These positions can quickly become firm contractures. Proper positioning is required to prevent early contracture development. The patient's other medical conditions and factors affecting local blood flow also influence the decision about when to begin early motion.

Deciding on how early motion should be applied involves determining the number of joints moved at one time, the type (active or passive) of motion, the duration of motion, and the safe arc of motion.

The time for initiation of early motion is the final option to consider. One must determine if the motion is intermittent or constant.[10]

The goal of an early motion program is to provide the minimum amount of stress to healing tissues while allowing for the right amount of excursion of soft tissues to prevent motion-limiting adhesions. "Minimum" and "right" amounts are different for each patient and injury. LaStayo[5] defined *early controlled motion* as active motion of the involved joint or previously immobilized structures and *early protected motion* as active or passive motion of the nonimmobilized joints. These terms are used throughout the chapter.

Precautions for Early Motion

The previously discussed information is intended to be a general guideline. The benefit and detriments of these stresses must be fully understood before initiating treatment. In managing complex injuries, the planning for early motion programs must not overload the weakest or most vulnerable tissue even if other structures involved in the injury are very stable. The consequences of inappropriate early motion must be understood.

In some instances, the injured joint actually requires immobilization up to 4 weeks whether treated with closed or open reduction. That period allows for the prolific fibroblastic stage of soft tissue healing to be completed, thus leading to increased joint stability that can eventually withstand active motion.

General Rehabilitation Goals

After the therapist performs a standard and comprehensive examination, problems are identified and goals are established. Outcome measures such as the Patient-Rated Wrist and Hand Evaluation (PRWHE)[16] are useful for understanding functional deficits and pain. The general goals for patients with joint injuries in the hand are listed in Box 33-1. Treatment planning begins by fully understanding the anatomy, injury, and potential complications; the surgical or nonsurgical management chosen; tissue tolerance for stress application; other medical conditions the patient may have that may affect fracture or soft tissue healing; the patient's ability to perform required therapeutic interventions; and the patient's goals and expectations. Full recovery may take several months.

Immobilization and Controlled and Protected Motion Phases

General therapy principles are applicable to most hand joint injuries and intra-articular fractures. Early edema control is accomplished through elevation, cold, compression, and manual edema mobilization.[17,18] Early reduction of edema is desirable to facilitate joint motion and tendon excursion and prevent contractures. Constant vigilance is necessary to evaluate and adjust orthoses as edema fluctuates. Pin care is essential for preventing irritation and infection. Pin care generally involves cleaning the skin surrounding the pin and then maintaining a dry, clean environment with appropriate

---

Box 33-1   Rehabilitation Goals in the Management of Intra-articular Fractures and Dislocations of the Hand

Reduce or control edema.
Obtain full wound closure of incisions and pin or external fixation sites and prevent infection.
Maintain joint stability and obtain complete fracture healing.
Restore joint range of motion and muscle tendon–unit length.
Complete activities with correct motor performance instead of using compensatory movement patterns.
Reduce or control pain.
Improve strength and function.
Independence is achieved in patient home program and educational information.

---

dressings. If the external hardware does not directly block joint ROM, then the surgeon is contacted regarding the stability of the involved joint in relation to the initiation of controlled motion.[5] Patient education is extensive and involves ensuring the patient understands the necessary precautions, the purpose of and reasoning behind the therapy program, and their expected participation. Precautions associated with all diagnoses must be fully understood to guide the specifics and timing for each technique. Early controlled motion generally begins with performing active short arc motion for the involved joint as well as placing the proximal and distal joints in positions that enhance tendon glide and excursion. Template orthotics allow specific desired degrees of motion. Blocking exercises do not imply resistance to the fracture and in fact, in some cases, provide support to the fracture site. One exception is the mobilization of a mallet finger injury, which generally begins with composite motion to prevent attenuation of the healing terminal extensor tendon. The importance of avoiding the development of an extensor lag cannot be overstated.

Early protected motion begins with isolated active and passive motion to the nonimmobilized joints as long as the structural stability of the injury can withstand this degree of motion. Motion then progresses to full isolated joint motion while always monitoring for extensor lag. As isolated motion improves, composite (flexion–extension of all joints for the involved digit) and tenodesis exercises are initiated.

Advancements in motion are not made if the patient experiences acute pain or a marked increase in edema occurs following a treatment intervention. Prompt referral back to the physician may be needed to ensure the injury remains stable. The cause of stiffness must be understood, as attempts to mobilize a malunited, unstable, or arthritic joint is contraindicated.

Motor reeducation strategies are employed to improve active motion. Early use of mirror imagery may limit cortical degradation.[19,20] Neuromuscular electrical nerve stimulation (NMES) for muscle reeducation and specific motor control strategies facilitate the correct activation of desired and isolated musculature. At times this may require extensive one-to-one observation and demonstration time spent with the patient. Performance of graded activity is very helpful in motor reeducation as long as the activity is structured to facilitate desired movement patterns. It is nonproductive to have patients performing graded activities if the desired motion and muscles are not being activated. In fact, poorly selected activities may end up reinforcing compensatory movement patterns instead of desired movement patterns.

Adapted and compensatory ADL strategies are reviewed based on individual patient needs followed by gradual return to functional tasks with the involved extremity.

Orthotics can improve active motion through positioning that allows for isolated joint movement and resisted motion. Orthotics can improve passive motion through application of low-load, prolonged-duration stress to shortened tissues.

Scar management includes mobilization combined with motion to restore movement between tissue planes, scar massage, and scar pads or silicone gel.

Passive motion techniques include joint distraction, heat modalities combined with positioning at the end ROM, composite stretch to shortened muscle tendon unit, and joint mobilization.

Desensitization, review of sensory precautions and sensory reeducation are rarely required in the management of these injuries. Pain control includes thermal or electrical modalities, edema reduction, and the resolution of stiffness.

If motion limitations persist, a thorough examination is performed to determine which tissue structures are responsible for the limitation, and appropriate therapeutic intervention is provided.

Guidelines for each specific type of joint injury and intra-articular fracture regarding immobilization, controlled and protected motion, anticipated problems and key exercises, therapeutic techniques, and orthoses are described on Tables 33-1 and 33-2. It is important to note that time frames vary for each case.

Text continues on page 435

Table 33-1 Protective Stage of Management Following Intra-articular Hand Fractures and Joint Injuries

PIP JOINT INJURIES		
Collateral Ligament Injury		
Degree of Injury	**Immobilization/Controlled Motion**	**Time Frame**
1. Grade I (stable through AROM and PROM)	Buddy-taping to adjacent digit above and below the PIPJ; a LF RCL injury is taped to the IF and LF UCL injury is taped to the RF. A RF RCL injury is taped to LF, and RF UCL is taped to the SF. The SF may need a custom-sewn buddy-strap due to length difference of the P1 and P2 of the adjacent RF. Buddy-straps may be padded to provide for neutral alignment of PIPJ.	2–4 weeks
	Modifications: If there is significant pain and swelling, a finger gutter with PIP and DIP in extension is used or an HB resting orthosis including MP in 70 degrees of flexion and IPs in full extension for involved and adjacent digit. Straps are used to control neutral PIP alignment. After approximately 1 week, replace orthosis with buddy-straps (Fig. 33-2)	Use orthosis for 1 week then replace with buddy-straps
2. Grade II (stable through AROM)	Finger gutter with PIP and DIP in extension or an HB resting orthosis, including MP in 70 degrees of flexion and IPs in full extension for involved and adjacent digit for 2–4 weeks. After initial period of rest for 2 weeks, replace orthosis with buddy-straps.	2 weeks full-time orthosis wear f/b intermittent use or buddy-straps
3. Grade III (unstable through AROM and PROM) non-op	See grade II. Controlled motion: FiB or HB static extension block or figure-of-8 orthosis to block arc of motion (usually limiting full PIPJ extension) where instability is present (Fig. 33-3). After orthosis is discontinued, use buddy-straps as described above for grade 1 injury.	2–3 weeks full time, f/b intermittent use
	Modifications: May require surgeon's observation using fluoroscopy to determine effectiveness of extension block orthosis	
Dorsal Dislocation (P2 Dorsal to P1): Volar Plate Injury: May Involve Fracture Fragment: Type I–III		
Management	**Immobilization/Controlled Motion**	**Time Frame**
4. Closed reduction	Controlled motion: Typically requires two buddy-tapes to adjacent digit placed around P1 and P2	2–4 weeks
	Modification: If additional protection is desired and FiB and HB dorsal PIP extension block or a figure-of-8 orthosis is used. Full active flexion is allowed by removing straps on the FiB orthosis. Exact degree of extension block is determined by the physician. The surgeon may use fluoroscopy to determine the effectiveness of the extension block orthosis, which can be alone or in conjunction with using buddy-tapes for AROM exercises (see Fig. 33-3).	1–2 weeks f/b buddy-straps until week 4
5. Extension block pinning	Controlled motion: FiB or HB static dorsal protective orthosis covering pin. Remove straps to allow for active flexion.	4 weeks
	Controlled motion: After pin removal, wean to a figure-of-8/FiB static dorsal extension block orthosis limiting hyperextension and allowing flexion as required	PRN

Continued

Table 33-1   Protective Stage of Management Following Intra-articular Hand Fractures and Joint Injuries—cont'd

Dorsal Dislocation (P2 Dorsal to P1): Volar Plate Injury: May Involve Fracture Fragment: Type I–III

Management	Immobilization/Controlled Motion	Time Frame
6. Hinged external fixation (often with associated fx)	Controlled motion: If an extension block is required, an FiB or HB static dorsal block orthosis accommodating the hinged fixation and allowing active and assisted flexion is fabricated. A protective HB radioulnar gutter can be used to protect the external fixator. An FiB orthosis can be used to provide additional protection and block extension (Fig. 33-4)	4–6 weeks
	Controlled motion: After the fixator is removed, the use of an orthosis depends on joint stability. If the joint has some instability, the patient will need to use figure-of-8 or FiB static extension block orthosis.	PRN

Volar Dislocation (P2 Volar to P1): May Injure Central Slip of Extensor Tendon

Management	Immobilization/Controlled Motion	Time Frame
7. Closed reduction—central slip intact	Controlled motion: Finger gutter with PIPJ in extension. The orthosis should allow for full DIP motion. Orthosis may be fabricated by using a circumferential design with a small opening laterally to accommodate changes in edema. The orthosis is removed for AROM of PIPJ.	2–3 weeks
	Modifications: For extra protection an exercise template volar finger gutter is used, allowing progressive degrees of PIPJ flexion when out of the protective orthosis. When there is significant stiffness, buddy taping to the adjacent digit can help guide motion of the involved digit during the day.	Beginning when ROM is started
8. Closed reduction—central slip rupture	Immobilization: Finger gutter as above. The PIPJ must be supported in extension full time especially when the orthosis is removed for hygiene. The patient is slowly weaned from the orthosis to avoid the development of an extensor lag.	4–6 weeks
	Controlled motion: A Capener-type (Fig. 33-5) or Fib/HB dynamic PIP extension orthosis is used during the day and a finger gutter is used at night if starting AROM of PIPJ at week 4 or if extensor lag is evident.	Beginning when ROM is started
9. ORIF/repair of central tendon	Immobilization: A finger gutter with PIP and DIP in extension; if no internal fixation, for controlled motion, two exercise template orthoses are used (Fig. 33-6)[21] (see Chapter 39) 1. PIP extension orthosis used to perform isolated DIP flexion exercises 2. Finger gutter allowing PIP flexion to 30 degrees, DIP flexion to 25 degrees. Advance at week 2 to 40 degrees PIP flexion Week 3 to 50 degrees of PIP flexion Week 4 to 80 degrees of PIP flexion. If extensor lag develops, advance more slowly. If active motion is not progressing, use a flexion orthosis intermittently at week 4. The avoidance of extensor lag greater than 30 degrees is critical.	6 weeks total

Intra-articular Fractures Condylar, Volar/Dorsal Lip of P2/Pilon

Management	Immobilization/Controlled Motion	Time Frame
10. Volar fx: less than 30% of joint surface: Nondisplaced and stable. Non-op	Controlled motion: FiB or HB static dorsal PIP extension block orthosis typically limits the last 30 degrees of extension. The orthosis allows for active flexion by removing straps. Frequent reexaminations by physician are necessary to ensure fracture remains stable in the orthosis with remolding/refitting as necessary.	0–4 weeks
11. Volar fx greater than 40% of joint surface/ condylar fx that are unstable: ORIF (lag screw/K-wire)	Controlled motion/immobilization: HB resting or gutter orthosis for the involved and adjacent digit(s) with MPJs in 70 degrees of flexion, DIP extension and PIP in position determined by fixation method (generally in full extension). May allow for active flexion based on stability of fixation.	0–3 or 4 weeks
	Modification: If pinned, provide pin protection as needed with bivalved orthosis/padded dressing or padded straps and PIPJ positioned as pinned.	4 weeks
12. Volar fx: hemihamate reconstruction	Controlled motion: FB static dorsal PIP extension block orthosis at 20–30 degrees of flexion for the involved digit. The straps are removed to allow for active finger flexion and extension to the limits of the orthosis.	Week 0–2
	Controlled motion: Finger based dorsal block or figure-of-8 orthosis to block full extension and buddy-straps for flexion exercises.	Week 3–4 (6)
13. Volar fx/pilon fx/ condylar fx that are unstable: Dynamic external fixation	Controlled motion: HB static dorsal extensor block orthosis to block full PIPJ extension when hinge is unlocked for exercises or with external fixator in place.	0–2 or 4 weeks
	Controlled motion: A HB radioulnar gutter can be fabricated as needed to protect the external fixator from unwanted stresses.	0–4 or 6 weeks
	Modification: A static mallet type orthosis with the DIPJ in extension if an extensor lag is present. The fixation may tether the lateral bands along P2	0–4 or 6 weeks
14. Dorsal lip fx. of P2 involving attachment of central tendon non-op and ORIF with K-wire	See item 8 above. Immobilization of PIPJ in extension. The orthosis protects pins as required.	6 weeks for non-op 4 weeks for post-op
15. Combined fracture–dislocation—Any management	Controlled motion/immobilization: FiB or HB static protective orthosis in a position depends on direction of dislocation (volar or dorsal), and the orthosis/exercise program may allow motion in the opposite direction (See items 4–9 above)	4 weeks
	Modification: In cases of persistent instability after fracture management, the PIPJ may be immobilized full time to prevent recurrent dislocation followed by several weeks of protective orthotic use, position dependent on the direction of the dislocation.	2 weeks
16. PIPJ arthroplasty	See Chapter 107	

Table 33-1 Protective Stage of Management Following Intra-articular Hand Fractures and Joint Injuries—cont'd

DIP JOINTS (INDEX-SMALL) AND THUMB IP JOINT		
Dislocation (Rare)		
Management	**Immobilization/Controlled Motion**	**Time Frame**
17. Closed reduction	Controlled motion: FiB IP/thumb IP static dorsal extension block orthosis in 20–30 degrees of DIPJ flexion allowing active flexion of DIPJ thumb IPJ. For all DIPJ injures, maintenance of PIPJ full ROM is important.	2–3 weeks
18. Open reduction	Immobilization: DIPJ/thumb IPJ static orthosis to protect DIPJ/thumb IPJ pinning.	4 weeks
Intra-articular Fractures		
Management	**Immobilization/Controlled Motion**	**Time Frame**
19. Mallet—Non-op (see Chapter 39) Extensor tendon	Immobilization: A DIP/thumb IPJ static extension orthosis is used (Fig. 33-7). The DIPJ is supported in extension when orthosis is removed for hygiene. The therapist performs weekly checks for orthosis fit, compliance, and skin breakdown	6–8 weeks
	Modification for mallet finger with significant PIPJ hyperextension (swan-neck-mallet finger): PIP joint extension block at 30 degrees of flexion and DIP joint maintained in extension; orthosis allows PIP joint flexion (Fig. 33-8)	Use for 2 weeks initially
20. Mallet/open fx s/p ORIF	Immobilization: A DIPJ/thumb IPJ static extension orthosis is used with pin protection	6–8 weeks
	Modification: As above (item 19). If extension block pin is used, the orthosis must protect the pin placed dorsally.	
21. Fx or fx/dislocation at palmar base involving flexor tendon (FDP) avulsion; s/p ORIF (see Chapter 36)	Controlled motion: FA-based static dorsal block orthosis with MPJs in flexion, PIP full extension. The DIPJ may be placed in 30 degrees of flexion with second orthosis and the thumb IPJ can placed in 20 degrees within the dorsal block orthosis for 3 weeks. (See Chapter 36)	6 weeks

MP JOINTS FOR INDEX-SMALL FINGERS		
Dislocations/Collateral Ligament Injuries		
Management	**Immobilization/Controlled Motion**	**Time Frame**
22. Collateral ligament grades I–II: Non-op	Immobilization: An HB static MPJ orthosis with the injured and adjacent MPJs in 70 degrees of flexion; volar resting or a radioulnar gutter design. The molding techniques/strapping or padding can provide extra protection by placing the healing ligament in a medial or lateral deviated position to decrease stress on the injured ligament.	0–3 or 4 weeks
	Modification: Controlled motion: The PIPJ and DIPJ can be positioned in extension with a dorsal block placed on the HB orthosis to provide for more protection from lateral stresses and resolve PIPJ flexion contractures.	
	Controlled motion: Buddy-tapes are used following initial immobilization. Buddy-taping three adjacent fingers with appropriately placed padding can assist with corrective positioning at the MPJ.	Up to week 12
	Modification: HB hinged MPJ support allowing MPJ motion and preventing lateral stresses can be used.	As needed
23. Collateral ligament grades III post-op	Immobilization: Orthosis as above (item 22)	4–6 weeks
24. MPJ dislocation: Closed/ spontaneous reduction	Controlled motion: An HB dorsal MPJ extension block orthosis at neutral to 30 degrees of flexion is used and allow for full MPJ flexion by removing straps. Modification to HB orthosis as above (item 22).	3–4 weeks
25. MPJ dislocation: ORIF	Controlled motion: HB dorsal MP block orthosis at 30–50 degrees of MPJ flexion Modification to HB orthosis as above (item 22). May allow for active MPJ flexion depending upon stability.	4–6 weeks
Intra-articular Fractures		
Management	**Immobilization/Controlled Motion**	**Time Frame**
26. MPJ intra-articular fx at MCPJ (base P1 or head MP), non-op	Immobilization: A HB resting or gutter orthosis with MPJ in flexion and generally with PIPs free. Adjacent digits(s) are included in the orthosis.	4 weeks
	Modifications: If the P1 fx is potentially unstable or if a PIPJ flexion contracture is evident, the PIPJ may be included in the orthosis. Intermittent controlled PIPJ motion may be considered. If there is malrotation at the MPJ, consider volar HB resting orthosis including PIP and DIP with straps to correct the malrotation.	4 weeks
27. MPJ intra-articular fx at MCPJ (base P1 or head MP) Post-op ORIF	Orthosis as above (item 26) with accommodation for pin. Initiation of MPJ motion and adjustments for rotation discussed with the physician. Modification to the HB orthosis as above (item 22)	4 weeks
28. MPJ intra-articular fx at MCPJ (base P1 or head MP) Post-op external fixation	Immobilization: An HB Resting orthosis with MPJs supported as positioned by external fixator. Modification to the HB orthosis as above (item 21)	4/6 weeks

Continued

Table 33-1 Protective Stage of Management Following Intra-articular Hand Fractures and Joint Injuries—cont'd

Intra-articular Fractures

Management	Immobilization/Controlled Motion	Time Frame
29. MPJ arthroplasty	See Chapter 107	6–12 weeks

CMC JOINTS INDEX-SMALL FINGERS

Dislocations of Ring and Small, Intra-articular Fractures for Index-Small

Management	Immobilization/Controlled Motion	Time Frame
30. Dislocation RF and SF and fx index-small, non-op	Immobilization: Wrist orthosis in neutral is used. Modifications: May use a FA-based ulnar gutter or MPJ extension block orthosis with wrist in neutral and MPJs at 70 degrees for extra protection.	4 weeks
31. Dislocation/fx ring and small post-op (ORIF—screws/pins)	Orthosis as above (item 30). The fit must accommodate for external pins; MPJs typically included in the orthosis following this procedure.	4–6 weeks

THUMB MP JOINT

Dislocations

Management	Immobilization/Controlled Motion	Time Frame
32. Volar–dorsal closed reduction, non-op	Immobilization: An HB thumb spica with MPJ in neutral with the IPJ free.	3–4 weeks
33. UCL/RCL grades I–II: Non-op	Immobilization: As above (item 32). One can carefully mold the orthosis to ulnarly deviate the MPJ to provide additional protection to the UCL and radially deviate the MPJ to provide additional protection to the RCL. Patient is very slowly weaned from the orthosis.	3–4/6 weeks
34. UCL/RCL grade III: Post-op	Typically the joint is pinned for extra protection. Immobilization: An HB/FB thumb spica is fabricated with MPJ position as pinned, and IPJ free. The patient is very slowly weaned from the orthosis.	4–6 weeks

Intra-articular Fractures

Management	Immobilization/Controlled Motion	Time Frame
35. Fx, non-op	Immobilization: An FB or HB thumb orthosis with wrist and MPJ in neutral and IPJ free.	4 weeks
36. Fx, post-op	Immobilization: An above (item 35). The orthosis must accommodate pin fixation	4 weeks

THUMB CMC JOINT

Dislocations (Rare)

Management	Immobilization/Controlled Motion	Time Frame
37. Non-op or closed reduction	Immobilization: An FB thumb spica with wrist neutral, CMC in palmar abduction, MPJ neutral and IPJ free is fabricated. Casting is an alternative for a complete tear.	4–6 weeks
38. Post-op	See above (item 37). The orthosis must accommodate pin fixation. If screw fixation is used, a controlled motion program may begin within the first 10 days.	4–6 weeks

Intra-articular Fractures

Management	Immobilization/Controlled Motion	Time Frame
39. Closed reduction and pinning and ORIF	Immobilization: As above (item 37)	4–6 weeks

Terminology:
Protected motion: Active or passive movement to the nonimmobilized joints.[5]
Controlled motion: Active controlled movement of the injured or previously immobilized joint(s).[5]
AROM, active range of motion; CMC, carpometacarpal; DIPJ, distal interphalangeal joint; Dyn, dynamic; FB, forearm-based; f/b, followed by; FiB, finger-based; fx, fracture; HB, hand-based; IF, index finger; IPJ, both PIP and DIP joints; LF, long finger; MCPJ, metacarpophalangeal joint; MP, metacarpal; ORIF, open reduction with internal fixation; ORL, oblique retinacular ligament; P1, proximal phalanx; P2, middle phalanx; P3, distal phalanx; PIPJ, proximal interphalangeal joint; PROM, passive range of motion; RCL, radial collateral ligament; RF, ring finger; SF, small finger; SP, static progressive; thumb IPJ, thumb interphalangeal joint; UCL, ulnar collateral ligament.

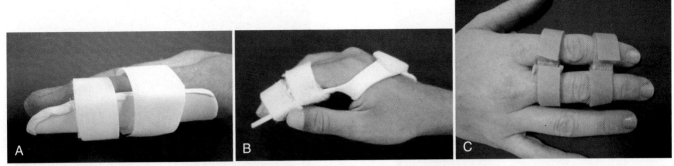

Figure 33-2 Orthoses used for PIPJ collateral ligament injury: **A,** Finger gutter with proximal interphalangeal and distal interphalangeal in extension. **B,** Hand-based resting orthosis including MP in 70 degrees of flexion and interphalangeals in full extension for involved and adjacent digit. After approximately 1 week, replace orthosis with buddy straps **(C).**

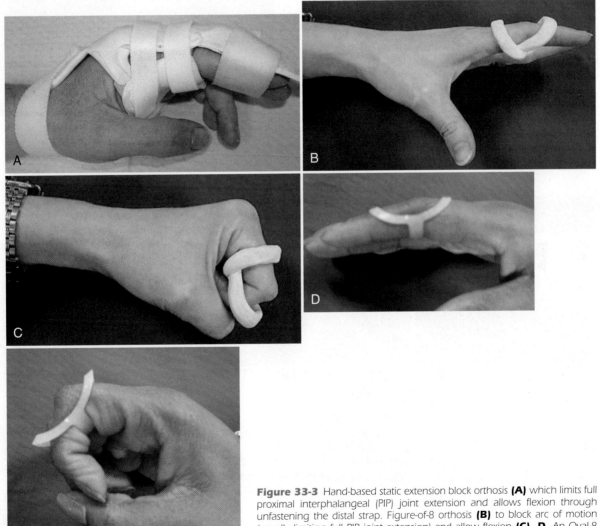

Figure 33-3 Hand-based static extension block orthosis **(A)** which limits full proximal interphalangeal (PIP) joint extension and allows flexion through unfastening the distal strap. Figure-of-8 orthosis **(B)** to block arc of motion (usually limiting full PIP joint extension) and allow flexion **(C). D,** An Oval-8 orthosis (3 Point Products) can be adjusted to block full PIP joint extension and **(E)** allow for full flexion.

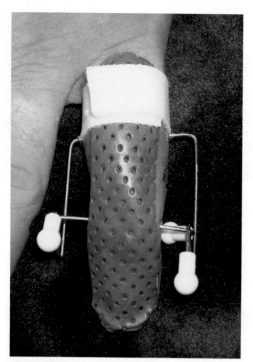

Figure 33-4 A finger-based orthosis can be used to provide additional protection and block extension with dynamic external fixation.

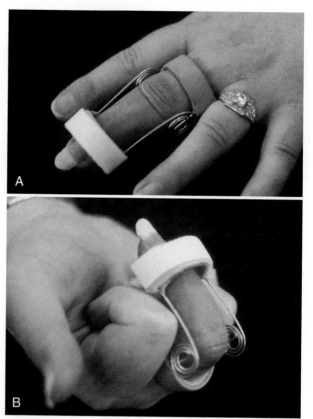

Figure 33-5 A Capener-type orthosis provides assistance for PIPJ extension **(A)** and allows flexion **(B).**

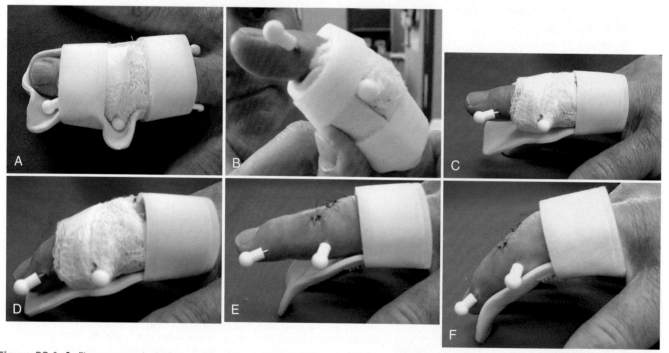

Figure 33-6 A, Finger gutter, including proximal interphalangeal (PIP) and distal interphalangeal (DIP) joints with pin protection. **B,** Exercise orthosis supporting the PIP joint in extension used to perform isolated DIP flexion exercises; **C–F,** An exercise template volar finger gutter is used and serially adjusted allowing PIP joint extension with progressive degrees of flexion in the case of central slip involvement according to Evans short arc motion protocol for repaired central slip injuries. (Evans R. Therapeutic management of extensor tendon injuries. In Hunter JM, Mackin EJ, Callahan AD, et al (eds): *Rehabilitation of the Hand*, St. Louis, CV Mosby, 1990, p 492.)

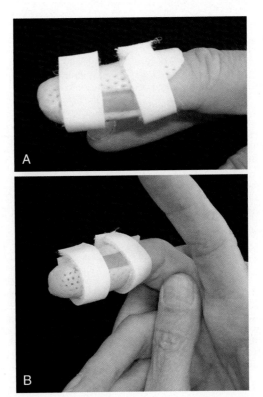

Figure 33-7 Mallet injury orthosis to maintain the DIPJ in extension **(A)** and allow PIP joint motion **(B).**

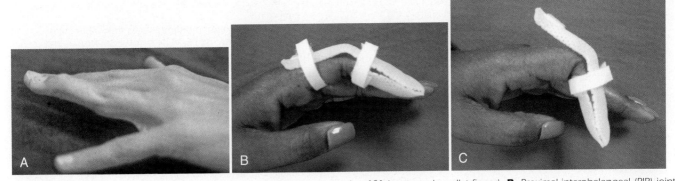

Figure 33-8 Modification for mallet finger with significant PIPJ hyperextension **(A)** (swan neck–mallet finger). **B,** Proximal interphalangeal (PIP) joint extension block at 30–35 degrees of flexion and distal interphalangeal (DIP) joint maintained in extension. **C,** Orthosis allows PIP joint flexion while maintaining DIP joint in extension.

Table 33-2 Mobilization Stage of Management*

PIP JOINT INJURIES

Collateral Ligament Injury

Anticipated Problems	Key Exercises/Techniques	Orthoses
1. Pain with lateral stress or joint lateral deviation. 2. Limited PIP joint active or passive flexion.	Buddy-straps to the adjacent finger used to control alignment at rest and with exercise Pinch activities are monitored to maintain neutral alignment at PIP joint. Blocking exercises for active PIP joint flexion—MCP joint blocked in neutral extension Gentle PROM for PIP joint flexion with maintenance of lateral stability Massage over collateral ligaments	A volar HB orthosis with straps to control PIP joint alignment. FiB orthosis molded to correct the deviation Custom hinged PIP joint orthosis to control lateral deviation Silver ring alignment orthosis (Fig. 33-9) Blocking orthosis to isolate PIP joint ROM during active exercises—orthosis blocks motion at the MCP and DIP joints to allow concentration of motion at the PIP joint (Fig. 33-10) Dyn/SP PIP mobilization orthosis, PIP joint elastic/web flexion strap or a PIP–DIP elastic flexion loop; monitor for extensor lag (Fig. 33-11)

Dorsal Dislocation

Anticipated Problems	Key Exercises/Techniques	Orthoses
3. Persistent instability: (PIP joint hyperextension or swan-neck deformity) 4. Limited PIP active/passive extension; PIP joint flexion contracture 5. ORL tightness	Isolated FDS strengthening especially during pinch tasks Blocking exercises for PIP joint extension with MCP joint positioned in flexion to direct action of the EDC to extend the PIP joint. ORL and lateral band stretching: DIP joint flexion with PIP joint held in extension. PIPJ mobilization techniques Isolated passive PIP joint extension while avoiding hyperextending the DIP joint DIP joint flexion with PIP joint held in maximum extension.	Figure-of-8 orthosis to limit PIP joint hyperextension during the day. Static PIP orthosis in slight flexion at night. Blocking orthoses to isolate PIP joint ROM during active flexion exercises–orthoses block motion at the MCP and DIP joints to allow concentration of motion at the PIP joint Blocking orthoses for PIP joint extension exercises: HB static orthosis with involved MCP joint in flexion (Fig. 33-12) or the Merritt Yoke orthosis to position adjacent MCP joint in extension and the involved digit MCP joint in relatively increased flexion to direct the force of EDC to extend PIP joint. DIP flexion orthosis worn while performing PIP joint active extension to retain lateral bands dorsal to PIP joint axis and triangular ligament taunt. PIP extension orthoses: (1) custom static PIP extension orthosis; (2) belly gutter extension orthosis, (3) prefabricated PIP extension orthosis (LMB/Capener/spring coil), (4) three-point extension orthosis, (5) Dyn/SP PIP extension orthosis, or (6) serial casting Exercise orthosis with PIP in maximal extension allowing DIP joint flexion (both active and passive) FiB orthosis with PIP joint in maximal extension and DIP joint maintained in passive flexion either with static or dynamic pull.

Volar Dislocation

Anticipated Problems	Key Exercises/Techniques	Orthoses
6. Limited PIP active or passive flexion 7. Limited PIP joint active extension (Central slip involvement with extensor lag at PIP joint) 8. ORL tightness	Blocking exercises are performed for PIP flexion while monitoring for extensor lag. Blocking exercises for PIP joint extension with MCP joint positioned in flexion to direct action of the EDC to extend the PIP joint. ORL and lateral band stretching: DIP joint flexion with PIP joint held in extension Isometric contraction of extensors during healing phase while PIP joint is held in an extension orthosis Balance exercises in favor of PIP joint extension; avoid stressing PIP joint flexion at the expense of extension; delay composite finger A/P flexion. See item 5	See item 2 above. Monitor for extensor lag when working on flexion Use of PIP joint extension orthosis: If less than 30 degrees: Intermittent daytime use of PIP joint extension orthosis and full-time night use. If greater than 30 deg: Full-time use of PIP joint extension orthosis with duration based on recovery of PIP joint extension. Remove for ROM exercises stressing active extension. PIP joint extension orthoses include: FiB static extension orthosis; FiB/HB Dyn. PIP or Capener type PIP joint extension orthosis for day use; HB static orthosis with MCP joint flexed; Merritt Yoke orthosis to position adjacent MCP joint in extension and involved digit MCP joint in relatively increase flexion. Kinesiotaping can be used on the dorsum of finger for day use. FiB static DIP orthosis in slight flexion to use for exercise. See item 5

Intra-articular Fractures: Non-Op and ORIF

Anticipated Problems	Key Exercises/Techniques	Orthoses
9. Potential for instability 10. Lateral deviation at PIP joint 11. Limited PIP joint active/passive flexion	Early in treatment, limit motion to a short arc within stable range for PIP joint Reduce frequency of exercise/arc of motion or hold initiation of motion. Consider delaying DIP joint AROM. See item 1. See item 2 Early short arc motion Focus on isolated joint motion before composite to avoid the development of an extensor lag	Regular monitoring of protective orthosis for secure fit Use template orthosis for exercise to guide patient with short arc motion program. See No. 1 If using a Dyn/SP PIP mobilization orthosis Insure mobilization orthosis line of pull does not contribute to deviation. Blocking orthosis to isolate PIP joint ROM during active exercises—orthosis blocks motion at the MCP and DIP joints to allow concentration of motion at the PIP joint Dyn/SP PIP mobilization orthoses, PIP joint elastic/web flexion strap and/or a PIP–DIP elastic flexion loop; monitor for extensor lag

Table 33-2 Mobilization Stage of Management*—cont'd

PIP JOINT INJURIES		

Intra-articular Fractures: Non-Op and ORIF

Anticipated Problems	Key Exercises/Techniques	Orthoses
12. Limited PIP joint active/passive extension	See items 4 and 7 For fxs involving reattachment of central tendon, begin careful PIPJ active isolated flexion at 4 weeks while monitoring for extensor lag	See 4 and 7
13. Stiffness of uninvolved joints due to necessary immobilization	Early AROM of MP may be allowed. AROM of DIP joint with P1, PIP, P2 manually supported in orthosis A/PROM of adjacent digits. Quadriga effect may limit uninvolved joint motion For involved finger, as injury stability increases advance to PROM of individual joints before composite motion. For severe cases, motor re-education including graded motor imagery and NMES.	Blocking orthoses as above to direct motion to individual joints As joint motion increases, composite joint flexion orthoses using Dyn/SP traction or flexion straps
14. Limited DIP Active extension (extensor lag at DIP joint)	Trial period of immobilization—see orthosis section. Avoid stressing DIP joint flexion and monitor to prevent this limitation rather than treat it after it develops. Stabilization of MCP joint and PIP joint in neutral/slight flexion to direct extensor force to the DIP joint	If less than 30 degrees: Intermittent rest in extension and night extension with static DIPJ extension orthosis If greater than 30 degrees: Trial of a full-time extension orthosis for a period of time determined by improvement or persistence of extensor lag as well as the degree of available flexion and ADL requirements Kinesiotape can be placed on dorsum of digit with the finger in extension to serve as a slight assist to extend to finger.
15. ORL tightness	See item 5 above	See item 5 above

Hemihamate Reconstruction

Anticipated Problems	Key Exercises/Techniques	Orthoses
16. Wrist AROM limitations	Wrist AROM exercises begin at week 2	No orthosis indicated
17. PIP joint A/PROM limits within the first 4 weeks.	Week 1: A/AA PIP flexion and active extension to limits of orthosis. Week 2: Full AROM allowed out of the orthosis and progress to gentle PROM into flexion only. Week 4: Consider gentle PROM into extension if PIPJ flexion contracture is greater than 20 degrees. Note: If used for initial fracture management, this procedure can provide for an excellent outcome. If used for delayed treatment, outcome is dependent on the resolution of longstanding soft tissue limitations.	A HB Dyn PIP joint flexion orthosis with very light traction can be considered if not progressing with exercises. See intra-articular fractures after 4–6 week time period.

Dynamic External Fixation Volar Lip Fractures

Anticipated Problems	Key Exercises/Techniques	Orthoses
18. Limited active flexion and extension within the first 6 weeks. See intra-articular fxs for other limitations (items 9–15)	Week 1: A/AA flexion. Active ext to limits of ext block orthosis/line drawn on Compass hinge. Can use Compass hinge to "drive" passive flexion or perform gentle PROM into flexion when edema decreases as tolerated. Progressive increased PIP joint extension depending on stability of joint. Week 4–6: Hinge removal. Can begin full active extension generally after hinge removal	Extension block orthosis at PIP joint if unstable Static extension orthosis at DIP joint if there is an extensor lag or there is a need to direct motion to the PIP joint. Stability of joint into extension must be determined by physician before using extension orthoses

Dynamic External Fixation: Pilon Fracture

Anticipated Problems	Key Exercises/Techniques	Orthoses
19. Post-traumatic arthritis See intra-acticular fxs for other limitations (items 9–15)	A/PROM and strengthening in pain-free range	Soft supports or taping for support during tasks requiring motion can be of some benefit. A static PIP orthosis in position of comfort is used at night and for resistive tasks (Fig. 33-13) The stability of the joint into extension must be determined by physician before initiating extension orthoses and passive extension

Table 33-2 Mobilization Stage of Management*—cont'd

DIP JOINTS (INDEX-SMALL) AND THUMB IP JOINT		
Dislocation (rare)/Fractures		
Anticipated Problems	**Key Exercises/Techniques**	**Orthoses**
20. DIP or thumb IP joint active and passive flexion and extension limits	Isolated joint blocking exercises and hook fisting Monitor for DIP joint extensor lag and change the program if this occurs. Resisted blocking with the PIP and MCP joints held in extension and reverse blocking with PIP joint held in slight flexion to increase DIP joint AROM The thumb MCP joint is placed in extension for blocking exercises for IP joint flexion and slight flexion for reverse blocking for IP joint extension.	Flexion: A static blocking orthosis with MCP and PIP joints in extension used during exercises; Dyn/SP DIP joint flexion orthosis, PIP–DIP joint flexion loop to increase DIP joint PROM in flexion Extension: Mallet type orthosis/finger gutter used intermittently; Kinesiotape can be placed on the dorsum of DIP joint while in extension to serve as a slight assist for extension. Thumb IP joint flexion: Blocking orthosis with MP in extension to focus effort at the IP joint during flexion exercise; Dyn/SP thumb IP joint flexion orthosis Thumb IP joint extension: Thumb mallet type orthosis; HB thumb extension orthosis including the MCP joint and IP joint; Dyn/SP thumb IP joint extension orthosis

MPJ JOINTS: INDEX-SMALL FINGERS		
Dislocations/Collateral Ligament Injuries/Intra-articular Fractures		
Anticipated Problems	**Key Exercises/Techniques**	**Orthoses**
21. MCP joint instability (collateral ligament)	Isometric strengthening of interossei, lumbricals, and EDC in direction opposite to instability	Prolonged use of protective orthosis, buddy tapes or HB hinged MCP joint orthosis with adjacent digit included to provide external stability Taping techniques/soft straps for limited support while allowing function
22. MCP joint limited active and passive extension	EDC extension and differential EDC glides (where adjacent digits are held in flexion and the injured digit performs MCP joint extension). EDC glides can be performed while mobilizing adherent scar on dorsum of the hand. Intrinsic and flexor stretching can resolve muscle tendon unit contractures to allow for improved MP extension.	FB/HB dynamic MCP joint extension orthosis or HB static MCP joint extension orthosis Blocking orthosis limiting the motion of the IP joints to isolate MCP joint extension, e.g., FiB cylinder orthosis with PIP and DIP joints in extension
23. MCP joint limited active and passive flexion	Blocking exercises for MCP joint flexion: wrist and CMC joint of the involved finger are stabilized in neutral extension to isolate MCP joint flexion exercise. Extensor tendon composite stretching exercises if shortening or adherence of the extensor tendon is apparent, monitoring for extensor lag. Lumbrical strengthening	Exercise blocking orthosis to stabilize the wrist and the CMC joint of the involved finger; or immobilizing PIP joints and DIP joint of the involved finger to direct motion to the MCP joint Passive: FB or HB Dyn/SP MCP joint flexion orthosis—requires proximal joint stabilization of the wrist and corresponding CMC joint, control for a 90-degree angle of pull from P1 to the attachment point on the base of the orthosis; an intermediate outrigger can be used to achieve the 90-degree angle with significantly decreased MCP joint flexion Composite flexion orthosis if extensor tendon tightness/shortening is a component of the problem
24. Intrinsic muscle tendon unit tightness	MCP joint held in full extension with active/passive PIP and DIP joint flexion	HB Dyn/SP Intrinsic stretching orthosis with MP in mamximal extension, flexing PIP joint and DIP joint (Fig. 33-14)
25. Flexor muscle tendon unit tightness	Obtain isolated joint passive extension f/b composite stretch to flexors (fingers and wrist in extension). Hand flat on table and elbow is raised; wall slides Thermal agents combined with end range/length positioning	FB serial static orthosis to increase length of the shortened flexor muscle tendon unit starting with neutral wrist and simultaneous extension of MCP, PIP, DIP joints. Orthosis is serially adjusted as increased length is achieved. Orthosis is adjusted to accommodate varying degrees of flexor tightness. Typically used at night
26. Extensor muscle tendon unit tightness	Isolated joint passive flexion followed by composite stretch to extensors (simultaneous finger and wrist flexion exercise) Monitor for extensor lag and adjust exercises as needed. Thermal agents combined with end range/length positioning	FB Dyn/SP orthosis with neutral wrist and simultaneous flexion of MCP, PIP, DIP joints

Table 33-2   Mobilization Stage of Management*—cont'd

CMC JOINT INJURIES INDEX-SMALL

Dislocations and Fractures

Anticipated Problems	Key Exercises/Techniques	Orthoses
27. Limited wrist, CMC and MCP joints active and passive flexion and extension	For ulnar digits, include fourth and fifth flexion at CMC joint to restore transverse metacarpal arch "hand cupping" exercise—patient attempts to touch hypothenar to thenar pad both actively and passively EDC glides (see item 22) Finger abduction and adduction exercises Intrinsic, flexor, extensor stretching is performed unless there is an extensor lag/crepitus (see items 24–26)	FB dyn/SP MCP joint mobilization orthosis to resolve passive MCP joint deficits. A wrist mobilization orthosis may be needed to resolve passive wrist deficts. Exercise cylinder blocking orthosis with PIP and DIP joints in extension to isolate MP active motion; proximal stabilization also required
28. Extensor tendon irritation/rupture	Limit repetitive extensor exercises and use Physical agents to reduce inflammation and calcific development	Maintain protective orthosis and consider including MPJ in extension.
29. Injury to motor branch of ulnar never	Physical agents to reduce inflammation Rest from provocative activity Nerve gliding Reeducation for ulnar innervated musculature	Continue with protective orthosis. HB anticlaw orthosis if ulnar claw deformity is present

THUMB MCP JOINT

Dislocation/MCP joint Collateral Ligament Injuries/Intra-articular Fracture

Anticipated Problems	Key Exercises/Techniques	Orthoses
30. Thumb IP joint active and passive flexion and extension limitations	Early IP joint AROM while in orthosis Blocking for IP joint flexion with MCP joint stabilized in extension; reverse blocking for IPJ extension with MCP joint stabilized in slight flexion Blocking with resistance	HB Dyn/SP IP joint flexion/extension orthosis. Traction is used to gain PROM. A dynamic component is used to perform resisted flexion–extension against elactic traction Exercise orthosis blocking the MCP joint to isolate IP joint flexion and extension
31. MCP joint active and passive flexion and extension limitations	Stability is preferred over painful mobility at this joint. Blocking and reverse blocking for MCP joint flexion and extension with the CMC joint stabilized Resistive blocking exercises Lateral stress to MCP joint should be avoided. Generally delay thumb pinch strengthening.	FB Dyn/SP MCP joint flexion–extension orthosis to gain PROM. Avoid lateral stress to the MCP joint with dynamic–static traction.
32. Webspace contracture	Massage to webspace Thermal agent combine with web stretch	HB static webspace stretcher. Attention needed to prevent stress to the thumb UCL (Fig. 33-15)
33. MCP joint instability	Multiple-angle isometric exercises for thumb intrinsics Compensatory strategies and adaptive equipment to reduce stress to MCP joint	Protective MCP joint orthosis or neoprene thumb support to provide stability (Fig. 33-16) An MCP joint figure-of-8 orthosis for MCP joint hyperextension

THUMB CMC JOINT

Dislocations (rare) and Intra-articular Fractures

Anticipated Problems	Key Exercises/Techniques	Orthoses
34. IP and MP active and passive flexion and extension limitations	See items 30, 31 above	See items 30, 31 above
35. Webspace contracture	See item 32 above	See item 32 above

*Specific problems associated with each injury are described with corresponding key treatments. The general approach to the management of joint injuries is described in the text.

Terminology:

Protected motion: Active or passive movement to the nonimmobilized joints.[5]

Controlled motion: Active controlled movement of the injured or previously immobilized joint(s).[5]

A/P, anteroposterior; AROM, active range of motion; CMC, carpometacarpal; DIP, distal interphalangeal; Dyn, dynamic; EDC, extensor digitorum communis; FB, forearm-based; f/b, followed by; FDS, flexor digitorum superficialis; FiB, finger-based; fx, fracture; HB, hand-based; IF, index finger; IP, both PIP and DIP; LF, long finger; MCP, metacarpophalangeal; MP, metacarpal; ORIF, open reduction with internal fixation; ORL, oblique retinacular ligament; P1, proximal phalanx; P2, middle phalanx; P3, distal phalanx; PIP, proximal interphalangeal; PROM, passive range of motion; RCL, radial collateral ligament; RF, ring finger; SF, small finger; SP, static progressive; thumb IP, thumb interphalangeal; UCL, ulnar collateral ligament.

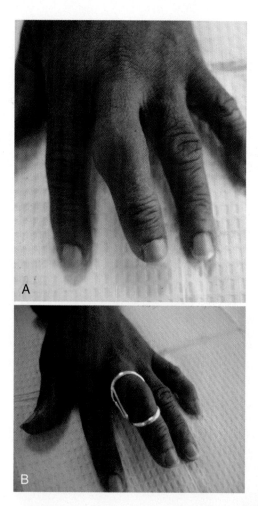

Figure 33-9 A, Proximal interphalangeal joint deformity with lateral deviation. **B,** Silver ring alignment orthosis.

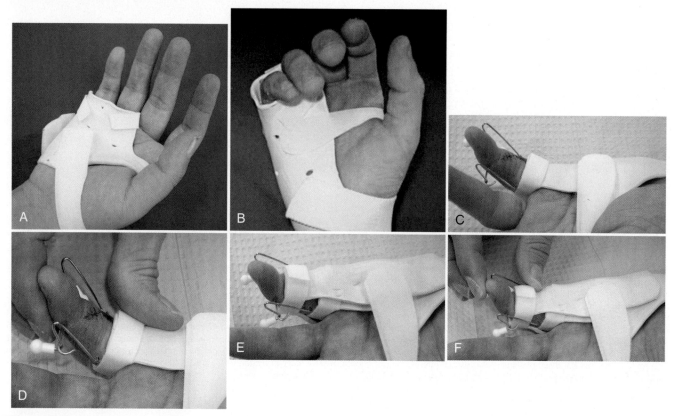

Figure 33-10 Blocking orthosis **(A, B)** to isolate proximal interphalangeal (PIP) joint range of motion (ROM) during active exercises; blocking orthoses **(C–F)** used with dynamic external fixation to allow isolated PIP and distal interphalangeal joint active and passive ROM exercises.

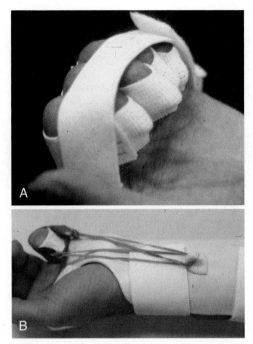

Figure 33-11 Orthoses to increase proximal interphalangeal flexion. **A,** Flexion strap with flexion loops. **B,** Metacarpophalangeal joint flexion orthosis used with flexion loop to achieve composite flexion.

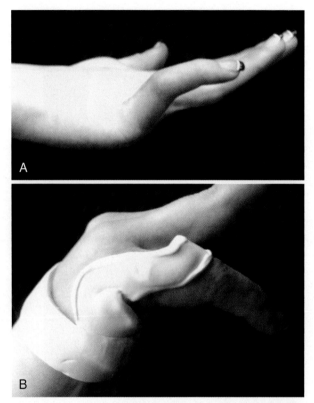

Figure 33-12 A, Proximal interphalangeal (PIP) joint extension lag with hyperextension of the metacarpophalangeal (MCP) joint. **B,** Blocking orthosis which blocks MCP joint hyperextension and allows concentration of extensor tendon action at the PIP joint.

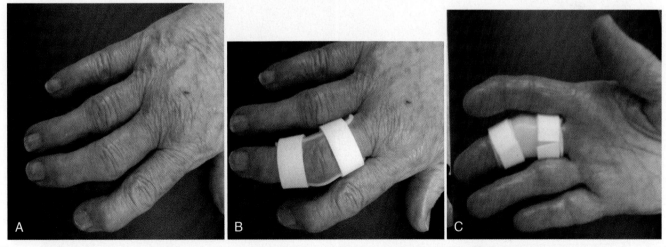

Figure 33-13 A, Traumatic osteoarthritis of a proximal interphalangeal (PIP) joint with lateral instability. **B, C,** Static orthosis in position of comfort is used at night and for protection during resistive tasks for PIP joint arthritis and chronic instability.

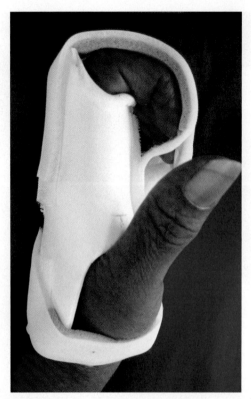

Figure 33-14 Hand-based, static progressive, intrinsic stretching orthosis with metacarpophalangeals in maximal extension, flexing proximal and distal interphalangeal joints.

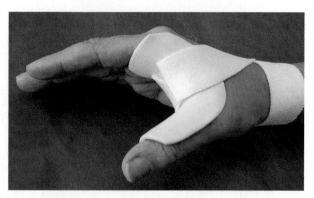

Figure 33-15 Hand-based static webspace stretcher. Attention is needed to prevent stress to the thumb MCP ulnar collateral ligament.

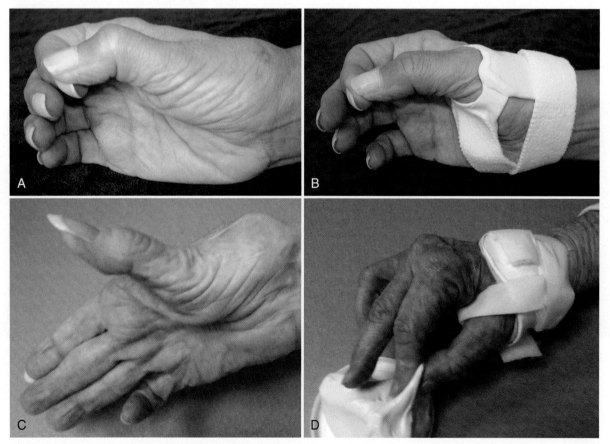

Figure 33-16 A, Thumb metacarpophalangeal (MCP) joint instability with hyperextension during pinch. **B,** Orthosis to stabilize the first metacarpal and carpometacarpal (CMC) joint to increase stability of the MCP joint during pinch. **C,** More severe thumb CMC and MCP joint instability. **D,** Orthosis to stabilize the first metacarpal and CMC joint to improve stability during pinch.

Strengthening and Return to Function Phase

During the first 2 weeks the patient is allowed to use the involved upper extremity as a gross functional assist without movement of the involved digit(s) for light ADLs (e.g., grooming, eating) with an orthosis or protective device in place. As fracture consolidation increases and joint stability is maintained, the patient can begin using the involved hand in normal patterns of use with the orthosis in place. When light resistance is tolerated at the site of injury, the patient is allowed to perform minimally resistive functional tasks without the orthosis. Examples of light functional activities include coin sorting, towel folding, and other tasks requiring ROM of the involved joints with minimal resistance. Resistive activity is generally not introduced until 8 weeks.

After 8 weeks or when the injury is determined to be stable enough for resistance, protective orthosis use is typically gradually decreased instead of abruptly discontinued. Light homecare, work tasks, or sport-specific activities are gradually reintroduced. In therapy, resistive activities begin without the orthosis. Close monitoring for poor tolerance of resistive tasks is important, and the resistive program is modified as indicated. Typically by 12 weeks, the patient should return to unrestricted work or sports under guidance from the physician. The time frames related to functional activity may need to be modified based on the severity of injury, extent of joint instability, length of immobilization, and mechanism of healing (primary vs. secondary).

Complications and Considerations

Fracture malunion or nonunion or joint instability require either use of a supportive orthosis or additional surgical intervention (or both). Stiffness in one joint can affect motion in proximal and distal joints in the involved finger as well as other digits due to the quadrigia effect. Kinematic chain disturbances such as pseudoboutonnière and swan-neck deformities can occur and require a corrective orthosis or surgery. Tendon adhesions or joint contractures that are not responsive to therapy interventions may require additional surgery. Active extensor lag of all joints is a difficult problem to manage either surgically or through therapy.

Summary

Injury to the joints of the hand may result in intra-articular fracture of the bones or damage to the supporting joint capsule and ligament systems. Absolute respect for the principles of bone and soft tissue healing is paramount in providing safe, yet progressive rehabilitation. This chapter offers treatment guidelines for creating individualized treatment plans. The time frames for each phase of rehabilitation are flexible because the immobilization period differs for each injury and each patient. Therefore, consistent communication between the surgeon and therapist is essential to safely progress the patient though each phase of treatment. Although the chapter focuses on early motion, the generalized goals and treatment guidelines remind the therapist of various concerns and treatment required to achieve an excellent result for the patient.

REFERENCES

The complete reference list is available online at www.expertconsult.com.

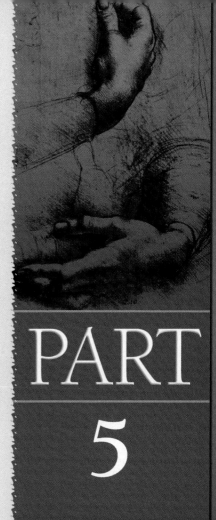

PART
5

Tendon Injuries
and Tendinopathies

Advances in Understanding of Tendon Healing and Repairs and Effect on Postoperative Management

PETER C. AMADIO, MD*

CHAPTER 34

SIGNIFICANCE OF TENDON INJURIES
TENDON HEALING
TENDON GRAFTING
AUGMENTATION OF INTRINSIC TENDON
   HEALING WITH STEM CELLS

TENDON REPAIR
EFFECT ON POSTOPERATIVE MANAGEMENT
SUMMARY

CRITICAL POINTS

Biology
- Motion aids healing and reduces adhesions.
- There is *no* evidence that loading, in the absence of motion, is helpful, or that, once the tendon is moving, more loading helps healing.
- We do know that loading may lead to failure of the repair.

Safe Zone
- Enough loading to initiate motion
- Not enough to risk the repair

Future Surgical Methods
- Gaps: Lubricated graft
- Slow healing: Cell-rich patch between tendon ends, with or without cytokines
- Stronger repairs: Newer sutures

Significance of Tendon Injuries

Upper extremity injuries are common, representing approximately one third of all traumatic injuries. Tendon injuries are among the most severe upper extremity injuries. The number of tendon injuries is difficult to quantify because epidemiologic studies have not been done, but estimates suggest that roughly 40,000 inpatient tendon repairs are done each year in the United States.[1] A much larger number of tendon surgeries are done on an outpatient basis. More importantly, these injuries occur almost exclusively in a young, working-age population and result in considerable disability. The typical tendon injury requires 3 to 4 months of rehabilitation, during which time the affected hand is unavailable for work use. Failure rates or residual impairment remain disturbingly high, in the 20% to 30% range in most series, despite ongoing attention to the problem. From 1976 to 1999, consistently between 7% and 8% of the articles in the *Journal of Hand Surgery* focused on tendon injuries.[2] Despite this evident importance and ongoing interest, translation of research results into meaningful clinical improvements have been limited. By most accounts,[3] the most significant improvement in tendon rehabilitation remains the institution of early passive motion therapy by Kleinert in the early 1970s.[4] Since then, quality improvements have been incremental. Tendon rupture rates continue to be cited at an incidence of 5% to 10%. These failures require complex secondary tendon reconstruction surgeries.[5-8] Better methods for improving intrinsic tendon healing and minimizing tendon adhesions are still needed so we can improve upon clinical outcomes, with the ultimate goal being the production of an adhesion-free tendon repair.

Tendon Healing

The extracellular matrix (ECM) is the principal component of tendon tissue and is responsible for its material properties.[9-11] The major constituents of the ECM are type I collagen; proteoglycans, principally decorin, but also aggrecan in the gliding regions;[12-15] fibronectin; and elastin. This matrix is synthesized by tendon cells, or tenocytes (Fig. 34-1). These cells are surrounded by the dense matrix; thus, although they

*Disclosure: The author has, with others, applied for a patent relating to the tissue engineering of tendon surfaces to reduce friction, but has no financial or other relationships with any commercial entities related to the subject of this chapter.

Extracellular Matrix in Tendon

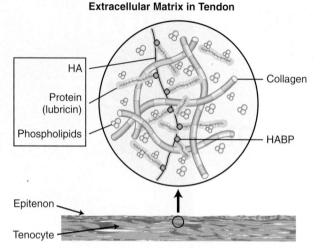

Figure 34-1 *Schematic of tendon matrix. HA, hyaluronic acid; HABP, hyaluron binding protein.*

are metabolically active, they do not participate much in the tendon-healing process. Instead, undifferentiated cells in the epitenon do the heavy lifting for tendon healing, and proliferating, migrating into the gap between the tendon ends, and finally uniting the cut tendon ends[16,17] (Fig. 34-2). Unfortunately, this process presents a bit of a dilemma; if these same cells migrate away from the tendon, toward the tendon sheath, they form adhesions that restrict tendon motion. Often this is indeed the case, as the relatively ischemic tendon is surrounded by better vascularized tissue, which sends out vascular buds under the stimulation of vascular endothelial growth factor (VEGF).[18-21]

After tendon injury, the ECM undergoes significant changes due to synthesis of new elements, such as type III collagen, by the tenocytes,[22-24] degradation of existing elements by various matrix metalloproteinases (MMP), and remodeling of the resulting combination, under the influence of cytokines such as transforming growth factor beta (TGF-β) as well as mechanical forces. Manipulation of these processes, to augment their action between the tendon ends while reducing them at the tendon's gliding surface, is the goal of much research, as described later.

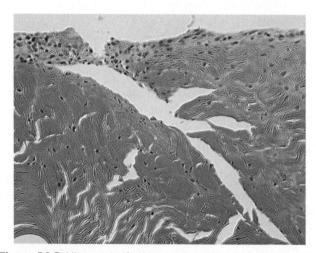

Figure 34-2 *Micrograph of epitenon cells migrating into the repair site 3 weeks after injury.*

Pharmacologic Manipulation of Tendon Healing

Various pharmacologic agents have been used in the past in an attempt to modify adhesion formation. Steroids, antihistamines, and β-aminoproprionitrile have not been shown to decrease scar formation clinically.[25,26] Ibuprofen and indomethacin, however, have been found to have a small beneficial effect.[27]

The ideal pharmacologic agent should have no systemic side effects, should be limited to a single application, and should be directed at growth factor expression and ECM production. Such a drug may be 5-fluorouracil (5-FU), an antimetabolite used not only as a cancer chemotherapeutic agent but also to prevent adhesions in glaucoma filtration surgery. The exposure of a surgical field to 5-FU produces a focal inhibition of scarring. Blumenkranz and colleagues have found that 5-FU inhibits the proliferation of fibroblasts in cell cultures and reduces retinal scarring.[28,29] Single exposures to 5-FU, for as short duration as 5 minutes, can have antiproliferative effects on fibroblasts for several days. The suppression of fibroblast proliferation has been observed for up to 36 hours without signs of cell death.[30,31] This time frame may be adequate to inhibit tendon adhesions prior to beginning postoperative motion protocols. Reversible prolonged inhibition of fibroblast function is attributed to the drug's inhibition of DNA and messenger RNA (mRNA) synthesis through thymidylate syntheses. More importantly, these effects appear to be focal to the site of application and titratable in terms of length of action.[32-34] A 5-minute exposure to 5-FU has been shown to significantly decrease postoperative flexor tendon adhesions in chicken and rabbit models.[35,36] This beneficial effect is felt to be due to the downregulation of TGF-β and modulation of MMP-2 and MMP-9 production.[37,38] The effect on surface lubrication is unknown. No adverse effect was noted on tendon healing in these studies. It is presumed therefore that the topical 5-FU does not penetrate to affect the cells below the tendon surface. Topical 5-FU may well have a role in improving the outcomes in selected cases of tenolysis.

Growth Factors

Growth factors are the chemical signals that direct the migration and proliferation of the tendon fibroblast during the healing process. The role of growth factors has been examined extensively in cutaneous wounds and other soft tissue processes, yet we are only beginning to know the specifics involved in flexor tendon healing.[11,39] The factors that appear to be involved include TGF-β, platelet-derived growth factor (PDGF), basic fibroblast growth factor (bFGF), insulin-like growth factor (IGF), epidermal growth factor (EGF), and VEGF.[21,40,41] These same growth factors have also been shown to optimize tissue-engineered constructs used for tendon repair.[21,40-44] Growth differentiation factor-5 (GDF-5), a member of the TGF-β superfamily, has also been shown to accelerate tendon healing in multiple animal models.[45-47]

TGF-β stimulates the formation of the ECM. It signals fibroblasts to produce collagen and fibronectin, decreases protease production, and increases the formation of integrins, which promote cellular adhesions and matrix assembly. In normal tissue, TGF-β becomes inactivated once wound healing is complete; however, it may remain active in tendon adhesion formation, continuing the cycle of matrix accumulation.[48,49] Excessive expression of TGF-β is detrimental to many tissues, resulting in tissue fibrosis in the heart, kidney, and liver.[49] Modulation of TGF-β has been reported to reduce the fibrotic process in glomerulonephritis, dermal wounds, and arthritis as well as decreasing peritendinous adhesions in a rabbit tendon model.[49-52] TGF-β levels can remain elevated for up to 8 weeks after tendon injury.[53,54]

Neuropeptides may also play a role in tendon healing.[55-58] During the early phases of healing, tendons exhibit nerve fiber ingrowth.[55] This nerve ingrowth is associated with the temporal release of substance P (SP). SP promotes tendon regeneration through the stimulation and proliferation of fibroblasts.[59-62] Further studies have found that tendon motion helps to modulate the release of SP.[56] The injection of SP into the peritendinous region of ruptured rat tendons improves healing and increases tendon strength.[63] Similarly, GDF-5 has a potential to stimulate bone marrow-derived stem cell (BMSC) proliferation and regulate BMSC differentiation to tenocytes.[64] Recent experiments have shown a beneficial effect of GDF-5 on tendon healing as well.[19,46,65]

Tendon Grafting

At one time, most flexor tendon injuries were treated with tendon grafts,[66,67] but today primary repair is used almost exclusively, with grafts being used primarily to reconstruct otherwise unbridgeable tendon gaps. This is a good thing, since tendons in the hand are intrasynovial and have a specialized gliding surface, whereas most tendon grafts, such as the palmaris or plantaris, are extrasynovial and have no such specialized surface.[68,69] The result is much more adhesion formation than would be the case if intrasynovial grafts were available. As noted later, in the future it may be possible to engineer such grafts to reduce friction and improve healing.

Augmentation of Intrinsic Tendon Healing with Stem Cells

Healing of flexor tendons in zone 2 depends on the ability of the injured tendon to recruit fibroblasts and other cellular components to the site of injury.[70] Normally these are circulating or locally derived undifferentiated (i.e., stem) cells that are recruited to the injury site by the expression of cytokines in the wound.[18,21,71-73] Cytokine stimulation is also important in converting these undifferentiated cells into the tendon phenotype, characterized by the expression of markers such as tenomodulin and scleraxis.[74,75] BMSC can also enter and participate in soft tissue healing.[76-78] BMSCs delivered on collagen sponges improve healing in animal models of tendon repair,[42,79] and stem cells from other origins have been shown to be effective in enhancing repair in several other tendon injury models.[80-83] Current research is focused on optimizing the isolation and differentiation of stem cells into the tendon phenotype. In the future, it is likely that cells derived from the patient's own bone marrow, fat, skin, or muscle will be used to augment tendon repair and to populate engineered

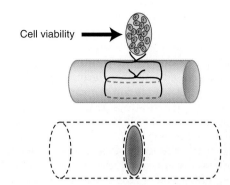

Figure 34-3 Conceptual model of stem cell patch to augment tendon repair.

tendon graft substitutes (Fig. 34-3). My colleagues and I are pursuing one such option in our laboratory now: a decellularized flexor digitorum profundus tendon allograft, reconstituted with stem cells from the patient's own tissues and lubricated with an engineered surface containing hyaluronic acid (HA) (Fig. 34-4) and lubricin.[84-87] Such a graft could be used to bridge flexor tendon defects and, finally, to replace like with like.

Tendon Lubrication: Hyaluronic Acid and Lubricin

In addition to collagen and structural proteoglycans, such as decorin, the tendon ECM also contains important lubricants for efficient flexor tendon motion (see Fig. 34-1). The synovial cells of the flexor tendon sheath secrete HA into the ECM, which may serve as a surface lubricant.[88] HA, a

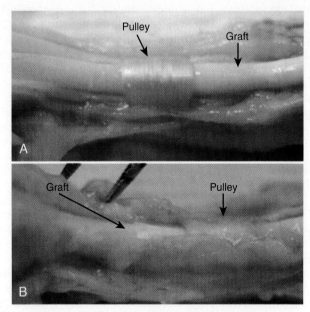

Figure 34-4 A, Graft treated with carbodiimide-derivatized hyaluronic acid at 6 weeks. Note marked reduction in adhesions. **B,** Tendon graft at 6 weeks. Note extensive adhesions. (Reprinted, with permission, from Zhao C, Sun YL, Amadio PC, et al. Surface treatment of flexor tendon autograft with carbodiimide-derivatized hyaluronic acid. An in vivo canine model. *J Bone Joint Surg Am.* 2006;88:2187, Fig. 8.)

polysaccharide, is found in all vertebrate tissues and body fluids. Various physiologic functions have been assigned to HA, including lubrication, water homeostasis, filtering effects, and regulation of plasma protein distribution.[89] HA is found in increased amounts during the first week after tendon repair.[90] After a tendon is treated with a hyaluronidase solution, which destroys HA, the gliding resistance between the tendon and pulley increases significantly.[91] This suggests that HA on the surface of the flexor tendons may play a role in the surface lubrication of the tendon–pulley system. In vivo results have demonstrated that HA may inhibit the proliferation of rabbit synovial cells, thus preventing cell adhesion between the sheath and the tendon.[92,93]

Recent studies indicate that lubricin, a proteoglycan found in the superficial zone of articular cartilage, may play an important role in preventing cellular adhesions in addition to providing the lubrication necessary for normal joint function.[94-97] Lubricin was originally isolated from articular cartilage.[98] It has since been identified on the surface of tendons[97,99-101] and plays an important role in tendon lubrication.[85] However, lubricin also inhibits cellular adhesion and so has the undesirable effect of inhibiting tissue repair.[102]

The expression of lubricin is modulated by interleukin-1 (IL-1), tumor necrosis factor (TNF-α) and TGF-β.[97] Little else is known about the expression or regulation of lubricin within digital flexor tendons, but its modulation may have a profound effect on the restoration of the flexor surface and the prevention of adhesions after tendon injury and repair (Fig. 34-5) and perhaps as a coating on a tissue-engineered tendon graft or tendon graft substitute, as discussed later.

Engineering the Tendon Surface

The effect of HA on flexor tendon repair has been investigated in animal and clinical studies.[103-107] Exogenously applied HA may prevent adhesion formation between the flexor tendon and surrounding tissue following tendon repair without affecting tendon healing,[108-111] although in vivo results have been contradictory.[93,106,112] As the half-life of HA in tissue is short, native HA is probably eliminated too rapidly to maintain a long-lasting physical barrier between opposing tissues.[113] Moreover, abrasion during tendon gliding constantly threatens to physically remove HA from the tendon surface.[114] Therefore, extending HA half-life and strengthening HA binding ability on the tendon surface are important to enhancing the clinical effect of exogenously administered HA.

The carbodiimide derivatization, a chemical modification of HA, has been developed recently for clinical use.[115-117] This modification of HA decreases the water solubility of HA, increases its intermolecular binding strength, and therefore increases tissue residence time.[118] Clinical studies of a proprietary form of this derivatized HA (Seprafilm or Seprafilm II, Genzyme Corp, Cambridge, MA, or Hyaloglide; ACP gel, Fidia Advanced Biopolymers, Abano Terme, Italy), fabricated as a cross-linked sheet to be inserted as a barrier between opposing surfaces where adhesion is undesirable, have shown that it can reduce postsurgical adhesions in gynecologic and abdominal surgery.[118-121] A variation on this theme, by doing the cross-linking reaction in situ to fix the HA directly to the

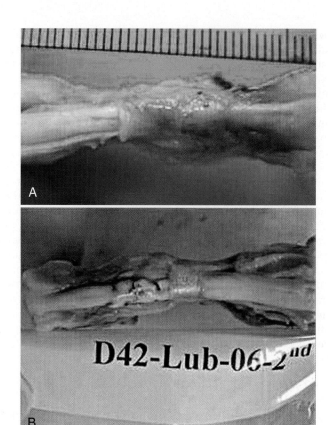

Figure 34-5 A, Tendon repair at 6 weeks. Note adhesions. **B,** Tendon repair treated with carbodiimide-derivatized lubricin, hyaluronic acid, and gelatin. Note marked reduction in adhesions.

tendon surface, using collagen as an intermediary (carbodiimide derivatized HA, or cd-HA), has had promising preliminary results in animal studies in vitro and in vivo.[122] The combination of HA and lubricin appears to have an additive effect.[85] Recent work has also shown, though, that although physicochemical and pharmacologic interventions can reduce adhesion formation, in both tendon grafts and tendon repairs,[122-124] there is a cost in terms of delayed or impaired tendon healing after tendon repair. Newer investigations are considering how to combine adhesion reduction and improved healing through the use of growth factors and stem cells.

Tendon Repair

Over the past 50 years, novel repair techniques have resulted in improved clinical outcomes following flexor tendon surgery.[125-129] The details of clinical tendon repair are covered in Chapter 35, but this chapter focuses on the effect of repair constructs on tendon healing and tendon kinematics.

Despite these advances in repair technique, adhesions continue to occur, and results can be less than adequate, particularly when the injury occurs in zone 2, the so called no-man's land, where the tendon resides within a fibro-osseous pulley system. Critical features related to tendon repair include a strong, minimally reactive repair that maintains strong tendon coaptation while permitting tendon gliding.[130-134] Two major problems continue to occur within the clinical setting: gapping with rupture at the repair site and adhesion formation within the flexor sheath.[70,135-137] Despite attempts at modifying rehabilitation, whether through increased levels of applied load or increased rates, tendon excursion methods have failed to increase early tendon core strength.[138-141]

Repair Biomechanics

The ideal tendon repair is strong, easy to perform, and does not interfere with either tendon healing or tendon gliding. Current methods are moderately strong and able to withstand the normal forces of light motion.[142-147] However, some of these constructs, especially those with multiple loops or knots on the anterior tendon surface,[133,148,149] also generate high-friction forces with movement and may abrade the pulley surface over time[150] (Fig. 34-6). Newer suture designs have incorporated features such as fewer surface loops, loops on the lateral rather than anterior tendon surfaces, and knots inside the repair rather than on the surface; all these features help reduce friction while having little effect on breaking strength.[151] Newer suture materials, such as FiberWire, a composite suture consisting of a monofilament polyethylene core surrounded by a braided polyester jacket (Arthrex, Naples FL), combine higher breaking strength, so that a smaller-diameter suture can be used, as well as providing low friction.[146,152]

The Effect of Friction on the Results of Tendon Repair

Animal studies over the past decade have shown convincingly that high-friction repairs result in abrasion of the tendon sheath (Fig. 34-7) and adhesion formation, even when factors such as rehabilitation method are optimized.[150,153,154] Thus, the goal should be to use a high-strength, low-friction repair construct and a low-friction suture material. Most recently I have been using 3-0 Ethibond and a modified Pennington design, but the recent data noted earlier on FiberWire is certainly intriguing.

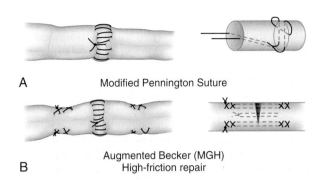

A   Modified Pennington Suture

B   Augmented Becker (MGH) High-friction repair

Figure 34-6 **A,** Modified Pennington suture. Low-friction, high-strength repair. [Modified, with permission, from Pennington DG. The locking loop tendon suture. *Plast Reconstr Surg.* 1979;63:(5)648-652; and Tanaka T, Amadio PC, Zhao C, et al. Gliding characteristics and gap formation for locking and grasping tendon repairs: A biomechanical study in a human cadaver model. *J Hand Surg Am.* 2004;29(1):6-14.]. **B,** Augmented Becker Massachusetts General Hospital high-friction, high-strength repair. [Reproduced, with permission, from Amadio PC. Friction of the gliding surface. Implications for tendon surgery and rehabilitation. *J Hand Ther.* 2005;18(2):115, Figure 4.]

Effect on Postoperative Management

Until the mid-1960s, most flexor tendon repairs were immobilized postoperatively for 3 weeks. This policy was based on the research of Mason and Allen,[155] who had shown that canine flexor tendon repairs decreased in tensile strength for 3 weeks postoperatively. Subsequent clinical work by Verdan,[156] Kleinert and Verdan,[157] and Duran and associates[158] showed that human flexor tendon repairs could be safely mobilized with a combination of active extension and passive flexion.

The use of early mobilization after tendon repair has resulted in improved outcomes.[4,156,158-161] In animal models,[153,162-167] earlier mobilization results in better final

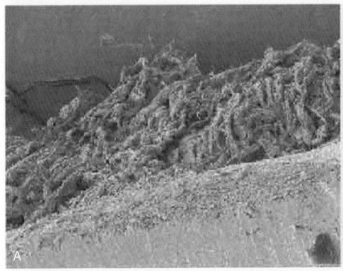
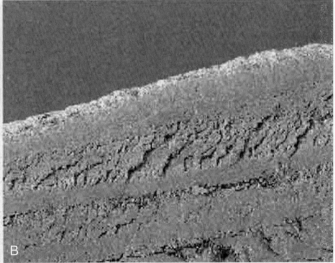

Figure 34-7 Scanning electron micrograph of tendon sheath in contact with **A,** high-friction Massachusetts General Hospital suture. **B,** Low-friction suture (modified Kessler technique). [Reproduced, with permission, from Zhao C, Amadio PC, Momose T, et al. Remodeling of the gliding surface after flexor tendon repair in a canine model in vivo. *J Orthop Res.* 2002;20(4):861, Fig. 6.]

tendon gliding and tensile strength. More recently, the fine details of mobilization have been studied, specifically the effect of timing[168-170] and the effect of differential motion of the wrist and finger joints on tendon loading and tendon gliding during the healing period.[153,171,172] Active motion protocols have also been used, although, interestingly, the clinical results are not reliably better than passive protocols.[5,125,173,174] Moreover, the addition of loading to motion in animal models has been shown to have little effect on the final result in terms of strength and motion.[166,172,175] Thus, the available evidence suggests that motion, not load, is the critical factor.

Of course, there must be some load on the tendon if it is going to move; at the very least, the load must be sufficient to overcome the forces of friction. It is for this reason that low-friction repairs are important—they minimize the load needed to initiate movement. Friction, though, is not the only concern. The force needed to overcome joint stiffness and to flex traumatized, edematous tissues must also be considered, as well as the weight of the distal digit itself; often these latter forces far outweigh the frictional ones in magnitude, especially in injured digits. So, the minimum force needed to load the tendon is a combination of the frictional force and the force needed to move the joints and soft tissues. This combination is often called the "work of flexion" of the unloaded digit.[169,176,177]

One might imagine that the maximum load that could be applied is the load that represents the breaking strength of the tendon, but that would be incorrect: long before the tendon breaks, it begins to gap, and gapping also increases friction, setting up a vicious cycle that can lead to later rupture. So, really, the upper bound is not breaking strength but the force needed to create a gap, which is usually much less.[161,178-187] The difference between the two forces—the unloaded work of flexion and the gapping force—represents the "safe zone" in which rehabilitation can occur[151] (Fig. 34-8). Early on, this safe zone is bounded by strictly mechanical parameters related to the anatomy and biomechanics of the repair. Over time, though, the effects of tendon healing are added in; the general effect is usually to gradually widen the safe zone, enabling the rational use of a graded resistance program as outlined by Groth.[188] The details of such programs are reviewed in Chapter 36.

Unfortunately, in some cases, early mobilization after tendon repair is not possible by any method. Common examples include situations with complex hand injury, in which motion might jeopardize bone, skin, nerve, or vascular integrity; patients who are uncooperative due to age or mental status; or situations where the tendon repair is deemed to be too tenuous to tolerate mobilization. In such cases, adhesions have been, up to now, inevitable. It is possible, though, that the application of a tissue-engineered, biocompatible adhesion barrier that is porous to nutrients might allow an immobilized tendon to heal without adhesions. We are currently pursuing research to address this issue, using cd-HA and lubricin, linked to collagen, as the proposed barrier, and hope to have an update in time for the next edition of this book!

Summary

In summary, considerable advances have been made in our understanding of tendon healing and both the biology and

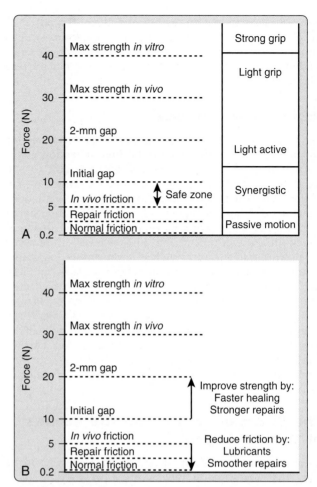

Figure 34-8 A, The "safe zone" concept [Reproduced, with permission, from Amadio PC. Friction of the gliding surface. Implications for tendon surgery and rehabilitation. *J Hand Ther.* 2005;18(2):115, Fig. 3.] **B,** Implications of tendon research on the safe zone.

biomechanics of tendon repair and reconstruction. The "safe zone" concept provides a good framework for thinking about the interaction among friction, repair strength, healing, and loading. Early motion, using the least load possible, is the key to better results, but early motion alone is usually not sufficient to prevent adhesions, without posing an undue risk of repair rupture. Thus, the ideal tendon repair of the future will probably need to include a combination of three features. There will always be a need for better, low-friction repair techniques. Lubricants bound to the tendon surface would further reduce friction, lower the loading requirements, and block adhesions. Cell and cytokine "patches" at the repair site can speed healing and allow a faster widening of the safe zone, which should result in fewer complications. This combination approach would appear to offer the best path toward the ultimate goal of predictable restoration of normal function after tendon injury.

REFERENCES

The complete reference list is available online at www.expertconsult.com.

CHAPTER
35

Primary Care of Flexor Tendon Injuries 📹

JOHN S. TARAS, MD, GREGG G. MARTYAK, MD, AND
PAMELA J. STEELMAN, CRNP, PT, CHT

ANATOMY	OPERATIVE TECHNIQUE
NUTRITION	TREATMENT OF ACUTE FLEXOR TENDON INJURIES
FLEXOR TENDON HEALING	REHABILITATION
ZONES OF INJURY	COMPLICATIONS
DIAGNOSIS	FUTURE
INDICATIONS AND CONTRAINDICATIONS	SUMMARY

CRITICAL POINTS

Surgical Timing

- For an injury less than 3 weeks old, nonemergent repair is indicated unless there is active purulent infection.
- An injury greater than 6 weeks old is a relative contraindication to attempt primary repair.

Pearls

- Multi-strand core suture technique with a running circumferential epitendinous suture is used
- A red rubber catheter should be ready if retrieval is required.
- The goal of repair and rehabilitation is a strong repair site that will not elongate beyond 3 mm with gentle active range-of-motion therapy designed to prevent adhesion formation.

Pitfalls

- Lacerations of the slips of the FDS require different suture techniques than do FDP lacerations.

Technical Points

- Enter sheath between distal A2 and proximal A4.
- Retrieve proximal stump: skin hooks, reverse Esmarch, Sourmelis, direct exposure.
- Deliver distal stump by passive DIP flexion
- Transfix tendons, once delivered through pulleys with 25-gauge needle.
- Use a minimum of a four-strand core suture (4-0 FiberWire) technique with a running 6-0 Prolene epitendinous suture (nonlocked, deep bites into tendon).

Postoperative Care

- Use graded active rehabilitation protocol under supervision of a qualified therapist.

Restoring digital function after flexor tendon injury continues to be one of the great challenges in hand surgery.[1-7] In recent years, important advancements in our understanding of tendon anatomy,[8,9] biomechanics,[10-12] nutrition,[13-18] adhesion formation,[19-23] and tendon repair techniques have led to enhanced results after flexor tendon repair. Despite the many gains, problems of stiffness, scarring, and functional impairment continue to frustrate the most experienced hand surgeons.

Anatomy

Appreciation of flexor tendon anatomy[10] as well as the flexor retinacular sheath[8,9,24-27] is critical to the surgeon's ability to deal with flexor tendon injuries. The flexor digitorum profundus (FDP) arises from the proximal volar and medial surfaces of the ulna, the interosseous membrane, and occasionally the proximal radius. Along with the flexor pollicis longus (FPL), the FDP forms the deep muscle layer in the flexor compartment of the proximal forearm. In the midforearm, the muscle belly separates into a radial bundle and an ulnar bundle. In the distal third of the forearm, the radial bundle forms the index finger profundus tendon, and the ulnar bundle forms the profundus tendon to the ulnar three digits. The profundus tendons pass through the carpal canal, occupying the floor of the tunnel.

After traversing the carpal canal, the profundus tendons diverge to the digits. The lumbrical muscles originate at this level. The profundus tendons enter the flexor sheath deep to the superficialis tendons at the level of the metacarpophalangeal (MCP) joint. At the midproximal phalanx level, the profundus tendon becomes more palmar as it passes through the bifurcating superficialis tendon. It continues distally to insert into the palmar base of the distal phalanx.

The anterior interosseous branch of the median nerve innervates the FDP to the index and occasionally the long finger. The ulnar nerve innervates the FDP to the ring and small fingers.

The flexor digitorum superficialis (FDS) originates from two separate heads. The humeroulnar head arises from the medial humeral epicondyle and the coronoid process of the ulna. The radial head arises from the proximal shaft at the radius. In the proximal forearm, it occupies the intermediate layer of the flexor compartment superficial to the flexor profundus. In the middle third of the forearm, four separate muscles are identified. Four distinct tendons are seen in the distal third of the forearm. Presence of the small finger superficialis varies and may be absent in 21% of patients.[28] At the carpal tunnel level, the long and ring finger superficialis tendons lie superficial and central to those of the index and small, which lie deeper and more peripheral.

At the level of the MCP joint, the superficialis tendon enters the flexor sheath palmar to the profundus tendon. At the proximal third of the proximal phalanx, the superficialis bifurcates around the profundus tendon. The two slips reunite deep to the profundus tendon at Camper's chiasm, with 50% of fibers decussating and 50% remaining ipsilateral. The superficialis tendon then inserts through the radial and ulnar slips onto the proximal metaphysis of the middle phalanx. The median nerve provides sole innervation of the superficialis muscle.

The FPL originates from the proximal radius and interosseous membrane. In the proximal third of the forearm, it lies radial to the digital flexors in the flexor compartment's deep layer. At the carpal tunnel level, the FPL lies on the radial floor. After traversing the carpal tunnel, it enters the palm by emerging between the adductor pollicis and the flexor pollicis brevis (FPB). The FPL is the only tendon that enters the thumb flexor sheath, and it inserts at the proximal palmar base of the distal phalanx. The anterior interosseous branch of the median nerve innervates the FPL.

The digital flexor sheath is a synovium-lined fibro-osseous tunnel. This system holds the flexor tendons in close opposition to the phalanges, ensuring efficient mechanical function in producing digital flexion. The flexor sheath is composed of synovial and retinacular tissue components, each with separate and distinct functions.[24] The synovial component of the sheath consists of a visceral, or epitenon, layer that envelops the flexor tendon and a parietal, or outer, layer that lines the walls of the flexor sheath. These two layers are contiguous at the ends of the sheath, creating a double-walled, hollow tube that surrounds the flexor tendons. In the index, long, and ring fingers, the membranous sheath begins at the MCP joint and ends at the distal phalanx. At the thumb and

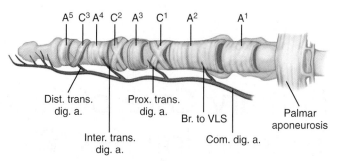

Figure 35-1 Flexor digital retinacular sheath and flexor tendon vascular supply. Br. to VLS; branch to the vinculum longus superficialis; Com. dig. a, common digital artery; Dist. trans. dig. a, distal transverse digital artery; Inter. trans. dig. a., interphalangeal transverse digital artery; Prox. trans. dig. a, proximal transverse digital artery.

small fingers, the synovial sheath continues proximally into the carpal tunnel as the radial and ulnar bursae, respectively.[8,25] The synovial sheath provides a low-friction gliding system and nutrition to the tendon.

The retinacular portion of the sheath is characterized by fibrous bands that overlie the synovial sheath in segmental fashion (Fig. 35-1).[8,9,26,27] Thickened transverse bands are termed *annular pulleys*, and thin flexible areas of criss-crossing fibers are termed *cruciate pulleys*. Stronger, broader annular pulleys provide mechanical stability to the system, ensuring optimal joint flexion for a given amount of tendon excursion. The more flexible cruciate pulleys permit flexibility to the system. The following pulleys have been identified: the palmar aponeurosis pulley, five annular pulleys, and three cruciate pulleys. The palmar aponeurosis pulley is formed from the transverse fibers[9,27] of the palmar aponeurosis. It is located at the beginning of the membranous sheath and is anchored on each side of the sheath by vertical septa that attach to the deep transverse metacarpal ligament. The first annular pulley (A1) arises from the volar plate of the MCP joint. The second annular pulley (A2) arises from the volar aspect of the proximal half of the proximal phalanx. The first cruciate pulley (C1) extends from the A2 pulley to the third annular pulley (A3), which arises from the volar plate of the proximal interphalangeal (PIP) joint. The fourth annular pulley (A4) arises from the middle phalanx and is connected proximally to the A3 pulley by the second cruciate pulley (C2). The fifth annular pulley (A5) arises from the volar plate of the distal interphalangeal (DIP) joint. It is connected proximally to the A4 pulley by the third cruciate pulley (C3). Not all of the elements of the flexor sheath can be identified as described, particularly A3 and A5, which can be indistinct or absent.

The pulley system of the thumb is distinct from that of the digits[25] (Fig. 35-2). One oblique and two annular pulleys have been identified. The first annular pulley of the thumb (A1) arises from the palmar plate of the MCP joint, and the second annular pulley (A2) arises from the palmar plate of the interphalangeal (IP) joint. The oblique pulley originates and inserts on the proximal phalanx in close association with the insertion of the adductor pollicis tendon.

Anatomic and clinical studies have demonstrated that the A2 and A4 pulleys are the most important components of the flexor sheath, their presence ensuring biomechanical efficiency of the system.[10,11,24] The A3 and the palmar

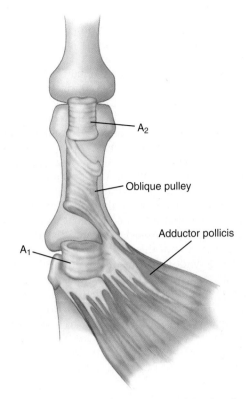

Figure 35-2 Flexor retinacular sheath of the thumb.

aponeurotic pulleys become important only when A2 and A4 have been damaged.[9,11,24,27] The loss of all or portions of the pulley system may lead to flexor bowstringing. This leads to an increased mechanical moment arm, which can create late flexion contractures. In addition, increased flexor tendon excursions are required to produce full digital flexion. In the thumb, the oblique pulley is the most important. Loss of the thumb oblique pulley results in decreased IP joint motion. Incompetence of both the A1 and oblique pulleys of the thumb leads to a 30% loss of IP joint motion.[25]

Flexor tendon excursion in the retinacular sheath zone in cadaveric specimens has been calculated.[29] DIP joint motion produces excursion of the FDP on the FDS of 1 mm for every 10 degrees of DIP flexion. PIP joint motion produces excursion of the FDS and the FDP together of 1.3 mm for every 10 degrees of PIP flexion relative to the retinacular sheath. Recently, postrepair clinical motion studies have demonstrated that this calculated excursion decreases.[30] DIP joint motion of 10 degrees produces excursion of the FDP of only 0.3 mm, and PIP motion of 10 degrees produces excursion of the FDP and superficialis of 1.2 mm. This may explain why DIP motion is often suboptimal after flexor tendon repair.

Nutrition

Flexor tendon nutrition appears to occur through both direct vascular supply[31-43] (see Fig. 35-1) and synovial diffusion.[16,17,27,44-50] Proximal to the digital sheath, a longitudinal

blood supply originates from within the proximal muscle tissue and is carried distally through the peritenon. Within the sheath, transverse branches of the digital arteries passing through the vincular system add segmental blood supply.[39] These branches include a proximal vessel to the vinculum longus superficialis, a proximal digital transverse artery, an IP transverse digital artery, and a distal transverse digital artery. As the transverse branches pass to the midline, they merge to carry palmarly into the tendons via the vincula. The vinculum profundus brevis is a short triangular pedicle supplying the profundus tendon near its insertion. A similar short vinculum supplies the superficialis tendon at the neck of the proximal phalanx, but here the vessels continue to form the vinculum longus to the profundus tendon. The superficialis receives additional blood supply from the vinculum longus superficialis at the base of the proximal phalanx. Both tendons receive additional blood supply from their distal osseous attachments. Throughout the sheath, vessels enter the tendon from the dorsal surface, with the palmar third remaining relatively avascular.[35] This anatomic fact has led to the surgical technique of palmar placement of sutures within the tendon to preserve blood supply. Finally, an avascular watershed zone of the FDP has been identified between the longitudinal and vincular vessels at the midproximal phalanx level.[34,35]

In addition to nourishment of the flexor tendons by vascular perfusion, experiments have demonstrated the importance of diffusional nutrition by the synovial fluid.[16,17,27,44-49] Radioisotope tracer studies suggest a greater role of diffusion than perfusion.[16,47] In addition, strong evidence has demonstrated that the superficial layers of isolated segments of tendon can heal in an isolated synovial environment without direct vascularity.[8,17,51] This finding has led some authors to recommend sheath repair to restore synovial fluid.[52-54] The relative significance of these dual nutritional pathways in the normal and repaired flexor tendon has yet to be completely clarified. Recent studies suggest that synovial diffusion associated with neovascularization of the healing site in the absence of ingrowth of peripheral vessels may play a role in the nourishment of the healing tendon.[13]

Flexor Tendon Healing

The subject of flexor tendon healing has traditionally been associated with controversy. Two theories have been proposed to help explain observed experimental phenomena. The first, the extrinsic healing theory, suggests that tendon healing occurs through cells extrinsic to the tendon through a fibroblastic response from surrounding tissue.[55-60] This theory presupposes the necessity of surrounding peritendinous adhesions to allow complete healing of the tendon; thus, immobilization after flexor tendon repair was encouraged. Experimental clinical evidence of adhesions at the repair site has supported this concept. The sequence of healing by extrinsic mechanism begins with an inflammatory phase from 48 to 72 hours, formation of collagen fibers from 4 to 21 days, and scar remodeling after 21 days.

The second theory, intrinsic healing, suggests that healing is possible in the absence of cells and tissue extrinsic to the tendon.[14,31,45,48,61-70] More recent experimental and clinical evidence to support this concept includes rounded ends of unrepaired tendons, tendon healing in the absence of adhesions, and in vitro healing of tendons in isolated, cell-free environments. Controlled mobilization of repaired tendons to allow healing but preventing peritendinous adhesions was the stated advantage of this healing theory. The sequence of intrinsic healing begins with the inflammatory phase, from 0 to 3 days after injury or repair with proliferation and thickening of epitenon cell layers. At 5 to 7 days, collagen formation and early vascular ingrowth ensue. A fibrous callus becomes visible by 10 days, and proliferation ingrowth of endotenon tenocytes occurs at 2 to 3 weeks.

Although the function of each type of tendon healing continues to require clarification, in the clinical situation, tendons probably heal by a combination of extrinsic and intrinsic cellular activity.[20,62,71] Theoretically, the more intrinsic healing occurs, the fewer peritendinous adhesions form. This concept forms the basis of controlled mobilization programs after tendon repair.

Zones of Injury

One must consider the level of injury when performing flexor tendon repair. Five anatomic zones of injury have been identified based on Verdan's original description of the flexor tendon system[7,72-75] (Fig. 35-3). The level of injury should be recorded in relation to the position of tendon laceration in the sheath, with the finger in the extended position.

Zone I extends from the insertion of the FDS at the middle phalanx to that of the FDP at the distal phalanx. Injuries in this level may involve lacerations or avulsions of the FDP. Zone II involves that region in which both the FDS and FDP travel within the flexor sheath from the A1 pulley to the

insertion of the FDS. This zone was termed "no man's land" by Bunnell because of the poor prognosis associated with treatment of flexor tendon injuries at this level.[1] A more descriptive term may be "some man's land" because the more experienced hand surgeon can obtain satisfactory results with appropriate care. Zone III comprises the area between the distal border of the carpal tunnel and the A1 pulley of the flexor sheath. In addition to the common digital nerves, vessels, and both flexor tendons, the lumbrical muscles reside in this zone. Zone IV consists of that segment of flexor tendons covered by the transverse carpal ligament within the carpal tunnel. Injuries concomitant to the median and ulnar nerves may be associated with flexor tendon injuries in this zone. Zone V extends from the flexor musculotendinous junction in the forearm to the proximal border of the transverse carpal ligament. Associated neurovascular injuries may compromise results in this region as well.

The flexor tendon system in the thumb is predicated on only one flexor tendon. Zone I is at the insertion area of the FPL. Zone II coincides with the flexor retinaculum of the thumb, from the neck of the metacarpal to the neck of the proximal phalanx. Zone III is the area of the thenar muscles. Zone IV represents the area of the carpal canal. Finally, zone V is the anatomic area from the musculotendinous junction of the FPL to the transverse carpal ligament.

Diagnosis

Knowledge of flexor tendon anatomy is necessary for diagnosing acute injury accurately. In the cooperative patient, diagnosis is usually not difficult. Because of the common muscle origin of the flexor profundi, FDS function can be assessed only by restraining the profundi by completely extending the other digits. An independently functioning superficialis is demonstrated by full flexion of the PIP joint of the affected finger. This test often is not applicable to the index finger because of the independent muscle belly of the FDP. The FDS to the index finger can be demonstrated through pulp-to-pulp pinch with the thumb and index finger.

Demonstration of index finger PIP joint flexion with the DIP joint fully extended or hyperextended confirms superficialis function to the index finger. As noted earlier, the presence of small-finger FDS varies and can be absent in 21% of patients.[28] FDP function is demonstrated by means of active flexion of the DIP. Active flexion of the thumb IP joint indicates an intact FPL. If, when performing these tests, the patient demonstrates motion but experiences pain, the surgeon must entertain the possibility of partial flexor tendon injury.

In the uncooperative or unconscious patient or a child, additional diagnostic signs may be helpful. In the normal hand, a cascade of flexion of the digits is noted, increasing as one proceeds from the index to the small fingers. Abnormal posture or change in the normal cascade can indicate flexor tendon injury (Fig. 35-4). In addition, squeezing the forearm musculature to demonstrate flexion of the digits may be helpful. Finally, assessing tenodesis of flexor tendons with the wrist in extension demonstrates loss of finger flexion if flexor tendons are severed.

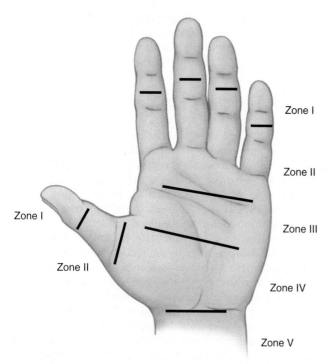

Zone I

Zone I

Zone II

Zone II

Zone III

Zone IV

Zone V

Figure 35-3 Zone classification of flexor tendon injuries.

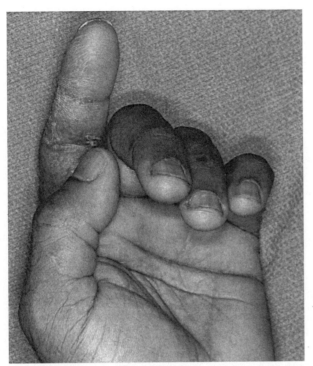

Figure 35-4 Laceration of the index finger. Posture of the index finger in extension suggests complete laceration of the flexor digitorum profundus and superficialis.

The examiner is responsible for determining that the flexor tendons are intact before discharging the patient. If the examiner is uncertain, exploration of the wound under operating room conditions may be required. The actual level of tendon laceration depends on the position of the fingers when the injury occurred. If the injury occurred with the finger in extension, the skin wound and both tendons will be lacerated at the same level. In fingers injured in flexion, the tendon injury will be distal to the skin wound. In addition, the FDP will be lacerated at a level different from that of the superficialis tendon because of their different excursions.

Indications and Contraindications

There has been controversy in the past over the efficacy of primary repair of flexor tendons, particularly in zone II,[1,2,68,76] yet immediate or delayed primary repair is currently advocated for flexor tendon injuries with few exceptions.[3-7,77-90] The advantages of primary repair over secondary grafting include less extensive surgery, decreased periods of disability, and restoration of normal tendon length.[74]

Specific contraindications to immediate or delayed primary repair include severe contamination where infection is a possibility.[3,5,85,87-89] In addition, loss of palmar skin overlying the flexor system generally precludes tendon repair,[3,5] although there have been some recent reports of concomitant tendon repair and soft tissue coverage procedures.[91] Another contraindication to primary repair is extensive damage to the flexor retinaculum, where pulley reconstruction and one- or two-stage tendon reconstruction probably is required.[92]

Concurrent fracture or neurovascular injury, however, does not necessarily contraindicate tendon repair. If fracture stabilization can be obtained, then flexor tendon repair generally should ensue.

Researchers have effectively demonstrated that repair of both the FDP and the FDS rather than the FDP alone, even in zone II injury, provides the best result.[7,75,77,78,93] The advantages of repairing and maintaining the FDS include maintenance of vincular blood supply to the FDP, retaining of a smooth gliding surface for the FDP, independent motion of the digit with stronger flexion power, and decreased possibility of hyperextension deformities of the PIP joint.

Schneider and colleagues[94] demonstrated that tendon repairs delayed as long as 3 weeks after injury exhibited outcomes similar to those of tendons repaired more immediately. Although not statistically significant, repairs performed within the first 10 days after injury tended to be superior. Recent animal studies also have supported improved tendon excursion with early repairs.[95] These studies demonstrate that, although tendon repair is not emergent, repair within the first few days after injury appears warranted.

Operative Technique

General Considerations

Flexor tendon repair is ideally performed by trained surgeons who know the anatomy of the flexor tendon system and the potential pitfalls of surgical repair. Repair is generally accomplished under regional or general anesthesia in a bloodless field. Traditionally, a tourniquet has been used. Recently, Lalonde and coworkers reported using elective injection of lidocaine with epinephrine into the operative field in the office setting. This "wide awake" technique creates a relatively bloodless field, without the need for a tourniquet, allowing use of local anesthetic only. They report the risk of digital infarction is remote, with the benefit of observing the repair with the patient's active movement.[96] Despite the appeal of performing surgery in the office, I have no experience with this technique.

The use of 2- to 4-power loupe magnification decreases inadvertent nerve or vessel injury. Lateral or palmar zigzag (Bruner's) incisions are performed, depending on the surgeon's preference. The Bruner incision, our preferred approach, offers excellent exposure but can cause scarring over the palmar surface of the digit.[97,98] The midlateral incision is technically more demanding and may interfere with transverse digital branches supplying the vincula but has the advantage of decreased scarring over the flexor surface, which can lead to improved rehabilitation.[78] Delicate use of instrumentation is required; pinching or crushing of the flexor tendon or sheath inevitably leads to suboptimal results.[1,2] We generally prefer to handle the tendon at its cut end only, avoiding grasping of the epitenon, which can create later epitendinous adhesions. Minimal debridement of tendon ends is not usually required but may be performed if necessary using a knife or nerve-cutting instrument. Many suture techniques have been described.[99-105] Traditionally, many surgeons have preferred a modified Kessler grasping-type

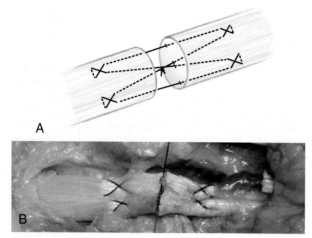

Figure 35-5 Preferred suture technique used in flexor tendon repairs first described by Seiler.

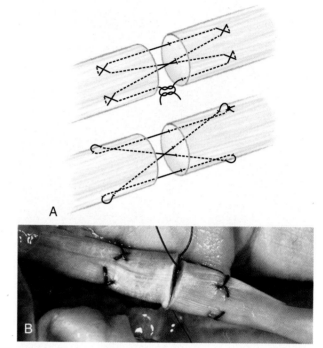

Figure 35-6 Four-stranded cruciate and locked cruciate repairs popularized by Wolfe.

two-strand core stitch based on the studies by Urbaniak and others.[106-108] Although 3-0 or 4-0 braided synthetic material placed in the volar third of the tendon has been the most popular core suture material, I prefer the more recently developed 4-0 FiberWire (Arthrex, Naples, FL) because it is stronger than braided synthetic suture of the same caliber and not too bulky when knotted. Most authors currently recommend a four-strand core repair, crossing the repair site with epitendinous suture augmentation to afford sufficient strength to support a program of early active motion rehabilitation. A variety of multistrand core suture designs have been described, ranging from four to eight strands crossing the repair site. My preferred technique uses a single suture to create a four-strand repair as first described by Seiler (Fig. 35-5). A four-strand cruciate flexor repair has been described by McLarney and colleagues[109] and is similar to my preferred suture technique (Fig. 35-6). Taras found that increasing suture caliber significantly increased the load to failure of core suture techniques. With 5-0 or 4-0 suture, the method of failure was suture rupture. With 3-0 and 2-0 suture, the failure was caused by suture pullout, clearly showing that repair technique with the modified Bunnell and double-grasping suture techniques securing the ends better than the modified Kessler technique.[110] Recent studies have demonstrated that epitendinous suture significantly increases the repair strength.[104,111-114] The epitendinous technique described by Silfverskiöld (Fig 35-7), employing a cross stitch has shown excellent results in reducing gapping by 10% to 50% at the repair site.[115] The superficialis tendon is preferably repaired with a four-strand core suture depending on the size of the tendon and the location of the laceration. A recent study by Tran and associates found that in vitro a four-strand Tajima technique with a Silfverskiöld epitendinous cross stitch was superior to a four-strand Tajima core suture with running locking epitendinous technique and capable of handling the rigors of an early active rehabilitation protocol.[116]

Several techniques are available to atraumatically retrieve retracted tendon ends. With the wrist and MCP joints placed in maximal flexion, flexor muscle bellies can be milked manually to deliver the tendon ends. If this fails, alternatives are available. If a tendon end is visible in the flexor sheath, one may use a skin hook. The hooked end is slid along the surface of the sheath until it has passed the tendons, and the hook is then turned toward the tendons, engaging the most superficial one. As the instrument is pulled distally, the tendons follow. The tendons then can be held in position by a Keith or 25-gauge hypodermic needle placed through the skin and A2 pulley area for later repair.

Another common retrieval technique uses a red rubber urologic catheter, pediatric feeding tube, Hunter rod, or IV tubing, which is passed distal to proximal alongside the flexor tendons, which are left in situ. The catheter is sutured to both tendons 2 cm proximal to the A1 pulley through a second palmar incision. The catheter is advanced distally to deliver tendon ends into the repair site. A 25-gauge hypodermic needle is passed transversely through the skin and A2 pulley to maintain tendon position. Core sutures are then placed. The catheter tendon suture is then cut in the palm and withdrawn.[117]

Another often-used technique uses a catheter that is passed from distal to proximal through the flexor sheath. A stitch is placed into the tendon end, and the other end of the suture is placed into the end of the catheter. The catheter and suture, followed by the tendons, are pulled distally through the flexor sheath. Further retraction of tendons is prevented again by transfixing them to the skin and A2 pulley with a 25-gauge hypodermic needle.

For all of these techniques, the anatomic relationship of the profundus to the superficialis tendons must be maintained.[53] One anatomic point that can aid the surgeon in maintaining this orientation and preventing tendon twisting is the fact that the vincula insert on the dorsal surface of the tendons.

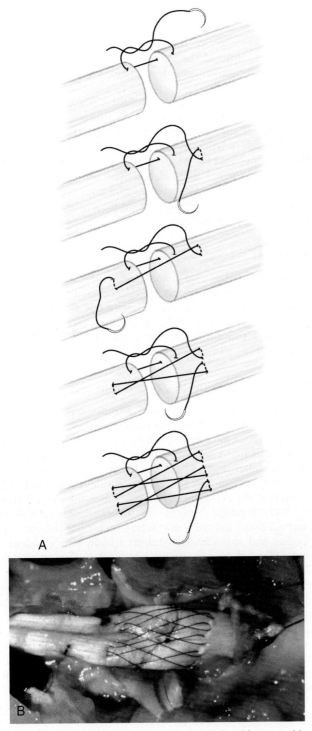

Figure 35-7 Silfverskiöld epitendinous cross stitch adds a surprising amount of strength to repair.

Every attempt is made to preserve all pulleys of the flexor retinacular sheath. Small surgical windows into the sheath often are required to identify tendon ends. Whether the sheath should be subsequently repaired is controversial.[19,23,31,41,54,118-120] Theoretical support for repair includes tendon gliding and nutrition. To date, no clinical studies have documented superiority of repair versus resection of the sheath.[31,54] In addition, one prospective study comparing the two techniques demonstrated no superiority of sheath repair.[119] Currently, we favor sheath repair when possible using 6-0 or 7-0 monofilament suture if there has been minimal loss of sheath substance and the repair can be performed easily without constriction of the sheath or the tendon repair.

Recently, a stainless steel device, TenoFix (Ortheon Medical, Columbus, OH) has been introduced for zone II flexor tendon repair. The authors reported similar results to a four-stranded core repair; however, smaller profundus tendons were unable to accommodate the device.[121]

Treatment of Acute Flexor Tendon Injuries

Zone I

In zone I, distal to the FDS insertion, only the FDP tendon is injured. The patient maintains PIP joint flexion but loses DIP flexion. Although adequate finger function can be maintained without repair in some circumstances, early direct repair is desirable. This is particularly true as one proceeds from the radial (precision grip) to the ulnar (power grip) side of the hand. In addition, the small finger superficialis is absent in a significant percentage of individuals, necessitating repair of the lacerated FDP tendon in that digit. With early repair, digital function can be near normal.

If more than 4 weeks have elapsed since the injury, direct repair usually cannot be performed due to FDP muscle contracture and degeneration of the lacerated ends of the tendon. Another pitfall in zone I is injury to the normally functioning FDS caused by excessive surgical manipulation. Finally, the surgeon must not advance the profundus tendon more than 1 cm at this level of injury to accomplish repair.[122] This leads, particularly in the ulnar three digits, to unacceptable flexion contractures of the affected digit as well as incomplete flexion of the neighboring digits—a condition termed *quadrigia syndrome*.[73]

Three patterns of laceration occur in zone I. The first occurs when the short vincula of the FDP remain intact. Although this pattern is rare, the FDP remains just proximal to its insertion. Direct repairs can be performed late with this pattern of injury. The second pattern presents with the long vincula of the FDP intact. The severed end of the tendon lies at the FDS decussation. The prognosis for early repair is good. The third laceration pattern occurs when the FDP retracts into the palm, rupturing both vincula and resulting in loss of vincular blood supply. This type of repair requires more extensive surgical dissection and early repair. When this pattern of injury is diagnosed late, alternative treatments such as observation, tendon graft, DIP tenodesis, and arthrodesis must be entertained.

Surgical Technique in Zone I Injuries

A volar zigzag incision from the PIP joint crease to distal to the DIP joint is utilized. Every effort is made to preserve the A4 pulley. If only a short distal stump of FDP remains, opening the tendon sheath at the C3-A5 pulley level may be required. If the proximal FDP stump has retracted to the level of the PIP joint, a window at the C2 pulley may be fashioned

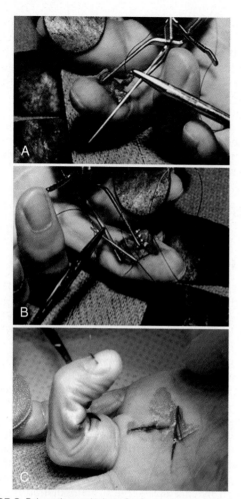

Figure 35-8 Reinsertion technique for flexor digitorum profundus avulsion at distal phalanx in zone I injury.

to retrieve it. If the proximal profundus has retracted to the level of the palm, the zigzag incision may be extended proximally, or a separate transverse incision in the palm proximal to the A1 pulley may be required. Retracted proximal FDP tendon ends are retrieved atraumatically as described previously. If the injury is recent, the FDP may be passed through the FDS decussation. In older lacerations, one slip of the superficialis may be sacrificed to facilitate passage of the FDP through a tight flexor sheath. Under no circumstances should a normal FDS be completely excised to repair the FDP.

Every effort is made to repair to the distal tendon stump to avoid overadvancement. As previously discussed, the FDP is not advanced more than 1 cm to permit repair. If the repair catches at the end of the A4 pulley, a small portion of the sheath may be vented.

If the distal stump is extremely short or nonexistent, the tendon must be repaired to the distal phalanx (Fig. 35-8). One develops a periosteal flap at the base of the distal phalanx, carefully avoiding the palmar plate of the DIP joint. The cortex is prepared with a curette to provide a bleeding bone surface that will encourage tendon-to-bone healing. A synthetic monofilament suture, such as 2-0 Prolene, is inserted into the tendon in "unlocked" fashion to facilitate later removal. The ends of the suture are threaded onto a Keith needle. Regardless of whether a short FDP stump is present,

I fasten the sutures using an "around-the-bone" technique. With the use of a needle holder, the Keith needles are passed around both sides of the distal phalanx to emerge through the middle third of the nail plate. Effort should be made to avoid the germinal nail matrix; the ideal point of exit through the nail plate should be 3 to 4 mm distal to the lunula and approximately 2 mm from the midline. The Keith needles are withdrawn, and the sutures are tied directly over the nail. The pullout suture is removed 6 weeks after initial repair. Alternatively, a bone anchor is reported to have been used at the distal phalanx level for this injury. The length of the bone anchor must avoid the nail bed. The use of a bone anchor technique has been reported to make no significant difference in outcome versus pullout suture technique without the morbidity of this method.[123]

Zone II

Classically termed "no man's land," injuries at zone II are associated with the greatest technical difficulties in obtaining maximal function. Atraumatic technique is nowhere more important than in zone II, where both flexor tendons are confined within the flexor retinacular sheath. Early repair of both the FDP and FDS is indicated when wound conditions permit.

Surgical Technique in Zone II Injuries

Preferred Technique. The area is exposed with a volar zigzag or midlateral incision incorporating the laceration. One identifies the flexor sheath, carefully protecting the neurovascular bundles. If nerve injury is identified, the nerve is prepared for repair after repair of the flexor tendons. Every effort must be made to maintain the annular pulleys, especially some portion of the A2 and A4 pulleys. If possible, repair should be made through windows in the cruciate–synovial areas through small lateral or transverse incisions. The distal profundus and superficialis tendons usually can be identified and delivered into the wound by acutely flexing the digit. The proximal tendons are atraumatically identified and delivered into the wound by one of the methods previously described. When retrieving the proximal tendons, one should maintain the superficialis and profundus tendons together so as not to interrupt their vascular connections. In zone II, the surgeon must understand the spiral nature of the FDS as it bifurcates around the profundus to reinsert on the middle phalanx at Camper's chiasm. If the superficialis is lacerated after its bifurcation, proximal and distal ends can rotate 180 degrees in different directions. If this anatomic orientation is not corrected, then profundus tendon excursion can be less than optimal.

After the tendons are delivered into the wound, a Keith or 25-gauge hypodermic needle is placed across the skin and annular pulley to maintain tendon position. A 3-0 or 4-0 core suture is placed in a four-strand single-cross grasp as described by Seiler and Noguchi et al.[124] Although traditionally the suture has been placed volarly in the tendon to avoid the blood supply, recent studies show some biomechanical benefit to dorsal placement.[125,126] The core suture is then tied with the tension being removed from the repair by flexing the distal joint of the digit. Then a 6-0 Prolene suture is placed in an epitendinous cross-stitch fashion as described by Silfverskiöld. "If the superficialis is lacerated distal to its birfurcation, two-strand locking sutures in each limb usually suffice. If the superficialis is lacerated proximal to the bifurcation, I prefer a four-strand core suture. Every attempt should be made to repair the superficialis tendons. However, if the superficialis tendon is too bulky to glide under the A2 pulley, we recommend resection of one slip of the superficialis tendon rather than resecting the A2 pulley." The flexor retinaculum is repaired with 6-0 or 7-0 Prolene if possible. If this cannot be achieved and a bulky repair is snagging on a pulley, a portion of the pulley should be vented with a lateral release to allow unimpaired motion after surgery. Finally, at the proximal level of the flexor sheath, one may consider converting a zone II to a zone III injury by excising the A1 pulley. This is particularly appropriate if a bulky repair is performed at the A1 pulley level. If pulleys require reconstruction, we currently favor staged tendon reconstruction at this level.

Zone III

Injuries in zone III carry a good prognosis because zone III is located out of the fibro-osseous sheath and is therefore less prone to adhesion formation. Injuries to the common digital nerves may accompany the tendon injury. Both superficialis and profundus tendons should be repaired. Delayed primary repair can be performed up to 3 weeks or more after injury because the proximal end of the profundus tendon is held by the lumbrical origin.

Surgical Technique in Zone III Injuries

The zigzag approach to the palm is used for surgical repairs in zone III. Excision of local palmar fascia may be necessary for exposure. Careful protection of associated neurovascular structures is essential. Repair of both tendons with 3-0 or 4-0 core suture and a 6-0 epitendinous Prolene suture is standard.

Zone IV

Flexor tendon injuries in zone IV (within the carpal tunnel) are less common because of the anatomic protection of the medial and lateral bony pillars as well as the stout transverse carpal ligament. Injuries to the median and ulnar nerves, ulnar artery, and superficial palmar arch are often associated because of their proximity to the flexor tendons. If possible, repair of all tendons should be undertaken. If swelling precludes repair of all tendons, the superficialis to the small finger can be excised. If anatomic confines preclude even further repair, all the superficialis tendons can be excised as necessary. Delayed primary repair should be performed within 3 weeks of injury because myostatic contraction prevents repair after this.

Surgical Technique in Zone IV Injuries

Zone IV injury is approached through a volar zigzag incision, incorporating a carpal tunnel–type incision. One may consider a Z-plasty lengthening of the transverse carpal ligament for later repair, although some authors have not found

bowstringing to be a problem if an appropriate postoperative orthosis is used with the wrist in neutral position.[78] If the motor branch of the ulnar nerve is lacerated, one should consider repairing it first because it is the deepest structure requiring repair in the wound. All zone IV flexor tendons are repaired with four strands of 4-0 FiberWire core suture. Frequently, swollen or hemorrhagic synovium must be resected to allow repair. Closing the transverse carpal ligament without Z-plasty lengthening is not wise because it may constrict the median nerve. After surgery, a controlled mobilization program with the wrist near neutral position and the MCP joints flexed to 70 degrees is maintained to prevent bowstringing and avoid placing stress on nerve repairs.

Zone V

Deep forearm lacerations proximal to the transverse carpal ligament typically involve multiple structures, including tendons, median and ulnar nerves, and the radial and ulnar arteries. Primary repair of all structures is recommended. Return of satisfactory motion is the rule in this zone, but it may take several months.

Surgical Technique in Zone V Injuries

A zigzag or curvilinear skin incision is used to expose the injured structures. Depending on the level of laceration, a carpal tunnel release may be performed. A four-strand core repair with 4-0 FiberWire or 3-0 Ethibond is favored based on the caliber of the tendons at this level. A surgical caveat in this zone applies; if multiple tendons and nerves are lacerated, it is prudent to identify and tag structures as one progresses from superficial to deep. This organization averts the mistake of mismatching proximal and distal tendon ends, because the proximal tendon ends can lose their normal anatomic alignment as the dissection is performed. Circumferential epitendinous suture can be performed if time permits, although it is not necessary if multiple tendons require repair during a long procedure.

Flexor Pollicis Longus

The anatomic differences between the FPL and the digital tendons and sheath have been described. The FPL spans only two digital joints and travels alone in its flexor sheath. These factors may explain improved results in FPL repair.[127-129] The FPL has only one vinculum and no associated lumbrical muscles; therefore, FPL lacerations in zones I and II are more likely to retract proximally to the palm or wrist level. Direct repair of the FPL is recommended at all levels as wound conditions permit if no more than 3 or 4 weeks have elapsed since the injury.

Surgical Technique for Flexor Pollicis Longus

Lacerations in zones I and II of the FPL are approached in a volar zigzag incision. The flexor sheath is identified, and windows are made for identification of the tendon ends as required. The A1 or oblique pulley must be maintained to prevent late bowstringing.

If the tendon is lacerated at its insertion, a pullout suture to the distal phalanx, as previously described, is used. More proximally in the thumb, if the proximal tendon end is easily identified, it is usually still being held by an intact vinculum. If the proximal tendon is not identified in the thumb, it is retracted into the palm or wrist. We prefer not to explore the carpal tunnel or thenar eminence to retrieve the proximal end for risk of damaging sensory or motor branches of the thumb; rather, a separate transverse or curvilinear incision in the distal forearm is used to identify the proximal tendon. Passing a tube or catheter from the distal incision to the proximal one, using one of the techniques described earlier, can atraumatically retrieve the tendon. Standard end-to-end repair is accomplished with an additional epitendon suture.

Partial Flexor Tendon Lacerations

The treatment of partial flexor tendon lacerations is controversial.[130-139] Early experimental studies demonstrated that if more than 60% of a tendon is transected, rupture is likely under applied stress.[133] Other reported complications of untreated partial flexor tendon lacerations include triggering, rupture, and entrapment.[131,134] On the other hand, several researchers have noted that placement of core sutures into a largely intact tendon weakens the tendon, increasing the likelihood of tendon rupture.[136,138] More recently, researchers have demonstrated that early protected mobilization after partial tendon laceration demonstrated improved tensile strengths. In addition, they recommended repair of partial flexor tendon lacerations when more than 60% of the width of the tendon is lacerated.[140-142]

Surgical Technique for Partial Flexor Tendon Lacerations

A volar zigzag approach is used to expose tendon injury, and the partial laceration is assessed. It has been our practice, based on the available data, to repair partial lacerations greater than 60% of the tendon's substance with a modified Kessler core suture followed by an epitendinous 6-0 suture. Lacerations of 25% to 60% of the tendon are repaired with a 6-0 running epitendinous suture. Partial lacerations of less than 25% of the tendon's diameter are treated by minimal handling of the tendon and beveling of sharp edges to prevent catching. A dynamic controlled mobilization program is used postoperatively.

Closed Rupture of the Flexor Digitorum Profundus Tendon

Rupture of the FDP is caused by forced extension at the DIP joint while the profundus muscle is maximally contracting. The injury commonly occurs in football or rugby players as they grab an opponent's jersey. The patient describes pain and swelling over the area of distal avulsion. Because the superficialis still provides function to the PIP joint, the injury is often missed, losing the opportunity for early repair. Radiographs should always be obtained because, occasionally, a fragment of distal bone is also avulsed, which can localize the profundus tendon end.

Although any digit, including the thumb, has been reported to be involved, this injury most often involves the ring finger. Several theories have been advanced to explain the propensity for ring finger involvement, including a lack of independent extension of the ring finger because of its junctura tendinae and another demonstrating that the ring finger has the weakest profundus insertion.[143]

Avulsion of the profundus tendon has been classified by Leddy[78] and Leddy and Packer[144] into three main types. In type I, the tendon retracts into the palm, where a substantial blood supply is lost because of vincular rupture. Tendon repair must be performed early, within 7 to 10 days, before it becomes contracted. In type II avulsions, the tendon retracts to the PIP joint. The vincula are intact, and some synovial nutrition remains. Although early repair is recommended, repair up to 3 months after injury can result in satisfactory results. Type III injuries involve a large bone fragment. The A4 pulley prevents retraction of the tendon. Early reinsertion or, with large fragments, open reduction and internal fixation (ORIF) provide satisfactory results. Finally, type IIIA injuries describe a simultaneous avulsion of the profundus tendon and a fracture fragment distally.[78,145,146] This injury requires ORIF of the bony fragment and reinsertion of the avulsed tendon.

If a case of flexor profundus avulsion is missed and left untreated beyond the period of repair, options for treatment include observation, tendon grafting, a DIP joint tenodesis, or arthrodesis.[78]

Surgical Technique for Closed Rupture of Flexor Digitorum Profundus Tendon

A palmar zigzag or midlateral incision is used, exposing the flexor sheath just proximal to the PIP joint to the insertion of the profundus tendon. For a type I injury, a transverse window is made just distal to the A2 pulley. If the tendon is not seen, it has retracted into the palm, and an additional incision is required in the palm proximal to the A1 pulley. The proximal tendon is atraumatically passed through the sheath and the superficialis decussation by one of the methods described previously. It is then reinserted to the distal phalanx with 3-0 nonlocking Prolene suture tied over a button on the nail plate distal to the germinal matrix. For type II injuries, the tendon end is noted at the incision just distal to the A2 pulley, held by its vincula. No palmar incision is required. The tendon is reinserted distally as described. For type III or type IIIA incisions, the bony fragment is noted just distal to the A4 pulley. A transverse sheath incision distal to the A2 pulley is not required. ORIF of the bony fragment usually provides satisfactory results. In the case of a IIIA injury, after ORIF of the bone fragment, the distal tendon is reinserted as described previously.

Rehabilitation

Adhesion is the most common complication of flexor tendon repair. The techniques employed in postoperative orthosis use and tendon rehabilitation contribute significantly to the functional outcome of flexor tendon repair. Historically, flexor tendon rehabilitation programs have evolved from postoperative protective orthotic immobilization to protect the repair and promote healing to controlled tendon activity to restore tendon tensile strength and promote tendon gliding. The reader is referred to Chapter 36 for a comprehensive discussion of postoperative tendon management.

It is currently generally accepted that a flexor tendon rehabilitation regimen depends on the strength of the surgical repair. Therapists are encouraged to contact the treating surgeon and obtain surgical reports, whenever possible, so that a tendon rehabilitation program formulated on the specific strength of the tendon repair can be instituted. In all cases, orthosis use and therapy should begin as early in the postoperative period as possible. The therapist should bear in mind that edema greatly increases the stress placed on the repaired tendon through movement and that premorbid conditions such as diabetes can alter individual tolerances for force placed on the postoperative tendon. If the repair technique is unknown to the therapist, it is advisable to institute a traditional protected range of motion (ROM) tendon program.

Preferred Therapy Regimen

Recently, we moved to the use of the pyramid model of tendon rehabilitation described by Groth[147] and Steelman and coworkers[148] for our patient population. No timelines are used to introduce activity according to this program. Instead, this program requires assessment of tissue response during each therapy session so that the patient can progress through the program as tissue response warrants. The program begins at postoperative day two or three. The patient is fitted with an orthosis like that described for the two previous flexor tendon rehabilitation programs discussed earlier. Therapy interventions begin at the base of the pyramid and progress upward to the apex. The major tissue response utilized to determine when the patient can progress through the steps of the pyramid is an active joint lag, which is defined as passive joint ROM that exceeds active joint ROM. When the ROM lag does not respond to treatment, the patient progresses up the pyramid (Fig. 35-9), one step per treatment session, until the desired treatment effect is achieved. When adverse reactions such as swelling or inflammation occur, the patient is backed down the pyramid accordingly. Patients demonstrating no active lag and acceptable ROM may be discharged, never progressing past active composite fisting. Conversely, a patient with significant scar adhesion may progress up the pyramid to isolated joint motion within a few treatment sessions. We have had excellent outcomes and few adverse reactions in our flexor tendon repair population using the pyramid model. It is an excellent tool to guide clinical decision making in flexor tendon rehabilitation for the experienced hand therapist.

Complications

Despite the use of stronger suture repair techniques and the application of early controlled mobilization, adhesion formation remains the most common complication after flexor tendon surgery. Surgical tenolysis is the preferred treatment if an appropriate period of therapy (3–6 months) has failed to restore tendon gliding.[71,149,150]

Tendon rupture after primary repair is uncommon. Although rupture can occur as late as 8 weeks after surgery,

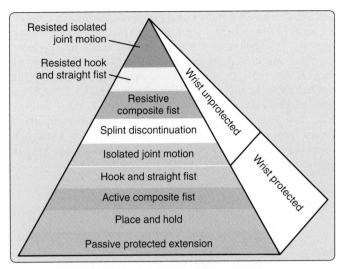

Figure 35-9 Tendon rehabilitation pyramid.

in my experience it is usually noted around the seventh to tenth postoperative day. Early reexploration and repair is the usual treatment of choice for tendon rupture.[78,151,152] If the FDP is advanced and repaired greater than 1 cm, quadrigia syndrome can develop.[73,121] This is based on the limited proximal excursion of the remaining FDP tendons, which have a common muscle belly. A flexion contracture of the affected digit is noted, and the patient often complains of a weak grasp because of lack of full motion of surrounding digits. Other less common complications include pulley failure and bowstringing, triggering, and swan-neck deformity.[153]

Summary

Early active mobilization or controlled active motion is now established as a reliable method for the postoperative management of flexor tendon repairs.[75,114,154] Several factors must be considered when these protocols are used in clinical practice. The tensile strength of the suture material must be adequate, and the design of the suture must enable it to withstand active mobilization without rupture or gapping. Several recent studies have addressed these issues.[102,155-165] It is clear from these studies that tendon repair strength is roughly proportional to the number of strands that cross the repair site.[166] Multiple-core suture designs have been described. It is believed that a core repair of at least four strands in conjunction with an epitendinous suture is required to withstand the rigors of an early active motion protocol. This knowledge must be tempered by the fact that the work of flexion is also proportional to the amount of suture material present at the repair site.[167] The epitendinous stitch has assumed an increasingly important role both in ultimate strength and prevention of gap formation after flexor tendon repair.[104,110-113]

Future

Current themes in flexor tendon research include understanding the healing process from the cellular, molecular, and genetic levels. Studies using mesenchymal stem cells on a scaffold to bridge tendon gaps have shown some promise.[168,169] Before the era of molecular medicine, researchers had attempted to modify adhesion formation with mechanical barriers, such as silicone, hydroxyapatite, and polyethylene, between the healing tendon and sheath. Others have tried chemical means, including corticosteroids, ibuprofen, 5-flourouracil, and hyaluronic acid; however, these media have not been adopted in clinical practice. Molecular techniques targeting cytokines such as transforming growth factor beta (TGF-β), which has been implicated in scar formation after repair, have shown promise in reducing adhesions and increasing ROM.[170] Other prospects include introducing a bone morphogenic protein (BMP-13) to improve tendon healing.[167]

REFERENCES

The complete reference list is available online at www.expertconsult.com.

Postoperative Management of Flexor Tendon Injuries

KAREN PETTENGILL, MS, OTR/L, CHT AND
GWENDOLYN VAN STRIEN, LPT, MSC

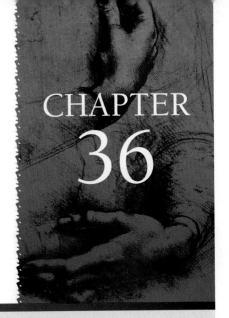

CRITICAL POINTS

- Know the specifics of both injury and surgery.
- Calculate the "safe zone" and recalculate as needed.
- Base your rehabilitation program on both your evaluation and the known data on tendon anatomy, healing, excursion, and repair strength.
- Each patient responds differently, so do *not* use the same approach with every patient, and do *not* adhere rigidly to a protocol.
- Change your approach if it is not working.
- Aggressive treatment progression is essential, but that does not require aggressively vigorous treatment.
- Before advancing the program, identify all the tissues involved, and target those tissues appropriately.
- If you recognize today that the program should be changed, don't wait until tomorrow because you're too busy!
- Measure what you're trying to change, for example, measure proximal interphalangeal (PIP) joint flexion contractures *passively*, because limited *passive* extension is the cause of limited active extension.

Postoperative management of the repaired flexor tendon requires a thorough understanding of the anatomy, physiology, biomechanics, and normal and pathologic healing not only of the flexor tendons but also of all adjacent injured structures. The therapist assesses tendon function through palpation, observation, and measurement. When the patient is referred for therapy, the surgeon communicates to the therapist the particulars of injury and of surgical and medical management; the therapist then questions both surgeon and patient to obtain any additional information. On the basis of this information, the therapist, in consultation with the referring surgeon, selects the appropriate therapeutic approach and modifies treatment when needed.

This chapter presents fundamental tendon management concepts and then reviews the aspects of flexor tendon anatomy, biomechanics, and mechanisms of nutrition and healing pertinent to postoperative management. Following that is a discussion of the three approaches to tendon management, with protocols or programs that exemplify each. Each protocol gives guidelines for management; all protocols should be evaluated and modified according to the patient's individual needs.

The next section covers techniques for treating or preventing commonly encountered problems. The most important part of the chapter is the section on clinical decision making and application of the scientific evidence to the healing tendon. The chapter concludes with consideration of two special cases: flexor pollicis longus lacerations and laceration of multiple tendons and nerves at the wrist.

Fundamental Concepts

Goal: A Strong Repair That Glides Freely

Normal tendon function requires free gliding of the tendon without hindrance from surrounding tissues. Each tendon glides through a given amplitude of excursion to flex the digit completely and with adequate power. Because so many structures lie in such a constricted space within the hand, scar adhesions between adjacent structures can occur very easily after injury or surgery. Tendon adhesions can limit excursion to such an extent that tendon function is seriously compromised; intertendinous adhesions can further decrease function.

As it glides, a tendon encounters a certain normal amount of resistance or drag from surrounding tissues. For the first weeks after a repair, that drag is increased considerably by normal post-traumatic or postoperative edema, lacerated tissues, and the extra bulk of sutures and newly forming scar. Given the low strength of a newly repaired tendon, extra care must be taken to allow for increased drag during all immediate postoperative exercise. The effect of such factors as edema and adjacent injuries is to increase the work of flexion (the work necessary for the tendon to overcome the gliding resistance encountered). Calculation of work of flexion should take into account both gliding resistance between tendon and sheath and external forces (e.g., joint stiffness, edema) impeding gliding.[1]

In addition to unobstructed gliding, the tendon repair requires enough strength to withstand the normal forces acting on the tendon during daily activity. If subjected to excessive stress during early phases of healing, the repair may rupture or the tendon ends may pull apart without complete rupture. The gap may be filled with scar, and not only will it be weaker than a healthy repair, the tendon will also elongate, in effect putting it on slack. An elongated tendon requires even greater excursion to function as it should. Gap formation also has been shown to provoke increased adhesion formation in immobilized tendon repairs, although the functional significance of such gaps appears to be less in the repair that was mobilized early.[2,3]

Therefore the goal is for the tendon to heal without rupture or gap formation, with sufficient strength and excursion for daily activities. The therapist must understand and plan treatment to address all of the impediments to glide and the dangers to the repair for each patient. In addition to this chapter, the reader is encouraged to read Chapter 34 for a more comprehensive discussion of the variables of healing, nutrition, and gliding resistance that dictate individualization of flexor tendon treatment. Near the end of this chapter is a discussion of how to plan treatment in light of all these variables.

Table 36-1   Adhesion Grading System

Absent	Less than or equal to 5-degree discrepancy between digital active and passive flexion
Responsive	Greater than or equal to 10% resolution of active lag between therapy sessions
Unresponsive	Less than 10% resolution of active lag between therapy sessions

Adapted from Groth GN. Pyramid of progressive force exercises to the injured flexor tendon. *J Hand Ther* 17:31, 2004.

Evaluating Tendon Function

To plan effective therapy, the therapist evaluates tendon function in several ways. The most obvious is measurement of active and passive range of motion (AROM and PROM, respectively). If passive flexion greatly exceeds active flexion, the tendon is not functioning adequately. The repair may have ruptured or elongated, or it may be adherent. Groth[4] has devised an adhesion grading scale to aid the therapist in determining the severity of adherence and the need to increase stress to the tendon to increase excursion (Table 36-1). She classifies adhesions as absent (≤5-degree discrepancy between active and passive flexion), responsive (≥10% resolution of active lag between therapy sessions), and unresponsive (≤10% resolution of active lag between therapy sessions). Using this scale, the therapist can evaluate the lag (number of degrees greater passive than active flexion) and assess response to intervention. If the lag is responsive, then the current program may be continued. If not, then the program should be stepped up to more vigorously address adherence. The presence and extent of adhesions alone is not enough information, however. The therapist now palpates along the course of the tendon to detect impediments to smooth gliding. Such impediments may be very subtle; patience and experience are needed to accurately assess glide, but this is one of the therapist's most valuable skills.

An adherent tendon usually exhibits some excursion, however limited, but the entire excursion may be taken up by flexion of a single joint. For example, an adherent flexor digitorum profundus (FDP) tendon may produce active flexion of the distal interphalangeal (DIP) joint when the PIP and metacarpophalangeal (MCP) joints are held passively in extension, but when the proximal joints are left free, the limited excursion may not be sufficient to produce flexion at all joints.

An adherent tendon also limits passive composite extension, because it is in effect tethered to tissues at one level or more and cannot passively glide and lengthen to allow full extension. Figure 36-1 illustrates this phenomenon. The therapist evaluating limitations in motion also differentiates between those caused by impaired tendon function and those caused by articular or periarticular involvement.

Three Approaches to Tendon Management

Each postoperative tendon management protocol falls within one of the following three categories:

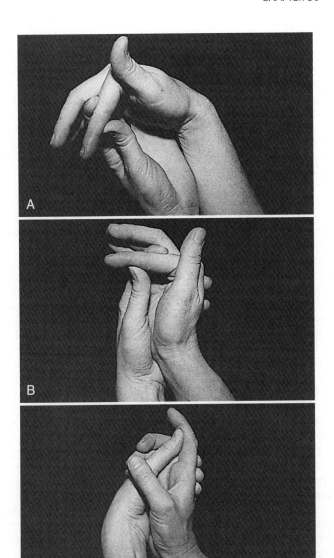

Figure 36-1 A, The proximal interphalangeal (PIP) joint can be extended completely when the wrist and metacarpophalangeal (MCP) joints are flexed. This means that there are no periarticular or articular restrictions to PIP joint extension. **B,** The PIP joint still can be extended completely when the wrist is extended, but we see the distal interphalangeal joint begin to flex, reflecting some tightening of the flexor digitorum profundus tendon. **C,** When the MCP joint and wrist are extended simultaneously, the PIP joint cannot be extended, indicating probable flexor tendon adhesions in the palm or at the level of the MCP joint or the proximal phalanx. (From Stewart KM. Tendon injuries. In: Stanley BG, Tribuzi SM, eds. *Concepts in Hand Rehabilitation.* Philadelphia: FA Davis, 1992;353–394.)

Immobilization. This approach involves complete immobilization of the tendon repair, generally for 3 to 4 weeks, before beginning active and passive mobilization.

Early passive mobilization. This approach involves mobilizing the repair early (usually within the first week, often within 24 hours), either manually (by therapist or patient) or by dynamic flexion traction. Passive flexion pushes the tendon proximally, and limited active or passive extension pulls the tendon distally.

Early active mobilization. This involves mobilizing the repair (within a few days of repair) through active contraction

of the involved flexor, with caution and within carefully prescribed limits.

Anatomy

Flexor tendon anatomy and zones were described in Chapter 1 and in Chapters 34 and 35. Following is a brief discussion of anatomic features according to the zone of injury pertinent to postoperative management.

Tendon injuries in zone 5 commonly become markedly adherent to overlying skin and fascia, but these adhesions are not generally problematic because adhesions form between the tendon and paratenon. Because the paratenon is a loose connective tissue, adhesions are not as restrictive as those that form between tendon and the firm, well-anchored flexor retinaculum or fibro-osseous tunnel.

Zone 4 injuries at the carpal canal are at risk for adhesion to synovial sheaths, to each other, and to the other structures lying within the constricted carpal tunnel space. As with zone 2 injuries, intertendinous adhesions limit differential glide and thus can severely limit hand function.

Zone 3 lacerations distal to the carpal tunnel are susceptible to adhesions to adjacent tendons, lumbricals, and interossei, and to overlying fascia and skin.

The anatomy of the flexor tendons in zone 2 is complex, and the reader is referred to Chapters 1 and 35 for a complete review.

With so many structures packed into the confines of the fibro-osseous tunnel, adhesions are highly likely between FDP and flexor digitorum superficialis (FDS); between tendon and sheath; and between tendon and bony, vascular, and other soft tissue structures. This risk is further compounded if both slips of FDS are repaired at the same level as FDP, as the bulk of the three sutures combine to increase gliding resistance. If only one slip of FDS was repaired, there is a risk of adherence to the unrepaired stumps of FDS, which may also catch on the edge of pulleys, thus impeding glide. The surgeon may minimize the risk by trimming stumps down and shaping the proximal end to remove the protruding unrepaired portion.

If tendons have retracted (in a repair delayed over 14 days, or if the finger was in flexion during injury so that muscle contraction pulled the proximal tendon stump into the palm), the tendon must be retrieved, inevitably contributing intraoperative trauma. In cases of delayed repair, the tendon may have shortened since injury and thus may be repaired under some tension.

In addition, damage to the pulleys may compromise tendon function, and injury to the vincula may compromise nutrition. Without the restraint of the pulleys, the tendon pulls away from bone with each muscle contraction, resulting in "bowstringing" (Fig. 36-2). Finally, loss of even a few millimeters of tendon excursion can mean a considerable functional deficit. It's no wonder that so much time and effort have been expended in designing postoperative techniques to control adhesion formation, facilitate adequate nutrition and healing, and attain maximum excursion in the zone 2 injury.

In zone 1, the tendon does not have great excursion (only 5–7 mm), so loss of even a small amount of excursion can

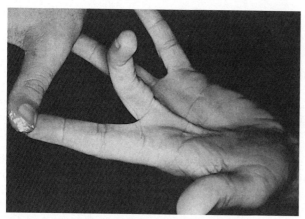

Figure 36-2 Bowstringing of the flexor tendons is illustrated in this patient with absent pulleys because of a childhood injury.

be functionally limiting. These injuries also are prone to adhesion of the repair to the A4 or A5 pulley and attenuation of the repair.

Nutrition

Flexor tendon nutrition is described in detail in Chapters 1 and 35.

It is important to note that in zone 2, where the tendons are surrounded by the pulley system and there are areas of relative avascularity, tendon nutrition comes from two sources: the blood supply and synovial diffusion.

Synovial fluid is apparently "forced" into the tendon under influence of high pressure against the pulleys during active flexion of the finger.[5,6] The pumping mechanism, under influence of pressure of the tendon against the firm resistance of the pulleys, has been compared to the mechanism of synovial diffusion in articular cartilage.

A delicate balance between the two nutritional pathways exists. Nutrition to relatively avascular areas is supplied mostly by diffusion from the synovium. When injury occurs in these areas, the balance is disturbed and excessive adhesion formation may be seen. The adhesions bring the additional blood supply to the tendon necessary for the healing process, yet they limit free tendon glide. Injury to the vincula themselves also affects the nutritional balance, compromises tendon healing, and causes adhesion formation.

Basic Concepts of Tendon Healing

Three phases are described for wound healing: the exudative or inflammatory phase, the proliferative or fibroplasia phase, and the remodeling or maturation phase. In reality these phases do not occur as separate events, but rather as an intricate process during which the phases overlap considerably and are modified by intrinsic factors and external forces. The process of tendon healing is described in detail in Chapter 34.

An essential characteristic of the healing of repaired tendon is the fact that the entire wound actually involves more than just the tendon. All surrounding tissues, such as skin, subcutaneous tissues, and underlying tissues, also are involved in the wound-healing process. In the immobilized tendon, during the first few days after repair, the wound is filled with a cicatrix, consisting of ground substance and many types of cells. Scar formed in the first 3 weeks "glues" all involved tissue layers together, and independent function is lost. This was described by Peacock[7] as the one-wound concept. The task of the therapist and surgeon is to restore gliding between soft tissues and thus recover their independent function.

Following are key events related to healing.

The exudative, or inflammatory, phase starts immediately after injury. Tensile strength of the *immobilized* tendon repair diminishes in the first 3 to 5 days because of softening of the tendon ends. As we shall see, this softening does not occur in tendons that have been mobilized in a controlled fashion during the first postoperative week.[2,8]

During the proliferative phase, fibroblasts migrate to the wound area and start production of tropocollagen approximately 5 days after injury. Tropocollagen is a triple-helix molecule with little tensile strength. After the weak hydrogen bonds of the tropocollagen molecule are replaced by stronger crosslinks between the three strands of the helix, collagen fibers are formed, and tensile strength starts to develop. The collagen molecules form a randomly oriented network, creating a bond between all tissues in the wound. From day 5 to day 21, tensile strength of the immobilized repair increases as the collagen matures and the intramolecular cross-linking continues. As we shall see, repairs that are subject to early controlled stress gain strength more rapidly.

In the third phase of wound healing (the remodeling phase), the tissues are differentiated, and dense, unyielding scar can be changed into more favorable scar. Scar remodeling is characterized by a balance between collagen production and collagen lysis. The randomly oriented collagen between tendon ends, under the influence of stress, is slowly replaced by newly formed collagen oriented along the long axis of the tendon, thus providing increased tensile strength. The randomly oriented fibers of the scar between tendon and surrounding tissues, however, must become loose and filmy to regain gliding function.

Extrinsic Versus Intrinsic Healing

It's well accepted that tendons heal through a combination of intrinsic and extrinsic mechanisms.[9-11]

Extrinsic healing depends on formation of adhesions between tendon and surrounding tissue. These adhesions provide the blood supply and the cells (in particular, fibroblasts) needed for tendon healing. Unfortunately, they also prevent the tendon from gliding.[12,13]

Intrinsic healing occurs between the tendon ends only, without formation of limiting adhesions. This type of healing relies on the synovial fluid for nutrition and does not result in restricted motion of the tendon. The cells needed for tendon healing are supplied by the epitenon and endotenon itself.[14-17]

Although experimental research demonstrates that tendon healing is possible by either intrinsic or extrinsic means, in actual practice adhesions are seen to varying degrees, and the healing response is probably a balance between intrinsic and extrinsic healing mechanisms.

Effects of Motion and Force on Tendon Healing

Beneficial effects of early mobilization and stress applied to tendon anastomoses have been demonstrated in a number of laboratory experiments. Although concluding that the risks outweighed the potential benefits, Mason and Allen,[8] in 1941, noted that motion created a stronger repair in the wrist flexor tendons of some of their canine subjects. Tensile strength increased after the seventh day, especially when mobilization was protected.

Gelberman and others[18-22] performed a series of experimental studies of early passive mobilization of tendons in dogs. The authors reported that compared with tendons subjected to immobilization or delayed mobilization, the tensile strength and excursion of mobilized tendons were superior, probably as a result of improved intrinsic healing and consequently restored gliding surfaces. These studies support the hypothesis that motion has a beneficial effect on tendon nutrition, tenocyte metabolism, or both.

In 1987, Hitchcock and colleagues[2] studied healing of chicken flexor profundus tendons, comparing immobilized tendons with those allowed immediate controlled mobilization. They found that the immobilized tendons healed as described by previous investigators,[8] with a decrease in strength as tendon ends softened during the exudative phase as early as 5 days after repair. In contrast, the mobilized tendons did not go through a definable exudative phase, and therefore the tendon ends did not soften as occurs with an immobilized repair. Instead, repairs gained strength, appearing to heal through intrinsic mechanisms, with a notable lack of adhesion formation. Numerous other studies have confirmed the benefits of early mobilization.[23-30]

The Future of Tendon Healing

Many researchers have attempted to improve the quality of tendon healing by influencing quantity and type of adhesion formation. To limit fixed adhesions, weak healing is needed between tendon and surrounding tissues. In contrast, strong healing is needed between the tendon ends to transmit muscle power. This type of differential wound healing seems necessary to recover a free-gliding and functioning tendon after flexor tendon repair.

Over the past 15 years research has increased dramatically on the influence of growth factors on tendon healing. Growth factors are molecules that influence various cellular functions, regulating various steps along the cascade of tendon healing. The actual clinical applications of this research in tendon healing is still unclear.[31-36] In an effort to decrease gliding resistance of the repaired tendon, recent studies have investigated the application of lubricants such as lubricin and hyaluronic acid.[37-39] This research is explored in Chapter 34.

Postoperative Management

Factors Affecting Healing and Rehabilitation

Many variables may affect the outcome of a tendon repair. Among these are individual patient characteristics, factors related to injury or surgery, and aspects of the therapy.

Patient-Related Factors

Age. The only documented age-related factor is the number of vincula, which decreases as the patient grows older.[6] As a result, larger areas within the tendon lack blood supply, with a consequent decrease in healing potential. In addition, in theory, cell aging could lead to decreased healing capacity of tenocytes.[5]

General Health and Healing Potential. In general, patients in good health heal well. Certain lifestyles or dietary habits, however, adversely affect healing. For example, a cigarette smoker often experiences delayed healing.[5,40-42]

Rate and Quality of Scar Formation. In practice, clinicians often observe that of two patients with virtually identical injury, surgery, and therapy, one may form scar rapidly and heavily and have great difficulty mobilizing the tendon as a result, but the other may form scar slowly and then form very light scar. The latter patient runs a greater risk of tendon rupture.

Patient Motivation. The patient's motivation and ability to follow the postoperative program are critical determinants of the end result of a primary flexor tendon repair. One cannot expect careful and conscientious performance of the therapy program by a patient who does not understand his central role in his own rehabilitation. Each patient's goal is different and often is dictated by his occupation. The therapist must identify the patient's goals and make them a part of the overall therapy goals.

Patient education can decrease the danger of rupture, prevent overzealous patients from exercising too much or too forcefully, and perhaps help less-motivated patients to understand the importance of adhering to the home program.

Socioeconomic Factors. A patient's family life, her economic status, and other socioeconomic factors can help or hinder in rehabilitation. The patient may have no health insurance and no income, or may be supporting a family but unable to work. Her family may be unsupportive of her rehabilitation efforts or may simply be unable to help her. She may live alone and be unable to handle all of the daily responsibilities while performing a complex home program. If these factors are not taken into account in planning treatment, therapy may fail.

Injury- and Surgery-Related Factors

Level of Injury. The effect of injury varies depending on the zone of injury. These variations were described earlier.

Type of Injury. The nature of the injury is another important determinant of final outcome. In an untidy laceration or crush injury, subsequent infection may prolong the inflammatory process and delay healing. Crushing or blunt injuries usually cause more associated injuries to surrounding tissues and lead to more scar formation. Crush injuries also frequently involve vascular injury, and this can impair healing, especially with injury to the vincula. When adjacent injured tissues must be protected (as with fractures or injuries to neurovascular bundles), treatment is modified, subsequently compromising the ultimate result.

An isolated FDP injury heals with fewer adhesions, partly because there is only a single repair rather than two contiguous repairs that are prone to intertendinous adhesion. If both slips of FDS were injured and repaired along with FDP, the added bulk may make excursion and intertendinous gliding harder to attain. If FDS is injured, there is likelihood of greater vincular damage, and vascularity is impaired, again increasing the risk of adhesion formation (Fig. 36-3, online)

The prognosis also may be better for a partial laceration than for a complete laceration, because vascularity is generally better preserved. There is controversy in the literature about whether to repair the partial laceration.[43-45] Triggering or entrapment may occur when the irregular surface of an untreated partially lacerated tendon catches on the sheath, and theoretically the unrepaired partially lacerated tendon may rupture. Some evidence indicates that partial lacerations may be better left untouched except for beveling to prevent gliding problems.[46]

If the finger was flexing powerfully when injured, the contracting muscle will pull the proximal portion proximally like a rubber band cut under tension. The vincula may be ruptured or stretched, impairing vascularity. The surgeon must retrieve the proximal tendon stump before repair. The very retrieval may be traumatic to the tendon and surrounding sheath.

Position of the finger when injured also affects outcome in that a given point on the tendon glides proximally during flexion and distally during extension. For example, suppose a test tube breaks in a patient's hand, lacerating the FDP and FDS of one finger. The finger is flexed when injured. If the digit is extended, the cut distal portion of each tendon could be pulled distally by as much as 3 or 4 cm, depending on the excursion of the tendon in that patient and the actual level of injury. Thought should be given to postoperative positioning to avoid resting the repair(s) adjacent to the original wound or other involved tendon.

Sheath Integrity. The sheath and pulleys often are involved in a zone 1 or 2 injury.

Injury to the pulley system decreases the mechanical advantage of the tendon.[47-50] Pulley injury also affects tendon nutrition because of the role the pulleys play in synovial diffusion.

Several studies have shown no advantage to sheath repair.[51-55] Apparently a single cell layer much like the sheath regenerates in the first postoperative days.[11,55] Many surgeons attempt to repair the sheath, however, to prevent the possibility of triggering of the tendon repair site on the open sheath.

Surgical Technique. Meticulous surgical technique can minimize the amount of additional tissue trauma and hematoma, thereby reducing the number of adhesions. Excessive postoperative hematoma causes increased inflammatory and cellular responses. An increase in the amount of hematoma therefore may increase the number of adhesions surrounding the repaired tendon.

Tissues Must Be Handled Delicately. Potenza[56] has demonstrated that even the marks of the forceps on the epitenon can trigger adhesion formation. The effect of different surgical variables on adhesion formation in repaired tendons also has been investigated. Matthews and Richards[57] demonstrated an increase in adhesion formation when suture material was added to a gliding tendon. Injury to the sheath and use of an orthosis were other variables investigated and found to increase adhesion formation. Sutures may "strangulate" the intratendinous vessels and provoke adhesion formation. In fact, sutures often are placed in the relatively avascular volar aspect of the tendon to avoid damage to the dorsally placed intratendinous vessels.

Suture Strength Is a Crucial Variable. It was only when both strong and atraumatic sutures were developed that early mobilization could be contemplated. The suture must be strong enough to prevent gapping while allowing gentle stress to the repair. The development of early active mobilization techniques depends even more heavily on adequate suture strength. Although a discussion of specific sutures is beyond the scope of this chapter, several recently developed sutures clearly are strong enough to withstand early active mobilization if performed with carefully controlled force. The literature indicates that given a grasping suture that is technically well placed, strength is directly proportional to the number of strands crossing the repair.[58-61] This is illustrated in Figure 36-4. Several studies also have indicated that a well-designed circumferential suture will add strength to any repair.[62-68] Suture knot placement may also affect strength.[69,70] Another consideration is the work of flexion, or resistance to gliding due to placement, bulk, or other design aspects of the core or circumferential suture.[62,71,72]

Timing of Repair. The longer a tendon repair is delayed, the more difficult the rehabilitation may be.[73] By 2 weeks after injury, the cut tendon ends have scarred down to surrounding tissues and must be dissected free before repair. In addition, the entire musculotendinous unit shortens and pulls the tendon proximally, which may place tension on the repair and increase the risk of gapping or rupture; shortening also increases the risk of later flexion contractures. Injury- and surgery-related factors are summarized in Box 36-1.

Therapy-Related Factors

Timing. As noted before, an immobilized tendon repair loses strength initially, whereas early mobilization strengthens the repair. Therefore, if early mobilization is to be used, therapy should begin as soon as possible. If mobilization begins at 1 week after repair, the repair will already have weakened enough to be at increased risk for rupture or deformation.

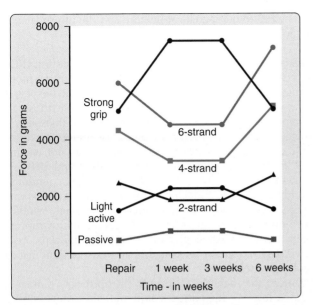

Figure 36-4 This graph plots the strength of two-, four- and six-strand repairs against the forces exerted by passive flexion, light active flexion, and strong grip, with a margin allowed for friction, edema, and stress. (From Strickland JW. Development of flexor tendon surgery: twenty-five years of progress. *J Hand Surg.* 2000 25A:214.)

Level of injury determines which anatomic, healing, and biomechanical features to consider in planning treatment.

Type of injury

Untidy laceration/crush injuries. Infection may prolong the inflammatory process and delay healing. Associated injuries may increase the risk of adhesions

Isolated FDP injury. Easier to regain gliding because only one tendon involved

Combined FDP/FDS injury/repair

Risk of poor gliding because of adhesions between repairs

Repair of separate FDS slips. Increased bulk, and increased risk of adhesions

FDS laceration. Chance of greater vincular damage leads to increased risk of adhesions

Partial laceration. Prognosis may be better, depending on surgical management

Position of the finger when injured

If finger injured when flexed tendon retracts proximally, retrieval is difficult and may cause more scarring.

Avoid positioning repair at original injury site to prevent adherence

Sheath integrity. Repair of sheath may not improve healing of repaired tendon but may improve gliding

Injury to the pulley system

Decreases mechanical advantage of tendon

Affects synovial tendon nutrition

Surgical technique

Tissue handling. Atraumatic surgical technique decreases risk of adhesions

Suture technique. Suture may strangulate intratendinous vessels and cause more adhesion formation

Suture strength. Is it appropriate for your chosen treatment approach?

Timing of repair. Delayed repair causes scarring of tendon ends or shortening of musculotendinous unit (or both), both increase risk of adhesions

FDP, flexor digitorum profundis; FDS, flexor digitorum superficialis.

Adhesions also will have begun to form, adding to the stress placed on the weakened repair. A 1995 study by Tottenham and coworkers[74] found better results in patients whose repaired zone II tendons were mobilized passively within 1 week than in those mobilized between 1 and 3 weeks after repair. However, in a severely edematous digit, starting early mobilization on the day of surgery would be dangerous. Inflammation and edema subside after a day or so of rest and elevation in the compressive postoperative dressing, which reduces the work of flexion.[75]

Another aspect of timing is progression according to tendon healing status. Although not always described as such, every protocol can be divided into three phases or stages. The early stage is a protective period that includes the inflammatory and proliferative or fibroplasia phases and sometimes the beginning of the remodeling phase of wound healing, when the repair is at its weakest. This lasts for 3 to 4 weeks. Next is the intermediate stage, when stress to the tendon is increased, either by mobilizing for the first time, or by decreasing protection during mobilization. The late stage generally begins at 6 to 8 weeks and continues to the end of therapy. Stress to the tendon is increased, and muscle strengthening and job simulation are added gradually.

Technique. As will be clear from the following discussion, the postoperative rehabilitation technique must be selected with care to match the needs of the patient. Not every tendon injury can be treated with the identical protocol, and often the best approach is a combination of techniques from various protocols.

Expertise. The therapist's expertise must be taken into account in selecting the postoperative rehabilitation approach. No therapist should undertake a treatment program without

sufficient preparation, experience, and any supervision needed. This may seem evident, but despite the multitude of available options for tendon management, many therapists attempt to use approaches that they simply do not understand, following rigid protocols without consideration of individual variables and the rationale for treatment. Nowhere is it more vital to fully understand the rationale for treatment than in tendon management.

The uninformed reader may be misled easily by results of various studies presented in the literature. In addition to evaluating research design, instrumentation, and other components of any study, the therapist must bear in mind the differences between the population in the study and the patient now being treated. For example, military patients are a "captive audience" and can be assumed to be more compliant than civilians. The health care delivery system may also make a difference in the outcome. Some studies involve patients who are hospitalized and therefore more closely supervised. If your patient is restricted by insurance coverage to one visit per week, your choice of approach may need to change or the way you educate the patient and monitor progress.

In addition, studies use varying means of assessing the results of flexor tendon repair. The interested reader is referred to Elliot and Harris' comprehensive review of the different methods of assessing results of tendon repair.[76]

Following are the rationale, indications, and representative protocols for each of the three basic approaches to flexor tendon management: immobilization, early passive mobilization, and early active mobilization. The discussion of immobilization is the most concrete and detailed, including concepts and techniques that may be used in other approaches.

Immobilization

Rationale and Indications

No matter how sophisticated our therapeutic and surgical care becomes, there will probably always be a need for immobilization of flexor tendon repairs in some circumstances. Early mobilization protocols are appropriate for alert, motivated patients who understand the exercise program and precautions. For that reason, immobilization is still the treatment of choice for patients who are too young, those with cognitive deficits, and those who for any other reason are clearly unable or unwilling to participate in a complex rehabilitation program. These patients benefit far more from protection of the repair until adequate healing and adhesion formation have taken place. Some tendons also must be immobilized to protect other injured structures. In some cases the patient is not referred to therapy for a postoperative orthosis but simply remains in the postoperative cast until sent to therapy at 3 to 4 weeks after surgery. Therefore all therapists must be prepared to treat the immobilized tendon with skill and care. It may be very difficult to mobilize these repairs because of heavy adhesion formation.

Treating the Immobilized Tendon Repair

The following guidelines are based on those developed by Cifaldi Collins and associates,[77] to ensure sufficiently aggressive therapy after immobilization. We describe here several techniques and concepts applicable to all flexor tendon management, regardless of the approach used.

Early Stage (from 0 to 3 or 4 weeks)

Orthosis. The dorsal forearm-based postoperative orthosis or cast holds the wrist in 10 to 30 degrees of flexion, the MCP joints in 40 to 60 degrees of flexion, and the interphalangeal (IP) joints in full extension.

Exercise. At home patients perform range-of-motion (ROM) exercises of uninvolved joints (elbow, shoulder) to prevent stiffness. The orthosis is worn 24 hours a day, except for therapy visits once or twice a week when the orthosis may be removed for gentle protected PROM by the therapist. For protected PROM, the therapist holds adjacent joints in flexion while extending and flexing each joint. Thus, for example, for PIP joint extension, the wrist and MCP and DIP joints are kept flexed to give some slack to the flexor tendons. If the adjacent MCP and DIP joints were allowed to remain extended during PIP joint extension, the slack would be taken up and PIP joint extension might stretch or rupture a repair at the proximal phalanx level. The concept of protected passive motion is applied in all flexor tendon management protocols.

During the therapy session the therapist may remove the orthosis to clean the patient's skin and, after the sutures are removed and the incision is well healed, perform massage to the scar. As the scar heals, massage may help modify both skin and tendon adhesions. Elastomer or other pressure dressings are helpful for flattening unusually bulky scars but generally should be used only at night, to avoid restricting mobility during the day. In some patients such pressure can be applied during the early stage without removing the orthosis.

Intermediate Stage (starting at 3 to 4 weeks)

Orthosis. At 3 to 4 weeks, the orthosis is modified to bring the wrist to neutral (0 degrees). The patient is taught to remove the orthosis hourly for exercise.

Exercise. With the wrist at 10 degrees of extension, the patient performs passive digit flexion and extension, followed by active differential tendon gliding exercises (Fig. 36-5). These exercises elicit maximum total and differential flexor tendon glide at the wrist–palm level.[78] The straight fist, with the MCP joints and PIP joints flexed but the DIP joints extended, elicits maximum FDS glide in relation to surrounding structures. The full fist, with the MCP, PIP, and DIP joints flexed, does the same for the FDP tendon. In the hook fist, with the MCP joints extended while the IP joints flex, maximum differential gliding between the two tendons is achieved. For the Cifaldi Collins and associates' protocol,

There are three ways of making a fist:

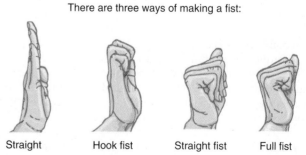

Straight   Hook fist   Straight fist   Full fist

Figure 36-5 The three different positions of tendon gliding exercises: hook fist, straight fist, and full fist.

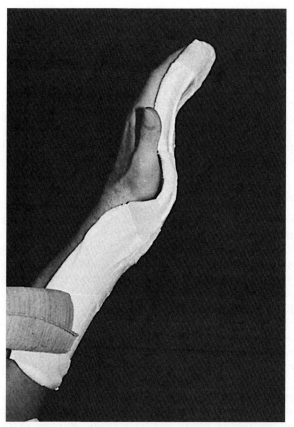

Figure 36-6 A forearm-based orthosis or plaster "stretcher" maintains maximum comfortable extension at night. It is serially remolded or remade to accommodate gains in extension.

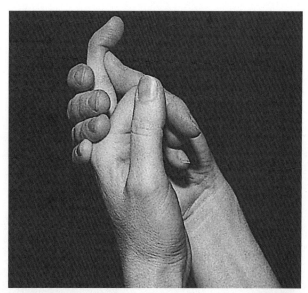

Figure 36-7 Blocking exercise for flexor digitorum profundus gliding. The proximal interphalangeal (PIP) joint is gently maintained in passive PIP joint extension to prevent flexor digitorum superficialis glide. Blocking exercises are performed carefully, avoiding forceful distal interphalangeal joint flexion that may apply excessive stress to newly healed tendons. (From Stewart KM. Review and comparison of current trends in the postoperative management of tendon repair. Hand Clin. 1991;7:447–460.)

the exercises incorporate synergistic wrist motion (SWM): the wrist extends when the digits flex, and flexes when the digits extend, to increase the excursion attained and prevent simultaneous full wrist and digit flexion.

After 3 or 4 days of these exercises, tendon function is evaluated. The therapist measures active and passive flexion, totaling the degrees of flexion achieved at the MCP and IP joints for total active and passive flexion. If there is a discrepancy of more than 50 degrees between total active and total passive flexion, poor gliding and heavy adhesion formation are assumed, and the patient is moved on to the next phase of therapy. According to the original published guidelines, if the discrepancy is less than 50 degrees, the patient continues with the current phase of therapy until 6 weeks after repair. The authors of this chapter do not wait until 6 weeks unless the discrepancy is far less (see also Groth's Pyramid of Force Progression,[4] discussed later on, and Fig 36-19).

Late Stage (starting at 4 weeks or later, depending on tendon glide)

Orthosis. The dorsal blocking orthosis is discontinued. If flexor muscle–tendon unit shortening is a problem, a forearm-based palmar nighttime orthosis may be worn, holding wrist and fingers in maximum comfortable extension (Fig. 36-6). The orthosis, made of plaster or thermoplastic material, is serially remade or adjusted to accommodate any improvements in extension.

Exercise. The patient begins gentle blocking exercises for isolated FDP and FDS glide. For isolated FDP gliding, the MCP and PIP joints are held in extension, thus preventing FDS glide, while the FDP functions alone to flex the DIP joint (Fig. 36-7). Some patients are unable to perform this exercise without exerting excessive force and risking rupture or repair deformation. Alternative interventions can be found discussed under the sections "Treating Adhesion Problems" and "Clinical Decision Making." For isolated FDS glide, the adjacent fingers are held in full extension, thus holding FDP tendons (which have a common muscle belly) at their full length and making it virtually impossible for them to assist as the FDS flexes the PIP joint (Fig. 36-8). The index finger often has a separate FDP muscle belly, allowing FDP glide even when the adjacent middle finger is held in extension, but often the patient can be taught to use only the FDS tendon, with extension of the middle finger as a cue.

If active flexion does not improve rapidly enough (in 1 week according to the original publication), the program is upgraded to include activities involving increased stress to the repair to elicit greater excursion. From there the program is gradually progressed to add greater stress as needed. If the patient begins to make faster progress, the progression of the program is delayed, to avoid excessive stress in the presence of improving tendon excursion.

Greater resistance to flexion elicits a stronger muscle contraction and therefore assists in elongating tendon adhesions and improving glide, but excessive resistance may rupture a tendon even as late as 3 months after injury. In general, the more adherent the tendon, the safer it is to apply resistance to glide. The tendon that is gliding well does not need that

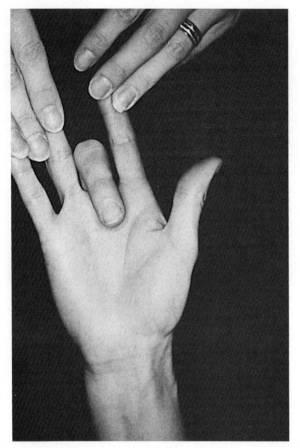

Figure 36-8 *Active isolated superficialis exercise—flexing one finger at a time at the proximal interphalangeal joint while holding the other fingers in extension with the uninvolved hand.*

additional resistance. Most tendons are not ready for heavy resistance (e.g., lifting over 10 pounds, using grip exercisers) and manual labor job simulation until 10 to 12 weeks.

Early Passive Mobilization

Rationale and Indications

If applied with care, early passive mobilization (starting within a few days of repair) has been shown to produce superior results, apparently because early mobilization inhibits restrictive adhesion formation, promotes intrinsic healing and synovial diffusion, and produces a stronger repair, preventing the decrease in tensile strength of repairs noted in immobilized tendons by Mason and Allen and by Urbaniak and colleagues.[2,8,15,20,26,79,80] In a study using metal markers in repaired flexor tendons, Silverskiöld and coworkers[81] demonstrated that measurable passive excursion occurs with passive IP joint flexion. Related studies by May and associates[82] and Silverskiöld and colleagues[83] found a significant correlation between early passive IP joint flexion and later active flexion measured in long-term follow-up. Drawing on the results of these studies and others,[21,84-88] Strickland[89] summarizes the passive excursion of the long finger flexors as follows: In uninjured flexors, passive MCP joint motion does not provide any excursion, while DIP joint motion provides 1 to 2 mm of FDP excursion per 10 degrees of joint flexion, and PIP joint flexion provides 1.5 mm of glide per 10 degrees of joint flexion. In contrast, in the case of repaired flexors, 10 degrees of passive DIP joint flexion produces only 0.3 mm of excursion (a substantial decrease), and 10 degrees of passive PIP joint flexion gives 1.3 mm of excursion (a much smaller decrease compared with the unrepaired tendon). Clearly the repaired tendon's excursion is affected by the increased bulk and other factors contributing to gliding resistance.

Published Protocols

There are two basic types of early passive mobilization programs. One approach is based on the work of Kleinert and colleagues,[90,91] and the other on that of Duran and Houser.[92] Hand specialists have worked many variations on these two approaches, and in fact, few experienced therapists adhere closely to one protocol or the other.[93-96]

In both approaches, a forearm-based dorsal orthosis blocks the MCP joints and wrist in flexion to place the flexor tendons on slack, and the IP joints are left free or allowed to extend to neutral within the orthosis. The orthosis allows passive flexion of the fingers but does not allow extension beyond the limits of the orthosis. Dynamic traction maintains the fingers in flexion, to further relax the tendon and prevent inadvertent active flexion. The dynamic traction may be provided by rubber bands, elastic threads, springs, or other devices; the traction is applied to the fingernail either by placing a suture through the nail in surgery, or by gluing to the fingernail a dress hook, Velcro, a piece of soft leather or moleskin, or the rubber band itself.

Duran and Houser

Early Stage (from 0 to 4.5 weeks)
   Orthosis. The wrist is held in 20 degrees of flexion and the MCP joints in a relaxed position of flexion.
   Exercise. Duran and Houser[92] determined through clinical and experimental observation that 3 to 5 mm of glide was sufficient to prevent formation of firm tendon adhesions; the exercises (six to eight repetitions twice a day) are designed to achieve this. With the MCP and PIP joints flexed, the DIP joint is passively extended, thus moving the FDP repair distally, away from an FDS repair. Then with the DIP and MCP joints flexed, the PIP joint is extended; both repairs glide distally away from the site of repair and any surrounding tissues to which they might otherwise form adhesions (Fig. 36-9).

Intermediate Stage (from 4.5 weeks to 7.5 or 8 weeks)
   Orthosis. After 4.5 weeks, the orthosis is replaced with a wristband to which rubber-band traction is attached (Fig. 36-10)
   Exercise. Active extension exercises begin within the limitations imposed by the wristband. Active flexion (blocking, FDS gliding, and fisting) is initiated on removal of the wristband at 5.5 weeks.

Late Stage (starting at 7.5 to 8 weeks). Resisted flexion waits until 7.5 to 8 weeks. The program is upgraded

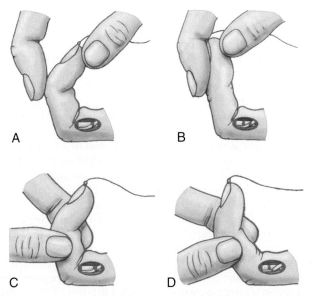

Figure 36-9 Duran and Houser's exercises for passive flexor tendon gliding. With the metacarpophalangeal (MCP) joint and proximal interphalangeal (PIP) joint flexed **(A),** the distal interphalangeal (DIP) joint is passively extended **(B),** thus moving the flexor digitorum profundus repair distally, away from a flexor digitorum superficialis repair. Then with DIP and MCP joints flexed **(C),** the PIP joint is extended **(D);** both repairs glide distally away from the site of repair and any surrounding tissues to which they might otherwise form adhesions. (From Duran RJ, et al: Management of flexor tendon lacerations in zone 2 using controlled passive motion postoperatively. In Hunter JM, et al, editors: *Rehabilitation of the Hand,* ed 3. St Louis: Mosby, 1990.)

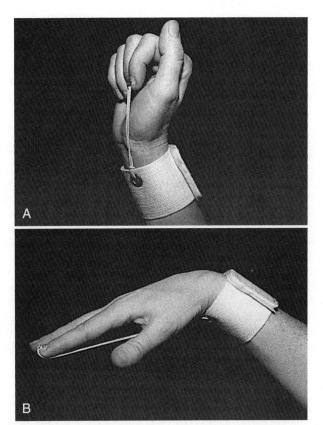

Figure 36-10 Elastic traction from the wrist band prevents simultaneous wrist and finger extension. **A,** When the wrist is extended, the fingers are passively flexed by the elastic traction. **B,** When the fingers extend, the wrist is passively flexed. (From Stewart KM. Tendon injuries. In: Stanley BG, Tribuzi SM, eds. *Concepts in Hand Rehabilitation.* Philadelphia: FA Davis, 1992;353–394.)

following the principles outlined under the section on "Immobilization."

Modified Duran

The Duran protocol is not frequently used in its standard form by hand therapists. Some therapists (including the authors of this chapter) now use what is often called a "modified Duran" approach. This applies a dorsal protective orthosis (we prefer 40–50 degrees of flexion at the MCP joints and from 20 degrees of extension to 20 degrees of flexion at the wrist, depending on the quality of the repair and other factors), but the rubber-band traction is omitted and the IP joints are strapped in extension between exercises or at night (Fig. 36-11). Patients perform passive individual and composite flexion and extension, and active composite extension exercises (manually blocking the MCP joint in greater flexion for more complete active IP joint extension) as well as the passive flexion and extension exercises advocated by Duran and Houser. Only during therapy is the orthosis removed for careful protected SWM exercises (passive or assisted simultaneous wrist flexion and finger extension, alternating with simultaneous wrist extension and finger flexion). Obviously performance of SWM exercises depends on the zone of injury and relative safety of this maneuver for the patient.

Kleinert

Duran and Houser use dynamic traction to rest the digit in flexion, but Kleinert and colleagues uses the rubber band to resist full active extension, based on findings of electromyographic silence in the flexors during resisted digit extension.[91,97] Others have questioned this finding in more recent research, as noted later.

The original protocol is not described in detail, as it is no longer used much in the original form.

Orthosis. In the original Kleinert protocol, the dorsal blocking orthosis blocked the wrist in 45 degrees of flexion and the MCP joints in 10 to 20 degrees (since modified to less wrist flexion [20 degrees] and more MCP joint flexion [40 degrees]). Rubber-band traction was directed to the

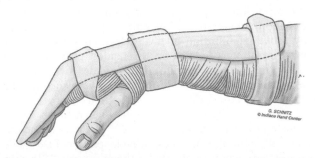

Figure 36-11 Dorsal blocking orthosis used for modified Duran protocol. Wrist and metacarpophalangeal joints are flexed, and fingers are strapped in interphalangeal joint extension when not exercising. (From Cannon N. *Indiana Hand Cen News.* 1993;1:13.)

fingernail from the wrist or just proximal to the wrist (more recently modified to direct traction through a palmar pulley, as we shall see in May's program discussed in the following section and later in this chapter).

Exercise. Every hour, the patient actively extends the fingers to the limits of the orthosis 10 times, allowing the rubber bands to flex the fingers.

At 3 to 6 weeks (depending on the quality of tendon glide) gentle active flexion may begin (intermediate stage), although resisted exercise waits until 6 to 8 weeks (late stage).

May and colleagues[95] published an early passive mobilization protocol that they called the "four-finger" method. The wrist is flexed 30 to 45 degrees and the MCP joints 50 to 70 degrees. The dorsal orthosis extends only to the PIP joints, to allow full active PIP joint extension. Rubber-band traction passes through a palmar pulley, and patients perform hourly active IP joint extension exercises. All four fingers are included in traction, even if not injured. Manual pressure to all four fingers is used to attain the final degrees of passive flexion during exercise. Patients use the uninvolved hand to decrease resistance from the rubber bands by pulling them distally during the active extension part of the exercises. At night the rubber bands are detached, and a volar component is added holding the IP joints in extension.

The orthosis is discontinued at 4 weeks, and active flexion and extension is initiated (intermediate stage).

As previously noted, all early passive mobilization programs use a dorsal blocking orthosis for at least 3 weeks, and all involve some form of passive flexion and active extension. Except for the Duran, all use frequent exercise: every 1 to 2 hours. Over the years, there has been a tendency to use less and less wrist flexion; severe wrist flexion angles are uncomfortable and may lead to difficulty regaining wrist extension. In the zone 4 or 5 injury, excessive flexion can lead to serious flexion contractures.

Early Active Mobilization

Rationale

Early mobilization is applied to recently injured, edematous tendons with added bulk at the suture sites. The tendons are mobilized within surrounding sheath or other structures that are also edematous and that often do not provide a smooth gliding surface. In early passive mobilization programs, the tendon is pushed proximally; as has been pointed out, this is akin to pushing a piece of cooked linguine down a tube. The tendon is likely to fold or bunch up rather than glide. Early active mobilization involves active contraction of the injured flexor muscle, pulling the tendon proximally, and logically this should produce better glide. Certainly the results of such programs so far have been very encouraging, supporting the observation made earlier that some of the best early passive mobilization results come when patients "cheat" and add a little active motion. Studies[81,87,98,99] have found that passive IP joint flexion does provide passive FDP glide. However, one study found that although passive PIP joint flexion "mobilized the tendon with an efficiency of 90%" compared with active motion, the efficiency of DIP joint flexion was only 36%.[100] This could mean a poorer prognosis

for zone II FDP injuries over the middle phalanx when managed with passive mobilization.

Kubota and coworkers,[26] investigating the breaking strength and increase in cellular activity produced by early mobilization and tension to tendon repairs, found that early mobilization without tension on the repair was not as effective as a combination of the two (such as would occur in active mobilization). We conclude that active mobilization produces a stronger repair with better excursion, especially at the level of the middle phalanx. Furthermore, if the tendon attains better excursion, the "milking" effect increases, thus enhancing the nutrition through synovial diffusion.

Repair techniques have improved vastly in recent years: we now have stronger, less bulky sutures that glide much more easily. Clearly, whenever feasible, early active mobilization is preferable to early passive mobilization. The literature is growing rapidly and contains a diversity of postoperative approaches.[24,58,94,101-109] It can be difficult to sort out the relative value of one approach over another, or to select the appropriate patient for early active mobilization. This should not stop the experienced therapist or surgeon from exploring this promising avenue, as long as we remember one caveat: Just as a piece of cooked linguine bunches up if pushed through a tube, it also tears if pulled too hard! Early active mobilization is only appropriate if both therapist and surgeon possess skill and experience in tendon management, if they communicate closely with each other, if the suture used was of adequate strength, and if the patient is highly reliable and understands the program thoroughly.

Published Protocols

Most early active mobilization programs were developed for zone 2 injuries. Almost all use a dorsal blocking orthosis like those employed for early passive mobilization. Exercises and exercise frequency vary, but all programs protect the tendon by limiting active flexion for the first 3 to 6 weeks. Following is a discussion of the distinctions between a few selected protocols. Some of these undoubtedly have been updated since publication. Wherever possible, changes have been incorporated in the following material.

Active Mobilization

Belfast and Sheffield. Authors from the United Kingdom have published a group of related early active mobilization programs. Two similar original protocols[102,107] were modified subsequently by other authors.[103,104,110,111] Following is one of the more detailed of the recently published versions by Gratton.[104]

Early Stage (from 0 to 4 or 6 weeks)

ORTHOSIS. The postoperative cast maintains the wrist at 20 degrees of flexion and the MCP joints at 80 to 90 degrees of flexion, allowing full IP joint extension. The cast extends 2 cm beyond the fingertips to inhibit use of the hand. A radial plaster "wing" wraps around the wrist just proximal to the thumb to prevent the cast from migrating distally. On initiation of therapy, the postoperative dressing is debulked to allow exercise.

EXERCISE. For zone 3 injuries therapy is initiated 24 hours after repair, but zone 2 repairs are allowed to rest until 48 hours after surgery to allow postoperative inflammation to subside. Exercises, performed every 4 hours within the orthosis, include all digits and consist of two repetitions each of full passive flexion, active flexion, and active extension. The first week's goal is full passive flexion, full active extension, and active flexion to 30 degrees at the PIP joint and 5 to 10 degrees at the DIP joint. Active flexion is expected to gradually increase over following weeks, reaching 80 to 90 degrees at the PIP joint and 50 to 60 degrees at the DIP joint by the fourth week. In actual practice these precise flexion measurements are not used; instead the patient is taught to place the four fingers of the opposite hand across the palm of the involved hand, with the little finger touching the palm. The patient is asked to flex the involved finger(s) to touch the contralateral index finger, which is closest to the tips of the involved fingers. To advance the program the patient progressively places three fingers in the palm instead of four (to set a new goal for increased flexion), then two fingers, and then one. This gives a gradually moving goal that progresses to flexion to the palm.[112]

Intermediate Stage (starting at 4 to 6 weeks)

ORTHOSIS. The orthosis is discontinued at 4 weeks if tendon glide is poor (not achieving expected goals given earlier), at 5 weeks for most patients, or at 6 weeks for patients with unusually good tendon gliding (full fist developing within the first 2 weeks). Three weeks after orthotic positioning is discontinued, any residual flexion contractures are treated with finger-based dynamic extension orthoses.

EXERCISE. The only exercise specified for this period is protected passive IP joint extension (with the MCP joint held in flexion) in the presence of flexion contractures. Presumably patients continue active flexion and extension exercises, and the program is progressed from this point as it would be for any tendon protocol. Small and associates[107] do speak of using blocking exercises to increase tendon glide at 6 weeks, and Cullen and colleagues[102] initiate progressive resistive exercise and heavier hand use at 8 weeks, with full function expected by 12 weeks.

Note that in published versions of this approach, the patients were hospitalized initially to ensure compliance. This is no longer the case for most patients in Britain. There are no published results for this program without hospitalization.

Active Hold/Place Hold Mobilization.

Strickland/Cannon. Various authors[24,80,113,114] have attempted to quantify the force or muscle tension of the flexors during such motions as passive and active flexion and flexion against varying amounts of resistance. Each author has used a different method and arrived at different numbers. For their early mobilization protocol, Strickland[115] and Cannon[101] assumed forces similar to those measured by Urbaniak and coworkers[80]: for FDP, 500 g for passive motion (Urbaniak and coworkers: 200–300 g) and 1500 g for "light grip" (Urbaniak and coworkers: 1500 g for flexion against moderate resistance). For FDS, the values are 15% to 30% of the values for FDP. Their protocol assumes that some margin must be allowed for postoperative edema and other factors, and they rely on tensile strength of 2150 to 4300 g during the first 3 weeks with the Tajima repair plus a horizontal

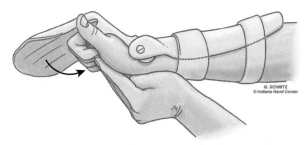

Figure 36-12 The patient extends the wrist actively with simultaneous passive digit flexion. (From Cannon N. *Indiana Hand Cen News.* 1993;1:13–17.)

mattress (or an equivalent four-strand suture[59]) and a running lock circumferential suture. They further decrease the load on the tendons by holding the wrist in extension and keeping the MCP joints flexed for active flexion exercise. This is based on work by Savage,[113] who found that the force required for active digit flexion (work of flexion) decreased when the wrist was held at 45 degrees of extension and the MCPs at 90 degrees of flexion.

This is properly speaking an "active hold" or "place hold active mobilization" program. The digits are passively placed in flexion, and the patient then maintains the flexion with a gentle muscle contraction. Patients learn to use only minimal force by practicing with the uninjured hand and also use biofeedback to monitor the strength of contraction (<10 mV on a Cyborg model biofeedback unit).

Early Stage (from 0 to 4 weeks)

ORTHOSIS. Two different orthoses are used. A dorsal blocking orthosis is worn most of the time, with the wrist at 20 degrees of flexion and the MCP joints at 50 degrees (Figs. 36-12 and 36-13). The exercise orthosis has a hinged wrist, allowing full wrist flexion, but wrist extension is limited to 30 degrees. Full digit flexion and full IP joint extension are allowed, but MCP joint extension is limited to 60 degrees. The orthosis used for distal FPL repairs (zone T1) is similar

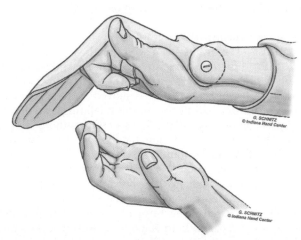

Figure 36-13 The patient maintains digit flexion with a gentle active muscle contraction. (From Cannon N. *Indiana Hand Cen News.* 1993;1:13–17.)

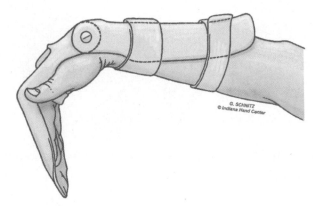

Figure 36-14 The wrist is allowed to relax into flexion with simultaneous digit extension (limited to 60 degrees at the metacarpophalangeal joints). (From Cannon N. *Indiana Hand Cen News.* 1993;1:13–17.)

but allows IP joint extension to only 25 degrees (as in the Evans zone 1 protocol) to prevent repair deformation and problems with glide deep to the A2 pulley. In current practice, the authors sometimes use only the exercise orthosis, adding a block between the two hinged components to maintain wrist flexion between exercise sessions.[116]

EXERCISE. Every hour patients perform the modified Duran exercises in the dorsal blocking orthosis, followed by place-and-hold digit flexion in the exercise orthosis. The patient extends the wrist actively with simultaneous passive digit flexion (see Fig. 36-12) and actively maintains digit flexion for 5 seconds (see Fig. 36-13). The patient then relaxes and allows the wrist to flex and digits to extend within the limits of the orthosis (Fig. 36-14). Note again the use of SWM to both protect the tendon and increase excursion.

Intermediate Stage (from 4 weeks to 7 or 8 weeks)

ORTHOSIS. The exercise orthosis is discontinued. The patient still wears the dorsal blocking orthosis except for active flexion exercises.

EXERCISE. The SWM exercises (Fig. 36-15) continue every 2 hours, but now flexion is active. The patient is instructed to avoid simultaneous wrist and digit extension. FDS gliding also may be added. At 5 to 6 weeks, blocking and hook fists may be added if needed to improve tendon gliding.

Late Stage (starting at 7 to 8 weeks)

ORTHOSIS. The orthosis is discontinued.

EXERCISE. Progressive resistive exercise is initiated. The patient gradually resumes activities of daily living, with no restrictions by 14 weeks. FPL is moved more aggressively than digit flexors, and flexors to the small finger are moved the least aggressively, in the light of the authors' clinical observation that repairs of these tendons are the most prone to deformation and rupture.[117]

Silfverskiöld and May.[118] These authors have added an active hold component to their previously published early passive mobilization protocol (see the May and colleagues' protocol,[95] discussed earlier) in patients whose zone II FDP tendons were repaired with a modified Kessler core suture and a new epitenon suture (the "cross-stitch"). The wrist is positioned in neutral instead of 30 to 45 degrees of flexion, but the orthosis is otherwise identical to the early passive

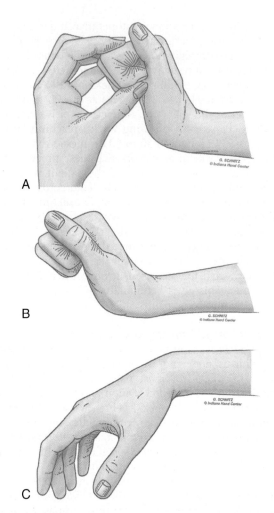

Figure 36-15 The exercise orthosis is discontinued at 4 weeks, but the patient continues tenodesis exercises. **A,** The wrist is extended, with passive digit flexion, maintained actively **(B). C,** The patient then allows the wrist to relax into flexion with simultaneous digit extension. (From Cannon N. *Indiana Hand Cen News.* 1993;1:13–17.)

mobilization protocol (MCP joints in 50–70 degrees flexion and orthosis extending only to the PIP joints). Exercises are similar to those outlined for the four-finger program, but after using the uninvolved hand to push the fingers of the involved hand into full flexion, the patient uses an active muscle contraction to maintain flexion of the involved fingers for 2 to 3 seconds. The program is progressed in the same manner as the four-finger protocol. In a prospective clinical study of 47 patients with 56 injured fingers, the authors demonstrated promising results. Note that in the original Swedish study, patients were hospitalized initially to ensure close compliance with the program. Nowadays Swedish patients performing this program are no longer hospitalized; there are no recently published results.

Evans and Thompson. Evans and Thompson[24] have examined the biomechanical aspects of early active hold mobilization using the concept of "minimal active muscle–tendon tension" (MAMTT), the minimal tension required to overcome the viscoelastic resistance of the antagonistic muscle–tendon unit. They calculated the drag encountered by each flexor tendon, the force necessary to overcome that drag, and the force normally exerted by the finger in flexion in various positions. Two central findings were that flexion forces increase dramatically at the end of the flexion range (in a full fist) and when digit flexion is combined with wrist flexion. The authors then surveyed currently used tendon repair sutures and designated guidelines for early place hold mobilization of the tendon with any suture used in combination with an epitenon running suture. They presented a retrospective review of 165 tendons (both flexor and extensor tendons) treated with their guidelines.

The MAMTT exercises are performed only under a therapist's supervision, while the patient follows an early passive mobilization program at home (which protocol is not specified by the authors; a dorsal blocking orthosis is used, without rubber band traction). For MAMTT exercise, the orthosis is removed. The wrist is passively placed in 20 degrees of extension and the finger passively flexed to 83 degrees at the MCP joint, 75 degrees at the PIP joint, and 40 degrees at the DIP joint. The patient is then asked to maintain the position with as gentle a muscle contraction as possible. The force of the muscle contraction is measured with a small (<150 g) Haldex pinch gauge. A loop of string passes perpendicularly around the gauge arm of the pinch meter and around the finger tip. The patient flexes the finger with a force of 50 g or less.

Unlike the Strickland/Cannon protocol, the Evans and Thompson guidelines suggest that few patients can perform this program at home. However, Evans[119] does state that she has patients perform active hold exercises with the uninvolved fingers at home, thus probably eliciting some active muscle–tendon tension in the involved fingers.

Assisted Active

Sandow and McMahon. These authors[120] take a rather unusual approach. They position the wrist in 20 degrees of extension to decrease passive extensor resistance to active flexion, and the MCP joints in 90 degrees of flexion, allowing full IP joint extension. They initiate assisted active flexion in the operating room. Exercises are performed hourly. The patient is seen weekly in therapy for adjustment to the program as needed. The orthosis is discontinued at 6 weeks, and buddy straps are applied for interim protection. The program is progressed in the same manner as other tendon management programs.

Timing of Initiation of Early Active Mobilization

Based on studies indicating that early motion increases repair strength,[2,22,26] most published protocols start motion at 24 to 48 hours after surgery. Several studies have now been published supporting a longer delay in initiating active motion. These studies all examine the work of flexion encountered during active motion at various points in the first week. Halikis and colleagues[75] compared immobilized repairs to those mobilized immediately, those mobilized at 3 days, and those mobilized at 5 days. They found that the work of flexion increased markedly in tendons mobilized immediately, whereas the work of flexion increased the least for tendons initiating active mobilization at 3 days. Other authors have recommended delaying initiation to 5 days[121,122] or 7 days.[123]

Treating Adhesion Problems

Restrictive adhesions are the most common complication after immobilization of the repaired flexor tendon. There are many techniques for mobilizing the adherent tendon, all aimed at gradually lengthening adhesions to allow greater glide. The object is not to break adhesions, because this internal trauma may lead to greater fibrosis and new adhesions.

The best way to treat adhesions is to prevent them or to catch them at a very early stage. To select the best method of treatment, the therapist first identifies the location and extent of adhesions, as described earlier. Precise identification of adhesions assists in planning precise intervention: if a single FDS tendon is adherent, exercise could focus on gliding of that single tendon, with or without resistance (see Fig. 36-8). If all FDS tendons are adherent, DIP joint extension orthoses may be worn during active and resistive exercises to aid in eliciting FDS glide.

A number of different exercises are designed to elicit greater excursion. A commonly used example is blocking exercises (as described earlier under "Immobilization") to isolate motion of a particular tendon. Blocking exercises can be dangerous for a newly healed tendon if not performed correctly. This is true particularly in the case of isolated DIP joint flexion. If the patient does not concentrate on flexing only the DIP joint but instead "fights" the fingers holding the PIP joint in extension, this active exercise becomes a strongly resisted exercise. When the finger is edematous and the FDP tendon is gliding poorly, the patient may have difficulty resisting the temptation to exercise too vigorously. Patient education includes the danger of rupture with overzealous blocking exercise; some patients may not be appropriate candidates for blocking until 2 or 3 weeks later, when the tendon repair is stronger.

Tendon gliding exercises (see Fig. 36-5) facilitate gliding of FDP and FDS as well as differential gliding to control intertendinous adhesions. If the patient has difficulty understanding how much force is safe to exert, light prehension with synergistic wrist motion may be helpful. If the patient does not understand the concept of synergistic wrist motion or appears to be flexing with excessive force, the following technique may be helpful. The patient sits with elbow on the table, wrist relaxed forward into flexion. He is instructed to extend the wrist while keeping the fingers relaxed. If he is able to do this, then the fingers automatically assume a midflexion position. If instead he extends his fingers along with his wrist, he is asked to extend the wrist while touching his fingers to his thumb or grasping a light object such as a pencil, held by the therapist. Often a functional grasp is much easier for an apprehensive patient to comprehend than a structured exercise.

Sustained grip activities such as dowel sanding, use of a rake or other garden implement, or bicycling elicit isometric flexor contraction. Some patients find it helpful to carry with them at all times a lipstick, a pill bottle, or other small cylinder that they can barely grip. Frequently throughout the day they grip the cylinder 10 times for 10 to 30 seconds.

Therapy putty squeezing or scraping resists tendon excursion and elicits stronger flexor contractions. Whenever possible, functional motions are used in place of exercise: "piano playing" on the tabletop, towel walking, paper crumpling, handling dice, grasping handfuls of packing "popcorn" or large beans, handling light objects of varying size and shape. The patient should be encouraged to resume daily activities as soon as it is safe, not only to facilitate reintegration of the involved fingers, but also to incorporate functional grasp activities to facilitate tendon excursion at home.

One of the most common mistakes made by patients is overdoing resistive exercise or a favorite activity, however light the resistance to flexion involved. This can provoke inflammation and lead to increased fibrosis and stiffness. Patients may develop trigger fingers (stenosing tenosynovitis) through excessive repetitive gripping or squeezing (as with putty exercise). The therapist must not only warn patients of this danger but also routinely palpate for triggering at the A1 pulley.

Neuromuscular electrical stimulation may be used to provoke a stronger muscle contraction; this is appropriate within 1 week of initiating resisted exercise. Ultrasound applied over the area of tendon adherence may be used to provide deep heat and when combined with passive extension active flexor tendon gliding can help to modify and lengthen adhesions. Interested readers are referred to Chapter 118 for further discussion. Superficial and deep scar respond well to soft tissue mobilization techniques such as cross-frictional massage. The patient also may actively contract the affected muscle while massaging over the adherent tendon; the tendon pulls proximally while the patient gently pushes the skin distally, stressing local adhesions.

If flexor adhesions limit extension, orthotic positioning and gentle passive extension may be necessary to regain functional extension. Orthotic options include dynamic and static-progressive extension orthoses for intermittent daytime use, and serial-static orthoses for night use.

Beyond Protocols: Clinical Decision Making

With all of the many tools and techniques at our disposal, the hardest decision is when to use which technique. All of the protocols described are meant to be guidelines rather than recipes. Following are examples of modifications to popular protocols, new directions in research, and new tools for assisting in application of rehabilitation techniques using clinical reasoning and integration of more recent research.

Prevention of Proximal Interphalangeal Joint Flexion Contractures

When the fingers are maintained in PIP joint flexion with dynamic traction, PIP joint flexion contractures often result. One solution is to remove the traction at night and strap the fingers in IP joint extension.[82,96,124] Therapists employ variations on night and intermittent day orthotic positioning to correct incipient PIP joint flexion contractures in both Kleinert and "modified Duran" protocols, particularly if a delicate digital nerve repair or other injury has mandated positioning the PIP joint in slight flexion initially.[124,125] A static PIP joint

extension orthosis may be inserted between the dorsal blocking orthosis and the dorsum of the finger to address this problem when it first develops. Prevention, however, is the best treatment.

Another reason for PIP joint flexion contractures may be the difficulty of extending the injured finger fully against excessive resistance. Recent studies[126,127] indicate that increasing the strength of dynamic flexion traction has no advantage; in fact, these electromyographic studies disagree with that of Lister and coworkers,[97] finding that flexor contraction is inconsistently inhibited no matter how great the resistance to extension (thus throwing some doubt on any use of resisted extension in early passive mobilization programs). Studies have shown that rubber bands offer increasing resistance as finger extension stretches the elastic further.[128-130] Burge and Brown[128] found that this increase could be moderated by use of a palmar pulley or by positioning the MCP joint in no more than 20 degrees of flexion. Patients may be instructed to manually release some rubber-band tension during exercise to ease extension as in the May and associates'[95] protocol.

Another proposed solution is to change the means of dynamic traction within the orthosis design. In the Washington regimen[93,129,131,132] (also known as modified Kleinert) two rubber bands are used, one of which is cut in half so that it forms a single strand. Before performing active extension exercises, the patient detaches proximally the intact rubber band so that only the single-strand elastic resists extension, making full extension easier to achieve. The finger rests in complete flexion to the distal palmar crease when not exercising. An orthosis design proposed by Werntz and colleagues[130] incorporates a coiled lever to offer a more constant resistance and make full extension easier to achieve. However, this orthosis is not commonly used, given the less expensive alternatives available.

Even in the absence of dynamic flexion traction, the patient may develop PIP joint flexion contractures if the volar wound and surgical incisions are allowed to limit PIP joint extension as they form scar and contract; if there is excessive edema; or if the patient has difficulty extending fully due to pain, apprehension, or an orthosis that blocks full extension. Unfortunately it is common for permanent PIP joint flexion contractures to develop. Any patient showing this tendency should be positioned in complete PIP joint extension as needed, using some combination of dynamic, static, or serial-static PIP joint extension positioning. If a patient is discharged from therapy with a residual PIP joint flexion contracture, night positioning in extension is crucial for the first few months to a year.

Force and Excursion Issues

Excursion

McGrouther and Ahmed[88] found that complete excursion of the FDP and differential excursion between FDP and FDS could be accomplished only through flexion of the DIP joint; later this principle was found to be true also for the flexor pollicis longus (FPL). In other words, to achieve glide of a repair, it is necessary to flex the joints distal to the repair. Horibe's cadaver study of FDP excursion in zone II confirmed the importance of distal joint flexion but also found that PIP

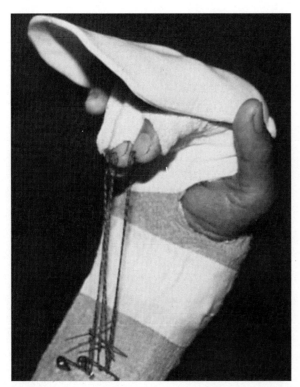

Figure 36-16 In the Kleinert orthosis as originally designed, the metacarpophalangeal joint and proximal interphalangeal joint are held in flexion by rubber-band traction, but the distal interphalangeal joint rests in almost complete extension.

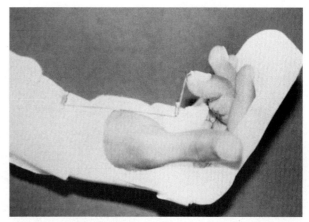

Figure 36-17 A simple palmar pulley can be provided by a safety pin attached to a palmar strap at distal palmar crease level. The line passes through the "eye" of the safety pin to direct the pull precisely.

joint flexion appears to produce the greatest excursion relative to the tendon sheath.[87] Silfverskiöld and colleagues, in their series of in vivo studies, initially found results agreeing with Horibe's.[100] Later, using a larger number of cases, they found a significant correlation between controlled passive DIP joint ROM and FDP excursion.[81] All of these studies taken together suggest that early passive mobilization programs should incorporate the greatest possible degree of flexion in the IP joints. Remember also the difference noted by Strickland and others[21,86-89,133] regarding the reduced passive excursion in the repaired flexor tendon.

In the standard dynamic flexion orthosis as first designed by Kleinert, the rubber-band traction is directed from the wrist or distal forearm to the fingernail. This flexes the MCP joint and to a lesser extent the PIP joint but leaves the DIP joint in virtual extension (Fig. 36-16). Slattery and McGrouther[134] proposed adding a palmar pulley to redirect dynamic traction and thus fully flex the DIP joint (Fig. 36-17). This orthosis innovation (also known as modified Kleinert) has become standard practice with zone II FDP injuries. Brown and McGrouther[84] later suggested that similarly, in FPL lacerations the thumb MCP joint be immobilized and efforts directed toward mobilizing the IP joint.

Evans[94] published her analysis of the excursion data and results of an early passive mobilization program specifically designed for zone I injuries, which are prone to excursion problems, given the limited excursion available in the uninjured zone I FDP. She keeps the DIP joint positioned in flexion with a small orthosis within the larger dorsal protec-

tive orthosis. She has also used a similar approach with early active mobilization.[135]

Cooney and others[87,98] conducted a cadaver study comparing the total FDP, total FDS, and differential FDP/FDS excursion obtained at three levels (zones II, III, and V) using three different methods. The first was original Kleinert traction directed from the distal forearm. The second was an orthosis with a palmar pulley (Brooke Army orthosis or modified Kleinert orthosis). Third was a new orthosis using SWM to produce a dynamic tenodesis effect: wrist flexion producing finger extension and wrist extension producing finger flexion. The study found that although all three orthoses produced adequate total excursion (judged according to Duran and Houser's recommended 3–5 mm), the Brooke Army orthosis produced more than did the Kleinert, and the SWM orthosis produced the greatest excursion of all. Surprisingly, in view of previously cited tendon excursion studies,[87,88,100] the traditional Kleinert orthosis produced more differential gliding than did the Brooke Army; the SWM orthosis again outperformed both of the other orthoses.

More recent studies have examined the relative excursion and force in varying combinations of wrist and finger motion. Several authors[136-140] have concluded the following: passive flexion and extension of the digits produces low excursion with low force to the repair if the wrist is held in flexion, high excursion with high force to the repair if the wrist is held in extension, and high excursion with low force to the repair if the wrist moves synergistically (wrist extends with finger flexion and flexes with finger extension).

In 2005 Amadio and Tanaka[141,142] each published studies that propose a modified SWM exercise for increased excursion with early passive mobilization (Fig. 36-18). The hand starts in full finger and wrist flexion. The first step is passive extension and flexion of the involved digit. The next is extension of the wrist with the fingers held in flexion. Finally, with the wrist still held in extension and the IP joints held in flexion, the MCP joint is extended as far as possible. Then the steps are reversed: MCP joint flexed, wrist flexed, and fingers extended. All of these steps are performed gradually and gently, with respect to soft tissue resistance and always

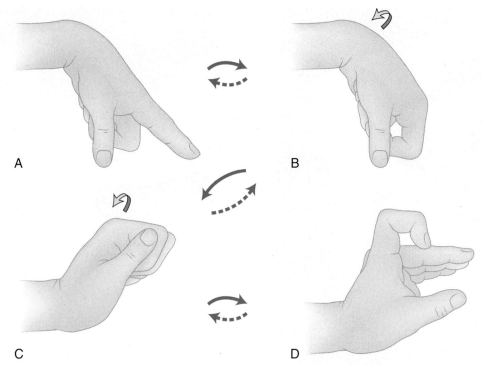

Figure 36-18 Modified passive synergistic wrist motion protocol. **A,** Passive full extension of metacarpophalangeal (MCP), PIP and DIP joints with wrist at 60 degrees flexion, to pull the tendon distally. **B,** Passive composite flexion of the finger, keeping the wrist flexed 60 degrees. **C,** Slow, careful wrist extension to 60 degrees (or maximum comfortable extension), with finger remaining flexed. **D,** Slow, careful MCP joint extension to 45 degrees hyperextension (or maximum comfortable extension). Steps are repeated in reverse order. (From Amadio PC. Friction of the gliding surface. Implications for tendon surgery and rehabilitation. *J Hand Ther.* 2005;18:112.)

following gentle and persistent protected joint passive range of motion and edema control measures.

Motion Versus Tension

There is an ongoing debate regarding the relative importance of the two different kinds of stress applied to the healing tendon: the motion imparted to the tendon and the tension or force placed on the repair. As noted before, Kubota and coworkers[26] found that the rate of cellular activity at the repair site was greater with either motion or tension than with neither, but greatest with a combination of the two.

Closer examination of excursion and force variables suggests that in a canine model, increased excursion (>1.7 mm) does not improve ultimate excursion or tensile properties of the repair.[138] This contradicts the earlier finding of Silfverskiöld and colleagues[81] that the greater the passive excursion (≤6–9 mm, after which the benefit is less) the greater will be the ultimate active excursion. Furthermore, high force (simultaneous extension and flexion of wrist and digits, or force increased from 5 to 17 N) does not appear to improve healing or increase the rate at which the repair gains strength.[143,144] As a result of these studies, the therapist must conclude the following: (1) synergistic wrist motion is the safest (high excursion and low force) means of attaining the highest excursion during exercise, whether active or passive; (2) although both motion and stress to the repair are responsible for the known benefits of early mobilization, there is no evidence that high force is

more effective than lower force in improving strength or excursion of the tendon; there is no definitive answer about how much early passive or active excursion is need for optimal results.

Choosing the Right Approach and Progressing the Program Appropriately

The most important question in therapy following flexor tendon repair is how to treat the patient in the first few weeks. Simplistically speaking, this boils down to immobilization, early passive mobilization, and early active mobilization. In a perfect world, with a perfect patient, surgeon, and therapist, early active mobilization is the treatment of choice. However, this is not possible for all patients. With a patient who is unable to follow an early mobilization program (because of youth, illness, or other factors), immobilization is the only choice. With a patient who can follow a complex program, early active or passive mobilization should be used. If early mobilization is the choice, then further decisions are dictated by a number of factors, including strength of repair; edema and other sources of resistance to tendon glide; the frequency with which patient can attend therapy; surgical preference; and the therapist's preference, clinical reasoning skills, and degree of autonomy in making decisions. A recent article by Groth[145] examines clinical decision making and therapists' autonomy in making clinical decisions regarding flexor tendon management.

Surgeon–therapist team A may decide to use early passive mobilization with a patient who appears able to participate

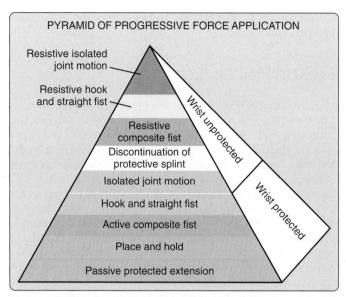

Figure 36-19 Progressive application of force to the repaired intrasynovial flexor tendon. (From Groth G. Pyramid of progressive force exercises to the injured flexor tendon. *J Hand Ther.* 2004;17:31.)

but a little overenthusiastic: a possible risk of rupture in the event of inadvertent "cheating" on an early active mobilization program.

Surgeon–therapist team B may decide on early active mobilization for their patient because the suture is strong, the edema well-controlled, and the patient apparently very cautious.

In both of these cases, either tissue response or patient response may not be as anticipated, and the plan may need changing on the subsequent visits. It's incumbent on surgeons and therapists to understand that just as not every patient can follow a certain protocol, many patients need a more nuanced approach to treatment, with the plan changing as needed in accordance with findings at each visit. In addition, using one or more of several available clinical decision-making models, the therapist and surgeon can carefully examine the available information and design a program that allows for increasing or decreasing force and excursion, switching from passive to active mobilization and otherwise upgrading the program in a logical and safe fashion.

Groth[4] devised the Pyramid of Progressive Force Exercises, a model for systematic evaluation and progression of stress applied to the healing tendon, based on existing studies of tendon excursion and loading. She used the concept of a pyramid with nine levels (Fig. 36-19) to illustrate the model. The broad base of the pyramid represents exercises applying the lowest force to the repair, and therefore prescribed most frequently; the apex of the pyramid represents exercises applying the highest force, and therefore prescribed least frequently. The nine levels are further divided into exercises performed with the wrist protected (the lowest five levels) and the wrist unprotected. The adhesion grading system discussed earlier (see Table 36-1) aids the therapist in determining when to progress the program. Essentially, the program is progressed when a flexion lag is present and does not respond adequately to current treatment.

A brief description of the nine levels and their rationale follows. Passive protected digital extension consists of passive flexion and extension of the IP joints, both independently and in composite motion, together with SWM to increase excursion and decrease force applied to the repair. The next level is place-and-hold finger flexion in 20 degrees of wrist extension and partial finger flexion, similar to the Evans and Thompson exercises, designed to gain composite active flexion with low stress. The third level exercise is full active composite flexion (increased force to the repair) with slight wrist extension. At the fourth level, hook and straight-fist exercises are added to increase total and differential tendon excursion. Isolated joint motion is the fifth level, adding blocking for FDP gliding, PIP joint flexion and FDS gliding to increase the force to the tendon repair. The remaining four levels, discontinuance of protective positioning, resistive composite fist, resistive hook and straight fist, and resistive isolated joint motion, all eliminate wrist protection (whether by incorporation of synergistic wrist motion or by holding a given wrist position during finger motion) and place successively increasing stress to the repair. Although excursion and force data are still limited, Groth's program uses what data are available to logically relate tendon response to treatment options. Thus she provides a useful tool for planning treatment according to tendon status, rather than according to a timed protocol. More recently von der Heyde presented her version of the pyramid, using essentially the same data to support synergistic wrist motion as proposed by Cannon.[146]

Another potentially useful tool is the concept of a safe zone, which the therapist and surgeon can use to balance surgical, patient, and therapeutic considerations in moving the tendon appropriately. This model, proposed by Amadio,[141] incorporates data on force, gliding resistance, and tendon repair strength, to illustrate the range of tendon loads that produce excursion but do not cause a rupture or tendon gap. In Figure 36-20 we see a narrow safe zone between forces (in newtons) capable of producing excursion and excessive forces with risk of gapping or rupture. Figure 36-21

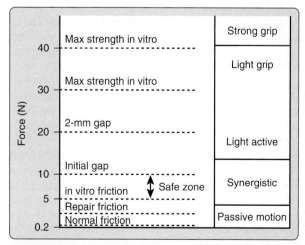

Figure 36-20 Small safe zone for a four-strand repair with 40-N (9-pound) breaking strength. (From Amadio PC. Friction of the gliding surface. Implications for tendon surgery and rehabilitation. *J Hand Ther.* 2005;18:112.)

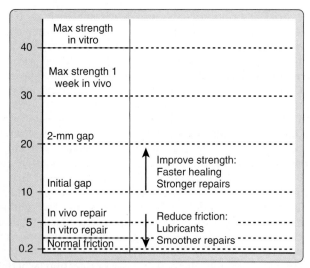

Figure 36-21 *Larger safe zone with increased suture repair strength and faster healing, and reduced friction through the use of lubricants and repairs with smooth gliding surfaces. (From Amadio PC. Friction of the gliding surface. Implications for tendon surgery and rehabilitation.* J Hand Ther. *2005;18:112.)*

illustrates how the safe zone is expanded with increased repair strength or reduction of resistance to gliding.

Groth's and Amadio's models can be used together. The clinician can determine the safe zone at initiation of therapy and then decide how to initiate motion while staying within that safe zone. If complications arise (e.g., unexpected increase in edema), the safe zone contracts, and therefore the plan must be modified to place less stress on the repair or to stay at the same level of stress until the safe zone can be expanded (e.g., if edema decreases). The adhesion-grading system helps the clinician decide when levels of stress must be modified, and the force pyramid gives a structured way to choose how to increase or control stress to the repair.

Although the steps delineated by Groth are appropriate, they need not be adhered to unquestioningly. For example, some patients have difficulty learning how firmly to stabilize the PIP joint when isolating DIP joint motion and may endanger the FDS repair by actually resisting FDS. The same patients may more easily apply an appropriate amount of stress using functional grasp activities such as picking up and transferring large pieces of polyester batting.

The force pyramid and the concept of the safe zone can be applied to existing programs such as the Indianapolis hinged orthosis program. There is no requirement that the patient delay active mobilization and start with passive mobilization. The therapist may choose active (place-and-hold) mobilization in a hinged orthosis, as long as the safe zone allows.

We prefer to start therapy with postoperative orthosis application as soon as possible after surgery. If we are using active mobilization, we start with gentle passive motion and edema control and delay initiation of active mobilization until 3 to 5 days after surgery to allow inflammation to subside somewhat and reduce the work of flexion. We always precede active flexion exercises with edema control measures and passive flexion to reduce tissue resistance and

always integrate a modified Duran approach with active mobilization.

Flexor Pollicis Longus

Management of flexor pollicis longus (FPL) repairs presents a different set of problems to the therapist, for several reasons. Lacerated FPL tendons tend to retract further and more quickly than do the finger flexors. This may be due to the lack of a lumbrical origin to restrain retraction, fewer interconnections with the adjacent tendons, or, as Elliot and Southgate have speculated,[147] to an inherent tendency of the FPL muscle itself to shorten rapidly. Even a short delay to surgery may require not only a separate proximal incision at or near the wrist to retrieve the proximal FPL, but also a repair performed under tension. Tendon-lengthening procedures can decrease tension on the repair, but additional adhesions may result from lengthening as well as from the proximal incision and the process of pulling the proximal stump into place for repair. To complicate matters further, there are often concurrent injuries to digital neurovascular structures, thenar muscles, and the branches of median and ulnar nerves in the thenar eminence. One study found that 74% of FPL injuries studied were in zone II, and 82% involved injury to one or both neurovascular bundles.[148] The challenges presented, therefore, are (1) to repair the tendon as early as possible, under as little tension as possible, and with the strongest suture feasible; (2) to restore motion with a program that is aggressive enough to produce functional excursion by preventing or modifying dense adhesions and yet cautious enough to prevent rupture; and (3), in the presence of irreparable digital nerve injury, to restore thumb function without return of full sensation.

As we plan our treatment, it's vital to understand the balance of muscle activity controlling the thumb and the functional results of residual strength and ROM deficits. An electromyographic study by Cooney and colleagues[149] found that the FPL was the primary muscle involved in isometric flexion and one of the primary muscles (along with adductor pollicis, flexor pollicis brevis and opponens pollicis) involved in key pinch, but it played a secondary role in other kinds of pinch. In addition, there remains disagreement as to the functional impairment posed by limited IP joint flexion, with some stating that limited IP joint extension (−25 degrees) and flexion (30 degrees) does not significantly impede function.[148]

Given the relative paucity of published studies on rehabilitation of FPL repairs, most therapists position the wrist in some degree of flexion, the thumb in mild carpometacarpal (CMC) joint flexion and palmar abduction, the MCP joint in flexion, and the IP joint allowed full extension. For passive mobilization, some use an adapted Kleinert technique, but others use a form of modified Duran. Whichever passive technique is used for zone I and II repairs, the therapist should incorporate immobilization of the MCP joint during passive IP joint flexion, based on the work of Brown and McGrouther,[84] who found no FPL gliding over the proximal phalanx with MCP joint flexion, compared with considerable glide with the MCP joint immobilized and the IP joint passively flexed and extended.

The published studies on rehabilitation of FPL repairs use a variety of means of mobilization and methods of assessing results, making them difficult to compare. The majority of studies examine immobilization or early passive mobilization (or both). Interestingly no studies have large enough populations to recommend one over the other.

A recent series of articles by Elliott, Sirotakova, and colleagues[103,147,150,151] have taken a systematic look at early active mobilization, raising some interesting questions. They compared four different groups of patients with variations on suture and postoperative management. Results improved with three specific elements: (1) immobilization of the fingers between exercise sessions (to prevent the inadvertent thumb IP joint flexion that accompanies grasp and may have increased the rupture rate), (2) wrist position in 10 degrees of ulnar deviation and 10 degrees of wrist extension (to reduce stress at the point where the FPL changes course at the distal border of the carpal canal), and (3) the stronger suture (four-strand core and cross-stitch circumferential suture). Although the authors note no evidence comparing early passive to early active mobilization, and therefore do not recommend one over the other, they do recommend a four-strand core and cross-stitch circumferential suture.

The active mobilization program as most recently published[147] involves active opposition of the thumb tip first to the tip of the middle finger in the first week, to the tip of the ring finger in the second week, and then as far as possible thereafter. Flexion was assisted and more vigorous passive flexion was added as needed.[112]

A Special Case: Multiple Tendon and Nerve Lacerations in Zone V

Laceration of multiple flexor tendons in zone V presents a special problem in management. As noted earlier, in zone V (from proximal edge of carpal tunnel to the musculotendinous junction) the flexor tendons lie in close proximity both to each other and to major nerves (median and ulnar) and arteries (radial and ulnar). This type of injury has been labeled "spaghetti wrist," "suicide wrist," and "full-house syndrome" by various authors.[111,152-156] As with all flexor tendon injuries besides those in zone II, there is very little in the literature to indicate the best postoperative management. However, to design the appropriate program, we can draw on experience, a good understanding of how the involved structures heal, and both specific and related literature.

The psychosocial ramifications of such injuries are significant, but luckily not insurmountable. A certain percentage of these injuries are due to suicide attempts, so that one might expect a poor prognosis due to psychological and emotional issues. However, some authors have found favorable results and improved psychological status after such injuries. Many sustain these injuries on broken glass, often when an angry young man punches his fist through a glass window. Again the immaturity and poor impulse control of the patient seem to predict compromised results, but youth is to the patient's advantage, with better results having been noted in younger patients by some authors.

These patients, correctly treated, generally attain satisfactory or full digit flexion, since the extrasynovial tendons can produce full flexion even with excursion limited by relatively heavy adhesions to the overlying skin and surrounding tissues. Independent FDS glide is difficult to achieve, but has not been found to impair function. In fact, recent research indicates that in the normal hand, FDS may not glide as independently as one might assume.[157] Wrist and digit extension are commonly limited to some extent by flexor adhesions. There may be limitations in isolated wrist extension as well as in composite wrist and digit extension. In most cases, either passive extension can be regained over time through diligent treatment, or the patient finds that the lack of extension is not a functional impairment.

A greater problem is reinnervation. Both sensory and intrinsic muscle reinnervation are needed for a full functional recovery. One small study suggests that ulnar nerve injuries may have a poorer prognosis than median nerve injuries.[156] In any case, in addition to impaired flexor tendon function, these patients lack part or all of their intrinsic muscle function (depending on which nerve is injured) as well as median or ulnar nerve sensibility. Unless and until reinnervation occurs, patients may injure their insensate fingers when attempting to use their hands normally and may have difficulty with prehension and strong grip due to lack of normal sensory feedback. They lack full grip strength and pinch strength in the absence of intrinsic muscle power and miss the control and balance afforded by the intrinsics for fine dexterity. Over time, if not carefully treated, they may develop deformities ("claw hand" or "ape hand," PIP joint flexion contractures, thumb adduction contracture) that are both unattractive and an impediment to function.

The literature includes both early passive mobilization[152-156,158] and early active mobilization[111] approaches. As always, the approach should be selected according to the individual patient's characteristics, with preference given to early mobilization of some sort. All of the published protocols keep the wrist in some flexion, but as with injuries at other levels, the recent trend is toward less wrist flexion. Too much wrist flexion can make it very difficult to regain extension with an injury so close to the wrist and to the flexor retinaculum, a prime source for flexor adhesions.

Our preference is to protect the patient with wrist as close to neutral as possible and the MCP joints flexed about 40 degrees. Holding the MCP joints in flexion might encourage some intrinsic tightness, which is a bonus when a long wait for return of nerve function is expected. Nerves repaired under tension must be very carefully protected with more wrist flexion.

Early management is similar to that for injuries in other zones, with the following special considerations. As soon as possible after active mobilization is initiated, the program should include differential tendon gliding. Because passive extension is so often a problem, these patients may need nighttime serial static extension positioning (see Fig. 36-6) as early as 4 weeks after repair, and dynamic extension positioning during the day beginning within the following week. Often the flexor tightness limits the "clawing" produced by intrinsic palsies, but if not, an "anticlaw" orthosis of some sort (preventing MCP joint hyperextension but allowing full wrist and finger flexion) may be needed to prevent development of a full-fledged claw deformity. The therapist may opt as well to forego intrinsic stretch exercises in the protective stage, so that some intrinsic tightness is allowed to develop as noted earlier.

Summary

This chapter has reviewed the fundamentals of tendon management and explored a range of management approaches. No single source can prepare the clinician to treat the repaired flexor tendon. Readers are urged to read both the original references cited in discussion of each protocol and the research that validates each approach.

As we study suture strength and gliding properties, measure muscle–tendon force, gather data, and choose the protocol based on scientific principles, we must not lose sight of the most important variable of all: the patient. After all, our job is patient care. Without a motivated patient who is able to participate fully in her rehabilitation, all our efforts are in vain. So understanding is really the key to effective postoperative management of the flexor tendon, understanding the scientific basis for our intervention, and understanding the patient herself.

REFERENCES

The complete reference list is available online at www.expertconsult.com.

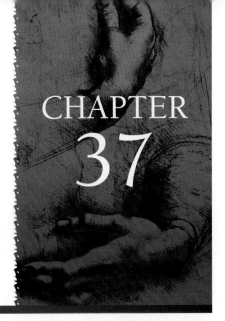

Staged/Delayed Tendon Reconstruction

EDWARD DIAO, MD AND NANCY CHEE, OTR/L, CHT

PART I: STAGED/DELAYED TENDON RECONSTRUCTION

If the acute flexor tendon repair and rehabilitation is one of the measurements for the successful interplay among surgical decision making, application of operative techniques, efficacy of therapy, and participation of patient, surgeon, and therapist, then delayed tendon reconstruction is perhaps one of the greatest challenges to the hand reconstruction and rehabilitation team.

Several factors are primary considerations in the decision making regarding delayed flexor tendon reconstruction. A delayed presentation due to missed injuries or owing to concomitant conditions is unavoidable for the treating team. The obvious considerations at the time of presentation and preoperative planning are the condition of the wound and digits and hand, including associated injuries, quality of skin and soft tissue coverage, presence of bone and joint injuries and nerve and vascular injuries, and overall medical condition of the patient. These can determine the quality of the tendon bed and are contributing factors to the overall success rate of the surgical reconstruction and the efficacy of the rehabilitation protocol. The length of time between injury and reconstruction is a determinant of the soft tissue changes in and around the fibro-osseous tunnel as well as the length–tension relationship of the severed muscle–tendon unit. Sometimes associated medical conditions, the overall condition of the traumatized patient, or healing soft tissue injuries may determine the eventual timing of delayed treatment.

At the time of reconstruction, the following factors play a direct role in surgical decision making:

1. Quality of the fibro-osseous tunnel
2. Status of the critical pulleys
3. The muscle–tendon excursion and length

The surgical choices available to the patient for delayed flexor tendon reconstruction include the following:

1. Direct repair after successful stretching of the proximal tendon and muscle unit to restore normal length–tension relationships
2. Direct repair after lengthening of the muscle–tendon unit proximally at the forearm, in the muscle belly and at the musculotendinous junction
3. Direct repair with Z-lengthening of the tendon proximally in the palm to restore normal length–tension relationships

4. Immediate tendon grafting using a short interposition graft between the proximal and distal ends of the separated tendon

5. Immediate tendon grafting with the distal junction at the connection to the distal stump, or at the flexor digitorum profundus (FDP) insertion, and the proximal end in the forearm level proximal to the palm using the original motor muscle–tendon unit

6. A superficialis finger in which proximal interphalangeal (PIP) joint motion is retained or reconstructed to be obtained and distal interphalangeal (DIP) joint active motion is sacrificed with tenodesis or arthrodesis of the DIP joint

7. Staged tendon reconstruction with placement of a silicon flexor tendon rod and, if necessary, pulley reconstruction followed by free tendon graft

The contemporary hand reconstructive surgeon should be prepared to employ any of these strategies to successfully reconstruct an injured digit. It is important for these possibilities to be discussed with the patient preoperatively so that the patient is prepared. This is particularly true if there is a possibility of a staged tendon reconstruction with at least two surgical reconstructions, both associated with rehabilitation protocols, with significant time intervals between the surgical events. The overall time required for the staged tendon reconstruction may be a year or more. If immediate or secondary tendon grafting is necessary, another decision needs to be made about the donor site for the tendon and whether this should be an extrasynovial or an intrasynovial tendon graft to be harvested from the lower extremity.

This chapter is written in two parts. We have preserved intact, in the online supplement, the chapter by James Hunter and Evelyn Mackin[1] on staged flexor tendon reconstruction, which remains accurate in large part to the present day. We offer some commentary on the role of this type of reconstruction. Because significant advances have been made in primary flexor tendon reconstruction techniques and results, the indications for staged flexor tendon reconstruction have narrowed to some extent. In cases of complex injury, significantly delayed treatment, and failed prior flexor tendon surgery, staged flexor tendon reconstruction remains an important technique. We focus on the other treatment options described earlier for both decision making and execution of surgery. A discussion of rehabilitation after flexor tendon reconstruction follows.

Direct Repair Approaches

Minimizing the time between injury and surgery is desirable. With the passage of time the likelihood of a tendon–muscle contracture is greater, complicating the surgical tactics. The passage of time also increases the likelihood that soft tissue changes at the fibro-osseous tunnel will interfere with successful gliding of a repaired or reconstructed flexor tendon. Nevertheless, in some instances a delay in repair is inevitable due to the timing of the referral, associated injuries, and other considerations. During the first several weeks after an acute flexor tendon injury, a direct repair is usually possible. However, the goal is restoration of the preinjury length–tension relationship of the injured flexor tendon. Therefore,

it behooves the surgeon to attempt to restore normal length–tension relationships prior to or during the repair surgery.

The simplest technique for restoring relationships in the contracted muscle–tendon unit is to retrieve the proximal end of the tendon and apply tension.[2] Retrieval of the proximal tendon is discussed in Chapter 35 on acute flexor tendon injuries. Retrieval can be performed (1) by carefully grasping the tendon within the fibro-osseous tunnel system proximally toward the wrist using a fine mosquito or tendon passer, (2) by making proximal "windows" in the fibro-osseous tunnel system until the proximal tendon end can be grasped and then sequentially delivered distally along the fibro-osseous tunnel system using surgical instruments, or (3) by passing suture into the proximal stump and delivering the tendon utilizing the suture from proximal to distal windows and eventually to the site of the distal stump. Sometimes a stainless steel wire loop or red rubber catheter can facilitate passage of the tendon and tendon suture.

Using an instrument such as Kelly's or Kocher's clamp, 5 minutes of manual tension by the surgeon can, in some circumstances, successfully restore the muscle–tendon unit to preinjury status and overcome early myostatic changes. If this is achieved, and the quality of the fibro-osseous tunnel is acceptable (in instances where the critical A2 and A4 pulleys are functioning and intact), the protocol for acute flexor tendon laceration with direct repair using multistrand techniques can be performed.

Myriad repair techniques are available. They should all take advantage of a multistrand core system, and the use of a peripheral suture to both improve gliding potential and add additional strength to the tendon repair.[3-5] If the tendon does not revert to its original length–tension relationship, the surgeon can consider several options.

Flexor Digitorum Profundus Avulsion Injuries

FDP tendon avulsion injuries fall into several injury categories. In Leddy type II injuries with modest retraction of the avulsed tendon to the level of Camper's chiasm, or in Leddy type III injuries with avulsions that stay at the DIP joint level, primary repair can generally be performed even if delayed past 6 weeks because retraction and length–tension changes are modest. In Leddy type I injuries, the avulsed FDP tendon retracts into the palm, and vincular injury, sheath hematoma, and myostatic contracture ensues. Generally after 6 weeks, primary repair is not possible, and the following described surgical techniques can be employed.[6-8] The decision in this situation is whether to perform delayed flexor tendon reconstruction for the FDP tendon, as outlined in the introduction, in the face of normal FDS function in order to improve overall digital function.[9,10]

Direct Repair with Lengthening at the Musculotendinous Junction

For direct repair with lengthening at the musculotendinous junction the surgeon makes a proximal incision in the forearm and identifies the affected flexor tendon. To identify the proper muscle–tendon units, one uses standard techniques with a sequential application of tension applied proximally in the forearm to the individual units, noting the end effect in the various digits. The lacerated unit has an abnormally blunted or complete lack of digital flexion effect, depending on the extent and location of laceration. Once the appropriate tendon has been identified, the musculotendinous juncture is carefully dissected with scissor technique while manual tension is applied on the distal portion of the muscle–tendon unit using a Kessler or Bunnell suture on the tendon to pull on the unit and provide some tension. By dissecting the fibers of the muscle as they insert on the tendon itself, approximately a centimeter of length can be achieved without full disruption of the muscle to the proximal tendon. If there are some concerns about the integrity of this juncture, sutures can be applied to reinforce the muscle relationship to the tendon using mattress-type sutures or a Bunnell weave. This technique works when approximately a centimeter of length or less will restore normal length–tension relationships. After this is achieved, a delayed primary repair of the flexor tendon can be performed.

Direct Repair with Z-Lengthening of the Tendon in the Palm

An alternative to the previously described technique is to perform the delayed primary repair of the muscle–tendon unit first by suturing the distal flexor tendon injury. In this case, the resting position of the digit exhibits abnormally increased flexion compared with its neighbors, and the normal "cascade" of the digits in a resting position is disrupted. At this point, after repair at this juncture, if the injury is in zone 1 or zone 2 of the fibro-osseous tunnel, a proximal lengthening can be performed by a Z-lengthening of the tendon in the palm level. A longitudinal split of approximately 3 cm is performed using a tongue depressor and a #15 or #11 blade. This allows increased length in the muscle–tendon unit proximal to the direct repair, which can be adjusted so that normal length–tension relationships are restored. Once the appropriate lengthening has been achieved, three nonabsorbable mattress sutures are placed to create a secure robust side-to-side repair between the two lengthened split limbs of the tendon. If planned appropriately, this juncture lies proximal to the fibro-osseous tunnel and distal to the carpal canal (Fig. 37-1).

Immediate Tendon Grafting

If the quality of the fibro-osseous tunnel is reasonable but the gap distance between the proximal and distal ends is quite long and cannot be overcome by the above-mentioned techniques, then immediate tendon grafting can be considered. Short-segment immediate tendon grafting can be performed by a repair to the proximal and distal junctures of the cut ends of the tendon. The type of suture used is dictated by the location of the injury. If the injuries are at the level of the fibro-osseous tunnel, then the standard zone 1 or zone 2 flexor tendon repair techniques are required. Alternatively,

the distal FDP tendon can be debrided and the tendon graft attached to the FDP stump and to the bone. There are several ways to do this.[11-13] In short-segment flexor tendon grafting, the proximal stump may lie proximal to zone 2, in the midpalm in zone 3, in which case a more bulky but stronger repair may be acceptable.

Depending on the placement of the proximal juncture or the amount of damage to the proximal muscle–tendon unit, the surgeon may elect to perform a long tendon graft and have the proximal tendon end come proximal to the wrist and be sutured into the muscle–tendon donor near the musculotendinous junction. This places the proximal repair far away from the zone of injury and where the bulk of the repair will not be affected either underneath the transverse carpal ligament or by the fibro-osseous tunnel constraints. Also, the repair can be performed as a tendon weave, and in this way a robust repair can be performed that is unlikely to rupture.[14-20]

Superficialis Finger

The surgeon and patient may elect to have a "superficialis" finger in any of the following circumstances: when there is significant damage to the FDP tendon, when the DIP joint is damaged, when the quality of the fibro-osseous tunnel from the PIP joint distally is severely compromised, when complex bone and joint injuries occur distal to the PIP joint, or when there is damage to the A4 pulley system. In this technique the function of digital flexion is provided by FDS only. When an isolated zone 1 injury occurs, which is the only flexor tendon injury, and a superficialis muscle–tendon unit is intact, tendon reconstruction is not required. In this case addressing the associated soft tissue problems is appropriate. Additionally, depending on the laxity of the DIP joint and the possibility of hyperextension or "joint collapse" with pinch, either tenodesis using a distal stump of FDP or arthrodesis using pin or screws across the DIP joint after preparation of DIP joint for arthrodesis can be performed. If the proximal FDP stump is tender to palpation or deep pressure when gripping functions are performed, excision of the proximal stump to shorten it so the proximal end lies in the proximal palm, carpal canal, or forearm is indicated. This may be an acceptable reconstruction, given the lengthy alternative of staged tendon reconstruction or when the expectation of success of staged tendon reconstruction is guarded given concomitant injury to the digit.

Pulley Reconstruction

Staged tendon reconstruction may be desirable in the face of simultaneous tendon and pulley damage since it is difficult to successfully reconstruct a critical pulley and a flexor tendon and to rehabilitate both simultaneously. In these cases a staged tendon reconstruction is an excellent choice, with formal pulley reconstruction being performed at the time of the index (stage one) operation. The benefit of this staged tendon reconstruction is that with passive tendon rods there is no significant tension on the pulley, which is given an opportunity to heal prior to passage of an active tendon unit, tendon rod, or tendon graft.

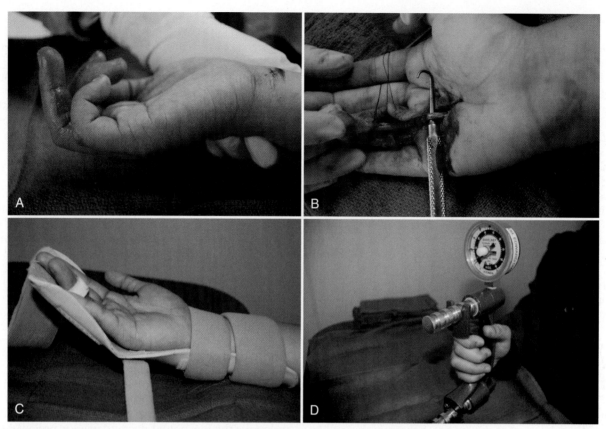

Figure 37-1 A, This 28-year-old woman sustained a work injury when she fell off of a ladder. She sustained a laceration to her fourth finger with loss of digital flexion at the distal interphalangeal (DIP) joint and loss of sensibility in the finger. The patient was taken to surgery 1 month after the injury due to authorization issues with her workman's compensation case. **B,** Intraoperatively, the proximal and distal tendon ends were identified and mobilized in zone 2 and repaired with a 3-0 Ticron suture ×2. Because of the chronic contracture despite stretching of the proximal muscle–tendon unit, the patient had loss of normal cascade. A decision was made to perform a Z-lengthening of the flexor digitoum profundus tendon proximal to the level of the repair to avoid the use of an interposition tendon graft or a Z-stage tendon reconstruction with silicone rod. **C,** The postoperative extension block orthosis is seen as well as the pulley ring to protect the A4 pulley. **D,** Postoperatively, the patient gradually regained normal motion of the proximal interphalangeal joint, and with gripping, excellent DIP joint motion and strength were restored as indicated on the dynamometer.

The traditional pulley reconstructions utilize flexor tendon remnants, either FDP for staged flexor tendon reconstruction in which flexor tendon is sacrificed or in situations where FDS can be removed for the purposes of tendon pulley reconstruction.

An alternative source can be extensor or flexor retinaculum from the wrist. This alternative has the advantage of thinner tissue, which still has good strength. The desired repair at the proximal phalanx level for the A2 pulley is to have a continuous loop of tissue that is passed dorsally underneath the extensor apparatus and between the extensor and the dorsum of the proximal phalanx bone and volarly at the level of the fibro-osseous tunnel. It can be sutured to itself and supplemental sutures placed to the surrounding soft tissue. Alternatively, remnants of the fibro-osseous tunnel attachment to the phalanx itself can be utilized to suture the graft, or used as a belt loop to pass the graft through. In this way, a non-360-degree circumferential pulley reconstruction can be performed. This can be a much weaker pulley reconstruction, however, and has a higher likelihood of failure than 360-degree circumferential pulley grafts.

At the level of the middle phalanx for the A4 pulley, the pulley reconstruction can have a 360-degree circumferential loop—in this case superficial to the extensor tendon mechanism dorsally as it goes into the terminal tendon insertion of the DIP joint level[21-39] (Fig. 37-2).

Intrasynovial Versus Extrasynovial Tendon Grafts

Work by Seiler and colleagues has demonstrated that intrasynovial tendon grafts behave differently from extrasynovial ones. Their method of incorporation and data on restoration of strength showed that tendons that start off as intrasynovial grafts when transplanted to the fibro-osseous tunnel sheath system incorporate more quickly than do extrasynovial tendon grafts. The papers describe techniques for harvesting intrasynovial tendon grafts from the lower extremity—from the flexor digitorum tendons in the sole of the foot[14,40-51] (see Fig. 37-2E, F).

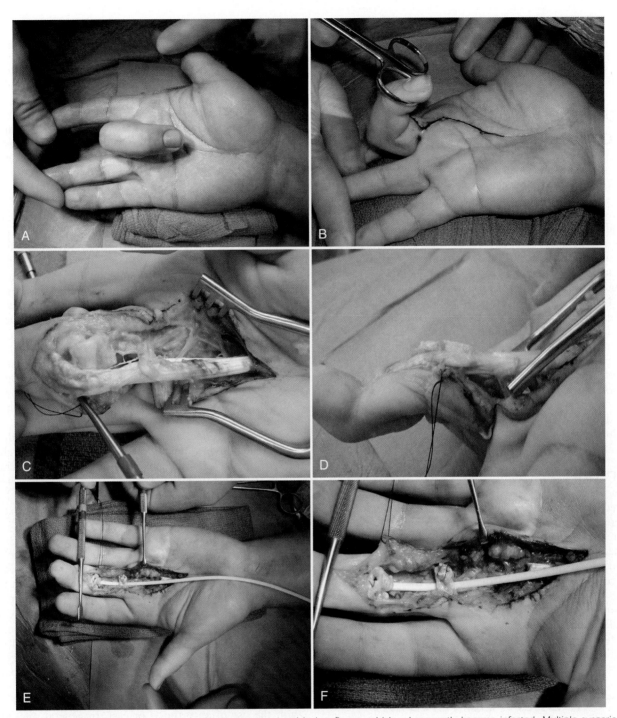

Figure 37-2 A, B, This 38-year-old woman had a puncture wound in her finger, which subsequently became infected. Multiple surgeries were performed, and the patient was referred with a fixed contracture. Other surgeons recommended amputation. My operative plan was surgical release and finger reconstruction. **C, D,** Intraoperative photographs showed proximal interphalangeal (PIP) joint contracture release with collateral ligament excision and demonstrated a volar plate insufficiency with PIP hyperextension. **E, F,** Because of the severe nature of the tendon dysfunction, a staged reconstruction was elected with use of flexor digitorum superficialis as pulley reconstruction and placement of a Silastic tendon rod.

Alternative Techniques: Flexor Digitorum Superficialis to Flexor Digitorum Profundus Transfer

In certain instances, digital injury of both flexor tendons may be reconstructed by taking the proximal FDS to be repaired distally to the FDP. This may be desirable when the level of the injuries to both tendons are favorable, and by performing this maneuver one may avoid having to do a flexor tendon graft or a staged tendon reconstruction. In performing this maneuver, a superficialis finger is converted to a finger that has both FDS and FDP function, active PIP and DIP flexion. The advantages are that a one-stage reconstruction can achieve active DIP flexion, using a working FDS motor–tendon unit. The disadvantage is the relative weakness of the FDS motor for both PIP and DIP flexion. However, this may not be much of a difference compared with single-motor FDP powering of both PIP and DIP flexion, as is the case in standard two-stage flexor tendon reconstruction.

Two-Stage Flexor Tendon Reconstruction

When the aforementioned strategies are unlikely to be successful due to damage to the fibro-osseous tendon sheath and pulley system or because of salvage situations with extensive injuries, a two-stage tendon reconstruction is recommended. Critical steps include careful planning of incisions to allow access to the fibro-osseous sheath with a combination of volar zigzag incisions (so-called Brunner's incisions) and midaxial lateral incisions. Proper planning allows for coverage and advancement flap choices at the first- as well as the second-stage surgeries. Preparation of the tendon bed involves dilation of the sheath system, preservation of as much tissue as possible including pulleys, and selection of the appropriate-sized tendon implant. If joint contractures are present, these should be addressed with appropriate releases.[52] If there are pulley deficiencies, the pulleys should be reconstructed, especially the crucial A2 and A4 pulleys. The methods were described earlier[9,53,54] (see Fig. 37-2). For more detail, see the chapter by James Hunter and Evelyn Mackin in the online version of this text.

Summary

Delayed or staged flexor tendon reconstruction remains a challenge for the surgeon, rehabilitation specialist, and, of course, the patient. By using the principles and guidelines outlined in this chapter, treatment can be customized to the individual patient and situation to increase the likelihood of a successful outcome. For the surgeon, having the proficiency to perform a number of reconstructive techniques is mandatory, including tendon repair, tendon lengthening, immediate tendon grafting, staged tendon reconstruction, and pulley reconstruction. Rehabilitation is dictated by the strength of the repairs and extent of reconstructed tissues.

PART II: DELAYED TENDON RECONSTRUCTION: POSTOPERATIVE THERAPY

NANCY CHEE, OTR/L, CHT

Advances in surgical technique have allowed for better treatment choices in postoperative management and care of tendon reconstruction patients, including earlier mobilization of tendons and joints. Choices of postoperative treatment depend on strength of repair (multistrand repair with peripheral suturing), quality of tendon (frayed versus clean), and whether tendon sheath repair is needed. When these factors are optimal, intensive rehabilitation can be applied. Communication and collaboration between the surgeon and therapist is particularly important following flexor tendon reconstruction, given the varying surgical procedures that may be performed.

The varying surgical choices for delayed tendon reconstruction have corresponding postoperative therapeutic approaches, including immobilization, early passive mobilization, and early active mobilization. Early controlled active motion has been found to enhance the tensile strength of repairs, improves tendon excursion, allows for increased joint mobility, restores the gliding surface, reorganizes extrinsic scar, decreases scar adhesions, and improves nutrition and intrinsic healing of the tendon repair. Decision making about which postoperative treatment approach is best must take into consideration the level and type of repair, surgical technique, experience of the therapist in postoperative tendon management, patient factors (age, cognition level), socioeconomic factors (finance, family support), and the patient's ability to follow through (motivation, compliance).[55,56]

Therapists have numerous choices in the rehabilitation approach following flexor tendon repair.[57-66] These choices are covered in detail in Chapter 36. Unique considerations in the postoperative management following flexor tendon reconstruction are covered in the following sections.

Immobilization

Immobilization after tendon reconstruction is seldom used except in specific circumstances. When flexor tendon reconstruction is associated with other injuries (fractures, soft tissue injuries, skin defects), immobilization may be required until conditions become more stable. Young children, noncompliant patients, and those with cognitive deficits may need immobilization to protect the repairs. Finances and limited insurance coverage may also interfere with a patient's ability to follow up with treatment.

Initially, immobilization is maintained for 3 to 4 weeks with the use of an orthosis or cast. In general, the wrist is positioned at 10 to 30 degrees flexion, metacarpophalangeal (MCP) joints at 40 to 60 degrees flexion, and PIP/DIP joints in extension. Specific positions may vary depending on any changes in the length–tension characteristics of the reconstructed flexor tendon and whether lengthening procedures have been performed. In this instance, communication between the surgeon and therapist is essential to avoid inappropriate positioning in the orthosis.

No exercises are done independently by the patient. Exercises are performed only under the direct supervision of the therapist and include passive range of motion (PROM) and protected active extension. Active range of motion (AROM) and tendon-gliding exercises may then begin at 3 to 4 weeks.[58]

Early Passive Mobilization

Early passive motion may be used when repairs are not optimal, including for delayed repairs, frayed tendon conditions, repair under tension, or if a patient's therapy referral is delayed and the patient is not seen until 1 week after repair or longer. Tensile strength of the tendon is diminished between 5 to 21 days after surgery, and this conservative method of treatment should be considered. Positioning within a dorsal blocking orthosis varies with the wrist in 0 to 20 degrees of flexion, MCP joints in 40 to 50 degrees of flexion, and PIP/DIP joints in extension. Exercises within the orthosis include manual passive mobilization of the affected digit into flexion and active extension in a protected flexed position.[59] Dynamic traction[62,63] may be used to bring fingers into flexion passively and allow finger extension within the orthosis. Active flexion is prohibited to avoid imparting tension to the repair site and risking disruption. Details of the postoperative orthoses and exercise programs may be found in Chapter 36.

Early Active Mobilization

When surgical repairs are optimal and other factors do not affect compliance and outcome, early active mobilization of the repair may begin within 3 to 5 days of repair. This approach allows for active contraction of the muscle of the repaired tendon, and tenodesis or synergistic wrist motion to promote improved tendon gliding. Splint positioning may vary,[57,61,64,66] with wrist flexion at 0 to 20 degrees, MCP joint flexion 50 to 80 degrees, and PIP/DIP joints in full extension. An additional exercise tenodesis or hinged orthosis[57,66] may also be considered. Initial exercises include passive placement of digits in a composite fist, gentle active muscle contraction, and holding of the digits within the orthosis. Details of these protocols, orthotic positions, and the rationale and supporting evidence for their use are covered in Chapter 36.

Staged Tendon Reconstruction— Postoperative Therapy

Passive Tendon Implant—Stage I (Hunter/Mackin)[1]

Immediately following the insertion of the passive tendon implant, treatment is initiated to allow protected movement of the affected digits. A minimally bulky dressing is applied with the fingers individually wrapped allowing for isolated finger movement. With this surgical treatment, there is no flexor tendon repair to protect. Rather the concern is to avoid kinking or irritation of the proximal end of the tendon rod into the wrist and to avoid an exaggerated inflammatory response, which could occur with unrestricted hand use or aggressive hand therapy following repair.

A dorsal blocking orthosis is applied with the wrist in 30 degrees of flexion, MCP joint at 60 to 70 degrees of flexion, and interphalangeal joints in full extension. The orthosis is worn at all times (24 hours/day). Within the first week, pro-tected exercises may begin with gentle passive flexion of the affected digit and finger trapping where the adjacent finger may actively assist the affected digit into flexion. Exercises may be done with 10 repetitions per session, four to six times a day as tolerated. Other therapeutic treatment may be done to address edema control and scar management after the wound has closed.

At 3 weeks following surgery, the dorsal protective splint may be removed and a Velcro trapper or buddy strap may be used to tie the affected digit to an adjacent finger. This allows for protection of the affected finger while permitting functional use of the hand for activities of daily living. In some cases, patients are able to return to work activities depending on job requirements.

Precautions and Complications

Early movement of a digit is designed to reduce adhesions and contractures. However, with early movement of the digit after surgery, a patient may be at risk for developing *synovitis*. Aggressive movement or overexercising may lead to increased pain, swelling at the incision site, and decreased PROM of the digit. The surgeon should be notified, exercises should be discontinued, and a resting orthosis used to immobilize the hand until the synovitis resolves. Persistent synovitis results in thickening of the sheath, loss of ROM, and development of contractures.

If a PIP or DIP *contracture* exists prior to surgery or begins to develop at any stage of treatment, it should be treated immediately with an orthosis to gradually regain full extension. Continual monitoring, orthotic adjustments, and use of a night orthosis for persistent flexion contractures may be needed through both stages of tendon reconstruction. Protected PROM may also be done with extension of the affected joint with flexion of the joints proximal and distal to the target joint. Persistent contractures may also be managed with a proximal joint wedge placed dorsally over the proximal phalanx, placing the MCP joint into greater flexion. Then, a Velcro strap is applied distally, pulling the contracted interphalangeal joint into gentle extension.

The goals of stage I tendon reconstruction are to maximize PROM, attain good joint mobility, prevent flexion contractures, and develop a viable gliding sheath for eventual tendon grafting.

Tendon Grafting—Stage II

The second stage surgical reconstruction is performed with the proximal end of the tendon graft attached to the remaining motor tendon and then distally to the bone. The distal attachment may be done with or without a button and wire and remains in place for a minimum of 6 weeks. After surgery and referral for therapy, the therapist must establish with the surgeon a treatment plan based on the strength and condition of the repair. If the repair is strong and the tendon sheath is in excellent condition, an *early active mobilization* program (refer to previous section) should be initiated within the first postoperative week. Passive composite fist and active flexion hold (place and hold) may be done within the confines of a protective orthosis. If the tendon graft repair and the sheath are not in optimal condition, an *early passive mobilization* program should be used as described[59] or one with dynamic traction.[62,63] Refer to Chapter 36 for guidelines in treatment for early passive or active mobilization programs. As in stage I, precautions should be taken to minimize development of synovitis or contractures.

Care is taken also at this time to monitor the amount of excursion a patient has within the first 3 to 4 weeks. Those patients with full excursion or approximately 70% of normal ROM for PIP or DIP motion may form minimal adhesions at the repair site and may be at greater risk of rupture. In such cases, the dorsal blocking orthosis is worn through 6 weeks and active exercises are progressed with caution. Also, if a button and wire was placed as a distal anchor, it may be kept in place longer (up to 12 weeks) to allow more time for healing.

Active Tendon Implant—Stage I

The placement of the active tendon implant is similar to the passive type, however, the proximal end is attached to an active motor tendon to allow for early mobilization and function. Therapy is initiated within 3 days after surgery and progresses as in stage II tendon grafting with early active mobilization.

If a *pulley reconstruction* is required, it is usually performed in stage I surgery, allowing for time to heal before stage II repair is done. With passive tendon implants in which the attachment is only distal, pulley repairs do not require protection because movements done are passive and therefore put less stress over the pulley. With active tendon implants, a pulley ring is needed because active movement of the implant stresses and damages the pulley repair. During the first postoperative week, a soft Velcro strap may be used or manual pressure from the patient's other hand applied over the pulley repair during active exercise to protect the pulley repair. As edema decreases in the finger, a thermoplastic pulley ring may be made to provide pulley protection during exercises and hand function. If protection is needed for longer, a thick metal ring may be used. Pulley repairs should be protected for at least 6 months.

Due to the strength of the active implant, exercises and activities may progress sooner. Gentle progressive resistive exercises, as with a foam roll or sponge, may begin at 3 weeks postoperatively and may progress to light resistive putty use at 4 weeks. The dorsal blocking orthosis may be discontinued at 6 weeks though an active patient may need additional protection for 2 weeks. From 8 to 12 weeks, patients are allowed full use of the hand for activities, except for restrictions of forceful gripping and lifting until 12 weeks. Patients are encouraged to progress with their strengthening exercises along with gradual return to work activities.

Tendon Grafting—Stage II

The active tendon implant may remain in place and functional for an indeterminate period. However, any contractures, adhesions, or ruptures that may occur warrant a more immediate stage II tendon grafting. Considerations for stage II tendon grafting are based on strength of the motor unit, optimal ROM, and suppleness of the soft tissues of the finger. Stage II tendon reconstruction for an active implant is similar to that for a passive implant, with removal of the implant, insertion of the tendon graft, and progression of postoperative therapy through early passive or active mobilization.

Summary

Rehabilitation following flexor tendon reconstruction requires close communication and collaboration between surgeon, therapist, and patient. It is critically important that the patient's lifestyle and circumstances be considered in addition to the specific details of the injury in the decision making about the surgical procedure to be performed. Rather than adhering to rigid timetables, the therapist must monitor the patient's response to the postoperative orthosis and exercise regimen and make adjustments based on the patient's progress and healing considerations in consultation with the surgeon.

REFERENCES

The complete reference list is available online at www.expertconsult.com.

The Extensor Tendons: Evaluation and Surgical Management

CHAPTER

38

ERIK A. ROSENTHAL, MD AND BASSEM T. ELHASSAN, MD

DORSAL FASCIA

WRIST EXTENSOR TENDONS

FINGER EXTENSOR TENDONS

EXTENSOR TENDON INJURIES ABOUT THE
METACARPOPHALANGEAL JOINTS (ZONE V)

EXTENSOR TENDON INJURIES ABOUT THE
PROXIMAL INTERPHALANGEAL JOINTS (ZONE III)

EXTENSOR TENDON INJURIES AT THE DISTAL
INTERPHALANGEAL JOINT (ZONE I)

SWAN-NECK DEFORMITY

THUMB EXTENSOR TENDONS

FRACTURES AND EXTENSOR TENDON DEFORMITY

EXTENSOR TENDON SEPARATION: CONFRONTING
THE TENDON GAP

PATTERNS OF RESTRAINT FROM SCARRED EXTENSOR
TENDONS

CRITICAL POINTS

- Treatment and rehabilitation of extensor tendon injury can be equally complex, demanding, time consuming, and disappointing as flexor tendon injury.
- The display of extensor tendons over the dorsum of the hand and digits offer disproportionally large surfaces that are susceptible to injury and restraint by scar.
- Preservation of a functional segment of the extensor retinaculum about the wrist is necessary to avoid tendon bowstringing with resulting distal extension lag.
- Suture technique for repair of extensor tendons should consider the dimensions and fiber direction of the tendon as well as consistency of the tendon bed and covering tissues.
- Early protected motion protocols have application in selected extensor tendon injury patients. Early motion should not be recommended after repair of the terminal tendon (Zone 1), repairs confined to the wrist extensor tendons, or repairs proximal to the musculotendinous junction in the forearm.
- Study of the functional anatomy of the digital extensor mechanisms is fundamental to acquiring insight into the pathomechanics and treatment of mallet, boutonniére, and swan neck deformities.
- Scar that restrains extensor tendons can disrupt balanced extension as well as flexion of distal segments. The location and dimension of the restraint can often be defined by careful clinical examination.

- Secondary surgery for release of scar, such as tenolysis, should not be pursued until maximum improvement has been realized with hand therapy, the patient is no longer improving objectively, and the repaired tendons are sufficiently healed to survive surgical dissection with separation from the supporting blood supply of surrounding tissues.

Normal hand function mirrors the integrity of the extensor tendons. Their contribution to the balance, power, dexterity, and range of hand activities is fundamental; any restraint on them is reflected in a proportional loss of function. The effect of an injury on the extensor tendons is often regarded as being less serious than a flexor tendon injury. The treatment and rehabilitation of the injury often are believed to be less intricate, less time-consuming, and associated with a relatively more favorable prognosis than that associated with flexor tendon injuries. Experience, however, demonstrates that injuries to the extensor tendons can be equally complex, time-consuming, frustrating, and disappointing. The extensor muscles to the digits are weaker, their capacity for work and their amplitude of glide are less than their flexor antagonists, yet they require a latitude of motion that is not necessary for flexor function. The extensor tendons distal to the extensor retinaculum are relatively thin, broad structures that present a disproportionately large surface vulnerable to injury and susceptible

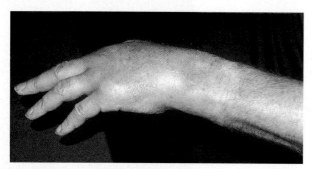

Figure 38-1 Distention of dorsal skin and fascia reverses transverse metacarpal arch and tethers digits in extension.

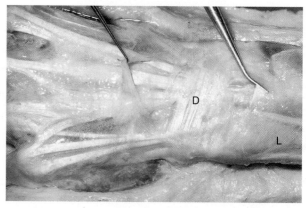

Figure 38-2 Anatomy of deep dorsal fascia. The probe elevates deep fascia proximally while the hook holds deep fascia distal to fibers of extensor retinaculum. Areolar peritendinous fascia, the paratenon, envelops extensor tendons distal to the extensor retinaculum. Fascia contributes to efficiency of tendon excursion and intrinsic tendon circulation. D, extensor retinaculum; L, linea jugata.

to the formation of restraining scar. The complex interrelationships within the intricately designed extensor tendons of the digits increase their susceptibility to functional disarray after injury. Any violation of the extensor tendons or their investments introduces the potential for a functional deficiency.

Dorsal Fascia

An appreciation of the fascial anatomy of the forearm and hand is helpful for the design of surgical procedures and for modification of a rehabilitation program after an injury.

The pliable skin over the dorsum of the hand lacks the fascial septa that stabilize the palmar skin. The skin redundancy associated with digital extension is consumed during grip. This tightening of the dorsal skin compresses the underlying dorsal veins and lymphatics, providing an efficient venous and lymphatic pump.

The superficial dorsal fascia of the hand is composed of a variable fatty layer and a deeper membranous layer that contains the dorsal veins, superficial lymphatics, and sensory branches of the radial and ulnar nerves. The superficial fascia is loosely attached to the deep fascia, with the interface representing a potential space. Dorsal subcutaneous bleeding and lymphedema tether the fingers in extension and the thumb in extension–supination. The pump mechanism is hampered, swelling increases, and grip is further restrained. Dorsal cicatrix also restrains normal grip mechanics. The penalty for uncontrolled dorsal swelling is secondary joint stiffness with tightness of the metacarpophalangeal (MCP) joints and dorsal fascia of the thumb web (Fig. 38-1).

The fascia of the forearm is divided into superficial (pars superficialis) and deep (pars profunda) layers.[1] The extensor retinaculum at the wrist level is composed of supratendinous and infratendinous layers that originate from the pars profunda of the forearm fascia (Fig. 38-2). The supratendinous portion consists of multidirectional woven fibers that wrap around the wrist. The proximal fibers of the supratendinous retinaculum on the radial side merge with the forearm fascia over the palmaris longus; the central fibers insert onto the distal radius, and the distal fibers attach to the thenar fascia. The supratendinous retinaculum on the ulnar side wraps around the distal ulna but does not attach to it. The proximal ulnar fibers of the supratendinous retinaculum pass over the flexor carpi ulnaris tendon and merge with the forearm fascia, the central fibers attach on the triquetrum and pisi-

form, and the distal fibers attach to the hypothenar fascia. Six vertical septa attach the supratendinous retinaculum to the distal radius and partition the first five dorsal compartments. These define fibro-osseous tunnels that position and maintain the extensor tendons and their synovial sheaths relative to the axis of wrist motion in the proximal pole of the capitate (Fig. 38-3). The brachioradialis tendon and periosteum of the distal radius cover the floor of the first compartment.[2] The periosteum of the radius forms the floor of the second and third. The infratendinous retinaculum forms the floor of the fourth and fifth compartments. The sixth septum separates the extensor digiti quinti (EDQ) from the extensor carpi ulnaris (ECU) and is attached proximally to the ulnar border of the distal radius but not to the ulna.[1,3] This radial attachment forms a fibrous nucleus with the origins of the dorsal distal radioulnar ligament and ulnocarpal complex,[3,4] a ligamentous confluence that is analogous to the assemblage nucleus described at the palmar corner of the

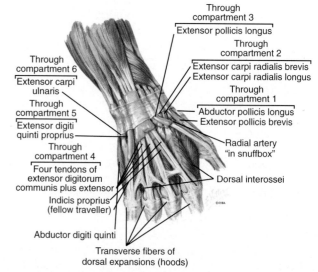

Through compartment 3
Extensor pollicis longus
Through compartment 2
Extensor carpi radialis brevis
Extensor carpi radialis longus
Through compartment 1
Abductor pollicis longus
Extensor pollicis brevis
Radial artery "in snuffbox"
Dorsal interossei
Through compartment 6
Extensor carpi ulnaris
Through compartment 5
Extensor digiti quinti proprius
Through compartment 4
Four tendons of extensor digitorum communis plus extensor
Indicis proprius (fellow traveller)
Abductor digiti quinti
Transverse fibers of dorsal expansions (hoods)

Figure 38-3 Extensor tendon anatomy. (Reprinted, with permission, from Lampe EW. *Surgical Anatomy of the Hand.* Summit, NJ: CIBA Pharmaceutical, 1969.)

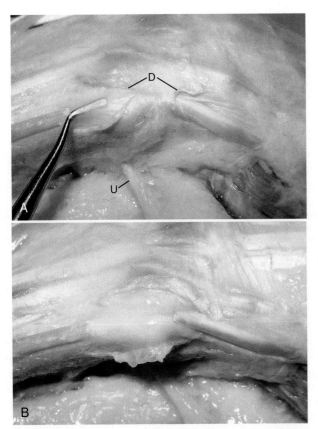

Figure 38-4 Sixth dorsal compartment. Supratendinous extensor retinaculum is superficial layer that hoods the compartment but is separate from the subsheath and extensor carpi ulnaris (ECU) tendon. **A,** Retinaculum incised proximally and distally, preserving central fibers. The spatula is within subsheath. ECU tendon fixed from base of ulnar styloid to triquetrum by subsheath, a synovial-lined tunnel of fascia derived from infratendinous retinaculum. The ECU inserts on fifth metacarpal to right. **B,** Angulation of tendon during supination increases ulnar displacement forces. The subsheath normally stabilizes ECU but does not restrict tendon glide. D, extensor retinaculum; U, dorsal sensory branch ulnar nerve.

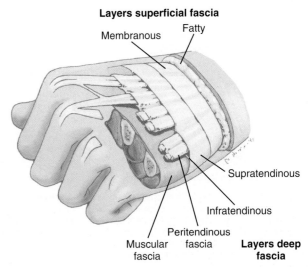

Figure 38-5 Dorsal fascia of the hand. (Redrawn, with permission, from Anson BJ, Wright RR, Dykes J. The fascia of the dorsum of the hand. *Surg Gyn Obst.* 1945;81:327–331.)

finger MCP joints.[3,5] The sixth compartment retinaculum is anchored by septal attachments, which are composed entirely of soft tissue and are not attached directly to bone. This compartment is relatively stiff, with a high failure load that is able to withstand tensile forces well because of its ability to stretch and deform. This is of clinical importance because of the occurrence of symptomatic volar displacement of the ECU tendon.[6]

The ECU, within the sixth compartment, is stabilized in a separate tunnel formed from the infratendinous retinaculum that is separated from the supratendinous retinaculum by loose areolar tissue. This lack of attachment to the supratendinous retinaculum permits unrestricted ulnar rotation during pronation and supination. The fixed tunnel, or *subsheath*,[4] exists only distal to the ulnar head[1,7] and attaches to the triangular fibrocartilage complex (TFCC),[8] triquetrum, pisiform, and fifth metacarpal. This tunnel maintains the straight course of the ECU between the ulnar styloid and the fifth metacarpal during forearm pronation and supination (Fig. 38-4). The ECU slips dorsal to the ulnar styloid and outside its groove during supination. The ECU is dynamically stabilized proximal to the fixed sheath by a fascial sling, the *linea jugata*, that tightens during supination and opposes further tendon displacement (see Fig. 38-2).[3]

The extensor retinaculum continues distally as the deep fascia over the dorsum of the hand. This deep fascia is composed of two layers: a dorsal supratendinous layer and a deep infratendinous layer. They define a closed fascial space bordered by the synovial sheaths of the extensor tendons proximally, the index and fifth metacarpals, and the metacarpal heads distally. The flattened finger extensor tendons course between these two layers of the deep fascia, invested in a vascularized film of peritendinous fascia—the *paratenon* (see Fig. 38-2). The infratendinous layer of the deep fascia rests on the interosseous fascia (Fig. 38-5).

The peritendinous fascia is represented in the embryonic hand and is believed to give rise to the extensor tendons. Anatomic variations in the extensor tendons may reflect developmental variations in the precursor of adult paratenon.[9-12] This transparent vascular membrane permits gliding of the extensor tendons within the small tolerances of the two layers of the deep fascia. The response to certain traumatic conditions demonstrates a prodigious capacity for generating scar tissue and adhesions (see later discussion of Secrétan's disease).

The extensor tendons receive their blood supply through vascular mesenteries—mesotendons that are analogous to the vincula of the flexor tendons.[13] Branches of the radial and ulnar arteries, perforating dorsal branches of the anterior interosseous artery, and vessels originating in the deep palmar arch are carried to the tendons in these flexible folds of delicate fascia. The mesotendons are longer and are adapted to a longer tendon excursion.[14] The intratendinous vascular architecture of the extensor tendons is similar throughout.[15] Synovial diffusion, which provides 70% of the nutrition, is the major nutritional pathway for the extensor tendons beneath the extensor retinaculum. Vascular perfusion through the mesotendons provides significantly less (30%) nutrition. No significant contribution is made by the longitudinal intratendinous vasculature.[16] The contribution of the deep fascia to the intrinsic nutrition of the extensor tendons may parallel the role of the fibro-osseous sheath in synovial diffusion of the flexor tendons.[13,16]

Loss Extensor Retinaculum

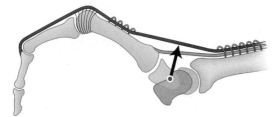

- Moment arm EDC increased
- EDC becomes wrist extensor
- Extension lag finger MCP joints

Figure 38-6 Loss of extensor retinaculum. Illustration depicts anatomic and biomechanical changes that result from loss of the extensor retinaculum. EDC, extensor digitorum communis; MCP, metacarpophalangeal. (Reprinted, with permission, from Rosenthal EA. Dynamics of the extensor system. In: Hunter JM, Schneider LH, and Mackin EJ, eds. *Tendon and Nerve Surgery of the Hand. A Third Decade.* St. Louis: Mosby–Year Book 1997, Plate 7.)

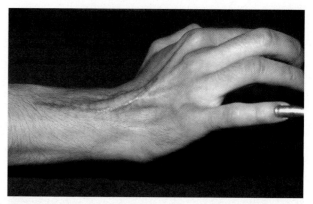

Figure 38-7 Dorsal bowing and reduced effective extensor excursion as result of removal of dorsal retaining layers. A portion of the extensor retinaculum must be retained to preserve normal function and avoid disfigurement.

The dorsal fascia contributes another function to the extensor tendons. The supratendinous layer constitutes a dorsal pulley that promotes efficient distal transfer of the inherent strength and tendon excursion of the extensor muscles. Selective removal of portions of the dorsal fascia is compatible with retained function. A portion of the extensor retinaculum should be retained at the level of the radiocarpal and ulnocarpal joints. The tendon excursion required to achieve a given degree of wrist extension is doubled by resecting the extensor retinaculum (Fig. 38-6).[4] Excessive removal results in unsightly bowing and altered extensor kinetics. Patients may compensate for bowstringing and decreased extensor power by suppressing their voluntary finger extension when the wrist is extended (Fig. 38-7).

Extensor tenovaginotomy of the first dorsal compartment for stenosing tenosynovitis should preserve the volar attachment of the extensor retinaculum to the distal radius and limit any fascial release distal to the radial styloid. Disruption of the volar attachment of the first compartment permits palmar displacement of the first compartment tendons during wrist flexion. An extended release distal to the radial styloid can introduce tendon bowing that changes normal thumb mechanics. First metacarpal abduction by the abductor pollicis longus (APL) is then weakened. Extensor pollicis brevis (EPB) bowing increases its moment arm for first metacarpal

extension but may also lessen thumb MCP joint extension (Fig. 38-8).

The dressing applied after an operative procedure should contribute to the control of hand edema and discourage hematoma formation. Sterilized Mountain Mist polyester batting (Leggett and Platt, Inc.), immersed in saline solution and applied wet about the wound, provides comfortable, gently compressive immobilization of the hand and promotes diffusion of expressed blood away from the wound. This buoyant, hydrophobic material allows wound aeration with moisture evaporation, which discourages skin maceration (Fig 38-9).

Eight extensor tendon injury zones were defined by Kleinert and Verdan[17]; Doyle added a ninth zone.[18] Zones I, III, V, and VII cover joints; zones II, IV, and VI cover shafts of tubular bones; zone VIII proximal to the extensor retinaculum covers the distal forearm; zone IX encompasses the remainder of the forearm proximally (Fig. 38-10).

Wrist Extensor Tendons

The wrist extensor tendons are the key to balanced hand function and the success of rehabilitation after injury. Positional grip depends on the selective stabilizing forces of the three wrist extensor tendons. The digital extensor tendons, in the absence of the wrist extensor tendons, can secondarily induce wrist extension. This substitution pattern, however,

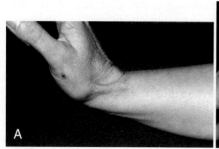
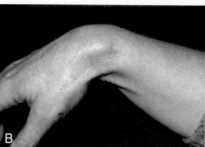
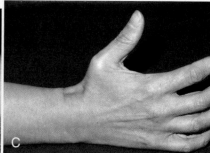

Figure 38-8 Thumb imbalance reflecting removal of extensor retinaculum and deep fascia that retains abductor pollicis longus and extensor pollicis brevis. **A,** Displacement of tendons and bowing with wrist extension. **B,** Wrist flexion. **C,** Exaggerated extension of first metacarpal with extension lag at metacarpophalangeal joint results from alteration of moment arms and decreased effective excursions of these tendons. Deep fascia about the distal radius should be retained when the extensor retinaculum is released over the first dorsal compartment; fascia distal to the radius need not be released.

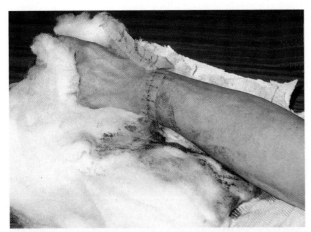

Figure 38-9 Wet polyester batting makes a comfortable, gently compressive dressing that disperses blood away from wound; buoyant material also discourages skin maceration.

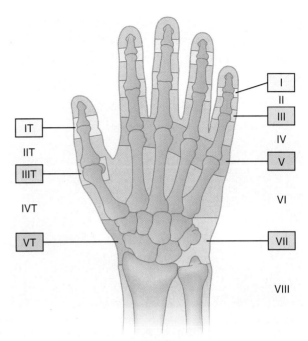

Figure 38-10 Extensor tendon injury zones in the hand and forearm. Zone VIII in the distal forearm is proximal to the extensor retinaculum. Zone IX encompasses the remainder of the forearm more proximally.

lacks normal power and is devoid of voluntary dexterity in spatial positioning of the hand. Wrist extension is then the obligate follower of finger extension, an unnatural functional sequence.

The stations of the extensor carpi radialis longus (ECRL), extensor carpi radialis brevis (ECRB), and ECU are fixed relative to the axis of wrist motion in the second, third, and sixth dorsal compartments, respectively, at the level of the distal radius and ulna (see Fig. 38-3). The three wrist extensor muscles have different masses, cross-sectional areas, fiber lengths, and moment arms.[19-22] These differences manifest in varying performances and contributions to wrist motion.*

The ECRB, with the longest extension moment arm and the largest cross-sectional area, is the strongest and most efficient wrist extensor. The ECRL extends proximal to the elbow, originates from the lateral epicondyle, inserts on the base of the second metacarpal, and has the longest muscle fibers and the largest mass. It thus has the greatest capacity for sustained work. It extends and radially deviates the wrist and opposes the flexor carpi ulnaris (FCU). The ECU has the longest moment arm for ulnar deviation but is most effective as an ulnar deviator with the forearm positioned in pronation. The radial wrist extensors have an amplitude of 37 mm during wrist flexion–extension; the ECU has an amplitude of 18 mm.[23] These three muscles with different anatomic endowments are cerebrally integrated to balance wrist extension and flexion, as well as ulnar and radial deviation.

The ECU is unique among the wrist extensor tendons. It exhibits some degree of contraction during all phases of wrist motion. Its variable potential for wrist extension depends on the position of forearm rotation. During pronation, the normal tendon rests on the medial (ulnar) side of the ulnar head and stabilizes the wrist. It is a strong ulnar deviator and balances the tension of all tendons radial to the axis of wrist motion (in the proximal end of the capitate) but is a relatively weak wrist extensor. When the forearm is supinated, the

*Mass or volume of muscle fibers is proportional to work capacity. Cross-sectional area of all fibers is proportional to maximum tension. Average fiber length is proportional to potential excursion. Moment arm is the perpendicular distance from the axis of motion.

ECU moment arm for wrist extension lengthens and it becomes a more efficient wrist extensor.[24]

The tendon of the ECU inserts distally on the base of the fifth metacarpal. The ECU is firmly stabilized distal to the ulnar head, from the base of the ulnar styloid to the triquetrum, by its own fibro-osseous sheath, a strong collar of synovial-lined deep fascia that is separate from the overlying supratendinous layer of the extensor retinaculum.[25,26] The ECU fibro-osseous sheath, or *subsheath*, has a broad, strong connection with the underlying TFCC. Release of the TFCC increases excursion and bowstringing of the ECU during wrist extension[8] (see Fig. 38-4).

Proximally, the ECU tendon is stabilized dynamically by a longitudinal thickened band of the forearm fascia, the *linea jugata,* that originates from the ulnar styloid and courses obliquely proximally and radially. The tendon assumes an ulnar-directed obtuse angle during supination. The apex of the angle is at the transition point between the proximal dynamic stabilizer, the linea jugata, and the distal fixed stabilizer, the subsheath. This angle becomes increasingly acute as forearm supination and ulnar wrist deviation increases. Contraction of the ECU, forearm supination, and ulnar wrist deviation increase ulnar-directed stresses on the ECU that are opposed by the subsheath, the extensor retinaculum, and the linea jugata (see Fig. 38-2).[3,27]

Attrition of the ECU from stress-induced tenosynovitis with partial tendon rupture is a source of chronic ulnar wrist pain.[28] The deep fascial tunnel of the ECU can rupture, permitting subluxation of the tendon during forearm rotation.[29,30] This painful condition reflects a specific anatomic deficiency. Reconstruction with a radially based flap from the extensor retinaculum is feasible in patients when symptoms persist despite conservative treatment.[27] Repair with suture anchors and deepening the ECU groove has also been reported.[31]

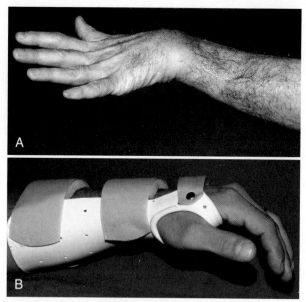

Figure 38-11 Loss of wrist extensor function after trauma. There was no direct insult to wrist extensors. **A,** Substitution pattern employing digital extensors to extend wrist. **B,** Early orthotic use and reeducation of wrist extensors are necessary.

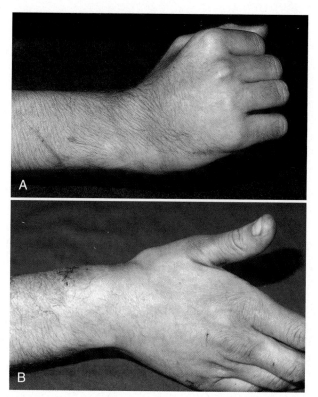

Figure 38-12 A, Interruption of extensor carpi ulnaris (ECU) introduces imbalance of wrist extensors. Therapy after repair requires awareness of multiple facets of normal ECU function. **B,** Laceration of radial wrist extensor tendons. Inability to deviate wrist radially introduces major deficiency in spatial positioning of hand and grip strength.

Rupture of the ECU tendon over the distal ulna from forced supination has been reported.[32] Erosion of the floor of the sixth extensor compartment from an ulnar osteophyte is a variable finding but may contribute to attrition of the tendon. The ruptured tendon can be reconstituted with an intercalary free tendon graft.

The ECU contributes a rare anomalous tendon slip to the EDQ extensor hood. This connection between two tendons with differential excursions can impede simultaneous flexion of the small finger and wrist and produce painful dysfunction. Resection of the anomalous tendon is then indicated.[33]

Wrist extensor function may deteriorate after an injury to the hand or wrist without direct trauma to the wrist extensor tendons. A wrist drop occurs, and a pattern substituting the digital extensors is adopted to implement extension of the wrist. This centrally mediated inhibition of the wrist extensor tendons should be detected early, and use of a supportive wrist orthosis should be initiated. The wrist is supported in slight extension, permitting digital flexion and extension while the wrist extensors are being retrained. Extending the wrist against resistance while the digits are fully flexed is helpful in this pursuit. The natural synergy between the wrist extensors and digital flexors facilitates recovery (Fig. 38-11).

Laceration of the ECU introduces a significant imbalance in some patients. The inability to balance the tension of the radial wrist extensors produces persistent radial deviation of the wrist. Extension in ulnar deviation is precluded, grip is weak, and most functions are performed awkwardly (Fig. 38-12A). Laceration of the radial wrist extensors also interferes with balanced spatial positioning of the hand and dexterity of grip (Fig. 38-12B). All three wrist extensor tendons contribute significantly to normal function, and each should be repaired after injury. Repair of all three wrist extensor tendons after a common injury may influence long-term

functional prognosis adversely with diminished grip and pinch strength.[34]

Finger Extensor Tendons

Proximal to Metacarpophalangeal Joints (Zones IX, VIII, VII, and VI)

The extensor tendons of the fingers are the extensor digitorum communis (EDC), the extensor indicis proprius (EIP), and the EDQ. The tendons of the EDC and EIP pass beneath the extensor retinaculum within synovial sheaths in the fourth dorsal compartment then diverge as they course distally, where they blend with the sagittal bands over the MCP joints of the fingers. They flatten distally between the layers of the deep fascia. The EDC contributes substantial tendons to the index, long, and ring fingers, giving a variable slip to the small finger (Fig. 38-13). Anatomic variations in the EDC tendons are common.[35] The anomalous *extensor digitorum brevis manus muscle* that usually originates on the dorsum of the hand radial to the third metacarpal and inserts with the extensor tendons to the index and long fingers may manifest as a gentle dorsal mass but has no clinical significance.[36]

Extension of the MCP joints of the long and ring fingers depends on the position of the adjacent fingers; independent extension is lacking.[37,38] Extensor autonomy is less in the long finger and least in the ring finger. Loss of extensor

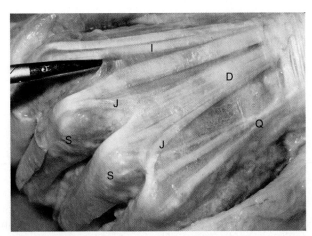

Figure 38-13 Extensor tendon anatomy. Deep fascia has been removed. Instrument lifts vestige of junctura tendinum to index extensor tendons. D, extensor digitorum communis (EDC); I, extensor indicis proprius (EIP); Q, extensor digiti quinti (EDQ); J, junctura tendinum; S, sagittal bands over metacarpophalangeal joint. Juncturae tendinum dynamically stabilize extensor tendons during grip.

autonomy has been attributed to fibrous connecting bands within the muscle belly of the EDC in the forearm[39] as well as to the integrity of the juncturae tendinum.[38] A separate muscle belly of the EDC to the index finger with individual nerve supply from the posterior interosseous nerve can preserve independent index finger extension after the EIP has been transferred.[40]

The EIP and EDQ have independent muscles that allow independent function. Extension of the index and small fingers is readily performed, irrespective of flexed positions of the other fingers (Fig. 38-14). The EIP and EDQ course ulnar to their respective EDC counterparts; the EIP is usually a single tendon, whereas the EDQ has two. The EIP may contribute a rare, anomalous tendon to the thumb: the *extensor pollicis and indicis communis* tendon.[9] An anomalous muscle originating from the dorsal compartment of the forearm and inserting into the extensor hood of the long finger, the *extensor medii proprius*,[41] is analogous to the EIP.[42] When the EIP splits and inserts into both index and long fingers, the anomaly is termed the *extensor indicis et medii communis.*[41]

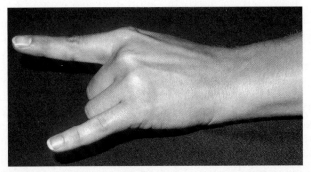

Figure 38-14 Extensor indicis proprius and extensor digiti quinti have independent function from separate muscles. No distal tethering exists with flexion of other fingers. The extensor digitorum communis to index finger may have a separate muscle belly with individual nerve supply.

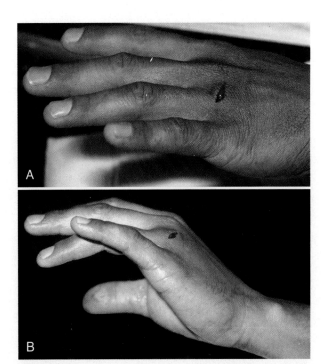

Figure 38-15 Laceration of extensor tendon to ring finger. **A,** No apparent deficit with wrist in neutral. Metacarpophalangeal joint extension accomplished through fascial connection. **B,** Deficit is apparent when function is tested with combined wrist and finger extension.

Excursion of the extrinsic finger extensor tendons approximates 50 mm: 31 mm with wrist flexion–extension, 16 mm with MCP joint motion, 3 to 4 mm with proximal interphalangeal (PIP) joint motion, and 3 to 4 mm with distal interphalangeal (DIP) joint motion.[43] DIP joint motion only imparts motion to the extensor tendon proximal to the PIP joint when that joint is restrained in neutral. Normally, terminal tendon excursion is dissipated at the level of the PIP joint by palmar migration of the lateral bands during interphalangeal (IP) joint flexion and does not affect the extensor tendons more proximally.

Juncturae Tendinum

The juncturae tendinum are broad intertendinous connections that diverge from the EDC tendon to the ring finger. These bands connect with the EDC tendons to the long, small, and, variably, index fingers (see Fig. 38-13). The EDQ commonly receives a significant contribution, but the EIP does not.[41,44] The connection with the EDC tendon to the index finger extensor tendons is frequently only a vestige. These bands assist extension of adjacent connected fingers by transferring forces during extension, enabling the extensor tendons to function as a unit.[37,41] Laceration of an extensor tendon proximally may be obscured by the contribution of these bands. Demonstration of a full range of potential motion with direct visualization of the injured tendon is required before the possibility of a lacerated tendon can be dismissed (Fig. 38-15). A junctura between the index EDC and extensor pollicis longus (EPL) is an anatomic variant. Thumb IP joint flexion restrains index finger extension when this variant exists.[45]

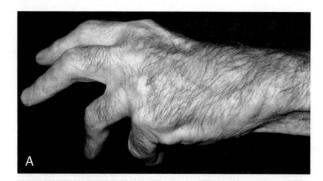

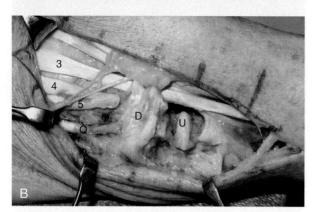

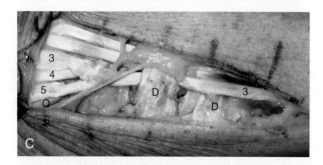

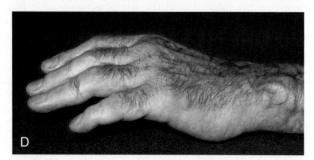

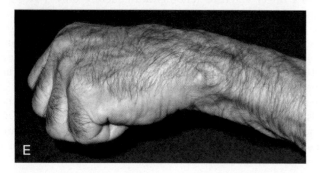

Figure 38-16 *Ruptured extensor tendons to ring and small finger in a 65-year-old-man with caput ulnae syndrome caused by rheumatoid arthritis.* **A,** *Active extension deficit.* **B,** *Distal ends of ruptured extensor digiti quinti (EDQ) and extensor digitorum communis (EDC) to the ring and small fingers lie distal to retained strip of extensor retinaculum. Deformed ulnar head has eroded joint capsule.* **C,** *Adjacent suture of the EDC from the ring and small finger into EDC to long finger, and EDQ into EDC to the small finger. Tendon junction is flat, and sutures are tied beneath tendon.* **D,** *Active extension 6 months after reconstruction.* **E,** *Finger flexion was retained. D, extensor retinaculum; U, ulnar head; 3, EDC to long finger; 4, EDC to ring finger; 5, EDC to small finger; Q, EDQ.*

The extensor tendons to the fingers diverge distal to the extensor retinaculum. During finger flexion these tendons glide distally and separate. The juncturae tendinum assume a more transverse orientation and develop increased tension as they displace distally. They dynamically stabilize the fingers by transmitting forces to the radial sagittal bands of the index and long fingers and to the ulnar sagittal bands of the ring and small fingers. Active grip thus contributes to the stability of the transverse metacarpal arch and to the centralization of the extensor tendons over the dorsum of the MCP joints.[46]

The role of the juncturae and the normal displacements of the finger extensor tendons are applied during reconstruction for extensor tendon ruptures. Distal ends of ruptured tendons are sutured to intact adjacent tendons. Tension at the tendon junction is adjusted with the fingers held in flexion: fingers with intact tendon in full flexion; injured finger(s) slightly less than full flexion. This ensures that the angle between sutured tendons is sufficiently acute for transmission of active extension forces and the tendons will not be tethered during finger flexion (Fig. 38-16).

Extensor Digiti Quinti

The extensor tendons to the small finger have significant anatomic features.[47] An oblique junctura from the ring finger permits continued extension of the small finger after interruption of the EDQ more proximally. The patient often is unaware of any deficit until decreased strength and loss of independent extension are demonstrated. This situation is seen commonly in patients with rheumatoid arthritis (Fig. 38-17).

The EDQ gains attachment to the abductor tubercle of the base of the proximal phalanx through insertion of its ulnar tendon into the abductor digiti quinti (ADQ) tendon. Some patients with ulnar palsy who are incapable of MCP joint hyperextension but do not develop a claw deformity acquire an abduction deformity of the small finger (Wartenberg's sign) from paralysis of the third palmar interosseous muscle. Their abducted small finger is associated with an oblique junctura from the ring finger, a weak biomechanical link. The EDQ is relatively unopposed and abducts the small finger. Patients who do not acquire this deformity have a transverse orientation of the junctura, a biomechanically forceful link that opposes the deformity (Fig. 38-18).[48]

Tendon Ruptures

The wrist and finger extensor tendons are exposed to entrapment by fractures of the distal radius[49-51] and dislocations

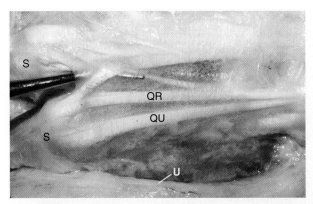

Figure 38-17 Extrinsic extensor tendons to the small finger. Deep fascia has been removed. Instrument lifts oblique junctura tendinum to small finger. This oblique connection can mask disruption of the extensor digiti quinti (EDQ) proximally. QR, radial tendon EDQ; QU, ulnar tendon EDQ; S, sagittal bands; U, dorsal sensory branch of ulnar nerve.

of the distal ulna.[52] Attrition with delayed rupture has been reported from multiple conditions, including anomalous extensor brevis manus muscle,[53,54] Madelung's deformity,[55] tophaceous pyrophosphate deposition,[56] rheumatoid tenosynovitis, traumatic dorsal subluxation of the distal ulna,[55] granulomatous tenosynovitis, extraskeletal osteochondroma,[57] Kienböck's disease,[57] nonunion scaphoid fracture,[55] instability of the distal ulna after excessive surgical resection,[58] fixation screws,[57] and nonunion fracture of Lister's tubercle.

Secrétan's Disease

Hard, brawny edema involving the dorsum of the hand has stimulated controversy since it was described in 1901.[59] The condition follows trauma to the dorsum of the hand, often pursues a protracted course, and has been associated with an unfavorable surgical prognosis.[60] It has been considered synonymous with factitious, or self-induced, edema.[61,62] Monetary gain and compensation award have been considered significant causative factors. The anatomy of the dorsum of the hand and the clinical observations at surgery support the contention that a specific pathologic entity is present involving peritendinous fibrosis about the extensor tendons and

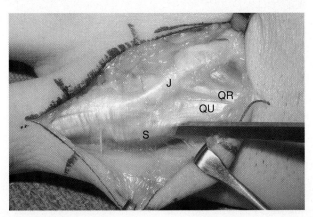

Figure 38-18 Extensor tendon insertion at metacarpophalangeal joint of the small finger. Extensor digiti quinti (EDQ) gains attachment to lateral tubercle of proximal phalanx through insertion of its ulnar tendon into abductor digiti quinti tendon. J, junctura tendinum; QU, ulnar tendon EDQ; QR, radial tendon EDQ; S, sagittal bands.

juncturae tendinum, within the confines of the layers of the deep fascia after trauma, which is different from factitious dorsal edema.[63,64] The form and distribution of the fibrosis conform to the fascial anatomy already described.[65] The inelastic peritendinous scar restricts excursion of the finger extensor tendons and their juncturae, blocking longitudinal and transverse tendon glide. Surgical, psychologic, and rehabilitative treatment are necessarily integrated. This condition presents a diverse spectrum of clinical challenges with a cautious prognosis.

Metacarpophalangeal Joints and Distal (Zones V, IV, III, II, and I)

The form and complexity of the extensor tendons change at the level of the sagittal bands that shroud the MCP joints of the fingers. Distally, they consist of a continuous sheet of precisely oriented fibers that transmit tension. This fiber array wraps the finger skeleton in the form of a bisected cone that is composed of a tendon system, which transmits tension and imparts motion, and a retinacular system, which stabilizes the tendon system. An alteration in the alignment or length of the proximal or middle phalanges of the fingers changes the normal adjustment of forces within the tendon systems and permits the retinacular system to foreshorten.[66] The imbalance within the tendon system establishes deformities; tightening of the retinacular system fixes these deformities and resists correction.

The broad, fibrous dorsal hood of the finger MCP joints consists of fibers from the juncturae tendinum, sagittal bands, and extensor tendon. The extensor tendon is nested between two layers of the sagittal bands: a thin, superficial layer and a thick, deep layer. These two layers blend laterally to form a single, substantial layer.[67,68] This blend of fibers is strong except in the long finger, where the superficial sagittal layer and the deep extensor attachments are relatively weak.[69] Ulnar displacement forces are greatest with the MCP joints in full extension, decrease during the first 60 degrees of flexion, then progressively increase with greater flexion. Relatively little force is needed to maintain a normally located extensor tendon. Significantly higher restraining forces are required to prevent added displacement of a tendon that is displaced ulnarward; an ulnar-displaced tendon tends to displace further with increased MCP joint flexion.[69] Sagittal band rupture can occur during full extension or with grip, is more likely with ulnar wrist deviation, and usually involves the radial sagittal fibers. Experimental section of the ulnar sagittal band does not cause extensor tendon instability.[70] In the long finger, the extensor tendon can separate from the underlying sagittal band and displace without sagittal band disruption (Fig. 38-19).[69]

The extensor tendons have a variable insertion on the base of the proximal phalanx that is not critical for extension of the fingers.[66,72,73] This insertion, if present, centralizes the extensor tendon but contributes little to the normal kinematics of finger extension. There is a linear relationship between excursion of the extensor tendons over the dorsum of the hand and the angle of motion of the MCP joints.[19,74] Extension of the MCP joint is achieved through the sagittal bands, vertically oriented fibers that shroud the capsule and collateral ligaments, which connect the extensor tendons with the

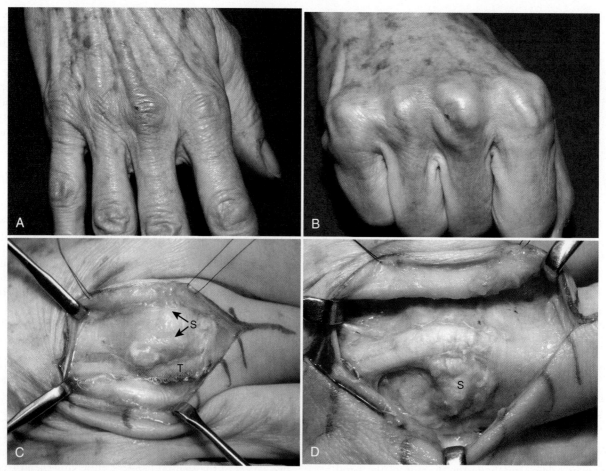

Figure 38-19 Traumatic ulnar dislocation of extensor digitorum tendon metacarpophalangeal (MCP) joint of the long finger. **A,** No swelling or tenderness. Tendon is centralized. Tendon instability not evident with MCP joint extended. **B,** Ulnar displacement of extensor tendon increases with MCP joint flexion. **C,** Operative findings: Extensor tendon displaced ulnar to MCP joint; sagittal bands are intact; normal channel for displaced tendon is evident. White deposits are crystalloid residue from steroid injection. **D,** Tendon repositioned anatomically and secured with interrupted, marginal, braided 5-0 white Mersilene (Ethicon, Johnson and Johnson Gateway LLC) sutures. T, extensor digitorum tendon; S, sagittal bands; *Black arrows,* normal channel for tendon.

volar plate and proximal phalanx on both sides of the joint.[75] These broad bands constitute functional slings that pass between the joint capsule and the intrinsic muscles. They cover the axis of joint motion during extension and pass distal to the axis of motion during flexion. They stabilize the extensor tendons over the dorsum of the MCP joints during flexion, complementing the juncturae tendinum.[5]

Laceration or closed rupture of the sagittal bands disrupts the stability of the extensor tendons over the MCP joints. The extensor tendon displaces ulnarward during flexion. Active extension then produces ulnar angulation of the MCP joint with supination of the finger. A painful snap may accompany extension as the extensor tendon relocates dorsally. Tightness develops that maintains the ulnar deviation deformity, prevents dorsal relocation of the extensor tendon, and precludes full active extension of the MCP joint (Fig. 38-20, online).

Distal to the sagittal bands, the lumbrical and interosseous muscles contribute proximal vertical and distal oblique fibers to the tendon expansion over the proximal phalanx (Fig. 38-21). The vertical fibers transmit flexor forces to the proximal phalanx, which flex the MCP joint. The oblique

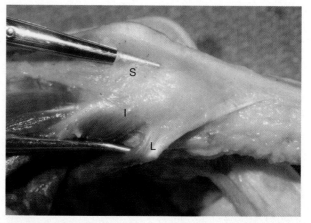

Figure 38-21 Extrinsic and intrinsic tendons merge about the radial side of the index finger metacarpophalangeal (MCP) joint. Sagittal bands affect MCP joint extension. Interosseous and lumbrical muscles transmit tension through the dorsal apparatus and lateral bands for MCP joint flexion and interphalangeal joint extension. S, sagittal bands; I, interosseous tendon; L, lumbrical tendon.

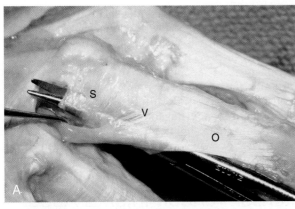

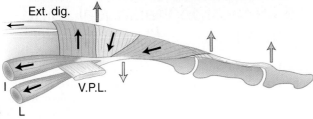

Figure 38-22 A, Dorsal apparatus of the fingers. Hook retracts the lumbrical muscle. Sagittal bands separate intrinsic muscles from the metacarpophalangeal (MCP) joint capsule. Delicate fibers are vulnerable to interference by scar. **B,** Vertical sagittal bands *(blue)* are extrinsic tendon fibers that extend MCP joint. Vertical intrinsic tendon fibers *(yellow)* flex MCP joint. Extrinsic and intrinsic tendons merge distally to form oblique fibers *(green)* that extend the interphalangeal joints and form the conjoined lateral bands. Ext. dig., extensor digitorum; S, sagittal bands; V, vertical intrinsic tendon fibers; O, oblique extrinsic and intrinsic tendon fibers; I, interosseous muscle; L, lumbrical muscle; VPL, intervolar plate ligament (deep transverse metacarpal ligament).

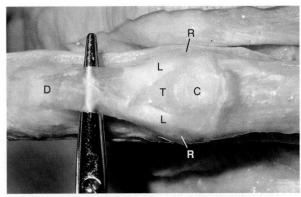

Figure 38-23 Extensor tendon anatomy about proximal interphalangeal (PIP) joint and middle phalanx. Central tendon (continuation of extrinsic extensor tendon) courses deep to proximal, transversely oriented retinacular fibers to insert on the dorsal base of the middle phalanx. More distal retinacular fibers (the triangular ligament) normally restrain descent of the lateral bands during PIP joint flexion. Scarring of these fibers can impair PIP joint flexion. Instrument lifts the merged conjoined lateral bands that insert as the terminal extensor tendon to the left. Dissection of the extensor tendon over the middle phalanx invites scarring that may restrict distal interphalangeal joint motion. C, central tendon; D, terminal tendon; L, conjoined lateral band; R, transverse retinacular ligament; T, triangular ligament.

fibers transmit extension forces to the PIP and DIP joints. This contiguous sheet of combined extrinsic and intrinsic tendon fibers about the MCP joint and proximal phalanx is appropriately termed the *dorsal apparatus* because it contributes to both extension and flexion.[39,76] The extrinsic extensor tendons are primarily extensors of the MCP joints. They are capable of secondarily extending the IP joints only if hyperextension of the MCP joint is prevented. The intrinsic tendons flex the MCP joints and extend the IP joints (Fig. 38-22).[77,78]

The extensor mechanism about the proximal phalanx is a complex assembly of multidirectional fibers that present a variable spatial orientation during PIP joint flexion. The fiber connections between the central tendon and lateral bands crisscross in separate layers. The fibers from the central tendon pass superficial to those from the intrinsic lateral bands. Descent of the lateral bands during flexion is accompanied by an increase in the longitudinal angle between these crossing fibers, analogous to the expansion of a taut mesh.[79] These geometric changes are caused by changes in the orientation of the fibers rather than by changes in the length of individual fibers.[80] The delicacy of this fiber interplay accentuates the vulnerability of the extensor tendons in the fingers to the restraints of scar. The extrinsic extensor tendon continues as the central tendon to insert on the dorsal base of the middle phalanx with medial fibers from the intrinsic tendons.

The conjoined lateral bands represent the continuation of the oblique fibers of the intrinsic tendons, supplemented by lateral fibers from the central extensor tendon. The lateral bands continue distally, converging over the middle phalanx as a single terminal tendon that inserts on the dorsal base of the distal phalanx proximal to the germinal matrix of the nail (Fig. 38-23).[81]

The lateral bands normally lie dorsal to the axis of motion of the PIP joints during extension and descend to cover the axis of joint motion during flexion. This shift of the lateral bands permits synchronized motion of both PIP and DIP joints by compensating for the difference in radii—or moment arms—of both joints. Normally IP joint motion is linked: The larger PIP joint with a greater range of motion flexes before the smaller DIP joint, which has less motion.[5] The smaller DIP joint would extend disproportionately relative to the PIP joint without the compensation provided by shifting of the lateral bands (Fig. 38-24).[5,82]

Retinacular Ligaments

The retinacular ligaments consist of fibers that encircle the finger obliquely about the PIP joint. They originate proximally from the flexor fibro-osseous sheath and palmar plate and course dorsally and distally about the joint. Their function is analogous to that of the sagittal bands about the MCP joints. Fibers palmar to the lateral bands—the transverse retinacular ligaments—contribute to axial stability of the PIP joint, restrain dorsal displacement of the lateral bands, and assist descent of the lateral bands during flexion. Dorsally, these fibers connect the lateral bands: Proximal fibers cover the insertions of the central tendon and medial fibers of the intrinsic tendons; more distal fibers connect the converging conjoined lateral bands. These distal fibers constitute the triangular ligament. Preservation of these dorsal retinacular ligaments after rupture or surgical division of the central

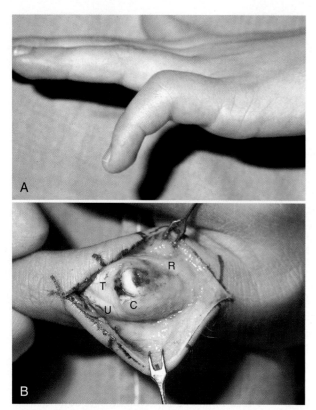

Figure 38-24 Closed rupture of extensor tendon about the proximal interphalangeal (PIP) joint. Active and passive extension were limited. There was no resistance to flexion of distal joint. **A,** Clinical posture of injured finger. **B,** Operative findings: central tendon ruptured with herniation of head of proximal phalanx; triangular ligament was preserved. Radial lateral band is trapped beneath condyle of proximal phalanx. Inability to passively extend PIP joint is indication for primary operative repair in extensor tendon injuries at this level. C, central tendon; R, radial lateral band; T, triangular ligament; U, ulnar lateral band.

tendon retains active extension of the PIP joint without development of a boutonnière deformity. Interruption of the transverse retinacular ligaments fosters dorsal displacement of the lateral bands with development of a swan-neck deformity (Fig. 38-25A, B).

The oblique retinacular ligaments originate from the flexor fibro-osseous sheath at the proximal phalanx, pass palmar to the axis of the PIP joint deep to the transverse retinacular ligament, and insert on the dorsal base of the distal phalanx adjacent to the terminal extensor tendon.[83] Distal fibers interdigitate with the terminal tendon before inserting, an important anatomic feature that influences the clinical presentation of the mallet tendon lesion[5,84] (Fig. 38-25C, D).

The terminal tendon alone is capable of completely extending the distal phalanx.[85] The dorsal rectangular segment of the collateral ligaments of the DIP joints can support the distal phalanx in 45 degrees of flexion. In the absence of the terminal tendon, the fully flexed distal finger joint passively returns to midflexion because of the collateral ligaments assisted by the dorsal capsule and oblique retinacular ligaments.[86]

The oblique retinacular ligaments probably contribute little to DIP joint extension in the normal finger.[87,88] The

position of its proximal fibers depends on the position of the PIP joint. They are below the joint axis only when the PIP joint is flexed. Passive extension of the PIP joint does not normally increase tension through the oblique retinacular ligaments.[89] They may stabilize the loaded fingertip when fully flexed under certain circumstances, such as the intrinsic-plus position with the DIP joint flexed during chuck pinch or when fingering the E string of a violin.[90] They can contribute significantly to deformity in the imbalanced finger or when they have been altered by scar (Fig. 38-26).

Extensor Tendon Injuries About the Metacarpophalangeal Joints (Zone V)

Closed soft tissue injuries about the MCP joints of the fingers jeopardize the extensor tendons, sagittal bands, dorsal joint capsule, collateral ligaments, and adjacent intrinsic tendons. Closed fractures of the metacarpal and sprain fractures of the MCP joints develop swelling and pain, which must be differentiated from soft tissue injuries by careful clinical and radiographic examination. Radiographs for assessing swelling and tenderness after injury of the finger MCP joints should include posteroanterior (PA), lateral, and Brewerton's* views to eliminate the possibility of occult marginal fractures.

Differential Diagnosis

Subluxation of the Extensor Tendon

Subluxation of the extensor tendon at this level was described in 1868.[91] It may result from chronic sustained forces,[92-94] tendon attrition, sudden exertion,[95,96] or direct trauma.[97] Rupture of the radial sagittal bands usually occurs.[98] Traumatic ulnar dislocation of the extensor tendon without sagittal band disruption does occur in the long finger, where the fibrous attachments of the extensor tendon to the underlying sagittal bands are significantly weaker than in the other fingers.[67,69] A partial arcuate tear in the ulnar sagittal bands with chronic pain and swelling over the MCP joint without displacement of the extensor tendon has been described.[99] Radial displacement of the extensor tendon is rare.[100] A chronically painful traumatic rupture of the dorsal capsule without rupture of the overlying sagittal bands can occur; repair of the capsule is then indicated.

Displacement of the tendon in the acute injury may be obscured by swelling. Extensor tendon subluxation with ulnar finger angulation of the index, long, or ring finger may not appear immediately and requires near complete disruption of the radial sagittal bands.[70] Ulnar angulation of the small finger is opposed by the junctura tendinum. Swelling,

---

*An anteroposterior tangential view of the metacarpal heads that is useful for visualizing the fossae of origin of the collateral ligaments. The dorsum of the extended fingers rests on the cassette, with the MCP joints in 65 degrees of flexion. The x-ray beam is perpendicular to the cassette and directed 15 degrees from the ulnar side.

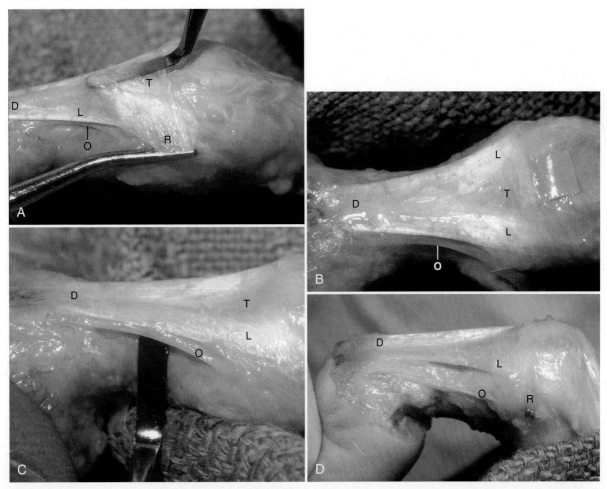

Figure 38-25 *Anatomy of the retinacular ligaments in the fingers.* **A,** *Vertical fibers about the proximal interphalangeal joint. These continuous fibers influence the descent and ascent of the lateral bands during flexion and extension.* **B,** *Fibers bridging the lateral bands dorsally restrain palmar migration during flexion. The blue insert is beneath the dorsal retinacular fibers and superficial to the central tendon insertion.* **C** *and* **D,** *Oblique retinacular ligament. Fibers are oriented in the axis of the finger. Proximal fibers pass beneath the transverse retinacular ligament palmar to the axis of the joint. Distal fibers mix with the lateral bands and terminal tendon. D, terminal tendon; L, lateral band; O, oblique retinacular ligament; R, transverse retinacular ligament; T, triangular ligament. (Adapted, with permission, from Rosenthal EA. Extensor surface injuries. In: Bowers WH, ed.* The Interphalangeal Joints. *London: Churchill Livingstone, 1987, p. 96.)*

tenderness, and ecchymosis are suggestive of significant fiber disruption in the acute case. Resisted finger extension with attempted deviation toward the examined sagittal band is a painful provocative test when the sagittal band is injured.[71]

Nonoperative treatment of the recent injury includes immobilization of the injured MCP joint for a minimum of 4 weeks.[101] Wrist immobilization is unnecessary. IP joint motion is permitted. A hand-based orthosis that supports the injured MCP joint in neutral position is comfortable and practical. A bridge orthosis that cradles the injured digit's MCP joint in 10 to 15 degrees greater extension than the adjacent supporting fingers for 8 weeks is an alternative.[101]

Surgery is appropriate in the acute case when complete rupture of the radial sagittal band is apparent (the extensor tendon has subluxated and the digit is angulated) and in the chronic recurrent case of ulnar tendon dislocation. Precise reconstitution of the normal anatomic relationships restores a balance that may be only wishful with closed methods (see Fig. 38-19).

Surgical repair of a sagittal band defect with extensor subluxation was first described by Haberern.[102] Repair of the radial[103] or ulnar[99] sagittal bands, anatomic relocation, and a variety of surgical tenodeses that maintain the centralized extensor tendon have been described for operative correction of imbalance and dysfunction that persist despite adequate nonoperative treatment.[37,57,104-108]

Saddle Syndrome

The interosseous and lumbrical tendons converge distal to the deep transverse metacarpal ligament radial to the MCP joint of the long, ring, and small fingers (Fig. 38-27). Consolidation of these tendons by restraining adhesions about the deep transverse metacarpal ligament after closed injuries has been descriptively termed the *saddle syndrome.*[109] This uncommon chronic condition is characterized by persistent pain with grip. Direct and compression tenderness between the adjacent metacarpal necks, painful active intrinsic function (MCP joint flexion with IP joint extension) against

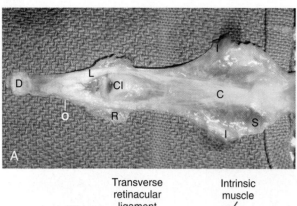

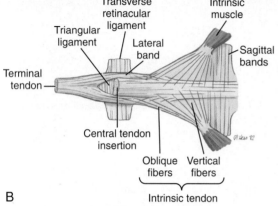

Figure 38-26 *Extensor tendons in fingers are represented by continuous sheet of specialized fibers that are stabilized by retinacular ligaments.* **A,** *Deep side of extensor tendon complex. Terminal tendon is at left.* **B,** *Schematic drawing of* **A.** *C, central tendon; CI, central tendon insertion; I, intrinsic tendon; L, lateral band; O, oblique retinacular ligament; R, transverse retinacular ligament; S, sagittal bands; D, terminal tendon.*

resistance, and pain with eliciting the intrinsic tightness test (passive flexion of the IP joints while the MCP joints are supported in extension) support this diagnosis. Intrinsic restraint can be lateralized by deviating the finger away from the side being tested. Intrinsic tenolysis, including resection of the distal margin of the deep transverse metacarpal

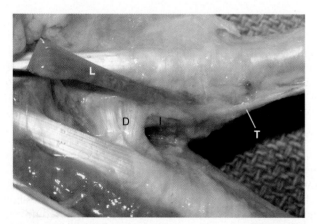

Figure 38-27 *Lumbrical and interosseous muscles merge distal to deep transverse metacarpal ligament: the anatomic basis of saddle syndrome. Hook lifts the third lumbrical muscle from the ligament connecting the palmar plates of the long and ring finger MCP joints. Adhesions between the ligament and intrinsic tendons may produce painful intrinsic dysfunction. D, deep transverse metacarpal ligament; I, interosseous muscle; L, lumbrical muscle; T, intrinsic tendon fibers of dorsal apparatus.*

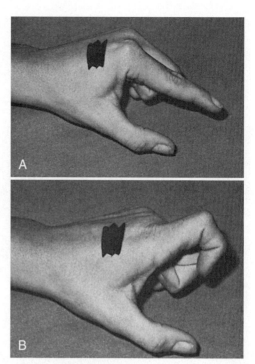

Figure 38-28 *Extensor-plus finger tenodesis caused by restrained extensor tendons proximal to the metacarpophalangeal (MCP) joints.* **A,** *Active and passive flexion of MCP joint produces passive tenodesis with extension of IP joints.* **B,** *Active or passive interphalangeal flexion passively extends MCP joints.*

ligament through a palmar incision, is indicated when symptoms persist.[109,110]

Collateral Ligament Rupture

Early diagnosis is apparent when the fully flexed MCP joint is unstable to lateral deviation. Normally, this joint is most stable in full flexion. Partial ruptures are painful when tested but retain stability. Radiographs are essential. Closed treatment is indicated initially for soft tissue injuries; significant joint fractures are replaced and internally stabilized. Closed sprains that continue to be painful after immobilization and supportive nonoperative treatment may require surgery. Early surgical repair has been shown to lead to earlier healing of the ligaments and earlier return to work in patients with complete ligaments' interruption.[111,112]

Chronic Tendon Adhesions

Inelastic adhesions between the extensor hood, intrinsic tendons, and underlying capsule may be the source of persistent painful swelling with loss of motion. Thickening of the dorsal joint capsule may develop beneath the scarred extensor hood. Chronic thickening of the extensor hood from repeated trauma, reported in students of karate, has been termed *hypertrophic infiltrative tendinitis* (HIT syndrome).[113] Painful active motion, an extrinsic tenodesis (the extensor-plus phenomenon [Fig. 38-28]), and positive intrinsic tightness test all are possible findings when adhesions consolidate the extrinsic and intrinsic tendons about the finger MCP joints.[114] Tenolysis that selectively defines the extrinsic and intrinsic tendon systems, in combination with a dorsal capsulectomy when necessary, liberates the tethered tendons (Fig. 38-29).

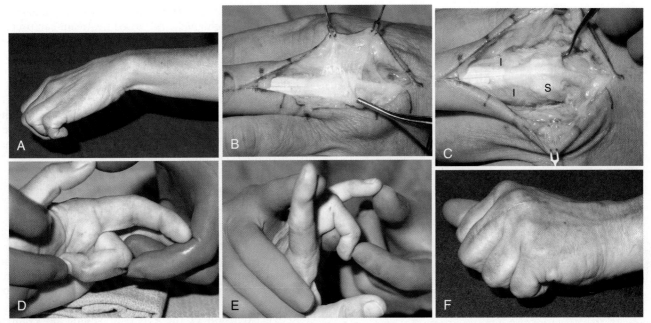

Figure 38-29 Extrinsic and intrinsic dysfunction from scarring caused by focal crush injury about the long finger metacarpophalangeal (MCP) joint in 54-year-old woman. **A,** Limited, painful grip 6 months after injury. **B,** Dorsal exposure over the MCP joint. Adhesions between skin flap and extensor hood are evident. **C,** Anatomic structures clearly defined after tenolysis. Instrument is beneath the radial sagittal bands of dorsal apparatus. **D,** Extrinsic tenodesis has been eliminated. **E,** Intrinsic tightness test is negative. **F,** Voluntary grip 10 weeks after surgery. S, ulnar sagittal bands; I, intrinsic fibers of dorsal apparatus.

Extensor Tendon Injuries About the Proximal Interphalangeal Joints (Zone III)

Interruption of the extensor tendons at the PIP joint may result from lacerations, closed trauma, burns, rheumatoid synovitis, or tightly applied casts and orthoses. The deformities that develop reflect a distortion of forces that are normally balanced by tendon and retinacular systems. Early deformities are reversed more easily than lasting ones that have developed ligament and tendon tightness. Persistent deformities become resistant to correction and influence the prognosis for treatment adversely.

Functional Anatomy

The central tendon is the primary extensor of the PIP joint. The intrinsic tendons contribute medial slips that insert on the dorsal lip of the middle phalanx adjacent to the central tendon and receive lateral slips from the extrinsic tendon to form the conjoined lateral bands The lateral bands normally descend during flexion and cover the axis of joint motion, where they are incapable of initiating extension. In this position, they do not transmit much tension and initially do not generate a significant deforming flexor moment to the PIP joint.[80] The central tendon alone is capable of initiating extension of the flexed joint. Tension through the lateral bands increases progressively as they migrate dorsally during extension; their contribution to PIP joint extension increases with dorsal displacement. Dorsally stationed lateral bands can maintain extension of the PIP joint. Normally, the lateral bands are relaxed when the PIP joint is fully flexed, tethered

by the central tendon and incapable of extending the DIP joint. In moderate (30- to 40-degree) PIP joint flexion, transfer of tension through the lateral bands to the DIP joint is weak but evident. This can be demonstrated clinically by holding the MCP joint in neutral and the PIP joint in moderate flexion: a weak active extension of the DIP joint is evident (Fig. 38-30).

The transverse retinacular ligaments and their dorsal fibers connect the lateral bands and are functionally similar to the sagittal bands about the MCP joint; they contribute to extension of the PIP joint. Translation of the lateral bands is controlled by the fibers of the retinacular ligaments. Descent is limited by the dorsal fibers of the retinacular ligament (the triangular ligament); dorsal displacement is restrained by the transverse retinacular ligament. The palmar plate and the flexor superficialis tendon resist hyperextension.

Pathologic Anatomy

Disruption of the central tendon interferes with normal active extension of the PIP joint. Initiation of extension of the flexed joint is lost. The final 15 to 20 degrees of active extension also is lost. This can be demonstrated by actively extending the fingers while the wrist and MCP joints are supported in flexion: It implies disruption of the central tendon with potential for development of a boutonnière deformity.[115] The positioned PIP joint can be maintained in extension by the lateral bands while they remain dorsal.

Release of the central tendon allows the finger extensor mechanism to slide proximally. This increases forces transmitted to the middle phalanx through the transverse retinacular ligaments and to the distal phalanx through the

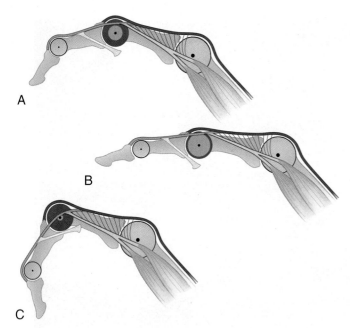

Figure 38-30 *Lateral band shift. The radius of the blue circle depicts extrinsic central tendon moment arm for the proximal interphalangeal (PIP) joint extension; radius of green circle depicts moment arm of lateral bands.* **A,** *There is balanced tension between the central tendon and lateral bands in the resting position. The interphalangeal joints are partially flexed. Intrinsic muscle tension through the lateral bands is diminished by partial lateral band descent. Active distal interphalangeal (DIP) joint extension is incomplete.* **B,** *The lateral bands rest dorsally during extension. Moment arm for extension of the PIP joint by lateral bands is maximum. Active DIP joint extension is strong. Even a single lateral band can maintain extension of the fully extended PIP joint.* **C,** *Moment arm of the lateral bands decreases progressively with PIP joint flexion; the moment arm of the central tendon does not. Only the central tendon can initiate extension of the fully flexed PIP joint normally. Active extension of the DIP joint is weak and incomplete. (Reprinted, with permission, from Rosenthal EA: Dynamics of the extensor system. In: Hunter JM, Schneider LH, Mackin EJ, eds. Tendon and Nerve Surgery of the Hand. A Third Decade. St. Louis: Mosby–Year Book, 1997)*

lateral slips, conjoined lateral bands, and terminal tendon. Active extension of the DIP joint then can be demonstrated while the MCP joint is held in neutral with the PIP joint in full flexion.[116] Hyperextension of the PIP joint is resisted by the transverse retinacular ligaments that restrain dorsal displacement of the lateral bands during extension and by the flexor superficialis tendon and palmar plate. These observations form the anatomic rationale for surgical tenotomy of the central tendon in selected patients with a mallet finger deformity.[107]

The dorsal fibers of the retinacular ligament (triangular ligament) significantly influence the sequence of events after rupture of the central tendon. Partial tears of the triangular ligament retain sufficient control of the lateral bands to ensure dorsal positioning during extension with a favorable prognosis for return of extensor function after closed treatment. However, partial tears extend if unprotected motion continues after an injury.[117] Complete tearing of the triangular ligament, combined with interruption of the central tendon, eliminates control of both joint extension and the lateral bands. This situation initiates an imbalance that results in a fixed deformity unless diligent treatment intervenes. Passive extension of the PIP joint implies that the

lateral bands have relocated dorsally, the retinacular ligaments have not tightened, and closed treatment can proceed.

The finger is vulnerable to combined tissue injuries that involve the extensor tendons, collateral ligaments, and palmar plate when the flexed PIP joint is subjected to torsional stress.[118] Axial instability with extensor tendon rupture after a closed injury is an indication for primary surgery. Loss of active and passive extension of the PIP joint occurs when a lateral band becomes trapped beneath the condylar flare of the proximal phalanx. This is another indication for primary operative intervention (see Fig. 38-24).

Examination of the Injured Proximal Interphalangeal Joint

The finger deformity and distribution of swelling are important indicators that infer the location and nature of the injury. Palpation with the fingertip or a pencil eraser can precisely locate tenderness. Radiographs should include posteroanterior, true lateral, radial, and ulnar oblique views of the injured finger.

Active extension of the PIP joint should be evaluated against gravity and against resistance with the MCP joint in neutral.[119] Only the central tendon can initiate extension of the fully flexed PIP joint. The lateral bands alone can maintain extension of the passively extended joint if they rest dorsal to the axis of joint motion, but they cannot initiate extension of the completely flexed joint. A single lateral band can maintain extension even when the other lateral band and the triangular ligament are torn. Inability to initiate active extension of the fully flexed PIP joint is consistent with interruption of the central tendon (see Fig. 38-30).

Integrity of the central tendon also can be tested by a tenodesis mechanism. The wrist and MCP joint are held in flexion, and active PIP joint extension is tested. A 15- to 20-degree extension lag at the PIP joint suggests injury to the central tendon with the potential for development of a boutonnière deformity.[115]

Assess DIP joint extension while the PIP joint is moderately flexed (30–40 degrees) and fully flexed.[116] The lateral bands normally do not transmit tension to the DIP joint when they have descended to the axis of joint motion during full PIP joint flexion; transmitted tension increases progressively as the PIP joint is extended. The lateral bands cannot extend the DIP joint while the PIP joint is fully flexed and only weakly extend the DIP joint when the PIP joint is partially flexed, unless the central tendon is interrupted. Relatively strong DIP joint extension, compared with adjacent normal fingers, with the PIP joint fully flexed or partially flexed is consistent with interruption of the central tendon and retention of at least one lateral band. DIP joint extension cannot be executed when both lateral bands have been interrupted.

The lateral bands are normally weak extensors of the DIP joint when the PIP joint is in full extension. Increased tension, compared with adjacent normal fingers, with passive flexion of the DIP joint while the PIP joint is fully extended implies interruption of the central tendon with proximal slide of the extensor tendons.

The therapist should assess axial stability for both sides of the joint as well as hyperextension stability. Axial instability is consistent with collateral ligament rupture. Oblique hyperextension can rupture the proximal attachments of the palmar plate with localized tenderness but with normal initial radiographic films. Early motion with a protective orthosis is required to prevent the development of a pseudoboutonnière deformity.[120,121] Axial instability combined with extensor tendon rupture defines a combined tissue injury and is an indication for primary operative repair.[118]

Boutonnière Deformity

The boutonnière deformity develops after an injury to the extensor mechanism and specifically denotes flexion of the PIP joint with hyperextension of the DIP joint. The head of the proximal phalanx herniates through a defect in the extensor mechanism after rupture of the central tendon and dorsal fibers of the retinacular ligament (triangular ligament).[28] An analogous deformity occurs in the thumb with MCP joint flexion and IP joint extension. The mechanisms of closed injury include involuntary forceful flexion of an actively extended digit, blunt trauma to the dorsum of the joint, and dislocation of the joint with tearing of the extensor tendons and stabilizing ligaments.

Interruption of the central tendon and triangular ligament permits proximal displacement of the extensor mechanism and palmar shift of the lateral bands. The unopposed flexor digitorum superficialis (FDS) flexes the PIP joint. The extrinsic extensor tendon, released from the middle phalanx, transfers forces through the sagittal bands that enhance extension of the MCP joint. Both extrinsic and intrinsic muscles transmit exaggerated forces through the conjoined lateral bands that extend the DIP joint. The transverse retinacular ligaments, oblique retinacular ligaments, and check ligaments of the palmar plate are loose early in the evolution of the deformity (Fig. 38-31A, B). The test for retinacular tightness is negative, and the deformity is reversible passively (Fig. 38-32A). The lateral bands return to their normal dorsal station and can maintain extension. Prognosis after orthotic application is most favorable during this early phase.

The lateral bands descend progressively, and the PIP joint cannot be maintained in full extension. An active extension lag develops that is passively correctable, whereas the transverse and oblique retinacular ligaments and palmar plate remain supple and have not foreshortened (see Fig. 38-31B).

The palmar-displaced lateral bands become fixed to the underlying collateral ligaments and joint capsule, and the retinacular ligaments and palmar plate tighten and oppose passive correction (see Fig. 38-31C). The DIP joint loses active flexion, develops hyperextension, and progressively loses passive flexion. The retinacular tightness test is then positive (Fig. 38-32B). The deformity is fixed and cannot be reversed without sustained effort. Treatment of the fixed deformity is complicated, and the prognosis is altered (Fig. 38-33).

Nonoperative Treatment

Closed extensor tendon injuries about the PIP joint must be accurately appraised and closely monitored. Prescribed treatment is designed for a specific injury. A palmar injury with potential for a pseudoboutonnière deformity is approached

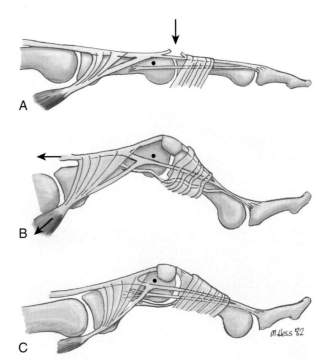

Figure 38-31 Development of boutonnière deformity. **A,** Injury involves insertion of central extensor tendon at the base of the middle phalanx with interruption of dorsal fibers of transverse retinacular ligament. **B,** Middle phalanx is pulled into flexion by the flexor digitorum superficialis. Lateral bands displace palmarward over the joint axis and become flexors of this joint. At this stage, palmar plate ligaments and oblique and transverse retinacular ligaments are loose. The deformity can be reversed with relative ease. **C,** Established deformity with shortening of extensor tendons, tightening of palmar plate ligaments and oblique and transverse retinacular ligaments. The retinacular tightness test is positive. Passive correction of deformity is resisted. Reversal of deformity at this stage is slow and represents a significant commitment by surgeon and therapist.

differently from a dorsal injury with potential for a classic boutonnière deformity. Swelling and dorsal tenderness should be considered an indication of an injury to the extensor tendons even when examination suggests intact structures. Partial ligament and tendon tears may extend unless the injured digit is protected.[117] The PIP joint is positioned

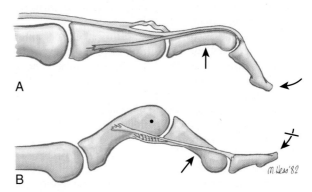

Figure 38-32 Testing for tightness of the oblique retinacular ligament. **A,** Passive extension of middle phalanx with passive flexion of the distal phalanx is performed without resistance in the normal finger: a negative test. **B,** Contracture of oblique retinacular ligament, with resistant flexion of the proximal interphalangeal (PIP) joint and hyperextension of the distal interphalangeal (DIP) joint. The DIP joint cannot be passively flexed when extension of PIP joint is passively increased: a positive test.

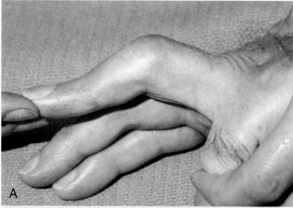
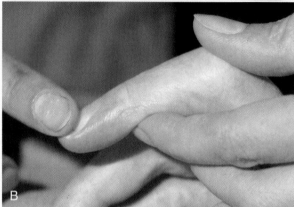

Figure 38-33 Established boutonnière deformity. **A,** Fixed flexion deformity of the proximal interphalangeal (PIP) joint with hyperextension of distal interphalangeal (DIP) joint. **B,** Resistant passive flexion of the DIP joint with attempted extension of the PIP joint from tightness of the retinacular ligaments augmented by tightness of the extensor tendons through displaced lateral bands.

Table 38-1 Treatment of Closed Injuries of the Extensor Tendons of the Proximal Interphalangeal (PIP) Joint

• Suggestive examination • Active extension • Passive extension • No fracture	• Active extension loss • Passive extension • No fracture	• Active extension loss • Passive extension loss • +/− Axial instability • +/− Fracture
Orthosis PIP joint Reassess in 1 week	Orthosis PIP joint 6 weeks ? Kirschner wire	Primary repair Open reduction fracture ? 2nd stage tendon reconstruction

Reprinted with permission, modified from Rosenthal EA. Extensor surface injuries at the proximal interphalangeal joint. In Bowers WH, editor: *The Hand and Upper Limb, Vol. 1—The Interphalangeal Joint.* London: Churchill Livingstone, 1987, p. 99.

in extension for an additional 2 to 4 weeks, when active motion is not being pursued. The requirements for continued support of the PIP joint reflect postural stability of the finger. Orthotic use is reinstituted if an extensor lag or boutonnière deformity recurs. An orthosis is recommended only at night, when PIP joint extension can be sustained and if there has been no deterioration during subsequent visits.

The time required for rehabilitation of the boutonnière deformity by orthotic positioning can be prolonged. Resistant cases can require attention and supervision for 6 to 9 months after injury. Tissue maturation with realization of the full potential function of the finger may not be achieved for a full year (Fig. 38-34).

Operative Treatment

Primary operative repair is indicated for the acute closed injury with loss of passive extension of the PIP joint and in combined tissue injuries when central tendon rupture is associated with joint instability. Severe soft tissue injuries associated with fractures may require staged reconstruction. The fracture is repaired primarily, then tendon restoration is performed as a separate procedure after the fracture has healed.

Electing surgery for the chronic boutonnière deformity is an individualized decision. A mild flexion deformity of the PIP joint (<30 degrees) has variable individual effect and may not significantly interfere with grasp or finger function. The cosmetic deformity is often disliked by patients but may not be sufficient to motivate a request for reconstruction. A comfortable, useful range of active flexion of both IP joints provides excellent function despite the persistence of a slight flexion deformity of the PIP joint.

More severe deformities do create functional impairments. A large portion of the handicap with an established boutonnière deformity reflects loss of distal joint flexion. Candidates for surgery should be selected carefully after evaluating their symptoms, deformity, anticipated improvement after treatment, and compliance. Selection as a candidate for surgery implies a willingness to participate in a closely supervised, often prolonged, rehabilitation program after surgery.

PIP joint flexion deformity should be reversed and active DIP joint flexion should be restored before surgery. The results from surgery are better when joint deformities are corrected preoperatively[11] (Fig. 38-35, online). Mature, hard, resistant scar occasionally demonstrates a surprising

in extension, and the digit is reassessed in 1 week. DIP joint motion is permitted during this period. A repeat normal functional examination of the finger implies that complete tendon rupture has not occurred. However, orthotic use is continued for an additional 2 weeks if swelling, tenderness, or ecchymosis is noted during reexamination. Orthotic use is discontinued after 3 weeks if the patient continues to demonstrate intact extensor tendons and no deformity has developed (Table 38-1).

A digital orthosis or QuickCast for a closed extensor tendon injury about the PIP joint treated without operative intervention immobilizes the PIP joint in neutral. The MCP joint and DIP joint are left free. Active distal joint flexion synergistically relaxes the intrinsic and extrinsic extensor tendon muscles. A 3- to 4-mm glide is imparted to the central tendon through the lateral bands while the PIP joint is restrained.[122] The oblique retinacular ligament also is exercised through continued distal joint motion.

An orthotic program for treatment of the established boutonnière deformity should be tailored to fit the tissue requirements of the patient. The physician and therapist should be familiar with the anatomy of the extensor tendons and the pathomechanics of the deformity being treated. Initial orthotic positioning supports the PIP joint in neutral while permitting active flexion of the DIP joint. Its use is continued without interruption for 6 weeks. Carefully monitored flexion of the PIP joint is then initiated. The PIP joint is supported

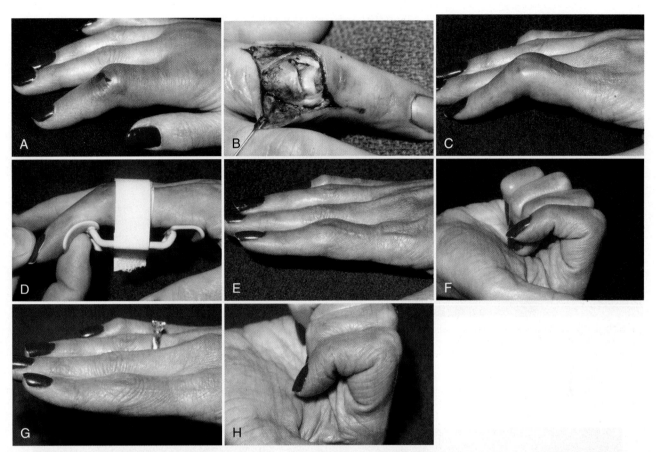

Figure 38-34 Conservative treatment of boutonnière deformity. Laceration of extensor tendons with delayed primary treatment and wound infection. **A,** Untreated laceration 5 days after injury. **B,** Operative findings: Complete division of the central tendon; palmar displacement of the lateral bands; Streptococcal pyarthrosis in the proximal interphalangeal (PIP) joint. **C,** 7 weeks after surgery: Fixed deformity with resistant flexion of PIP joint and extension of distal interphalangeal joint. **D,** Supervised use of a serial static orthosis designed to reestablish extension of proximal and flexion of distal joint deformities. (Extension Finger Splint marketed by COSCO, Redding, Cal.) **E,** Active extension with normal power 5 months after program instituted. Tissue softening is progressing. Dorsal bump represents cosmetic disfigurement. **F,** Active flexion after 5 months. **G,** Complete extension with mature soft tissues and reduced disfigurement after 3 years. **H,** Active flexion after 3 years.

plasticity when subjected to tension for long periods of time. Extensor tendon reconstructions alone do not improve the passive correction that preoperative treatment has gained (Fig. 38-36). Fingers that cannot be corrected by means of orthosis and supervised therapy require extensive surgical releases that introduce new imbalances capable of promoting additional future deformity (Fig. 38-37).

The method for operative repair is determined by the condition of the central tendon and lateral bands. Elliott's anatomic reconstruction requires an adequate central tendon and both lateral bands.[104,123] Littler and Eaton restored PIP joint extension by reefing both lateral bands over the dorsum of the PIP joint and central tendon remnant. The lumbrical tendon and oblique retinacular ligament were preserved to maintain DIP joint extension.[108] Matev's method has application when the central tendon is deficient; this method permits rebalancing of both PIP and DIP joints[124] (Fig. 38-38). Other innovative techniques have been promulgated to replace variable deficiencies of the skin–subcutaneous envelope, central tendon, and lateral bands when correcting the boutonnière deformity. Intact lateral bands may be mobilized then approximated centrally over the dorsum of the PIP joint without interrupting the terminal tendon when there has been loss of substance of the central tendon.[125,126] Mobilized lateral bands can be reinforced by folding both transverse retinacular liga-

ments dorsally.[127] A lost central tendon also can be replaced by reinserting a single lateral band[128]; distally reversing the segmental tendon graft from the proximal extensor tendon[129]; transferring a lateral band from an adjacent finger[130]; bridging the central tendon insertion with a free tendon graft using proximal extrinsic extensor tendon[131,132] or an intrinsic tendons[133]; interposing the FDS tendon that is passed dorsally through the normal insertion of the central tendon[134]; intercalary palmaris longus free tendon grafting that includes the deep forearm fascia[135]; and an arterialized tendocutaneous flap containing a lateral band.[136] The use of suture anchors has been advocated recently in the reconstruction of chronic boutonnière deformity.[137] The works by Burton[138] and Rosenthal[43] are recommended for expanded discussions of operative management of deformities from extensor tendon injuries about the PIP joint.

Extensor Tendon Injuries at the Distal Interphalangeal Joint (Zone I)

Mallet finger is synonymous with interruption of the extensor tendon mechanism at the level of the DIP joint. The term is

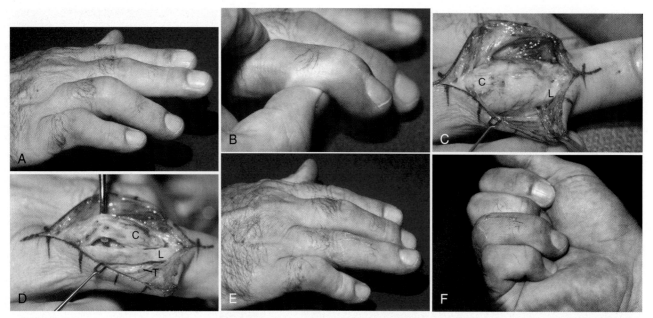

Figure 38-36 Chronic boutonnière deformity with functional impairment. Closed ring finger injury in a 67-year-old man initially treated with 2 weeks of orthotic use. Regression followed removal of the orthosis. **A,** Posture when first evaluated. Passive correction the proximal interphalangeal (PIP) joint was achieved with orthotic use. **B,** Active distal interphalangeal joint flexion with the PIP joint in neutral position confirms reversal of tendon and ligament tightness. **C,** Normal tendon anatomy about the PIP joint transformed by scar; subluxated ulnar lateral band is adherent to the capsule. **D,** Elevator lifts central tendon created from scarred tissue. Lateral bands were surgically defined. Thick transverse retinacular ligaments were incised. Proximal and distal joint extensor tendons were functionally rebalanced. **E,** Active extension 7 months after surgery lacks 20 degrees. **F,** Active flexion at 7 months. C, central tendon; L, lateral band; T, transverse retinacular ligament.

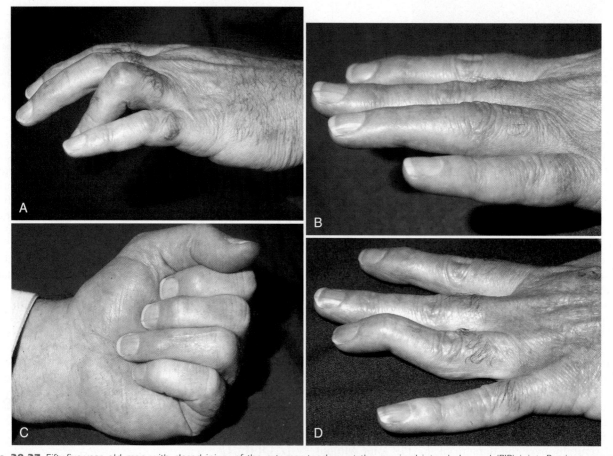

Figure 38-37 Fifty-five-year–old man with closed injury of the extensor tendons at the proximal interphalangeal (PIP) joint. Previous unsuccessful surgery 3 months after injury for uncorrected boutonnière deformity. Surgery included suture of the lateral bands dorsally with terminal tendon tenotomy. **A,** Fixed deformity when first seen 4 months after surgery. **B,** Clinical extension 6 months after anatomic reconstruction of the central tendon, palmar plate release, and resection of accessory collateral ligaments of PIP joint. The extensor tendon over the middle phalanx was not disturbed. **C,** Active flexion 6 months after surgery. **D,** Posture 9 years after reconstruction. Swan-neck deformity has developed from hyperextension instability of the PIP joint. The distal interphalangeal joint flexed actively. Mature scar retains some plasticity when subjected to chronic tensions. Extensive surgical releases introduce a potential for imbalances beyond those in original deformity.

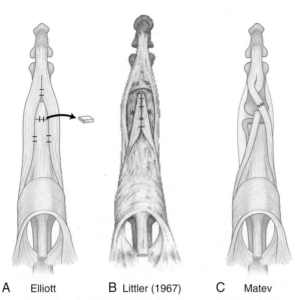

A Elliott   B Littler (1967)   C Matev

Figure 38-38 *Operative methods for reconstruction of the chronic boutonnière deformity.* **A,** *Anatomic reconstruction described by Elliott.* **B,** *Replacement of the central tendon with lateral bands that are folded dorsally and inserted on the base of the middle phalanx, described by Littler.* **C,** *Matev's method for reconstructing the central tendon and adjusting the terminal tendon using both lateral bands. (Reprinted, with permission, from Rosenthal EA. Extensor surface injuries at the proximal interphalangeal joint. In: Bowers WH, ed.* The Hand and Upper Limb, *Vol. 1,* The Interphalangeal Joints. *London: Churchill Livingstone, 1987.)*

not descriptive but has gained universal acceptance for the deformity that results (Fig. 38-39).

The terminal extensor tendon represents the distal extension of the merged lateral bands that insert on the dorsal base of the distal phalanx. The more central fibers of the tendon are bordered by the distal extensions of the oblique retinacular ligaments that insert on the lateral base of the distal phalanx adjacent to the terminal tendon.[5] The interweaving of adjacent tendon and ligament fibers before insertion contributes to the success of treatment of central fiber injuries at this level.

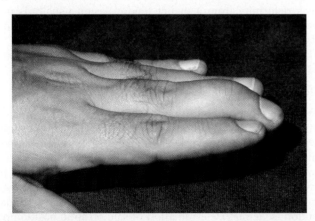

Figure 38-39 *Mallet finger with hyperextension deformity of the proximal interphalangeal joint. Interruption of the terminal tendon concentrates extension forces at the middle phalanx. Swan-neck deformity with mallet tendon lesion has wide ranges of severity.*

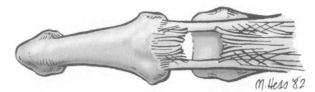

Figure 38-40 *Mallet tendon lesion. Shredding or tearing of the terminal tendon occurs proximal to its insertion, over the trochlea of the middle phalanx. Central fibers that insert on the dorsal beak of the distal phalanx have the greatest moment arm for distal joint extension, are subject to greater tension during passive distal joint flexion, and rupture first. More lateral fibers that insert closer to the axis of joint motion are less efficient extensors, are subject to less stress, and may be preserved. Interweaving between lateral extensor tendon fibers and the oblique retinacular ligament may maintain some continuity of the extensor tendon with the distal phalanx.*

Patterns of injury

The patterns of closed injuries depend on the position of the DIP joint at the time of injury and the direction of the injuring force. The treatment depends on the type of injury.

Passive flexion of the distal phalanx is resisted by tension through the terminal tendon through the initial 45 degrees of DIP joint flexion. The oblique retinacular and collateral ligaments are normally relaxed through this range. Direct trauma to the partially flexed distal phalanx ruptures (frays) the central fibers of the terminal tendon over the trochlea of the middle phalanx.[84] These central fibers, which insert on the dorsal beak of the distal phalanx, have the largest moment arm for distal joint extension and are the most efficient terminal tendon fibers for active extension. Lateral border terminal tendon fibers that insert on the distal phalanx closer to the axis of joint motion are less efficient distal joint extensors, are subject to less stress during passive joint flexion, and may be preserved. The oblique retinacular ligaments are not under tension and remain intact. The interwoven border fibers of tendon and ligament retain some anatomic continuity with the base of the distal phalanx. Partial distal joint extension that is often retained by these patients exists from preservation of lateral terminal tendon fibers. Recoil of the passively flexed distal joint is by the collateral ligaments of the joint and retinacular ligaments.[86] The extension lag is passively correctable. This is a pure tendon lesion (Fig. 38-40).

Both the terminal tendon and the oblique retinacular ligaments are under tension when the DIP joint is flexed beyond 45 degrees. Passive flexion of the distal phalanx while tension is transmitted through the terminal tendon produces a dorsal avulsion fracture with total interruption in the functional continuity of the extensor tendon[139] (Fig. 38-41).

A longitudinal impaction force that hyperextends the DIP joint creates a large articular fracture of the base of the distal phalanx[140] (Fig. 38-42A). This is a significant joint injury. The effect on extensor tendon function is often small, without a mallet deformity. The large dorsal fragment retains collateral ligament attachments to the middle phalanx. Dorsal fractures of more than one third of the base of the distal phalanx may be unstable.[141,142] Subluxation was not observed when the fracture fragment measured less than 43% of the joint surface but consistently occurred when the fragment measured greater than 52%.[143] The degree of instability relates to

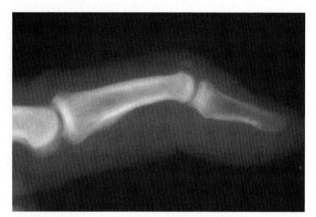

Figure 38-41 Total interruption of terminal extensor tendon insertion with adjacent retinacular ligaments may be associated with a small dorsal avulsion fracture. This produces a mallet deformity. Residual extension of the distal interphalangeal joint results from retained lateral tendon fibers.

disruption of collateral ligament attachments to the distal fracture fragment. A stable distal fragment flexes; the unstable distal fragment is pulled proximally by the flexor profundus with volar displacement (Fig. 38-42B). Patients are inclined to dismiss the injury as trivial and may not seek early treatment.

Development of Deformity

Interruption of the terminal tendon insertion permits retraction of the extensor tendons proximally. This transfers

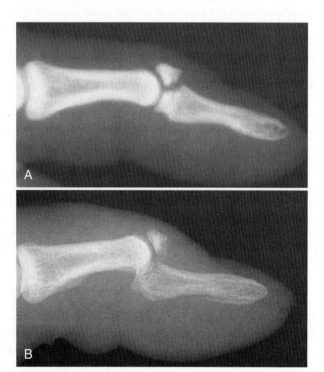

Figure 38-42 Impaction hyperextension injury produces major articular fracture with potential instability of the distal interphalangeal joint, usually without mallet deformity. **A,** Radiograph at the time of injury. **B,** Six weeks after injury: Persistent palmar subluxation is evident; traumatic arthritis is established. Major articular distal joint injuries are potentially unstable. Despite significant potential for remodeling, operative reduction with internal stabilization is more predictable and preferable.

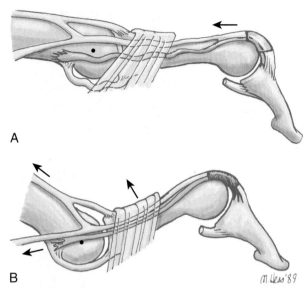

Figure 38-43 Development of mallet deformity. **A,** Interruption of the extensor tendon over the distal interphalangeal joint permits unopposed flexion of the joint by the flexor digitorum profundus (FDP) tendon. Loss of distal restraint permits proximal slide of the extensor tendons. Oblique retinacular ligaments and lateral bands become slack. Palmar plate at the proximal interphalangeal (PIP) joint resists hyperextension. **B,** Concentration of extension forces from extrinsic and intrinsic muscles transmitted through the central tendon, lateral bands, and transverse retinacular ligaments produces hyperextension at the PIP joint. Hyperextension increases as the palmar plate yields. Transposed dorsal lateral bands and tight oblique retinacular ligaments resist flexion until forced palmar over the condylar flares of the proximal phalanx from extreme flexion of the distal joint by the FDP tendon.

tension to the central tendon and conjoined lateral bands. The central tendon (via its bony insertion) and the lateral bands (via the transverse retinacular ligaments) concentrate extension forces on the middle phalanx. The palmar plate resists hyperextension of the PIP joint. The retinacular ligaments are initially lax. Hyperextension of the PIP joint develops if the palmar plate is lax. The flexor digitorum profundus (FDP) flexes the DIP joint, creating a mild swan-neck deformity. The severity of the deformity is inversely proportional to stability of the palmar plate at the PIP joint. The swan-neck deformity from a mallet tendon lesion usually is not severe enough to impair finger flexion unless hyperextension of the PIP joint is advanced (Fig. 38-43).

Treatment

Closed Injuries

The mallet tendon lesion without fracture should be treated with uninterrupted immobilization of the DIP joint in slight hyperextension for 6 weeks.[18,139] The PIP joint is not immobilized. The classical treatment proposed by Smillie,[144] which immobilized the PIP joint in flexion and the DIP joint in hyperextension, is no longer advocated. Hyperextension may produce dorsal skin blanching with cutaneous and terminal tendon ischemia. Determination of safe orthotic positioning is individualized; dorsal skin should not blanch in the immobilized position.[145] Reliable patients can be treated with an orthosis; others may require Kirschner-wire (K-wire) pinning. Some patients require adjustment of the attitude of the positioned joint as the swelling of injury subsides and further extension is tolerated.

Carefully supervised treatment is successful in restoring DIP joint extension and reducing extension lag when treatment is initiated early (within 2 weeks of injury) or is delayed (beyond 4 weeks of injury).[146] A favorable prognosis is more predictable with earlier treatment than with delayed treatment even though successful delayed treatment has been reported. K-wire pinning under metacarpal neck block anesthesia with mini C-arm control is the most secure and predictable treatment for mallet tendon injuries. The risk of pin tract infection increases the longer the pin is retained and the more actively the patient uses the digit during the treatment period. Cutting the distal end of the pin beneath the skin is a worthwhile precaution that lessens the risk of infection and permits more normal function. However, this precaution requires a secondary operative procedure to remove the pin.

Numerous designs for mallet orthoses have been promoted. Variations in digital contour, distal joint extensibility, and swelling after injury justify use of orthoses that are individually crafted for each injured finger. A carefully molded digital QuickCast2 (Sammons Preston, Inc., Bolingbrook, Ill.) that immobilizes only the DIP joint is a stable immobilizing method that avoids risk of positional lapses during orthotic changes. These casts reduce swelling, but are even more effective when applied over Coban (3M Health Care, St. Paul, Minn.). The cast needs to be replaced periodically to ensure skin hygiene throughout immobilization (Fig. 38-44). A dorsal orthosis of the DIP joint with a foam-padded aluminum orthosis does not encroach on the tactile palmar surface of the finger and avoids localized pressure over the site of tendon injury. A better orthosis can be made by thinning the foam of commercially available material. Cloth adhesive tape between the foam and skin reduces maceration. The orthosis may be changed periodically by the insightful patient; other patients require more frequent visits to the physician or therapist (Fig. 38-45, online). The traditional Stack orthosis[147] has been windowed to enhance moisture evaporation and permit pulp contact during orthotic use, but these remain less desirable than QuickCast2 or aluminum orthoses. Perforated thermoplastic orthoses with Velcro straps also are available.[148,149] A bent, semitubular, small fragment plate with Steri-Strips (3M, St. Paul, Minn.), and Mexican hat orthosis, have also been used successfully.[150,151] Active motion of the PIP joint is continued throughout the period of orthotic use; this flexion reduces tension at the site of injury. Distal joint motion is begun after 6 weeks of continuous positioning in an orthosis. Night orthotic positioning of the distal joint is continued for an additional 2 to 4 weeks after distal joint motion is begun. Full-time orthotic use should be reinstituted if clinical regression occurs after active distal joint motion is begun (Fig. 38-46).

Loss of active extension—an *extension lag*—and decreased distal joint flexion from terminal tendon scarring are both complications from closed treatment of the mallet tendon lesion.[152] Dorsal skin maceration or necrosis is a complication of improper use of an orthosis. A 45% incidence of complications associated with closed treatment of mallet finger injuries has been reported.[153]

The clinical result may not be realized for at least 6 months after injury.[154] An early extension lag can decrease as the healing tendon scar contracts.[147] Pulvertaft observed that

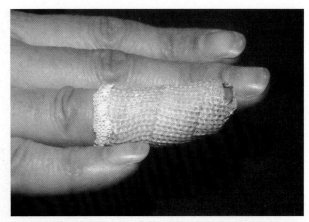

Figure 38-44 Digital QuickCast2 for a mallet finger. Cast may be applied over Coban to reduce swelling and may be split to facilitate removal for skin care. Digital cast provides more predictable immobilization without the jeopardy posed by positional changes associated with changing removable orthoses.

60% of patients obtained satisfactory results with use of an orthosis and 20% more of injuries improve sufficiently over time to be acceptable.[155]

Treatment of the distal tendon avulsion fracture is the same as that described for a pure tendon lesion. Positioning the distal joint in slight extension returns the distal phalanx to the small proximal fragment. Success can be monitored by comparing lateral radiographs taken before and after orthotic positioning. Calcification of the bridging callus may form a dorsal beak that nonetheless represents functional continuity of the extensor tendon and usually is not symptomatic.

Nonoperative treatment of larger articular fractures of the distal phalanx has been recommended because of the significant capacity of the distal phalanx to remodel its articular surface and the incidence of complications after surgery.[142,156,157] Satisfactory results are reported in cases with involvement of more than one third the articular surface of the distal phalanx with or without subluxation.[158] The most common impairment after open reduction of a major articular fracture of the distal phalanx is decreased flexion of the DIP joint from a scar tenodesis over the middle phalanx.[159] Additional complications from surgery for this injury are wound infection, thinning of the dorsal skin, joint injury, nail bed injury, pulp fibrosis, pain, and dysesthesias.[160,161] A 53% incidence of complications after operative treatment of mallet fingers has been reported[153] (Fig. 38-47C, online).

Despite the capacity for these injured joints to remodel with nonoperative treatment,[162] an accurate approximation of the fracture fragments has merit.[140,141,163] Reapproximation of the distal phalanx to the retracted proximal fragment can be performed through a transverse incision localized over the fracture site without disturbing the terminal tendon proximal to the joint. The dorsal capsule proximally should not be disturbed. An oblique 0.028-inch K-wire compresses the fracture site and prevents proximal retraction of the terminal tendon.[164] The palmar surface of the dorsal fragment can be notched to accommodate the pin that stabilizes the distal joint in neutral position.[165,166] This delicate procedure is demanding technically and represents a challenge in precision. The wires are removed and active motion is begun after 6 weeks. Night use of an orthosis is continued for 2 to

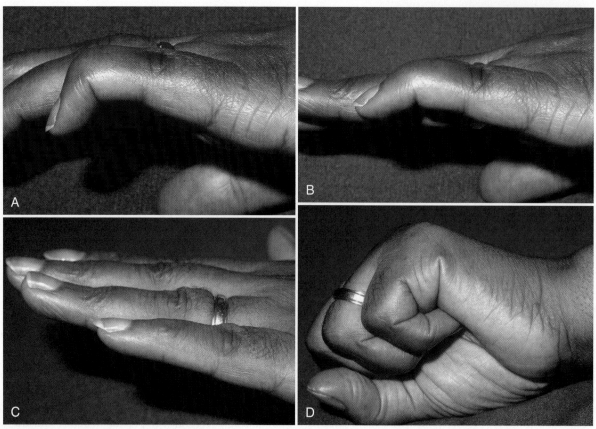

Figure 38-46 Chronic mallet deformity from blunt injury in a 54-year-old female. **A,** Resting attitude of 70 degrees. **B,** Active extension to 55 degrees, suggesting potential benefit from use of an orthosis. **C,** Active extension after 7 weeks of uninterrupted orthotic use and an additional 4 weeks of a night orthosis. **D,** Active flexion.

4 weeks until absence of an extension lag is ensured (Fig. 38-48). Other methods of operative treatment include percutaneous fixation by the "umbrella handle" technique,[167] pull-in technique,[168] hook plate,[169] open reduction with screw fixation,[170] and external fixation.[171]

A chronic mallet finger deformity may implicate only the DIP joint or may manifest with an imbalance collapse of the entire finger—a swan-neck deformity. Favorable results have been reported after secondary suture repair and also with plication of the terminal tendon scar, a *tenodermodesis*.[172,173] The terminal tendon has a small excursion, and the tenodesis

that is created may restrict distal joint motion. This procedure is contraindicated in the presence of a fixed flexion contracture, joint instability, or osteoarthritis. Operative correction of chronic mallet finger by reattaching the extensor tendon to the distal phalanx with a Mitek Micro Arc bone anchor has been successful.[161] If the distal joint is unsightly or intrusive, arthrodesis of the DIP joint in neutral position with a single pin is a reliable procedure that provides a painless, stable, cosmetically improved finger.[174] DIP joint fusion in neutral position is as functional and more acceptable cosmetically than DIP joint fusion in flexion.[175]

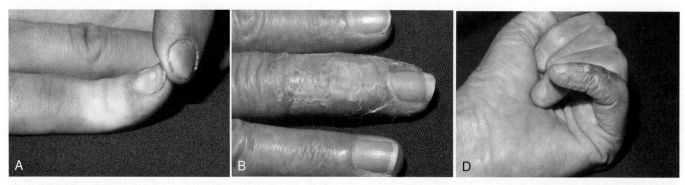

Figure 38-47 Complications of treatment for mallet finger deformity. **A,** Dorsal skin blanching signifies ischemia of subcutaneous tissues and terminal tendon. **B,** Maceration of dorsal skin beneath orthosis from neglect. Secondary infection can develop. **D,** Tenodesis of the extensor tendons with osteomyelitis of the middle phalanx after surgery. Distal joint is subluxated.

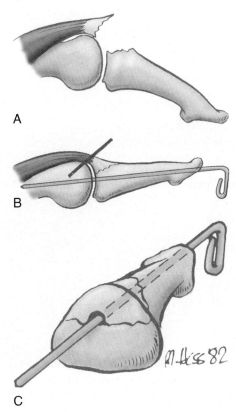

Figure 38-48 Operative method for major articular fracture of the distal interphalangeal joint. **A,** Injury represents significant interruption of the articular surface with potential instability. Effect on extensor tendons may be small. **B,** Accurate reduction of fracture fragments. Longitudinal wire stabilizes the distal joint in neutral or slight extension. Oblique buttress wire compresses fracture site and prevents retraction of proximal fragment by extensor tendon. **C,** Palmar surface of proximal fragment may be notched to accommodate the Kirschner wire.

The chronic mallet finger with a swan-neck deformity represents a more complex problem. Surgery to rebalance the finger should not be considered unless both joints are healthy and the joint deformities are passively correctable. The finger can be rebalanced by tenotomy of the central tendon insertion at the PIP joint.[87,175,176] The lateral slips to the intrinsic tendons and at least one of the transverse retinacular ligaments must be preserved. The lateral slips maintain terminal tendon continuity with the extrinsic extensor tendon. The transverse retinacular ligaments resist PIP joint hyperextension from dorsal displacement of the lateral bands. Both transverse retinacular ligaments can be preserved by releasing the central tendon through a longitudinal incision in the extensor tendon proximal to the dorsal fibers of the retinacular ligament. An extensor tenolysis over the middle phalanx is needed if distal joint position is not improved after the tenotomy. The extension lag noted at the PIP joint after this procedure can be reduced with appropriate orthotic use. Ultimate improvement may not be realized for a full year[177] (Fig. 38-49).

Swan-neck deformity in a mallet finger with significant hyperextension of the PIP joint may be rebalanced with reconstruction of an oblique retinacular ligament using a free tendon graft.[178,179] The tendon graft passes from the dorsum of the distal phalanx around the digit palmar to the flexor sheath and is attached proximal to the PIP joint. This reverses both distal joint flexion and proximal joint hyperextension.

Open Injuries

Lacerations of the terminal tendon should be approximated. Intramedullary K-wire pinning of the DIP joint in slight hyperextension coapts the tendon ends in tidy wounds without the need for tendon sutures.[180] Divided tendons that require suture repair are approximated with fine 5-0 or 6-0 braided, white, nonabsorbable sutures. Interrupted figure-of-eight or horizontal mattress sutures are used, depending on the consistency of the tendon ends. A relatively avascular critical zone exists in the terminal tendon 11 to 16 mm proximal to the osseotendinous junction, where the tendon is compressed over the head of the middle phalanx during flexion. This may influence healing after repair in this area.[181] The DIP joint is pinned because the repair initially depends on the integrity of the sutures. Motion is begun after 6 weeks. The distal joint is supported with an orthosis between active motion sessions for an additional 2 weeks. Development of an extensor lag indicates the need for further supportive orthotic use. There is no compelling rationale for an early motion protocol after repair of zone I or II extensor tendon injuries at this time.

Swan-Neck Deformity

The collapse deformity of the fingers that is metaphorically called the *swan-neck* deformity is a postural deformity with numerous causes. The deformity results from an imbalance of forces within the finger that creates an instability with collapse between the proximal, middle, and distal phalanges. Hyperextension of the PIP joint with flexion of the DIP joint—the swan-neck deformity—is the postural deformity that results.

The swan-neck deformity that follows the mallet finger tendon injury is one example of such an imbalance (see Fig. 38-43B). However, the pathomechanics of swan-neck deformity from other causes result in similar distortions of the finger extensor tendons and retinacular and capsular ligaments. The initiating factor may be increased forces through the extensor or intrinsic tendons, PIP joint instability, loss of the FDS tendon, or release of distal extensor attachment.

The basic mechanism in the swan-neck deformity was discussed relative to the mallet finger. The severity of this deformity increases and is more difficult to reverse when resulting from other causes: the transverse retinacular ligaments stretch, triangular ligament fibers shorten, and the lateral bands displace dorsally where they are tethered. The hyperextended PIP joint then resists flexion. A self-sustaining deformity is established as the oblique retinacular ligaments displace dorsally and shorten. Contracted oblique ligaments and lateral bands cannot traverse the condyles of the proximal phalanx during flexion. PIP joint flexion, which normally anticipates flexion of the distal joint, is then preceded by distal joint flexion: Synchronized IP joint flexion is halted. Distal joint flexion proceeds without flexion of the PIP joint until sufficient force develops in the FDP tendon to

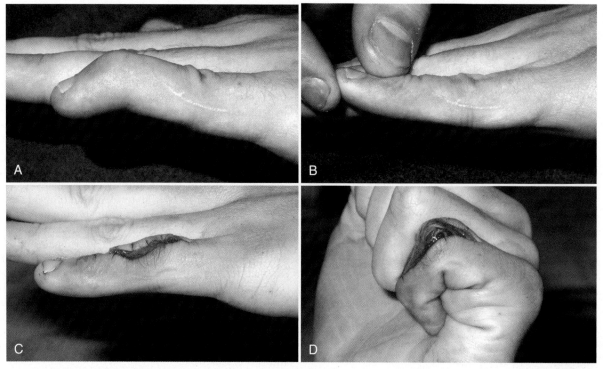

Figure 38-49 Tenotomy of the central tendon insertion on the middle phalanx for treatment of selected patients with a passively correctable mallet deformity. Tenotomy permits readjustment of tensions through the extensor tendons, reversing extensor deficiency at the distal interphalangeal (DIP) joint and reducing hyperextension forces at the proximal interphalangeal joint. **A,** Preoperative view of patient with a history of three ruptures of the terminal tendon while playing football and two previous surgical attempts at anatomic reconstruction. **B,** Passive correction attests to integrity of the DIP joint, a prerequisite for tenolysis. **C,** Active extension after tenotomy of central tendon with tenolysis over the middle phalanx. Both transverse retinacular ligaments were preserved. **D,** Active flexion.

overcome resistance by the structures dorsal to the PIP joint. Abrupt flexion occurring as the lateral bands snap over the condyles of the PIP joint are the pathomechanics of an established swan-neck deformity. Joint deterioration from rheumatoid synovitis or injury hinders treatment further.

The numerous causes of swan-neck deformity may be grouped anatomically by the pathway through which the deformity is initiated:

- Extrinsic tendon tightness
- Intrinsic tendon tightness
- Articular
- Distal tendon release

Normal Variants

People with normally hypermobile IP joints can produce swan-neck deformities of all fingers voluntarily by contracting their finger intrinsic muscles. Aside from the curiosity they may attract, these hands represent normal variants and do not need treatment.

Extrinsic Tendon Tightness

Tightness through the central tendon hyperextends the middle phalanx. Cerebral palsy with spasticity of the EDC is a dynamic cause in this category.

Flexion deformity of the wrist and subluxation of the finger MCP joint both tighten the extrinsic extensor tendon by lengthening the dorsal skeleton. MCP joint subluxation can result from rheumatoid synovitis, intrinsic contracture, or excessive surgical release of the collateral ligaments. In each instance, PIP joint hyperextension (resistance to passive flexion) increases with MCP joint flexion. This is an important distinction from intrinsic tightness.

Extensor tendon scarring over the dorsum of the hand that produces an extensor plus tenodesis increases tension through the central tendon while the MCP joint is flexed (see Fig. 38-28).

Treatment of swan-neck deformity caused by conditions in this category is incomplete unless the proximal abnormality is corrected. Hyperextension of the PIP joint is a distal deformity that stems from a more proximal imbalance.

Intrinsic Tendon Tightness

Increased tension through the intrinsic tendons can produce palmar subluxation of the MCP joint and hyperextension of the PIP joint in the fingers. Deformity is resisted by the glenoidal segments of the collateral ligaments at the MCP joint and the palmar plate and FDS at the PIP joint. Spasticity in cerebral palsy, rheumatoid arthritis, ischemic intrinsic muscle contracture, and post-traumatic intrinsic tightness all produce deformity by increasing tightness through the intrinsic tendons. Tendon transfers for weakness or claw deformity in the ulnar palsied hand can initiate swan-neck deformity by this same pathway. Less severe tightness exhibits a positive distal intrinsic tightness test (Fig. 38-50). Advanced tightness affects the MCP joint in addition to the PIP joint.

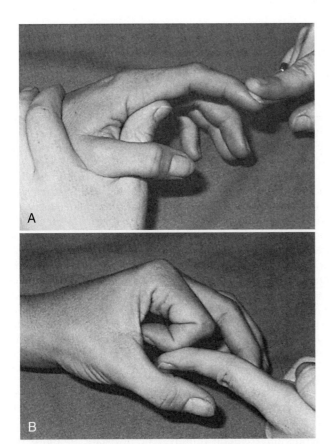

Figure 38-50 Intrinsic-plus test. **A,** Passive flexion of interphalangeal (IP) joints while the metacarpophalangeal (MCP) joint is supported in neutral tests for tightness through the distal intrinsic tendons. The radial and ulnar intrinsics can be individually tested by deviating the finger away from the side being tested. **B,** MCP joint flexion relaxes intrinsic muscles, lessens tension through extensor tendons, and decreases resistance to passive IP joint flexion.

Treatment of conditions in this category is directed toward release of the intrinsic tightness and rebalancing of the deformities. The procedures selected depend on the stage of the condition and the joints that are deformed. For example, flexor tenosynovectomy combined with distal intrinsic resections may suffice in rheumatoid disease with stable MCP joints. Otherwise, proximal intrinsic tenotomy with MCP joint arthroplasty also may be necessary to rebalance the fingers.

Articular Causes

Rupture of the palmar plate of the PIP joint permits hyperextension, which may progress without early protective orthotic use. The treatment is reattachment of the palmar plate that has avulsed distally. This is feasible in longstanding ruptures and has been successfully performed as long as 10 years after injury.

Synovitis of the MCP or PIP joints can destabilize fingers. Rheumatoid and psoriatic arthritis are the most commonly seen forms. Lupus arthritis results in joint deformity by a different mechanism but does not develop synovitis with cartilage erosion. Periarticular inflammation stimulates adhesions to the tendons, sagittal bands, and retinacular liga-

ments. This category of swan-neck deformities is difficult to treat because deteriorated joints are involved with adherent, displaced extensor tendons.

Distal Tendon Release

Release of the terminal extensor tendon concentrates extensor tension on the middle phalanx through the central tendon after a mallet tendon lesion. Hyperextension deformity with fracture of the middle phalanx has the same result; the distal extensor tendon is functionally lengthened. Prognosis for distal joint motion after fracture repositioning is guarded in cases that develop a tenodesis over the fracture site.

Loss of the FDS tendon eliminates an important stabilizer of the PIP joint. The severity of the deformity that results depends on the inherent stability of the palmar plate. This tendon should be divided as far proximally as possible when used for tendon transfer to preserve maximum tendon attachments within the flexor fibro-osseous sheath proximal to the PIP joint.

Thumb Extensor Tendons

The EPL is the most mobile of the digital extensor tendons. Its 58-mm longitudinal excursion exceeds that of the other digital extensor tendons.[19] (The EPL has a total excursion of 58 mm: 35 mm with wrist motion, 15 mm with MCP joint motion, and 8 mm with flexion–extension of the IP joint.) A 13-mm mediolateral translation of the tendon distal to the radius occurs with flexion–extension of the first metacarpal. The EPL supinates and adducts the thumb, extends the thumb MCP joint with the EPB, extends the thumb IP joint with the dorsal hood fibers from the thumb intrinsic muscles, and is the only tendon capable of hyperextending the IP joint. Hyperextension of the IP joint normally precedes extension of the MCP joint when the EPL is activated.[11]

The APL and EPB tendons are secured over the lateral border of the distal radius within the first dorsal fibroosseous compartment. Distal to the extensor retinaculum they pass beneath the superficial layer of the deep fascia (see Fig. 38-2). Fasciotomy distal to the extensor retinaculum during surgery to treat stenosing tenosynovitis of the extensor tendons (de Quervain's disease) may alter the balance of forces about the thumb.[182] Radial bowing of the APL and EPB tendons produces an exaggerated extension of the first metacarpal with an extension lag of the MCP joint (see Fig. 38-5). Release of the first dorsal compartment by a longitudinal incision of the extensor retinaculum along its dorsal border with loose coaptation of the release by fine absorbable sutures resists bowing and palmar subluxation of the released tendons. Use of a wrist orthosis for 3 to 4 weeks is advised routinely. The "Omega" pulley plasty entails periosteal elevation of the anterior attachment of the first extensor compartment pulley that expands the tunnel volume, effectively decompressing the tendons without a fasciotomy.[183]

Extensor tendon anatomy about the MCP joint resembles that of the finger PIP joint. Transverse fibers, similar to the transverse retinacular ligaments, shroud the capsule and attach to the flexor fibro-osseous sheath.[106] The adductor pollicis on the ulnar side and the abductor pollicis brevis on

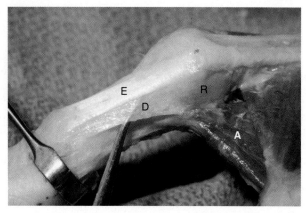

Figure 38-51 Extensor apparatus of the thumb. Adductor pollicis (AP) contributes to dorsal expansion and assists extension of the interphalangeal joint. Vertical fibers about the metacarpophalangeal joint represent the transverse retinacular ligament fibers in the thumb. A, adductor pollicis muscle; R, fibers representing homolog of transverse retinacular ligament; D, dorsal expansion from the AP and retinacular fibers; E, extensor pollicis longus over the proximal phalanx.

the radial side contribute dorsal expansions that stabilize the extensor tendons and transfer extension forces to the IP joint (Fig. 38-51). The intrinsic muscles of the thumb thus are able to extend the IP joint to neutral but are not capable of hyperextension.

The EPB usually inserts on the dorsal base of the proximal phalanx but commonly has a second insertion into the EPL.[7] It extends the first metacarpal and the MCP joint. Interruption of the EPB introduces extension weakness at the base of the proximal phalanx. As the MCP joint flexes, increased tension develops through the EPL, which hyperextends the IP joint (Fig. 38-52).

The EPL can extend the MCP joint through the fibers of the dorsal apparatus. Diastasis or rupture of these fibers permits palmar displacement of the tendon. The tendon flexes the MCP joint when displaced below the axis of joint motion, which exaggerates extension forces at the IP joint. This extrinsic-minus deformity, common with rheumatoid arthritis, is analogous to the boutonnière deformity of the finger.

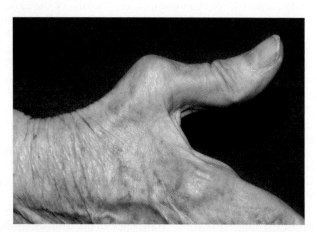

Figure 38-52 Rupture of the extensor pollicis brevis and dorsal fibers of the extensor apparatus produce loss of metacarpophalangeal (MCP) joint extension. Displacement of the extensor pollicis longus (EPL) may accentuate flexion of the MCP joint and contributes to hyperextension of the interphalangeal joint. The EPL tendon is identified clearly.

Closed Injuries

Rupture of the Extensor Pollicis Longus

The EPL is subject to continued stress during performance of normal activities. Tenosynovitis has been attributed to overuse in the classic drummer's palsy. Musicians with impairment of this tendon experience difficulty with dexterous maneuvers. Thumb-under transpositions on the piano keyboard or manipulations of a string-board are severely hindered with a painful affliction involving the EPL.[184]

The tendon usually ruptures at the level of the distal radius beneath the extensor retinaculum. Rheumatoid synovitis and fractures of the distal radius, often undisplaced, are common predisposing conditions[185]; surgery of the distal radius,[186] uremia, diabetes, and local steroid injections are less commonly implicated.[187] The cause of the rupture is believed to be ischemia of a segment of the tendon that normally has poor vascularity. Microangiographic studies suggest that pressure from the effusion that accompanies synovitis or a fracture impedes the intrinsic nutrition in this tendon segment.[188] Ultrasound examination has shown thickening about the EPL 6 weeks after distal radius fracture that lends further support to this hypothesis.[189] Oral anabolic steroids have been associated with tendon fiber dissociation with calcification and rupture.[190]

The most disabling impairment after rupture of the EPL is extension lost at the MCP joint (Fig. 38-53, online). The origin of the EPL is long, and the muscle retains some contractility after tendon rupture. The myostatic tightness that develops with attritional rupture can be overcome by strong thenar and thumb flexor antagonists after reconstruction. Successful rehabilitation with an intercalated free tendon graft that bridges the ruptured tendon ends depends on the potential function of the retracted muscle.[191] EIP tendon transfer (rerouted superficial to the deep fascia distal to the extensor retinaculum and sutured to the EPL at the MCP joint of the thumb) is technically easier, requires only one tendon repair, and simulates the normal vectors of the EPL.[185,192] The EIP and EPL have comparable mean fiber length and tension fraction.[20,21] The index finger usually retains independent extension from the EDC after transfer (Fig. 38-54).

Rupture Insertion of the Extensor Pollicis Longus

Closed rupture of the EPL mimics the mallet tendon injury of the finger. Loss of full active extension of the IP joint with localized dorsal swelling occurs. Incomplete extension after flexion is from intact lateral tendon fibers. Treatment is by uninterrupted use of a dorsal orthosis with the IP joint in hyperextension for 6 weeks. Subsequent use of a night orthosis for an additional 2 to 4 weeks is usually recommended. The position of the orthosis should not create skin blanching.[193-195]

Fractures and Extensor Tendon Deformity

Metacarpals

Fractures initiate deformity through the extensor tendons by mechanically fixing the tendon, disrupting normal tendon

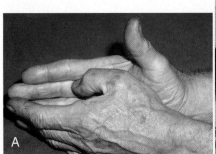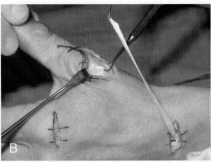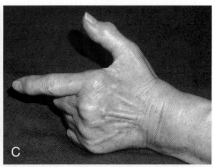

Figure 38-54 Rupture of the extensor pollicis longus (EPL). **A,** Loss of metacarpophangeal (MCP) joint extension and interphalangeal joint hyperextension. **B,** Reconstruction with extensor indicis proprius (EIP) transfer. The EIP has excursion comparable to EPL. Course of the tendon transfer simulates normal vector of ruptured tendon. Transfer is rerouted distal to the extensor retinaculum to tendon fibers over the MCP joint (insertion elevated by instrument). **B,** Active thumb extension 10 weeks after transfer. Independent index finger extension by extensor digitorum has been retained.

mechanics, and promoting adhesions. Skeletal architecture and the disposition of the extensor tendons about the skeleton influence fracture displacement and predetermine the deformity that results. The metacarpals and phalanges arch dorsally. Transverse fractures of the metacarpals flex because of the interosseous muscles. Spiral fractures flex and rotate, and the distal fragment displaces palmarward. The flexed metacarpal head positions the MCP joint in hyperextension. The dorsal fracture apex mechanically alters zone VI tendons. The lengthened dorsal skeleton increases tension transmitted distally by the extrinsic extensor tendons. MCP joint hyperextension is accentuated by increased tension through the extensor tendon. The PIP joint then reciprocally flexes; this is an extension lag. If the dorsal capsule and MCP joint collateral ligaments shorten, a dorsal MCP joint contracture ensues. The deformity is an extensor-plus claw deformity (Fig. 38-55, online).

Proximal Phalanx

The extrinsic extensor tendon and the distal fibers of the digital extensor mechanism are situated dorsally about the proximal phalanx. Transverse fractures of the proximal phalanx develop hyperextension at the fracture site. Segmental fractures permit linear shortening caused by loss of bone support. In spiral fractures, the distal fragment rotates, migrates proximally, and tilts dorsally, a combination of angular and linear shortening. Each condition relaxes the extensor mechanism, functionally lengthens the tendons, and weakens IP joint extension. An extension lag of the PIP joint results. The MCP joint then hyperextends by the sagittal bands as the extensor mechanism shifts proximally in a compensatory effort to achieve PIP joint extension through the central tendon. The ability of the extensor mechanism to compensate for proximal phalangeal shortening—the *extensor tendon reserve*—is limited by the volar attachments of the sagittal bands. Extensor tendon reserve has been 2 to 6 mm in cadaver studies[196] (Fig. 38-56). Fractures of the proximal phalanx and associated adhesions may also impede flexor tendons within the fibro-osseous sheath. Realignment of the proximal phalanx restores balance to the extensor mechanism and reverses MCP joint hyperextension. It is difficult to balance a finger through the tendons without restoring skeletal length and alignment first. Preservation of proximal

phalangeal length and alignment remains a primary objective after injury (Fig. 38-57).

Middle Phalanx

The middle phalanx hyperextends after transverse fractures because of the dorsally situated extensor tendons and oblique retinacular ligaments. Proximal fragment flexion is accentuated by the insertion of the FDS tendon. Spiral fractures permit skeletal shortening that relaxes the extensor tendon distally. The resulting deformity is an extension lag of the DIP joint with increased PIP joint extension. Flexion of the proximal fragment increases the extension moment by the central tendon and accentuates PIP joint extension. The deformity is resisted by the palmar-stabilizing ligaments of the PIP joint. PIP joint hyperextension results in a swan-neck deformity.

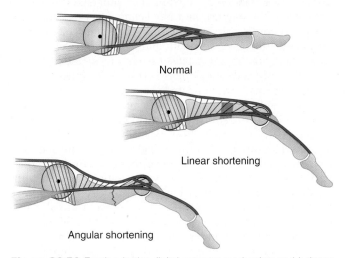

Figure 38-56 Tension in the digital extensor mechanism and balance between the extrinsic and intrinsic tendon fibers are maintained normally by integrity of the proximal phalanx. Segmental bone loss produces linear shortening. Unstable fractures of the proximal metaphysis and shaft permit dorsal angulation that results in angular shortening. Both conditions functionally lengthen the digital extensor mechanism with extension lag at the interphalangeal joints. The ability to compensate for shortening—the extension reserve—is limited. The intrinsic tendons have small excursions, and the extrinsic tendon is restrained by the sagittal bands that attach to the palmar plate and proximal phalanx.

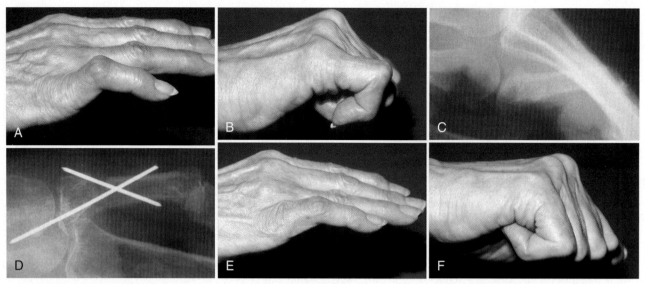

Figure 38-57 Deformity and extensor tendon dysfunction from malunion fracture of the proximal phalanx. Hyperextension of the proximal phalanx fracture functionally lengthens the extensor tendons, creating extension lag of the proximal interphalangeal joint with reciprocal hyperextension of the metacarpophalangeal (MCP) joint in this 72-year-old woman. **A,** Active extension 6 months after injury. **B,** Active flexion. Longstanding hyperextension has created a dorsal MCP joint contracture that blocks flexion. **C,** Hyperextension malunion fracture of the proximal phalanx. **D,** Correctional osteotomy of the proximal phalanx with removable pins. **E,** Active extension 6 months after osteotomy demonstrates improved extensor tendon balance. **F,** Active flexion.

Extensor Tendon Separation: Confronting the Tendon Gap

Disruption of a tendon is normally followed by a phased healing sequence. Blood vessels and fibroblasts capable of collagen production migrate into the wound. Protein aggregates and collagen fibers unite the tendon ends by approximately day 4. Tendon remodeling then progresses under the influence of biophysical and biochemical factors. The ideal flexor tendon repair reestablishes continuity of collagen fibers and establishes a smooth gliding surface. The requirements for a functioning extensor tendon repair are less stringent. Bridging collagen alone is necessary for function.[197]

Investigators have pondered the balance between immobilization and controlled motion after extensor tendon repair. Mobilization of repairs after 1 day of orthotic use stretched the repair sites and produced an extension lag. Immobilization for 3 weeks produced stiffness and decreased flexion. Ten days was once considered optimal immobilization.[198] Long-term results of extensor tendon lacerations treated with repair and conventional orthotic use for 3 to 4 weeks have been disappointing. Good to excellent results (total active motion, 230 degrees) were achieved in 64% of patients without associated injuries, but in only 45% with associated injuries. Injuries in distal zones I to IV had significantly poorer results than those in proximal zones V to VIII. The percentage of fingers that lost flexion exceeded the percentage that lost extension.[199] Modification of the biophysical environment of the healing tendon through controlled tension has improved the quality of tendon healing and clinical results. Experience with early protected motion after flexor tendon repairs was applied to extensor tendon injuries

with improved results.[200-207] Methods that were effective in proximal extensor zones V to VIII have been refined and successfully adapted for more distal zones III and IV.[122] The biomechanical[208] and electrophysiologic[209,210] rationale for the success of these early motion protocols has facilitated the implementation of these methods in the clinical arena. At this time there is still no justification for an early motion protocol after extensor tendon repair in zone 1 or 2 or after repair of a wrist extensor tendon.

The tensile strength of tendon has been compared with that of steel. The strength at the musculotendinous junction approximates 10% of the strength of tendons. Tensile strength of a healed tendon approximates that of the musculotendinous junction.[211] The junction of the repaired tendon remains the weakest link in the muscle–tendon unit. Separated tendons resist passive approximation after the healing process has begun; distal joint repositioning is not a predictable means of reapproximation (Fig. 38-58). A larger gap heals slower than a smaller one and is weaker when healed. Treatment strives to minimize the effect of the tendon gap.

Muscle Lacerations

Muscle belly lacerations without repair result in a gap that disrupts the parallel arrangement of endomysial tubes, prevents muscle regeneration, and heals by scar formation. Excessive gapping increases resting muscle length and decreases effective contraction. Completely lacerated muscles in animals recover 50% of their ability to produce tension and 80% of their normal excursion.[212] Through-and-through, free tendon grafts are effective approximators of lacerated muscle bellies: 41% of treated patients regained grade 5 muscle strength after repair.[213]

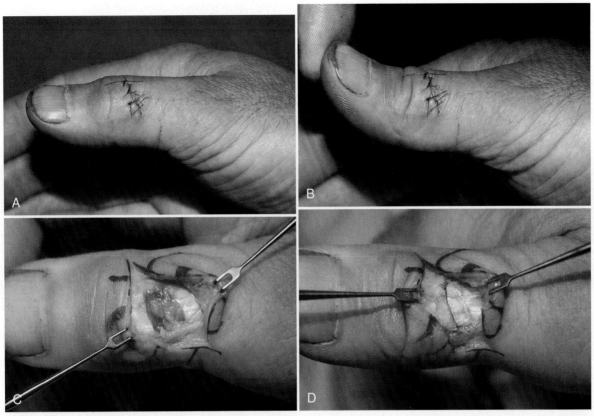

Figure 38-58 Laceration of the extensor pollicis longus (EPL) tendon in the thumb at zone II 10 days after primary wound repair without tendon repair. **A,** Active extension of the interphalangeal (IP) joint lacks hyperextension capability because of loss of the EPL. **B,** Joint mobility demonstrates the passive potential. **C,** Tendon gap is bridged by early elements of tendon healing. The tendon ends will not accurately approximate by passive positioning of the IP joint distally. **D,** The tendon gap has been evacuated and the tendon ends accurately approximated. Tendon strength is improved and adhesions are diminished by minimizing the tendon gap.

Extensor Tendon Repairs

Accurate repair aspires to minimize the tendon gap. There have been significant problems with the strength and quality of extensor tendon repairs. Sutured extensor tendons are roughly 50% as strong as flexor tendons, largely because of reduced tendon dimension and lack of collagen cross-linking. All tested repair techniques in zone VI cadaver tendons produced tendon shortening with restrained MCP joint motion caused by the repair. The Kleinert modification of the Bunnell method and the Kessler techniques were the strongest.[214]

Selection of suture caliber and method is determined clinically by the cross-sectional configuration and stiffness of the tendon. Braided, white, nonabsorbable sutures are preferred. Pigmented, monofilament, nonabsorbable sutures are unattractive when visible beneath thin skin, and their hard knots can create erosive lesions.[215] Knots are tied deep to the extensor tendons when there is a paucity of subcutaneous fat or the skin is thin. A Kessler peripheral grasping or Bunnell weave suture is used for round or oval tendons, such as the EPL, EIP, or EDQ. A horizontal mattress suture is weaker and gaps when tested[214] but is nevertheless useful for small, flat tendons, such as the juncturae tendinum, lateral bands

about the PIP joint, and the distal EPL. The baseball stitch[211] has been modified to pass through the tendon ends and is preferred for broad, thin tendons, such as the EDC in zone VI (Fig. 38-59, online). The extensor hoods over the MCP joints are substantial structures composed of longitudinal tendon and transverse sagittal band fibers that hold simple or figure-of-eight sutures well. The central tendon and terminal tendon insertions are structurally stiffer than other fibers in the finger extensor apparatus[216] and can be sutured securely. Large gaps may be unavoidable without introducing intolerable tension and must then be bridged. Interposition free tendon grafts, described for the EPL,[191] have broader application (Fig. 38-60).

The Functional Pseudotendon

Dehiscence of a tendon repair or failure to repair a tendon creates a large void between the tendon ends. The gap fills with scar that bears little physical resemblance to a normal tendon. This pseudotendon lacks the glide and physical characteristics of a normal tendon but may have sufficient structural integrity to function adequately after it has been surgically liberated (Fig. 38-61).

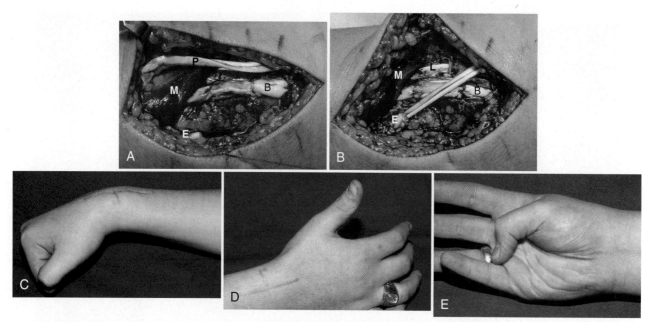

Figure 38-60 Lacerated extensor carpi radialis brevis (ECRB) and extensor pollicis longus (EPL) tendons (zone VI) in a 15-year-old boy 4 weeks after injury. The extensor carpi radialis longus (ECRL) was not injured. Tendon gaps from myostatic tightness bridged with free tendon grafts. Tendon grafts bridge gaps in lacerated tendons thus avoiding tendon repair with excessive tension. **A,** Tourniquet released. Intercalary graft from ECRL bridges the ECRB gap. **B,** Doubled palmaris longus graft bridges the EPL gap. **C,** Wrist flexion 7 months after repair. **D,** Active thumb extension. **E,** There is no restriction of thumb flexion. B, ECRB; E, proximal EPL; L, ECRL; M, extensor pollicis brevis muscle; P, palmaris longus grafts to distal EPL.

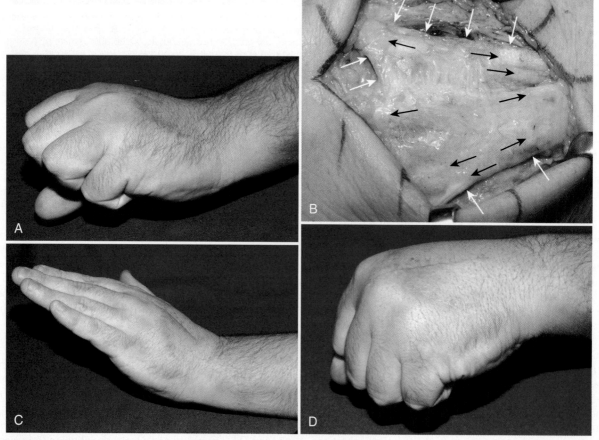

Figure 38-61 The functional pseudotendon. Restricted grip in a 33-year-old man seen 10 months after primary repair of extensor tendons to the index, long, and ring fingers in zone VI. **A,** Grip lacks combined metacarpophalangeal and proximal interphalangeal joint flexion, an extensor plus tenodesis. **B,** Extensor tenolysis has defined a functional sheet of scar—the pseudotendon—that bridges the dehisced ends of the repaired extensor tendons. Black monofilament sutures are visible in the tendons retracted proximally to the right. Tendon individuality had been lost but potential for unified finger extensor function was retained. **C,** Active extension 9 weeks after tenolysis. **D,** Active flexion. *Black arrows,* ends of dehisced tendon repairs; *white arrows,* margins of surgically defined pseudotendon after tenolysis.

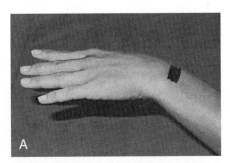

Figure 38-62 Tendon restraint proximal to extensor retinaculum. **A,** Wrist flexion extends digits prematurely because of extensor tenodesis.

Patterns of Restraint from Scarred Extensor Tendons

Injured extensor tendons are prone to restraint from scar formation and can be difficult to rehabilitate. Their disproportionately large surface area and comparatively smaller excursion, strength, and capacity for sustained tension compared with flexor tendons introduce special challenges after injury and reparative surgery.

Sites of blockage from tendon adhesions can be localized by comparing active and passive ranges of motion.[217] Skin adherence, localized induration, and dimpling reliably indicate the location of restraining scar. The following discussions relate to the extensor tendons and retinacular systems. These principles cannot be applied unless the joints are passively mobile.

Proximal to Extensor Retinaculum

Scar adhesions of the finger extensor tendons proximal to the extensor retinaculum restrain combined wrist and finger flexion. A reciprocal wrist extension/finger flexion grip pattern may develop; active finger flexion passively extends the wrist while active wrist extension permits the fingers to flex further by reducing the distance between the blockage and the extensor tendon insertions. Passive wrist flexion initiates a tenodesis that passively extends the fingers. Only wrist flexion is impaired when the wrist extensor tendons alone are involved (Fig. 38-62A; 38-62B, C, online).

Distal to Extensor Retinaculum

Neither active nor passive wrist motion is impaired. The pattern of scar restraint at this level depends on whether the scar glides, as with a bulky tendon repair, or is anchored to the deep fascia. Gliding scar limits motion because of its inability to pass beneath the deep fascia or extensor retinaculum. Combined wrist and finger extension is restricted. Wrist extension may be enhanced by flexing the fingers first. This pulls the impeding scar distally, farther from the distal edge of the abutting ligament, and permits additional wrist extension before the scar is again blocked by the extensor retinaculum proximally (Fig. 38-63).

Anchored scar fixing the digital extensor tendons to the deep fascia produces an *extensor-plus phenomenon*. This tenodesis passively extends the IP joints of the finger as the MCP joint is flexed. As the IP joints flex, the tenodesis is transferred proximally and the MCP joints passively extend. Active and passive reciprocity exists between the MCP and IP joints. Combined MCP and IP joint flexion is prevented (see Fig. 38-28).

Intrinsic Tightness Versus Tendon Scarring

Tightness of the intrinsic muscles and adhesions adjacent to the extensor hood about the MCP joint that involve the intrinsic tendons both can interfere with finger flexion. Active and passive flexion may be painful with either condition. Scar involving the extensor hood can produce a clinical picture that is indistinguishable from an intrinsic contracture by clinical testing. Intrinsic tightness is tested by passively extending the finger MCP joint while flexing the IP joints—the intrinsic tightness test described by Finochietto.[218] The radial and ulnar intrinsic muscles of each finger may be evaluated separately by deviating the finger away from the side being tested. Intrinsic restraint suggested by testing may be the result of muscle contracture or adhesions of the intrinsic tendons distally (see Fig. 38-50). Careful clinical examination often can differentiate scarring about the intervolar plate ligaments—the *saddle syndrome*—from scarring about the extensor hood at the MCP joint. The location of swelling and tenderness is helpful in differentiating these conditions. The discernment may not be absolute before surgery; it is then made at the time of tenolysis (see Fig. 38-29).

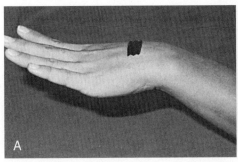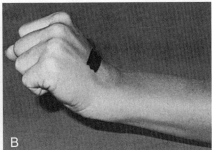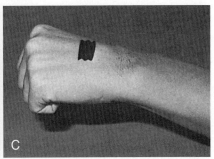

Figure 38-63 Gliding scar distal to extensor retinaculum. **A,** Bulky scar abuts extensor retinaculum, preventing simultaneous wrist and finger extension. **B,** Finger flexion before wrist extension increases potential for wrist extension. **C,** Wrist and finger flexion may not be impaired.

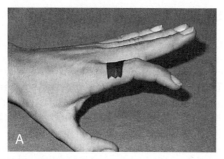

Figure 38-64 *Scar restraint of dorsal apparatus.* **A,** *Active extension beyond resting position is prevented.*

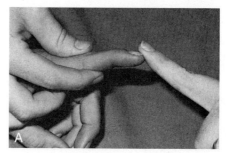

Figure 38-66 *Retinacular-plus test or intrinsic intrinsic-plus finger.* **A,** *Oblique retinacular ligament tightness is tested by passively flexing the distal joint while the proximal interphalangeal joint is supported in neutral. Resistance is relative and should be compared with normal fingers. Relative resistance indicates a positive test.*

Proximal Phalanx

Scarring of the extensor tendons over the proximal phalanx can restrict the extrinsic central tendon, intrinsic expansions, or the entire dorsal apparatus. The resting position of the PIP joint reflects the position of the extensor tendons when motion is finally arrested. Active extension of the PIP joint beyond the resting position is lacking (Fig. 38-64A). Frequently, an extension lag is present, and passive correction to neutral is possible. Active and passive flexion of the PIP joint is blocked; there is often an elastic or springy quality of restrained joint motion during testing (Fig. 38-64B, C, online).

Flexion of the PIP joint also can be blocked by scarring of the triangular ligament. This restrains the lateral bands dorsally and can consolidate the lateral bands with the central tendon insertion. Proximal IP joint flexion is blocked in both instances: in the first, palmar descent by the lateral bands is prevented; in the second, a tenodesis with the central tendon

exists. Flexion of the DIP joint is usually restricted when flexion of the PIP joint is blocked by these conditions.

Middle Phalanx

Scarring of the extensor tendon over the middle phalanx restrains flexion of the DIP joint. Active and passive flexion restraint that is unrelated to the position of the PIP joint implies scarring of the extensor tendon. The retinacular ligaments usually are involved also (Fig. 38-65A; 38-65B, online). These ligaments have little influence on the normal finger but play a significant role in the scarred or imbalanced finger by limiting distal joint flexion and fostering deformity. A tight oblique retinacular ligament produces a positive *retinacular-plus test* (*Haines' maneuver*)[5,90] also called an *intrinsic intrinsic-plus* finger.[104] Normally, there is some passive flexion of the DIP joint while the PIP joint is supported in extension. Shortening or scarring of the oblique retinacular ligament restrains distal joint flexion. This restraint depends on the position of the PIP joint (increased PIP joint extension diminishes DIP joint flexion), which differentiates this from fixation of the extensor tendon. Capsular contracture and ankylosis of the DIP joint can also restrict distal joint motion that is independent of PIP joint position. An integrated assessment of the history, clinical findings, and radiographic films assists in compiling a definitive appraisal (Fig. 38-66A; 38-66B, online).

REFERENCES

The complete reference list is available online at www.expertconsult.com.

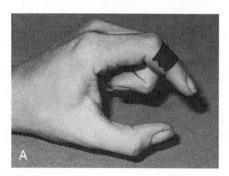

Figure 38-65 *Extensor tendon restraint over the middle phalanx.* **A,** *Active distal joint flexion is lacking. Extension lag may be present.*

Clinical Management of Extensor Tendon Injuries: The Therapist's Perspective*

ROSLYN B. EVANS, OTR/L, CHT

GENERAL CONSIDERATIONS
CLINICAL MANAGEMENT OF EXTENSOR TENDON
   INJURIES
SUMMARY

CRITICAL POINTS

- Extensor tendons in all zones except digital I and II and thumb TI and TII tolerate controlled active tension by the third post-operative day with precise orthotic positioning and controlled arcs of motion.
- The concepts of immediate tension at the repair site(s) are supported by experimental, biomechanical and clinical studies.
- Orthotic position, position of exercise, and angles of allowed flexion are dependent on the level of injury and status of adjacent tissues.
- Extension should be regained before flexion in all zones.
- Early intervention is critical to the ability of the therapist to manage edema, inflammation, impending joint problems, and tendon excursion during the first three weeks of wound healing.

Problems that accompany the complex extensor tendon injury or mismanagement of the simple extensor injury are well known to the hand specialist. Most functional problems in tendon systems are associated with the tendon's response to injury and repair, and despite decades of research on the subject, the problem of restrictive scar formation remains one of the most unpredictable factors contributing to postoperative morbidity.[1] Over the past three decades, the techniques

---

*Author's note: This chapter provides an update on extensor tendon rehabilitation as an addendum to the previously published chapter authored by myself in edition 5. For the most part my techniques of rehabilitation for early active motion are unchanged, based on clinical experience and updated literature review. New to this chapter are (1) my technique for early short arc motion (SAM) for the closed (boutonnière) zone III, IV injury, (2) a review of the relative extension orthotic positioning technique described by Wendell and Howell, and (3) postoperative management suggestions for sagittal band repairs. Evidence to support the therapist's interventions following extensor tendon repair with literature review are summarized, and references for all sections are updated.

of early controlled motion initially applied to flexor tendon management have been slowly incorporated into standard postoperative care for the extensor system. We have learned, with clinical studies and experience, that

1. Extensor tendons in all zones (except zone I) tolerate controlled *active* motion.
2. Gapping and rupture are rarely an issue in carefully applied postoperative regimens that control forces and excursion.
3. More digital joint motion can probably be allowed with injury in zones V through VII than had previously been thought possible.
4. Wrist position is critical to decreasing resistive forces from the flexor system and is a factor in true tendon excursion gained with digital motion.
5. These tendons have most likely been moving *actively* all along within the confines of their dynamic orthoses.
6. Early referral to therapy with attention to orthosis geometry and applied stress is a critical variable to outcomes.

Although experience and literature review continue to support the use of early postoperative controlled motion, some investigators report similar results with postoperative immobilization protocols.[2-4] However, for the most part, studies published in the past 5 years on postoperative management technique basically verify earlier studies, which demonstrated that extensor tendons respond well to the application of controlled motion with the use of both dynamic orthoses and exercise.[5-12] The only difference in protocols is simply some variation in orthosis design and in attempts to incorporate an active component into postoperative regimens. The principles of treatment are the same as for the previous edition of this text: Initiate therapy by postoperative day 3, rest the tendon short (the repair site proximal to its normal resting position), and control excursion with an orthosis design that allows at least 5 mm (or more) of motion at the repair site.

A literature search for extensor tendon rehabilitation (randomized controlled trials) from 2004 to 2009† produced only

---

†The literature search included the following url and databases www.ncbi.nlm.nih.gov/sites/entrez, Cochrane Library, MEDLINE, PEDro, EMBASE, and CINAHI.

one study that systematically reviewed available evidence comparing the effectiveness of different rehabilitation regimens on repaired extensor tendons.[13] The results of this systematic review, which included four randomized controlled trials and one other design study, found that short-term outcomes after immobilization were inferior to early motion programs, and that there was some limited support for early controlled mobilization over early active mobilization at 4 weeks. No conclusive evidence was found, however, regarding the long-term (12 weeks) effectiveness of the different rehabilitation protocols.[13]

The positive biomechanical effects of mechanical stimulation to a repair site continue to be supported with basic science research,[14-17] and further study of the mechanism for the loss of mechanical properties associated with mechanical unloading (cast immobilization) in the tendon continues to support previous studies that have demonstrated a rapid and significant decrease in material properties associated with immobilization of tendon and ligament.[18] Buckwalter and Grodzinsky[19] point out that one of the most important concepts in orthopedics in this century is the understanding that loading accelerates healing of bone, fibrous tissue, and skeletal muscle,[19] and thus we can surmise that early controlled motion to the healing tendon, as just noted, remains our best current treatment for tendon repair.

The concept of tissue engineering, which is the focus of much current research, is based on the manipulation of cellular and biochemical mediators that will positively affect protein synthesis and improve tissue remodeling. Woo and colleagues[20] have predicted that the combination of cell therapy with growth factor application via gene transfer will offer new opportunities for improving tendon and ligament healing. Although basic science studies continue to explore the healing of connective tissue through tissue engineering and the effects of mechanical stress, early intervention with edema control, precise orthosis geometry, and short arc motion designed to glide the repair site in a controlled range remain our most reliable techniques for producing excellent functional results. Even though these new biologic therapies show much promise for facilitating bone and fibrous tissue healing in the future,[21,22] others remind us that none has been proven to offer the beneficial effects comparable to those produced by the loading of healing tissues.[19]

Most basic scientific and clinical research on tendons has been focused on the synovial flexor tendon, which has posed the most problems with restoration of functional gliding after repair. Clinicians have perhaps been too liberal in their application of some of these basic science studies to clinical application in the extensor system. Nonetheless, despite the histologic, metabolic, and nutritional differences between the two tendon systems[23] and within the different levels of the extensor system,[24] the fact is that all tendon is a type of dense connective tissue that functions to transmit muscle force to the skeleton, and to perform its work requirement, all tendon must glide relative to its surrounding tissues.

After injury to tendon at any level in either the flexor or the extensor system, the wound response and subsequent problems of maintaining tendon excursion are the same.[25] A blood clot forms, a nonspecific inflammatory response occurs, the clot becomes populated with fibroblasts and advancing capillary buds, and collagen and ground substance are produced that will heal the deficit but that also may limit the tendon's normal gliding ability.[25,26] Loss of fiber gliding of tendon and neighboring connective tissues with resulting functional deficits of strength, mobility, and coordination impede the tendon's ability to transmit muscle force to bone with mechanical efficiency.[27] Rehabilitation of a healing tendon is simply reestablishing its ability to glide and transmit force without creating gapping or rupture at the repair site.

The purpose of this chapter is to define the problems that follow injury at the different extensor tendon levels and to offer solutions to these problems based on current experimental and clinical research in the areas of tendon repair techniques, tendon healing, true tendon excursions, and the application of force to the healing extensor tendon. Anatomy, clinical evaluation, and surgical management of the extensor tendons are addressed in this edition by Pratt (see Chapter 1) and Rosenthal and Elhassan (see Chapter 38) and elsewhere.[28]

The serious student, inexperienced or not, is encouraged to study the exquisite review of extensor tendon anatomy and management by Rosenthal and Elhassan in Chapter 38 of this text.[29]

The first section, *General Considerations*, is dedicated to a current literature review of basic science and clinical studies that support early motion for the healing tendon. Although this material may seem complex to the student or inexperienced therapist, it is essential information for any therapist or physician who assumes the responsibility of caring for an injured tendon. Treatment by protocol is appropriate only if there are no variables. Unfortunately, in the real clinical situation we are required to treat tendons with associated injury to bone, joint, nerve, and vessel in patients with associated metabolic, immunosuppressive, or personality problems, often referred by the nonspecializing surgeon, whose surgical technique and timing further complicate the case. This requires the therapist to be able to adjust treatment parameters based on a solid knowledge of wound healing, tendon repair tensile strength, and the effects of immobilization and early motion on the biochemistry and biomechanics of the healing tendon.

The questions once posed to me as a young therapist by Dr. Paul Brand (When? How often? How far? and How much?) when applying stress to healing connective tissue—are addressed in this chapter. These questions should be a part of the hand clinician's clinical decision-making process with each tendon case if optimal care is to be delivered.

The second section, *Clinical Management of Extensor Tendon Injuries*, is dedicated to management by level of injury. Within this section, general guidelines for treatment by immobilization, early passive motion, and early active motion are defined in terms of orthosis positioning and stress application.

General Considerations

Characteristics of the extensor tendon vary at each level, dictating variations in treatment. The committee on tendon injuries for the International Federation of the Society for Surgery of the Hand defines extensor tendon injury by delineating seven zones for the extrinsic finger extensors and five zones for the thumb extensors[30] (Fig. 39-1).

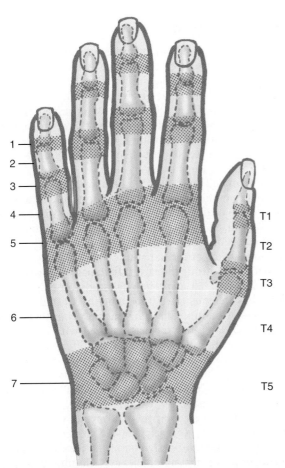

Figure 39-1 Extensor tendon zones as defined by the Committee on Tendon Injuries for the International Federation of the Society for Surgery of the Hand. (From Kleinert HE, Schepel S, Gill T. Flexor tendon injuries. *Surg Clin North Am.* 1981;61:267–286.)

Schedules for immobilization, the application of controlled stress, and progressive resistive exercises depend on the tensile strength of the repair technique and the stage of wound healing as they relate to the physiologic and biomechanical differences of the tendon in its different zones or anatomic levels. Guidelines for treatment based on the biochemical and biomechanical requirements of this system must be altered to accommodate the circumstances of the individual patient and injury. The surgeon should apprise the therapist of the quality of the repair, the type of repair, alterations in tendon length, the integrity of the tissue, the status of surrounding tissues, and any additional pathologic conditions that might alter the amount of controlled stress that the healing tendon can accommodate. The patient should be evaluated in terms of anticipated compliance. This information will influence any variation from suggested timing of immobilization and mobilization schedules. Therapeutic management should be considered in terms of the biochemical and biomechanical events of wound healing and the effects that our management techniques have on these events. Management of the inflammatory state; timing of stress application; the judicious application of controlled stress; and the effects of active versus passive motion, orthosis geometry, the position of exercise, external load application with stress application, and the duration of exercise all influence either positively or negatively the healing and remodeling of this fibrous connective tissue.

Controlling Inflammation

The importance of early repair,[31] nontraumatic surgery, prevention of infection, and edema control as a means of minimizing the inflammatory response after injury is well documented in the literature. The fibroblastic response and ultimately the amount of collagen produced at the wound site is proportional to the local inflammatory response.[32] Complex dorsal injuries are accompanied by significant edema and may require bulky, compressive dressings between therapy sessions for the first 5 to 7 days, but injuries with less tissue response can be lightly dressed and placed in early motion orthoses by 24 hours after surgery. The digits should be individually wrapped with a single layer of 2-inch Coban to control digital edema for as long as any extra volume of fluid is present about the proximal interphalangeal (PIP) joint, a time that may exceed 8 to 12 weeks after repair for the digital injury. Elevation for 24 hours, motion for the uninvolved joints, and controlled motion for the involved joints help control edema but require precise participation by the patient. Patient education (complete with explanations of anatomy, wound healing, and precautions) is a critical component of rehabilitation. Most people want to get well and will comply if they understand the importance of their actions; however, a recent study examining patient compliance with orthosis use and home program following tendon repairs found through an anonymous self-reported questionnaire of 76 subjects that 67% of patients did not adhere to their orthosis regimen; there was no significant correlation between patient profile and nonadherence.[33] Along those same lines in a study of causative factors to identify the reasons for zones I and II flexor tendon ruptures, it was found that half of the ruptures studied were due to "acts of stupidity."[34] The experienced clinician knows full well that patient compliance depends on instruction that requires time, patience, knowledge, and firm control on the part of the health care provider.

Proper management of the untidy, open, or cleanly incised and sutured wound is the first important component of preventing infection and controlling the inflammatory response. Careful cleansing, protection of the wound microenvironment, and proper dressing speed epithelialization and enhance macrophage activity so that time in the inflammatory stage is minimized. Exposed wounds tend to be more inflamed and necrotic than occluded wounds.[32] In the later stages, the dermis of exposed wounds is more fibroblastic, fibrotic, and scarred.[32,35]

Position of Immobilization

The tendon repair site, through the use of an orthosis, should be positioned proximal to the tendon's normal resting position during the first 3 weeks of healing to minimize stress at the repair site and thus decrease the chances for gap formation. Gap formation has been associated with increased adhesion formation and poorer clinical results[36-40] (Fig. 39-2). It has been demonstrated (in an experimental flexor tendon study) that gapping of more than 3 mm at a repair site does not increase the prevalence of adhesions or impair range of motion (ROM), but it does prevent the increase in strength and stiffness that normally occurs with time.[41] Any gapping at the repair site can result in elongation of the tendon callus,

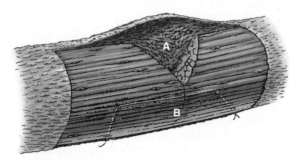

Figure 39-2 *Schematic drawing of a tendon repair. Area A represents the epitenon, where increased extrinsic healing is associated with gap formation. Area B represents the endotenon, where increased intrinsic tendon healing is associated with precise coaptation at the repair site. (Redrawn from Gelberman RH, Vandeberg JS, Manske PR, Akeson WH. Early stages of flexor tendon healing: a morphologic study of the first fourteen days. J Hand Surg. 1985;10A:776–784.)*

which is particularly critical in zones I to IV, where the tendon moment arms and excursions are small.[42] Extensor lag in any zone at 3 or 4 weeks is much more difficult to overcome than extensor tightness and can be prevented by precise positions of immobilization.[43,44]

Effects of Immobilization

Biomechanical and biochemical changes in immobilized connective tissue (tendon, ligament, and cartilage) have been studied primarily in the animal model in various joints.[18,45-51] We must interpret the information gained from these experimental studies with caution as we attempt to alter clinical treatment based on basic science studies in the nonhuman model and more often than not on synovial flexor tendon.

The negative effects of total immobilization during the inflammatory and fibroblastic stages of healing on tendon biochemistry are a loss of glycosaminoglycan concentration, loss of water, decreased fibronectin (FN) concentration, and decreased endotenon healing. Biomechanically, the immobilized tendon loses tensile strength in the first 2 weeks after repair,[18,52-55] and it loses gliding function by the first 10 days after repair.[45,51,56-58]

Effects of Controlled Stress

Many elegant studies have demonstrated the positive influence of stress on healing tendon, with documented improvement of tensile strength, improved gliding properties, increased repair-site DNA, and accelerated changes in peritendinous vessel density and configuration. Motion may enhance the diffusion of synovial fluid within the tendon in synovial regions.[46,59] Stress-induced electrical potentials may increase the connective tissue healing potential.[60-62] Studies have demonstrated that early passive motion in a clinically relevant tendon-repair model increases FN concentration[63] and fibroblast chemotaxis[64] at the tendon repair site. The positive biomechanical effects of mechanical stimulation to a repair site continue to be supported with basic science research.[14-17] Recent clinical studies continue to demonstrate the benefit of controlled motion over immobilization for the repaired extensor tendon.[5-12]

Effect of Timing

Time from injury to repair of intrasynovial flexor tendons, considered as an isolated variable, has been demonstrated to have a significant effect on the function of tendon in dogs. Tendons repaired immediately were significantly improved over tendons repaired at 7 or 21 days with respect to angular rotation and linear excursion, but there were no significant differences in total concentration of collagen at the sites of repair or in the levels of reducible Schiff base cross-links in tendons from the three groups.[31]

Gelberman and colleagues[45,65] demonstrated in the canine model that immobilized tendons become bound by adhesions by the tenth day after repair but that tendons that are immediately mobilized have early restoration of gliding surface without adhesion in-growth.

Preliminary experimental studies indicate that timing in relation to stress during the early inflammatory stage of wound healing is critical. An experimental study on chicken flexor tendons has demonstrated that tendons treated with controlled passive motion have significantly improved tensile strength by 5 days after repair compared with digits treated with immobilization.[53] The magnitude of difference in strength between the two groups increased with time. The authors of that study concluded that immediate constrained digital motion after repair allows progressive tendon healing without the intervening phase of tendon softening or weakening described in the classic study by Mason and Allen in 1941.[54]

In another study of early tensile properties of healing chicken flexor tendons, early controlled passive motion was found to improve healing efficiency.[66] Results of this study indicated that controlled passive-motion tendons had significantly greater values for rupture load, stress, and energy absorbed than immobilized tendons.

FN, which appears to be an important component of the early tendon repair process, has been localized in a clinically relevant tendon repair model. Fibroblast chemotaxis and adherence to the substrate in the days after injury and repair appear to be directly related to FN concentration.[67] Early passive motion has been correlated with an increased FN concentration in the tendon repair model of the previous study.[63] FN concentration in mobilized tendon was found to be twice that of immobilized tendon by 7 days after surgery. Iwuagwu and McGrouther[68] have determined that load applied the first 5 days postoperatively resulted in better orientation and fewer fibroblasts in repaired tendons. Zhao and coworkers have demonstrated in the canine model that starting controlled motion at day 5 following tendon repair is advantageous over day 1 because gliding resistance associated with postoperative surgical edema and other factors is diminished.[69]

We still have no studies on the effect of immediate motion on the healing of the in vivo human tendon, and one must recognize that most of the experimental tendon work is performed on the synovial flexor tendon in animal models. However, these basic science studies offer some documentation that increased cellular activity and strengthening occur with very early motion during the immediate postrepair period and emphasize the critical relationship between the application of force and timing. "Early motion" at 7 to 10 days after surgery may indeed not be early motion at all. By the end of the first week, the window of time may have been lost for the biochemical advantages of immediate motion, and by the tenth day after surgery, the immobilized tendon may be surrounded by dense adhesions.

Duration of Exercise

The duration of the daily controlled passive-motion interval has been determined to be a significant variable in a clinical study of repaired flexor tendons. A prospective multicenter clinical study of 51 patients with flexor tendon repair has determined that greater durations of daily controlled passive motion after flexor tendon repair resulted in increased active interphalangeal (IP) joint motion at a mean time of 6 months after surgery.[70] Two groups of patients treated with continuous passive motion (CPM) and traditional early passive motion were compared in terms of IP motion. The authors concluded that the duration of the daily controlled motion interval is a significant variable in postrepair flexor tendon excursion.[70]

In a related study, designed to determine the effects of frequency and duration of controlled passive motion on the healing flexor tendon after primary repair, adult mongrel dogs were studied as two groups based on the frequency of passive motion.[71] Results indicated that gliding function in both groups was similar, but tensile properties, as represented by linear slope, ultimate load, and energy absorption, were significantly improved in the higher-frequency group. The authors concluded that the frequency of controlled passive motion in postoperative tendon management protocols is a significant factor in accelerating the healing response after tendon repair, and higher-frequency controlled passive motion has a beneficial effect.[71]

These studies offer some proof that "more is better" in the early healing phase. However, in my clinical experience, the patient who exercises excessively may develop inflammation and synovitis within the synovial areas of both flexor[72] and extensor systems if tendon gliding is limited by adhesions that increase friction or if the tendon is still swollen from increased metabolic activity associated with healing. Patient compliance is a significant and often difficult-to-control variable with these postoperative regimens. Dobbe and associates[73] have developed a device to record duration of exercise that is attached to the postoperative orthosis. This concept may prove to have clinical relevance by improving patient compliance, but to date no practical use has been reported. In fact, recent studies have reported that the biggest cause of tendon rupture is "stupidity"[34] and, as noted in a previous section, noncompliance.[33]

Extensor Tendon Excursion

Tendon excursion in the early healing phases of tendon rehabilitation should be limited to a range that is great enough to provide the stress necessary to stimulate biochemical changes at the repair site and to provide some proximal migration of the repair site to control the collagen bonds as they form in the peritendinous region, yet small enough that it does not create gapping or rupture at the repair site. Researchers have raised the question of actual tendon excursion with passive motion.[74-78] Some tendon researchers

believe that a component of controlled active motion may be necessary to create some proximal migration of a tendon repair site and that passive motion may only cause the repair site to fold or buckle instead of glide proximally. This is the rationale for controlled early active motion as opposed to controlled passive motion in postoperative management of the repaired tendon. References to tendon excursion in the next section with cadaveric measurement, measurement by radians, and intraoperative measurement all refer to the relationship of passive joint motion to tendon excursion.

The tendon migration necessary to maintain functional glide and stimulate cellular activity may be in the range of 3 to 5 mm. Duran and Houser[79] recommended this passive excursion range for the flexor tendons in the digital sheath and thought that 3 to 5 mm was sufficient to prevent dense adhesions. Gelberman and colleagues,[37] in an earlier study, suggested that 3 to 4 mm of passive excursion is necessary to stimulate the intrinsic repair process without creating significant repair-site deformation with flexor tendons. More recent studies have indicated that 1.7 mm of tendon excursion is sufficient to prevent adhesion formation in canine tendon and that additional excursion provides little added benefit.[80] Early active and passive motion allowing an estimated 5 mm of excursion has proven to be successful with extensor tendon repairs in zones V through VII, T-IV, and T-V,[81-84] and approximately 4 mm of active excursion with extensor repair in the digital zones III and IV.[43,85]

To safely apply stress to a healing tendon, the therapist must understand tendon excursion as it relates to joint motion and understand tendon tensile strengths as they relate to suture techniques and healing schedules. This requires either a general working knowledge of tendon excursions as cited in the literature or the ability to calculate individual tendon excursions with Brand's technique of using the radian concept and corresponding joint moment arms.[86]

Literature Review of Extensor Tendon Excursions

Reported extensor tendon excursions vary but occur within a consistent range. Differences may exist between the individual extensor digitorum communis (EDC) tendons, as well as from person to person. Variation is also found in the method of study, as well as the size of the hand or joint being examined.[42,86] Cadaveric studies are limited by the absence of normal biochemistry and muscle tone.

Bunnell's cadaver studies of excursions[87] provide detailed information and closely correlate with those described by Brand.[86] Bunnell assigned values for individual finger tendons at each metacarpophalangeal (MCP), PIP, and distal interphalangeal (DIP) joint, with the wrist in a neutral position[87] (Table 39-1). The excursions become smaller as the joint size (and thus the tendon moment arm) decreases.

Excursions for the digital extensor in zones III and IV are small but may be slightly more than those reported by Bunnell, who calculated the EDC excursion to be 2 mm for the index finger, 3 mm for the long finger, 3 mm for the ring finger, and 2 mm for the small finger.[87] In other cadaveric studies, Tubiana[88] cites 8 mm, Valentine[89] cites 7 to 8 mm, Zancolli[90] cites 6 mm, and DeVoll and Saldana[91] cite up to 5 mm of tendon excursion at this level.

Table 39-1 Excursions for Digital Extensor Tendons as Reported by Bunnell

	Total (mm)	Wrist (mm)	MCP (mm)	PIP (mm)	DIP (mm)
Extensor Digitorum Communis					
Index	54	38	15	2	0
Long	55	41	16	3	0
Ring	55	39	11	3	0
Small	35	20	12	2	0
	Total	Wrist	CMC	MCP	IP
Extensor Pollicis Longus					
Thumb	58	33	7	6	8

CMC, carpometacarpal; DIP, distal interphalangeal; IP, interphalangeal; MCP, metacarpophalangeal; PIP, proximal interphalangeal.
From Boyes JH. *Bunnell's Surgery of the Hand.* Philadelphia: JB Lippincott; 1970.

An and coworkers [92] calculated tendon excursion and the moment arm of cadaver index finger joints during rotation and found that excursion and joint displacement were not always linear. Excursion of the extensor digitorum at the PIP level with a mean motion of 89.5 degrees was 5.58 mm. Micks and Reswick [93] determined that the extensor moment arm at the PIP joint is not constant and increases with the position of flexion.

Elliot and McGrouther [94] investigated the mathematic relationship between extensor tendon excursion and joint motion in seven cadaver hands and found this relationship to be linear for all joints in all five rays of the hand. They found that excursion of the middle slip over the proximal phalanx is in effect the excursion of the extensor digitorum that accompanies PIP joint movement. They calculate excursion per 10 degrees for each joint with all other joints immobile and all surrounding structures released. The mean motion per 10 degrees was 0.8 mm for the index, long, and ring PIP joints and 0.6 mm for the small PIP joint. This translates to 2.4 mm of excursion for the index, long, and ring fingers; 1.8 mm of excursion for the small finger; and 1.8 mm of excursion for the small finger per 30 degrees of PIP motion. Their findings are contrary to those of An and coworkers. [92,93]

Calculating Excursions with Radians and Moment Arms

Brand [86] describes a constant relationship between joint motion and tendon excursion at both the MCP and PIP joints. A fairly constant extensor tendon moment arm (the perpendicular distance from the joint axis to the extensor tendon) exists at both joint levels. Although not precisely constant, the extensor tendon moment arm does not change dramatically with joint motion. [86] Brand calculated the mean moment arm for the index MCP joint to be 10 mm in cadaver studies and for the middle finger PIP joint to be 7.5 mm. [86] The moment arm varies with joint size, but these figures give us a working base to calculate approximate extensor tendon excursion.

Tendon excursion can be calculated geometrically with radians. [86] A radian is the angle that is created when the radius laid along the circumference of a circle is joined by a line at each end to the center of the circle (Fig. 39-3). This angle always equals 57.29 degrees (1 radian). This segment of the

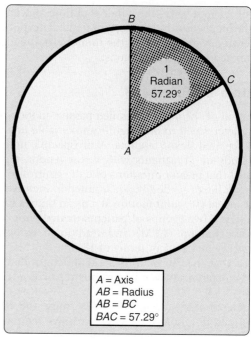

Figure 39-3 A radian is the angle that is created when the radius laid along the circumference of a circle is joined by a line at each end to the center or axis of the circle. Angle *BAC* equals 1 radian, or 57.29 degrees. (From Brand PW, Hollister A. *Clinical Mechanics of the Hand*, 2nd ed. St. Louis: Mosby; 1993: 62–91.)

circumference of the circle is always equal to the radius of the circle when the working angle is 57.29 degrees.

To calculate extensor tendon excursion at the MCP joint level, consider the head of the metacarpal in terms of a circle (Fig. 39-4A). The moment arm of the extensor tendon (or the perpendicular distance between the MCP joint axis, or center of the circle, and the extensor tendon) is equal to the excursion of the extensor tendon if the MCP joint is moved through 1 radian, or 57.29 degrees. Using Brand's figure of 10 mm for an average extensor tendon moment arm in the index finger, [86] MCP joint motion of 57.29 degrees yields 10 mm of extensor tendon excursion (see Fig. 39-4A). To obtain the 5 mm of excursion suggested by Duran and Houser [79] and Gelberman and associates [37] to minimize extrinsic adhesions, the joint must be moved through 0.5 radian, or 28.64 degrees, of rotation [83] (Fig. 39-4B).

Because joint size varies, the therapist must consider that it is the constant relationship of tendon excursion to angular rotation and the length of the moment arm that is important. A smaller joint with a smaller moment arm produces less tendon excursion with the same joint motion. For example, if the MCP joint of the small finger has a moment arm of 7.5 mm, angular change of 0.5 radian, or 28.64 degrees, will produce 3.75 mm of glide. To obtain the necessary excursion to maintain tendon glide in the smaller ulnar joints or in smaller hands, one must move these joints through more than 0.5 radian of rotation. [83]

Calculation by Simple Equation of Safe Parameters for Controlled Motion

Evans and Burkhalter [83] proposed a simple equation for determining excursion of the extrinsic finger extensors in zones

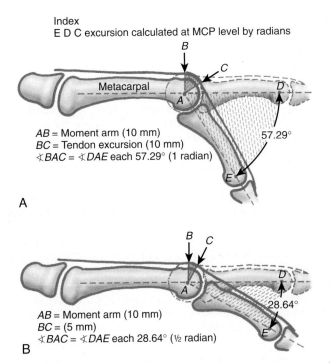

Index
E D C excursion calculated at MCP level by radians

AB = Moment arm (10 mm)
BC = Tendon excursion (10 mm)
∡BAC = ∡DAE each 57.29° (1 radian)

A

AB = Moment arm (10 mm)
BC = (5 mm)
∡BAC = ∡DAE each 28.64° (½ radian)

B

Figure 39-4 A, If the head of the metacarpal is considered in terms of a circle, the moment arm of the extensor tendon is equal to the radius of that circle. If metacarpophalangeal joint motion equals 57.29 degrees, or 1 radian, extensor tendon excursion is equal to the moment arm, or *AB* = *BC*. If the moment arm equals 10 mm, angular change of 57.29 degrees effects 10 mm of extensor tendon excursion. **B,** Angular change of 0.5 radian, 28.3 degrees, effects the 5 mm of extensor tendon excursion recommended for the early passive motion program. (**A,** From Evans RB, Burkhalter WE. A study of the dynamic anatomy of extensor tendons and implications for treatment. *J Hand Surg.* 1986;11A:774–779.)

Box 39-1	**Calculation for Extensor Digitorum Communis Excursion at the Metacarpophalangeal Level**

Index = 5.66 degrees per mm × 5 mm = 28.3 degrees
Long = 5.5 degrees per mm × 5 mm = 27.5 degrees
Ring = 8.18 degrees per mm × 5 mm = 40.9 degrees
Small = 7.66 degrees per mm × 5 mm = 38.33 degrees

From Evans RB, Burkhalter WE. A study of the dynamic anatomy of extensor tendons and implications for treatment. *J Hand Surg.* 1986;11A:774–779.

V through VII in the initial biomechanical study supporting early passive motion in these zones: Joint motion divided by tendon excursion for that particular joint is equal to the number of degrees of motion required to *effect* 1 mm of tendon glide.

Joint motion (degrees)/Tendon excursion (mm) = degrees of motion per millimeter of excursion

Application of this equation is contingent on total joint motion and total tendon excursion for each individual finger at the MCP level and the amount of excursion considered safe and effective for providing controlled stress to the healing tendon.

The suggested equation is applied with these average values for MCP joint motion: 85 degrees index; 88 degrees long; 90 degrees ring; and 92 degrees small finger.[83] Excursions used were those described by Bunnell,[87] because he measured each finger separately (see Table 39-1). Controlled stress allowing 5 mm of passive glide, as suggested by Duran and Houser[79] and substantiated by intraoperative measurements in the pilot study,[83] was determined to be a safe and effective excursion (Box 39-1).

Extensor tendon excursions were investigated in eight fresh cadaveric limbs.[78] The authors found that if the wrist is extended more than 21 degrees, the extensor tendon glides

with little or no tension in zones V and VI throughout a full simulated grip to full passive extension. On the basis of this cadaveric study, the authors recommend that up to 6.4 mm of tendon can be safely debrided in these zones and that full grip can be permitted postoperatively if the wrist is positioned in more than 45 degrees of extension. Their study emphasizes the importance of wrist position to tendon excursion, but their conclusions based on cadaveric study should be applied to the clinical situation with caution.

Intraoperative Measurement

Evans and Burkhalter[83] measured extensor tendon excursion intraoperatively and found by gross measurement that 30 degrees of MCP motion effected 5 mm of extensor glide in zones V through VII, supporting our calculations by radians with the previously described equation. This more limited amount of motion has worked well in my 34 years of clinical experience with early motion of extensor tendons, but others[78,95] believe that full digital flexion should be considered safe within the confines of orthoses that hold the wrist in extension and fingers controlled in dynamic extension traction.

Cadaveric studies and mathematical equations do not consider biology. No study to date describes extensor tendon excursion after repair in vivo to give us accurate measurements for passive or active motion; it would seem that intraoperative measurement may be more accurate than cadaveric study.

Excursion of the Central Slip Measured in Radians

The same calculation techniques can be applied to the PIP joint and central slip excursion and are used to establish safe parameters for immediate early active motion for central slip repairs (discussed later).[43] Biomechanically, the excursion of the extensor tendon at the level of the PIP joint is proportional to angular changes of the joint.[86] The mean moment arm for the extensor tendon of the long finger PIP joint has

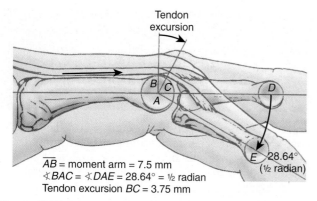

$\overline{AB}$ = moment arm = 7.5 mm
∢BAC = ∢DAE = 28.64° = ½ radian
Tendon excursion BC = 3.75 mm

Figure 39-5 Excursion of the central slip (zone III) as calculated by radians. AB = the moment arm of the central slip. Angle BAC = 0.5 radian, or 28.64 degrees. If the proximal interphalangeal joint is moved through 0.5 radian, the central slip excursion will equal one half the moment arm, or 3.75 mm. The average moment arm of the middle finger central slip is 7.5 mm as measured by Brand and Hollister.[20] (From Evans RB, Thompson DE. An analysis of factors that support early active short arc motion of the repaired central slip. J Hand Ther. 1992;5:193.)

been determined to be 7.5 mm.[86] Therefore PIP joint motion of 57.29 degrees, 1 radian, effects 7.5 mm of excursion in the freely gliding tendon. One half (0.5) radian, or 28.64 degrees, effects 3.75 mm of excursion[43] (Fig. 39-5).

There is some disagreement in the literature regarding the extensor moment arm at the PIP joint. Micks and Reswick[93] determined that the extensor moment arm at the PIP joint is not constant and increases with flexion. Brand[86] found the moment arm of the extensor to be fairly constant at this level, unchanging with motion. An and coworkers[92] found that excursion and joint displacement were not always linear at the PIP joint, but Elliot and McGrouther[94] found that relationship to be linear.

The protocol for early motion for the extensor zones III through VII[43,83-85] requires only 30 to 40 degrees of joint motion at the respective MCP or PIP joints; therefore the changes in the extensor moment arms are small and unlikely to be significant enough to alter the calculation of excursion.

Excursion of the Extensor Pollicis Longus

Excursions for the extensor pollicis longus (EPL) tendon vary in the literature from 25 to 60 mm.[87,96,97] The simple angular arrangement of the flexion–extension axis at the MCP level of the fingers does not exist for the EPL in zones T-IV and T-V. Calculating excursion mathematically is complicated by the oblique course that the tendon takes at Lister's tubercle, by the moments of adduction and external rotation at the carpometacarpal (CMC) level, and by the fact that alterations in thumb position alter the moment arms at each joint.[86,98] Evans and Burkhalter[83] measured EPL excursion intraoperatively to determine the amount of joint motion necessary to create 5 mm of glide for the early motion pilot study and found that with the wrist neutral and the thumb MCP joint extended, 60 degrees of IP joint motion effected 5 mm of tendon excursion at Lister's tubercle.

True Tendon Excursion

The question of actual tendon excursion with passive motion has been raised.[74,76,77] Experimentally (intact fresh frozen cadaver specimens), passive motion in flexor tendons has been demonstrated to be almost half that of theoretically predicted values under conditions of low tendon tension;[75] investigators have shown that actual tendon excursion is equal to the predicted tendon excursions of earlier studies[79,99] only when more than 300 g of tension is applied to the repair site.[75] Similar studies correlating in vivo tendon tension and tendon excursion for the extensor system have not been performed, but cadaver studies suggest that the tendons may buckle only in zones V through VII with digital joint motion from flexion to extension.[78]

The concept of using immediate active motion after tendon repair is simply an attempt to ensure that the repair site does glide proximally. Some clinicians now think that an as yet undefined degree of active tension at a repair site may be necessary to create a proximal migration of the healing tendon and that passive motion may only cause the tendon to buckle, fold, or roll up at the repair site.[76,78] The use of immediate active motion as a means of restricting the limitation posed by adhesions and improving tendon gliding is neither new[100-103] nor widely accepted in clinical practice, but it is now the subject of renewed interest in tendon management programs. Stronger suture techniques that are designed for active motion have been developed for flexor tendon repairs and for extensor system repairs.[104,105] Favorable clinical results with active motion programs have been reported for both the flexor system and the extensor system.[5-13,85,106-111]

Tendons rehabilitated in dynamic extension orthoses intended for passive motion programs in reality probably move actively throughout the early healing phases, so the discussion of "active versus passive" tendon excursion is most likely a moot point for extensors in zones V through VII when rehabilitated in such orthoses. Newport and Shukla[112] performed electromyographic (EMG) studies on a group of normal volunteers to determine the level of activity present in the EDC within the confines of a dynamic extension orthosis. Their study validates what most therapists observe clinically—that most patients actively move their repaired and positioned extensor tendons within the dynamic extension orthosis and within the exercise regimen that is intended to provide active flexion and passive extension. They found that if the MCP joints were positioned in 0 degrees of extension, the EDC tendons were active within the dynamic extension orthosis; however, if the MCP joints were positioned in modest flexion (20 degrees), the extensor tendons were quiescent during the active flexion exercise.[112] The authors of that study use this information to recommend that the MCP joints be positioned in 20 degrees of flexion to prevent active motion of the repaired tendon. I use their information to support dynamic positioning of the MCP joints at 0 degrees of extension to facilitate some physiologic active motion at the repair site. I believe that the MCP joints should be positioned at 0 degrees, not only to prevent extensor lag but also to create some active tension and true proximal migration of the repair site.

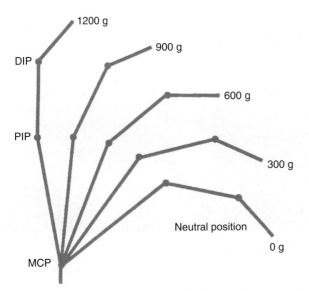

Figure 39-6 This schematic demonstrates the force analysis of the extensor digitorum communis (EDC) in various joint angles with the wrist extended. Note that with the metacarpophalangeal (MCP), proximal interphalangeal (PIP), and distal interphalangeal (DIP) joints in a neutral position, no force (0 g) is transmitted to the EDC, but that as extension angles for these joints increase, the forces are elevated to as much as 1200 g. With the wrist flexed, these forces are greatly diminished. (From Evans RB, Thompson DE. The application of stress to the healing tendon. *J Hand Ther.* 1993;6:270.)

Application of Force

Force application is the sum of muscle contraction and viscoelastic drag of the tissues. Viscoelastic drag is the sum of the antagonistic muscle tension, resistance from the periarticular support systems, edema, and adhesions.[42] Resistance from Coban wraps or bandaging also must be considered as an increased force application in early active motion programs. A safety margin must be established in which the force application (or the stress applied to the tendon) is less than the tensile strength of the tendon with all early motion programs.

Force Application at the Repair Site

Internal tendon forces as they relate to various joint angles and applied external loads are defined for the flexor and extensor tendons in two scientific articles on early active motion for both tendon systems.[43,84] The results of these biomechanical analyses are presented in a series of mathematical models that negate resistance from the antagonistic muscle–tendon group and any other drag and apply a known external force. The force analysis of the EDC with the wrist in an extended position and no external load is calculated so that conservative estimates of tendon forces can be made (Fig. 39-6). With the digital joints in a neutral position, tensions on the EDC are zero, but as the digits are extended, the forces rise to 1200 g. These forces would drop dramatically if the wrist were placed in 20 degrees of flexion (the position recommended for early active controlled motion) because resistance from the flexor tendons would be reduced by wrist position.[43,84,113] The force applied to the extensor tendon at both the MCP and PIP joint levels with active extension of

30 degrees of flexion to 0 degrees of extension (at either joint) has been calculated mathematically to be approximately 300 g if the wrist is positioned at 20 degrees of flexion.[43,84]

Tensile Strength of Extensor Tendon Repairs

The tensile strength of freshly sutured tendon depends on the strength of the suture material, the suture method, the balance between the strands and knot, the number of strands, the size of the tendon, and the addition of a circumferential suture to a core suture. Several studies[104,114-119] have investigated the mechanical strengths of tendon repair techniques and suture materials for the extensor system. Newport and Williams[115] reported on the biomechanical characteristics of extensor tendon suture at 2-mm gapping and at failure. The mattress suture gapped 2 mm at 488 g and failed at 840 g; figure-of-eight suture gapped at 587 g and failed at 696 g; the Kessler suture gapped at 1353 g and failed at 1830 g; and the Bunnell suture gapped at 1425 g and failed at 1985 g.[115] A comparative study of four extensor tendon repair techniques demonstrated that strength to 2-mm gapping for the modified Becker suture technique (56.0 ± 9.2 N) and the modified Kessler technique (48.6 ± 12.6N) was significantly better ($p < 0.05$) than for the six-strand double-loop and figure-of-eight techniques.[117]

Most studies on repair tensile strengths report the strength in newtons (N), but as therapists, we usually calculate the forces of dynamic orthoses and torque ROM and the force of motion in grams. Evans and Thompson[84] reviewed a large number of studies on the strengths of the various repairs and translated newtons into grams to assist therapists as they assess the strength of the particular repair they are treating (1 kg = 9.8 N, or 1 g = 0.01 N; conversion of newtons to grams: N divided by 9.8×1000 = g). Comparisons of these studies are difficult because of the many variables (subject, material, technique of repair, and method of testing) studied.

The load at which a tendon gaps is the number that we must recognize, particularly with the controlled active motion programs. Gap formation has been associated with increased adhesion formation and poorer clinical results. Although most surgeons believe that gapping above 1 to 3 mm is incompatible with a good result,[36-40] investigators have demonstrated in an in vivo study that gaps of up to 10 mm in a repaired flexor digitorum profundus (FDP) are compatible with a good functional ROM when passive motion programs are used.[120] Gelberman and colleagues[41] have demonstrated that a gap at a repair site of more than 3 mm does not increase the prevalence of adhesions or impair ROM but does prevent the accrual of strength and stiffness that normally occurs with time.

Adjusting the Equation

The equations for force application and tensile strength just described must be adjusted to consider the increased resistance from postsurgical edema, stiff joints, and bandaging and to allow for a possible drop in tensile strength in the repaired tendon. The estimated tensile strength of the repair may decrease as much as 25% to 50% by postoperative day

5 to 15 in the unstressed tendon;[99,121] however, tendon subjected to immediate or very early controlled motion may not experience this drop in tensile strength.[52,53,63,67,122] The estimated force application to the repair site with the early active motion protocols may need to be doubled to account for the resistance from drag.[123]

Effect of Complex Injury

The relationship between the amount of tissue damage and the biological response is a basic phenomenon of wound healing.[32] Increased inflammation associated with severe injury increases the work requirement of the macrophage, and the number of macrophage cells necessary to meet the metabolic demands of the injury determines the number of fibroblasts that are signaled into the wound for repair. Collagen deposition can be expected to be proportional to the number of fibroblasts, or collagen-producing factories, present in the wound bed.[32]

Rothkopf and coworkers[57] studied mechanical trauma and immobilization in the canine flexor tendon model to study adhesion formation associated with complex injury. These researchers defined *complex tendon injury* as one associated with crush injury, concomitant nerve injury, or tendon injury treated with immobilization. Their experimental model demonstrated significant decreases in tendon excursions and an increase in work requirement to effect tendon excursion in the complex injury. This experimental model in the animal flexor tendon may have implications for the human flexor or extensor tendon.

We all have observed clinically that the more complex injury can be expected to cause more complications associated with increased fibroblastic response and that immobilization of the complex injury adds to those complications. Many authors have endorsed the use of early motion with the complex injury,[43,83,124-126] but there are few clinical reports in the literature on early motion for the complex tendon injury, and most clinical results refer to clean lacerations. Koul and associates recently published the results of 21 complex extensor tendon injuries in zones V through VII treated with single-stage reconstruction, including soft tissue reconstruction rehabilitated with immediate active motion. They reported excellent functional results (total active motion [TAM] 202.6 degrees at 6 weeks and 249.5 degrees at 12 weeks, and 75% grip at 12 weeks) and reduced morbidity and cost of treatment with single-stage reconstruction and early active motion.[127]

Clinical Management of Extensor Tendon Injuries

Zones I and II

A lesion of the terminal extensor tendon results in a flexion deformity of the DIP joint, commonly referred to as the *mallet*, or *baseball*, finger. Treatment and prognosis of the mallet finger depend on associated tissue injury and age of the lesion before treatment.[126,128] These injuries may be open or closed, with or without associated fracture or fracture dislocation. In many cases, conservative treatment with

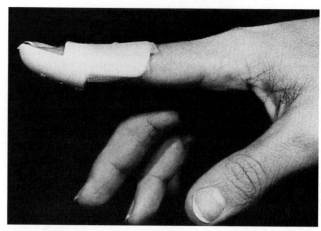

Figure 39-7 A stack orthosis for zone I extensor tendon injury immobilizes the distal joint in slight hyperextension. (From Evans RB. Therapeutic management of extensor tendon injuries. *Hand Clin.* 1986;2:157–169.)

orthotic immobilization is sufficient to restore tendon continuity.[126,128,129] However, open injury, associated fracture, or chronic deformity may require direct repair or Kirschner wire (K-wire) fixation[126,129,130] (see also Chapter 38).

Most authors recommend approximately 6 to 8 weeks of continuous extension positioning with a static orthosis for the middle and distal phalanx only with both conservative and operative treatment.[126,129,130] Dagum and Mahoney[131] have recommended that the wrist be positioned with a simple wrist control orthosis in addition to the distal joint orthosis to prevent gapping in zone I; however, in my clinical experience this does not seem to be necessary. Katzman and associates,[132] in a cadaveric study of gap formation in mallet fingers, determined that joint motion proximal to the DIP joint and retraction of the intrinsics did not cause a tendon gap in a finger with a mallet lesion, supporting the concept that positioning one joint is sufficient for these injuries. Honner[133] recommends some limited active flexion at 4 weeks, with continuous positioning between exercise periods for an additional 4 weeks. The DIP joint can be immobilized with commercially available Stack orthoses, aluminum-padded orthoses, or molded thermoplastic orthoses (Fig. 39-7). Orthosis application is most often volar to the level of the PIP joint. A wide plastic tape placed across the dorsal aspect of the DIP joint acts as a counterpressure and holds the DIP joint in complete extension. I prefer to use Transpore tape by 3M with a small square of moleskin lining the portion of the tape that is directly over the DIP joint. Dorsal immobilization permits more freedom of the PIP joint and allows the fingertip its sensory function; however, in the hands of my patients, dorsal positioning (Fig. 39-8) has not been as effective as volar positioning. Clinical experience teaches that early intervention for the zone I extensor lesion with orthotic positioning yields the best results in terms of extensor lag and time required for immobilization; however, Jablecki and Syrko recently made the point in a review article that "the period of time for which conservative treatment can be prolonged and still be effective is still being extended, and the absolute outside time limit remains unknown."[129]

Orthosis position and skin integrity should be monitored carefully. The distal joint should be immobilized at 0 degrees

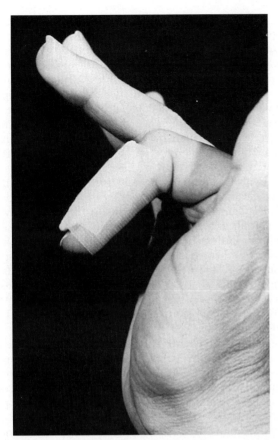

Figure 39-8 Dorsal immobilization of the distal joint permits more freedom of the proximal interphalangeal joint and allows the fingertip its sensory function. (From Evans RB. Therapeutic management of extensor tendon injuries. *Hand Clin.* 1986;2:157–169.)

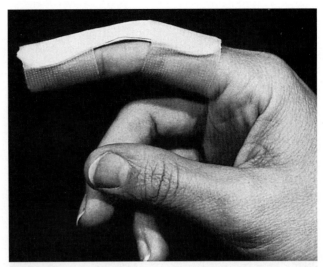

Figure 39-9 The proximal interphalangeal joint should be positioned in slight flexion in the mallet finger that develops a swan-neck posture to advance the lateral bands. (From Evans RB. Therapeutic management of extensor tendon injuries. *Hand Clin.* 1986;2:157–169.)

of extension or slight hyperextension.[130,134] Extreme hyperextension jeopardizes circulation to the dorsal skin by stretching the volar vasculature, which provides nutrition to the area distal to the termination of the dorsal vessels, and may create skin necrosis.[135] Rayan and Mullins,[134] in a study of skin necrosis complications associated with mallet finger positioning, suggested a position of hyperextension less than the angle that causes skin blanching, a precursor of skin necrosis. They determined the average total passive hyperextension of the distal joint to be 28.3 degrees and found that circulation to the dorsal skin was compromised when the distal joint was positioned at more than 50% of its total hyperextension. Orthosis immobilization that allows even slight flexion results in extensor lag because the tendon callus heals in an elongated position.[136]

Skin maceration is a problem with these injuries. It is difficult for patients to keep the affected hand dry for 6 to 8 weeks, and most patients find it irksome to be so limited by a one-joint injury. Patients must be instructed in proper orthotic application, skin care, technique for maintaining the DIP joint in extension during cleansing (I usually teach them to use the ipsilateral thumb to hold the DIP joint in hyperextension while cleansing with the contralateral hand), orthotic positioning, and orthotic adjustment to make sure that the distal joint always rests in complete extension. The orthoses can be lined with moleskin to absorb perspiration, and patients should be instructed to change the lining if it

becomes damp. The DIP joint must be held in hyperextension while the patient changes the orthosis lining. I provide two distal joint orthoses; one can be worn while showering. The orthosis must be adjusted as edema decreases to provide a precise fit.

During the immobilization phase, the patient should be seen weekly for wound care when necessary, for adjustment of the fit of the orthosis, and for maintenance of motion in the unaffected joints. The distal joint must be held in extension continuously during orthotic adjustments to prevent attenuation of the healing tendon.

If the PIP joint develops a posture of slight hyperextension, the PIP joint should be positioned at 30 to 45 degrees of flexion while the DIP joint is held in complete extension (Fig. 39-9). This position advances the lateral bands and may assist in closer approximation of the torn extensor tendon at the DIP joint.[137] Doyle[130] describes a treatment for the mallet finger with plaster casting of the PIP joint at 60 degrees and the DIP joint in slight hyperextension. He points out that in most cases, PIP immobilization is not necessary for these injuries but that casting both the PIP and DIP joints is a workable solution for patients who are unreliable or who are unable to understand or perform the correct application of an orthosis.[130] Bunnell explained the rationale for the 60-degree flexion angle of the PIP. In this position, the lateral bands are advanced a distance of 3 mm.[87] This much flexion could result in flexion contracture of the PIP joint, and clinically 45 to 60 degrees of PIP flexion has worked well for me. Flexion contracture of the PIP joint has not been a problem with PIP flexion positioning at these angles in my practice. Positioning the PIP joint may not be necessary beyond the first few weeks, after which the long orthosis can be exchanged for a shorter one-joint orthosis for the DIP. The most effective combination is a P[2], P[3] orthosis taped firmly over the DIP joint with an interlocking dorsal orthosis that holds the PIP joint at 45 to 60 degrees of flexion. The patient exercises the PIP joint to full flexion six times per day (15 repetitions) while the DIP joint is held immobile in the volar orthosis to ensure full motion of the PIP joint.

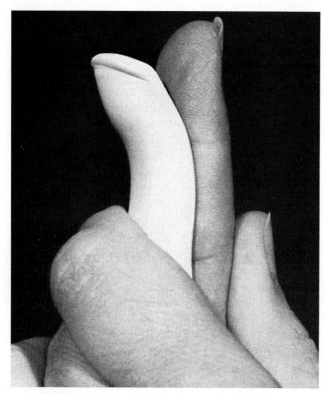

Figure 39-10 A template exercise orthosis sets limits for graded flexion and prevents overstretching of the terminal extensor tendon in the overly ambitious patient. (From Evans RB. Therapeutic management of extensor tendon injuries. *Hand Clin.* 1986;2:157–169.)

After 6 weeks of uninterrupted positioning in extension, very gentle active flexion exercises are initiated. The opposing FDP is a powerful musculotendinous unit and easily overpowers the more fragile terminal extensor tendon. Brand and Hollister[86] calculated the work capacity of the extensors to be less than one third of that of the flexors; therefore flexion increments should be obtained gradually with the initial emphasis on active extension. Because the moment arm of the extensor tendon at this level is small, so also is extensor tendon excursion.[86,87,96,97]

Instructions to the patient should be very specific. During the first week of mobilization, no more than 20 to 25 degrees of active flexion of the distal joint should be allowed. Exercise duration is empirically prescribed at 10 to 20 repetitions every couple of hours. During the second week, if no lag has developed, distal joint flexion to 35 degrees may be allowed. The overly ambitious patient benefits from a template exercise orthosis with specific angles of motion preset to prevent overstretching of the terminal tendon (Fig. 39-10). If the distal joint is tight in extension, the oblique retinacular ligaments (ORLs) may need to be stretched by manual immobilization with the PIP joint at 0 degrees of extension while the DIP joint is actively or passively flexed.[130]

If an extensor lag develops, repositioning is indicated and exercises are delayed for a few weeks.[126,130] Positioning between exercise sessions is recommended during the first 2 weeks of mobilization (a total of 8 to 10 weeks after injury), and night positioning with a volar static orthosis should be continued for an additional 4 weeks after intermittent daytime positioning has been discontinued.

Early active or passive motion has not been accepted practice for the tendon at this level, where excursions are small and where the tendon tissue becomes stiffer and more cartilaginous.[24,86] However, because of inconsistent clinical results with these injuries and problems of loss of both flexion and extension, earlier motion techniques have been investigated. Nakamura and Nanjyo[138] published their experience with surgical intervention with a wire implant and K-wire pinning for 3 weeks in 15 patients with freshly injured mallet fingers (average time from injury to surgery, 19.4 days) without associated fractures. The K-wire is removed at 3 weeks, and distal joint motion in gradually increased increments is allowed. The wire in the tendon stumps is removed at 5 weeks. Nakamura and Nanjyo[138] report improved ROM and fewer complications with this technique, which also reduces immobilization time. Zlatkov reported improved results for the zone I and II extensor tendon operated with "a "special tendon suture" and treated with early active motion (62.5% excellent, 20.8% good, 12.5% satisfactory, and 4.2% unsatisfactory) over those treated with immobilization (45.7% excellent, 22.9% good, 20% satisfactory, and 11.4% unsatisfactory).[139]

Prehension and coordination activities should supplement ROM exercise. Desensitization of a painful fingertip may be necessary with crush injuries or nail bed injuries before the patient incorporates the digit into prehension activities. Exercise may gradually proceed to resistive grasp and pinch activities. Flexion angles should be increased only if complete extension is maintained, and full flexion should not be attempted before 3 months.

Therapy for the zone I and II extensor tendon injury is primarily educational. If the patient understands the nature of the injury and the rationale for treatment, he or she should be able to perform most of the therapy independently. I typically monitor these patients once a week for correct orthosis position, compliance, motion at the PIP joint, and skin issues. This is a very irritating injury for most patients. I find that most patients with zone I and II injury need a great deal of encouragement to stay with the program and to be precise with positioning and motion protocols.

One systematic review was found in a Medline search questioning evidence to support interventions on the zone I and II extensor tendon injury. The results of the four randomized controlled studies, "all of which had methodological flaws," determined that there was insufficient evidence to support either customized or "off the shelf" orthoses and that there was insufficient evidence to determine when surgery is indicated.[140]

Zones III and IV

Extensor injuries in zones III and IV may result in a boutonnière deformity (see Chapter 38). The natural progression of the zone III extensor injury is well defined in the literature. Untreated, the lacerated middle band retracts, allowing the lateral bands to carry the full force of the extrinsic extensor tendon. The lateral bands migrate palmarward, act as flexors of the PIP joint, and with an increase in effort to extend the PIP joint, actually hyperextend the DIP joint. With time, the tendon and the retinacular tissues tighten and accommodate to the change in joint posture, tightening to a point where they resist even passive correction of the deformity. The relationship of the zone III tendon over the PIP joint and the zone IV tendon over the proximal phalanx to the lateral bands does differ, creating different tensions in these two zones as the distal joint is flexed;[27,43,90] however, for all practical purposes, I treat both zones with the same positioning and motion techniques and hereafter will refer to this injury as a zone III or central slip injury.

Traditional Management of the Zone III Tendon Injury

The literature contains conflicting opinions concerning direct repair and immobilization with K-wire versus conservative management of the open zone III injury. However, most authors recommend conservative treatment of the acute closed injury at this level with uninterrupted immobilization of the PIP joint at 0 degrees for 6 weeks.[126,130,141] Open and repaired injuries are mobilized as early as 3 to 4 weeks by some authors, with protective orthotic use between exercise sessions and graded increments in ROM allowed between 3 and 6 weeks;[81,142,143] however, most authors recommend continuous positioning for 6 weeks before motion is initiated.[66,130] Traditional management of this injury often calls for immobilization of the more proximal joints in extension as well as the PIP joint; however, I have never immobilized more than the digit (PIP and DIP joints) unless the zone IV injury is very proximal, approaching zone V, and have not found this to be a problem clinically. With either operative or nonoperative treatment, it is critical that the orthosis position of the PIP joint be at absolute 0 degrees; otherwise, there is some tension at the repair site, possibly creating some gapping, which may result in tendon healing in an elongated position.[43,85]

The PIP joint can be immobilized with a volar static thermoplastic orthosis with a counterpressure directly over the PIP joint applied with 1-inch Transpore tape (Fig. 39-11) or with a circumferential finger cast (Fig. 39-12A). The finger cast is always the treatment of choice with the closed injury, especially if the PIP joint is tight in flexion or if the digit is swollen. The circumferential pressure decreases edema, and the pressures that the cast imposes serve to elongate the tight

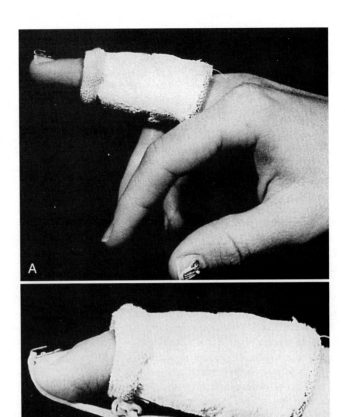

Figure 39-12 A, A cylinder plaster cast immobilizes the proximal interphalangeal joint at 0 degrees of extension. The circumferential pressure of the cast is effective in reducing digital edema. **B,** Gentle intermittent traction can be incorporated into the digital cast to stretch the distal joint periarticular structures if the oblique retinacular ligaments are tight. (From Evans RB. Therapeutic management of extensor tendon injuries. *Hand Clin.* 1986;2:157–169.)

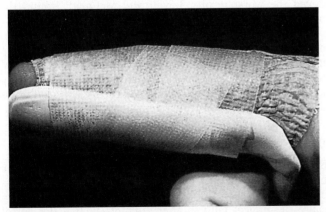

Figure 39-11 The involved digit is positioned in a volar static thermoplastic orthosis, immobilizing the proximal and distal interphalangeal joints at absolute 0 degrees. Dorsal pressure is applied over both joints with 1-inch Transpore tape (Velcro straps do not maintain as much pressure).

volar structures.[144] The finger cast is preferable when noncompliance is possible.

Finger casting is an art and requires some practice before this treatment is imposed on a patient (see Chapter 125). Casting material can be applied directly to the skin with the closed injury and encouraged to remain there with an application of benzoin to the skin before casting. With the open wound, a sterile contact layer and tube gauze dressing are applied first. If the wound area or skin is fragile, a small square of closed-cell adhesive foam can be applied directly over the PIP joint to disperse pressure before the fast-setting plaster is applied. Circulation should be monitored during cast application and for at least 20 minutes before the patient leaves the clinic. Casted digits that are cool, slightly discolored, or throbbing should be recast before the patient leaves the clinic. The patient should be instructed that if the finger swells or becomes painful at home, the cast should be removed by soaking the casted digit in warm water until the material softens and can be slipped off the digit. A digital static extension orthosis supplied by the therapist as a backup should then be applied until the next therapy appointment. To ensure a proper fit, finger casts must be removed and replaced during the first 7 to 10 days for wound care and as edema decreases.

If the lateral bands require no surgical repair, the distal joint is left free to prevent distal joint tightness, loss of extensibility of the ORL, and lateral band adherence.[90] Distal joint motion should be encouraged. If the lateral bands are repaired, the DIP joint also can be immobilized for 4 to 6 weeks;[130] however, this can result in significant loss of distal joint motion, so I start lateral band gliding exercises by the third week.

Active distal joint flexion, combined with static positioning of the PIP joint in extension and the DIP joint in flexion, or intermittent traction into flexion provides improved extensibility to the ORL for the digit with limited distal joint flexion (Fig. 39-12B).

Mobilization schedules for treatment by immobilization vary from 3 to 6 weeks for the open and repaired injury to 5 to 6 weeks for the closed boutonnière deformity. Proponents of this approach recommend progressive gentle flexion exercises between weeks 3 and 6 with protective extension positioning between exercise sessions.[126,130] PIP joint flexion exercises for both the open and repaired central slip or the closed boutonnière deformity should be initiated with caution because the immobilized extensor tendon has little tensile strength and is most likely adherent over the proximal phalanx (P^1), limiting gliding and elevating tension at the level of repair. The first week of mobilization (regardless of whether motion is started at week 3, 4, 5, or 6) should emphasize active PIP joint extension with an exercise position of the MCP joint at 0 degrees of extension and PIP flexion to no more than 30 degrees. If no lag develops, motion can progress to 40 to 50 degrees by the second week of motion, thereafter adding 20 to 30 degrees per week. Forceful flexion exercises are not appropriate, and development of lag should be addressed with increased extension positioning and decreased increments of flexion (Fig. 39-13).

If there is no extensor lag, flexor forces can be directed to the stiff PIP joint by (1) applying a forearm-based dynamic orthosis that blocks the MCP joint in extension and applies a light traction (<250 g) to the middle phalanx (P^2) level; (2) applying a hand-based exercise orthosis that blocks the MCP joint in extension and encourages PIP joint flexion in the hook fist position; or (3) positioning the distal joint with a P^2, P^3 volar orthosis, manually supporting P^1, and actively flexing the PIP joint (Fig. 39-14).

Digital swelling can be controlled with 2-inch Coban wraps. Scars can be softened with massage and silicone gel sheeting (SGS) or elastomer molds applied with pressure. Exercises should emphasize blocking of individual joints and grasping activity. Osteoarthritic IP joints with flexor tendon inflammation and incomplete hook fist position should not engage in repetitive grasping activity that requires acute composite flexion because this may encourage triggering in the flexor system.[72]

The chronic or fixed boutonnière deformity requires orthotic use and exercise to regain passive motion for both IP joints before surgery.[141] Treatment for the chronic boutonnière deformity is well described by a number of authors.[130,137,141,143]

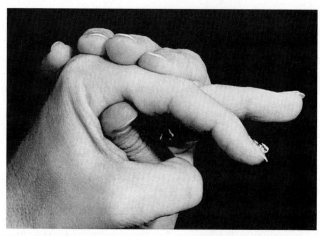

Figure 39-13 The proximal phalanx of the affected digit is held manually in flexion as the patient relaxes the proximal interphalangeal (PIP) joint into mild flexion and then actively lifts the joint to full extension. With the metacarpophalangeal (MCP) joint flexed, PIP joint extension is primarily effected through the interossei,[168,169] possibly with some contribution from the lumbrical,[89] but with little contribution from the extensor digitorum communis.[166] Tension on the central tendon is decreased with MCP flexion because of sagittal band distal migration.[90] PIP exercise should also be performed with the MCP held at 0 degrees of extension to direct increased forces to the central slip.

Immediate Active Short Arc Motion for the Repaired Central Slip

The acutely repaired central slip injury treated traditionally with 4 to 6 weeks of immobilization is often compromised by problems of extensor tendon lag, insufficient extensor tendon excursion, joint stiffness, and loss of flexion. Newport and colleagues,[145] in a report of long-term results of extensor tendon repair, found that extensor tendon injuries within the digit treated with immobilization had higher percentages of fair and poor results than those of more proximal injuries; they also found that injuries in zones III and IV had higher percentages of resultant extensor lag (35%) and loss of flexion (71%). They note that there is little margin for adhesion formation or shortening of the extensor tendon on the dorsum of the digit if a reasonable result is to be obtained.[145] Verdan[55] observed that extensor injury over the proximal phalanx produced the worst results; Lovett and McCalla[146] found the highest percentages of extensor lag in zones III and IV.

The following factors may negatively influence the final outcome of the acutely repaired and immobilized central slip injury: (1) the broad tendon–bone interface in zone IV, (2) resting of the tendon at less than absolute 0 degrees of extension during immobilization, and (3) the effects of stress deprivation on the connective tissue (tendon, cartilage, ligament) of the PIP joint.[43,85]

Broad Tendon–Bone Interface in Zone IV

Brand and associates[42] have noted that no other area in the human body has a ratio of tendon to bone as unfavorable as over P^1. This adverse ratio has been credited as the primary cause of surgical failures after attempts to free the dorsal expansion.[42] The broad tendon–bone interface, along with the intimacy of the periosteum and the extensor tendon and the complex gliding requirements of the extensor system in

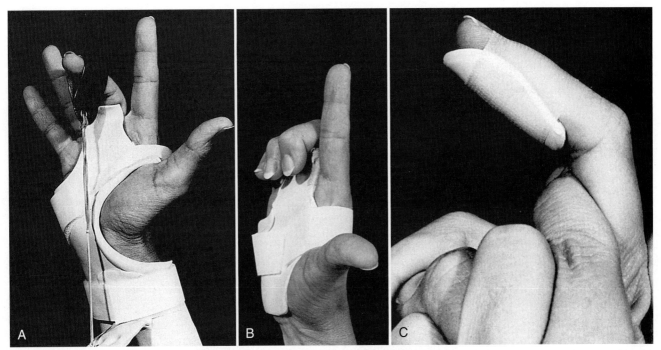

Figure 39-14 Flexion forces are applied to the proximal interphalangeal joint with a dynamic orthosis that blocks the metacarpophalangeal (MCP) joint in extension and applies a light traction of less than 250 g to the midphalanx level **(A)**; a hand-based static exercise orthosis that blocks the MCP joint in extension and encourages acute proximal interphalangeal (PIP) joint flexion in the hook fist position **(B)**; or a distal joint-blocking orthosis that negates profundus force, manual blocking of the MCP joint, and active flexion of the PIP joint **(C).**

zones III and IV, results in functional problems associated with adhesions.[147]

Zone III injuries tend to be complex, which compounds the problems of scar formation. In a clinical series of open and repaired central slip injuries of 64 digits that I treated from 1985 to 1992, 79.6% were associated with injury to adjacent soft tissue, the PIP joint, or the distal joint.[85] My experience from 1992 to 2009 remains the same. Other clinicians have reported similar findings.[126,145,147] We all have observed clinically, and investigators have demonstrated experimentally,[57] that the complex injury treated with immobilization can be expected to produce problems associated with increased fibroblastic response.

Considering these factors, we may hypothesize that a major problem in mobilization of the zone III extensor tendon injury is tendon-to-bone adherence in zone IV. The immobilized repair in zone III devoid of the benefits of greater intrinsic healing and strengthening associated with early motion may attenuate or gap when motion is initiated at 4 to 6 weeks because its proximal segment in zone IV is nongliding (Fig. 39-15). This increased resistance or drag from adhesion in zone IV elevates the extensor tension in zone III, which may exceed the tensile strength of the repair. This can be observed clinically in the immobilized central slip that begins to lose motion in extension as flexion is gained with late mobilization programs.

Resting the Tendon at Functional Length During Immobilization

The anatomy of the PIP joint favors flexion.[148] The normal resting position of the PIP joint is between 30 and 40 degrees of flexion.[42] In this position, the central slip, with a larger moment arm, and the lateral bands, with a smaller moment

arm, are at equal tension.[42] An edematous PIP joint postures in 30 to 40 degrees because in this position the joint more comfortably accommodates the increased volume from edema. A schematic drawing on the effects of edema on the dorsal PIP joint and overlying skin can help us visualize the effect of effusion or edema under the central slip[86]

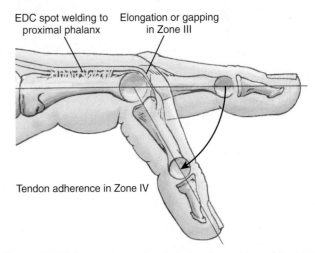

Figure 39-15 Schematic drawing illustrating the problem of tendon-to-bone adhesions after injury to the dorsal digital extensor mechanism. The broad tendon–bone interface in zone IV and the intimacy of periosteum and extensor tendon yield functional gliding problems in the zone III injury. The zone III portion of the tendon (the repaired central slip) may gap or attenuate in late mobilization programs because its more proximal segment is adherent and nongliding. The increased resistance in zone IV increases force application in zone III and may exceed the tensile strength of the repair. EDC, extensor digitorum communis tendon. (From Evans RB, Thompson DE. An analysis of factors that support early active short arc motion of the repaired central slip. *J Hand Ther.* 1992;5:190.)

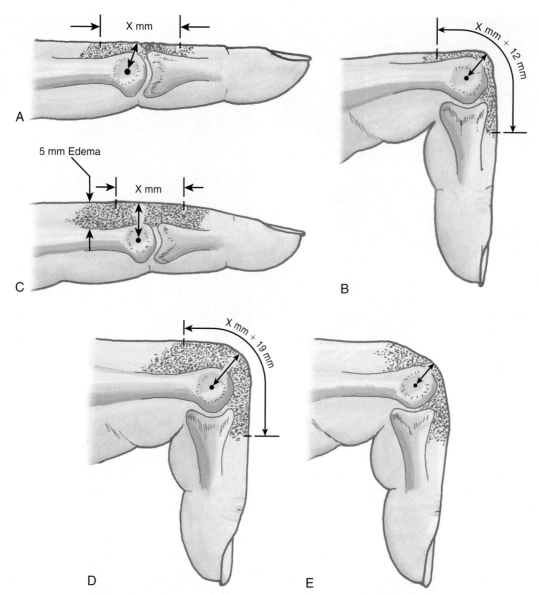

Figure 39-16 Schematic drawing by Brand illustrating the effects of a 5-mm increase in the diameter of a finger from edema and its effect on the dorsal skin. **A** and **B,** Dorsal skin requires 12 mm of lengthening for 90 degrees of flexion. **C** and **D,** With 5-mm thickness of edema, skin requires 19 mm of lengthening for 90 degrees of flexion. **E,** With continuing torque, slowly applied, the edema fluid moves around, permitting the skin to cross closer to the joint axis requiring less stretch. This illustration helps the reader visualize the effects of protein and cellular edema that may collect under the central slip, which would increase the moment arm of the tendon and possibly contribute to attenuation of the repair or a resting posture of slight flexion. (From Brand PW: *Clinical Mechanics of the Hand.* St Louis: Mosby; 1985.)

(Fig. 39-16). The increase in volume could increase the moment arm of the central slip and thus tension on the repair.[42,86]

A common problem with these injuries is inaccurate orthosis position that allows some flexion of the PIP joint during the healing phase, resulting in extensor lag. Alumafoam orthoses with adhesive tape proximal and distal to the PIP joint encourage swelling and allow the joint to rest in flexion; finger casts that are not checked frequently allow the PIP to rest in flexion as edema decreases. In my experience, unmonitored orthotic use is more often than not ineffective.

The orthosis position necessary to prevent gap formation and attenuation of the repair is absolute 0 degrees of extension. This position brings the repair site proximal to its normal resting position and reduces repair-site tension (see Fig. 39-11).

Connective Tissue Stress Deprivation

Total immobilization for 4 to 6 weeks can impose injury on uninjured cartilage and ligament. Although biochemical and biomechanical changes in immobilized connective tissue have been studied primarily in the animal model in various joints,[18,48,149] results of these studies have influenced our thinking on the subject of stress application to healing connective tissue in the human. The information gained from these experimental studies must be interpreted with caution as we attempt to alter clinical treatment based on basic science studies in the nonhuman model.

The biochemical and biomechanical effects of stress deprivation versus controlled motion for tendon are briefly reviewed in the first segment of this chapter. Similar changes take place in immobilized ligament and cartilage.[149] Stress deprivation for ligament results in alterations in collagen cross-linking synthesis and degradation, as well as in loss of water and proteoglycan content.[60,150-152] Nonligamentous injuries treated with immobilization can produce ligament-length problems, and there is evidence that ligament structures can shorten, limiting joint motion.[60,153] Investigators have demonstrated that ligaments under no tension are associated with the contractile protein actin and actually shorten over time.[148,154] It has been postulated that immobilization may decrease the normal stress-generated electrical potentials in the dense connective tissue of ligament, which signal the fibroblast as a signal to degrade the older collagen molecules and synthesize newer, shorter collagen molecules, thereby shortening the ligament structure.[60]

The relationship between motion and cartilage metabolism cannot be ignored. Joint motion is important to maintaining articular cartilage homeostasis. The substances required by the chondrocytes for normal metabolism are derived from synovial fluid.[155,156] The transport of these nutrients through cartilage occurs by diffusion, convection, or both, and the combination of motion and joint loading is essential to nutrient transport by convection.[155-158] Joint immobilization then decreases nutrient transport to cartilage. Prolonged immobilization results in decreased mechanical properties, disorganized ultrastructure, and biochemical alterations similar to those noted in ligament.[150,151] Experimentally, CPM has been found to produce a tissue that histochemically and morphologically resembles hyaline cartilage in healing rabbit cartilage.[159,160] Therefore immobilization at the PIP joint level, where cartilage is the thinnest of any joint in the body, should be avoided if possible.

Anatomic Considerations for the Short Arc Motion Program

The exercise position for the short arc motion (SAM) program is 30 degrees of wrist flexion, 0 degrees of MCP joint extension, and PIP joint motion from 0 degrees of extension to 30 degrees of flexion and active return to 0 degrees of extension. Only the digital joints (PIP and DIP) of the affected digits are immobilized between the active component of the exercise, allowing complete motion of the wrist and MCP joints. The distal joint is flexed from 25 to 30 degrees while the PIP joint is held at 0 degrees if the lateral bands are repaired and to full flexion while the PIP is at 0 degrees if the lateral bands are not repaired.

The elastic components of the surrounding soft tissue, as well as the active muscle forces, must be considered when calculating active force and resistance to a repaired tendon in the healing phase. Tubiana[161] makes the point that the coordination of motions in the hand depends on active and passive factors of the more proximal joints. The passive factors include the restraining action of the ligaments and muscular viscoelasticity, and the active factors include the dynamic balance between antagonistic muscles.[161] Therefore we must consider the effect of joint positional changes and contributions from the surrounding soft tissues when reducing or increasing the work requirement of the EDC.

Anatomic influences for the zone III extensor tendon have been analyzed in detail in the support paper for SAM[43] and are only briefly reviewed here.

The action of the middle or central extensor tendon, which inserts on the base of the P^2, functions in some regard to extend all three phalanges. It extends P^2 on which it inserts except when the MCP joint is in hyperextension, it contributes to extension of P^1 when the PIP joint is flexed, and it contributes to distal joint extension through the coordinating action of the ORLs.[161,162]

Wrist position influences tension in the extrinsic tendons because of the viscoelasticity of the antagonist muscle–tendon unit.[86,113,161,163,164] Passive tension is minimal when the muscle is short and increases as the muscle lengthens.[113] The movements of wrist flexion and finger extension are synergistic; finger extension is effectively increased as the wrist flexes.[90,162] The position of wrist flexion reduces the passive tension of the digital extrinsic flexors.[123] Although this position may increase passive tension in the extensor system as the muscle–tendon unit lengthens, the actual force required of the extensor communis to extend the digital joints is reduced by the reduction of viscoelastic flexor forces.[113] The action of the interossei muscles with the wrist flexed may further reduce work requirement of the digital extensor mechanism in active extension of the IP joints. Close and Kidd[165] have concluded that the interossei do contract with IP joint extension even when no resistance is applied if (1) all fingers are extended simultaneously or (2) the finger is extended with the wrist flexed.

Active wrist extension is synergistic with finger flexion. With the digital orthosis taped in place between exercise sessions, unrestricted motion can take place in the wrist and MCP joint. As the wrist extends, the MCP joint flexes because of the viscoelastic pull of the flexors. The sagittal bands glide distally with MCP flexion, actually reducing tension on the central slip.[90] Tubiana[161] states that the movement of the phalanges can be independent of wrist position through the action of the interossei.

Based on these anatomic considerations, the recommended position for the wrist with the SAM protocol is 30 degrees of flexion during PIP exercise. This position reduces flexor resistance, facilitates interossei function to extend the PIP, and thus reduces the work requirement of the EDC with active extension of the PIP joint.

MCP joint positional changes from complete extension to complete flexion glide the sagittal bands and interosseous hood proximal and distal by 16 mm[162] to 20 mm.[90] As the sagittal bands glide distally with MCP joint flexion, the EDC is able to transmit virtually no force distal to the MCP joint because of its insertion on the dorsal hood/sagittal band complex.[166] Tension on the central tendon is decreased with MCP flexion because of sagittal band distal migration.[90] This same observation has been noted by others in a study of central slip tension measured intraoperatively.[167] With the MCP joint flexed, PIP extension is affected primarily through the interossei,[168,169] possibly with some contribution from the lumbrical,[89] but with little contribution from the EDC.[166] A recent study on the effect of finger posture on the tendon force distribution within the finger extensor mechanism supports these previously noted biomechanical studies.[170]

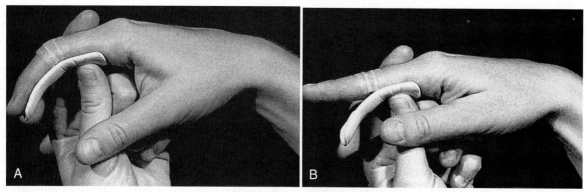

Figure 39-17 A and **B**, Template orthosis 1 allows 30 degrees at the proximal interphalangeal (PIP) joint and 20 to 25 degrees at the distal interphalangeal joint, preventing the patient from stretching the repair site by allowing only the precalculated excursion of the central slip. The wrist is positioned in 30 degrees of flexion, the digit is supported at the proximal phalanx by the contralateral hand, and the PIP joint is actively flexed and extended in a controlled range of motion. (From Evans RB. Early active short arc motion for the repaired central slip. *J Hand Surg.* 1994;19A:992–997.)

The sagittal bands glide proximally with MCP joint extension.[90] The attachment of the dorsal hood with the MCP joint extended is slack and allows distal transmission of power to the central slip region.[166] Long[168,169] has determined by EMG that the lumbrical is electrically active with the MCP joint extended, thus contributing to IP joint extension. Indirectly, the lumbrical contributes to IP joint extension by reducing the viscoelastic resistance of the FDP. Lumbrical contraction pulls the profundus distal, reducing the work requirement of the antagonistic extensor. Thus the lumbricals neutralize the viscoelastic tension of the profundi during digital extension.[166,168,169]

Although Long[168,169] used EMG to determine that the interossei are silent with the MCP extended, Valentine[89] determined by anatomic dissection that if the MCP joint is extended, contraction force of the interossei is transmitted directly to the lateral bands, which in turn extend the IP joints. As mentioned, Close and Kidd[165] have demonstrated that the interossei contract if all the MCP joints are extended simultaneously or if the wrist is in flexion.

Thus the position of MCP extension facilitates transmission of EDC force distal to the central slip region with proximal migration of the sagittal bands[90,166] while minimizing the work requirement of the EDC through the contribution of the lumbricals and interossei.[89,168,169]

Distal joint motion is an important aspect of this protocol for maintaining excursion of the lateral bands and of the ORLs. The DIP joint is unrestrained during the active PIP exercise of 30 degrees. With simultaneous flexion of the PIP and DIP joints, gliding of the terminal tendon is not transferred to the EDC but is taken up by the volar slide of the lateral bands.[162] The terminal tendon slackens through the action of the lateral band migration when the PIP joint is flexed, facilitating DIP flexion. Zancolli[90] observed in two cadaveric dissections that when the FDP acts, both IP joints flex (linked flexion); the middle phalanx flexes before the distal phalanx; and during the course of flexion, the angle of flexion of the middle joint is greater than that of the distal joint.

Distal joint extension is facilitated by combined action of the EDC, action of the lateral bands, and tenodesis of the ORL.[162,171] Active PIP joint extension, which is initiated by the long extensor, creates tension in the ORL, which assists DIP joint extension. DIP joint extension then is completed as the lateral bands rise dorsally and finally reach the same tension as the central tendon.[171]

Therefore the moderate flexion of 30 degrees in the PIP joint with the DIP joint unrestrained in the SAM protocol may create no more than an estimated 1 to 2 mm of excursion of both lateral bands and the terminal tendon, based on lateral band excursion cited by Zancolli[90] and by Littler and Thompson.[171]

If the lateral bands are repaired, DIP joint flexion to 30 degrees with the PIP joint held at 0 degrees of extension facilitates a minimal excursion for these structures. If the lateral bands are not repaired, the DIP joint may be flexed fully with the PIP joint held at 0 degrees of extension. Flexion of the DIP joint with the PIP restrained imparts 3 to 4 mm of distal migration to the EDC in zone IV through the action of the lateral bands in their attachment to the EDC proximal to zone III. This exercise position then actually reduces tension at a zone III repair site while creating distal migration of the zone IV tendon.

Clinical Application of Immediate Active Short Arc Motion for the Repaired Central Slip

Based on the assessment of problems associated with the immobilized zone III and IV repaired extensor tendon, I developed an early motion protocol in 1988 that uses immediate active SAM for the repaired central slip. The protocol is as follows.

Except during exercise, the involved digit is immobilized in a volar static thermoplastic orthosis that immobilizes only the PIP and DIP joints (see Fig. 39-11). The orthosis is taped directly over the PIP and DIP joints with 1-inch Transpore (3M) plastic tape to ensure that both of these joints rest at absolute 0 degrees extension.

Two exercise template orthoses are used by the patient during exercise sessions to control stress application and excursion for the repaired central slip. Template orthosis 1 (Fig. 39-17) for PIP joint motion is a volar static orthosis fabricated with a 30-degree flexion angle for the PIP joint and a 20- to 25-degree angle for the DIP joint. The template orthosis 2 (Fig. 39-18) for DIP joint flexion is a volar static

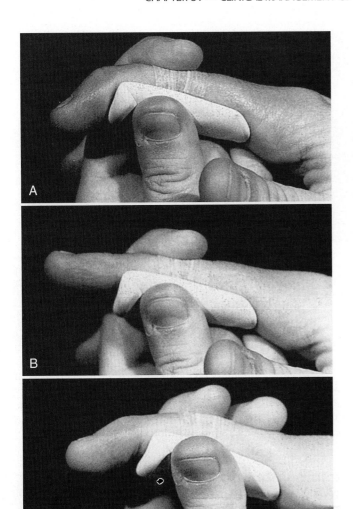

Figure 39-18 A to **C,** Template orthosis 2 immobilizes only the proximal interphalangeal joint, allowing isolated distal joint motion to create gliding of the lateral bands. If the lateral bands are not repaired, the distal joint is fully flexed and extended **(A, B).** If the lateral bands are repaired, the distal interphalangeal joint is flexed only to 30 to 35 degrees **(C).** (From Evans RB. Early active short arc motion for the repaired central slip. *J Hand Surg.* 1994;19A:993.)

orthosis for P^1 and P^2 with the PIP joint at 0 degrees and the DIP joint free.

The patient is instructed to remove the immobilization orthosis every waking hour for an empirical 20 repetitions of PIP and DIP joint exercise. The wrist is positioned at 30 degrees of flexion, and the MCP joint is positioned at 0 degrees of extension to very slight flexion. The patient is instructed to manually support the MCP joint in template orthosis 1, which allows the PIP joint to flex to 30 degrees and the unrestrained DIP joint to flex to 20 to 25 degrees. The patient actively flexes and extends the PIP joint through this 30-degree range with 20 repetitions (see Fig. 39-17). The patient is instructed that each repetition should be performed slowly and sustained briefly in a fully extended position. Template orthosis 2 is then applied with manual pressure to stabilize the PIP joint at 0 degrees (see Fig. 39-18A). If the lateral bands are not repaired, the distal joint is flexed fully and extended (see Fig. 39-18A, B); if the lateral bands are

repaired, the distal joint is flexed only to 30 to 35 degrees (visually monitored by the patient) with active extension emphasized (see Fig. 39-18C).

The patient is instructed in a technique of controlled active motion that applies very low internal tendon tension with the active extension exercise. For the program to be effective, the patient must understand that the exercise must be performed in the prescribed position (wrist, 30 degrees flexion; MCP joint, 0 degrees to slight flexion; with PIP and DIP joints moving within the guidelines of the template orthoses), that the repetitions are to be performed slowly and frequently, and that the position of the immobilization orthosis must be absolutely precise with the PIP and DIP joints resting at 0 degrees.

The application of force in this position with only the weight of the finger as resistance and no allowance for drag from tight joint structures or edema is approximately 300 g.[43,84] When the PIP joint is moved actively through the 30-degree range (approximately 0.5 radian, 28.65 degrees), extensor tendon excursion in zones III and IV is approximately 3.75 mm[43] (see Fig. 39-5).

At 2 weeks after surgery, the template orthosis 1 is altered to allow 40 degrees at the PIP joint if no extensor lag has developed. The PIP joint angle can be changed to 50 degrees by the third postoperative week and up to 70 to 80 degrees by the end of the fourth week if the PIP joint is actively extending to 0 degrees. If an extensor lag develops, flexion increments should be more modest and active extension exercise and extension positioning should be emphasized. In my clinical experience, by 4 weeks after surgery, the average PIP joint moves actively approximately 60 to 70 degrees, and by the sixth week, from 3 degrees of extension to 88 degrees of flexion. The stiff PIP joint at 4 weeks can be positioned intermittently into flexion, but static extension positioning for the digit should continue until week 5 or 6. By the fifth week, composite flexion exercises and gentle strengthening are appropriate; PIP joints treated with the SAM protocol often are ready for discharge by week 6, and the patient is allowed to strengthen with a home program.

The wrist joint, MCP joint, and uninvolved digits are free to move through a ROM with a natural tenodesis effect taking place (wrist extension and finger flexion, and wrist flexion and finger extension), with only the affected PIP and DIP joints of the injured digits immobilized (Fig. 39-19). General practices for wound care and edema control with Coban wraps, ice, and elevation should be followed. Controlled mobilization with active exercise and gentle distraction techniques to avoid cartilage–cartilage abutment, and dynamic flexion traction with less than 250 g of tension, help elongate periarticular structures, promote tendon glide, and ultimately reestablish PIP joint motion at the fourth and fifth postoperative weeks. Flexion must not be regained at the expense of losing extension; therefore increases in stress application and flexion angles should not be attempted unless extension is complete.

Comparison Study of Immobilization and Short Arc Motion

The results of open and repaired central slip injuries (64 digits, 55 patients) that I treated from 1985 to 1992 with two

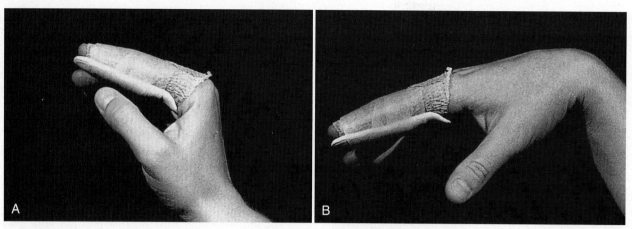

Figure 39-19 A, B, The wrist and metacarpophalangeal joints, as well as the uninvolved joints, are free to move through all available ranges of motion. The natural tenodesis action of wrist extension and finger flexion, as well as wrist flexion and finger extension, creates proximal and distal migration of the sagittal bands but places minimal stress on the repair site, which is protected by the position of proximal interphalangeal joint extension. (From Evans RB. Early active short arc motion for the repaired central slip. *J Hand Surg.* 1994;19A:993.)

entirely different protocols were analyzed.[85] Group I was treated with 3 to 6 weeks of immobilization (defined in the section on traditional management of zone III and IV injuries), and group II was treated with SAM (as described in the immediately preceding paragraphs), initiated between days 2 and 11. The two groups were further subdivided into simple injury (only tendon) or complex injury (associated injury to bone, cartilage, or DIP joint). The results of this preliminary study are summarized in Table 39-2 and continue to be supported by my clinical experience with these injuries treated since that time (2009). The conclusion from the clinical study[85] is that open and repaired central slip injuries treated with SAM yield statistically superior results compared with those treated by 3 to 6 weeks of immobilization in regard to extensor lag, TAM (Strickland-Glogovac formula,[172] which calculates only the PIP and DIP joint motion), and treatment time ($p < .01$; *t*-test). The greater extensor lag in the immobilization group may be due to improper positioning during the immobilization phase and attenuation of the repair during

mobilization because of extensor tendon adherence in zone IV.

Kalb and Pommersberger have reported similar results in a study of my SAM protocol with a slightly less satisfactory PIP extension deficit (8.5 degrees) and state that they have adopted this protocol at their hospital.[7] Others continue to support 6 weeks of immobilization.[8]

Immediate Short Arc Motion for the Closed, Nonoperated Boutonnière Deformity

Although traditional treatment recommends 4 to 6 weeks of uninterrupted orthotic use for the closed and nonrepaired central slip lesion, I have success over the past 20 years in treating these closed injuries with serial finger casting and immediate SAM with the same parameters described in the preceding section on early SAM for the repaired central slip.

Table 39-2 Final Results and Statistical Analysis for SAM and Treatment by Immobilization for the Repaired Central Slip

Results	Group I (Immobilization)	Group II (SAM)	Statistical Significance of *t*-Test	Statistical Significance of Chi-Square Test
Number of digits	38	26		
Mean age	39.9	42.2	>0.5, NS	
% Male sex	86.8%	80.8%		>0.5 NS
% Complex injury	76.3%	76.9%		>0.5 NS
Mean day motion initiated	32.9	4.59	<0.001, significant	
Mean day injury to discharge	76.07	51.38	<0.001, significant	
PIP extension lag on first motion day	13 degrees	3 degrees	<0.01, significant	
PIP extension lag on discharge day	8.13 degrees	2.96 degrees	<0.01, significant	
PIP motion at 6 weeks	44 degrees	88 degrees	<0.001, significant	
PIP motion at discharge	72 degrees	88 degrees	<0.01, significant	
Total active motion (PIP and DIP) at discharge	110.7 degrees	131.5 degrees	<0.01, significant	
DIP motion at discharge	37.63 degrees	45 degrees	<0.01, significant	

From Evans RB. Early active short arc motion for the repaired central slip. *J Hand Surg* 1994;19A:994.
DIP, distal interphalangeal; NS, not significant; PIP, proximal interphalangeal; SAM, short arc motion.

Results of 36 cases treated over a 20-year period support the concept that these injuries can be treated with a combination of casting, positioning with custom orthoses, and early SAM with resulting satisfactory functional ROM, minimal PIP extensor lag, and with rehabilitation times that are improved over the traditional 6-week immobilization schedule. The rationale and progressive limits for motion are precisely the same as for the treatment previously described for open and repaired tendons at this level. Thirty-six cases (1988 to 2008) in this series that were initially treated within 3 to 4 weeks of injury (while joint motion was passively correctable) recovered PIP flexion to an average of 92 degrees of flexion; the average extensor deficit at the PIP was 6 degrees; the average DIP flexion at the end arc of composite flexion was 47 degrees. Patients were treated an average of two times per week for an average total time of 8 weeks. The protocol is initiated with a circumferential finger cast including only the PIP joint immobilized in full extension, with the DIP joint left free. Patients are instructed to manually support the PIP within the cast with the contralateral hand and to slowly flex the distal joint 10 to 15 times every 2 hours to maintain excursion of the ORLs, and to advance the lateral bands. The cast is changed two times per week for 2 to 3 weeks depending on the active extension of the PIP joint noted during therapy sessions and expected patient compliance. The circumferential pressures of digital casting reduce edema requiring cast changes at least twice a week in the initial phase. Under direct supervision in therapy the PIP joint is allowed 30 to 40 degrees of controlled flexion and active extension; the DIP is allowed full flexion while the PIP joint is held in full extension by the therapist; no composite flexion is allowed. Although no clinical studies have been published that support modality intervention in these cases, heat, ultrasound (US) to the dorsal PIP joint, and retrograde massage are utilized to theoretically facilitate connective tissue healing and have been found to decrease edema. At the end of the second or third week, if edema is under control and the PIP joint extends to at least 10 to 15 degrees actively, casting is discontinued and the digit is wrapped with 2-inch Coban, positioned in full extension with a PIP digit orthosis, and given a template orthosis to work on SAM for the zone III to IV tendon independently as described previously. Motion is progressed on the same schedule as for the open and repaired central slip. The PIP joint is positioned in full extension for a total of 6 weeks with the exception of the exercise sessions six times per day.

Zones V and VI

Extensor tendons in zones V and VI can be managed postoperatively by immobilization,[130,173] controlled passive motion,[83,95,174,175] or the controlled active tension technique.[84] Considering the previously described benefits of controlled motion for the healing tendon, I could not recommend total immobilization for tendon at any level except zone I and II and T-I, T-II extensor. However, total immobilization may be necessary with the very young or noncompliant patient and may be acceptable treatment for the simple injury for a period of 3 weeks. The abundant and mobile soft tissue that characterizes the dorsum of the hand facilitates the reestablishment of tendon glide in this area and creates a forgiving

environment for simple tendon injury treated with total immobilization. Total immobilization should not be considered with extensor tendon injury associated with crush injury where the paratenon is extensively involved, with injury to the periosteum or adjacent soft tissues, or in hands with osteoarthritic or rheumatoid joints.[83]

Atraumatic surgical technique, preservation of the paratenon,[176] and proper postoperative immobilization minimize problems in the rehabilitation phase. Edema control is important for decreasing such complications as adhesion formation and shortening of periarticular structures that may result from the accumulation of protein and fluid in the extravascular space.[177] The extensor tendons have 11 to 16 mm of excursion in zones V and VI,[87] requiring protection of both wrist and digital joints within the immobilizing or controlled-motion orthoses to prevent excessive tension at the repair.

Treatment by Immobilization

During the first 3 postoperative weeks after extensor tendon repairs treated by immobilization, the therapist's concerns are for wound care, edema control, and proper postoperative immobilization to protect the repaired structures from rupture or elongation. The position of immobilization should be 35 to 40 degrees of wrist extension, 0 to 20 degrees of MCP joint flexion, and 0 degrees of IP joint flexion. Many authors[130,173,178,179] recommend positioning the MCP joints in mild flexion to retain the integrity of the collateral ligaments. However, in my clinical experience, positioning the MCP joints in mild flexion with the immobilization technique results in MCP extensor lag. The early motion programs that position the MCP joints at 0 degrees between exercise sessions yet allow some MCP joint motion solve the problem of collateral ligament tightness versus extensor lag.[83]

Simple laceration to the extensor indicis proprius (EIP) and extensor digiti minimi (EDM) requires immobilization of only the repaired tendons.[162,180] However, with the EDC, one must consider the juncturae tendinum, which, while functioning to dynamically stabilize the MCP joints, also limits independent function of these tendons[181,182] (see also Chapter 38). If the repair site is proximal to the interconnecting tendon, all fingers should be positioned in extension. If it is distal to the interconnection, the adjacent fingers can be immobilized in 30 degrees of flexion (Fig. 39-20A). The latter position permits advancement of the proximal end of the severed tendon by a force of the intertendinous connection, thus actually reducing tension on the anastomosis[182] (Fig. 39-20B).

The therapist should assess the digital joints in the immobilized hand for stiffness during dressing changes and orthosis rechecks during the first 3 postoperative weeks. The therapist should manually place the wrist in full extension while supporting all digital joints at 0 degrees. The therapist then can carefully assess the feel of each MCP joint by gently moving the index and long fingers from slight hyperextension to 30 to 45 degrees of flexion, and the ring and small fingers from hyperextension to 40 to 50 degrees of flexion (Fig. 39-21). This protected motion creates approximately 3 to 6 mm of tendon excursion and does not jeopardize the repair.[83] These excursions are calculated mathematically by radians and are explained in Box 39-1. If the MCP joints seem

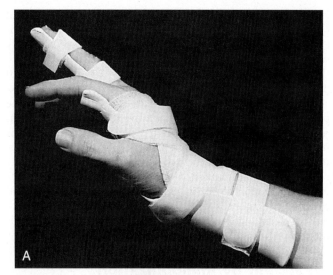

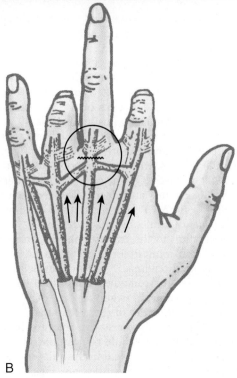

Figure 39-20 A, Repair to the extensor digitorum communis (EDC) distal to the juncturae in the long finger can be adequately protected with an orthosis that rests the long metacarpophalangeal (MCP) joint at 0 degrees and adjacent MCP joints at 30 degrees of flexion. This position relieves tension at the repair site while maintaining some extensibility of the collateral ligaments of the uninvolved fingers. **B,** Tension can be reduced on the anastomosis of the EDC when the repair site is distal to the juncturae tendinum if the adjacent fingers are held in mild flexion. This position advances the proximal end of the severed tendon by a force of the intertendinous connection. (From Beasley RW: *Hand Injuries,* Philadelphia: WB Saunders; 1981.)

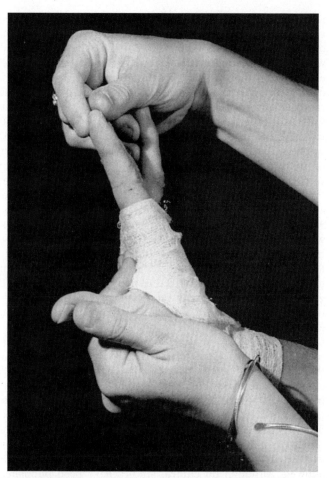

Figure 39-21 The hand treated with immobilization techniques should be assessed during the first and second postoperative weeks to determine whether excessive stiffness is developing at the metacarpophalangeal (MCP) or proximal interphalangeal joint levels. The wrist and digits are held passively in maximum extension as the therapist passively moves the MCP joints from hyperextension to 30 degrees of flexion for the index and long fingers, and 40 degrees for the ring and small fingers. Unyielding periarticular structures may require a change in orthosis position or in treatment approach to early passive motion.

excessively stiff and do not easily tolerate this much motion, the surgeon and therapist should consider passive motion during supervised therapy sessions or dynamic positioning instead of static positioning to allow some controlled passive motion by the patient.[81,83]

The PIP joints can be assessed with the wrist and MCP joints held in extension. Little excursion is created in zones V and VI with IP joint motion.[86,87] An extensor tendon amplitude study on eight cadaver hands demonstrated that if the wrist is held in more than 21 degrees of extension, the extensor tendon glides with little or no tension in zones V and VI throughout full simulated grip to full passive extension.[78] The authors of that study suggest that full passive flexion is safe with these injuries if the wrist is extended. However, I do not think that this much excursion is necessary, and I outline another approach to maintaining tendon excursion in the section on early passive motion. Each IP joint can be passively and individually moved through a complete ROM while the wrist and MCP joints are held in extension.[83] A solution to the problem of stiff IP joints associated with arthritis or swelling from the more proximal injury, when treatment by immobilization is chosen, is to cut away the immobilizing orthosis under each PIP joint to allow active and passive motion at this level (Fig. 39-22A). These joints should rest in extension between exercise sessions to prevent

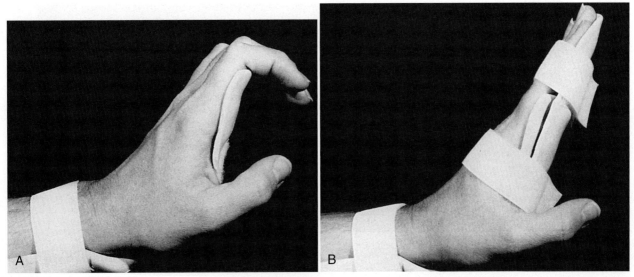

Figure 39-22 A, A static extension orthosis that immobilizes the wrist and metacarpophalangeal joints in extension allows motion of the proximal and distal interphalangeal joints without jeopardizing repairs in zones V through VII. **B,** A removable extension component is applied between exercise sessions to prevent volar plate tightness and extension lag—problems that are associated with swollen proximal interphalangeal joints that rest in flexion.

problems of extensor lag and PIP flexion contracture, a sequela of resting the swollen PIP joint in flexion. A removable volar component can be applied to the orthosis to rest the IP joints in extension between exercises (Fig. 39-22B).

Guarded active motion should be initiated by the third postoperative week. The immobilized tendon at 3 weeks should be considered to have little tensile strength from endotenon healing,[52-54,99,122] but some strength from peritendinous adhesions associated with immobilization.[45,183] The patient should be instructed to protect the repair by proper joint positioning during exercise and orthosis protection between exercise sessions.

As with any hand injury, one begins treatment by cleansing and softening the skin and instructing the patient in self-care. The hand may be washed or debrided in a small portable whirlpool in which the wrist and fingers can be supported in extension. The patient is instructed in retrograde massage techniques to reduce edema and to soften the scar. SGS or Otoform can be used to soften the scar (see Chapter 18). Micropore paper tape worn continuously on dry skin in a longitudinal fashion from approximately 2 weeks until 2 months after surgery reduces hypertrophic scarring by minimizing wound tension. This technique has been found to be as effective as the use of SGS and is much less expensive.[184,185]

Gentle active and active assistive exercise during the third to fourth week should emphasize extension at the MCP joint with the wrist in a neutral to slightly flexed position to decrease elastic resistance from the antagonistic flexor system,[84] and MCP joint flexion from 40 to 60 degrees should be performed with the wrist held in an extended position to maintain MCP collateral ligament extensibility without overstressing the anastomosis. This synergistic play of simultaneous wrist flexion and MCP joint extension, and wrist extension with MCP joint flexion, allows for active tendon excursion and ligament excursion without placing excessive force on the repair site. The IP joints may be exercised through a complete range with the wrist and MCP joints

extended. The repairs can be protected between exercise sessions with a dynamic extension orthosis that supports the wrist at approximately 20 degrees of extension and the fingers dynamically at 0 degrees (Fig. 39-23).

Duration of exercise is for the most part an empirical decision. As discussed in the first section of this chapter, one clinical study on management of flexor tendon injuries demonstrates improved motion with increased duration of motion,[70] but there is no such study on the extensor tendon.

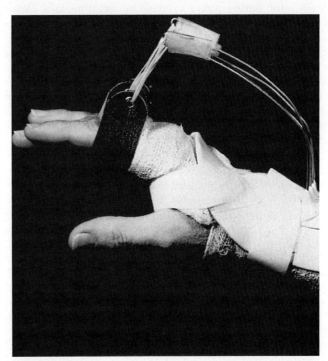

Figure 39-23 A dorsal dynamic extension orthosis that rests the metacarpophalangeal joints at 0 degrees and allows controlled flexion prevents excessive stress at the repair site while encouraging joint motion and increased tendon excursion.

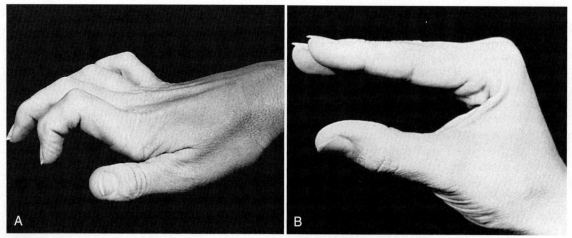

Figure 39-24 A, The intrinsic-minus or "claw position" isolates the extrinsic extensors during exercise. **B,** The intrinsic-plus position directs force to the metacarpophalangeal collateral ligaments without placing excessive stress on repairs in zones V, VI, or VII if the wrist is extended during exercise.

I usually instruct the patient to perform each exercise with 10 to 20 repetitions every waking hour. Patients are warned not to overexercise because this may cause inflammation of the tissues.

By the fourth week, composite flexion can be attempted with the wrist extended. Individual finger extension exercise and the "claw," or intrinsic-minus, position directs controlled stress to the extrinsic extensors[162,180] (Fig. 39-24A). Dynamic flexion orthosis for application of stress to the stiff MCP or PIP joints should be initiated as early as the third week if joint motion is less than 30 to 40 degrees with a "hard end-feel," and by the fourth week with motion limited in the range of 50 to 60 degrees. Force can be directed to the stiff MCP joint during active exercise by negating long flexor forces (Fig. 39-24B) or with volar digital extension orthoses taped directly over the PIP joint during intrinsic-plus exercise. Stiff IP joints should be positioned with a separate orthosis that blocks the MCP joints in extension between the third and fourth weeks to direct forces to the periarticular structures, but by the fourth to fifth week combinations of both MCP and PIP joint traction (MCP flexion cuffs and nail traction) can be used to direct forces along the length of the extensor tendons.

Composite finger flexion can be facilitated with the use of graded dowels between 4 and 5 weeks. By the sixth week, postoperative composite finger and wrist flexion exercises are tolerated by the repaired tendon, and mild strengthening can be added to the exercise regimen. A 1-pound weight for wrist flexion–extension exercise and for pronation–supination can be used for several weeks to increase the tensile strength of the tendons and also to strengthen the extensor carpi radialis brevis (ECRB) and flexor carpi ulnaris (FCU). These muscles, weakened by immobilization and disuse, make the patient who returns to sports activities or manual labor without strengthening prone to develop lateral or medial epicondylitis. Forearm strengthening should be performed with fewer repetitions (10 repetitions, three times per day, with gradual increments over a 2- to 3-week period, to 20 repetitions four times per day). The Baltimore Therapeutic Equipment (BTE) work simulator or other computerized exercise equipment can be used for mild strengthening but should be supple-

mented with a home program. In today's medical-economic climate, it is often not possible to follow a patient with a repaired tendon for 6 weeks, and treatment by immobilization that usually produces more complications of tendon adherence and joint stiffness should be considered only when the health care provider believes no other option is available. The patient should be advised that strong resistive exercise should be delayed until the 10th to 12th week, when the tendon has regained near-normal tensile strength.

The modalities of heat, cold, high-voltage galvanic stimulation, or whirlpool can be used as hand volume and joint stiffness dictate. Functional electrical stimulation (FES) on a light setting can be used by the fourth week as a type of biofeedback and applied with more force directed to the extensor muscle by the fifth week, and even to the flexor system by the fourth to fifth week when composite flexion becomes a goal. At present, the use of US with the healing tendon is still questionable,[186] although basic science studies indicate that US may have a limited role at low intensity during the earliest stages of wound healing.[187,188] The use of US during the early stages of wound healing has been shown to increase ROM, decrease scar formation, and to have no adverse effect of decreased strength in an experimental study of surgically repaired flexor tendons in zone II in the white leghorn chicken animal model.[188] However, the effect of US on the healing human tendon has not yet been established, although clinical studies are currently under way. Systematic reviews of the use of physical agents in the treatment of a repaired tendon could not be found as of this writing.‡

Treatment with Early Passive Motion

I established a controlled early passive motion program for the healing extensor tendon in zones V through VII in 1979 to reduce the postoperative problems associated with the complex injury. Precise guidelines for correlating tendon excursion with joint motion were defined in a study of the biomechanics and excursions of the extensor system[83] and are outlined in the first segment of this chapter. The rationale

---

‡Consult www.ncbi.nlm.nih.gov/pubmed.

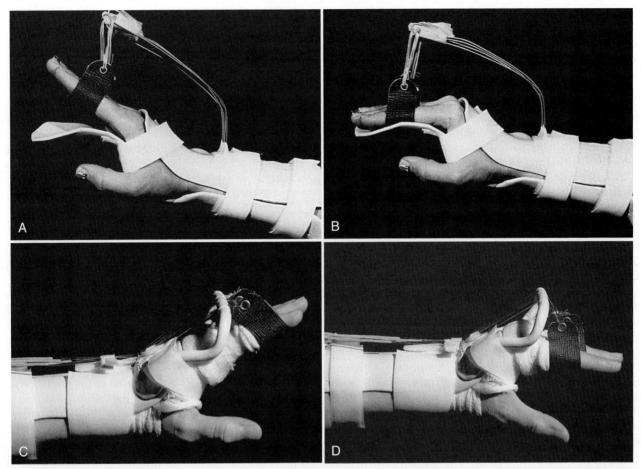

Figure 39-25 A, A dorsal forearm-based dynamic extension orthosis immobilizes the wrist at 45 degrees of extension and rests all finger joints at 0 degrees to position the repair site proximal to its normal resting position to prevent gapping and extensor lag. A volar block permits only the predetermined metacarpophalangeal (MCP) joint flexion, allowing slightly more flexion for the ulnar digits to achieve the necessary tendon excursion. **B,** The patient actively flexes the digits to the volar block an empirical 20 repetitions each waking hour to create approximately 5 mm of passive excursion for the extensor tendons. Dynamic traction returns the digits to 0 degrees, but most patients inadvertently actively extend within the slings as well. **C,** Low-profile dynamic orthosis that rests the digital joints at 0 degrees. **D,** The desired motion at the MCP joint is controlled by a stop bead that limits rubber band and monofilament line excursion. (**A,** From Evans RB, Burkhalter WE: A study of the dynamic anatomy of extensor tendons and implications for treatment. *J Hand Surg.* 1986;11A:774–779.)

for applying controlled stress to the healing extensor tendon is the same as that for the flexor tendon: to promote intrinsic healing and to encourage longitudinal reorientation of adhesions associated with extrinsic healing.[26,65,76,183,189,190]

Although the simple dorsal injury often is neglected at this level, significant problems of adherent tendon and extensor lag can result from immobilization, improper orthosis position, and inattention during the first 3 weeks of healing. Rosenthal[137] discusses the inflammatory response of the extensor paratenon (characterizing the extensor tendons in the extrasynovial zones V and VI) when disturbed, especially in the complex extensor tendon injury, and notes that the paratenon has a prodigious capacity for generating scar tissue and adhesions. Peacock,[47] in a study of the effects of enveloping tendon transfers with paratenon, observed that transplanted paratenon abounds in collagen-synthesizing cells. The observed physiologic response of the disturbed paratenon is an increased production of adhesions in surrounding tissues.[47,88,183] This increase may explain proliferative adhesion formation in the extrasynovial extensor tendon injury in zones V and VI, particularly with crushing injury in which the enveloping paratenon is widely disturbed.

Although in my earlier reports I suggested using early passive motion in these zones only for extensor injuries associated with periosteal injury, crush, or associated soft tissue injury,[81,83] I now recommend early motion for simple injury as well. Clinically, we observe that even the simple injury treated with immobilization can become problematic, and the biochemical and biomechanical benefits of early motion cannot be disputed.

Clinical Application

Controlled stress is applied to the extrinsic tendons 24 hours to 3 days after surgery by allowing the repaired tendons to glide 5 mm within a forearm-based dynamic extension orthosis. Stress is relieved at the repair site for the finger extensors by positioning the wrist at approximately 40 to 45 degrees of extension. Positioning the wrist in a neutral position, as suggested by Minamikawa and colleagues,[78] rests the repair site distal to its normal resting position and may result in extensor lag. The MCP and IP joints rest at 0 degrees in dynamic extension slings (Fig. 39-25A). I prefer to use a moving high-profile outrigger made of spring steel (as opposed to a static outrigger, which provides motion only through rubber band or monofilament), which is bent at a right angle at the point of attachment and applied to the orthosis proximal to the dorsal retinaculum. The counterforce from the resistance of the weight of the fingers is then proximal to the wound, and the moving outriggers offer less resistance to active flexion than would a static outrigger (Fig. 39-25B). The use of a high-profile outrigger, as opposed to a low-profile one, is supported by the work of Boozer and coworkers.[191] An interlocking palmar blocking orthosis permits only the predetermined angular changes at the MCP joint level (see Box 39-1).

The patient is instructed to actively flex the digits at the MCP joint until the fingers touch the volar orthosis and then to relax the digits, allowing the extensor outrigger to passively return the finger joints to 0 degrees (see Fig. 39-25A, B). The patient is instructed to repeat this exercise at least 20 times each waking hour. If the patient has difficulty flexing the fingers at the MCP joint level or if the proximal IP joints do not rest at 0 degrees within the extension slings, a volar digital extension orthosis should be fitted to each problematic digit and slipped inside each finger cuff to ensure that motion takes place at the MCP joint. A low-profile outrigger with stop beads to control excursion can be used, but for the reasons stated previously, I prefer to use a high-profile, moving outrigger (Fig. 39-25C, D).

The patient is seen in therapy for wound care, orthosis adjustments, controlled passive motion for the IP joints, and wrist tenodesis exercises. With the wrist and MCP joints fully extended, minimal excursion takes place at the IP joint levels, and each digital joint can be moved passively through a complete ROM without creating excessive stress or gapping to repairs at any level from zone V and proximal. Isolated exercise for the digital joints is especially important with the edematous or arthritic hand. Cooney and associates[75,163] have emphasized the importance of wrist tenodesis exercises with flexor tendon protocols to increase passive excursion of the repair site. I have applied their concept of tenodesis to the extensors with these parameters: The joints are moved passively in supervised therapy sessions with simultaneous maximum wrist extension and MCP joint flexion to 40 degrees, followed by simultaneous wrist flexion to 20 degrees with all digital joints held at 0 degrees. This concept of wrist tenodesis can be supported by the previously mentioned cadaver study on extensor tendons,[78] in which investigators demonstrated that if the wrist is extended more than 21 degrees, the extensors glide with little or no tension in zones V and VI throughout full simulated grip to full passive extension.

One must take care to ensure that the ulnar MCP joints do not rest in hyperextension, compromising the transverse metacarpal arch or creating problems for MCP joint collateral ligament extensibility. The patient may be instructed to remove the dorsal outrigger component and to secure the volar component by repositioning the Velcro straps to simplify dressing activities. The digits must rest at the 0-degree position at all other times, however, to prevent gapping or elongated tendon callous healing and extensor lag. I occasionally fit the patient with a second volar static extension orthosis with the MCP joints positioned at 0 degrees for sleeping. The patient follows the active-flexion, passive-extension exercise regimen at home within the confines of the dynamic extension orthosis and volar block.

This regimen is followed for 21 days, at which time the volar block is removed and increased digital joint motion and tendon excursion are permitted within the dynamic extension orthosis. Orthotic protection is necessary for another 2 to 3 weeks, with the dynamic extension component only in the daytime and the static volar component at night. The protocols for exercise, modalities, and dynamic flexion orthotic positioning as outlined in the section on management by immobilization can be followed at the 3-week period for tendons treated with early passive motion. In my clinical experience, these patients have composite finger flexion by the fourth to fifth week and composite finger and wrist flexion by the sixth week with no lag.

Treatment by Immediate Active Tension

The application of force with minimal active tension as a means of managing the repaired extensor tendon postoperatively is divided into two exercise components:[84,107] (1) Slow, repetitious passive motion should be performed until passive torque[192] at the end arc of extension is less than 200 to 300 g of force, before the active component of exercise is employed. Slow passive force reduces resistance and helps displace the high-molecular-weight fluids of edema[123] (Fig. 39-26). (2) The "active hold" component is then performed with the hand passively placed by the therapist in a position of 20 degrees of wrist flexion with all digital joints at 0 degrees, and the patient is asked to gently maintain this position to create some minimal active tension in the extensor system. The MCP joint is moved actively, from 30 degrees of flexion to 0 degrees of extension, while the wrist is held in 20 degrees of flexion, with all repairs at the MCP level and proximal. A calibrated small Haldex pinch meter (<150 g) can be used to demonstrate to the patient how gentle the forces of extension must be and can also provide the therapist with a repeatable and reliable technique for applying force to a tendon repair site. A string applied to the gauge arm of the pinch meter at a 90-degree angle and then around the digit at a 90-degree angle can be used to measure external load application[84] (Fig. 39-26B). The external force should be applied in the range of 0 to 25 g with joint angles as previously described. Force applied to repair sites in zones V through VII with these joint angles and with no external load except the weight of the finger has been calculated mathematically to be in the range of 300 g when drag is excluded.[84] The active component of treatment should be performed in the hands of the therapist after passive exercise in extension to reduce resistance of the antagonistic flexors. The active component is usually performed in my hands 20 or so times during a therapy session, three times per week for the first 3 weeks, and by the patients for their home program if they are deemed reliable.

Active motion is supplemented in therapy with wrist tenodesis exercises as described earlier. Patients are allowed to remove their protective orthoses at home for the active component or wrist tenodesis exercise only if they can reproduce the exercise regimen without cue and are reliable. The active component of this regimen is supplemented by the patient with the same dynamic orthosis (see Fig. 39-25A, B, or C, D) and passive protocol described in the previous section on passive motion. Digits held in extension slings are moving actively to some degree, inadvertently or otherwise,[84,112]

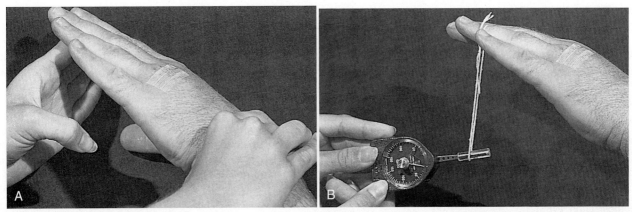

Figure 39-26 A, Passive extension for repairs in extensor zones V through VII with the wrist slightly extended to reduce the drag from edema, tight joints, and the antagonistic flexors. **B,** The active hold component (minimal active muscle–tendon tension, MAMTT) is carefully controlled. External load is measured with a small calibrated Haldex pinch meter in the active hold position with the wrist flexed to 20 degrees and the digital joints extended. The patient is allowed to apply active force in the range of 25 to 50 g in the prescribed joint position under therapist supervision. (From Evans RB, Thompson DE: The application of stress to the healing tendon. *J Hand Ther.* 1993;6:276.)

so one can assume that the tendon does experience some proximal migration within the dynamic extension orthosis. Treatment between 3 and 12 weeks with a gradual increase in excursion and resistance is the same as that outlined in the section on treatment by immobilization for zones V and VI.

Timing is a critical component of active motion programs. I prefer to see these patients 24 hours after surgery. The initial visit is important for initiating wound care, reducing edema, setting up the proper orthosis geometry, and giving instruction. It is safer to incorporate the active component by the third to fourth day when the early postoperative edema and inflammation[193] are diminished and before the tensile strength of the repair has decreased. At this early stage, suture is strong[99] and no collagen bonds have formed that would limit tendon glide.[31] Experimentally, investigators have demonstrated that very early stress at a repair site may prevent the anticipated drop in tensile strength associated with early healing.[52,53,63,67,122] Initiating therapy at day 7 to 10 when peritendinous adhesions have already formed

elevates tension at the repair site and increases the risk of rupture.

Clinical Results

I have compared the results of tendons treated with controlled active motion with tendons referred to me late that were treated with immobilization, and also to tendons treated from 1979 to 1990 with the passive motion technique (Tables 39-3 and 39-4). Tendons treated with wrist tenodesis and active motion demonstrated modest improvement (average, 9 degrees of TAM) compared with those treated with passive motion in a series that included both simple and complex injury but demonstrated significant improvement compared with treatment by immobilization (average improvement in TAM, 56 degrees[84]). The similarity in the results of active and passive techniques again is probably because tendons treated with the "passive" technique do, in fact, move actively at times. In a continuous series from 1993 to 2009, no extensor tendon treated with the active hold technique has ruptured.

Table 39-3 Clinical Results, Primary Repair of the Extensor System

Zone	No. of Patients	No. of Tendons	Mean Age	% Male	% Complex	Days from Surgery to Discharge	ROM Strickland-Glogovac	TAM* ROM	Extensor Lag
Immediate Minimal Active Muscle Tendon Tension									
III, IV	28	32	42	80%	77%	51	135 degrees		3 degrees
V, VI	14	24	40	56%	41%	50		249 degrees	0 degrees
Immobilization[†]									
III, IV	30	38	40	87%	76%	77	111 degrees		8 degrees
V, VI	8	15	50	86%	60%	80		193 degrees	31 degrees
VII	1	4	38	100%	100%	50		210 degrees	20 degrees
T-III, T-IV, T-V	6	6	38	100%	50%	53		120 degrees	5 degrees

From Evans RB, Thompson DE. The application of stress to the healing tendon. *J Hand Ther.* 1993;6:278.
ROM, range of motion; TAM, total active motion.
*TAM = MP + PIP + DIP − extensor lag.
[†]1990, 1991, 1992, 1993.
No tendon seen early in this time tx only c̄ passive motion.

Table 39-4 *Clinical Results of Extensor Tendons as Reported in Two Earlier Clinical Studies*

Zone	Early Passive Motion* (Pilot Study, 1986)			
	No. of Patients	No. of Tendons	% Complex	TAM
IV, V, VI	36	66	100	210 degrees
Multicenter Study 1989 (Early Passive Motion)†				
V, VI	32	50	0	240 degrees
V, VI	16	35	100	237 degrees
VII	8	17		242 degrees
T-IV, T-V	8	8	56	116 degrees
(Immobilization 1989)				
V, VI	6	9	100	185 degrees, 30 degrees extensor lag
VII	3	12	100	188 degrees

From Evans RB, Thompson DE. The application of stress to the healing tendon. *J Hand Ther.* 1993;6:281.

*Evans RB, Burkhalter WE. A study of the dynamic anatomy of extensor tendons and implications for treatment. *J Hand Surg.* 1986;11A:774.

†Evans RB. Clinical application of controlled stress to the healing extensor tendon: a review of 112 cases. *Phys Ther.* 1989;6B:1041.

Sagittal Band Injury

The sagittal band (SB) functions to maintain the EDC in proper alignment. Rupture or attenuation results in subluxation of the involved EDC (usually ulnarward and most often to the long finger) into the intermetacarpal region, resulting in altered EDC moments and loss of active extension with symptoms of pain and swelling at the MCP joint. In an anatomic and biomechanical study of the SB, Young and Rayan determined that the average pressure was greatest (50 mm Hg) with full MCP joint flexion and least (30 mm Hg) during MCP flexion of 45 degrees. When MCP joint radial or ulnar deviation force was added, the greatest pressure (57 mm Hg) was in neutral MCP position and the least (35 mm Hg) in 45 degrees of MCP flexion. They concluded that the greatest forces are imposed on the SB in full extension, and less

frequently in full flexion; that SB rupture is most common in the long digit, less so in the small digit; that proximal rather than distal SB injury contributes to extensor tendon instability; and that wrist flexion contributes to extensor tendon instability after SB disruption and may exacerbate the severity of the injury.[194]

Sagittal band reconstruction is supported in the literature.[195,196]

These injuries are most often treated with surgical repair or reconstruction; however, some investigators have reported success with conservative management with an MCP joint extension orthosis if the injury is recognized and treated early. Catalano and associates describe a static extension orthosis, which they term "the sagittal band bridge."[197] This orthosis actually is a design similar to the "relative extension" yoke orthosis described by Howell and colleagues for postsurgical treatment of the repaired zone IV through VII extensor tendon.[198] The orthosis differentially holds the injured MCP in 25 to 35 degrees of hyperextension relative to the adjacent MCP joints, with full motion allowed at the PIP joints. Based on the results of their retrospective review of 10 patients with 11 acute MCP dislocations due to SB ruptures in the nonrheumatoid hand, the authors recommend nonsurgical treatment of these injuries with early intervention.[197]

Inoue and Tamura report on 27 patients treated with SB rupture. Twenty-one cases were treated surgically and six were treated within 2 weeks of injury with positioning of the uninvolved MCP joint. They report excellent results in all cases with no recurrent subluxations and recommend that patients seen within 2 weeks of injury be treated conservatively with positioning.[199]

Partial SB ruptures or those treated in the immediate postinjury phase may respond to conservative treatment with immobilization of the MCP joint in extension, or hyperextension; however, surgical repair produces the most reliable results with frank subluxation of the EDC digital angulation.[29] I have limited positive experience with conservative management with a static hand-based extension orthosis holding the involved digit and adjacent digit at 0 degrees extension for 4 weeks, with protection for 6 weeks, and controlled progressive exercise (Fig. 39-27A). Repaired SB inju-

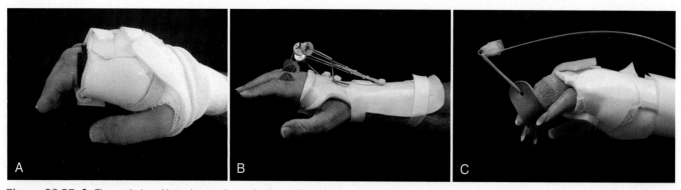

Figure 39-27 A, The static hand-based extension orthosis positions the involved digit and adjacent digit at 0 degrees extension for 4 weeks, with buddy tape protection for 6 weeks, and controlled progressive exercise as an early conservative intervention for closed sagittal band rupture. **B,** Repaired sagittal band injuries, a more reliable treatment, are positioned dynamically with controlled flexion at the metacarpophalangeal (MCP) joint with the same protocol that I utilize for extensor tendon repairs treated with immediate active tension, or **C,** in some cases with static MCP joint extension with dynamic traction at the proximal interphalangeal (PIP) joint level to protect a more tenuous repair while promoting tendon excursion and joint motion at the PIP joint level.

Table 39-5 Excursions for the Wrist Extensors as Reported by Bunnell

	Flexion (mm)	Extension (mm)	Radial Deviation (mm)	Ulnar Deviation (mm)
ECRL	16	21	8	16
ECRB	16	21	4	12
ECU	14	4	3	22

ECRL, extensor carpi radialis longus; ECRB, extensor carpi radialis brevis; ECU, extensor carpi ulnaris.
From Boyes JH: *Bunnell's Surgery of the Hand.* Philadelphia: JB Lippincott; 1970.

ries, a more reliable treatment, are positioned dynamically with controlled flexion at the MCP joint with the same protocol that I utilize for extensor tendon repairs treated with immediate active tension with progression to buddy tapes at 4 to 5 weeks (Fig. 39-27B), or in some cases with static MCP joint extension with dynamic traction at the PIP joint level to protect a more tenuous repair while promoting tendon excursion and joint motion at the PIP joint level (Fig. 39-27C).

A dynamic extension orthosis for attenuated SBs in the rheumatoid hand has been suggested by Chinchalkar and Pitts to facilitate active MCP joint extension to improve function and to retard secondary conditions such as swan-neck deformity.[200]

Zone VII

The extensor tendons are synovial at the wrist, where they pass through six fibro-osseous canals as they gain entrance to the hand.[130,137,201] The synovial sheaths and dorsal retinaculum act as pulleys, maintaining the relationship of tendon to bone while allowing for changes in direction. The synovial sheaths also may be important to tendon nutrition at this level.[202-204]

The moment arms and consequently tendon excursions are greatest for the digital extensor tendons at the wrist level[86] (Table 39-5). EDC excursions, as measured by Bunnell, at the wrist level vary as much as 20 mm from the small finger to the radial three fingers (see Table 39-1). The wrist extensors also vary significantly from tendon to tendon and with lateral motion as opposed to flexion and extension[87] (see Table 39-5). Note the large excursions with the ECU in ulnar deviation as opposed to radial deviation and extension.

The relationship between tendon excursion and joint motion has been shown to be approximately linear for the long extensors at the wrist and at the finger joints.[86,94] Elliot and McGrouther[94] have provided a set of values for the long extensors that serve as a basis for calculating tendon excursions as we establish controlled motion and positioning protocols. The excursions of the EIP and the EDC to the index finger were found to be indistinguishable during movement of the wrist and MCP joints, as were the EDM and EDC for the small finger.[94] At the wrist joint, the slips of the EDC to the long and ring fingers are bound closely together, moving in unison[94] and obligating us to position both of these fingers even when only one tendon is repaired.

The extrinsic digital tendons at this level can be treated with any of the three techniques described for zones V and

VI. Problems of adhesion formation in this synovial level are much the same as for zone II flexor tendons; therefore treatment by early passive motion or controlled active motion is especially important in this region. The wrist should be positioned in at least 40 to 45 degrees of extension and the digits held in dynamic traction at 0 degrees to allow the tendons to rest proximal to their normal resting position between exercise sessions to prevent extensor lag (see Fig. 39-25A, B). Wrist tenodesis exercises should allow the wrist to come to only approximately 10 degrees of flexion for the repaired EDC and to no more than 20 degrees of extension for the repaired wrist tendons to prevent excessive stress at the repair site(s) during the first 3 weeks of healing. Multiple repairs of the EDC require differential tendon-gliding exercises from the earlier described treatments. One can accomplish this by moving one digit at a time into flexion at the MCP joint level while all other digits are held in extension, but it may be important to move the long and ring fingers together because of their interconnection at the wrist.[94] The MCP joints can be moved from 30 to 40 degrees during the first 3 weeks, progressing to 40 to 60 degrees by week 4, and 70 to 80 degrees by week 5 while the wrist is extended. Very moderate wrist flexion with approximately 50% composite finger flexion is added to the excursion exercises by the fourth week, progressing to attempts at simultaneous composite finger flexion and complete wrist flexion by 6 weeks after surgery. Again, time schedules for duration of orthotic use, exercise, and the application of force for excursion and strengthening are as outlined in detail in the section on zones V and VI. The extensor tendon at this level is fairly large; therefore it has more tensile strength after repair than would a smaller tendon at a more distal level. The work requirement of the wrist tendons also is greater than that of digital tendons at a more distal level; therefore return to normal loading for the wrist tendons should be delayed a few weeks beyond the schedules outlined for digital extensor tendons.

If treatment by immobilization is chosen, both the wrist and MCP joints must be positioned in extension for repair of the digital tendons (Fig. 39-28). To prevent PIP joint tightness, extensor lag, or excessive force with active extension, a removable component such as the one described in Figure

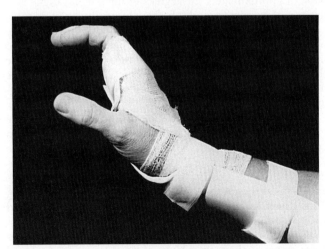

Figure 39-28 Repair of the digital extensors in zone VII treated by immobilization requires immobilization of the wrist and metacarpophalangeal joints.

39-22 can be used. Active extension with the wrist held in extension elevates force at the repair site dramatically,[84] and forces in this position may exceed the tensile strength of the repair. Extension of the PIP joints with the wrist and MCP joints held in extension should be passive; active extension is safe if the hand is removed from the orthosis and the wrist is held in a neutral position to slightly flexed position.[84]

Treatment by immobilization undoubtedly leads to tendon adherence to the synovial sheaths. Problems of limited tendon excursion and increased friction from adhesions that limit excursion may cause inflammatory problems with hand-intensive activities and often lead to long rehabilitation programs, the need for combined wrist and digital flexor orthotic positioning, and tenolysis.

Adhesions proximal to the dorsal carpal ligament restrict combined wrist and digital flexion because the tendons cannot glide distally under the dorsal pulley. Wrist flexion creates an exaggerated tenodesis effect of the digital extensors, depriving the patient of power grip. Scar distal to the retinaculum permits composite wrist and digital flexion but prevents composite wrist and digital extension because the tendons cannot glide proximally under the dorsal pulley. These problems can be minimized by proper postoperative orthotic positioning and early motion programs that use dynamic orthoses and controlled wrist tenodesis exercises. Micropore paper tape (3M) prevents tension to the cutaneous incision line and is extremely effective in preventing hypertrophic scar if worn continuously from week 2 until week 8.[184,185] SGS, applied very early, as soon as the skin wound is epithelialized, appears to discourage scar formation and to reduce the density of subcutaneous adhesion. This physiologic mechanism is as yet unexplained, but I have had excellent clinical results with this material, especially when applied during early wound healing. Dense scar also can be treated with elastomer molds applied with pressure or with mechanical stress applied to the tendons in all arcs of motion by the sixth week with either exercise or dynamic orthosis.

Treatment with early passive motion or controlled active motion is as described for the zone V and VI repair, with orthotic positioning and the active hold component. With repairs to the digital tendons, the therapist may position the wrist at approximately 20 degrees of flexion and digits at 0 degrees of extension while the patient gently maintains this position. However, if a wrist extensor tendon is involved, the wrist should not be moved beyond approximately 10 to 20 degrees of extension, and then the therapist should realize that forces at the repair site are increased with this change in wrist position because of increased resistance of the antagonistic flexors.[84]

Chinchalkar and coworkers have described a technique for encouraging relative excursion of repaired tendons in zones VI through VIII, which they term double reverse Kleinert technique. This very clever dynamic orthosis promotes differential tendon gliding to control intertendinous adhesions as they are formed in the early postoperative phase. This design encourages both independent and combined wrist and digital motion[9] (Fig. 39-29).

Disruption or extensive excision of the dorsal carpal ligament increases the moment arm of the extensor tendons and decreases mechanical efficiency.[86,161,202,205] Bowstringing of the extensor tendons at the wrist level translates to an exten-

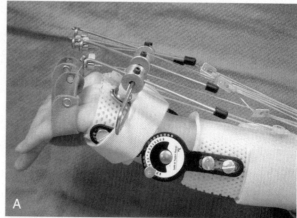
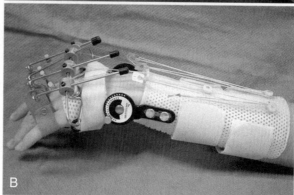

Figure 39-29 A, B, A custom-fabricated dynamic extension orthosis allows controlled excursion for the zone VI, VII, and VIII repairs. This "double reverse Kleinert extension orthosis" described by Chinchalkar and Ah Yong was designed to promote graduated excursion of the extensor tendons at the retinacular level through a wrist tenodesis action. (Borrowed with permission from Chinchalkar S, Yong SA. A double reverse Kleinert extension splint for extensor tendon repairs in zones VI to VIII. *J Hand Ther.* 2004;17:424–426.)

sor lag at the MCP joint (Fig. 39-30). Boland[202] correlated loss of the extensor retinaculum with extensor lag of only 2 to 4 degrees at the wrist level, but as much as 70 degrees at the MCP joint level, depending on the width of the retinacular fascia lost. With decreased mechanical efficiency, the workload of the extensor tendons is increased, especially during activities requiring sustained wrist and finger extension. Therefore the therapist should be aware that (1) with an absent or diminished dorsal retinaculum, it may not be possible to correct lag at the MCP joint with therapy, and (2) altered biomechanics resulting from adhesions or lost pulley may result in cumulative trauma problems. Treatment should be adjusted appropriately.

The work capacity and load requirements for the wrist extensors are great, requiring protective positioning for as long as 8 weeks.[86] Tendon excursion of the three wrist extensors as it relates to flexion–extension and radioulnar deviation determine the parameters for controlled motion programs (see Table 39-5). The wrist tenodesis exercises were previously described for the first 3 weeks of healing. By the third to fourth week, repaired wrist tendons, which may be expected to have approximately 25% to 30% of their tensile strength,[54,99] may be moved actively from 0 degrees to full extension with gravity eliminated. Larger tendons with more

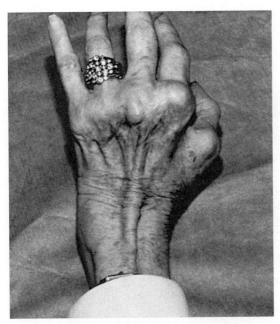

Figure 39-30 Disruption of the dorsal carpal ligament increases the moment arm of the extensor tendons, resulting in lost mechanical efficiency and an extensor lag at the metacarpophalangeal joint.

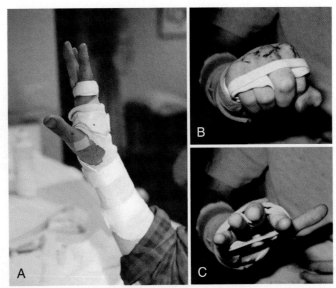

Figure 39-31 The immediate controlled active motion (ICAM) orthotic design positions the involved digit (digits) in relative hyperextension to the uninjured digits to relieve stress at the repair site. The orthosis design has two components: a simple yoke orthosis to control the metacarpophalangeal (MCP) joints, and a second wrist control orthosis. The current edition of the ICAM orthosis positions the wrist control component at 25 to 30 degrees of wrist extension, and the MCP of the involved digit (digits) in 15 to 20 degrees of relative hyperextension **(A)**. The patient is allowed immediate full active flexion within the ICAM orthosis **(B)**, and full active extension **(C)**. (From Howell JW, Merritt WH, Robinson SJ. Immediate controlled active motion following zone 4-7 extensor tendon repair. *J Hand Ther.* 2005;182–190. With Permission.)

surface area for suturing have more tensile strength than repairs at the more distal levels. The EDC tendons may be used to assist the wrist tendons during the first week of active exercise to bear some of the external load and possibly decrease stress at the wrist tendon anastomosis.

Increments in wrist flexion should be added slowly from week 5 to week 8. The same caution should be used with lateral motions. For example, the ECU has 22 mm of excursion in ulnar deviation, 3 mm in radial deviation, 4 mm in extension, and 14 mm in flexion.[87] To effect maximum excursion of the ECU, the wrist should be exercised into ulnar and radial deviation, with the forearm both supinated and pronated.[87,161,178] The patient may develop a tendency to lift the wrist with the EDC tendons, much like the pattern that we see after wrist fractures. Stress during exercise in the later stages of rehabilitation must be directed to the wrist tendons by excluding finger extension during exercise or functional electrical stimulation.

Relative Motion Orthotic Positioning or Immediate Controlled Active Motion for Zones IV to VII

Howell and associates have employed active motion and allowed for more tendon excursion in their immediate controlled active motion (ICAM) technique for the repaired zone IV through VII extensor tendon since the mid-1980s and have published their technique and results supporting the same.[198] They state that they have found the programs for early motion described by others "to be overly cautious and laborious." Their orthosis design positions the involved digit (digits) in relative hyperextension to the uninjured digits to relieve stress at the repair site. The orthosis design has two components: a simple yoke orthosis to control the MCP joints, and a second wrist control orthosis. The third edition

of the ICAM orthosis positions the wrist control component at 25 to 30 degrees of wrist extension, and the MCP of the involved digit (digits) in 15 to 20 degrees of relative hyperextension (Fig. 39-31). Their protocol is applied to injuries involving multiple adjacent digits as long as at least one digital extensor tendon is intact. The program includes three phases: Phase 1: The program during postoperative days 1 to 21 includes both orthoses worn continuously, wound and edema treatment, scar management when the sutures are removed, and full active and passive motion within the confines of the orthosis. Phase 2: Patients with full digital flexion and extension within the orthosis between days 22 and 35 can progress to wearing the yoke only for lighter activity and the two orthoses for any heavy activity. Wrist motions progress if no extensor lag is present. Phase 3: By days 36 through 49 the patient discards the wrist control component completely and is weaned from the yoke orthosis to buddy tapes as composite digital and wrist flexion and extension are regained. Their technique is supported by intraoperative measurement, a review of 140 cases, continued experience,[198] and a recently published biomechanical study.[206] The number of therapy visits required, lack of complications, and final ROM measurements with their ICAM technique are impressive.

Thumb

The thumb extensor tendons are divided into five zones[30] (see Fig. 39-1). Injuries in T-I and T-II are treated similarly

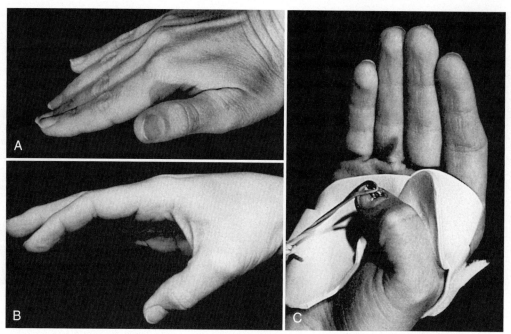

Figure 39-32 **A,** The thumb should be exercised from complete retropulsion with the wrist extended to, **B,** simultaneous abduction and flexion with the wrist flexed to obtain complete excursion of the extensor pollicis longus tendon by the sixth week. **C,** Combinations of abduction and flexion orthotic positioning may be necessary for the thumb positioned incorrectly with adduction of the carpometacarpal joint and hyperextension of the metacarpophalangeal joint during the immobilization phase.

to injuries of zones I and II of the finger.[126,130,207] Reports in the literature on the mallet thumb indicate that the injury is rare, and opinions differ concerning surgical repair versus conservative treatment with orthotic positioning.[130,207-210] Zone T-I injuries require that the IP joint be positioned for 8 weeks continuously at 0 degrees or slight hyperextension with conservative management, and 5 to 6 weeks with operative repair. Both approaches require an additional 2 to 4 weeks of orthotic immobilization between exercise sessions. Increments in flexion as mobilization is initiated should be no more than 20 degrees per week and delayed if extensor lag develops. IP joint extension orthotic positioning should be continued between exercise periods and at night for an additional 2 to 3 weeks. Pinching and gripping activity with mild resistance can be initiated between the sixth and eighth weeks, depending on the duration of immobilization. Elliot and Southgate make the point that the zone I extensor pollicis longus (EPL) tendon is not equivalent to the mallet finger because of the size of the EPL, which accommodates repair with a core suture without dehiscence. They make the observation that K-wiring of mallet thumbs frequently increases morbidity by causing increased adhesion and loss of flexion.[12]

Zone T-II injuries are immobilized with a hand-based static orthosis that immobilizes the MCP and IP joints at 0 degrees and radially extends the thumb. Active motion can be initiated in the short arc (25 to 30 degrees) by the third week, progressing slowly with more joint motion for the next 3 weeks. The problems of tendon-to-bone adherence are similar to those of the digit over the proximal phalanx. Orthotic protection between exercise sessions is needed for a total of 6 weeks.

Injuries in zones T-III and T-IV should be positioned with the thumb MCP joint at 0 degrees and slight abduction and the wrist in 30 degrees of extension. Care must be taken that the MCP joint does not rest in hyperextension or that the immobilizing orthosis does not migrate distally, hyperextending this joint. Regaining flexion at the MCP joint level is difficult in either case and may extend required rehabilitation. If the MCP joint is tight in hyperextension, dynamic positioning for the MCP joint with a gentle traction and joint mobilization techniques that use simultaneous axial distraction and flexion helps elongate the periarticular structures so that flexion can be regained.

Zone T-V injuries create difficult rehabilitation problems. Dense adhesions frequently limit excursion of the EPL at the retinacular level.[83] Improper immobilization in which the MCP joint is hyperextended or in which insufficient webspace is maintained creates extension contracture of the MCP joint, first-web contracture, and problems in regaining ligamentous extensibility and tendon glide.[83,126] Dynamic flexion positioning of the MCP joint with the wrist and first metacarpal extended is appropriate treatment for MCP joint extension contracture between weeks 3 and 4 if the rubber band traction is less than 250 g and the anastomosis is protected from excessive stress by proper orthotic positioning of the proximal joints. Combinations of abduction and flexion positioning and exercise are appropriate between weeks 4 and 5 for excursion problems at this level (Fig. 39-32).

Early Motion

Repair of the EPL in zone T-V always should be considered complex because the tendon at this level is synovial. The anticipated problems of maintaining excursion should be addressed with some type of controlled early motion–passive, controlled active motion, or combinations of both.

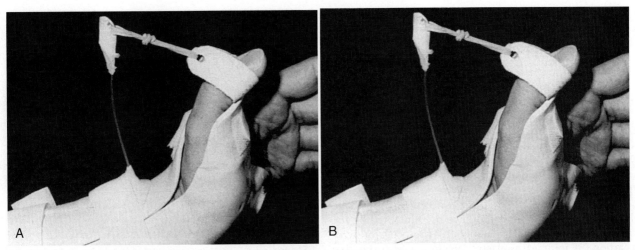

Figure 39-33 A, The repaired extensor pollicis longus tendon in zones IV and V is positioned with the wrist extended, carpometacarpal joint in neutral, metacarpophalangeal joint at 0 degrees, and interphalangeal joint resting at 0 degrees of extension in the dynamic traction. **B,** The patient actively flexes the distal joint through its available range (not to exceed 60 degrees) intermittently every hour to effect the 5 mm of glide at the level of Lister's tubercle. (From Evans RB, Burkhalter WE: A study of the dynamic anatomy of extensor tendons and implications for treatment. *J Hand Surg.* 1986;11A:774–779.)

Excursions for the EPL vary in the literature from 25 to 60 mm and are subject to many variables.[86,87,97] Excursion of this tendon cannot be calculated by the radian technique because the ratio of tendon excursion to joint motion is not linear. The simple angular arrangement of the flexion–extension axis at the MCP joint level of the fingers does not exist for the EPL in zones T-IV and T-V. Calculating excursion is complicated by the oblique course that the tendon takes at Lister's tubercle, by the moments of abduction and external rotation, and by the fact that alterations in thumb position alter moment arms at each joint.[86,98] Therefore Evans and Burkhalter[83] measured the EPL intraoperatively and determined that, with the wrist in a neutral position and the thumb MCP joint extended to 0 degrees, 60 degrees of IP joint motion effected 5 mm of tendon excursion at the level of Lister's tubercle. Extending the wrist beyond approximately 30 degrees most likely changes the excursion with IP motion. Tendon gliding for the EPL was recently studied in zone IV during passive motion in four different wrist positions in 25 healthy female volunteers using high-resolution US in a frame-by-frame cross-correlation analysis. It was determined that the mean gliding distance of the EPL tendon was 1.79, 2.45, 1.09, and 1.36 mm with the wrist positioned in neutral, 30 degrees of extension, 30 degrees of flexion, and 20 degrees of ulnar deviation, respectively. Wrist extension was found to induce the greatest magnitude of EPL tendon gliding.[211]

The early passive motion technique requires dynamic orthotic positioning that immobilizes the wrist in extension, the MCP joint at 0 degrees, and the IP joint at 0 degrees in dynamic traction. The volar component of the orthosis is cut away at the IP joint, allowing the prescribed 60 degrees of IP motion to take place (Fig. 39-33). I have altered my original approach to these injuries by adding other motions while the patient is in my hands. Passive motion by the patient is supplemented in therapy with controlled passive motion to the MCP joint of approximately 30 degrees while the wrist is held in maximum extension and the IP joint is held at 0

degrees; by abduction and adduction motions for the CMC joint in a 50% to 60% range; and by wrist tenodesis exercise in which the wrist is moved to a 0-degree position while the thumb kinetic chain is held in maximum extension, the thumb is relaxed, and the wrist is moved to full extension. To ensure that the tendon repair site is truly migrating proximally, I also add a component of "active hold." After the passive exercise, which helps minimize drag by reducing the resistance of edema and joint stiffness, the wrist is placed in 20 degrees of flexion while the CMC, MCP, and IP joints are held in extension and the patient is asked to gently maintain this position. The wrist position of minimal flexion reduces the elastic drag of the antagonistic flexor pollicis longus (FPL) tendon and thus reduces the internal force applied to the repair with the active hold portion of the exercise.[84] The patient may remove the protective orthosis during exercise and for showering during the third to fourth weeks, but orthotic protection should be maintained otherwise. Each joint should be moved actively into graded increments of flexion while all other joints in the thumb and the wrist are held in extension during the third and fourth weeks. By the fifth week, composite thumb flexion and opposition exercises may be initiated. Modalities and schedules for adding resistance for the tendon at this level are the same as for the digit. Continuous repetitive motions or overuse of therapy putty may inflame the tendons in the first dorsal compartment, creating a de Quervain's tendinitis in the overambitious patient trying to regain flexion.

Considerations for the Rheumatoid Tendon

Tendon rehabilitation in the rheumatoid hand is complicated by altered biomechanics created by lost pulleys, subluxed tendons, SB ruptures, imbalances between the intrinsic and extrinsic tendon systems,[212,213] the effects of immobilization on the diseased joints, and the integrity of the tendon before rupture or laceration.[213,214]

The type of repair (end-to-end anastomosis, suture of the distal stump to an adjacent tendon, or tendon transfer) affects the immobilization and early motion schedules. The therapist should estimate the tensile strength of the repair based on the type of suture used,[84] adjust this number to accommodate a decrease in strength that may be associated with each postoperative day, and adjust again for delayed healing that could be associated with poor tissue or steroid use. I have used the SAM program successfully for extensor reconstruction in the rheumatoid hand in zone III and have used early motion with the stronger repairs in zones V through VII, and T-V (e.g., a modified Kessler or Bunnell suture with an epitenon stitch, or a Pulvertaft weave with tendon transfer). The concepts and excursions described for immediate SAM for the repaired central slip have been adopted by the Mayo Clinic group for their postoperative protocols for pyrolytic carbon PIP joint arthroplasty[215] to effect a safe excursion for the zone III, IV extensor tendon following reconstruction at this level.

The application of force with passive motion or active motion should be calculated as outlined earlier in this chapter and then applied only if there is a safety margin between the tensile strength of the repair and the application of force with controlled motion. Early motion to the distal joints is especially important in these hands to prevent a loss of joint motion. These patients often have more problems with postsurgical bleeding or hematoma because of their medications, so again early motion is important to control adhesions as they form. Extensor lag with all zones is more of an issue in the rheumatoid hand, so it is especially important to allow these tendons to heal with no tension in the position of immobilization. The duration of orthotic protection probably should exceed that cited earlier for normal tendons by a few weeks.

Repairs in zones V through VII associated with intrinsic tightness should be positioned with the MCP joints at 0 degrees and the fingers free at the PIP joints and distal during the immobilization stage. This position protects the repairs but puts the digits in a position for intrinsic stretch. If the dynamic extension orthosis for early passive motion is used and there are swan-neck deformities, the digits should be positioned within their slings with a dorsal static two-joint orthosis that positions the PIP joints in 30 degrees of flexion (Fig. 39-34). This orthotic arrangement allows proximal joint flexion, inhibits the swan-neck deformity, and helps transmit the forces of passive motion to the more proximal zones. This same digital orthotic arrangement should be continued in the active stages of rehabilitation. The goal with extensor repair in the more proximal zones associated with swan-neck defor-

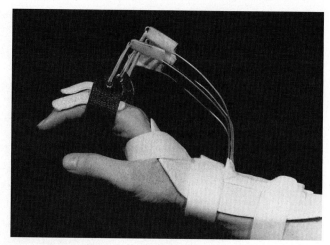

Figure 39-34 Swan-neck deformities should be counterbalanced with digital positioning to help transmit extensor forces to the zone V and VI levels when active extension exercise is initiated.

mity is to facilitate MCP extension, PIP joint flexion, and intrinsic stretch.

Summary

Extensor tendon management after surgery has changed dramatically over the past three decades, from prolonged periods of immobilization to shorter periods of immobilization, controlled passive motion programs, and minimal active muscle–tendon tension programs. Investigators have demonstrated clinically that extensor tendon in all zones except I, II, T-I, and T-II benefit from immediate short arc motion at the joint associated with the repair and some controlled motion at the wrist level. The concepts of immediate motion are supported biochemically in experimental studies, biomechanically through excursion studies, through mathematical analysis of excursion and force application, and through analysis of tendon repair tensile strengths. Meticulous care in the control of edema, postoperative positioning, and controlled motion programs greatly improves the results of both the simple and complex extensor tendon injury not only in terms of function achieved but also in terms of time and expense.

REFERENCES

The complete reference list is available online at www.expertconsult.com.

Flexor and Extensor Tenolysis: Surgeon's and Therapist's Management

RANDALL W. CULP, MD, FACS, SHERI B. FELDSCHER, OTR/L, CHT, AND SERGIO RODRIGUEZ, MD*

CRITICAL POINTS

Indications

- The patient suffered the injury or underwent repair 3 months ago, and therapy progress has plateaued, leaving the patient with immobile adhesions.
- Passive range of motion (PROM) exceeds active range of motion (AROM).
- AROM equals PROM, but grip strength is unsatisfactory.

Preoperative Evaluation

- The tenolysis candidate must be highly motivated, have healed fractures and wounds, soft, supple tissues, maximal PROM, and good strength.
- Preoperatively the patient is instructed in the surgical procedure, postoperative treatment, and the need to work through postoperative discomfort.
- The extensor tenolysis patient must be cautioned that some loss of extension with the recovery of flexion is not uncommon.

Priorities and Pearls

- Tenolysis demands immediate AROM.
- Intraoperative ROM must be achieved during the first 2 to 3 weeks following surgery.

Technical Points

- Tenolysis is performed under local anesthesia to allow for active patient participation and to enable the surgeon to determine when lysis is complete.

Pitfalls

- If the procedure is unsuccessful, the patient's hand may show no improvement or may even be worse.

- The risk of further decreasing the circulatory supply and innervation to an already deprived finger is a real one.
- Rupture of the lysed tendon, a disastrous complication, is another hazard of tenolysis.

Precautions

- Tendons of poor integrity have an increased likelihood of rupture and require protective orthoses and a protected ROM program designed to maximize excursion and minimize stress.
- Tenolysed extensor tendons must be protected from overstretching during the first few postoperative weeks.

Postoperative Care

- Week 1
  - Treatment includes wound care, AROM, place and hold exercises, PROM, edema control, and orthotic positioning as indicated.
  - Transcutaneous electrical nerve stimulation (TENS) units or marcaine catheters (or both) may be used to manage postoperative discomfort.
  - The home exercise program includes 5 to 10 repetitions of each active exercise performed hourly; gentle PROM, 10 repetitions four times a day; and overhead pumping 10 times per hour.
  - If necessary, neuromuscular electrical nerve stimulation (NMES) may be initiated at the end of the first week in patients having good tendon integrity to increase tendon excursion.
- Weeks 2 to 3
  - Treatment continues with upgrades as tolerated.
  - Moist heat, ultrasound (US), and scar management are initiated as indicated.

*The authors gratefully acknowledge Lawrence H. Schneider for his invaluable contributions to this work in both the present and past.

- The home program includes massage four to five times a day; light activities of daily living (ADL) at 2 to 3 weeks after surgery; and sustained gripping exercises at 3 to 4 weeks.
- Weeks 4 to 6
  - Progressive resistive exercises (PREs), graded grip strengthening, whole-body conditioning, or aerobic exercise may begin at 6 weeks.
- Weeks 7 to 8
  - The focus shifts toward preparing for return to work with job simulations and work hardening/work conditioning.
  - Heavy resistive exercises may be initiated at 8 weeks.

Return to Work
- The goal is return to work at 8 to 12 weeks.

Tenolysis is a salvage procedure intended to disrupt nongliding adhesions that have formed along the surface of a tendon after injury or repair. Tendon adhesions occur whenever the surface of a tendon is damaged either through the injury itself, be it laceration or crush, or by surgical manipulation.[1,2] At any point on the surface of a tendon where violation occurs, an adhesion forms in the healing period.[3,4] Whenever these adhesions cannot be mobilized by therapy techniques, tenolysis should be considered. This procedure is as demanding as tenorrhaphy itself and cannot be undertaken lightly. Tenolysis represents another surgical insult in an area of previous trauma and surgery. If the procedure is unsuccessful, the patient's hand may show no improvement or may even worsen. The risk of further decreasing the blood supply and innervation to an already deprived finger is a real one. Rupture of the lysed tendon, a disastrous complication, is another hazard of tenolysis. This chapter reviews preoperative evaluation and treatment for tenolysis, timing of surgery, surgical technique, technical points for flexor and extensor tenolysis, postoperative management of each, and expected clinical outcomes.

Preoperative Evaluation for Tenolysis

Several criteria must be strictly adhered to in order to provide the best prognosis. Patient selection is a vital aspect in successful tenolysis. The patient should have been in an adequate therapy program combining active motion techniques with gentle passive motion exercises for approximately 3 months after tendon repair or injury, and progress should have reached a plateau. The patient's level of cooperation in a postoperative program also can be assessed during this interval. A patient unable to wholly commit himself or herself to the program should be rejected for lysis. At 3 months after the injury or original surgery[5] if the range of movement (ROM) attained is regarded by patient and surgeon as inadequate, discussion begins regarding the risks and rewards of lysis in view of the functional demands and needs of the patient. A realistic picture must be drawn. A cold, insensate finger cannot be improved even if a full ROM could be regained. The decision to perform tenolysis is often subjective. For example, 50% of a normal ROM may be reasonable to accept, especially in an aged person, a person with a low functional demand, or one who has concurrent joint surface injury or degenerative arthritis.

Other prerequisites for a successful tenolysis include (1) the presence of adequate skin coverage, meaning stable soft scar and supple skin, (2) well-healed fractures in anatomic alignment, (3) intact tendon systems, and (4) good muscle strength.[6]

Ideally, the patient best suited for tenolysis is one whose repaired tendon had a localized adhesion that limited gliding. On release, a full ROM is regained. However, this is an uncommon situation. More commonly, the adhesions involve a long segment of the involved tendon and require extensive exposure for release. Joint contracture, which can occur secondary to the tendon fixation, also may require simultaneous correction and thus further complicates the surgery and the patient's recovery.[7]

Timing of Surgery

The patient should have been in an adequate hand therapy program incorporating PROM and AROM exercises for approximately 3 months following tendon repair or injury and have reached a plateau in which no improvement has occurred over the preceding 6 weeks. This time interval allows for wound healing while the patient is trying to elongate the already formed adhesions. Proceeding with tenolysis earlier than 3 months after the original event is believed to jeopardize the tendon's blood supply, thus increasing the risk of rupture.

Surgical Technique

Once the patient has been found to be an appropriate surgical candidate, meeting all the prerequisites, tenolysis can be offered. We prefer performing the tenolysis under local anesthesia to allow full evaluation during the procedure itself.[8] It is through this technique that one can determine whether release of the offending tendon system adhesions is adequate to restore motion or whether the patient also requires surgical release of the joints.

The local anesthetic agent used is 1% or 2% lidocaine, infiltrated locally in the skin or as a digital block at the metacarpal level. Nerve blocks at the wrist also can be used, but with resultant paralysis of the intrinsic muscles, some benefits of this technique are sacrificed.

The administration of IV medication relieves anxiety and alleviates tourniquet pain. Many anesthetic agents that can be administered intravenously have been useful in achieving sedation and comfort while allowing active participation in the operative procedure. This medication is given as needed for the patient's comfort and as allowed by the patient's condition. Monitoring of the vital signs by experienced anesthesia personnel in an operating room environment is essential.

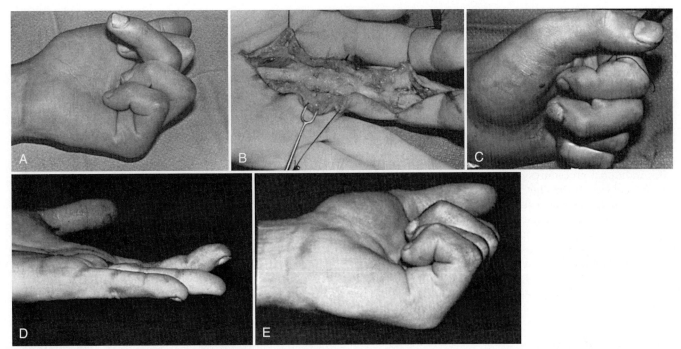

Figure 40-1 Flexor lysis. A 17-year-old boy severed both flexor tendons in his left long finger. After primary repair of his flexor digitorum profundus, he had minimal pull-through of his flexor system at 4 months after repair. **A,** Attempted flexion of the left long finger. **B,** During tenolysis, massive adhesions were found at the repair site. **C,** After lysis under local sedation, he obtained excellent active flexion with hand lying on a table. **D, E,** Through an active therapy program, he maintained the gains accomplished through surgery. Photographs of extension and flexion taken at 3 months after surgery.

Careful titration of the medication is also necessary because excessive amounts of sedatives reduce the patient's ability to cooperate. With proper dosage, the tourniquet can be tolerated for as long as 1 hour.

The tenolysis can truly be a test of the surgeon's dexterity. Many techniques and instruments have been designed. We prefer the use of Meals tenolysis knives (George Tiemann and Co., Hauppauge, NY). The dissection should proceed rapidly, from the unaffected proximal area to the affected distal tendon, and the patient's ROM is repeatedly evaluated until tourniquet paralysis intervenes at 20 to 25 minutes. If further dissection is needed, it is continued as necessary and evaluation is carried out after the tourniquet is released and hemostasis is obtained. If additional surgery is deemed necessary, the tourniquet is reinflated and dissection continued until completed. The surgeon can directly determine whether the tendon motor actually is effective and flexor pulleys are adequate. This is one advantage of using local anesthesia. If, however, general anesthesia is used, adequacy of the tenolysis can be assessed by pulling on the tendon. Careful inspection determines whether the lysed tendon appears healthy or whether a tendon graft, usually conducted in two stages, is advisable. When tenolysis has successfully restored AROM that is deemed acceptable, the wounds are closed and a dressing is applied.

Flexor Tenolysis

We prefer a wide exposure of the flexor tendons using a Bruner zigzag-type incision. This approach allows us complete visualization of the flexor tendon anatomy as well as the pulley system. When dealing with crush injuries, it is often necessary to turn the hand over and release the opposing tendon system as well. This is especially common when associated phalangeal fractures are present. All patients for flexor tenolysis have given their informed consent for a possible staged tendon reconstruction if a reasonable flexor mechanism cannot be salvaged.[9,10]

Summary of Technical Points for Flexor Lysis[10-12]

1. Make a zigzag (Bruner) incision; if needed, be prepared to expose the entire course of the tendon.
2. Preserve pulleys as possible (especially A2 and A4).
3. Release joints if significant contractures exist.
4. Meticulously examine the site of the tendon repair or injury. The surgeon should be wary of a gapped tendon that has filled in with scar tissue. Although one may succeed in carving a tendon-like structure out of this scar tissue, when a large gap is present, the tendon is too long and will develop mechanical insufficiency, increasing the chance of rupture (see item number 5).
5. Obtain preoperative informed consent from the patient for a possible staged tendon reconstruction to be done at the same sitting when tenolysis is recognized as unlikely to succeed.[9,10,13]
6. Flexor tenolysis (Fig. 40-1) after failed direct repair has been more successful than after failed tendon graft, a finding that further stresses the advantages of direct repair, done early, in flexor injuries when wound conditions allow.[2,14]

Postoperative Management of Flexor Tenolysis

The procedures surrounding the tenolysis operation are as vital as the lysis itself. Complications are not uncommon, but they can be minimized when a knowledgeable postoperative hand therapy program is implemented. Referral information should include

1. The integrity of the lysed tendon
2. Intraoperative AROM, if available
3. Intraoperative PROM
4. Additional procedures performed (e.g., capsulectomy)
5. Vascularity of the digit
6. The surgeon's prognosis for motion

This information then dictates the postoperative treatment program. For example, tendons of good integrity can undergo more vigorous postoperative therapy programs, whereas those of poor quality have an increased likelihood of rupture and require a protected ROM program designed to maximize tendon excursion while minimizing the stress applied to the lysed site.[10-12,15]

Tendons of Poor Integrity

Cannon[16] and Strickland[17-19] have described their "frayed exercise program" for use with patients having poor tendon integrity intraoperatively who require protection against rupture. This protected ROM program involves place-hold exercises (Fig. 40-2C) performed in full flexion, followed by active extension to 0 degrees to passively maximize excursion of the long flexors. Place-hold exercises are the only active flexion exercises performed. These exercises apply less tensile loading on the operated tendon than other active exercises, yet they provide the same tendon excursion that is produced when the patient actively flexes the digit to end range. The benefits of this program include decreased pain, decreased rupture rate, and ease in maintaining excursion of the lysed tendon. This program also may be used with patients experiencing crepitus or synovitis postoperatively when rupture is a concern. As the tendon heals and gains in strength, gentle active exercises may be added progressively to the program when indicated by the surgeon.

Tendons of Good Integrity

Recently, the timing of the initiation of therapy following tenolysis has become debatable. All agree that early active motion is desirable. Some clinicians start immediate motion on the first postoperative day while others advocate waiting 3 to 5 days for inflammation and subsequent friction between tendon and sheath to diminish and the gliding environment to improve, thus decreasing the work of flexion, before beginning rehabilitation.[20,21] Still others, such as Foucher and colleagues[22] and Goloborod'ko[23] have published their postoperative technique after tenolysis in which they briefly immobilize the operated fingers in flexion to allow soft adhesions to form between the lysed tendon and surrounding tissues, then passively extend the fingers to break these adhesions. We advocate immediate AROM that is compatible with wound healing.

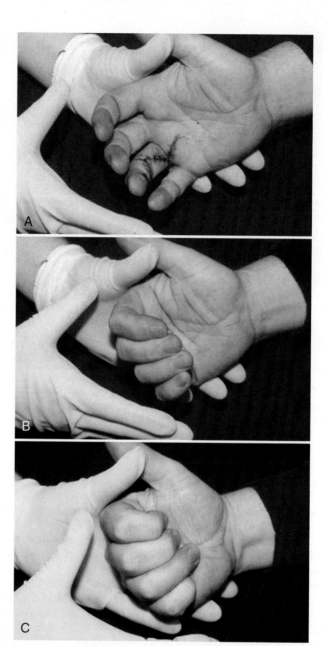

Figure 40-2 "Place-hold" exercises are performed by the patient placing his fingers into slight flexion **(A)**, moderate flexion **(B)**, or full flexion **(C)**, using the uninvolved hand. The patient maintains the fist, using his own muscle power.

Postoperative Week 1

Tenolysis demands immediate AROM.[7] It is initiated in the operating room and recovery area on the day of surgery. When possible, the patient is also seen in therapy on the day of surgery. A more detailed therapy program is initiated on the first postoperative day. Ideally, the patient is seen in therapy daily for the first 5 postoperative days.

The first 5 days are crucial to the postoperative management. Inflammation occurs during the process of tissue healing and may result in associated edema and discomfort. Intraoperative ROM should be achieved in therapy as soon as possible in an effort to prevent the recurrence of binding adhesions.

Evaluation

Universal wound precautions must be implemented at all times. Evaluation and treatment are performed with the involved hand on a sterile drape. The therapist wears sterile gloves. Initial evaluation includes assessment of the wound, edema, AROM, PROM, and level of discomfort.

The bulky dressing applied at surgery is removed; the adherent dressing covering the incision is left undisturbed to protect the wound. The status of the wound is noted. At the end of the treatment session, a dry sterile gauze pad is reapplied to the incision. This is held in place by a tube bandage if a digit is involved and a gauze wrap if the incision extends into the palm or forearm. The newly applied dressing should not be removed until the next treatment session with the therapist. Postoperative dressings should be protective but nonrestrictive. Full AROM must be possible within the confines of the dressing.

Circumferential measurements for edema are recorded with a tape measure over the dressing. Measurements of AROM and PROM also are taken. The distance from the fingertips to the distal palmar crease is recorded during active flexion.

The patient's subjective reports of discomfort may be assessed with one of the many available pain assessments or outcomes measures such as the DASH, which is a valid, reliable, and responsive questionnaire that evaluates symptoms and physical function.[24] Such assessments provide valuable information regarding the patient's level of function and pain tolerance and her ability to participate fully in the program.

Treatment

Initial treatment includes AROM, PROM, edema control, pain management, orthotic positioning if necessary, and home program instruction. Techniques to enhance muscular activity and the use of continuous passive motion (CPM) are also discussed.

Active Range of Motion. Preoperatively, patients should have been instructed in the postoperative therapy regimen. They are warned that the postoperative therapy program will begin immediately after surgery and that it will be vigorous. Despite such warning, patients are often reluctant to exercise the recently operated finger because of discomfort. The therapist must be supportive, understanding, and encouraging. Both the patient and therapist must work together, giving forth their best effort to achieve a maximal result. The patient must understand that if he or she exercises consistently and frequently, each exercise session will get easier as ROM improves and stiffness begins to decrease.

Gentle active exercises begun during the first postoperative visit include tendon gliding exercises (TGEs)[25-27] and place-hold exercises. Occasionally, digital blocking exercises and individual flexor digitorum superficialis (FDS) glides may be added, but they are usually reserved until the second postoperative week.

1. TGEs (Fig. 40-3A) include full extension and a hook-fist, a full-fist, and a straight-tip-fist position.[27] A tabletop position is included to maximize metacarpophalangeal (MCP) joint motion. The hook fist requires

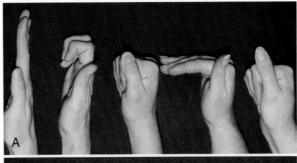
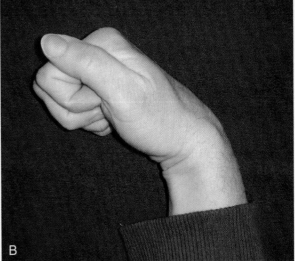
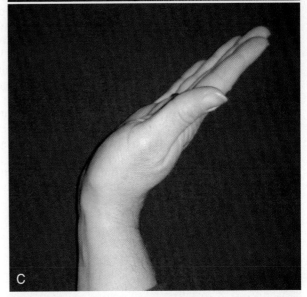

Figure 40-3 A, Tendon gliding exercises allow for the flexor tendons to glide to their maximum potential. **B, C,** Incorporation of wrist range of motion further increases tendon excursion.

maximal differential gliding of the flexor digitorum profundus (FDP) and FDS tendons; the full fist requires maximal glide of the FDP; and the straight fist requires maximal glide of the FDS. TGEs are performed to minimize potential adhesions between the tendons and between the tendons and bone. Initially, these exercises are performed with the wrist in a neutral position;

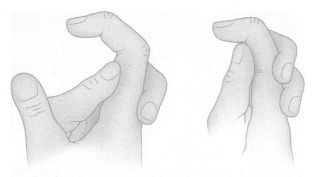

Figure 40-4 Blocking exercises increase active range of motion by better directing the available tendon excursion to the target joint.

all TGEs begin from a position of neutral wrist and finger extension. Composite wrist and digit flexion (Fig. 40-3B) are followed by simultaneous wrist and digit extension (Fig. 40-3C), which may be added later to increase tendon excursion.

2. Place-hold exercises (see Fig. 40-2) are performed by having the patient place his fingers into three positions—slight flexion, moderate flexion, and maximal flexion—using the uninvolved hand. At each position, the patient releases the "helping" hand and maintains the fist, using his own muscle power.

3. Two different blocking exercises (Fig. 40-4) are performed on each digit in turn: (1) active flexion of the proximal interphalangeal (PIP) joint while holding (blocking) the MCP joint in extension, and (2) active distal interphalangeal (DIP) joint flexion while holding (blocking) the MCP and PIP joints in extension. Blocking exercises increase AROM by allowing the available tendon excursion to be better directed to the target joint.

4. Isolated FDS glides (Fig. 40-5) are performed with the patient's hand supinated on a flat surface. The therapist manually holds all the digits in extension except the digit being flexed. The patient is instructed to actively flex the PIP joint into the palm. This exercise requires isolated function of the FDS and enhances

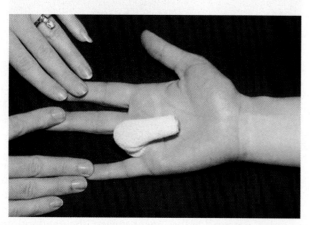

Figure 40-5 Flexor digitorum superficialis (FDS) glides allow for isolated function of the FDS tendon and promote differential gliding between the FDS and flexor digitorum profundus tendons.

differential tendon gliding between the FDS and FDP tendons.

Passive Range of Motion. Gentle passive exercises are incorporated into the exercise program when joint stiffness is present. Caution must be used when performing these exercises. Overly vigorous ROM can result in increased pain and inflammation that only impedes recovery.[28-30]

Edema Control. Edema, a normal reaction to trauma, must be controlled early because persistent edema may result in significant tissue scarring and fibrosis.[30] Uncontrolled edema leads to restrictions in ROM and tendon excursion.

Edema control includes elevation of the hand above the level of the heart to minimize limb dependency.[29] If elevation does not control edema sufficiently, other measures may be considered. Cold packs may be applied to the involved extremity three to four times a day for approximately 15 to 20 minutes with the hand in elevation. When one is applying cold packs, the wound must be kept dry and sterile and vascular status must be monitored.

A self-adherent elastic wrap (Coban) is applied without tension in a figure-of-eight, distal-to-proximal fashion to digits with good vascularity. Coban may be worn full-time (if needed), except during wound care. If ROM is impeded by Coban, it should be removed during exercise.

Therapeutic (Isotoner) gloves may be worn by patients (with good digital vascularity) who have excessive edema present throughout the hand.

An exercise that is very effective in controlling edema and in promoting active tendon excursion is overhead pumping. This exercise entails the patient elevating the involved extremity overhead and making a firm fist 10 times per hour.

Pain Management. TENS (Fig. 40-6A) may be applied to the involved extremity immediately after tenolysis to manage postoperative discomfort.[31] Presterilized, disposable electrodes are placed along the peripheral nerve distribution supplying the affected area. The patient is instructed in the operation of the unit at home. After pain relief has been achieved, the daily wearing time is gradually reduced and the patient is weaned from the unit.

Another method to reduce postoperative discomfort is an indwelling polyethylene catheter (Fig. 40-6B) that provides a local anesthetic.[32] The catheter is inserted at the time of the surgical procedure, proximal to the incision, over the sensory nerve branches.[11-13,15] The patient slowly instills small amounts (1–2 mL)[11,29] of local anesthetic (bupivacaine 0.25% or 0.5%)[32] into the area every 4 hours.[11,29] At each dressing change, an antibiotic ointment is applied to the catheter entrance site. The catheter is left in place for approximately 5 to 7 days, during which time the patient is on a regimen of oral antibiotics.[29] Although this technique is effective in reducing postoperative discomfort, we have found that it is being used with less frequency in recent years due to the risk of wound complications.[10]

Orthotic Positioning. Orthotic positioning may be required to achieve or maintain the ROM gained in surgery, to rest violated tissues between periods of exercise to allow

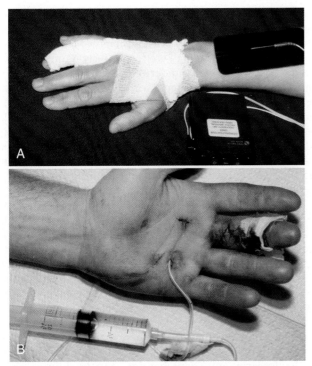

Figure 40-6 Transcutaneous electrical nerve stimulation **(A)** or bupivacaine hydrochloride (Marcaine) catheter **(B)** may be used to manage the postoperative discomfort that in some cases prevents the patient from exercising.

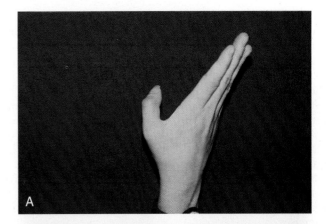

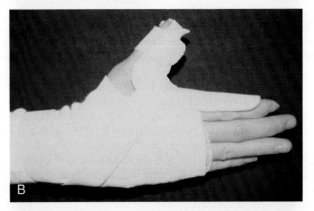

healing to occur, or to protect weakened tendons or repaired pulleys.

Patients who have had flexion contractures released at the time of tenolysis require static extension positioning of the involved joint(s) (Fig. 40-7). Extension orthoses initially may be worn full-time, except during exercise and wound care. As extension improves, the daily wearing schedule may be gradually reduced, but nighttime extension orthotic positioning may be necessary for up to 6 months.[29] Orthoses designed to increase or maintain PROM must be monitored carefully. Too much stress applied too early can increase pain and inflammation.

Tendons of poor integrity usually require positioning in the form of a dorsal block orthosis to protect the weakened tendon. The orthosis is worn full-time and the patient is instructed in the "frayed exercise program."

Pulleys are rarely reconstructed at the time of tenolysis. On occasion when they are, they require protective positioning. Before any active motion is initiated, a pulley ring, con-

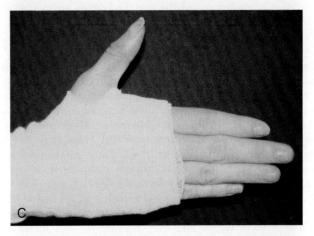

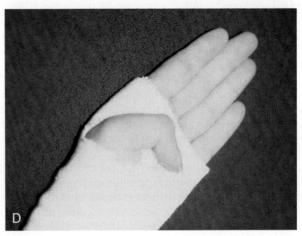

Figure 40-7 This 30-year-old right-hand-dominant bartender slipped and fell at work. This resulted in lacerations of her right flexor pollicis longus tendon in zone III; median nerve, proximally from the palm to digit I; radial and digital nerves to digit I; and radial digital nerve to digit II. **A,** At 3 months after primary repair, thumb active range of motion (AROM) was metacarpophalangeal 20 degrees/65 degrees and interphalangeal 30 degrees/55 degrees. **B,** A web stretcher was fabricated after lysis and worn nightly to maintain the gains achieved in range of motion. **C, D,** The patient was discharged at 8 weeks after surgery with AROM within normal limits.

structed of felt and Velcro, is applied over the reconstructed pulley. After edema subsides, a thermoplastic ring is fabricated. Some patients elect to wear a metal ring instead of the thermoplastic ring for greater durability and improved esthetics. Direct pressure applied over the reconstructed pulley by the patient's uninvolved hand during exercises also may be used to protect the pulley. The pulley ring is worn full-time for 6 months after repair.

When dynamic or serial static extension positioning is required, two pulley rings are fabricated to maintain adequate protection of the repaired pulley. One pulley ring is fabricated with the orthosis in place to counteract the passive extension forces of the extension outrigger; the second is fabricated without the orthosis in place and is worn during exercises.[29]

Home Program Instruction. The patient is instructed in a home program consisting of 5 to 10 repetitions of each active exercise performed hourly. Exercises are upgraded according to patient tolerance and progress. Patients who are unable to tolerate the exercise program because of persistent discomfort require a modified program consisting of a decreased number of repetitions and frequency of exercises (i.e., three repetitions performed every other hour). This allows continued tendon gliding through the lysed area without further increasing discomfort. Patients are instructed to actively hold the end position of each exercise for 10 seconds to increase total end-range time and to extend and flex the digits fully and strongly to maximize tendon excursion.[25] Gentle passive exercises at each joint of the involved digits are performed for 5 to 10 repetitions, four times per day. Edema control is included in every home program.

Enhancement of Muscular Activity. NMES may be implemented after tenolysis to increase tendon excursion, muscle strength, and AROM via the facilitation of muscle contractions.[16,33,34] It may be initiated by the end of the first postoperative week if the patient is not independently demonstrating strong active muscle contractions, if PROM exceeds AROM, and if the surgeon reports that tendon integrity is good.

Verification of tendon integrity is essential if NMES is being considered. NMES at high intensities is equivalent to the performance of resistive exercises. A weakened tendon may be unable to tolerate such strong muscle contractions before 6 to 8 weeks and may rupture if such tension is applied too soon. Caution also must be used with NMES to avoid overexercise, which could result in an inflammatory response and further impede recovery. NMES is continued until the goal of full AROM is achieved or when progress reaches a plateau.

Electromyographic (EMG) biofeedback[35,36] may be used in conjunction with electrical stimulation to further enhance muscular activity, restore functional coordinated movement, motivate the patient, redirect attention away from postoperative discomfort, or facilitate muscular relaxation.

Continuous Passive Motion. McCarthy and coworkers[37] studied CPM as a treatment adjunct to tenolysis. They found that CPM was associated with an increase in tendon rupture and in the terminal force necessary to flex the phalanx actively. Histologically, it appeared that the passive motion

elicited a hypergranular response that weakened the tendons and decreased the motion. In their study, CPM was continued for 5 consecutive days without removal for AROM.

Schwartz and Chafetz[38] retrospectively compared two groups of patients who underwent tenolysis (or capsulectomy). One group (15 patients with 22 involved fingers) was treated with CPM immediately following surgery. The second group (21 patients with 26 involved fingers) was treated with a standard exercise program. They found no statistically significant difference between the groups in terms of ROM gained. They concluded that CPM did not significantly alter the total active motion (TAM) gained during the course of therapy, nor did it reduce the treatment duration.

Tenolysis protocol demands immediate AROM to maximize tendon excursion and enhance tensile strength and nutrition of the muscle–tendon unit.[16,25,39,40] CPM may be used following tenolysis as a treatment adjunct, not as a replacement for AROM. The device is worn when the patient is not actively exercising. Cannon[16] has identified indications for initiating CPM following tenolysis. These include PROM that is not fully supple preoperatively; pain or edema that persists longer than expected with the initial injury; excessive scarring following the initial injury; the need for extensive tenolysis from the digital level proximally to the muscle belly in the forearm; and apprehension and fearfulness about moving the digit. Nothing is more important than active motion in the postoperative therapy program following tenolysis.

Postoperative Weeks 2 to 3

As the proliferative phase of wound healing begins, scar tissue forms and the wound begins to rapidly gain strength. Gains in AROM may become more difficult to achieve or maintain if adhesions begin to reform. At this stage, edema and discomfort are decreasing, and ideally, intraoperative AROM should have been achieved.

Evaluation

Evaluation includes assessment of the wound or scar, edema, AROM, PROM, discomfort, ADL performance, and sensibility (if necessary). After the wound is well healed, the scar is assessed for thickness and mobility. Thickened, immobile scars restrict tendon gliding and require immediate intervention. Edema may be assessed using either circumferential or volumetric measures after the wound is well healed. AROM, PROM, and discomfort are assessed as previously described. ADL performance may be assessed via observation, patient interview, or outcome measures such as the DASH. When used intermittently throughout treatment, the DASH has the potential to monitor changes in physical function and symptoms.[24] Sensibility may be assessed using Semmes–Weinstein monofilaments.

Treatment

Treatment goals now include maintenance of AROM as collagen bonds begin to form, edema control, scar management, functional use of the involved hand, and independence with ADLs. Following wound healing and suture removal, the treatment plan is progressed.

Moist Heat. Moist heat may be initiated to increase collagen tissue extensibility, decrease stiffness, and assist in the resolution of inflammatory infiltrates.[41] US may be initiated to increase collagen tissue extensibility and blood flow, decrease pain, improve joint mobility, and enhance tendon gliding.[41-43] When used in conjunction with hot packs, US may provide greater elevation of tissue temperature.[44]

Ultrasound. Studies on tendon healing suggest that the time at which US is initiated in the course of tendon healing is critical.[16,42,45-48] Gan and associates[46] compared the effects of early and late US treatments. They found US to be beneficial early in the healing process of flexor tendons. Other findings indicate that US may increase rate of repair, collagen synthesis and maturation, and breaking strength of healing tendons.[49,50] Many of the available studies on US have been conducted in various animal models using a variety of parameters, making it difficult to draw conclusions and make applications to the clinical setting.

Dosage parameters for US vary throughout the literature. A frequency of 3.0 MHz is recommended for treatment of the hand[51] and in treating tissues 1 to 2 cm from the skin surface.[42,43] A frequency of 1.0 MHz is used to affect deeper structures.[42,43,52] The strength of a US beam is determined by its intensity. The weakest beam or lowest possible intensity that produces the desired effect should be used when treating patients. To enhance tissue healing, US[52] should be used in the range of 0.1 to 0.5 W/cm.^{2} An intensity of 0.5 W/cm^2 may be used with acute and subacute injuries.[42] A continuous or pulsed-wave mode is selected, depending on the stage after injury and the desired therapeutic effect. Continuous-wave US is appropriate for use once the surgeon has determined that it is safe to perform a strong active contraction of the lysed tendon.[13] Continuous-wave US may be contraindicated if circulation is compromised, sensibility is altered, or edema is uncontrolled and a thermal effect is not desirable. The literature indicates that low-intensity pulsed US may be most appropriate to resolve acute and subacute inflammation; promote healing of open wounds; promote tissue healing; and enhance repair in tendon, nerve, and bone.[45,51,52] Recent findings in the literature suggest that pulsed US is able to accelerate the healing of ruptured tendons in the early healing process more effectively than continuous US.[53,54] More research is needed to determine optimal dosage parameters to achieve maximal benefits of US following tenolysis.

Scar Management. Deep friction massage is initiated once wounds are healed to help soften the scar and maintain tissue mobility as collagen bonds form and gain in strength. An elastomer or Otoform mold is fabricated or silicone gel sheeting is worn nightly to help soften thickened, immobile scars.

ROM. AROM exercises are continued with upgrades as tolerated. PROM exercises are continued, if necessary, for persistent joint stiffness.

Edema Control. Once the inflammatory phase of wound healing has ended and fibroplasia has begun, manual edema mobilization (MEM) may be added to the program if needed to further decrease edema. The reader is referred to Chapter 65 for more details regarding this very effective technique.

Orthotic Positioning. Orthotic positioning techniques are continued as previously described, with modifications as needed to account for increasing AROM and decreasing edema.

Home Program. The home program now includes deep friction massage performed four to five times per day along the scar line. Deep friction massage is performed to help soften the scar and maintain tissue mobility as collagen bonds form and gain in strength. The patient may be taught a home program of MEM to be performed several times per day if needed to decrease edema. Light ADL may be initiated to encourage functional use of the involved hand.[29]

Postoperative Weeks 4 to 6

The proliferative phase of wound healing is now ending, and scar remodeling is in process. During scar remodeling, the pattern of the collagen fibers becomes more organized and forms parallel to the wound surface. The wound should now be well healed, scars are beginning to soften, edema and discomfort are decreased or absent, AROM is equivalent to or greater than that achieved during surgery, and strength is improving.

Evaluation

Evaluation includes assessment of the scar, edema, AROM, PROM, and grip and pinch strength. In tendons of poor integrity that are being treated with a frayed exercise program, grip and pinch strength testing is delayed, possibly as long as 10 to 12 weeks.

Treatment

Treatment goals are to maintain AROM as collagen bonds continue to form and gain in strength, to continue scar management, and to increase grip and pinch strength.

AROM, PROM, and orthotic use are continued, with upgrades as tolerated. Edema control continues as indicated. Scar management techniques are continued to influence remodeling. If the surgeon reports that tendon integrity is good, sustained gripping exercises may be initiated at 3 to 4 weeks after surgery, and later progressed to increase resistance.[29] Some examples of these activities are dowel squeezes, foam squeezes, and isometric exercises. If tendon integrity is poor, sustained gripping exercises are added to the program only when indicated by the surgeon.

Home Program. The home program now includes sustained gripping exercises in addition to active exercises, deep friction massage, and light ADL. Passive exercises and edema control techniques are continued if needed. The home program should be reevaluated regularly, and exercises that are no longer needed should be eliminated from the program.

Strengthening. At 6 weeks, graded grip strengthening exercises and PREs are initiated during treatment and at home.

Whole-body conditioning must now be considered as return to work is approaching. Aerobic exercise such as walking or bicycle riding is recommended to increase whole-body strength and endurance.

Postoperative Weeks 7 to 8

The focus of treatment now begins to shift toward preparation for return to work via job simulation, work hardening, and on-site job visits.

Evaluation

Evaluation includes assessment of ROM and strength. In addition, the patient's abilities in comparison with job demands are functionally assessed. Such evaluation may include assessment of lifting, carrying, pushing/pulling, and reaching. In addition, prehension skills, material/tool handling, and endurance may be assessed.

Treatment

The treatment goals include maintaining ROM and maximizing strength while initiating light job simulation. The goal is to return the patient to work at approximately 8 to 12 weeks after tenolysis, depending on job requirements.

Heavy resistive exercises may be initiated at 8 weeks.

Outcomes Data

A review of the literature reveals varying results with respect to findings and methods of reporting data. Schneider and Hunter[12] in 1975 reported that 72% of 60 patients achieved improvement in AROM to the distal palmar crease with 48% good or excellent results. Four ruptures were reported, using a modification of Verdan's scale. Strickland[19] reported a 50% improvement in TAM in 64% of tenolysed digits. Fifteen percent of patients gained fair function; 20% did not benefit from the surgery; and 8% had ruptures.

Several researchers have reported similar, favorable results following flexor tenolysis, documenting 78% to 85% improvement in active motion with 50% to 65% of the patients categorized as having good or excellent results.[14,55-57] Birnie and Idler[58] examined flexor tenolysis performed in 26 children younger than 16 years. They achieved similar results in children aged 11 to 16 years. In children 10 and younger they obtained no good or excellent results, leading them to conclude that children younger than age 11 are not good candidates for flexor tenolysis.

Few studies report on complex cases. Jupiter and colleagues[59] report their results in 37 replanted digits and 4 thumbs requiring tenolysis. Mean TAM increased 58 degrees. Using the Strickland formula of assessment,[60] they report 13 excellent results, 11 good, 6 fair, and 11 poor. They support tenolysis after replanted fingers but not thumbs. Eggli and coworkers[61] report on 23 patients treated with tenolysis following repair of complex zone II injuries. They report significant functional improvement in 88% of the digits. TAM increased a mean of 51 degrees after dorsal tenolysis, 55 degrees after palmar tenolysis, and 63 degrees after combined tenolysis. Using the Buck–Gramcko scoring system they documented 15 excellent results, 8 good, 4 fair, and 5 poor. All patients returned to work. They report three ruptures

occurring after flexor or combined tenolysis but none following extensor tenolysis and conclude it to be a safe procedure. This is the only study that reports grip strength, documenting improvement from 45% to 75% contralateral strength. Another study by Hahn and associates[62] documented a decrease in improvement as severity of trauma increased. They reported a 110 degree increase in TAM in 84% of 36 patients and 80% good, excellent, or fair results using the Buck–Gramcko classification.

Foucher and colleagues[22] and Goloborodko[23] have published their specialized postoperative techniques and results following tenolysis. Foucher and colleagues[22] reported their results in 78 fingers, documenting a 68-degree increase in TAM in the fingers and a 50-degree increase in the thumb in 84% of the cases. No improvement was noted in four digits. Nine fingers were made worse, averaging a loss of 25.4 degrees of motion and there were two ruptures. Goloborod'ko[23] reported his results on 20 fingers, according to Strickland's formula. Results were excellent in 18 fingers, fair in 1, and poor in 1. Complications, including complete or partial ruptures and flexion contractures, were noted in five fingers.

Extensor Tenolysis

The need for tenolysis following extensor tendon repair has decreased with the use of early mobilization protocols.[63] More frequently extensor tenolysis is needed following metacarpal and phalangeal fractures that damage the extensor mechanism and result in adhesion formation and often accompany implant removal.[63-65]

These adhesions may limit flexion in addition to extension by acting as a tether on the dorsum of the finger. If both flexor and extensor surfaces require tenolysis, the extensors are released first to allow full PROM flexion before flexor tenolysis.[61,63,65]

Preoperative Management

Preoperatively, maximum PROM must be achieved. The patient only gains active extension equal to preoperative passive extension unless surgical contracture release is performed; more flexion may be gained as the tethering adhesions are removed. The patient must be cautioned that some loss of extension with the recovery of flexion is not uncommon.[15]

Surgical Technique

Through a dorsal longitudinal incision, the extensor mechanism is exposed. The dissection should begin in a nontraumatized area of the hand and proceed to the affected area.

The tenolysis technique involves mobilizing the lateral bands along its volar edge from the MCP joint up to the PIP joint. A Freer elevator should be passed volar and dorsal to the intermetacarpal ligament to provide complete lysis of any adhesions that might have formed along the lumbrical (volar) and interosseous (dorsal) tendons.

At the level of the PIP joint, the transverse retinacular ligament should be released along its volar aspect.

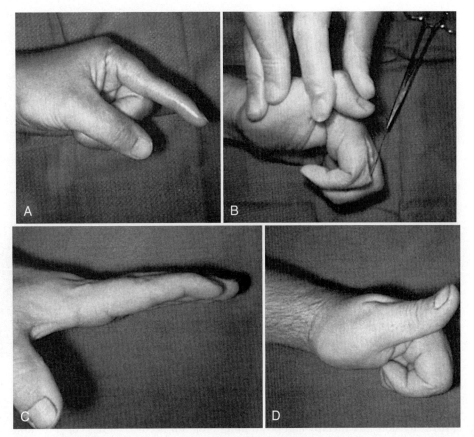

Figure 40-8 Extensor lysis. A 42-year-old man severed his extensor mechanism over the proximal interphalangeal (PIP) joint of his left index finger. After repair, extension contracture persisted despite an active exercise program. **A,** Fixed extension posture of the finger before lysis. **B,** On an operating table, after lysis of tendon adhesions and release of dorsal capsule of the PIP joint, he could flex actively to 90 degrees. **C, D,** Range of motion was retained with therapy as shown at 3 months after tenolysis.

Extreme caution should be taken to avoid damaging the insertion of the central slip into the base of the middle phalanx or damaging the triangular ligament while performing the tenolysis of the extensor mechanism.

After completion of the extensor mechanism, the patient is asked to actively flex and extend the digit. If limited flexion is still present, an intrinsic tightness test should be performed. This is done by assessing the PIP joint flexion while the MCP joint is held in extension. When intrinsic tightness is present, PIP joint flexion is limited when the MCP joint is held in extension, but if the MCP joint is flexed, the PIP joint is able to flex. If intrinsic tightness is present, intrinsic release should be performed.

If ROM is still limited, a dorsal capsulotomy of both the PIP and DIP joints should be performed. Following dorsal capsulotomies, the motion is assessed once again; if there is still some tightness, a release of the cord portion (most dorsal portion) of the collateral ligament should be performed.

If, when evaluating the motion following a capsulotomy, there is no gliding of the surfaces over each other, rather an opening dorsal wedge, it may be necessary to release the volar plate, which has most likely scarred.

Summary of Technical Points for Extensor Tenolysis[10-12]

1. Make a curvilinear incision over the adherent area (Fig. 40-8).
2. Perform tenolysis, attempting to preserve continuity of the tendon.

3. Tendon incisions between the central slip and lateral bands may be helpful for exposure.
4. Joint releases, particularly dorsal capsulotomies, are often needed.
5. Try to preserve some segment of the dorsal retinaculum at the wrist.
6. When both flexor and extensor tendons are involved in adhesions, the prognosis is notably poorer, but fingers can occasionally be salvaged (Fig. 40-9).

Postoperative Management

Following extensor tenolysis, the main principles and therapy techniques are the same as those described earlier for flexor tenolysis (see Critical Points list). Some differences are highlighted as follows.

Precautions

The extensors must be protected from overstretching during the first few postoperative weeks. Overstretching of the extensor tendon mechanism can result from an overemphasis on passive flexion exercises and can result in an active extensor lag. The extensor tendons are significantly weaker than the flexors and they may have been further weakened by being stretched prior to surgery. Active extension must be closely monitored. It is important to regain flexion but not

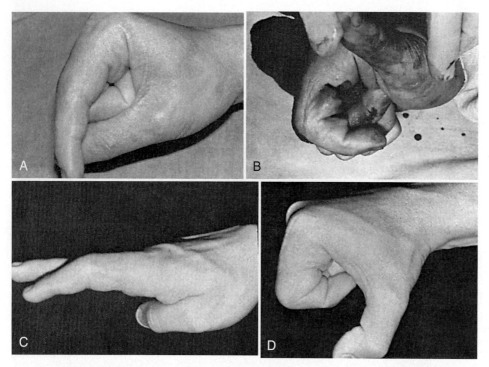

Figure 40-9 Combined extensor and flexor lysis. A 35-year-old man sustained a crush injury to his right index finger. His extensor system primarily was involved. His finger became contracted in extension, and he had only 20 degrees of flexion from a straight position at the proximal interphalangeal joint (PIP). **A,** Maximum active flexion at the PIP joint. **B,** Lysis of extensor tendon system with release of PIP joint dorsal capsule returned passive flexion, but active flexion was not regained until volar exposure revealed adhesions of the flexor tendons. With release of these adhesions, he regained active flexion as shown here. **C,** Active extension was maintained at 4 months. **D,** Active flexion also was possible at 4 months.

at the expense of extension. If the patient gains in flexion but loses extension, the therapy and positioning program needs to be adjusted to balance efforts in favor of extension.

Orthotic Positioning

Extension orthoses are used when a preoperative flexion contracture or extension lag was present. Initially, orthoses may be worn full-time with removal for AROM, wound care, and hygiene. Continued night extension positioning may be needed for up to 6 months. Orthotic use is gradually weaned as the patient demonstrates the ability to independently maintain gains in ROM.

Orthotic positioning interventions vary depending on the zone of injury. Zones I and II may require static DIP extension orthoses. Zones III and IV may require a dynamic hand-based PIP joint extension orthosis to increase motion (Fig. 40-10A). These orthoses provide low-load, prolonged stress to increase passive PIP joint extension; augment extrinsic extensor tendon function (by instructing the patient to actively extend with the rubber band traction); and allow active flexion against light resistance to increase flexor pull-through. For especially stiff PIP joints, a static progressive force (Fig. 40-10B) may be added to this same orthosis for night use to further improve PIP joint extension. Glasgow and coworkers[66] found that a daily total end-range time of more than 6 hours per day facilitated contracture resolution at a faster rate. Zones V and proximal may require dynamic MCP joint extension orthoses to support the MCP joint in extension, prevent lengthening of the extensors, and allow for full flexor excursion. If the wrist is included, the orthosis must be removed intermittently for wrist AROM.

Following extensor tenolysis, flexion positioning may be needed to increase passive flexion. Flexion positioning may be in the form of flexion gloves, dynamic or static progressive MCP or PIP joint flexion orthoses, web straps, PIP/DIP straps, or combinations of these orthoses. Such positioning must begin gently with minimal force application and be closely monitored to prevent overstretching of the extensor mechanism and subsequent extensor lags.

Passive Range of Motion

Each exercise session begins with passive extension to ensure that the tenolysed tendon is not working against tissue resistance. Caution must be taken when performing passive DIP flexion if the original injury included zone I or II.

Active Range of Motion

Active exercises must emphasize full excursion of the tenolysed extensor and possibly flexor tendons. For those patients with limited flexion, blocking is initiated cautiously, one joint at a time. The progression to full fists depends on the patient's pain level and tissue resistance.

Conditions such as extrinsic tendon tightness and intrinsic tightness must be assessed and corrected with the exercise program as well as orthotic positioning.

Some active exercises specific to the extensor tendon include the following.

1. Often called "reverse blocking," active PIP joint extension is performed while holding (blocking) the MCP joint in a hyperflexed position with the uninvolved hand (Fig 40-11). The hyperflexed MCP joint facilitates PIP joint extension. This exercise is performed to encourage PIP joint extension when the PIP joint has a flexion contracture or an extension lag and is at risk of developing a contracture.

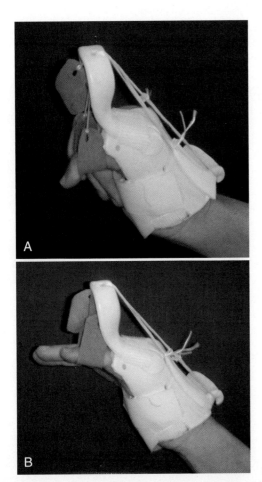

Figure 40-10 This orthosis incorporates dynamic traction and a static progressive force in one orthosis to increase motion. **A,** This dynamic proximal interphalangeal (PIP) extension orthosis may be worn daily to provide low-load prolonged stress to increase passive PIP joint extension, augment extrinsic extensor tendon function, and allow active flexion against light resistance to increase flexor pull-through and excursion. **B,** For especially stiff PIP joints, a static progressive force may be added to this same orthosis for night use to maximize total end-range time and further improve PIP joint extension.

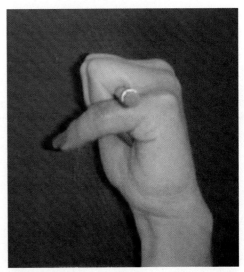

Figure 40-11 "Reverse blocking" facilitates proximal interphalangeal (PIP) joint extension in patients having a PIP joint flexion contracture or those at risk of developing a contracture. This exercise may be performed using the uninvolved hand to position the metacarpophalangeal joint in hyperflexion or a pencil as shown.

2. In Extensor Digitorum Communis (EDC) gliding exercises the patient assumes a fisted position and then moves into a hook fist and finally into full digit extension (Fig. 40-3A).

3. EDC gliding exercises in which the patient makes a fist and holds this position for 10 seconds and then moves directly into a hook fist and holds this position for 10 seconds. Then the hand returns to a fisted position. This sequence is repeated 10 times.

4. In active MCP joint extension exercises, the patient places his hand flat on the table with the MCP joints hanging over the edge. The patient is instructed to lift his fingers until they are even with his hand and hold the position for 10 seconds.

Brown and associates[67] have published their technique for achieving maximal tendon excursion in zones IV through VI (for use with tendons of good integrity) designed for the specific purpose of overcoming extensor lags at the PIP and MCP joints. Their technique involves placing the extensor tendon under load with isometric contraction in full joint flexion. The reader is referred to their article for more details.[67]

Strengthening

When extension lags are present, extensor strengthening should begin first, followed by resisted flexion exercises.

Outcomes Data

Creighten and Steichen[64] report on their series of extensor tenolyses performed after phalangeal fractures. They found TAM improved an average of 54 degrees and the active extension lag improved by 50% in patients requiring tenolysis alone. No improvement in active extension was noted in patients requiring tenolysis and dorsal capsulotomies, although TAM improved 34 degrees. They found that improvements in motion plateaued at 6 months after extensor tenolysis with dorsal capsulotomy.

Landi and coworkers[68] reported on their series of tenolyses performed after tenorrhaphy, grafting, and closed trauma. Excellent results (MCP active flexion >80 degrees, PIP flexion >90 degrees, and no extension deficit) were achieved in 19.35% of the cases. Good results (MCP flexion >70 degrees, PIP flexion >90 degrees, extension deficit <30 degrees) were achieved in 32.25%. Satisfactory results (MCP flexion >50 degrees, PIP flexion >60 degrees, and extension deficit <30 degrees) were achieved in 22.5%. Poor results (MCP flexion >50 degrees, PIP flexion <60 degrees, and extension deficit >30 degrees) were achieved in 6.5% of the cases.

Chinchalkar and associates[69] statistically analyzed the results of extensor tenolysis with dorsal capsulotomy for PIP joints with extension contractures. They analyzed 26 PIP joints in 25 patients and found that superior results were achieved by using a posterior approach to perform extensor tenolysis and dorsal capsulotomy. They reported an average gain of 38.3 degrees following this procedure.

Summary

Tenolysis is a very demanding procedure both surgically and therapeutically. In some cases, it is the final option for patients. For this procedure to be successful, the patient, surgeon, and therapist all must work cooperatively and diligently to achieve a freely gliding tendon.

REFERENCES

The complete reference list is available online at www.expertconsult.com.

Management of Hand and Wrist Tendinopathies

MARILYN P. LEE, MS, OTR/L, CHT, SAM J. BIAFORA, MD,
AND DAVID S. ZELOUF, MD

STENOSING TENDOVAGINITIS
INSERTIONAL TENDINOPATHIES
TENOSYNOVITIS ASSOCIATED WITH SYSTEMIC
    DISORDERS AND INFECTION

CONGENITAL TRIGGER DIGIT
SUMMARY

CRITICAL POINTS

- Wrist and hand tendinopathies are more common in women than men and may be attributed to increased exposure to forceful repetitive gripping or pinching.
- Patients with diabetes mellitus, rheumatoid arthritis, and other metabolic conditions have a higher incidence of wrist and hand tendinopathies, often with multiple tendon involvement.
- Nonoperative management includes nonsteroidal anti-inflammatory drugs (NSAIDs), corticosteroid injections, hand therapy, and ergonomic counseling.
- Surgery is most often indicated for patients who present with anatomical anomalies, space-occupying lesions, metabolic disorders, severe degenerative changes, and for those unresponsive to nonoperative management.

Tendons transmit forces from muscle to bone and help accomplish the movement and stability required for hand function. Tendons are subjected to tensile stresses by contraction of their respective muscles and by passive stretch. They also undergo compressive and shear stresses as they move through tight fibro-osseous tunnels en route to their insertions. These fibro-osseous tunnels maintain the tendon in close proximity to the bones to prevent bowstringing and to maximize tendon excursion.[1] Most wrist and hand tendinopathies occur in these tunnels—specifically, at the first annular (A1) pulleys in the hand and at the flexor and extensor retinacula in the wrist. These conditions are called stenosing tendovaginitis or tendon entrapment.[2] Less common in the hand and wrist are insertional tendinopathies that affect tendons at their insertions into bone, for example, the

radial wrist extensors as they insert onto the metacarpal bases.

Thickening occurs in both the tendon and the retinacular sheath. The fibro-osseous tunnel then becomes a source of constriction that results in pain and impaired tendon gliding. Systemic conditions that affect connective tissues can aggravate these conditions. For example, patients with diabetes are four to five times more likely to develop carpal tunnel syndrome (CTS) or trigger digits[3] than patients without diabetes. Patients with rheumatoid arthritis develop a proliferative synovitis that involves the synovial lining and that may invade the tendon itself. Pregnancy and its associated hormonal fluctuations can result in fluid retention, which may increase the pressure in the fibro-osseous tunnels.

In this chapter, we use *tendinopathy* as the inclusive term for all tendon pathologies, embracing acute and chronic, as well as inflammatory and noninflammatory conditions (i.e., tendinitis and tendinosis). Primary tendinopathies, resulting from local degenerative processes or overuse, are discussed first, followed by those that are secondary to systemic diseases and infection. The chapter concludes with a review of congenital trigger digit.

Stenosing Tendovaginitis

Pathology

Stenosing tendovaginitis describes the condition of the tendon and its overlying retinacular sheath that both hypertrophy, causing stenosis and constriction.[4-6] The retinacular sheath undergoes fibrocartilaginous metaplasia in which a deep layer of irregular connective tissue forms, consisting of small collagen fibers and abundant extracellular matrix (Fig. 41-1).[7] The thickness of this sheath can increase up to threefold.[8] This thickening can cause secondary changes within

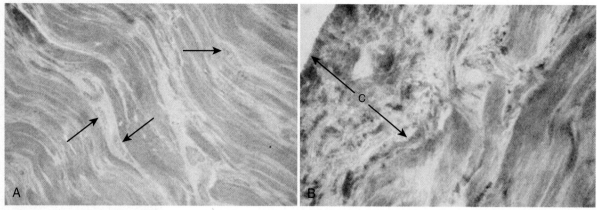

Figure 41-1 A, Specimen from a normal pulley. Among the fibers are seen spindle-shaped fibrocytes (*arrows*) (Semithin section, toluidine blue stain). **B,** Specimen from a pathologic pulley. The inner layer (C) is formed by a thin sheet of irregular connective tissue that faces the flexor tendons (Semithin section, toluidine blue stain. Original magnification ×250). (From Sbernardori MC, Bandiera P. Histopathology of the A1 pulley in adult trigger fingers. *J Hand Surg.* Eur Vol. 2007;32(5):557.)

the tendon substance, resulting in a palpable nodule. This "nodule" is often a combination of retinacular sheath thickening and intrasubstance changes within the tendon. Except in some systemic conditions, inflammation of the synovial sheath usually does not occur. In patients with tendovaginitis, biopsies demonstrate that synovial proliferation is uncommon, and that degeneration is limited to the retinacular sheath. In chronic cases, adhesions can develop between the tendons, synovium, and pulleys. Blood flow and nutrition are compromised by both constriction and thickening of tissue layers, which increases the distance for diffusion.[9] Although pain typically is present, it is not a ubiquitous symptom; for example, a patient can experience pronounced but painless triggering. The source of pain is unclear; some authors suggest that it may be the innervated tenosynovium.[10,11]

Demographics and Etiology

Tendovaginitis is more common in women than in men. Lapidus and Fenton[12] reports a female/male ratio of 4 to 1. Occupation and lifestyle may play a role, but the problem usually is multifactorial. Tendinopathies tend to cluster in some individuals. Often, multiple conditions coexist, such as CTS, trigger digits, de Quervain's disease, lateral epicondylitis, and rotator cuff disease. Over the past century, anecdotal reports and research studies have debated the role of trauma and repetitive stress in the development of tendovaginitis.[4,13]

More recently, Armstrong and colleagues[9] stated that the risk of hand and wrist tendinopathy in persons who perform highly repetitive and forceful jobs is 29 times greater, according to epidemiologic data. Assemblers, musicians, and meat cutters are vulnerable. Of 100 musicians treated at the Mayo Clinic, onset of symptoms was associated with dramatic increase in practice time; more than half presented with symptoms of tendinopathy.[14] Keyboard players stress multiple tendons at the wrist and digits[15] as they play up to 24 notes per second[16] with pronated forearms; repetitive radial and ulnar deviation of the wrist; hyperabduction of the small finger; and digital flexion, extension, and abduction. Guitarists are prone to multiple tendinopathies affecting both wrist and digital flexors as they assume extreme wrist flexion

and sustained finger pulp pressure on the left hand and sustained pinch or thumb movement on the right hand.[15] A high incidence of trigger digits has been found in meatpackers.[17] When holding knives with small, slippery handles and wearing work gloves in cold environments, the hand tends to grip more tightly, thereby increasing stress in the fibro-osseous tunnels.

Assessment

Assessment begins with a thorough history, including exploration of provocative activities and associated medical conditions that may predispose the patient to tendinopathies. The pain, which is generally localized, can be provoked with direct pressure, stretch, or resistance to the affected tendons. Acutely, there may be concomitant swelling and erythema. In subacute or chronic cases, crepitus may be palpable. At the A1 pulley, triggering or locking may be detected. Active motion that is significantly less than passive motion, may indicate poor tendon pull-through or, in rare cases, tendon rupture. When the diagnosis is unclear, some physicians recommend auscultation[15] or a transducer[18] on the premise that certain mechanical disorders produce distinctive, reproducible patterns of vibrations. Wallace notes that harsh, high-pitched rubbing sounds often are heard in stenosed, as compared with unaffected, tendon tunnels.[18]

Postoperatively, the clinician should assess wound status, edema, sensation, as well as tendon excursion and quality of gliding. As healing progresses, surgical scars should be monitored for hypersensitivity and adherence.

General Principles of Management

Although often controversial, treatment of these tendinopathies has evolved over the past century. Howard[5] advocated "adequate, complete immobilization of [the] joints ... moved by the affected ... tendons [as] the logical and most effective treatment." He stated that "baking, heat, massage, elastic compression or strapping are makeshifts and are utilized without a true understanding of the pathological changes existing." Griffiths[19] concurred that massage, heat, and cold were "useless." In subsequent decades, surgery was

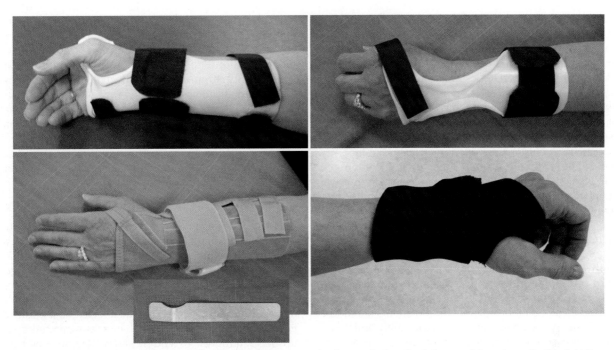

Figure 41-2 Orthotic positioning options. Clockwise from top left corner: volar thermoplastic orthosis for complete rest; semiflexible light thermoplastic dorsal-based design allowing partial wrist motion and tactile feedback on the palm; flexible neoprene wrap; prefabricated elastic wrist brace with removable bar.

advocated. Lapidus and Fenton[12] operated on 354 of 423 (84%) patients with wrist or digital tendovaginitis. They stated that, "although spontaneous recovery may occur, operative release is preferable, particularly when symptoms are present more than one month." With the advent of steroid injections in the 1950s, a decrease in the frequency of surgery followed. Lapidus and Guidotti[20] reported a 67% success rate with injection of trigger digits and the first extensor compartment of the wrist. Hand therapy also offers nonoperative interventions to resolve symptoms of hand and wrist tendinopathies and to prevent recurrence.

Reduction of Pain and Inflammation

Rest. In the acute phase, rest of the involved muscle–tendon units is indicated until symptoms subside,[19,21] and pain-producing movement should be eliminated or minimized. A rigid orthosis may be used initially for complete immobilization to abate acute symptoms; a softer, semiflexible orthosis is indicated as symptoms subside or when rigid immobilization is impractical (Fig. 41-2). Orthotic use should be gradually tapered according to symptom response and prolonged immobilization should be avoided.

Nonsteroidal Anti-inflammatory Drugs and Corticosteroids. In addition to reducing inflammation, NSAIDs may promote healing by accelerating the formation of cross-linkages between collagen fibers.[22] NSAIDs include aspirin, ibuprofen, naproxen, and the newer cyclooxygenase-2 agent inhibitors (e.g., celecoxib [Celebrex]).

Corticosteroids inhibit the inflammatory process by preventing prostaglandin synthesis and by reducing migration of white blood cells to the injured area.[23] Sampson and coworkers[24] suggest that corticosteroids may act to reduce

the fibrocartilaginous metaplasia that occurs in tendovaginitis. Steroids inhibit collagen synthesis and therefore can weaken tendons, if used in excess.[25] Corticosteroids also should be given with caution in immunocompromised patients because they interfere with the immunologic defense mechanisms.[26] Steroids can be administered orally, transcutaneously, or by injection.

Injection. In general, one or two injections of corticosteroid may be offered to the patient. These are given several weeks to months apart. If the tendovaginitis is secondary to a systemic condition such as diabetes mellitus or rheumatoid arthritis, the patient is informed that the chance of success with injection alone is reduced. Under strict sterile conditions, a mixture of lidocaine (plain with no epinephrine) and a soluble corticosteroid solution are placed in a 3-mL syringe. Generally, our preferred corticosteroid is Celestone (betamethasone). A small 27- or 25-gauge needle is used for injection. The needle should be placed in close proximity to the tendon or into the sheath, but not into tendon substance. Controversy exists about whether the efficacy of the steroid is altered by placement into or outside of the sheath, but in general, we attempt to inject the corticosteroid/lidocaine combination within the sheath. Complications include depigmentation, skin and subcutaneous atrophy, and infection, especially in the immunosuppressed patient. Patients with diabetes mellitus should be warned that a transient elevation in blood glucose may occur after the injection.[23] Wang and Hutchinson[27] reported blood glucose levels in type I and type II diabetic patients increased to 73% more than average in the first morning following trigger finger injection.

Physical Agents. Cryotherapy, thermotherapy (superficial heat and ultrasound [US]), phonophoresis, and iontophoresis are typically utilized in the rehabilitation of wrist and hand tendinopathies to reduce pain and inflammation. To date, only a paucity of evidence supports the use of these physical agents; mostly because there is a lack of well-designed studies. Anecdotal reports suggest that they may be helpful in the temporary relief of impairments such as pain, edema, and decreased range of motion (ROM). However, they should be used along with a plan of care that includes patient education, ergonomic counseling, and therapeutic exercise. Physical agents should be discontinued if no measurable benefits such as pain reduction or increased mobility are observed or cannot be attributed directly to the use of the physical agent.[28,29] The selection of the appropriate physical agent depends on patient status, equipment availability, and potential precautions or contraindications. In the future, evidence to support best practice for the use of physical agents with tendinopathies will contribute to clinical decision making.

Cryotherapy techniques may be easily applied in the clinic or as part of a home program. Ice bags or commercial cold packs are commonly used, but ice massage[30] may work best for the focal area of pain or inflammation. Patients should be advised about overuse and reinjury immediately following the application of cold because it may "mask" pain until tissue temperature increases.[31] Due to the high incidence of wrist and hand tendinopathies in patients with diabetes and rheumatoid arthritis, cold should be used with caution or avoided as these individuals often present with cold sensitivity symptoms or Raynaud's phenomenon.[32]

Thermotherapy agents such as superficial heat (hot packs, paraffin, and Fluidotherapy) and US enhance blood flow, increase soft tissue extensibility, and decrease pain.[31] Ultrasound has been shown to increase collagen synthesis, tissue repair, and tensile strength of tendons.[33-35] As previously stated, evidence to support the use of physical agents in this population is limited; however, Klaiman and associates[36] reported a significant short-term decrease in pain with the use of US in four patients with de Quervain's disease.

There is limited evidence to support the use of US as an enhancer of transdermal application of medications or other substances by increasing the kinetic energy of the local tissue. Cameron and Monroe[37] reported that betamethasone in aqueous US gel transmitted 88% of the US energy, whereas hydrocortisone lotions and creams transmitted less than 30%. To maximize delivery, Byl[33] recommends using topical agents that transmit US, pretreating the skin by warming or trimming hair (or both), and using an occlusive dressing after treatment to retain the US gel over the target tissue. Selection of US intensity should be appropriate for the phase of tissue healing. In acutely inflamed tissues, a low intensity of 0.1 to 0.2 W/cm^2 avoids a thermal effect.[28] Recommendations for optimal duty cycle vary in the literature. Some authors suggest that a low duty cycle, for example, 20%, ensures a nonthermal effect. Others believe that the continuous mode (100% duty cycle) is more efficacious.

The depth of penetration is at least 1 cm[26] for iontophoresis, so it is a convenient way to administer dexamethasone to superficial hand and wrist tendons, especially for patients who cannot tolerate injections. Research suggests that dexamethasone sodium phosphate administered iontophoretically is effective in controlling pain and inflammation, but more controlled studies are needed, especially with wrist and hand tendinopathies.[26,38-40] Preparation strength of dexamethasone sodium phosphate is typically 4 mg/mL. No optimal parameters for current dosage (mA-min) have been established for tendinopathies, but typically iontophoresis is applied until 40 mA-min is delivered.[38] Patient tolerance to current amplitude is typically the determining factor. All commercial units within the United States have maximum current amplitude of 4 mA. Recently, battery-driven electrodes have been developed that use a very low current amplitude (0.1 mA) and perform iontophoresis over several hours. Anderson concluded that this new delivery method is more effective with enhanced patient tolerance.[41]

Enhancement of Tendon Healing and Mobility

Massage. Massage is purported to improve tendon function by increasing circulation and tendon nutrition and by remodeling hypertrophic tendons, thus reducing tissue bulk at the pulleys.[36,42,43] Evans and colleagues[44] advocate massage of the entire tendon sheath and adjacent areas. Cyriax[42] popularized transverse friction massage (TFM), in which the clinician moves the patient's skin over the affected area perpendicular to tendon fiber orientation, with increasing pressure, working up to 15 minutes. If tendon and pulley are involved, they state that the clinician should hold the tendon taut and mobilize perpendicular to the sheath. Other than anecdotal reports, no controlled studies demonstrate the efficacy of TFM in the hand and wrist, particularly for stenosing tendovaginitis.[45] TFM is a vigorous technique that is not always well tolerated by the hands of the patient or the clinician performing it.

Gliding and Stretching. Gliding and stretching of the affected tendons can prevent or reduce adhesions and enhance nutrition by synovial diffusion. When the length of a muscle–tendon unit is increased, strain during joint movement is decreased.[46] Superficial thermotherapy before or in conjunction with ROM can be used to enhance tissue extensibility. Tendons should be mobilized gently, progressively, and in pain-free ranges. Tendon gliding may be used to glide both flexor and extensor tendons of the fingers (Fig. 41-3, online). Composite elbow, wrist, and digital extension brings the flexors of the wrist and digits to their full length, whereas elbow extension with composite wrist and digital flexion stretches the extensors of the wrist and digits (Fig. 41-4, online). The components of Finkelstein's maneuver can be performed in stages to glide and lengthen the tendons in the first dorsal compartment involved in de Quervain's (Fig. 41-5, online). The therapist can augment the patient's efforts at muscle–tendon lengthening by providing manual tension at the muscle bellies (Fig. 41-6, online).[47,48]

Progressive Strengthening

Strengthening may be initiated when acute symptoms have subsided. When performed in a graded, symptom-free manner, it can accelerate tenocyte metabolism, speed repair, and prepare the patient to meet the physical demands of daily activities.[49,50] Strengthening may be done in isometric, isotonic, and isokinetic modes. Isometric contractions are initiated at a muscle's resting length (roughly midrange). Lowe[51] recommends starting with brief repetitive isometric exercise for hand and wrist musculature: specifically, five repetitions,

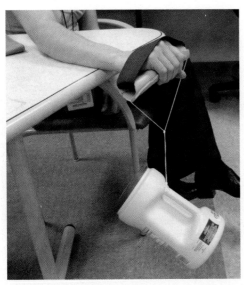

Figure 41-8 *Homemade weight for wrist strengthening with larger handle and water bottle reduces undesired tight grip and allows gradual progression of weight.*

for 6 seconds each, performed once daily. When isometrics can be performed at multiple joint angles, isotonic exercise can be added concentrically or eccentrically. Eccentric strengthening may be helpful in cases of chronic tendinitis.[46] Exercise programs should be tailored to an individual's functional needs. For a racquet ball player who requires sudden recruitment of wrist extensors for a backhand stroke, progressive resistive exercises may be most appropriate. For a typist or pianist, more frequent, submaximal repetitions may be indicated. Putty, free weights, and resistive bands are practical for home use (Fig. 41-7, online; and Fig. 41-8).

Return to Activity and Lifestyle Modifications

Activities should be resumed gradually and performed in a pain-free manner. Ergonomic modifications, including altering technique to prevent recurrence, may be required for work or sports tasks as well as for playing a musical instrument (Box 41-1). Gloves may be helpful to distribute pressure and reduce shear forces, but they may cause the wearer to grip harder in attempting to overcome fabric stiffness and compensate for impaired sensory feedback.[52] Working with the forearm in neutral or supination and the wrist in neutral or slight extension optimizes muscle efficiency and takes stress off tendons as they cross the wrist.[49,53] The motto, "bend the tool, not the wrist," has materialized into a variety of adapted equipment ranging from ergonomic keyboards to pistol grips (Fig. 41-9, online). In their randomized, placebo-controlled study, Tittiranonda and coworkers[54] found that computer users with symptoms of CTS or wrist/hand tendinitis reported the greatest relief of symptoms after 6 months of using the Microsoft Natural Keyboard (Fig. 41-10) compared with three other keyboards. Zecevic and associates[55] reported similar findings. Other strategies include using larger joints to accomplish the task, reducing task frequency and duration, and diversifying work. Finally, the clinician should encourage general health and fitness by teaching the patient principles of good nutrition; cardiovascular conditioning; and how to balance work, leisure, and rest. The effect of lifestyle choices, such as smoking, on tissue health should be explained.

Surgical Intervention and Postoperative Management

In general, surgery includes the release of constricting fibrous pulleys and, in some systemic conditions, excision of hypertrophied tenosynovium. Specific operative procedures are discussed in the following sections under their respective conditions.

After surgery, the wrist and affected digits are usually immobilized in a plaster dressing for up to 1 week postoperatively. Gentle active and passive motion are initiated by the end of the first week with the goal of achieving full joint motion and tendon glide. The clinician should also monitor wound status, edema, and sensation, as well as initiate edema reduction techniques. Thermotherapy may assist with desensitization, remodeling, and mobilization of scar. During heating, shortened tissues can be placed on stretch, followed by tendon gliding and additional lengthening[32] (Fig. 41-11, online; and Fig. 41-12). Massage, application of silicone elastomer sheeting or molds, and use of compressive wraps are indicated for hypersensitive and hypertrophic scars (Fig. 41-13). During the 3 to 6 weeks after surgery, strengthening is typically initiated as is gradual resumption of functional activity. Between the 6th and 12th weeks, the patient may return to work or sports according to his or her progress and the physical demands of the tasks in question.[56]

Types of Stenosing Tendovaginitis

Stenosing tendovaginitis can affect any of the 23 extrinsic tendons that power the wrist and hand. The digital flexor tendons are susceptible to compression and shear at the level of the wrist and the metacarpophalangeal (MCP) joints where they enter fibro-osseous tunnels. The wrist flexors, which are enveloped in synovial sheaths as they cross the carpus, occasionally are affected. Most extensor tendinopathies occur at the extensor retinaculum of the wrist. The six compartments, formed by tough fibrous septations of the extensor retinaculum and the underlying radius and ulna, collectively contain at least 12 tendons that extend the wrist or digits (or both).

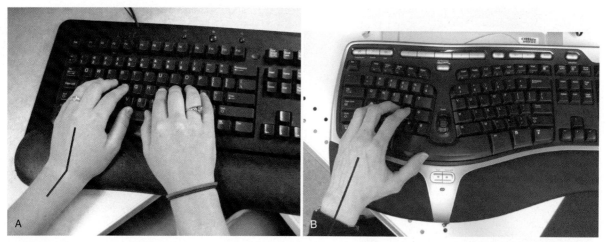

Figure 41-10 Keyboards. **A,** Standard keyboard forces wrists into ulnar deviation. **B,** Ergonomic design allows for neutral wrist position and reduces extreme forearm pronation.

The compartment containing the abductor pollicis longus (APL) and extensor pollicis brevis (EPB) tendons is by far the most commonly affected dorsal compartment, followed by the sixth compartment, which contains the extensor carpi ulnaris (ECU) tendon. Insertional tendinopathies of wrist extensors and interosseous tendons occur infrequently and are discussed in a separate section.

Flexor Tendinopathy in the Carpal Tunnel

CTS, which is discussed in depth in Chapters 48 and 49, results from compression of the median nerve at the wrist. Frequently, a source of this compression is hypertrophy of the flexor tenosynovium at the carpal tunnel deep to the nerve. Conservative management includes positioning the wrist in neutral with a wrist orthosis, flexor tendon and median nerve gliding, and activity modification. Steroid injection usually does not provide lasting relief. Success rates reported in the literature are low.[57,58] Surgical treatment includes an endoscopic or open (standard, mini, or two-incision) release of the transverse carpal ligament. When tenosynovial proliferation is a source of compression, a tenosynovectomy is performed in addition to an open release. In these cases especially, therapy should include management of pain and edema, scar control, flexor tendon gliding, and isolated exercises for flexor digitorum superficialis (FDS) and flexor digitorum profundus (FDP) tendons. These patients

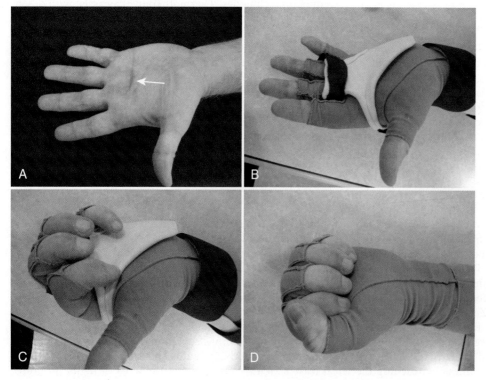

Figure 41-12 This patient had similar loss of long flexor tendon pull-through as did patient in Figure 41-11 following long and ring finger trigger finger releases **(A).** Forearm-based metacarpophalangeal blocking orthosis with compression glove **(B, C)** enhanced edema resolution as well as flexor digitorum superficialis and flexor digitorum profundis gliding and return of full fist **(D).**

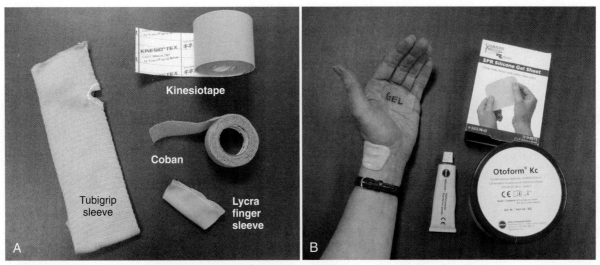

Figure 41-13 Materials for edema **(A)** and scar **(B)** management.

may require prolonged use of a wrist orthosis; a soft support can be added at night, which places the digits in relative extension to assist with resolution of digital pain and edema, and to maintain flexor tendon length.

Trigger Digits

Anatomy and Pathomechanics. Triggering of the digital flexor tendons most commonly occurs at the fibro-osseous tunnel formed by the metacarpal neck dorsally and the A1 pulley volar to the MCP joint at the distal palmar crease. In rare cases, triggering also may occur at the A3 pulley[59] or at the proximal part of A2.[60,61] At the thumb MCP joint, the sesamoid bones, on which the flexor pollicis brevis inserts, also may be a site of constriction. The FDS is generally affected because it lies directly underneath the A1 pulley.[6,58] Other authors implicate the FDP tendon,[62,63] and some speculate that adhesions between the two tendons may contribute to triggering in more advanced cases.[64,65] The tendon swells and thickens, and its fibers bunch up at the distal end of the pulley similar to strands of a thread as it is pushed through a needle's eye.[66] As first described by Notta in 1850,[62] a palpable nodule develops with an hourglass restriction adjacent to this bulbous enlargement.[12] In addition, the poor tendon vascularity between the A1 and A2 pulleys renders the tendons more susceptible to degenerative changes[67] (Fig. 41-14). A correlation between the frequency of triggering and the absence of vinculi has been documented.[68] Triggering at the A1 pulley can also occur following carpal tunnel release; bowstringing of the flexor tendons at the wrist after transverse carpal ligament transection may create more tension at the A1 pulley.[69]

During pinch activities in which forces are applied at the distal end of the digits, flexor tendons are subjected to maximal stress at the proximal end of the fibrous sheath (A1 pulley overlying the MCP joint) because the resistance arm is the longest. In addition, as MCP joint flexion increases, so does the tension on the pulley (Fig. 41-15). Gripping, pinching, or pressing with the fingers or thumb involves exertions that require tensile loading of the flexor tendons of the digits. Therefore, activities that require high tensile loading with a

flexed MCP joint over sustained or repetitive time periods, are most detrimental.[2] Direct compression at the A1 pulley from blunt trauma or sustained tool use also can be a source of injury.

Demographics. Primary trigger digit, which occurs in otherwise healthy individuals, affects women two to six times as frequently as men,[4,6,13,70] with a mean age of 58 years.[63] The thumb, ring, and long fingers are most frequently involved. The index and small fingers are involved infrequently.[12,71]

Diagnosis. The quality and ease of digital motion varies with progression of the disease, from sluggish movement on rising only, to locking and flexion contracture of the proximal interphalangeal (PIP) joint. Pain may or may not accompany the abnormal tendon gliding. When present, pain is typically at the A1 pulley and sometimes at the PIP joint. Dorsally based PIP joint pain may result from extensor overpull.[72] For more precision in classification, the quality of tendon gliding

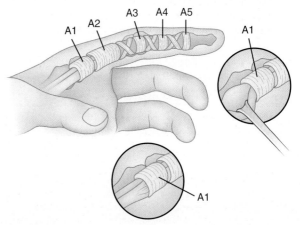

Figure 41-14 Anatomy of the flexor tendon pulley system. *Top inset,* flexor digitorum profundus nodular thickening. *Bottom inset,* flexor digitorum superficialis fraying. A1–A5, annular pulleys. (From Tara S, Miskovsky C. Nonoperative Management of trigger digits. *Atlas Hand Clin.* 1999;4:1.)

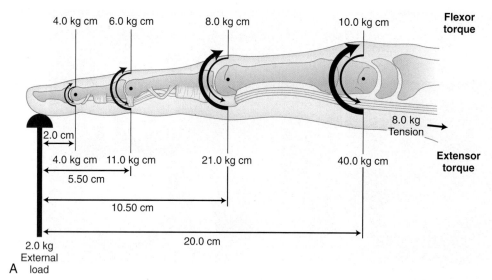

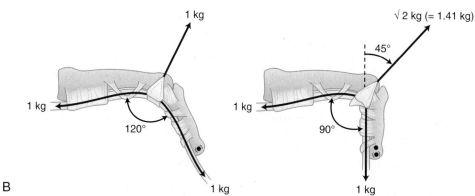

Figure 41-15 Biomechanics of stresses at the A1 pulley. **A,** The further away from a joint that force is applied, the higher the torque required to oppose that force. Thus, when an extensor force is applied to the finger tip, the flexor torque required to oppose that force is greatest at the wrist and metacarpophalangeal joints and is least at the interphalangeal joints. **B,** Tension in the flexor pulley system increases with joint flexion. (Modified from Brand P, Hoolister A. *Clinical Mechanics of the Hand.* 2nd ed. St Louis: Mosby, 1993.)

can be graded (Table 41-1). Differential diagnosis of trigger digit includes loose bodies, anomalies of sesamoid bones,[73] sesamoiditis,[74] Dupuytren's contracture, and flexor tendon masses (i.e., ganglia, tumors, and lipoma).[75]

Conservative Management. A poorer outcome with conservative measures is associated with multiple digit involvement, duration of symptoms greater than 4 to 6 months,[76,77]

Table 41-1   *Grading of Stenosing Tendovaginitis at the A1 Pulley (Trigger Digit)*

Grade	Description	Characteristics
I	Pretriggering	Pain; history of catching but not apparent on physical exam; point tenderness over A1 pulley
II	Active	Demonstrable catching but full active movement
III	Passive	Demonstrable catching:
A.	⟶	• Which requires passive extension, or
B.	⟶	• Results in an inability to flex
IV	Contracture	Demonstrable catching with a fixed flexion contracture of the PIP joint

PIP, proximal interphalangeal.
Adapted from Wolfe SW. Tenosynovitis. In: Green DP, ed. *Operative Hand Surgery.* Vol. II, 5th ed. Philadelphia: Churchill Livingstone, 2005, p. 2142.

diffuse tendon thickening versus a discrete nodule,[70] and the presence of marked triggering.[13] Many of these characteristics are present in patients with secondary trigger digit associated with connective tissue disorders.

Corticosteroid Injection.

EFFICACY. Success rates reported in the literature vary between 50% and 94%.[6,11,58,71] Success generally is defined as complete resolution of symptoms, or only minimal and occasional symptoms that do not interfere with function. Some studies do not specify duration of the symptom-free period following the injection or patient characteristics such as coexisting medical conditions. In general, success rates are much lower in individuals with comorbidities such as diabetes (50%)[78] as compared with the general population (72%–93%). In a study of 235 nonrheumatoid patients with 338 trigger digits, Newport and colleagues[76] reported that 77% resolved or improved after one to three injections. Follow-up time averaged 3 years with no orthotic positioning or other treatment given. Baumgarten and coworkers[79] performed a prospective, randomized, double-blinded study comparing the results of corticosteroid injection in patients with and without diabetes. They reported 86% success rate after one or two injections in patients without diabetes. Their group of patients with diabetes achieved a 63% success rate after one or two injections of corticosteroids compared with a 53%

success rate in their placebo group of patients with diabetes receiving 1% lidocaine alone. No statistical significance was found between the diabetic groups. Patients with systemic manifestations of diabetes (nephropathy) had fewer successful responses to corticosteroid injections. Kazuki and associates[80] prospectively studied extrasynovial steroid injection in 129 trigger fingers. Pain and snapping were relieved in 98% and 74%, respectively. Recurrence occurred in about half of their patients. Some controversy does exist about the need for intrasynovial injection for trigger finger. Taras and Miskovsky[65] performed a prospective randomized study to determine the accuracy of attempted intrasheath injection and whether true intrasheath injection offers superior outcomes over injection into subcutaneous tissue overlying the A1 pulley. Radiopaque dye was used to identify accuracy on postinjection radiographs. In the attempted intrasheath group, steroid solution was completely within tendon sheath in 19/52 (37%) fingers. Nine (17%) digits showed no evidence of steroid within the sheath. In the all sheath group, 9 fingers (47%) had good results. In the subcutaneous group, 45 fingers (70%) had good results. Although the power of this study did not achieve statistical significance, the results demonstrated a trend in which extrasynovial injections proved as effective as intrasynovial injections in treating trigger fingers. Despite the results of this study, we continue to attempt intrasynovial injection of corticosteroid. Delayed FDS and FDP ruptures after steroid injection for a trigger finger have been reported.[81]

AUTHOR'S (DZ) PREFERRED TECHNIQUE. Injection techniques vary,[58,76,81,82] but we generally use a combination of 0.2 mL of 2% lidocaine (plain without epinephrine) with 1.0 mL of a soluble corticosteroid (betamethasone). With the patient's hand prepped and the affected digit slightly extended, the surgeon palpates the metacarpal head and introduces the needle directly into the flexor tendon sheath. If necessary, placement of the needle can be confirmed by asking the patient to flex and extend the digit; it moves if it is properly located. The needle should be withdrawn slowly, and when it emerges from the tendon into the sheath, resistance is reduced. As the corticosteroid/lidocaine solution is injected, a fluid wave may be palpated proximally or distally to the injection site. Godey and coworkers[82] describe a technique using US for accurate injection of steroid in treatment of trigger finger.

Orthoses. There is a dearth of literature on using orthoses on trigger digits. Rhoades and associates[77] reported a 72% success rate with orthoses and injection; therefore, no conclusion could be drawn about the efficacy of the orthosis alone. The affected digits were positioned with MCP and interphalangeal (IP) joints in 15 degrees of flexion continuously for 3 weeks. Eaton[21] advocated a similar orthotic design for night use primarily. He stated that the orthosis draws the tendons distally, reducing the redundancy and swelling at the pulley entrance, thereby allowing the tendons to glide more easily in the morning. Based on a similar rationale, in 1988 Evans and colleagues[44] introduced a hand-based orthosis that rests the MCP joints at 0 degrees, leaving the IP joints free. They reported a 73% success rate in 55 fingers of 38 nonrheumatoid patients with daily use of the orthosis and hook fisting exercises for 3 to 6 weeks. PIP flexion contractures were treated with nighttime PIP extension orthoses. Results

were best in patients with a symptom duration of less than 4 months. Patel and Bassini[11] used an orthotic design and extrinsic tendon gliding protocol similar to that of Evans and colleagues.[38] They reported a success rate of 66% in 50 digits treated with a 3- to 9-week course of full-time positioning and exercise alone, as compared with 84% in another 50 digits treated with injection alone. Fingers fared much better with orthoses than did thumbs: 70% versus 50% success rates, respectively. The authors did not include information about coexisting medical conditions in their sample. Most recently, Rodgers and colleagues[63] positioned 31 fingers in orthoses, of meatcutters who had symptoms of pain or triggering but not locking. They reported a 55% success rate, with an average of 8 weeks of positioning only the distal interphalangeal (DIP) joint in extension. In contrast to other authors, they hypothesized that the FDP is involved in the pathogenesis of trigger finger and by decreasing its excursion, the synovitis or nodule may resolve. In summary, extension of one or more of the digital joints may be necessary to reduce or eliminate symptoms. A simple way to guide the clinician's orthosis selection is to hold a given joint of an involved digit in extension while allowing the other joints to flex, noting the effect of each position on pain and smoothness of tendon glide. The least restrictive orthosis that accomplishes this goal should be used.[83] For trigger fingers, we recommend an MCP joint extension orthosis with IP joints free to promote flexor tendon gliding and nutrition as well as resolution of intrinsic tightness. However, for thumbs, a small extension orthosis on the IP joint is most practical for hand function and usually eliminates triggering while being worn (Fig. 41-16).

Exercise and Activity. According to Wehbé and Hunter,[84] tendon gliding exercises are helpful in improving tendon nutrition and in resolving nodules and adhesions. In the hook-fist position, differential gliding between the FDS and FDP tendons is maximal, and triggering usually does not occur. Evans and colleagues[44] advocate hook-fisting 20 times in an orthosis and place-holding in a full fist every 2 hours while awake (see Figs. 41-3D and 41-16A), augmented by massage to the entire digital tendon–sheath unit. As stated previously, full and repetitive fisting should be avoided while symptoms persist. Resistive exercises can be performed in alternative hand positions, such as hook-fisting, and a modified intrinsic-plus position (see Fig. 41-7). This also is important in patients with CTS both preoperatively and postoperatively, as overzealous exercise can precipitate triggering at the A1 pulley.

Surgery. Surgery may be indicated when conservative treatment has failed, as well as in patients with significant fixed flexion contractures. Cure rates reported in the literature range from 60% to 100% and are usually at least 85%.[64,85-88] Various techniques for percutaneous trigger finger release have been described.[64,83,89-97] Authors report excellent results ranging from 73.7% to 100%.[64,89,91-94,96,97] In a prospective randomized trial of open versus percutaneous release in 100 trigger fingers, Gilberts and coworkers[98] successfully treated 98% of cases using the open technique and 100% of cases using a percutaneous technique. These results were not statistically significant.

TECHNIQUE. Trigger digits can be released via open or percutaneous means. The open technique is performed under

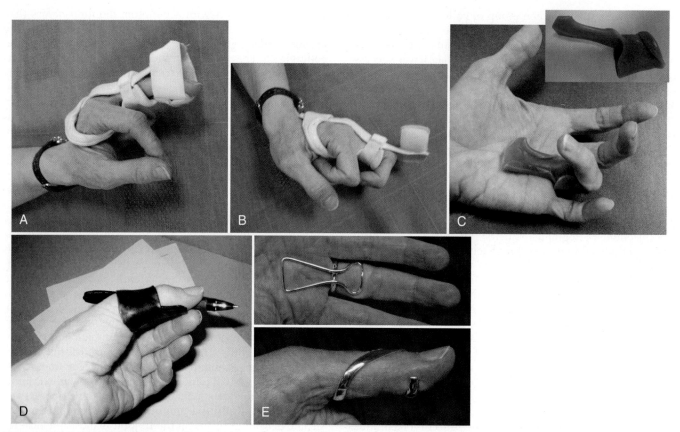

Figure 41-16 Orthotic positioning options for trigger digits. **A,** Hand-based metacarpophalangeal (MCP) extension orthosis. **B,** For proximal inter-phalangeal flexion contracture, dorsal component for static progressive extension. **C,** Paddle design blocks MCP flexion but allows extension; slip-on design allows for easy donning and doffing (based on design by Linder-Tons and Ingell, 1998). **D,** Slip-on thumb interphalangeal flexion block orthosis. **E,** Silver ring orthoses for chronic triggering (photographs courtesy of Silver Ring Splint Company, www.silverringsplint.com).

local anesthesia with or without sedation. A tourniquet is typically utilized. A 1.0- to 1.5-cm transverse incision is made over the metacarpal head of the affected finger. We typically utilize an incision within the MCP flexion crease. Blunt dissection is carried down through the subcutaneous tissues and the palmar fascia to the flexor sheath. The proximal edge and the entire A1 pulley is identified. The proximal edge of the A2 pulley also is identified. The entire A1 pulley and the palmar aponeurosis pulley are incised. Care is taken not to damage the A2 pulley. We most often excise the central portion of the A1 pulley to prevent recurrent or persistent triggering. The patient is asked to actively flex and extend the finger to ensure that the triggering has been eliminated. In cases with continued triggering despite adequate release of the palmar and A1 pulleys, we check for adhesions between the FDS and FDP tendons or hypertrophic tenosynovium. Surgical options for the complex trigger digit include partial sublimis resection, full sublimis resection, or reduction flexor profundus tenoplasty.[72] A small hand dressing is then applied, leaving the fingers free.

Percutaneous release has been advocated by some surgeons. This is performed with sterile technique in the office. After a local anesthetic is infiltrated into the region, a 19-gauge needle is placed in the A1 pulley, and, with a sweeping motion, the A1 pulley is released. The finger must be trigger-ing for this to be performed in the office. Complete release is confirmed by asking the patient to actively flex and extend the digit. Some surgeons are performing percutaneous release of thumb and index trigger fingers. We do not advocate this because of the risk of injury to neurovascular structures. It also should not be used in cases of complex trigger digit in which additional procedures, such as debulking of the bulbous nodule (i.e., reduction flexor tenoplasty) and release of adhesions between the FDS and FDP, may be required[72] (Fig. 41-17).

COMPLICATIONS. Complications include digital nerve injury, stiffness, and inadvertent sectioning of the A2 pulley, which can result in bowstringing of the flexor tendons and subsequent loss of full-finger flexion as well as full PIP joint extension. Recurrent and/or persistent triggering and scar hypertrophy have also been reported.[90,91,99] Bowstringing or tendon or neurovascular injury has not been reported in percutaneous trigger release.[83,89-91,94,96,97] If digital nerve injury does occur, the patient should undergo prompt surgical exploration and repair or reconstruction. Individuals with significant preoperative PIP joint flexion contractures most often do not regain full motion despite surgical release and postoperative therapy.

POSTOPERATIVE MANAGEMENT. Active motion can be initiated on the day of the procedure.[6] Patients who fail to regain

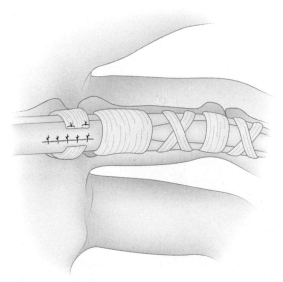

Figure 41-17 Surgical release of A1 pulley: reduction flexor tenoplasty for complex trigger digit. (From Osterman AL, Sweet S. The treatment of complex trigger digit with proximal interphalangeal joint contracture. *Atlas Hand Clin.* 1999;4:9.)

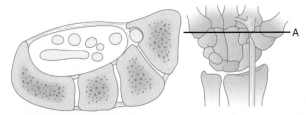

Figure 41-18 Anatomy of the flexor carpi radialis (FCR) tendon tunnel. *Left,* Cross section of the FCR tunnel at the distal aspect of the trapezium. The FCR tunnel consists of the trapezial crest palmarly, the trapezial body radially, the trapezium-trapezoid joint and trapezoid dorsally, and the retinacular septum ulnarly. The tendon occupies 90% of the available space in the tunnel. *Right,* Insertions of the FCR tendon (A). (From Bishop AT, Gabel GT, Carmichael SW. Flexor carpi radialis tendinitis. Part I: Operative anatomy. *J Bone Joint Surg.* 1994;76A:1011.)

full, smooth ROM by the third postoperative day,[62] those with PIP flexion contractures, or those who develop hypertrophic or hypersensitive scars should undergo formal hand therapy. Initial hand therapy should include wound and edema management and tendon gliding. An orthosis supporting the MCP in extension can protect the incision while allowing IP joint motion. When PIP flexion contractures are present, a dorsal piece can be added for static progressive PIP joint extension (see Fig. 41-16B). Strengthening usually can be initiated after 3 weeks, but resumption of forceful composite fisting should be delayed or minimized by patients who are prone to triggering in multiple digits.

Flexor Carpi Radialis Tendinopathy

Etiology and Pathology. The flexor carpi radialis (FCR) tendon is prone to both primary stenotic tendovaginitis and injury secondary to degenerative changes or trauma of the carpus. The FCR tendon occupies 90% of its fibro-osseous tunnel, which is formed by the ridge of the trapezium and the carpal ligament (Fig. 41-18). The FCR tendon runs a sharply angulated course around the trapezium to its primary insertion on the base of the index metacarpal, also sending slips to the trapezial tuberosity and the base of the third metacarpal.[100] FCR tendinopathy can be confused with ganglion cysts, basal joint degenerative arthritis, scaphoid fractures and nonunions, and de Quervain's disease. Traumatic or degenerative changes of the carpus, particularly at the scaphotrapezial joint, may coexist with FCR tendinopathy, particularly in older women. Parellada and associates[101] have described the anatomic and functional relationship between the FCR tendinopathy and scaphotrapezium trapezoidal osteoarthritis demonstrated by MRI. Fitton and colleagues[102] have proposed that an underlying degenerative process may be responsible for the attritional changes seen in and around the tendon. These include fraying or rupture of the tendon,

hyperemia of synovial tissue, thickening of the sheath, adhesions, and exostosis formation.

Symptoms. Pain over the proximal wrist crease and at the scaphoid tubercle is common. The pain may radiate distally to the thenar eminence or proximally into the forearm.[103] Localized swelling may be evident. Pain can be provoked with resisted wrist flexion and radial deviation. Passive wrist extension, which stretches the tendon, also may provoke discomfort.

Management. The initial treatment for FCR tendinopathy consists of nonoperative measures. The options include immobilization with a forearm-based supportive wrist orthosis, NSAIDs, and corticosteroid injection.[103] Gabel and coworkers[104] state that conservative treatment usually is effective for primary FCR tendinopathy, but surgery often is necessary for other local lesions. Attritional rupture may occur if the underlying pathologic condition is not addressed. Surgical procedures include release of the sheath, decompression of the tunnel, and excision of a ganglion or exostosis, if present. The tendon usually is approached through a longitudinal incision over the tendon that extends proximally from the wrist crease. Injury to the palmar cutaneous branch of the median nerve and the thenar branches of the radial sensory nerve must be avoided. The sheath is opened proximally and then followed distally beyond the trapezial tunnel. The tendon should be inspected thoroughly. Osteophytes along the trapezial ridge should be removed, and the tendon sheath should be left open. A conforming dressing is applied, and wrist motion is encouraged postoperatively. In two studies reviewed, success rates postoperatively ranged between 80% and 90%.[102,104]

Flexor Carpi Ulnaris Tendinopathy

Symptoms and Provocation. The flexor carpi ulnaris (FCU) is the most common wrist flexor involved in tendinopathy.[103,105] FCU tendinopathy may also accompany pisotriquetral arthrosis. Symptoms generally are localized to the FCU insertion into the pisiform and hypothenar fascia. Pain can radiate both proximally to the forearm and medial elbow, and distally to the ulnar side of the hand. In their patients with FCU tendinopathy, Budoff and associates[106] describe the point of maximal tenderness to be approximately 3 cm proximal to the FCU insertion into the pisiform. The pain can be provoked by resisted wrist flexion and ulnar deviation. Passive stretching of the FCU (e.g., wrist extension and radial deviation) also may provoke discomfort. FCU tendinopathy is often bilateral.[107] Activities that can provoke FCU tendinopathy include golf, racquet sports, and badminton.

Management. Treatment for FCU tendinopathy usually is nonoperative. In the acute phase, NSAIDs and a resting orthosis in slight wrist flexion are used. Surgery is indicated rarely; however, for individuals with chronic FCU tendinopathy, a subperiosteal pisiform excision, which preserves the continuity of the FCU tendon, and a Z-plasty tendon lengthening may provide relief.[108] Budoff and associates[106] describe six cases of FCU tendinopathy that failed nonoperative management. These patients underwent debridement of degenerative tissue, which appeared to occur preferentially in the deep surface of the FCU tendon. Angiofibroblastic hyperplasia (i.e., tendinosis) was diagnosed in all cases. Of the five patients available for follow-up, all reported complete relief or near-complete relief of their symptoms at an average period of 20 months.

De Quervain's Disease

Fritz de Quervain, a Swiss surgeon, described stenosing tendovaginitis of the first dorsal compartment in 1895. In the 1893 edition of *Gray's Anatomy*, a similar condition named washerwoman's sprain was described.[6] De Quervain's stenosing tenosynovitis is a common condition; in two series reviewed, it made up more than one third of all cases of tendovaginitis affecting the hand and wrist.[12,109]

Anatomy and Pathology. The APL and EPB tendons pass through the first dorsal compartment of the extensor retinaculum, which is approximately 2 cm in length (Fig. 41-19). However, the synovial sheaths encasing the tendons are of much greater length. There is a great deal of anatomic variation between individuals. In fact, fewer than 20% of individuals may have the "normal" anatomy. The EPB is always thinner than the APL and may be absent in 5% to 7% of people. The APL often has two, three, or more tendinous slips that may insert into the base of the first metacarpal, trapezium, volar carpal ligaments, opponens pollicis, or abductor pollicis brevis. The EPB may occupy its own compartment.[110] In a study of 300 cadaveric wrists, 40% had a septation between the APL and the EPB. In contrast, in two studies of surgical patients with de Quervain's syndrome, 67% to 73% had this septation.[111,112] As in other types of tendovaginitis, the fibrous retinaculum hypertrophies. The synovial membrane is thickened except at the point of constriction. The tendons may have an hourglass appearance and can be bound together by fine adhesions.[107,113] In their review of 23 patients treated surgically for de Quervain's disease, Clarke and colleagues[114] observed thickening of the tendon sheath and an accumulation of mucopolysaccharide, indicating myxoid degeneration. Myxoid degeneration within the intracellular matrix of the tendon sheath in the absence of active inflammation was the characteristic finding in their series.

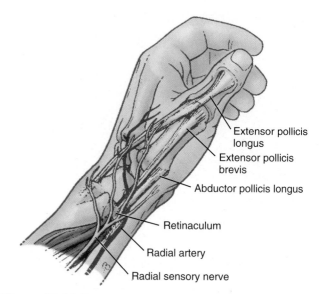

Extensor pollicis longus

Extensor pollicis brevis

Abductor pollicis longus

Retinaculum

Radial artery

Radial sensory nerve

Figure 41-19 First extensor compartment, radial nerve and artery. (From Bednar JM, Santarlasci PR. First extensor compartment release and retinacular sheath reconstruction for De Quervain's tenosynovitis. *Atlas Hand Clin.* 1999;4:39.)

Etiology and Associated Factors.

Cumulative Microtrauma. Forceful, sustained, or repetitive thumb abduction and simultaneous wrist ulnar deviation may contribute to the development of de Quervain's tendovaginitis. Opening jars, wringing the hands, cutting with scissors, holding surgical retractors, playing the piano, and doing needlepoint are a few examples of provocative activities.[6,16,19,113,115] In contrast to Finkelstein,[113] Muckart[110] suggested that radial deviation with pinch is more stressful than thumb abduction with ulnar deviation because the APL and EPB tendons are taut and sharply angulated at the wrist and trapeziometacarpal joints. This results in a "tearing strain" at the distal edge of the pulley. Muckart also argued that friction is not a significant factor, citing Thompson and associates,[116] who studied 419 cases of peritendinitis crepitans in factory workers, of whom only 2 developed de Quervain's disease.

Sex. As in other conditions of stenosing tendovaginitis, women are more susceptible to de Quervain's disease than men by at least a 4 to 1 ratio.[58,107,110,112] The incidence is high in persons 35 to 55 years of age. Women in the third trimester of pregnancy and those with young children also are vulnerable.[110,117,118] Increased acute angulation of the tendons in women may be a predisposing factor.[119]

Acute Trauma. Although less common, acute injuries to the first dorsal compartment can occur. A sudden wrenching of the wrist and thumb while trying to restrain an object or person, or a fall on an outstretched hand, can precipitate injury.

Diagnosis and Physical Examination. The most common complaint of de Quervain's tendovaginitis is radial-sided wrist pain, specifically at the first dorsal compartment over the radial styloid, which can radiate to the thumb or distal forearm. The pain is aggravated with movement of the thumb. Typically, increased tensile load on the EPB or APL (i.e., stretching or contraction) intensifies the pain. Finkelstein's test is typically positive: with the thumb held in the palm and

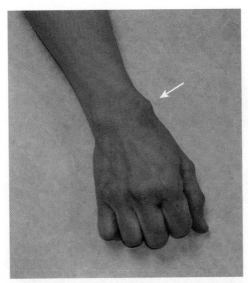

Figure 41-20 Note visible prominence (*arrow*) in patient with de Quervain's disease.

the wrist ulnarly deviated (see Fig. 41-6E), the patient often experiences sharp pain because the tendons are simultaneously stretched and compressed over the radial styloid.[113] Wrist flexion and extension can be added to this maneuver; flexion should intensify the pain and extension should relieve it.[24] Resisted thumb extension is usually painful and reproduces symptoms. Other symptoms include swelling, occasionally a visible prominence (Fig. 41-20), and, very rarely, pseudotriggering (approximately 1% of cases). Additional sources of radial-sided wrist pain must be considered; these include trapeziometacarpal arthritis, scaphoid fractures, arthritis of the radioscaphoid or scaphotrapezial trapezoidal joints, scapholunate instability, intersection syndrome, and radial neuritis (Wartenberg's syndrome).[6,13] Some of these conditions can coexist with de Quervain's disease. Radiographic studies should be performed to rule out many of the aforementioned conditions. MRI may show increased fluid in the first extensor compartment (Fig. 41-21).

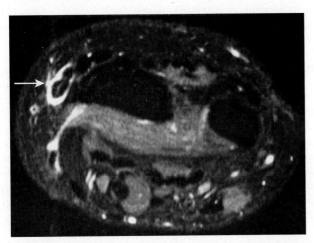

Figure 41-21 MRI showing increased fluid in the first extensor compartment.

Nonoperative Management.

Activity Modification and Orthotic Positioning. Adapted or alternative equipment that minimizes ulnar deviation at the wrist and substitutes power grip for pinch can be used. Examples include ergonomic keyboards, tools with a pistol grip, and a key holder. Strong evidence in the literature to support the efficacy of wrist orthoses is lacking.[110] Stern[107] recommended a 3-week trial of positioning, with the wrist in neutral and the thumb radially abducted in a wrist orthosis. Witt and colleagues[112] reported a 62% satisfactory outcome with injection and placing the wrist in 20 degrees of extension and the thumb MCP and IP joints in extension within an orthosis. Weiss and coworkers[120] reported only a 30% success rate with orthoses alone in 37 patients, as compared with a 69% success rate for injection alone and 57% for the injection plus orthosis. They concluded that the use of orthoses provided no additional benefit when combined with cortisone injection. Avci and associates[121] studied de Quervain's disease of pregnancy and lactation in 18 patients. All nine patients who received injections alone reported complete resolution of pain. None of the nine patients who wore orthoses had complete relief of pain; however, at the end of the lactation period, eight had spontaneous resolution of symptoms. Lane and colleagues[122] advocate steroid injection as the initial treatment in patients whose symptoms are severe enough to interfere with activities of daily living. In our clinical experience, the use of a wrist orthosis in the acute phase can assist with symptom control; the orthosis can be removed for brief periods of movement in pain-free ranges. As pain subsides, the patient can progress from a rigid support to a flexible support (Fig. 41-22).

Injection. Success rates ranging from 50% to 90% are reported in the literature following one to two injections.[6,58,117] In Medl's series,[13] patients with a symptom duration of less than 2 months had a success rate of 90%.

TECHNIQUE. The area over the radial styloid is prepped. The APL and EPB can be palpated easily as the patient abducts and extends the thumb. The two tendons are bracketed by the gloved index finger and thumb of the examiner proximal to the radial styloid. The needle is introduced into the tendon sheath. Initially, resistance may be felt. The needle is withdrawn slowly while pressure is maintained on the plunger of the syringe. When the resistance lessens, half the corticosteroid and lidocaine solution is injected. A fluid wave should be palpable both proximally and distally to the injection site. The needle then should be redirected more ulnarly in an attempt to infiltrate the sheath of the EPB (which may be in a separate compartment).

Operative Management.
Surgical release of the first dorsal compartment is indicated after failed conservative management and pain relief following diagnostic injection.[6] Patients with pseudotriggering respond poorly to conservative measures and very often require surgical release.[123] Success rates are typically high; most recently, Ta and coworkers[124] reported that 91% of 43 surgical patients were satisfied and had complete symptom resolution. Yuasa and Kiyoshige[125] stressed the importance of release of the EPB subcompartment. Seventy-three percent of their patients with de Quervain's disease were found to have an EPB subcompartment. Release of this compartment alone in these

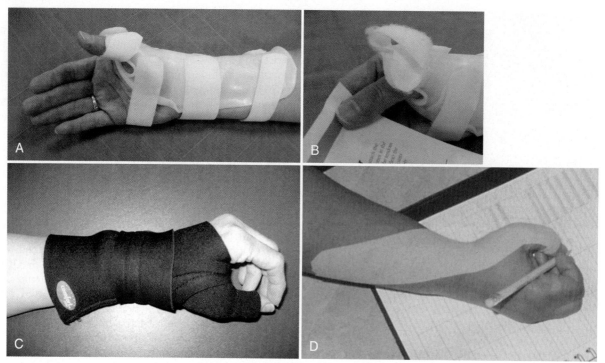

Figure 41-22 Positioning and taping options for de Quervain's syndrome. **A,** Thermoplastic forearm-based thumb orthosis providing complete rest for the abductor pollicis longus and extensor pollicis brevis. **B,** With removable strap to allow metacarpophalangeal flexion. **C,** Flexible neoprene thumb/wrist orthosis. **D,** Kinesiotape.

patients completely relieved their symptoms. Although we do not advocate release of this subcompartment alone, its presence should not be overlooked.

Technique. The procedure is typically performed under local anesthesia in conjunction with IV sedation. A pneumatic tourniquet is placed on the upper arm. We typically utilize a longitudinal incision over the first dorsal compartment approximately 1 cm proximal to the radial styloid. A longitudinal incision as opposed to a transverse incision improves visualization and also affords less retraction on the branches of the superficial radial nerve. Great care is taken to identify and protect these sensory nerve branches as injury can result in prolonged pain and dysfunction. These branches cross the compartment obliquely and are just deep to the dermal layer. The annular ligament covering the compartment should then be incised along its dorsal margin. Complete excision of the sheath should be avoided as palmar subluxation of the tendons may ensue. It is important to look for a separate compartment for the extensor brevis tendon and to fully release it if present. A tenosynovectomy is recommended if necessary. The tendons are explored individually and are lifted out of the tunnel to ensure complete decompression from the musculotendinous junction to a point at least 1 cm distal to the retinaculum. Once the procedure is completed, the wrist is passively flexed and the tendons inspected for palmar subluxation. If present, a portion of the retinaculum can be used to prevent palmar subluxation. Care is taken to ensure that the reconstructed sheath is not too tight (Fig. 41-23). Hemostasis is attained after deflation of the tourniquet and the skin is closed. A bulky hand dressing is applied, followed by a plaster thumb spica orthosis.

Complications. Complications include iatrogenic injury to the radial sensory nerve, which can result in painful neuroma formation. Vigorous retraction of the nerve may produce a neuroma-in-continuity. Other complications include reflex sympathetic dystrophy, scar hypersensitivity or adhesion, incomplete release, and tendon subluxation.[126] Incomplete relief of pain is not uncommon. Other associated diagnoses, including carpometacarpal (CMC) joint arthritis, should be considered. In cases of persistent pain, the possibility of a separate, unreleased EPB compartment should be considered. Louis[127] states that in such cases, pain can be reproduced by placing the patient's thumb in radial abduction and passively flexing the MCP joint: In this maneuver, the EPB is stressed while the APL is placed on slack. Symptomatic tendon palmar subluxation occasionally requires reconstruction using a portion of the brachioradialis tendon.

Postoperative Management. The hand is maintained in an orthosis for the first 7 to 10 days. If a primary reconstruction of the sheath has been performed, a static orthosis maintaining the wrist joint in about 20 degrees of extension is typically utilized for 3 weeks. If the sheath has not been reconstructed, a forearm-based thumb spica orthosis is used during the first 2 to 3 weeks to control postoperative pain and swelling. Gentle active ROM and tendon gliding should be initiated in the first few days postoperatively. The goal is full, pain-free excursion of the APB and EPB, approximating Finkelstein's test position. Grip and pinch strengthening starting at approximately 2 weeks can be progressed gradually. By 6 weeks, the patient usually is able to resume heavier activities.[128]

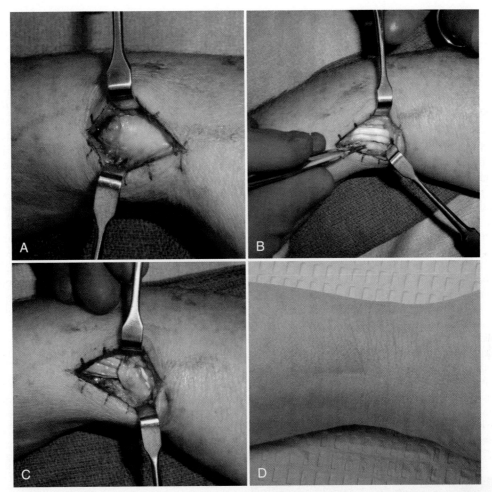

Figure 41-23 Surgical release of first extensor compartment. **A,** Typical thickened retinaculum in de Quervain's disease. **B,** Retinaculum has been released along its dorsal margin. **C,** Retinacular reconstruction with local tissue to prevent volar subluxation of extensor pollicis brevis/abductor pollicis longus tendons. **D,** Mature longitudinal incision for first dorsal compartment release.

Intersection Syndrome

As its name suggests, intersection syndrome occurs at the intersection of the radial wrist extensor tendons as they pass underneath the muscle bellies of the APL and EPB approximately 4 cm proximally to Lister's tubercle[10] (Fig. 41-24). Intersection syndrome has been variably described as stenosing tenosynovitis of the second dorsal compartment with pain and swelling of the overlying muscle bellies of the APL and EPB;[6] exertional compartment syndrome of the APL and EPB muscles;[103] and peritendinous bursal inflammation, or "squeaker's wrist."[129] According to Wolfe,[6] it is the synovium of the second dorsal compartment tendons that becomes inflamed rather than a separate bursa. It is seen frequently among athletes, particularly weightlifters and rowers. Findings include localized pain and swelling 4 cm proximal to wrist, and in more severe cases, redness and painful crepitation with thumb and wrist movements. Grip and pinch are often painful and weak. The patient may report a history of repetitive wrist or thumb activities.[129]

Conservative management is similar to that for de Quervain's syndrome. A steroid injection into the second dorsal compartment; use of a forearm-based wrist or thumb spica orthosis; and activity modification, including avoidance

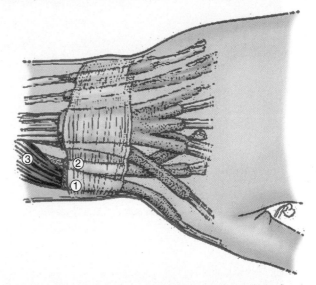

Figure 41-24 Anatomy of intersection region includes (1) the first dorsal compartment, (2) the second dorsal compartment, and (3) the muscles bellies of the first dorsal compartment tendons (abductor pollicis longus, extensor pollicis brevis) overlying the second dorsal compartment tendons (extensor carpi radialis longus, extensor carpi radialis brevis). (Reproduced with permission from Kirkpatrick WH. Intersection syndrome. *Atlas Hand Clin.* 1999;4:55.)

of repetitive wrist flexion and extension, typically relieve symptoms. For recalcitrant cases, the second dorsal compartment can be released surgically and inflamed bursa can be removed, if present.[6,10,103] Postoperatively, an orthosis supporting the wrist in slight extension can be worn for 1 to 2 weeks, followed by progressive mobilization.

Tendovaginitis of the Digital Extensors

The long extensor tendon of the thumb, extensor pollicis longus (EPL), found in the third dorsal compartment, angulates sharply around Lister's tubercle. The EPL tendon can be affected adversely by degenerative or inflammatory conditions of the wrist, distal radius fractures, or a hypertrophied muscle belly extending into the third dorsal compartment.[6,103] In their report of two cases of tendovaginitis of the third dorsal compartment, Mogensen and Mattsson[130] found the muscle of the EPL to extend into the third dorsal compartment. Their dissections of 15 cadaveric specimens revealed the musculotendinous junction ending within the compartment in 27%. Provocative activities, though rarely causative, include repetitive wrist and thumb motions, especially in extreme excursions. Musicians who play drums, accordions, and other keyboards are susceptible as are writers who hold their pens in dorsiflexion and radial deviation.[4] Symptoms include pain, swelling, tenderness, and often crepitus at Lister's tubercle. Pain may radiate proximally or distally.[4] Both active and passive flexion of the IP joint may elicit pain. Conservative management includes NSAID use and forearm-based thumb orthosis, with the IP joint included. In recalcitrant cases, a corticosteroid injection may be required. Surgical release of the third dorsal compartment occasionally is necessary to prevent attritional rupture of EPL tendon.[105] A 2-cm incision centered over Lister's tubercle is utilized, with care taken to avoid injury to the branches of the radial sensory nerve. The third dorsal compartment is identified and incised. The EPL is transposed radial to Lister's tubercle, and the retinaculum is then closed to prevent resubluxation of the tendon into the groove. Wolfe[6] states that postoperative positioning is unnecessary, and the patient can begin using his or her wrist and hand as tolerated.

The extensor tendons of the fingers, which include the extensor indicis proprius (EIP) and the extensor digitorum communis (EDC) found in the fourth dorsal compartment, and the extensor digiti minimi (EDM) found in the fifth compartment, rarely are involved in primary stenosing tendovaginitis. Of these, the EDC to the index and small fingers are involved most commonly because they angulate more acutely at the distal edge of the extensor retinaculum. Isolated EIP tendovaginitis has been described secondary to the presence of muscle within the retinacular sheath and following a Colles' fracture.[6] Clinically, swelling and tenderness are present over the affected compartment, and pain may be increased with resisted MCP extension of the affected digit with the wrist flexed. Treatment consists mainly of nonoperative measures, including rest, activity modification, ice, NSAIDs, and in some cases, corticosteroid injections. An orthosis supporting the wrist in slight extension as well as the affected MCP joints may be helpful (Fig. 41-25).

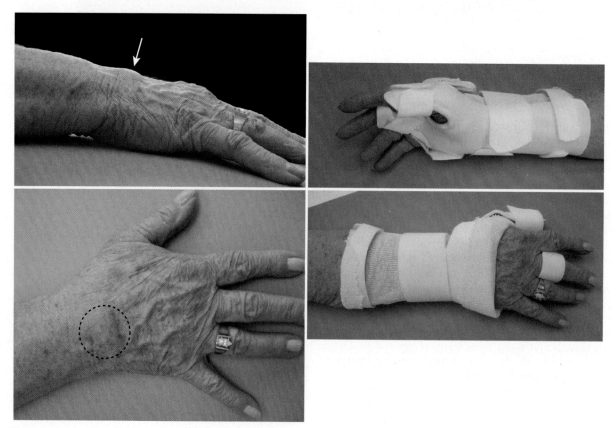

Figure 41-25 Extensor tenosynovitis (nonrheumatoid). Symptomatic digits positioned in extension. Arrow points to section in circle.

Tendovaginitis of the Extensor Carpi Ulnaris

The sixth dorsal compartment, which contains the ECU, is the second most frequently involved extensor compartment. The floor of the ECU sheath is thick and forms part of the triangular fibrocartilage complex (TFCC), which helps stabilize the distal radioulnar joint (DRUJ). ECU tendinopathy can occur in isolation or in association with other conditions, such as destabilizing injuries to the TFCC.[129,131] Precipitating events can include repetitive snapping motions of the wrist, which can occur while playing tennis, golfing, or weightlifting.[103,129,131] Abrupt twisting injuries, particularly hypersupination with wrist flexion, can result in a tear in the ulnar border of the fibro-osseous tunnel overlying the ECU tendon with resultant ECU instability and tendinitis. Symptoms include diffuse ulnar-sided wrist pain with wrist and forearm motions, which is intensified by resistance to ulnar deviation and wrist extension, or by passive stretch into radial deviation and flexion.[132] To rule out instability, the extended, supinated wrist can be moved into flexion and ulnar deviation. If the ECU tendon is unstable, it will subluxate volarward with or without audible snap.

Conservative measures include use of NSAIDs and ice, wrist orthoses, and injection, although injection rarely provides lasting relief.[6] Futami and Itoman[132] report a high success rate with nonoperative treatment in patients with a history of repetitive overuse, but not violent trauma, instability, or TFCC involvement: Of 43 patients, 40 were symptom-free with use of an elastic bandage or wrist brace, NSAIDs, or steroid injections. Activities such as turning a screwdriver or wringing a cloth should be avoided because they require forceful, repetitive wrist and forearm motions in combination.

Surgical Management. The need for surgical intervention in tendovaginitis of the ECU is rare. However, when conservative measures fail, the sixth compartment can be released on the radial side. A 3-cm incision is made over the DRUJ, with care taken to protect the branches of the dorsal sensory ulnar nerve. The sixth fibro-osseous tunnel then is completely released. Retinacular repair is controversial. Kip and Peimer[131] and Wolfe[6] report that postoperative instability has not been a problem. Complications include injury to the dorsal ulnar sensory nerve. Postoperatively, the wrist should be positioned in neutral for 1 to 2 weeks, after which therapy can be initiated to restore tendon gliding and strength. The patient can work on isolated uniplanar motions first (i.e., wrist flexion–extension, then radial–ulnar deviation, and finally, pronation–supination) before doing them in combination.

Insertional Tendinopathies

Radial Wrist Extensors

Activities that subject the radial wrist extensors to sudden, forceful, or sustained exertion can result in microtears of the extensor carpi radialis longus (ECRL) and brevis (ECRB) tendons. Provocative activities include forceful gripping; sports, such as racquetball, tennis, and golf, in which the wrist is subjected to sudden acceleration or deceleration; or sustained hyperextension of the wrist such as with harp playing.[16,129] Pain may be elicited with resisted radial wrist extension or with palpation of the second dorsal compartment just radial to Lister's tubercle. Over time, the insertion points of ECRL and ECRB on the bases of the second and third metacarpals, respectively, can hypertrophy and undergo degenerative changes, a condition called CMC boss. Most CMC bosses are not symptomatic. In those who are, management includes rest from, or modification of, activity; wrist support; and NSAIDs. In some patients, a corticosteroid is injected, but oral medication is preferable because an injection may, in rare cases, result in tendon rupture. Sports equipment, musical instruments, and other tools should be modified when possible, as should body mechanics and playing technique. For a tennis player, adjusting the racquet handle and string tension, taping the wrist, and modifying hitting technique may reduce stress to the radial wrist extensors and prevent recurrence.[105] In recalcitrant cases, a wedge excision of the involved CMC joints can be excised surgically. This procedure is not entirely predictable, however, and some surgeons advocate CMC fusion. We recommend fusion in highly selected cases.

Interosseous Tendons

Sudden, forceful, or repetitive radial or ulnar deviation at the MCP joints can stress the interosseous tendons. Symptoms are vague but generally occur at the level of the MCP joint or intermetacarpal region. Pain may be provoked with a handshake or with pressure at the tubercle of the proximal phalanx, the bony insertion of the interosseous tendon.[105,129] In addition to the usual conservative measures, the involved MCP joints can be positioned in approximately 70 degrees of flexion with a hand-based orthosis. As symptoms resolve, buddy-strapping at the proximal phalanges allows MCP joint flexion and extension while preventing lateral motions.

Tenosynovitis Associated with Systemic Disorders and Infection

Several systemic disorders alter connective tissues and can predispose an individual to stenosing tendovaginitis. Tendons, their synovial sheaths, fibrous retinacula, or local vasculature may be affected adversely, depending on the condition.

Diabetes Mellitus

Diabetes mellitus is a disease caused by altered glucose metabolism. This leads to abnormal accumulation of stable endproducts of collagen glycosylation, which are thought to be responsible for increased cross-linking, packing, and stiffening of collagen.[3] The resulting proliferation of fibrous tissue in the tendon sheath is responsible for the stenosis of tendon tunnels. Diabetes also produces a microangiopathy, which is believed to be responsible for many of its deleterious effects, including resistance to nonoperative measures. Because the disease process is diffuse, it is not uncommon

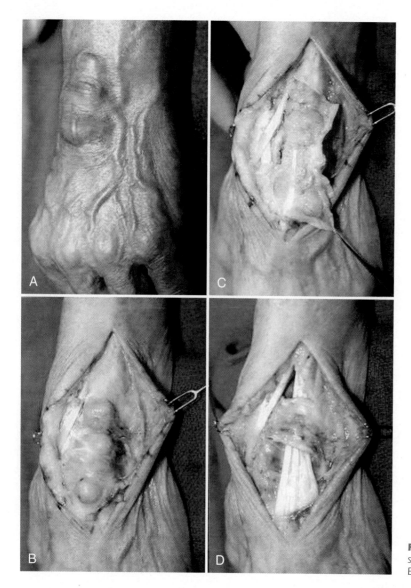

Figure 41-26 Surgical excision of rheumatoid extensor tenosynovitis. **A,** Preoperative presentation. **B,** Skin incision. **C, D,** Extensor tenosynovectomy.

for patients with diabetes to have multiple sites of involvement. Patients with diabetes are four to five times more likely to develop stenosing conditions of the tendons, such as CTS and trigger digits, especially if they are insulin-dependent.[3] They also are more likely to have multiple digit involvement and bilateral disease.[133] Griggs and associates[78] reported a 59% incidence of multiple digit involvement in patients with insulin-dependent diabetes as opposed to only 28% for patients with non-insulin-dependent diabetes. They suggested that patients with more severe disease might have a diffuse rather than nodular type of tendon hypertrophy, as well as poor microvasculature and a greater fibroblast response. If conservative therapy is chosen as an initial course of treatment, the patients must be advised to carefully monitor glucose levels because these can vary greatly after a corticosteroid injection. For many, surgical release is inevitable, particularly for those who are insulin-dependent (56% as opposed to only 28% for patients with non-insulin-dependent diabetes).

Rheumatologic Disorders

Rheumatoid arthritis, psoriatic arthritis, and lupus can adversely affect tendons. More than 65% of patients with rheumatoid arthritis will develop tenosynovitis of the hand or wrist, most commonly at the extensor retinaculum[6] (Fig. 41-26). Proliferative tenosynovitis may begin with inflammation of the synovial lining of the tendon sheath or may invade the tendon from the adjacent joint. The tenosynovium proliferates not only at the tendon–pulley interface but diffusely along the entire sheath. Entrapment of the profundus at the superficialis decussation may account for up to 22% of trigger digits in patients with rheumatoid arthritis. Because of increased bulk and destructive enzymes, the tendons and pulleys adjacent to the diseased tenosynovium can become adherent, weaken, or rupture. Preventing rupture is the most important goal in treating rheumatoid arthritis. Medical management, including disease-modifying agents, is essential to attempt to control the active disease. Orthoses that rest the affected tendons and support unstable joints can provide symptomatic relief. For patients with chronic or multiple trigger digits, three-point orthoses are a practical choice (see Fig. 41-16E). In addition to pharmacologic management, surgical measures, including extensive tenosynovectomy and tendon transfers in cases of rupture, may be necessary. The A1 pulley is left intact or released on its radial border only, to prevent ulnar subluxation of the flexor tendons.

Hypothyroidism

Musculoskeletal disorders such as joint stiffness, Dupuytren's contracture, CTS, and trigger finger often accompany thyroid disorders. Cakir and colleagues[134] reported that trigger digits were present in 10% of patients with subclinical hypothyroidism.

Crystalline Tendinopathies

Deposition of crystalline substances in the enclosed space of the tendon sheath can incite an acute inflammatory response characterized by intense pain, swelling, and erythema. Gout is a disorder of urate metabolism in which the patient has hyperuricemia and hyperuricosuria. Monosodium urate crystals are deposited into the joints or tendons, resulting in synovitis. Gouty involvement of the flexor tenosynovium has been associated with CTS.[135,136] In the treatment of gouty tophi, positioning and pharmacologic management usually suffice. Medications include colchicine and anti-inflammatory agents. In severe or untreated cases, surgical procedures, such as synovectomy, excision of intratendinous tophi, and tendon transfer, may be necessary.

Calcific tendinitis can result from the release of calcium salts. Calcific deposits usually respond to positioning, corticosteroid injection, and NSAIDs; rarely are surgical excision and tenolysis required. Calcium pyrophosphate deposition disease (pseudogout) rarely causes a fulminant tenosynovitis within the carpal tunnel, producing symptoms of median-nerve compression.[6]

Deposition Diseases

Amyloidosis is a disorder that results in the deposition of a serum protein, β_2-microglobulin, in bones and soft tissues. Thick, plaquelike material is deposited on tendons, leading to poor gliding, triggering, and ruptures. The condition occurs as either a primary enzymatic defect or as part of a secondary syndrome in individuals with renal failure on dialysis. Involvement in the hand is usually in the form of cystic lesions in the carpal bones and destructive arthritis. A case of primary amyloidosis manifesting as extensor tenosynovitis has been reported.[137] Treatment is surgical; tenosynovectomy is effective in relieving the symptoms of CTS and stenosing tenosynovitis.[138]

Ochronosis is a rare genetic defect in tryptophan metabolism. Deposits of homogentisic acid, a darkly pigmented protein, often are found in joints, intervertebral disks, and tendons. Surgical release may relieve cases of stenosing tendovaginitis.[6]

Box 41-2	**Kanavel's Four Cardinal Signs of Flexor Tendon Sheath Infection**

- Digit uniformly swollen
- Digit rests in a flexed posture
- Tenderness to palpation over the tendon sheath
- Painful passive extension of the digit

Sarcoidosis

Sarcoidosis is a systemic granulomatous disease that is immune-mediated. It primarily affects the lungs, spleen, and lymph nodes. Approximately 25% of cases have bone and joint or tenosynovial involvement. Sarcoidosis may precipitate secondary gout. Involvement of the hand is extremely uncommon, and fewer than 20 cases have been reported in the English literature.[138] Treatment options include use of systemic corticosteroids and tenosynovectomy.[108] Tenosynovectomy alone without subsequent medical management with steroids leads to recurrence.[139]

Septic Tenosynovitis

Infectious agents can spread to the digital flexor tendon sheath from a deep laceration or puncture wound. Needle sticks or animal bites are common causes. Immunocompromised individuals or those with severe diabetes are most vulnerable. Kanavel's four cardinal signs of flexor tendon sheath infection are likely present in the affected digit (Box 41-2). Management within the first 48 hours of onset includes aspiration of the sheath, followed by appropriate antibiotic coverage. In unresponsive or established cases, surgical drainage is indicated. Postoperatively, the hand should be rested in a forearm-based orthosis with the digits in the intrinsic-plus position. The wrist should be included when infection is present more proximally. When the infection is under control, mobilization and tendon gliding can be initiated. In cases of persistent contracture and adhesion, low-load prolonged stress applied with dynamic, serial static, or static progressive orthoses, may be necessary.[140]

Congenital Trigger Digit

The term *congenital trigger digit* technically is a misnomer because the condition is not diagnosed until after birth, and children so affected present with an IP joint flexion contracture of the involved digit, not triggering. Rodgers and Waters[141] found no trigger digits in 1046 newborns prospectively examined, and of 73 children with "congenital trigger digit," none presented before 3 months of age. Slakey and Hennrikus[142] also found none in 4719 newborns, prospectively examined; of 15 children with the condition, none presented at younger than 3 months of age, 14 of 15 were diagnosed after 1 year of age, and 10 of 15 after 2 years of age. Therefore, acquired flexion contracture is a more accurate description.[142] Incidence in the general population is 0.05%[6] and almost equally divided between males and females. The thumb is involved most frequently; occurrence is rare in the fingers.[143] The cause is unclear; some parents report antecedent trauma or thumb-sucking. Acquired IP joint flexion contracture can occur in association with trisomy.

The pathology of congenital trigger digit also differs somewhat from the adult form. Tendon and synovium are involved, not the fibrous sheath. A firm, nontender nodule is found on the flexor pollicis longus over the MCP joint (Notta's node),[6] and the IP joint typically is contracted in 20 to 75 degrees of flexion, although it occasionally is locked in extension.[70] Other conditions that can result in a flexed thumb include cerebral palsy, arthrogryposis, and hypoplasia of thumb extensors.[144] If the IP joint can be extended with the MCP joint held flexed, IP joint pathology can be ruled out.[145]

According to Dinham and Meggitt,[143] if the condition is diagnosed early in the first year of life, there is a 30% chance of spontaneous resolution. Therefore, their recommendation is to wait a year before deciding to operate. If diagnosed between 6 and 30 months of age, the digit can be watched for 6 months because there is a 12% chance of spontaneous recovery. If there is no resolution, a surgical release is indicated.[6,70,143] Delay in treatment beyond 3 years of age may prolong recovery and result in residual deformity.[144]

Some authors have recommended positioning of the thumb IP joint in an orthosis. Tsuyuguchi and coworkers[146] reported that 75% of cases completely resolved with continuous IP extension positioning using a spring-wire coil orthosis for an average of 9 months. Nemoto and associates[147] reported only a 56% success rate with a static extension orthosis worn at night and during nap times for an average of 10 months. Approximately 23% dropped out of treatment. It is our opinion that prolonged use of an orthosis is impractical and restrictive, particularly for this young age group.

Following surgical release of the A1 pulley, parents should be instructed to keep a clean and dry postoperative dressing on for 2 to 3 days, after which time a bandage should be sufficient. Most authors believe that normal activity is sufficient to restore full motion, and that formal therapy is unnecessary.[6] However, if full active MCP and IP thumb extension are not achieved within the first postoperative week, hand therapy and corrective positioning with orthoses should be provided.

Summary

Tendinopathies of the hand and wrist are a common source of pain and dysfunction. They are often manifestations of aging, systemic disease, and predilection to pathologic fibrosis, although they also can be precipitated by overuse in otherwise healthy individuals. Women are more susceptible than men because of hormonal, anatomic, and occupational factors. In some individuals such as the young child with acquired IP flexion deformity, the cause is not clear. The hand surgeon or therapist should take a thorough history, explore precipitating factors, and assess the nature of the symptoms and their effect on the individual's occupational roles. Intervention varies according to the duration of symptoms and the patient's age, lifestyle, and comorbidities. In the acute phase, corticosteroids and resting orthoses can be helpful in reducing pain and inflammation. As symptoms are controlled, pain-free tendon gliding can be initiated with progression to strengthening, if needed. When conservative management fails, surgical release of constricting fibrous pulleys cure the problem for most patients. Patients with rheumatoid arthritis are an exception; they may require extensive tenosynovectomies and, occasionally, tendon transfers. Finally, the therapist should teach the patient how to modify provocative activities, select appropriate ergonomic equipment, and use semiflexible supports to control symptoms or minimize the chance of recurrence.

REFERENCES

The complete reference list is available online at www.expertconsult.com.

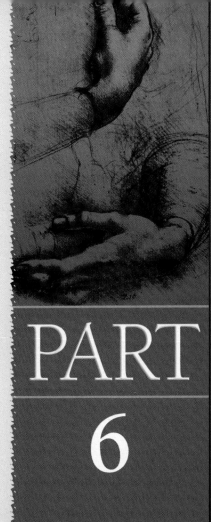

Nerve Lacerations

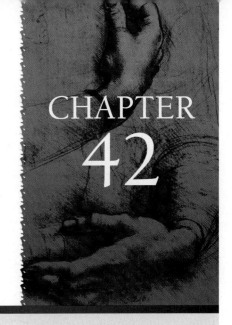

CHAPTER 42

Basic Science of Peripheral Nerve Injury and Repair

MARY BATHEN, BS AND RANJAN GUPTA, MD

RELEVANT DEVELOPMENTAL AND FUNCTIONAL
ANATOMY
CLASSIFICATION OF NERVE INJURY
TRAUMATIC/ACUTE NERVE INJURY
HEALING OF ACUTE NERVE INJURY:
REGENERATION AND REMYELINATION

CHRONIC NERVE COMPRESSION INJURY AND
HEALING
SUMMARY

CRITICAL POINTS

- **Neuron:** The primary cell of the PNS, which is polarized and has dendrites to receive information and axons to transmit information
- **Nerves:** Bundles of axons enclosed in specialized connective sheaths
- **Schwann cell:** Glial cell that supports and myelinates PNS axons
- **Endoneurium:** Collection of collagenous tissue that surrounds each individual axons and their associated Schwann cell
- **Perineurium:** The blood nerve barrier, which is composed of concentric layers of fibroblasts that form a sheath around each fascicle
- **Epineurium:** The collagenous connective tissue layer that surrounds the outer limits of the peripheral nerve, protecting it from external stress
- **Monofascicular:** Nerve section composed of one large fascicle
- **Oligofascicular:** Nerve section composed of a few fascicles
- **Polyfascicular:** Nerve section composed of many fascicles of varying sizes
- **Neurapraxia:** Nerve injury characterized by a reduction or complete block of conduction across a nerve lesion
- **Axonotmesis:** Nerve injury characterized by conduction block and interruption of axonal continuity
- **Neurotmesis:** Nerve injury characterized by conduction block, interruption of axonal continuity, and connective tissue damage

The human nervous system arguably defines the very nature of humanity. Through this complex and intricate system, effective communication and response is possible within the body and to the environment. This system has evolved to allow complex, coordinated movements while maintaining basic reflexes. These capabilities are facilitated by a variety of cells that make up the central nervous system (CNS)—brain and spinal cord and the peripheral nervous system (PNS). The PNS, the focus of this chapter, provides the mechanism for relaying information between the CNS and the environment.

One of the central paradigms of neuroscience has long been that the PNS, in contrast to the CNS, possesses the capacity of self-regeneration after traumatic injury. Despite advances in peripheral nerve repair techniques, however, complete functional recovery is seldom achieved in adults. In order for clinicians to better understand some of the limitations associated with the current treatment protocols for neural injuries, they need to be aware of the basic science behind peripheral nerve anatomy, injury, and healing. These topics are the focus of this chapter.

Relevant Developmental and Functional Anatomy

The origin of the PNS is from the ectodermal layer of the blastocyst, with most of the PNS cells being derived from the neural crest. The primary cell of the PNS is the neuron—a polarized cell with dendrites to receive information and axons to send information. Nerves are bundles of axons enclosed in specialized connective sheaths. Within the nerve, there are several different satellite cells known as glial cells, including Schwann cells, macrophages, and fibroblasts. Peripheral nerves can thus be defined as heterogeneous composite structures composed of neurons, Schwann cells, fibroblasts, and macrophages.

In 1839, Theodor Schwann identified the cell that now bears his name. Schwann cells, derived from the neural crest, are glial cells that support and myelinate PNS axons.

A mature, myelinating Schwann cell is responsible for extending a process of its plasma membrane to wrap an axon in myelin. As such, myelin is a multilamellar, membranous sheath that surrounds the axons of CNS and PNS nerves. Myelin itself acts as an insulator around the axon, reducing the dissipation of the action potential into the surrounding medium as it propagates through the axon. The myelin sheath has discontinuities along the nerve fiber known as nodes of Ranvier, which create distinct morphologic and biochemical domains along PNS nerves (Fig. 42-1). Nodes of Ranvier contain high concentrations of voltage-gated sodium channels. The arrival of an action potential at a node depolarizes the membrane, opening the sodium channels to induce a massive influx of sodium ions into the axon. This generates an electrical pulse that is propagated down the axon to the next node of Ranvier, a process termed *saltatory conduction*. Saltatory conduction allows not only for an increased speed of nerve impulse transmission, but also reduces the energy requirement.

Unmyelinated and myelinated nerves are bundled together in fascicles, with three main layers of tissue: the endoneurium, perineurium, and epineurium (Fig. 42-2). The endoneurium is a collection of collagenous tissue that surrounds each individual axon and their associated Schwann cells. The perineurium is an extension of the blood–brain barrier and is known as the blood–nerve barrier. It is composed of concentric layers of fibroblasts that form a sheath around each fascicle. Prominent basement membranes and numerous tight junctions control the intraneural environment by restricting diffusion into the fascicles. The perineurium is the neural layer most resistant to longitudinal traction and thus provides the peripheral nerve's elastic properties. The epineurium is the collagenous connective tissue layer that surrounds the outer limits of the peripheral nerve protecting it from external stress. The epineurium is divided into two layers: the internal and external. The internal epineurium cushions the fascicles within the nerve, while the external epineurium protects the nerve from external environment.

Fascicular patterns are divided into the following three types: monofascicular, oligofascicular, and polyfascicular.[1] Monofascicular patterns consist of one large fascicle, whereas oligofascicular patterns consist of a few fascicles; polyfascicular patterns consist of many fascicles of varying sizes that can be arranged with or without groupings of fascicles (Fig. 42-3). Nerves found in the upper arm are routinely polyfascicular. In its course from the upper arm to the fingertips, a peripheral nerve undergoes changes from a polyfascicular pattern in the upper arm, oligofascicular in the elbow region, and monofascicular in the hand and fingers. For example, the ulnar nerve is polyfascicular as it exits the brachial plexus until just before the elbow, at which point it becomes oligofascicular. After the division into the motor branch at the

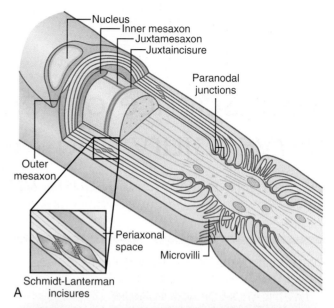

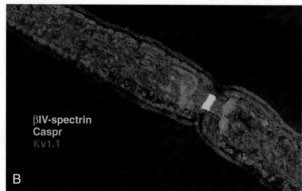

Figure 42-1 *Morphology of domains of myelinated axons in the peripheral nervous system.* **A,** *Schematic organization of a peripheral myelinated nerve is shown. Cross section through a myelinated axon (gray) surrounded by two myelin sheaths is illustrated, demonstrating the node of Ranvier (red), to which Schwann cell microvilli project; the paranodal loops and junctions (green); the juxtaparanodal region (purple); Schmidt-Lanterman incisures, which form gap junctions (shown at higher magnification in the inset); compact myelin (light blue); and the inner (IM) and outer (OM) mesaxons. The axon diameter is reduced in the region of the node and paranodes, with more tightly packed neurofilaments and accumulation of membrane vesicles and mitochondria. The intranodal axonal specializations, the juxtamesaxon, and juxtaincisures are also shown. The entire structure is surrounded by a basal lamina (not illustrated).* **B,** *Confocal immunofluorescence microscopy of teased sciatic nerve fiber illustrating axonal domains. The node is stained for βIV-spectrin (green), the paranodes for Caspr (blue), and the juxtaparanodes for Kv1.1 (red); juxtamesaxonal staining of Kv channels is also seen in the lower right. The field was photographed with differential interference contrast microscopy to illustrate the overall dimensions of the myelin sheath. (Figure borrowed from Salzer JA. Polarized domains of myelinated axons.* Neuron. *2003;40:297-318.)*

wrist, the pattern is monofascicular. These patterns may help to determine which type of nerve repair is appropriate for a particular nerve injury. In surgical nerve repair, proper identification of fascicular arrangement is crucial to maximizing the chances for a successful outcome.

Peripheral nerves are extensively vascularized with separate yet interconnected microvascular systems in the epineurium, perineurium, and endoneurium.[2,3] The vascular pattern

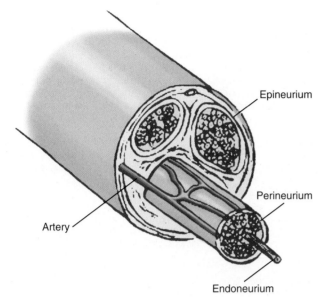

Figure 42-2 *Anatomy of the nerve. Unmyelinated and myelinated axons are bundled together into fascicles. The individual axons are surrounded by the endoneurium. The entire fascicle is ensheathed by the perineurium, which forms the blood–nerve barrier. The epineurium surrounds the entire nerve, holding these structures together.*

of the peripheral nerve is characterized by longitudinally oriented groups of vessels, with a great number of communicating anastomoses. The vasculature is composed of an intrinsic vascular system consisting of vascular plexa in the epineurium, perineurium, and endoneurium and an extrinsic system derived from closely associated vessels running with the nerve. The role of the intraneural microvascular system is vital in regard to the effects of chronic irritation, compression, mobilization, stretching, and transection, and

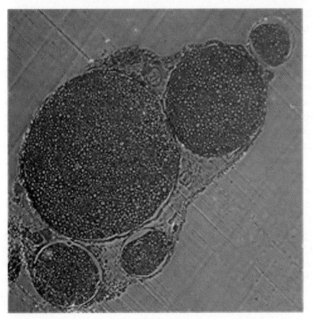

Figure 42-3 *Toluidine blue–stained polyfascicular cross section of a normal murine sciatic nerve (×10).*

should be considered in determining the proper surgical technique.

Classification of Nerve Injury

Nerve lesions are usually described using the standard classification schemes of Seddon[4] or Sunderland[5] (Table 42-1). In 1943, Seddon distinguished between three grades of damage: neurapraxia, axonotmesis, and neurotmesis.[4]

Neurapraxia is the simplest form of nerve injury and is characterized by a reduction or complete block of conduction across a nerve lesion, with preservation of conduction both proximal and distal to the lesion and conservation of axonal continuity.[4] Neurapraxic conduction blocks are caused by localized segmental demyelination.[4] Such demyelination is often mediated by progressive dysfunction of the Schwann cells, common in chronic nerve compression (CNC) disorders such as carpal tunnel syndrome. The prognosis for neurapraxic injuries is good.[4]

Axonotmesis is a more severe form of nerve injury, which is characterized by interruption of axonal continuity with preserved integrity of the nerve sheath.[4] Following injury, Wallerian degeneration occurs. Nerve crush injuries exemplify axonotmetic injuries.[4]

Neurotmesis is the most severe form of nerve injury and occurs when the axon, myelin, and connective tissue components are damaged and disrupted or transected.[4] In neurotmesis, recovery through regeneration cannot occur without surgical intervention.[4] Such an injury can be created by incision, fracture, or laceration and is classified as neurotmesis.[4]

In 1951, Sunderland devised a five-grade classification scheme, which is now more widespread than Seddon's three-grade system.[5] Roughly, grades I and II correspond to Seddon's neurapraxia and axonotmesis, respectively.[5] Sunderland further divided Seddon's category of neurotmesis injuries into grades III, IV, and V, based on the extent of damage to the axonal supporting structures.[5] In grade III injuries, axon continuity is disrupted by loss of endoneurial tubes, but the perineurium is preserved.[5] In grade IV injuries, nerve fasciculi (axon, endoneurium, perineurium) are damaged and intraneural scarring occurs, but nerve sheath continuity is preserved.[5] In grade V injuries, the endoneurium, perineurium, and epineurium are completely divided, and substantial perineural hemorrhage and scarring occurs.[5]

Although not routinely used, additional modifications to the classification scheme have occurred more recently. In 1988, Mackinnon and Dellon presented a grade VI injury that represented a complex peripheral nerve injury, involving combinations of Sunderland's grades of injury.[1] Furthermore, in 1992, Millesi amended Sunderland classification to include the extent of associated fibrous tissue proliferation (type A fibrosis, type B fibrosis, type C fibrosis).[6]

Traumatic/Acute Nerve Injury

Although the preceding classification scheme is helpful to the clinician, the basic science researcher classifies nerve

Table 42-1 Seddon and Sunderland's Classification of Nerve Injuries

Injury	Pathophysiology	Exam Findings	Nerve Studies	Prognosis	Example
Neurapraxia (Seddon)	Reversible conduction block	Motor paralysis: complete but reversible	Distal nerve conduction: present	Good	Chronic nerve compression (CNC) injury
1st Degree (Sunderland)	Localized segmental demyelination	Muscle atrophy: minimal	Motor unit action potential: absent	Full recovery usually within days to 2–3 weeks	e.g., Carpal tunnel syndrome
	Schwann cells dysfunction	Sensory alteration: minimal	Fibrillation: sometimes detectable		
Axonotmesis (Seddon)	Interruption of axon continuity	Motor paralysis: complete	Distal nerve conduction: absent	Fair	Crush injury
2nd Degree (Sunderland)	Preserved nerve sheath	Muscle atrophy: progressive	Motor unit action potential: absent	Full recovery possible without surgery	
	Wallerian degeneration	Sensory alteration: complete	Fibrillation: present	Recovery at 1 mm/day	
3rd Degree (Sunderland)	Endoneurium disrupted Epineurium and perineurium intact	Same as 2nd degree	Same as 2nd degree	Same as 2nd degree	
4th Degree (Sunderland)	Endoneurium and perineurium disrupted Epineurium intact	Same as 2nd degree	Same as 2nd degree	Same as 2nd degree	
Neurotmesis (Seddon)	Axon, myelin, and connective tissue damaged	Same as 2nd degree	Same as 2nd degree	Poor	Transection injury
5th Degree (Sunderland)	Disruption of endoneurium, perineurium, and epineurium			Surgery required Full functional recovery often not possible	e.g., Lacerations

injuries as simply acute or chronic. Acute and chronic nerve injuries lead to disparate physiologic and histopathologic changes to the involved nerve and its adjacent tissue, including demyelination, degeneration, remyelination, and regeneration.

Acute peripheral nerve injuries have a sudden onset, as in nerve crush and transection injuries. Almost immediately, the injured nerve undergoes a process known as Wallerian degeneration (WD), whereby the damaged segment of the nerve is phagocytosed, beginning at the first intact node of Ranvier and progressing distally to allow for regrowth to begin.[7] Granular disintegration of the axonal cytoskeleton, the hallmark of WD, is triggered by increased production of axoplasmic calcium and proceeds in an anterograde fashion down the axon. By 48 to 96 hours after the injury, axonal continuity is lost and impulse conduction is blocked.[8] By 36 to 48 hours afterward, myelin disintegration is well advanced.[8] The clearance of axonal and myelin debris creates an environment hospitable for regeneration.

Schwann cells and macrophages play pivotal, intertwined roles in degeneration and regeneration after acute peripheral nerve injury. Soon after injury, activated Schwann cells secrete chemotactic factors to recruit hematogenous monocytes to the site of injury, where they differentiate into macrophages. The macrophage is the primary phagocyte of myelin and accumulates by 72 hours. Early on, the macrophages express major histocompatibility complex class II antigen 1a and are not phagocytic.[9,10] Later, the hematogenously derived macrophages penetrate the basal lamina, lose 1a expression, become phagocytic, and produce interleukin-1 (IL-1).[9,10] IL-1 stimulates Schwann cells to produce nerve growth factor (NGF), which is required for regeneration of axons and myelin formation.[9]

Schwann cells play yet another role in regeneration. Whereas normal adult Schwann cells do not divide, Schwann cells within the distal segment divide within 24 hours of injury with peak response by 72 hours. They form Bünger's bands, which are cytoplasmic processes that interdigitate and line up in rows under the original basal lamina of the nerve fiber. Regenerating axons travel within these channels to reach their target end-organ.

By 5 to 8 weeks after the injury, the degenerative process is usually complete; all that remains are nerve fiber remnants composed of Schwann cells within an endoneural sheath.[8] Nonetheless, in more severe injuries, a more significant local reaction occurs, whereby hemorrhage and edema lead to a vigorous inflammatory response.[8] Fibroblasts, glial cells that help maintain the extracellular matrix, proliferate, and a dense fibrous scar causes a fusiform swelling of the injured segment.[8] In addition, interfascicular scar tissue develops, permanently enlarging the nerve trunk.[8] While denervated, the endoneurial tubes begin to shrink, reaching a minimum size at 3 to 4 months after injury.[11,12] Concurrently, the endoneurial sheath progressively thickens secondary to collagen deposition along the outer surface of the Schwann cell basement membrane.[11,12] In severe injuries, numerous endoneurial tubes do not receive a regenerating axon, and progressive fibrosis ultimately obliterates them.[11,12]

Changes in the neuronal cell bodies and nerve fibers proximal to the site of injury depend on the severity of the injury and the proximity of the injured segment to the cell body.[8] In extreme cases, in which the cell body degenerates, the entire proximal segment undergoes WD and is phagocytosed.[8] Arguably, the cell body and axon depend on each other for recovery: the cell body does not fully recover without the reestablishment of functional peripheral connections, and the final axonal caliber greatly depends on the recovery of the cell body.[8] In response to axonal injury, the nucleus of the nerve cell body undergoes a process referred to as chromatolysis, whereby the nucleus migrates to the periphery of the cell and Nissl's granules (nerve rough endoplasmic reticulum) break up and disperse.[8] It is believed that chromatolysis somehow signals the perineuronal glial cells to proliferate and extend processes that interrupt synaptic connections and isolate the neuron for recovery.[8] In addition, chromatolysis reprograms the metabolic machinery to enable the cell body to increase lipid and protein production necessary for regeneration.[8] The reversal of chromatolysis is one of the earliest signs of regeneration.[8]

In mild injuries the regenerative and repair processes begin almost immediately, but in more severe injuries nerve regeneration begins only after WD has run its course. One of the early signs of regeneration is the sprouting of new axons (growth cones) by myelinated and unmyelinated nerve fibers proximal to the injury site. Axons that successfully reinnervate the distal stump will mature. Magill and colleagues found that when the mouse sciatic nerve was crushed, 100% of motor end plates are denervated 1 week after crush, with partial reinnervation at 2 weeks, hyperinnervation at 3 and 4 weeks, and restoration of a 1:1 axon to motor end plate relationship 6 weeks after injury.[13] Schwann cells help guide the regenerating axonal sprouts to the denervated motor end plates, reforming neuromuscular junctions.[14] Depending on the size of the defect and extent of injury, axons may regenerate and begin to remyelinate at 6 to 8 weeks; however, the original thickness is never achieved.[4] On average, axonal growth occurs at a rate of 1 to 2 mm/day with a decreased rate in distal regions. Nevertheless, in more serious injuries, prolonged denervation is observed, which can lead to muscle atrophy. Denervated muscle fibers atrophy quite rapidly (on average, 70% reduction of cross-sectional area by 2 months).[8] Although not common, occasional dropout of muscle fibers does occur as a late phenomenon, between 6 and 12 months after denervation.[8]

Healing of Acute Nerve Injury: Regeneration and Remyelination

Unlike CNS nerves, peripheral nerves are capable of spontaneous regeneration after injury. Regeneration occurs when the environment is permissive and the intrinsic growth capacity of neurons is activated. Functional regeneration requires both axon regrowth and remyelination by Schwann cells.

That functional recovery is often suboptimal for a number of reasons: (1) The correct organ does not innervate in the correct location. (2) The end organ may be degenerated by the time the axon reaches the target. (3) An incorrect receptor may be innervated. (4) The receptor may be in the wrong location. (5) Axon continuity may not be maintained.

Many of these issues are related to the surgical coaptation. Even under the ideal surgical conditions, results are suboptimal. As such, most surgeons recognize that molecular mechanisms for regeneration are not effective at producing normal functional regeneration without advances in medical intervention.

Regeneration

Activation of Intrinsic Growth Capacity

The activation of the intrinsic growth capacity is best studied in the dorsal root ganglion (DRG) primary sensory neurons. DRG neurons are pseudobipolar neurons that have only one axon stemming from the cell body, which branches out to two axons: the peripheral branch innervates the sensory organs in the peripheral tissues, whereas the central branch enters the spinal cord and ascends the dorsal column to terminate in the brain. Largely due to disparate environments, the peripheral branch spontaneously regenerates after injury, while the central branch does not. However, if the peripheral branch is injured before the central branch, a phenomenon known as a conditioning peripheral lesion occurs, whereby the central branch can regenerate beyond the injury site, in the inhibitory environment of the spinal cord.[15,16]

The intrinsic growth capacity is controlled by a number of genes and gene products, proteins. Myelin-associated glycoprotein (MAG) is an important constituent of myelin in the PNS, where it is expressed primarily by promyelinating glial cells and plays a key role in the early stages on myelination. MAG has a biphasic function: early in development it enhances axonal growth, but in adults it inhibits axonal regeneration and neurite outgrowth. In adults, the binding of either myelin or MAG to the Nogo receptor (NgR)-p75 neurotrophic receptor complex activates the Rho pathway, which in turn inhibits cytoskeleton assembly.

In vitro experiments have shown that MAG inhibits DRG outgrowth.[17] However, in vitro as well as in vivo experiments have shown that when the peripheral branch is lesioned, the DRG axons sufficiently activate the intrinsic growth capacity to overcome the inhibitory effects of MAG.[18,19] Two independent studies argue that disinhibition occurs because of the increased postlesional intracellular cyclic adenosine monophosphate (cAMP) levels.[18-20] cAMP is synthesized from adenosine triphosphate and is a well-known second messenger, used for intracellular signal transduction. cAMP's significance was discovered when injection of dibutyryl-cAMP (a cAMP analog) into a nonlesioned DRG resulted in regeneration of the central branch of DRG neurons.[18-20]

The action of cAMP proceeds through protein kinase A (PKA). PKA refers to a family of enzymes whose activity is dependent on cAMP levels. Experiments have shown that if PKA is blocked, lesion-induced growth of neurons that have been plated on MAG is blocked.[15,19] The effects of both cAMP and PKA are transcription-dependent and are regulated by the cAMP response element binding (CREB) proteins.[21,22] CREB proteins are transcription factors that bind to certain sequences of DNA (Cre elements) to increase or decrease transcription of certain genes. When PKA triggers gene expression through CREB, the transcription of regeneration-related genes, such as *Arginase I,* is upregulated.[21] Arginase I, the liver isoform of arginase, is an enzyme involved in

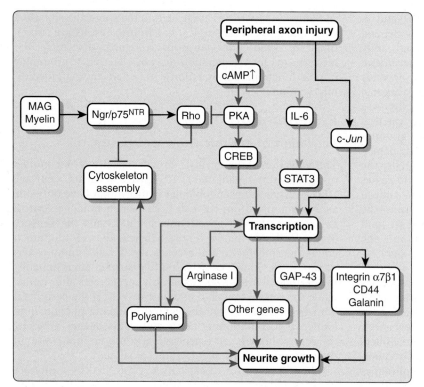

Figure 42-4 Activation of intrinsic growth capacity by peripheral nerve injury. Peripheral nerve injury elevates intracellular cyclic adenosine monophosphate levels, which activates protein kinase A (PKA). PKA triggers gene expression through cAMP response element binding (CREB), resulting in transcriptional up-regulation of regeneration-related genes such as *Arginase I. Arginase I* promotes the synthesis of polyamines, which may directly regulate cytoskeleton assembly or further induce gene expression necessary for regeneration. Activation of PKA also inhibits Rho antagonizing myelin-associated glycoprotein (MAG) or myelin-induced Rho activation and inhibition of neurite growth. Elevated cAMP levels also up-regulate interleukin-6 (IL-6), which, through signal transducers and activators of transcription-3 (STAT-3), induces regeneration-related genes such as the one that produces growth-associated protein-43 (GAP-43). Peripheral injury additionally induces c-*Jun* transcription factor-dependent regeneration-related gene expression, such as for integrin-α7β1 CD44 and galanin. Activation of the intrinsic growth capacity is regulated mainly at transcriptional level. (Figure borrowed from Chen ZL. Peripheral regeneration. *Annu Rev Neurosci.* 2007;30:209-233.)

polyamine synthesis (the urea cycle), and it has been discovered that cAMP disinhibition of MAG is ineffective when polyamine synthesis is blocked.[21] It is hypothesized that polyamines may induce expression of other regenerative genes or may directly affect cytoskeleton organization.[21] In sum, cAMP increases the transcription of *Arginase I* through PKA activation of CREB (Fig. 42-4).

A few additional pathways may play significant roles in regeneration. cAMP also directly upregulates interleukin-6 (IL-6) and inhibits myelin-associated Rho activation.[23] Moreover, Raivich and coworkers discovered that c-*Jun* knockout mice show impaired induction of several molecules involved in regeneration, including CD44, galanin, and integrin α7β1.[24]

Environmental Factors in Peripheral Axon Regeneration

Many argue that environmental differences can explain why PNS regeneration succeeds while CNS regeneration does not. CNS axon regeneration is made especially difficult by myelin-associated inhibitory molecules and the formation of a glial scar.[23] The PNS response to injury prevents accumulation of myelin-associated inhibitory proteins.[25] Following an injury in the PNS, Schwann cells and macrophages rapidly remove myelin debris and Schwann cells dedifferentiate and down-regulate myelin proteins.[25] Moreover, Nogo-A, a strong inhibitor in the CNS, is not normally expressed in the PNS.[26] A glial scar does not form in the PNS after injury because astrocytes, the glial cells that form glial scars, are absent in the PNS.

Successful regeneration may also depend on axon guidance cues, including extracellular matrix (ECM) proteins and neuronal adhesion molecules. One ECM protein, laminin,

has attracted significant attention in recent years, for it has been shown that laminin plays an important role in neurite outgrowth in vitro. Laminins are heterotrimeric glycoproteins composed of a α-, β-, and γ-chains and are major components of the basal lamina. Substantial evidence shows that laminin plays an important role in neurite outgrowth in vitro (for review, see Luckenbill-Edds 1997[27]). Of the 15 known laminin isoforms, laminin-2 and laminin-8 are expressed in the endoneurium of peripheral nerves[28] and are up-regulated after peripheral nerve injury.[29-31] Because laminin can directly promote neurite extension[32] and Schwann cells are dramatically affected by laminin knockout mice,[33] it is believed that laminin effects axonal regeneration by directly serving as a substrate for elongation or by indirectly supporting Schwann cell function, or both. Although the exact mechanism by which laminin supports regeneration is not completely understood, in vitro studies have shown that laminin plays a critical role in axon establishment through the PI/AKT signaling pathway.[34-36] Laminin binding to receptors (e.g., integrins, dystroglycan) triggers phosphorylation and activation of PI (phosphoinositide) 3-kinase. PI 3-kinase activation triggers the activation of AKT.[34-36] Active AKT then phosphorylates and inhibits glycogen synthase kinase-3 beta (GSK-3β) activity, triggering cytoskeleton-binding proteins to organize cytoskeleton elongation.[34-36]

Other Factors Affecting Peripheral Nerve Regeneration

Several neurotrophic factors, cytokines, and transcription factors may play a significant role in creating a permissive environment for regeneration. Neurotrophic factors prevent neuronal death and thus make axon regeneration possible. One major group of neurotrophic factors is the neurotrophins, four structurally related proteins: nerve growth factor (NGF), brain-derived neurotrophic factor (BDNF), neurotrophin-3 (NT-3), and neurotrophin-4 (NT-4). Neurotrophin signaling is mediated by two types of receptors: three high-affinity Trk receptor kinases (each neurotrophin-specific) and a low-affinity p75[NTR] (which binds all neurotrophins with similar affinity).

NGF, BDNF, and NT-3 are all believed to be involved in peripheral nerve regeneration. NGF is the first neuronal growth factor to be discovered, is specific for a subset of primary sensory neurons and for sympathetic neurons, and is involved in nerve cell survival and maintenance in the normal state. Because NGF messenger RNA expression is greatly increased following peripheral nerve injury, it appears that NGF is an important component of the nerve repair process. Although NGF has been shown to bind to both low-affinity (p75) and high-affinity (TrkA) receptors, studies have shown that only neurons that express the high-affinity receptor (TrkA) are affected by NGF. Because motor neurons do not express TrkA, regeneration in motor nerves is likely not affected by NGF,[37,38] although some studies contest this.[39]

In addition to NGF, BDNF and NT-3 are being explored as potential mediators of peripheral nerve regeneration. Both BDNF and NT-3 (as well as NT-3 and NT-4/5) undergo receptor-mediated retrograde transport to neurons to prevent neuronal death,[40] promote survival and differentiation of motor neurons in vitro,[41] and regulate the function of developing neuromuscular synapses.[42] Taken together, these qualities suggest that BDNF and NT-3 could potentially be used to promote regeneration. Two studies recently reported that BDNF promotes functional recovery after peripheral nerve injury,[43,44] but others present seemingly conflicting results.[45,46] Moreover, NT-3, which is down-regulated following peripheral nerve injury, was recently shown to enhance peripheral nerve regeneration through fibronection mats.[47]

Cytokines are also thought to be involved in peripheral nerve regeneration. Cytokines are similar to neurotrophins, except cytokines are inducible, whereas neurotrophins are constitutively expressed. Arguably the most widely studied cytokine is ciliary neurotrophic factor (CNTF). CNTF has a broad range of functions in the nervous system and has a trophic effect of denervated muscle. The neuronal specificity of CNTF overlaps considerably with that of the neurotrophins; however, its cellular localization, receptor structure, and signaling pathway are distinct.[48-50] In normal peripheral nerves, CNTF expression is abundant and localized in the cytoplasm of myelinating Schwann cells.[51,52] After axotomy, CNTF promotes survival of motor neurons in vitro and in neonatal animals, and it is hypothesized that CNTF acts as an "injury factor," being released by glial cells in response to injury.[53] Moreover, CNTF has been shown to protect denervated muscle from atrophy.[54] A second cytokine involved in peripheral nerve regeneration is interleukin-6 (IL-6). IL-6 acts as both a proinflammatory and anti-inflammatory cytokine (cellular communication protein). IL-6 mRNA is induced in the DRG sensory neurons after injury and at degeneration sites during WD after sciatic nerve crush. In IL-6 knockout mice, the adult mouse shows sensory defects and delayed regeneration of sensory axons after crush injury. Another cytokine, leukemia inhibitory factor (LIF), is induced after sciatic nerve crush. LIF can be retrogradely

transported to DRG sensory neurons to induce gene expression changes to promote regeneration, and LIF knockout mice show impaired peripheral nerve regeneration. In addition to the effects mentioned earlier, elevated cAMP levels following nerve injury causes IL-6 and LIF to activate the transcription factor STAT-3 (signal transducers and activators of transcription 3),[55] which results in the transcription of regeneration-related genes like growth associated protein-43 (GAP-43).[56] STAT-3 conditional knockout mice show that STAT-3 is required for motor neuron survival. Additional neurotrophic factors are thought to be linked to peripheral nerve regeneration, but a complete discussion of each is outside the scope of this chapter (for a review, see Terenghi 1999[57]).

Remyelination

Functional recovery is only possible if, in addition to regeneration, Schwann cells remyelinate the regrown axons. At any time, Schwann cells can only be in one state: dedifferentiated–proliferating or differentiated–myelinating. Schwann cells destined to myelinate differentiate to promyelinating Schwann cells and extend cytoplasmic bundles to form a 1 to 1 ratio with individual axons (radial sorting) and enwrap them in myelin sheath.[58,59]

The process by which multipotent neural crest cells differentiate into mature, myelinating Schwann cells is not well understood; however, it is known that the establishment of axonal contact triggers Schwann cell development and the absence of contact leads to degeneration. β-Neuregulin, a protein product of neuregulin-1 (see section on Neurotrophic Factors and Peripheral Remyelination), is thought to play a pivotal role in this contact-mediated effect. Moreover, it has been discovered that the rate of differentiation is positively regulated by fibroblast growth factor and negatively by endothelin. When Schwann cells receive promyelinogenic signals from the axon, they produce large amounts of plasma membrane and up-regulate several proteins that give them the ability to myelinate, including MAG, periaxin, P0, myelin basic protein (MBP), and PMP22. Two transcription factors, Oct-6 and Krox-20, have been shown to promote and mediate the phenotypic transition from promyelinating to myelinating. Oct-6, which is expressed in Schwann cell progenitors but not in mature myelinating Schwann cells, is a strong repressor of the end-stage myelin-specific genes *P0* and *MBP*. Krox-20, which is expressed only in mature myelinating Schwann cells, promotes the Schwann cells' withdrawal from the cell cycle.

As previously mentioned, Schwann cells undergo phenotypic changes following nerve injury, and these changes play pivotal roles in degeneration–demyelination as well as regeneration–remyelination. Stoll and Muller showed that the loss of Schwann cell–axon contact following nerve injury leads to Schwann cell dedifferentiation followed by a series of proliferations.[60] Once the Schwann cell recontacts a regenerated axon, Schwann cell redifferentiation is triggered. As in normal development, Oct-6 expression is followed by Krox-20 expression and the reinduction of myelin-specific genes.[61-63]

In recent years, secondary to research into demyelinating diseases, it has been discovered that the Schwann cell phenotype is also largely influenced by ECM proteins, neurotrophic factors, and hormones.

Extracellular Matrix Proteins and Peripheral Remyelination

Bunge and associates have provided substantial evidence that Schwann cells require the formation of a basal lamina to properly ensheath and myelinate axons.[64,65] The basal lamina is a layer of ECM that envelops the Schwann cell–neurite units. Laminins, as discussed earlier, are major components of the basal lamina that are especially important to myelination. In fact, recent studies have shown that signals from laminins, and not the assembly of a continuous basal lamina per se, are required for myelination.[66] Yang and colleagues[67] and Yu and coworkers[68] showed that disruption of laminins in the PNS results in aberrant Schwann cell differentiation, a lack of radial sorting of axons, and severe hypomyelination. Yu and coworkers disrupted the *laminin-γ1* gene, which is one of the most abundant laminin chains and is present in all known PNS isoforms.[68] The results indicated that Schwann cells lacking laminin do not extend processes required for axonal sorting and mediating axon–Schwann cell interaction.[68] In a related study, Yang and colleagues found that combined laminin-2/laminin-8 deficiencies caused nearly complete amyelination.[67] A close analysis of the data revealed that laminin-2 and laminin-8 have a dominant role in defasciculation, and that laminin-8 promotes myelination without basal lamina.[67]

Laminin's ability to significantly affect myelination depends on its ability to bind to the appropriate receptor. Therefore, laminin receptors are now being explored as possible means of promoting myelination. Laminin receptors include integrin receptors and other plasma membrane molecules, such as dystroglycan. Integrins are cell surface receptors that interact with ECM and mediate various intracellular signals. Structurally, integrins are obligate heterodimers with two distinct chains, composed of α- and β-subunits. Two laminin-binding integrins expressed by Schwann cells are α6β1- and α6β4-integrins. Dystroglycan, on the other hand, is one of the dystrophin-associated glycoproteins that, in skeletal muscle, acts as a transmembrane linkage between the ECM and the cytoskeleton. Lefort and associates[69] and Masaki and colleagues[70] showed that remyelinating Schwann cells up-regulate expression of β1-integrin and dystroglycan.[69,70] Later studies revealed that β1-integrin is necessary for proper sorting of axons,[71] whereas dystroglycan maintains the myelin sheath and regulates myelin thickness.[72] Curiosity over how basal lamina components on the Schwann cell outside surface transduce a signal to influence axon sorting (a process affecting the inner and lateral surface) led to the discovery that laminin signaling activates the Rho family GTPase Rac1 in Schwann cells, which leads to radial sorting and subsequent myelination of axons.[73,74]

In addition to laminins and their receptors, extracellular proteases (e.g., plasmin) also regulate remyelination. Plasmin is an important blood enzyme that degrades fibrin. Studies have revealed that fibrinogen infiltrates the nerve following nerve injury. Fibrinogen is converted to fibrin, which accumulates and prevents two crucial steps to regeneration: migration and remyelination of Schwann cells.[75,76] In response to fibrin accumulation, Schwann cells produce tissue plasminogen activator (tPA),[77] which activates the fibronolytic cascade, paving the way for Schwann cell remyelination.

Neurotrophic Factors and Peripheral Remyelination

Originally, attention was drawn to neurotrophic factors for their role in neuron survival and regeneration. However, recent studies have revealed that neurotrophic factors also significantly affect Schwann cell differentiation and myelination.

As discussed earlier, one major group of neurotrophic factors, the neurotrophins (e.g., NGF, BDNF, and NT-3), are thought to play a significant role in remyelination following peripheral nerve injury. One study revealed that the addition of endogenous BDNF or depletion of exogenous NT-3 enhances myelination, suggesting that BDNF is a positive modulator and NT-3 is a negative modulator of peripheral nerve regeneration.[78] Another study showed that inhibition of TrkB (specific for BDNF) did not prevent myelination, whereas blockage of p75[NTR] showed inhibitory effects on myelination.[79] This result implies that p75[NTR] is necessary for proper myelination. Not surprisingly, the down-regulation of NT-3 and the up-regulation of both BDNF and p75[NTR] promotes remyelination following nerve injury. Further analysis of neurotrophin expression and transport may help direct the innovation of a therapeutic intervention. For instance, one interesting study recently revealed that sensory neurons of the DRG are a major source of BDNF, and DRGs transport and secrete endogenous BDNF along the surface of axons in the anterograde fashion.[80] Understanding the mechanism of expression is a key step to successfully harnessing the intrinsic ability to promote myelination.

Beyond the neurotrophins, a number of other neurotrophic factors affect Schwann cell differentiation, but a review of each is outside the scope of this paper. Neuregulin-1 (NGR-1) and transforming growth factor-β (TGF-β) are the two major neurotrophic factors under active investigation. Neuregulins are a family of four structurally related proteins that are part of the epidermal growth factor (EGF) family of proteins. The NRG-1 family includes more than 15 EGF-like ligands that interact with ErbB receptor tyrosine kinase to control many aspects of neural development. During development, NRG-1 isoforms positively regulate Schwann cells at multiple stages of cell lineage.[81] NRG-1 type III isoform is the principal regulator of early Schwann cell lineage (including precursors), and a threshold level of NRG-1 type III triggers Schwann cell myelination.[82] Additionally, NRG-1 type III regulates myelin sheath thickness to match axon caliber.[82] Carroll and associates revealed that neuregulin and ErbB expression increased after axotomy of the sciatic nerve.[83] Nevertheless, a recent study showed that disruption of ErbB2 in mature Schwann cells does not impair regeneration after injury, diminishing the enthusiasm for the potential use of NRG-1 to promote remyelination.[84] Notably, this study emphasizes that the developmental process of Schwann cell differentiation is not identical to Schwann cell differentiation after injury.

During development, TGF-β maintains the nonmyelinating, proliferating state of Schwann cells and regulates Schwann cell survival.[81] Scherer and colleagues demonstrated that following sciatic nerve injury, TGF-β1 mRNA in the distal nerve stump increases, whereas TGF-β3 mRNA falls

(TGF-β2 is not detected).[85] This shows that Schwann cells alter expression of TGF-β1 and TGF-β2 in response to nerve injury.[85] Studies have demonstrated that, as in development, TGF-β blocks Schwann cells differentiation–myelination after injury. TGF-β exerts its effects by preventing the expression of *Ski*, a proto-oncogene that coordinates the transition from Schwann cell proliferation to differentiation.[86] *Ski* expression is decreased 4 days after nerve injury, but returns to preinjury levels following complete regeneration and remyelination. It would be interesting to explore the manipulation of *Ski* expression to promote remyelination after peripheral nerve injury.

Hormones and Peripheral Remyelination

Beyond ECM proteins and neurotrophic factors, studies have shown that myelination and remyelination are affected by a number of hormones, including progesterone, thyroid hormone (triiodothyronine, T_3), and erythropoietin. Progesterone, a steroid hormone secreted by the adrenal glands, is involved in the female menstrual cycle, embryogenesis, and pregnancy (supports gestation). Koening and coworkers found that blockage of the effects of progesterone decreases the thickness of myelin sheaths of remyelinating axons after injury, whereas administration of exogenous progesterone to the injury site promotes myelin sheath formation.[87] The thryoid hormone T_3, a tyrosine-based hormone produced by the thyroid gland, plays an integral role in regulating metabolism and homeostasis. Voinesco and associates discovered that administration of T_3 to an injured rat sciatic nerve increased nerve regeneration and increased the number, diameter, and myelin thickness of remyelinated axons.[88] Erythropoietin (EPO), a glycoprotein hormone, regulates red blood cell production and is expressed in PNS axons and Schwann cells.[89] Recent studies suggest that EPO may facilitate peripheral nerve regeneration by increasing Schwann cell proliferation and decreasing tumor necrosis factor-alpha (TNF-α) mediated injury and death.[90,91]

Chronic Nerve Compression Injury and Healing

CNC injuries, such as carpal tunnel syndrome, cubital tunnel syndrome, and spinal nerve root stenosis, affect millions of individuals. In contrast to acute nerve injuries, CNC injuries develop over the course of weeks to months. Until recently, they were considered variants of acute nerve injuries that developed over time and had a similar pathogenesis. Much of the earlier literature described compression neuropathies as the by-product of mild WD that occurred at the site of injury. Recent research using both in vivo and in vitro modeling systems has called that notion into question. Active research into chronic nerve compression injuries has revealed important details about their unique pathogenesis and corresponding repair mechanisms. Chapter 46 provides additional information on the pathophysiology of nerve compression, whereas this section focuses on Schwann cell changes.

Chronic nerve compression injury induces both Schwann cell proliferation and apoptosis, with minimal morphometric evidence of early axonal pathology.[92] Design-based stereologic techniques revealed that Schwann cell number increased sixfold relative to the normal site of compression at 1 month and then slowly declined toward control levels.[92] Assays of apoptosis revealed extensive Schwann cell apoptosis at 2 weeks after compression, demonstrating a concurrent Schwann cell proliferation and apoptosis that was confirmed with counts of bromodeoxyuridine-labeled Schwann cells.[92] Electron microscopic analysis confirmed that these dramatic changes in Schwann cells occurred in the absence of axon degeneration and axonal swelling and before there was any detectable alterations in nerve conduction velocity.[92] Although WD is known to trigger Schwann cell proliferation, alternative hypotheses exist such as mechanical stimuli providing Schwann cell mitogenic signals.[92] An in vitro model to deliver shear stress in the form of laminar fluid flow to pure populations of Schwann cells confirmed that mechanical stimuli do, indeed, induce Schwann cell proliferation.[92] These findings suggest that CNC injury induces Schwann cell turnover with minimal axonal injury and support the idea that mechanical stimuli have a direct mitogenic effect on Schwann cells.[92]

As Schwann cells undergo marked cellular turnover in the early stages of CNC injury, it is possible that demyelination and remyelination occur at the same time.[93] Through nerve teasing techniques and unbiased stereology, myelination in nerves 1 month and 8 months after compression was recently assessed.[93] Evaluations of myelin thickness and axonal diameter using design-based, unbiased stereology revealed a dramatic decrease in the average internodal length (IL) and an increase in the proportion of thinly myelinated axons, indicative of remyelination.[93] The mean IL was reduced after 1 month of chronic nerve injury with no further decrease in IL at 8 months.[93] There was limited change in average axonal diameter at both 1 and 8 months.[93] Measures of myelin thickness revealed a sixfold increase in the number of axons with very thin (<5-μm thickness) myelin sheaths, as well as a proportional decrease in the number of axons with the thick myelin sheaths characteristic of normal nerve.[93] These results confirm that an early consequence of CNC is local demyelination and remyelination, which may be the primary cause of alterations in nerve function during the early postcompression period.[93]

In addition to stimulating Schwann cell proliferation, in vitro mechanical loading alters the phenotype of many different cell types.[94] After exposure to sustained shear stress, Schwann cells decreased their mRNA expression and protein levels of MAG and MBP. The mRNA expression of MAG and MBP was down-regulated 21% and 18%, respectively, whereas the Western blot showed down-regulation in MAG and MBP protein expression by 29% and 35%, respectively.[94] The data suggests that down-regulation of myelin-associated proteins may be a direct response to physical stimulus that is not secondary to axonal injury.[94] Immunohistochemistry data analysis revealed significant axonal sprouting at early time points, when MAG and MBP is down-regulated.[94] Thus, the data suggest that down-regulation of MAG and MBP may create an environment permissive to axonal sprouting.[94]

Quantititative microscopic techniques helped to define the nature of this sprouting response and explore whether down-regulation of MAG by proliferating Schwann cells induces local sprouting.[95] In the outer regions of CNC nerves, axonal sprouting was observed without evidence of WD.[95] Immunolabeling and Western blot analysis revealed a local down-regulation of MAG protein within the site of injury, and local delivery of purified MAG protein abrogates the axonal sprouting response.[95] These data demonstrate that CNC injury triggers axonal sprouting and suggest that a local down-regulation of MAG within the peripheral nerve secondary to CNC injury is the critical signal for sprouting response.[95]

Within the region of CNC injury, studies have shown that, in addition to Schwann cell changes, vascular permeability and neural vascularity increase.[96] Vascular endothelial growth factor (VEGF) is a potent mitogen for endothelial cells and promotes blood vessel sprouting and vascular permeabilization.[96] VEGF mRNA and protein expression increased within Schwann cells as early as 2 weeks after compression and peaked by 1 month, with a subsequent marked increase in the number of blood vessels.[96]

In addition to changes that result from Schwann cell phenotypic changes, CNC injuries vary markedly from acute injuries in terms of macrophage recruitment.[97] In acute injuries, there is an immediate recruitment of macrophages, with a peak as early as 24 to 96 hours after injury.[97] In CNC injuries, macrophage recruitment occurs slowly.[97] Moreover, at 1 month after compression, macrophages are mainly localized in the outer third cross-section, to diffuse out later.[97]

After injury, hematogenously recruited macrophages express inducible nitric oxide synthase (iNOS), which generates localized increases in nitric oxide (NO).[97] NO is a free-radical gas that acts as a free messenger and plays an integral role in regeneration by inhibiting neurotoxins.[97] The majority of the iNOS expression is in the perineurium not the periphery, suggesting that iNOS up-regulation is due to ischemia regulated at the blood–nerve barrier.[97] Macrophages also secrete Schwann cell mitogenic factors.[97] In macrophage-depleting experiments, it was clearly shown that the hematogenously derived macrophages that are recruited to the region of CNC injury are integral to the alteration of the blood–nerve barrier, but had no detectable influence on Schwann cell proliferation after CNC injury.[97]

Summary

Clinicians should understand the basic science behind peripheral nerve anatomy, injury, and healing. It is equally important to recognize that recent research has revealed that the pathogenesis and recovery of acute and chronic nerve injuries differ in numerous and significant ways. A strong basic science background may improve the functional recovery, which is rarely complete today.

REFERENCES

The complete reference list is available online at www.expertconsult.com.

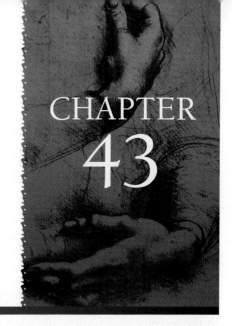

CHAPTER 43

Nerve Response to Injury and Repair

KEVIN L. SMITH, MD, MS

END-ORGAN DENERVATION CHANGES
MECHANISMS OF NERVE INJURY
FACTORS THAT INFLUENCE REGENERATION
REINNERVATION
PERIPHERAL NERVE RECONSTRUCTION
SUMMARY

CRITICAL POINTS

- Peripheral nerve end-organs *require* innervation to stay viable. The loss of the trophic stimulus of the nerve axon dooms the end-organ to atrophy and eventual death.
- Denervated muscles can be made to function by external electrical stimulation, and this can prevent some of the changes caused by denervation.
- Nerve injuries can result from many different mechanisms. They can result from compression by internal forces (e.g., tumors, fracture, callus) or by external forces (tourniquet or "crutch palsy"), or from ischemia, traction, x-radiation, inadvertent injection injury, or electrical injury.
- Regeneration of the peripheral nerve after injury is influenced by mechanical forces, delay to repair, the patient's age, and the level of the injury.
- The nerve axon has the greatest likelihood of accurate regeneration when minimum scar is interposed between the severed nerve ends and if there is accurate alignment of the fascicles.
- The most commonly used technique for peripheral nerve microcoaptation is the *epineurial repair* technique.
- Electrophysiologic studies supported the use of grafts in lieu of coaptation under tension and showed excellent recovery even in the face of two suture lines.

There are many diverse causes of peripheral nerve dysfunction, and most treatments are outside the scope of the hand surgeon and therapist. Although some of the sequelae of nerve dysfunction can be treated surgically (e.g., tendon transfer or decompression), essentially only traumatic peripheral nerve injuries—transection, crush, compression, and stretch—can be repaired or reconstructed surgically. Because each particular type of nerve injury carries with it a different prognosis, it is important to fully appreciate the effects of each kind of nerve injury and the extent to which they affect the nerve cell, axon, and target organ. With this knowledge, the surgeon and therapist can offer the patient reasonable advice regarding prognosis and the expected results of surgical reconstruction.[1] For a complete discussion of the basic science of nerve injury and repair, refer to Chapter 42.

End-Organ Denervation Changes

As long as a nerve cell body remains alive, it has an unlimited potential for regeneration. This is not the case for the sensory or motor end-organ. Peripheral nerve end-organs *require* innervation to stay viable. The loss of the trophic stimulus of the nerve axon dooms the end-organ to atrophy and eventual death. However, this deterioration does differ in time for each kind of end-organ, and the understanding of the pathophysiology of end-organ degeneration will help determine the time constraints for surgical reconstruction.

Sensory End-Organs

The response of the sensory end-organ to denervation varies along the continuum from atrophy to frank degeneration and disappearance. This response not only is time dependent but also depends on the life cycle of the receptor in question. Muscle spindles, which undergo no further division after differentiation, respond to denervation by atrophy. Other cell types that are characterized by a short life cycle and high turnover—such as the taste bud—respond to denervation by degeneration and complete disappearance within 1 to 2 weeks.[2] The integrity of sensory receptors apparently depends on an intact nerve fiber, although there need not necessarily be efferent impulses. Spinal ganglia, severed of their connections with the spinal cord, are able to maintain sensory structures as long as the axon is intact.[3]

The three most common sensory end-organs—the Meissner corpuscle, the Merkel cell–neurite complex, and the Pacinian corpuscle—have similar responses to denervation. As a result of Wallerian degeneration, the axon terminal progressively degenerates over time and is absent by 9 months. The lamellar components of the Meissner corpuscles and the Pacinian corpuscles become atrophic but never completely disappear, as do the supporting structures of the Merkel cell–neurite complex.[4-8] The Merkel cells seem to reduce in number, become atrophic, and possibly even become differentiated into transitional cells or keratinocytes after denervation.[9] If the sensory receptor does proceed to complete degeneration after long-term denervation, it is lost to the receptor pool because the adult mammal appears to have lost the ability to form new sensory receptors de novo.[10,11] The muscle spindle, innervated with both motor and sensory fibers, responds in a similar fashion. When the γ-innervation is severed, the polar regions become atrophic, while the central sensory component (nuclear bag or chain regions) remains intact. When the dorsal roots, which supply the sensory portions, are injured, the central regions decrease in size, lose their equatorial collections of nuclei, and are eventually replaced by striated muscle.[2]

Motor End-Organs

After the denervation of skeletal muscle, many changes are apparent. Clinically, the muscle ceases to function and there is gross muscle atrophy. Muscle atrophy after nerve injury results in a decrease of total muscle weight, a loss of total protein, and an overall reduction in muscle cross-sectional area.[12] There is not a decrease in the number of individual muscle fibers, even though there is a relative increase in the amount of connective tissue stroma.[13] Rates of atrophy can vary widely, with reports of as much as a 40% decrease in muscle mass within 1 to 3 weeks of denervation.[3] This does not represent an irreversible degradation, however, and anecdotal reports have documented successful restoration of function after 22 years of denervation.[14] Realistically, however, functional reinnervation is unlikely after 2 years of denervation. Denervated muscles can be made to function by external electrical stimulation, and this can prevent some of the changes caused by denervation.[15-19] However, the role functional electrical stimulation plays in the reconstruction and rehabilitation of the peripheral nerve injury remains to be seen.

Mechanisms of Nerve Injury

Whenever a patient has sustained a peripheral nerve injury, the treating physician and therapist must fully understand the nature of the injury and the mechanism by which the nerve was injured. Each different type of injury carries with it a different prognosis, and at the time of acute injury, the clinical findings of numbness, paralysis, paresthesia, or pain shed little light on the pathophysiology and ultimate prognosis. By knowing the mechanism of the injury and the pathologic changes produced by that injury, the clinician may better predict the outcome and be better able to plan the care and ultimate reconstruction of the patient's nerve injury.

Nerve injuries can result from many different mechanisms. They can result from compression by internal forces (e.g., tumors, fracture, callus) or by external forces (tourniquet or "crutch palsy"), or from ischemia, traction, x-radiation, inadvertent injection injury, or electrical injury. Although each mechanism represents a different type of injury, all of the injuries result from mechanical deformation, ischemia-induced metabolic failure, or both.

Mechanical deformation lesions encompass the entire spectrum of nerve injury, from first-degree neuropraxic injuries to fifth-degree injuries. In general, the effects of mechanical deformation depend on the rate of application of the deforming forces, the area of the nerve over which they are applied, and the magnitude of the forces. The regional anatomy of the nerve and its adjacent structures, as well as the nerve's proximity to underlying bone and unyielding fascial bands, must be considered. Internal nerve anatomy also is important.

Peripheral nerves organized as a single fascicle are much more vulnerable to injury than nerves consisting of many fascicles surrounded by a larger amount of protective connective tissue. The mechanisms of injury creating mechanical deformation include acute and chronic compression, crush, and stretch. All of these lesions involve some degree of vascular injury. Occlusion of the supporting vasculature accompanies any deformation and may remain after the release of the deforming force.[20] Recovery may depend on the degree of resultant ischemia that persists. When a peripheral nerve is subjected to a severe, abruptly applied deforming force, three grades of injury may result. There may be a rapidly reversible physiologic block, a local demyelinating block, or Wallerian degeneration.[21] Although it is not completely understood which mechanism—mechanical deformation or ischemia—causes the injury, each factor has some role, and they are probably additive.[22]

Acute Compression

Acute compression injuries are especially amenable to experimental examination and can be reproducibly created by the use of a pneumatic tourniquet.[23] At low pressures (up to 30 mm Hg), impaired venular flow is observed[20] and endoneurial fluid pressures are seen to be up to three times normal.[24] Physiologically, decreased nerve conduction velocities are noted.[25] At pressures of 60 mm Hg, nerve fiber viability is endangered by the creation of a local metabolic block, secondary to ischemia. In addition, at this level of compression, mechanical deformation within the nerve fiber is seen. At higher levels of compression (90 mm Hg and higher), there is even greater mechanical deformation of the axon and the supporting structures (Schwann cells), as well as collapse of the intraneural microcirculation, which is likely to persist upon the release of the deforming force.[24,26]

Application of a tourniquet at pressures above systolic but at levels insufficient to cause cellular damage results in progressive centripetal sensory loss and paralysis within 30 to 40 minutes.[27] In these first-degree neuropraxic injuries, the earliest pathophysiologic change is the inability of the nerve to transmit repeated impulses. Although the exact defect is unknown, ischemia from compression surely creates anoxic block of ionic and axonal transport. In addition, compression at high levels causes narrowing of the involved axons, increased endoneurial fluid pressure, and subsequent intra-neural edema.[28,29] The classic examples of acute neuropraxic compression neuropathy include the transient conduction block, typified by paresthesias, that results from local pressure on a peripheral nerve. This causes the familiar sensation that one's leg or arm "goes to sleep." The conduction block rapidly recovers when the pressure is relieved or posture altered. When a motor nerve is involved, the sensation is one of "pseudocramps."[30] With extended tourniquet application at suprasystolic pressures, motor deficits and mild sensory losses occur. There is a higher degree of impairment in faster-conducting larger axons (primarily motor, proprioceptive, and light-touch fibers), whereas the smaller and nonmyelin-ated axons (pain, temperature, and autonomic function) are spared.[31] Higher levels of compression yield a longer-lasting conduction block caused by focal demyelination without dis-ruption of axonal continuity. This local conduction block is caused by mechanical deformation (nodal intussusception).[21,32] Higher levels of pressure on a nerve create further mechanical deformation, which results in the shearing of the mesaxonal Schwann cell from the adaxonal portion of the cell. This damages the myelin, which then degenerates and leaves an area of exposed axon. Conduction is not restored until remyelination is complete,[21,32,33] and function returns in most cases by 3 to 6 weeks.[33] Because axonal continuity is maintained, there is little, if any, target-organ degeneration. Because of the differential susceptibility of axons, complete paralysis (large fibers) can occur without loss of cutaneous sensibility (smaller myelinated and unmyelinated fibers).[34]

Long periods of compression or high levels of pressure over a relatively small area of a peripheral nerve can produce a crushing injury that may be second, third, or even fourth degree. These are *lesions-in-continuity,* and the prognosis for recovery depends on the magnitude of the intraneural dis-ruption. When the crush injury is axonotmetic, the axonal basement membrane remains intact, and regeneration pro-gresses with an exact target-organ match and good recovery. Although recovery can be delayed, most patients have achieved 50% return by 4 months.[23] When the crush injury is neurotmetic (third or fourth degree), function is mildly or moderately reduced by the failure of some axons to achieve a proper end-organ match. Axonal admixture as well as increased amounts of intraneural scar prevents complete return of function, and budding axons can become lost in the interposed scar and develop a neuroma-in-continuity.

Chronic Compression

Injury created by low-grade chronic compression differs from the acute compression injury in all aspects of etiology, histol-ogy, and clinical presentation. The susceptibility of periph-eral nerves to chronic compression is a function of internal anatomy. Proximal nerves, which contain many fascicles and an abundant amount of supportive connective tissue, are much less vulnerable to compression than distal nerves. Within each nerve, peripheral fascicles are more affected

than central fascicles, and within each fascicle, peripheral axons are more likely to be injured than the central ones.[35] There is also a greater susceptibility to compression if the patient is afflicted with malnutrition, alcoholism, diabetes, or renal failure.

Histologic assessment of chronic nerve compression shows myelin sheath asymmetry, epineurial fibrosis, perineu-rial thickening, and, in severe stages, endoneurial fibrosis. Larger fibers appear to "drop out." There is some Wallerian degeneration, and simultaneous regeneration of axons is seen.[35] In contradistinction to the acute compressive neu-ropathy that creates nodal intussusception, the terminal loops of the inner lamellae of the thinned myelin near the entrapment become detached from the axon at the node and retract. An abundance of myelin appears at the opposite end of the internode, which produces bulbous paranodal swell-ing. The detachment and subsequent myelin retraction leave multiple consecutive internodes demyelinated. This partially accounts for the reduced conduction velocity seen in nerves injured by chronic compression. The conduction block seen in acute compression injuries is rarely seen in these chronic lesions.[36]

Chronic compression also affects the vascular supply of the involved segment. In pressures as low as 30 mm Hg, impaired venular flow is observed, ultimately leading to con-gestion and anoxia. This induced ischemia leads to further vascular dilation, nerve swelling, and more compression, beginning a vicious cycle.[37] The rapid reversibility of some chronic compression injuries supports the vascular etiology.[38]

Axoplasmic flow is decreased in chronic compressive inju-ries, and even when the force is insufficient to create a demy-elinating lesion, there is a profound effect on the function of the nerve. Distal to the compressive force, the nerve becomes more sensitive to low levels of pressure. Multiple subclinical levels of compression along any given nerve can lead to symptoms of compressive neuropathy. This *double-crush syn-drome* implies that serial constraints of axoplasmic flow are additive in nature.[39,40]

Histologic changes are observed in nerves subject to chronic compression. Epineurial fibrosis and perineurial thickening are noted, and there is a decrease in the number of large axons in the periphery of the affected fascicles. There is proteinaceous intraneural edema from the loss of the blood–nerve barrier, within which fibroblasts proliferate and ultimately render the nerve segment permanently scarred and potentially anoxic.[41] *Late* chronic compression injuries are more likely to require extensive external neurolysis (and sometimes even internal neurolysis) than early lesions because of the extensive nature of the *intraneural* scar. Patients with chronic compression injuries often report the sensation of pain, but this can arise along any area of the affected nerve's course and is often a misleading diagnostic sign. A more useful diagnostic sign that correlates with the site of compression is the Tinel's sign.[42] At surgical explora-tion, the affected nerve often is seen to be swollen, edema-tous, and hyperemic proximal to the area of compression. The nerve underlying the compression is often pale and narrow.[43] At the time of surgical decompression, almost all patients obtain relief of their pain, although improvement in conduction delay takes weeks or months to return.[41]

Stretch Injury

Peripheral nerves must incorporate within their structure the ability to accommodate changes in joint position. To do this, nerves have the inherent ability to stretch, recoil, and glide within their beds on their loose mesoneurial attachments.[44-47] Under conditions of minimal tension, the nerve fibers assume an undulating course within the fascicle. As longitudinal tension is applied to the nerve, the nerve slides within the bed and begins to take up the load and become stressed. The epineurium—an elastic structure—begins to elongate by "stretch" and the fascicles within completely straighten out. Upon release of the longitudinal tension, the nerve recoils and resumes its natural resting length.[35,44,48,49] As long as the nerve remains free to glide within its bed, significant stretch can be tolerated without injury. Normal excursions of nerves vary greatly, from a maximum of 15.3 mm (average for the brachial plexus) to a minimum of 1.15 mm (average for a digital nerve).[45-47]

When a nerve is injured (through compression, scar, entrapment, or adhesions) and is subsequently anchored by scar tissue to its bed, it can be subjected to "overstretch" traction injury during normal physiologic demands. There are also certain traumatic states that can exceed the normal nerve excursion or limits of elasticity and therein create injury.[47] A nerve achieves its strength through the perineurium. This layer has three orientations of collagen fibers in its outer sheath: circumferential, longitudinal, and oblique.[49,50] As longitudinal tension is applied the perineurium lengthens, but at the expense of the cross-sectional area. This creates an increase in the intrafascicular pressure along the entire length of the nerve.[47-51] As long as the perineurium remains intact, the nerve maintains its elastic characteristics, but intraneural damage occurs far below the point of mechanical failure.[51] The elastic limit, or allowable stretch limit, is about 20%. At that level there can be one or many areas of intraneural tearing, with axonal and fascicular disruption and areas of hemorrhage. Fibroblastic proliferation follows, which ultimately leads to intraneural scarring.[44,52,53]

Although the true incidence of nerve stretch injuries is unknown, these injuries are commonly associated with traumatic events, such as fractures, dislocations, obstetric trauma, and occasionally inadvertent retraction during surgery. Of nerve injuries associated with fractures, 95% occur in the upper extremities, and of the five most commonly injured nerves, 58% are radial, 18% ulnar, 16% peroneal, 6% median, and 2% sciatic.[54] In a prospective study of 648 nerve traction lesions in which the nerve was seen to be in continuity at the time of surgery, Omer[55] reported that 70% achieved spontaneous recovery. In low-velocity gunshot wounds, 69% recovered after 3 to 8 months. Patients with high-velocity gunshot wounds also recovered from nerve lesions 69% of the time, but recovery required up to 9 months. In patients with nerve injuries associated with fractures and dislocations, 83% recovered spontaneously in 1 to 4 months, and in patients with nerve traction (stretch) injuries, 86% recovered in 3 to 6 months.[55]

Not all traction injuries are traumatic. Some are the result of attempts to overcome an excessive nerve gap during reconstruction. This may be by stretch on the nerve stumps to achieve coaptation or by positioning the joints in flexion and creating the traction by the progressive postoperative extension of the joints. The progressive extension may lead to an ischemic injury or even exceed the elastic limits of the nerve.[56] It has been shown that some length can be gained with slow stretch over time.[51] This finding has been exploited using tissue expansion techniques that allow progressive nerve lengthening before nerve reconstruction to overcome nerve gaps. When caring for a patient with a major traction injury, we must be aware that the injury can affect the entire length of the nerve. The most clinically significant injury may be remote from the actual site of extremity injury, and this may test even the most astute diagnostician.

Ischemic Injury

The peripheral nerve requires a continuous and adequate supply of oxygen for aerobic metabolism to drive the normal functions of axoplasmic transport; maintain cell integrity; and remain primed for the generation, maintenance, and restoration of the membrane potentials necessary for conduction of impulses. To accomplish this goal, the nerve has an elaborate dynamic plexus of blood vessels composed of two integrated but functionally independent systems.[57] The peripheral nerve can survive relatively long anoxic periods with a rapid recovery of function,[58-60] but longer periods of acute ischemia or chronic hypoxia may produce irreversible injury. Muscle weakness, pain, paresthesias, hypersensitivity, and sensory deficits all are symptoms of ischemic nerve lesions.[13,61,62]

Ischemic injury may result from three different pathologic processes. There may be large-vessel occlusion, arteriolar angiopathy, or nutrient capillary disease. Large-vessel occlusion caused by conditions such as trauma or embolism is amenable to medical management or direct surgical reconstruction. Arteriolar and capillary disease is indirectly approached by attempts at improving the nerve environment (e.g., flap reconstruction of the nerve bed) or by release of the offending perineurial and intraneural scar (or both).[63,64] Some of the pathologic states that affect the arteriolar (50 to 400 mm in diameter) vessels are necrotizing angiopathic disorders such as polyarteritis nodosa, rheumatoid arthritis, Churg-Strauss syndrome, Wegener's granulomatosis, and thromboangiitis obliterans (Buerger's disease). All of these disease states affect the epineurial arterioles and result in patchy occlusion and ischemic nerve damage.[63,65-67]

The length of time the ischemic insult persists is the most important determinant of anoxic damage. Within the first 10 minutes of nerve ischemia, there is a rapid decrease in the membrane resting potential and electrical resistance. By 15 minutes, the action potential decreases and there is a further decrease in the resting potential, which blocks conduction.[68] There is a complete loss in conductivity by 30 to 40 minutes.[21] Reoxygenation brings recovery within 1 to 2 minutes, and recovery is usually complete by 10 minutes. This implies that the pathologic insult of ischemia is a metabolic phenomenon and not a morphologic one. In chronically ischemic nerves there is segmental demyelination,[66,69,70] and irreversible axonal infarction may occur.[71,72] If regeneration occurs there is a favorable prognosis, because the intraneural destruction leaves the axonal basement membrane intact. This ensures directed axonal regrowth and proper nerve end-organ connectivity.[73]

The question of tolerance to ischemia becomes very important when the issue of replantation or free-tissue transfer is raised. A normal nerve apparently can tolerate up to 8 hours of warm ischemia (room temperature) and suffer little morphologic damage. Nutrient blood flow is rapidly restored upon revascularization. After 8 hours there is a breakdown of the blood–nerve barrier, and the resultant influx of proteinaceous fluid negatively affects nerve regeneration by ultimately stimulating fibroblastic proliferation and subsequent intraneural scarring.[60]

For more proximal amputations in which there is a significant amount of muscle involved, the tolerance to ischemia of the nerve is not of clinical importance, because the target organs suffer irreversible damage before the nerves. However, injured nerve fibers are more susceptible to induced ischemia than are normal nerves. This may be because there is a reduction in axoplasmic flow in the injured nerve (especially if severed).[74]

Electrical Injury

An electrical injury to the upper extremity can run the gamut from minor to life-threatening and is associated with a significant percentage of resultant amputations (32.5%).[75] The severity of these injuries depends on the current pathway and the relevant features of voltage level, tissue resistance, and current duration. The neurologic defects following electrical injury are usually immediate in onset and, for reasons incompletely understood, more commonly involve motor nerves. Most injured nerves show some recovery over time, but complete resolution of significant injuries is rare.[76]

The major pathologic change in the electrically injured nerve is one of coagulation necrosis resulting from the generation of heat energy. The electrical current follows the path of least resistance, and resistance to flow increases in various tissues in the following order: nerve, blood vessel, muscle, skin, tendon, fat, and bone.[77,78] The electrical injury therefore preferentially follows the neurovascular bundles and creates deep-tissue destruction along these pathways. Flash thermal burns at the entrance and exit sites accompany these injuries. In 22% of reported cases of electrical burns, direct nerve destruction was the initial result of the injury.[75] In nondestructive lesions, electrical injuries are found to cause an increase in threshold stimulus and a loss of amplitude of the response to supramaximal stimulation. Although some of these changes were reversible, the electrical injury left a persistent increase in latency and decreased conduction velocity.[79] Severe injuries can lead to patchy necrosis of the entire nerve as well as central necrosis. Hemorrhage and subarachnoid bleeding also are common.[75,78,80-82]

If the nerve is not destroyed, total demyelination in a multifocal distribution is seen, and blood vessels in the vasa nervorum sustain significant damage, thus creating a late ischemic injury. Complicating electrical injury are violent tetanic contractures that can result in hemorrhage, muscle rupture, and broken bones. Late changes principally result from chronic ischemic changes associated with vascular damage and progressive perineurial fibrosis. Unlike the previously mentioned vascular pathology, this chronic ischemic injury may respond to neurolysis and revascularization of the nerve (e.g., muscle flap, omental transfer).[77,82]

Radiation Injury

As radiation treatment becomes more precise and refined, its use as a treatment modality in the therapy for cancer is increasing. With it come increasing survival rates for patients with cancer and also greater opportunity to observe the late effects of radiation injury on surrounding soft tissues and nerves. In the past, orthovoltage radiation (less than 1 million volts) was the standard, and this technique had very shallow tissue penetration. There were marked skin changes that limited the total dose of radiation before significant nerve damage could result. Today, megavoltage radiation (1 million to 35 million volts) has allowed increased penetrance to deeper tissue planes with minimal apparent skin damage, and the result is a much higher dose of radiation to the adjacent structures within the field.[83]

Radiation injury to the peripheral nerve is poorly understood. Injury results from direct cell injury and indirectly from damage caused to the supportive vascular and connective tissues. These injuries are synergistic.[84] Fortunately for neural tissue, there is relative stability in cellular population (i.e., there is little mitotic activity, and therefore little biologically significant damage occurs at the genetic encoding level) until attempts at neural regeneration.[85,86] Cellular damage is more pronounced if the radiation follows a nerve injury that stimulates the cellular supportive proliferation.[87]

Radiation injury is permanent and does not seem to abate with time. Histologically, there is axonal dropout and patchy loss of myelin within the radiated segment. Attempts at Schwann cell proliferation yield a decreased total number of cells that produce abnormally thin myelin sheaths. An increased nerve cross-sectional area implies that there is persistent intraneural edema associated with abnormal endoneurial vessel permeability. Late examination reveals marked intraneural and perineurial fibrosis with apparent fibrous replacement of fascicles and a marked amount of thick pale scar.[83,84,87,88]

Because of the common use of radiation in the treatment of cancers of the breast, brachial plexus radiation injury has been the most extensively studied type of radiation injury. The incidence of brachial plexopathy varies greatly, depending on the mode of delivery and the total dosage. In one series, using 4-MV radiation, 15% of patients developed neurologic symptoms after 5775 rads (5.775 Gy); after 6300 rads (6.3 Gy) the percentage increased to 73%.[83] After radiation given by a 15-MV betatron, 22% of patients receiving between 400 and 5000 rads (0.4 and 5 Gy) developed an actinic plexopathy, increasing to 47% after 550 to 6600 rads (0.55 to 6.6 Gy).[89] The latent period between radiation and the onset of symptoms of plexopathy has ranged from as short as 5 months to as long as 20 years, with a mean latency of 4.25 years.[88,90] Pain is by far the most common presentation of brachial plexopathy, with as many as 80% of patients reporting some amount. Fifty percent of patients describe their pain as severe. Sixty-six percent of patients presented with muscle weakness and atrophy, and this sign was often associated with marked upper extremity lymphedema. Most of the patients with sensory and motor deficits presented with median and ulnar involvement.[88,90]

The typical patient who presents to the hand surgeon with upper extremity pain and who has had radiation for the treatment of a carcinoma presents a diagnostic dilemma. The problem is in distinguishing an actinic plexopathy from local recurrence or metastatic involvement of the nerves by tumor. Both present with like signs and symptoms and have the same mean onset. Both progress steadily over years, but progression of the plexopathy without the development of other metastatic sites is the best presumptive evidence for a radiation-induced lesion. In all surgical cases, absence of metastatic disease must be confirmed by liberal biopsy.[90-93]

The strongest indication for surgical intervention in radiation-induced nerve injury is intractable pain, but surgery should not be approached in a cavalier fashion. Downgrading of function is a likely outcome, because the compromised nerves will not tolerate much surgical manipulation. The goals of surgical intervention should be to gently excise the strangulating fibrotic scar and to improve the vascularity of the involved nerves by transposition to an improved bed or by flap reconstruction.

Injection Injuries

The peripheral nerve is vulnerable to direct injection in many circumstances, and this can result in permanent damage to the nerve. It is common to inject various substances in the immediate vicinity of nerves when administering local anesthetic agents for regional anesthesia or injecting steroid preparations for the local treatment of inflammatory conditions. In addition, the intramuscular injection of materials such as antibiotics can result in inadvertent injection into an underlying peripheral nerve. Most of these injuries could be avoided by knowledge of the surface and underlying anatomy.[94] When a nerve injection injury occurs, the patient can experience severe pain at the site of injection that radiates to the distribution of the nerve. This is often associated with a neurologic deficit—sensory, motor, or both.[95-98]

Injection injury was thought to be caused by mechanical needle injury, allergic neuritis, ischemia, and the development of circumferential scar, as well as the intraneural deposition of neurotoxic substances. Several studies have shown that only the intraneural injection of neurotoxic substances causes significant nerve fiber injury. Only with diazepam, chlordiazepoxide, chlorpromazine, and benzylpenicillin was extrafascicular injection associated with nerve injury. The most severe injuries were related to the intrafascicular injection of meperidine, diazepam, chlorpromazine, hydrocortisone, triamcinolone hexacetonide, procaine, and tetracaine. Less severe, but still significant, injuries were produced by gentamicin, cephalothin, methylprednisolone, triamcinolone acetonide, lidocaine (worse if with epinephrine), and bupivacaine hydrochloride with epinephrine.[97-101] Several of these drugs contain similar buffers, and these may be the offending agents.[102,103]

Acutely, axonal dropout and Wallerian degeneration are seen. Alterations of the blood–nerve barrier change the normal endoneurial environment and may lead to late changes caused by the attendant swelling, ischemia, and

intraneural scar. By 8 weeks after injury, there is severe intraneural fibrosis associated with minimal external scar.[96,99]

When a peripheral nerve injection injury occurs, observation is indicated for the first 3 months, with electrophysiologic studies obtained about 6 weeks after the injury.[97] Early surgical exploration with irrigation of the offending agent or external neurolysis is not recommended. Because the damage is intraneural, extraneural manipulations do not address the pathology. If there is no clinical recovery by 4 months, exploration is indicated. An internal neurolysis procedure should be done to decompress the scarred fascicles, and several months should be allowed to elapse to see what functional recovery follows. If little improvement is gained, one should perform resection of the neuroma incontinuity, followed by reconstruction.[97,104,105]

Laceration Injury

Nerve laceration is likely to be one of the most common injuries that the peripheral nerve surgeon treats. Lacerations are either complete or partial, and all are fifth-degree neurotmetic lesions. A sharp instrument causes most such injuries, but some are associated with sharp bone fragments in a closed fracture. All are associated with a clearly defined neural motor or sensory deficit that will not improve without surgical intervention. Approximately 20% of all nerve lacerations that appear to be complete are in fact only partial lacerations, with contusion and stretch being responsible for the neuropraxic or axonotmetic deficit of the remaining intact fascicles.[105] Nerve lacerations are essentially low-velocity crush injuries isolated to very small areas of the involved nerve. Even under ideal conditions, a divided nerve will have some component of crush injury in the proximal and distal stumps, which must be treated by careful debridement at the time of surgical reconstruction.[106]

Factors that Influence Regeneration

Peripheral nerve reconstruction is built on a foundation of principles that, when followed, facilitate the natural regenerative process of the nerve. Regeneration of the peripheral nerve after injury is influenced by mechanical forces, delay to repair, the patient's age, and the level of the injury.

Mechanical interference to nerve regeneration is in the form of scar tissue and inappropriate topographic orientation. The nerve axon has the greatest likelihood of accurate regeneration when minimum scar is interposed between the severed nerve ends and if there is accurate alignment of the fascicles. This increases the probability that the regenerating axons will enter their native nerve fibers and achieve appropriate connectivity.[107]

Delay before reconstruction is another important factor. The capacity for a nerve cell body to regenerate is essentially unlimited as long as cell death does not occur. It is the passage of time, however, that eliminates the possibility for regeneration by time-related changes in the distal nerve segment (scar and progressive decrease in diameter) and in the target organs (atrophy and degeneration).[13]

There is little question that there is a consistently better functional return in the young after nerve injury.[108] Rates of nerve regeneration are age-related. They decline with increasing age and may be related to the decreasing rates of slow-axonal transport with age.[109] In addition, trophic mechanisms seem to function over greater distances in the young, and this may facilitate more accurate end-organ connectivity.[107] The differences in the quality of return of sensibility between the young and old may be attributable to the diminution in receptor populations that occurs naturally in the old (at least for populations of Meissner corpuscles).[110] Finally, the consistently better functional outcomes in the young may result from greater central plasticity. This is the cortical ability to relearn or reorganize spatially disrupted input and thereby overcome the inexact peripheral connectivity.[111]

The injury level (proximal versus distal) is one of the greatest factors in determining the prognosis for successful outcome of regeneration. Proximal injuries generally carry a worse prognosis than distal injuries. In a proximal injury, regenerative demand on the cell body is greater because the axon must regenerate for a greater distance. Also, in proximal injuries there is a greater likelihood of neuronal death.[36,112] Second, if the injury is proximal, there is a greater distance to the target organ, and in the time the axon takes to regenerate over the great distance to the end-organ, considerable atrophy or degeneration may have occurred.[105,112,113] Intraneural topography also plays an important role. The more proximal the nerve, the greater the fascicular heterogeneity. In higher level injuries, there is more axonal mixing during regeneration; this makes appropriate target-organ connectivity difficult if not impossible.[13]

The cause of the nerve injury is important, and the associated structures—skin, bone, joint, and vascular system—must be stabilized before any definitive reconstruction. Devitalized tissues must be debrided, bones must be stabilized, and blood vessels (when injured) must be repaired. Severe injuries may result in multilevel nerve lesions from traction, compression, or ischemia. As an injury increases in severity, there is more scarring around the nerve and its bed, thereby decreasing the quality of regeneration. In addition, a patient in an unstable condition may require delay in the repair. Nerve repair or reconstruction should not be performed in the absence of good skin cover, skeletal stability (ideally with supple joints), and without correction of vascular insufficiency. Infection should be aggressively treated, and adjunctive procedures such as flap coverage should be performed if they will facilitate earlier nerve reconstruction.

Reinnervation

Reinnervation of a target organ involves much more than just axonal regeneration and connectivity. After an axon reaches the target organ, neuromuscular junctions and the axon terminus of sensory receptors must be reestablished, and this does not occur if there is an axon target-organ mismatch.

Because of the randomness of regeneration for all of the higher level injuries, there are five potential outcomes of regeneration. An axon may achieve exact reinnervation by establishing continuity with its native target organ. If the end-organ is not irreversibly damaged, return of function can be essentially normal. If the end-organ has degenerated, there will be no useful return of function. The wrong receptor may be reinnervated within the proper territory, resulting in improper input, or the axon may achieve connectivity with the appropriate receptor in the wrong territory and create false localization. Finally, the axon may be frustrated and not achieve end-organ connectivity, thereby rendering the results of regeneration fruitless.

When a regenerating motor axon reaches a denervated muscle, reinnervation generally occurs at old motor end plates.[3,114,115] The axon then sprouts and reinnervates contiguous muscle fibers, creating histochemically uniform *giant* motor units.[116] Recovery of motor function does not immediately occur upon reestablishment of the neuromuscular junctions. There is an 18-day delay before nerve stimulation will produce contraction, and another 5 days elapse before functional reflex activity can occur.[117] Recovery of *functional* activity best correlates with the return of the γ-*efferent control* of the intrafusal fibers.[118] Without adequate γ-return, the muscle function is downgraded clinically by imprecision of motion despite good return.[119]

The recovery of sensibility occurs in a repeatable orderly sequence that correlates with the morphology of the reinnervated receptor populations. The perception of pain and temperature precede the return of touch, and the touch submodalities recover in the following sequence: 30-Hz frequencies, moving touch, constant touch, and finally 256-Hz stimuli.[10]

Peripheral Nerve Reconstruction

Over the past 20 years, the therapeutic approach toward the patient with nerve injury has significantly changed, facilitated by new technologies of intraoperative electrodiagnosis, by better instruments and magnification, and by better understanding of peripheral nerve structure and function. *Atraumatic* nerve handling and suture techniques have improved the potential for nerve reconstruction. Awareness of fascicular anatomy has made the results of nerve repair more precise, and the appreciation of the untoward effects of tension at the repair site has made nerve interposition grafting commonplace. After reconstruction, knowledge of the patterns of sensory recovery has led to elaborate schemes of sensory reeducation that enable more functional use.

Timing

There are no absolute rules regarding the timing of nerve repair, and the decisions should be made after careful consideration of the nature of the injury, the condition of the patient, and the status of the associated injuries. Nerve injuries can be divided into two broad categories. First are those injuries in which there is a suspected transection. These must be handled with primary reconstruction if all conditions permit. Second are those injuries in which the nerve is expected to be in continuity or in which there are multilevel lesions or marked contusion. These injuries require secondary reconstruction. By definition, primary repair is that which is done within 48 hours of injury. Early secondary repairs are those performed within the first 6 weeks, and late secondary repairs are performed after 3 months.[105,106,120,121]

If the limits of the nerve injury can be delineated, there is a definite advantage to performing repair or reconstruction primarily. If the repair is performed within 4 days, electrical stimulation can be used to identify distal fascicles and nerve stump retraction is limited. If the repair is delayed beyond 4 days, Wallerian degeneration has progressed and electrical stimulation is not possible. If the wound is contaminated or if there is a soft-tissue deficit or fracture, nerve repair must be delayed until a clean stable wound can be obtained. With adequate debridement, soft-tissue reconstruction, and fracture stabilization, the nerve repair can be done simultaneously. If a primary nerve repair fails because it is done under poor conditions, the patient is likely to obtain a worse result than if repair had been delayed until a secondary repair could be done under good conditions.

There are times when the surgeon should delay repair or reconstruction after an injury. These are when there is an expected first-, second-, or third-degree injury. No surgical reconstruction can provide a better result than an intact fascicle that has healed on its own, and time should be allowed to elapse for the resolution of low-grade lesions. It is appropriate to allow 8 to 16 weeks for the resolution of nontransecting blunt or stretch injuries.

The greatest advantage of primary nerve reconstruction is the saving of time.[121] The great disadvantage is the inability to detect the precise extent of the nerve injury, especially if there is an undetected traction or multilevel injury. If repair is done under the latter circumstances (undetected injury), some function can return with time, but the surgeon is then faced with the decision to reoperate in hopes of achieving greater return or to wait for improvement that is not likely to come. A great advantage of all secondary repairs is that the surgeon and the operating team can perform the surgery electively, without fatigue, and under proper operating room conditions, making it perhaps easier to achieve a more meticulous microcoaptation.

Nerve Repair Technique

Exploration after an injury always should be done under tourniquet control if possible. This allows for more accurate dissection and identification of the lesion. Nerve microcoaptation does not require a bloodless field as long as the structures are properly positioned and tagged. In fact, it is sometimes preferable to deflate the tourniquet before the microsurgical repair to obtain homeostasis, because this can be difficult to accomplish after a nerve repair without jeopardizing the coaptation.

Nerve lesions should be approached with wide exposure, proximal and distal. The nerve is dissected from the uninjured to the injured areas of the nerve, with attempt made to preserve all vascular attachments. For lacerations, high magnification is used to determine the fascicular pattern of the nerve; this allows the orientation of both the proximal and distal ends of the nerve to be appreciated. High magnification also should be used to perform the fascicular dissection for lesions that are in continuity. As the lesion is reached, fascicles that do not contribute to the neuroma can be carefully freed from the offending scar and involved fascicles. Electrical

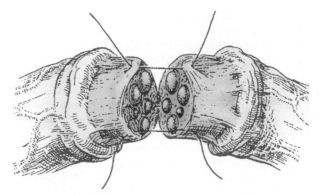

Figure 43-1 Epineurial repair. Diagrammatic representation of the microcoaptation. The outer epineurium is resected proximally and distally. After careful alignment of the nerve stumps, sutures are placed in the inner epineurium. Two or three tension-relieving sutures can be used if necessary, using 8-0 nylon, and the coaptation is completed using 10-0 nylon. (From Terzis JK, Smith KL. *The Peripheral Nerve: Structure, Function and Reconstruction.* New York: Raven Press, 1990.)

stimulation or intraoperative electrodiagnosis can be used to determine which of the fascicles retain sufficient conduction and can be spared. The fascicles that contribute to the neuroma then can be resected and repaired or reconstructed with interposition grafts.

End-to-End Coaptation

The most commonly used technique for peripheral nerve microcoaptation is the *epineurial repair* technique (Fig. 43-1).[122] This technique is applied to the completely transected nerve, and its advantages are simplicity, rapid execution time, and minimal requirement for magnification.

The cut nerve end is debrided carefully and serially sectioned until the axoplasmic outflow mushrooms under positive intrafascicular pressure and the fascicular pattern is identified and is relatively free of scar.[123] The same is done for the distal stump, and then, with the nerves lying without tension next to one another, the magnification is increased to 25× and 10-0 nylon sutures are placed in the epineurium, as one carefully realigns the fascicular bundles to achieve exact coaptation. A minimum number of sutures are used to complete the repair. Usually, 8 or 10 sutures are necessary for a large nerve and as few as 2 sutures for a small one. If the nerve gap is so large that the first 10-0 suture cannot hold the nerve ends in apposition, one or two guide sutures of 8-0 can be used.

The leading causes of failure of the epineurial repair are gapping, overriding, buckling, and straddling of the fascicle ends. Even slight tension can create a significant intraneural gap, which is quickly filled with scar tissue, making regeneration difficult at best.[124-126]

The second common technique of peripheral nerve reconstruction is the *perineurial repair* (Fig. 43-2). A great deal of discussion focuses on whether an *epineurial repair* or a *perineurial repair* (fascicular repair) is the preferred method of peripheral nerve reconstruction, but numerous articles report no difference in the regeneration and functional recovery associated with either technique.[127-130] When significant debridement is required before microcoaptation, fascicular

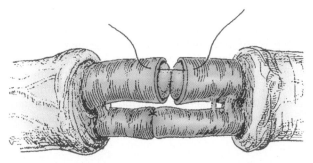

Figure 43-2 Perineurial (fascicular) repair. Diagrammatic representation of the microcoaptation. The outer and inner epineurium is dissected from the proximal and distal stumps. Fascicles and fascicular groups are aligned, and the coaptations are performed with the minimum number of 10-0 nylon sutures necessary (as few as two). Note the care taken to place the sutures within the inner epineurium or perineurium and not to violate the endoneurium. (From Terzis JK, Smith KL. *The Peripheral Nerve: Structure, Function and Reconstruction.* New York: Raven Press, 1990.)

matching is improved with this technique; it is also used extensively when interposition grafts are indicated.

Under high magnification, the nerve ends are prepared and the epineurium is dissected away. Fascicles are separated, and coaptation is performed between matching fascicles, with sutures placed into the inner epineurium. Sutures are carefully placed so as not to enter the endoneurium. The great advantage of the perineurial technique is the accurate coaptation of similar-size fascicles. The greatest disadvantage is the stimulation of greater amounts of intraneural scar by increased dissection and foreign material (suture).[130-133]

Tension and Nerve Grafting

After any nerve injury in which there is a gap between the nerve endings, either after trauma or as required by debridement, the surgeon faces a dilemma. Should the nerve gap be bridged by extensive mobilization and stretch (with the nerve repair under tension); should the defect be bridged with a nerve graft, forcing the axons to cross two coaptations[134]; or should the limb be postured in flexion to bring the nerve ends together and then slowly returned to full extension in hopes of stretching the nerves out to length?

Tension at the site of coaptation invites the proliferation of scar tissue at the repair. As the scar matures, it tends to constrict the regenerating axons within.[105] If the joints are flexed, mobilization can create a second traction lesion in the already injured nerve. If the regenerating axons manage to cross the suture line and grow down the nerve fiber, they are unlikely to achieve functional reinnervation in a great number of cases. Studies have shown that repeated stretching of a sutured nerve fails to result in its elongatation, and instead, repetitive traction injuries result.[56,135]

Comparing the results of nerve grafting with those of coaptation under tension, Millesi determined that there was little interposed scar at the coaptation if the nerve was repaired without tension, with or without a graft. Electrophysiologic studies supported the use of grafts in lieu of coaptation under tension and showed excellent recovery

even in the face of two suture lines.[43,136,137] Nerve grafting is approached surgically like any nerve exploration. The nerve ends are exposed and prepared, and a suitable donor nerve (commonly the sural nerve) is harvested and cut to length. Depending on the caliber of the injured nerve, the number of interposition grafts is chosen to match the cross-sectional area. Fascicular matching is conducted, and the perineurial repairs are done.

Alternatives to Nerve Grafting

Autogenous nerve grafting is no longer the only approach available to reconstruct the nerve gap. The nerve gap can be mechanically shortened by nerve-lengthening techniques (tissue expansion or nerve distraction)[138] or bridged by tubes of biologic or nonbiologic materials.

To avoid donor-site morbidity from autogenous nerve harvest, interest has been rekindled in various tubulization techniques and in homografting (transplant). Like an autogenous nerve graft, the nonneural tube offers a conduit for the budding axons, and growing nerves can be directed across a nerve gap to achieve connectivity with the distal nerve stump. Examples of conduits currently in use are those constructed from polyglycolic acid, autogenous vein, and amnion.[139,140] Results of reconstruction with conduits of short nerve gaps (less than 3 cm) in digital nerves show functional results equal to tensionless coaptations, thereby making this technique quite advantageous in view of the elimination of donor-site morbidity.[141] However, the maximum gap that can presently be bridged with a conduit seems to be 3 cm, and reconstruction with conduits requires 2 to 3 weeks of orthotic positioning in the postoperative period.

Promising results have also been obtained with tissue-expansion techniques. Slow expansion of Wallerian-degenerated nerve results in accelerated Schwann cell proliferation and increased vascularity that seem to facilitate nerve regeneration.[142] Promising results have also been obtained with tissue-expansion techniques. Slow expansion of Wallerian-degenerated nerve results in accelerated Schwann cell proliferation and increased vascularity that seem to facilitate nerve regeneration.[142] Permanent elongation of 30% could be achieved with expansion techniques yielding results of repair equal to tensionless primary nerve coaptation. However, the proximal segment tolerated expansion better than the distal segment.[143]

With successful repair, the progressing Tinel's sign can follow regeneration as the budding axons travel along the nerve. It is important to follow the punctum maximum, because this delineates the most distal extent of the majority of axons. If the Tinel's sign fails to progress and remains at the site of coaptation, this is an indication for reexploration and repair. If Tinel's sign stalls distally to the repair, one must assume there is a second lesion previously unknown.

After the nerve repair, it is important that the nerve coaptation be protected for 7 to 10 days by immobilization. Then, during the period of nerve regeneration, therapy should concentrate on keeping the affected areas supple, mobile, and ready to accept the growing axons. As soon as sensory reinnervation is seen, sensory reeducation programs should begin.

Summary

Over the last decades, peripheral nerve reconstructive surgery has evolved from rather crude reapproximation of severed nerve ends performed without much regard for tension or topographic orientation, to technically precise methods of surgery for which better understanding of the intraneural anatomy has allowed better fascicular alignment and has led to improved results. These still fall below the ideal of axon-to-axon realignment, however. Perhaps in the future, new understanding of tropic and trophic manipulations will allow us to achieve even better results and achieve exact target-organ reinnervation, and techniques of tensionless sutureless coaptation, and scar manipulation will serve to eliminate fibrotic interference with regeneration. Today, we can appreciate that the nerve cell has an essentially unlimited regenerative capability. It is the job of the surgeon to perform as precise a repair after a nerve injury as possible, and it is the job of the therapist to assist the patient in the maintenance of the end-organs by protective orthotic positioning, range-of-motion therapy, massage, and modalities as indicated, to achieve the best possible functional results after nerve injuries and repair.

REFERENCES

The complete reference list is available online at www.expertconsult. com.

New Advances in Nerve Repair

CHAPTER

44

DAVID J. SLUTSKY, MD, FRCS(C)

BASIC CONSIDERATIONS
NERVE REPAIR

NERVE GRAFTING
ALTERNATE METHODS OF NERVE
RECONSTRUCTION

CRITICAL POINTS

Indications
- Motor or sensory loss with open wound
- Crush or stretch injury without progressive motor or sensory recovery after 3 to 6 months.
- Irreparable nerve damage

Priorities
- Acute primary nerve repair without tension to achieve best outcomes
- Nerve graft with more than 10% loss of nerve substance
- Conversion of open dirty wounds to clean closed wounds before repair

Pearls
- Electrical fascicle identification useful for median/ulnar nerve repairs in the forearm
- Acceptable to substitute conduits for nerve grafts with sensory nerve gaps less than 3 cm
- Nerve transfers within 6 months following high median/ulnar nerve lesions or upper trunk plexus injury

Healing Times and Progression of Therapy
- Volar/dorsal block orthosis with short arc motion for 3 weeks following primary nerve repair
- Immobilization of limb in extension for 8 days after nerve graft, followed by unrestricted motion
- Sensory reeducation crucial for good outcomes after sensory nerve reconstruction or transfer
- Motor reeducation with emphasis on co-contraction of donor muscle following nerve transfer

Pitfalls
- Nerve repair under tension should be avoided
- Nerve graft through a poorly vascularized bed should not be attempted

Precautions
- Communication with surgeon regarding optimum position for limb immobilization essential

Timelines for Return to Work and Activities of Daily Living
- Activities of daily living to commence after 3 to 4 weeks in most cases
- Because motor and sensory recovery continue past 2 years, long-term job modification may be necessary

Basic Considerations

Although the techniques of nerve repair have been refined to a considerable degree, they remain relatively crude from the nerve's perspective. There have been few advances in the practical aspects of a basic nerve repair over the past 20 years, but there have been exciting discoveries that harness the nerve's regenerative capacities following injury and these have led to new methods for nerve reconstruction. Techniques that have been commonplace for brachial plexus surgery are now migrating into the arm, including end-to-side repairs, nerve conduits, and nerve transfers.

Nerve Anatomy

The science and rationale behind nerve reconstruction is built upon an understanding of nerve anatomy, physiology, and the basic science of nerve injury and healing. The reader is referred to Chapter 42 for a detailed discussion of this topic.

611

Nerve Biomechanics

A normal nerve has a longitudinal excursion that subjects it to a certain amount of stress and strain in situ. A peripheral nerve is initially easily extensible. Elasticity decreases by as much as 50% in the delayed repair of nerves in which Wallerian degeneration has occurred.[1] Experimentally, blood flow is reduced by 50% when the nerve is stretched 8% beyond its in vivo length. Complete ischemia occurs at 15%. Suture pull-out does not occur until a 17% increase in length has occurred. This suggests that ischemia and not disruption of the anastomosis is the limiting factor in acute nerve repairs.[2] Nerve is a viscoelastic tissue, meaning that when low loading in tension is applied over time the nerve elongates without a deterioration in nerve conduction velocity. Intriguing experimental work has been done with gradual nerve elongation to overcome nerve gaps using tissue expansion and external fixation,[3] but this cannot as yet be considered an accepted standard of treatment.

The Nerve Gap

There is a difference between a nerve gap and a nerve defect. A nerve gap refers to the distance between the nerve ends, whereas a nerve defect refers to the actual amount of nerve tissue that is lost. With simple nerve retraction following division, the fascicular arrangement is similar. With increasing nerve defects between the proximal and distal stumps there is a greater fascicular mismatch between the stumps, which leads to poorer outcomes, especially if the gap exceeds 5 cm.

Nerve Repair

The location of fascicles varies somewhat within a nerve, and there are cross-connections between them as fibers migrate from one fascicle to another. The use of intraoperative motor and sensory nerve differentiation can diminish the risk of fascicular mismatch when repairing or grafting a nerve.

Electrical Fascicle Identification

Motor and sensory fascicles can be differentiated by direct stimulation up to 72 hours.[4] The median and ulnar nerves in the distal forearm are most amenable to this technique.[5] A low-amperage stimulator is applied to the major fascicles of the proximal nerve end in a systematic manner with the patient under local anesthesia. Sensory fascicles will elicit pain and may be localized to a specific digit. Motor fascicles elicit no response at lower intensities and poorly localized pain at higher intensities. A cross-sectional sketch of the proximal stump is made. The sensory fascicles are tagged with 10-0 nylon and the patient is placed under general anesthesia. The distal stump is then stimulated in a similar fashion. The reverse picture will be seen, with motor fascicles eliciting a muscle twitch and sensory fascicles being silent. A cross-sectional map is again made and used to match the proximal and distal motor and sensory fascicles.

Alternatively, this author has used nerve action potentials (NAPs) in place of the muscle twitch to map the distal stump.[6] The compound motor action potential (CMAP) dis-

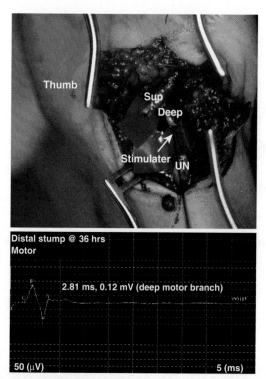

Figure 44-1 Intraoperative stimulation of ulnar nerve at wrist. **A,** Stimulation of deep motor branch. **B,** CMAP with normal latency but low amplitude (recorded from ADM).

appears at 7 to 9 days, whereas the sensory nerve action potential (SNAP) disappears at day 10 to 11.[7] In chronic injuries the NAPs are no longer present; hence, it is necessary to dissect the distal motor branch, and then follow the motor fascicles proximally to the nerve stump (Fig. 44-1).

Indications

The principal indication for surgery is a patient who presents with a laceration and a nerve deficit that does not recover within 1 week. A tension-free repair is the goal for any nerve anastomosis. When there is a clean transection of the nerve and the gap is caused by elastic retraction, an acute primary repair is indicated.

Contraindications

Nerve repair cannot be performed in an infected wound. If the degree of the longitudinal injury cannot be determined, nerve repair should be delayed.

Types of Repair

External Epineurial Suture

This technique is appropriate for small nerves containing only one or two fascicles, such as digital nerves. Since they only contain sensory fibers, matching is not a problem. Epineurial repairs are also indicated for mixed nerves where separate motor and sensory fascicle identification is not possible.

Group Fascicular Suture

The motor and sensory groups of fascicles are identified as described. In a major nerve such as the median or ulnar, four

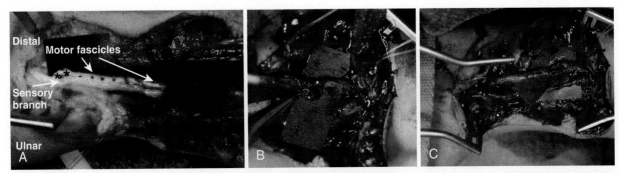

Figure 44-2 A, Ulnar nerve motor fascicles traced from the distal stump to the deep motor branch (*) in the palm. **B,** Group fascicular repair of motor group fascicles (*). **C,** Epineurial repair of remaining sensory fascicles.

or five groups may be chosen for suture. These are then matched appropriately with the opposite end and approximated with sutures in both the internal and external epineurium.

External Epineurial Splint

Jabaley has employed the external epineurium as a splinting device.[8] The external epineurium is incised longitudinally on its superficial surface and dissected away from the underlying fascicles. The epineurium is left attached on the deep surface, several millimeters from each nerve end. A few interrupted sutures with 8-0 nylon are used to join the ends of the external epineurial strips on the deep surface only, completing the construction of the splint. This maneuver provides for a coaptation of individual fascicles or groups of fascicles with little or no tension (Fig. 44-2).

Postoperative Rehabilitation

After nerve repair the rehabilitation focuses on three areas: initial immobilization to protect the repair; joint mobilization to promote longitudinal excursion of the nerve; and motor and sensory reeducation. Before wound closure, the adjacent joints are placed in various degrees of flexion and extension so as to determine the optimum limb position that unloads the repair site. This position is maintained with a blocking orthosis for 3 weeks but a protected short arc of motion may be instituted to provide some nerve gliding. The reader is referred to Chapter 44 for a detailed discussion of postoperative management and rehabilitation.

Nerve Grafting

Indications

When treatment of a nerve laceration is delayed, fibrosis of the nerve ends prevents approximation; hence, nerve grafting is required, even though there is no loss of nerve tissue. Nerve grafting to repair a defect is indicated when the length of the gap to be bridged would require more than a 10% elongation of the nerve.[1] This is a better indication for grafting than the nerve gap per se, although 4 cm is often used as a critical defect threshold.

Contraindications

Since the graft is vascularized from the tissue bed, nerve grafting cannot be performed in burned or irradiated tissue.

Role of the Nerve Graft

The nerve graft provides a source of empty endoneurial tubes through which the regenerating axons can be directed. A normal nerve can compensate for the change in length with limb flexion and extension because it is surrounded by gliding tissue that permits longitudinal movement. A nerve graft becomes welded to its recipient bed by the adhesions through which it becomes vascularized. As a consequence the nerve graft is exquisitely sensitive to tension because it has no longitudinal excursion. The harvested length of the graft must be long enough to span the nerve gap without tension while the adjacent joints are extended. This is also the position of temporary immobilization. If the limb or digit is immobilized with joint flexion, the graft will become fixed in this position. When the limb is then mobilized at 8 days, the proximal and distal stumps will be subject to tension even though the graft was initially long enough. Early attempts at lengthening the graft will lead to disruption of the anastomosis.

Considerations for Donor Nerve Grafts. Small-diameter grafts spontaneously revascularize, but thick grafts undergo central necrosis with subsequent endoneurial fibrosis that ultimately impedes the advancement of any ingrowing axon sprouts. The donor-site defect must also be acceptable for the patient. For these reasons most of the available grafts are cutaneous nerves. Typical donor nerves include the medial and lateral antebrachial cutaneous nerves and the sural nerve. The distal terminations of the anterior and posterior interosseous nerves are suitable for digital nerve grafts at the distal interphalangeal joint level.

Surgical Technique

Millesi has written extensively on this subject.[9] If the recipient nerve is the approximate diameter of the graft, the two stumps are transected until normal-appearing tissue without fibrosis is seen; the graft is then inserted by an epineurial repair. Multiple nerve grafts are used to completely cover the cross-sectional area of each fascicle in a 1 to 2 or 1 to 3 ratio (Fig. 44-4). If there is no group fascicular arrangement, interfascicular dissection is not performed. Graft insertion is then guided by the intraneural topography of the nerve for that specific level of injury.

Outcomes Following Repair or Graft

Most series report the results of nerve repair using the British Medical Research Council grading system, which has been

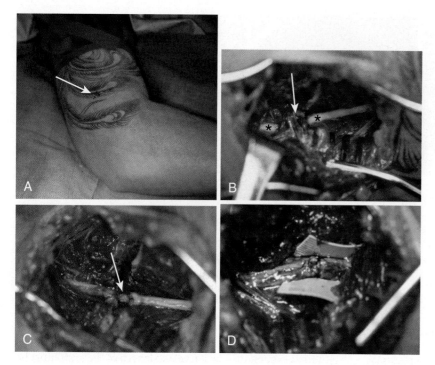

Figure 44-3 A, Miniscute exit wound (*arrow*) following a stabbing with a knife from the medial arm. **B,** Knife tract (*arrow*) with separation of proximal and distal nerve ends (***). **C,** Strip of posterior epineurium is sutured (*arrow*) to take the tension off the repair. **D,** Completed epineurial repair. (From Slutsky DJ. A practical approach to nerve grafting in the upper extremity. In: Slutsky DJ, Hentz VR, eds. *Peripheral Nerve Surgery: Practical Applications in the Upper Extremity.* Philadelphia: Elsevier, 2006, with permission.)

modified by Dellon and MacKinnon.[10] In this classification, scores of S0 and M0 represent absent sensory and motor function, respectively, while scores of S1 or S2 and M1 or M2 represent detectable but less useful function. S3 equates to recovery of pain and touch sensibility, with two-point discrimination of greater than 15 mm, while S3+ equates to two-point discrimination of 7 to 15 mm; an S4 is normal sensation. A grade of M3 equates to a recovery of muscle strength that is sufficient to overcome gravity. M4 is strength with gravity and added resistance, while M5 is normal. As noted below, however, many other classifications are also in use, adding to the difficulty of interstudy comparison.

Ruijs et al. performed a meta-analysis after microsurgical nerve repair of 623 median or ulnar nerve injuries. Motor and sensory recovery were significantly associated. In ulnar nerve injuries, the chance of motor recovery was 71% lower than in median nerve injuries.[11] Kallio and co-authors evaluated 132 patients (mean age 28 years) with injuries to the median nerve at an average 10.4 years after repair. Most of the nerve lesions were sharp or blunt injuries.[12] Division was total in 87 cases, and most were at the wrist level. Secondary repair was performed in 34 cases and fascicular grafting in 98 cases. The average gap width was 5.8 cm. Excellent or good results were obtained in only 49.2%. The result of nerve repair was poor in patients aged over 54 years, when the level of the injury was more than 56 cm proximal to the fingertip, if the preoperative delay was more than 24 months, or if the graft length was more than 70 mm.[12]

Secer et al. reported the results of 407 ulnar nerve injuries caused by gunshot wounds. A good outcome was noted in 15% of patients who underwent high-level repair, 29% of patients who underwent intermediate-level repair, and 49% of patients after low-level repair. The critical period for surgery was within 6 months of injury. Although the optimal graft length was found to be 5 cm, this finding was not statistically significant.[13] Kim and co-authors examined 45 patients following surgically treated posterior interosseous

nerve entrapments[14] or injuries.[15] Seven underwent suture repair, seven were grafted, and the rest underwent neurolysis. Most muscles achieved Louisiana State University Health Sciences Center grade 3 or better.[16]

Kallio studied 95 patients with 254 completely divided digital nerves at an average of 12.4 years after repair.[17] Secondary epineurial suture was used in 53, fascicular grafting in 37, and fascicular suture in 5. Useful sensory function was recovered in 79% of the nerves operated on with epineurial or fascicular suture and in 56% with fascicular grafting.[17]

It is commonly accepted that the results are far better in children than in adults. Tomei et al. evaluated 25 nerve repairs at the wrist in children under age 15 years with a minimum follow-up of 12 months. The sensory results were often excellent (S4 or S3+ in 23 of 25 cases), whereas motor recovery ranged between M2 and M3.[18]

Frykman and Gramyk reviewed eight studies of nerve grafting published before 1990.[19] This included 167 patients who underwent median nerve grafting. In this pooled dataset 81% achieved a grade of M3, while 79% achieved S3. In a more recent series from Daoutis et al., M3 or better was achieved in 68% and S3 or better in 75% of 47 patients with median nerve grafts.[20] Kim et al. reported M3/S3 in 72% of 50 patients.[21] Milessi achieved M4 or better in 61% and S3 or better in 42%. For the ulnar nerve, he reported M4 or better in 49% and S3 or better in 27%, whereas he reported S3+ or better in only 22% for digital nerve repairs.[9]

Alternate Methods of Nerve Reconstruction

End-to-Side Repairs

Experimental data in both rabbit and primate models have shown that intact donor nerves have the ability to sprout lateral branches from their axons that can grow through endo-, peri-, and epineurium and reinnervate target organs with functional sensory and motor results.[22,23] A standard end-to-side anastomosis involves suturing the recipient nerve into an epineural window that is created in the donor nerve. An advantage of this technique is that the donor nerve does not lose any function (Fig. 44-5).

End-to-side repairs cannot replace a sound primary repair, but they have been used as an adjunctive procedure in the following situations: intact nerve to the musculocutaneous to neurotize the biceps muscle; distal stump of the ulnar nerve to the median nerve at the wrist in high ulnar nerve palsies or vice versa; and ulnar digital nerves to intact median sensory nerves. The limb is positioned for 3 weeks so as to minimize tension, followed by motor and sensory reeducation. The procedure is best done early (within 6 months), since the results deteriorate if delayed beyond that. In Mennen's series of 56 patients, which included 33 ulnar-to-median and 7 median-to-ulnar repairs, M3/S3 was achieved in 56%.[24]

Neurotization

Brunelli pioneered the concept of direct neurotization of denervated muscles in situations where the motor nerve has been avulsed and direct nerve suture or grafting is not possible.[25] They demonstrated in rat and rabbit models that an axon that is in contact with a denervated muscular fiber can form a new neuromuscular junction. The motor end plate is actually not an anatomic formation but instead a functional alteration of the axon endings and the muscular fibers that develop with direct contact. A prerequisite for this procedure is that there is some residual trophism of the muscle. This is manifested by the presence of fibrillation potentials on the electromyogram. The procedure is contraindicated if there is muscle atrophy without fibrillation potentials or if there is extensive scarring or joint stiffness.

A sural nerve graft of adequate length is harvested and sutured end to end to the donor nerve. The distal part of the nerve graft is freed from the epineurium and is divided into as many artificial fascicles as possible. The artificial fascicles are then implanted into the muscle, held in place with fibrin glue and epineurial sutures, and immobilized for 15 days, followed by mobilization. In Brunelli's series of 80 patients, M4/M5 motor strength was achieved in 72 of the cases.[26]

Nerve Conduits

Neurotrophism is the ability of chemotactic hormonal or growth factors to enhance the rate of nerve regeneration. *Neurotrophic* factors produced by the target end-organ undergo retrograde axonal transport and help support the cell body. *Neurotropism* describes the directional accuracy of that regeneration. The growth cone is attracted to *neurotropic* proteins that are derived from the distal degenerating nerve segment after nerve transection. These phenomena have been exploited through the use of synthetic or natural conduits to bridge the nerve gap. Histologically, fibrin clot develops inside the tube within hours. Within the first week longitudinally oriented fibrin matrix bridges span the nerve gap. In the second week, fibroblasts, Schwann cells, macrophages, and endothelial cells permeate the matrix. Axon sprouts from

proximal nerve reach the distal stump and become myelinated by the fourth week. The axons elongate down intact inside the distal endoneurial tubes and reinnervate the target organs. Nondegradable tubes out of silicone were initially used. More recently, natural prosthetic tubes have included freeze-thawed muscle (which contains a basal lamina) and autogenous vein grafts. Biodegradable synthetic material includes polyglycolic acid, caprolactone, and collagen. The postoperative rehabilitation includes early mobilization of the part—since tension on the repair site is not a consideration—followed by appropriate sensory and/or motor retraining.

Lundborg compared tubulation using a silicone conduit, after intentionally leaving a 3- to 4-mm nerve gap (11 cases), with a conventional microsurgical repair of transected median and ulnar nerve repairs (7 cases) in the forearm. The results showed no significant differences between the two techniques, although the silicone tubes had to be removed at a later date, due to compression of the re-formed nerve.[15] Chiu et al. did a series of animal experiments bridging gaps of 1.0 to 6.0 cm using autogenous vein grafts.[27] The technique includes suturing a reversed vein graft in place distally so that the valves in the vein cannot collapse and block axonal migration. The proximal repair is performed after filling the vein with saline to prevent clot formation that would produce scarring and could obstruct the axons (Fig. 44-6). In their clinical series, Chiu and Strauch reported comparable results to those obtained with nerve repair and grafting for sensory nerve defects of less than 3 cm.[28]

Weber et al. performed a randomized prospective multicenter evaluation on 98 subjects with 136 nerve transections

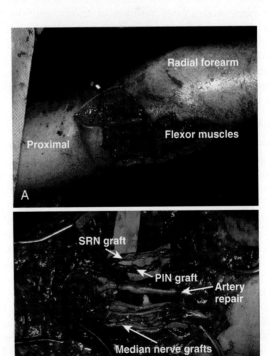

Figure 44-4 Proximal median and radial nerve grafts. **A,** Laceration through antecubital fossa. **B,** Multiple fascicular grafts to median nerve, superficial radial nerve, and posterior interosseous nerve. PIN, posterior interosseous nerve; SRN, superficial radial nerve.

in the hand, comparing a polyglycolic acid conduit with either end-to-end repair or a nerve graft for nerve repair. There were 56 nerves repaired in the control group and 46 nerves repaired with a conduit available for follow-up. The overall results showed no significant difference between the two groups as a whole. Nerves with gaps of 4 mm or less had better sensation when repaired with a conduit; the mean moving two-point discrimination was 3.7 ± 1.4 mm for poly-glycolic acid tube repair and 6.1 ± 3.3 mm for end-to-end repairs ($P = 0.03$). All injured nerves with deficits of 8 mm or greater were reconstructed with either a nerve graft or a conduit. This subgroup also demonstrated a significant difference in favor of the polyglycolic acid tube. The mean moving two-point discrimination for the conduit was 6.8 ± 3.8 mm, with excellent results obtained in 7 of 17 nerves, whereas the mean moving two-point discrimination for the graft repair was 12.9 ± 2.4 mm, with excellent results obtained in none of the eight nerves ($P < 0.001$ and $P = 0.06$, respectively).[29] Bertleff et al. examined the results of using a caprolactone tube versus primary repair in 34 digital nerve lesions with gaps greater than 2 cm. The results with the conduits were equal to those of repair as evaluated by the pressure-specified-sensory testing device and two-point discrimination.[30]

Nerve Transfers

One of the most exciting recent developments in peripheral nerve reconstruction has been the use of nerve transfers. They are indicated when there is a need to direct a large number of motor axons quickly to the denervated muscle in situations where there is insufficient time for axonal ingrowth. For motor nerves, an expendable donor nerve with pure motor fibers and a large number of axons near the target muscle is selected. It is preferable if the donor muscle is synergistic to the target muscle. Motor reeducation is crucial and involves the recruitment of the donor muscle and then contraction of the reinnervated muscle. Sensory nerve transfers require sensory retraining. Some specific examples of upper limb nerve transfers are described below.

Biceps Reinnervation

In 1994, Oberlin described a series of four patients who had undergone successful nerve transfer using redundant fascicles to the flexor carpi ulnaris (FCU) from the ulnar nerve to the motor branch of the musculocutaneous nerve for biceps reinnervation.[31] His group then modified this by performing a double fascicular nerve transfer using redundant fascicles of the median and ulnar nerve to reinnervate the biceps and brachialis muscles.[14] These transfers are indicated in C5–C7 plexus lesions where direct nerve reconstruction is not possible. Mixed plexus injuries can also be treated by this method if there is adequate clinical recovery in the lower roots. Since the neurorraphy is placed close to the target muscles, this nerve transfer is particularly useful in patients who have had a delay in surgical treatment. Successful restoration of elbow flexion has been reported even in cases done one year after injury. The absolute contraindication for this nerve transfer is a global brachial plexus palsy with no recovery of ulnar nerve function since the transfer requires intact function of the C8 and T1 nerve roots.

Following an isolated Oberlin transfer the patient is treated with a sling for the initial 2 weeks followed by passive elbow motion. Once there is evidence of reinnervation the patient is started on muscle reeducation and isometric strengthening. Elbow flexion is enhanced by activation of the FCU, which is achieved by having the patient grip while simultaneously trying to flex the elbow. In their review of the literature, Sharpe and Stevanovic identified a total of 100 cases. Eighty percent of patients recovered better than M4 motor strength for elbow flexion, 9% recovered M3 function, and 11% achieved less than M3 recovery. Clinical evidence of biceps reinnervation was seen at an average of 3 months, with a range of 2 to 7 months. Recovery of M3 function ranged between 4 and 13 months. For those patients who recovered M4 motor function, the range of elbow flexion strength was between 0.5 and 7 kg.[32]

Wrist and Finger Extension

Tung and Mackinnon et al. have demonstrated that redundant median nerve branches to the flexor digitorum sublimus (FDS), flexor carpi radialis (FCR), or palmaris longus (PL) may be used for transfer. In a dissection of 31 cadaver arms, they noted that double innervation of the FDS was found in 94% of the specimens.[33] They described two successful cases of transfer of the FDS fascicles to the pronator teres branch to restore pronation. They subsequently reported the use of this transfer to the extensor carpi radialis brevis (ECRB) branch and the posterior interosseous nerve (PIN) in a case of a high radial nerve palsy and a brachial plexopathy with excellent results.[34] In a separate study this group noted that the FCU branch of ulnar nerve can also be used, but this required a second incision.[35]

Proximal to the elbow, the median nerve condenses into three bundles. Branches arising from the anterior bundle can be seen innervating the FCR and pronator teres (PT). The FDS branches along with the FCR, and PL fascicles arise from the middle group. They are carefully differentiated from

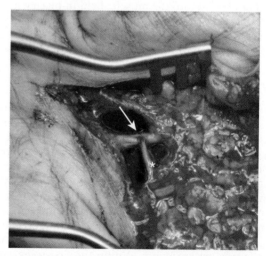

Figure 44-5 High ulnar nerve palsy. End-to-side repair of common digital nerve of the small finger (*) to the median derived common digital nerve to the third web (arrow).

the hand intrinsics using a hand-held stimulator. The radial nerve is isolated through the same incision. It can be found between the brachioradialis and brachialis as it divides into the superficial sensory nerve branch and the PIN branch. Mackinnon recommends use of the PL and the FDS or FCR branches to the PIN and the ECRB branch. The redundant median nerve fascicles are harvested in close proximity to the PIN to avoid undue tension on the repair site. An end-to-end coaptation is then performed. If necessary a short nerve graft can be interposed. Postoperatively an above-elbow orthosis is applied with the elbow at 90 degrees and the shoulder, wrist, and fingers free. Gentle elbow flexion is started after the first week, followed by gradual elbow extension. Motor retraining is akin to tendon transfers. The patient is instructed in active sublimus contractions, which will ultimately produce wrist and finger extension.

Published clinical series on this transfer are still lacking. In Mackinnon's series a 51-year-old male with a proximal left radial nerve palsy underwent transfer of the nerve branch to the PL and the FDS to the PIN and ECRB branch, respectively. He achieved 4/5 power (strength with gravity and added resistance) for wrist extension but lacked simultaneous finger extension at 14 months postoperatively. The second patient was a 24-year-old female following an iatrogenic radial nerve injury at the plexus level. The nerve branch from the PL and FDS were transferred to the PIN. A second FDS branch was transferred to the ECRB. The patient achieved 4/5 power (strength with gravity and added resistance) of wrist and finger extension.[34]

Intrinsic Muscle Reinnervation

The only donor nerve for intrinsic muscle reinnervation that fulfills all of the requirements for nerve transfer is the distal anterior interosseous nerve (AIN). It may be used to neurotize either the recurrent motor branch of the median nerve or the deep motor branch of the ulnar nerve. It is almost purely a motor nerve save for proprioceptive fibers to the wrist capsule, and it is expendable since there is minimal functional loss resulting from denervation of the pronator quadratus muscle. Just before entering the pronator quadratus muscle, the axon count of the AIN is equal to 75% of the deep motor branches of the median and ulnar nerves. With sufficient proximal interfascicular dissection of the distal median or ulnar nerves, direct coaptation of the transected distal AIN to the fascicular origins of the thenar branch of the median nerve or the deep motor branch of the ulnar nerve is possible.[36]

For thenar reinnervation, Wood has noted that a transfer of the distal AIN may be used only in those patients with median nerve loss distal to the origin of the AIN and with sparing of the entire AIN branch.[37] This technique should be considered in those patients who are unlikely to recover median innervated thenar motor function by a median nerve repair or reconstruction. Similarly, for intrinsic muscle reinnervation, transfer of the distal AIN should be considered in any patient with an ulnar nerve transection at or proximal to the upper forearm because in such patients recovery of intrinsic motor function with ulnar nerve repair or reconstruction is both poor and unpredictable, especially if there is a nerve gap. In either case the injury should not be so distal as to interfere with identification of the median or ulnar nerve motor fascicles. The procedure should be carried out within 6 months from the date of injury.

Sensory Nerve Transfers

The goal of nerve transfers for digital sensation is to redirect intact sensory input from less critical to more critical contact points. The distal thumb, radial side of the index, and ulnar side of the small finger have priority with regard to sensory reconstruction from a functional standpoint. Anesthesia in the thumb and index finger limits pinch and fine motor tasks, whereas anesthesia in the small finger causes a loss of proprioception of the hand. The adjacent sides of the third and fourth webspaces are by comparison relatively expendable. When a nerve transfer is indicated for a proximal median nerve injury, a failed distal median nerve repair or graft, or an upper trunk (C5, 6) injury, the ulnar-innervated fourth-webspace nerves can be transferred into the first-webspace nerves in an end-to-end manner to restore thumb and index finger sensation. In the case of ulnar nerve loss, the median-innervated third-webspace nerves are selected as donors for transfer to the small finger. The donor-site sensory loss may be treated with a secondary series of end-to-side transfers into the existing sensory nerve supply, which may provide at least protective sensation. For example, after the fourth-webspace nerves are transferred to the first webspace using end-to-end repair, the distal end of the fourth-webspace nerves are coapted end-to-side into the intact ulnar proper digital nerve of the small finger. With proximal median and ulnar nerve injuries, the superficial radial nerve is the only available sensory donor. Ducic et al. reported two cases of superficial radial nerve transfer to the ulnar digital nerve of the thumb and the radial digital nerve of the index finger in a proximal median nerve injury with recovery of

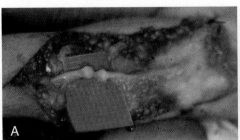
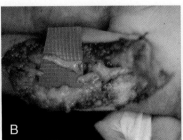
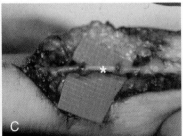

Figure 44-6 Digital neuroma. **A,** Neuroma of radial digital nerve. **B,** Resection back to healthy fascicles and reversed autogenous vein graft interposition. **C,** Completed repair.

protective sensation.[38] Similarly with a C6, 7 injury the dorsal cutaneous branch of the ulnar nerve provides an additional source of sensory axons.

Timing is not as crucial for sensory nerve reconstruction owing to the lack of a motor end plate; hence, this can be performed at the surgeon's and patient's discretion. As nerve regeneration progresses, specific training for sensory localization is integral to the outcome. Stocks et al. reported a recovery of S3+ or S4 in 85% of patients. Some tip sensibility returns within 3 to 4 months, with gradual maturation continuing past 2 years after nerve transfer.[39] In Mackinnon's experience, recovery of at least protective sensation can be expected following end-to-end coaptation of primary nerve

transfers for digital sensation.[40] Using the "ten test" evaluation designed by Strauch et al.,[41] sensory recovery even in the absence of sensory reeducation will be approximately 6/10 following end-to-end repair and 3/10 following end-to-side repair.[42] Localization of sensory stimuli to the donor digits persists for 2 to 3 years, with localization to the recipient digit improving with time, use, and sensory reeducation.

REFERENCES

The complete reference list is available online at www.expertconsult.com.

Therapist's Management of Peripheral Nerve Injury

SUSAN V. DUFF, EdD, PT, OTR/L, CHT AND
TIMOTHY ESTILOW, OTR/L

ADAPTATION TO INJURY
PRESENTATION OF SPECIFIC NERVE INJURIES
INTERVENTION
ENHANCING NEURAL RECOVERY AND
  PREHENSION

CASE STUDY
SUMMARY

CRITICAL POINTS

- After a peripheral nerve lesion, muscle denervation and sensory loss contribute to upper extremity prehensile limitations, leading to incoordination and maladaptive strategies.
- The key to successful rehabilitation is to adhere to precautions initially to protect the nerve after repair, then provide carefully designed therapeutic activity and exercise as the individual progresses through the phases of recovery.
- Greater emphasis placed on fostering neural reorganization and recovery of sensorimotor control may enhance achievement of flexible and efficient prehensile skill following nerve injury and repair.

Prehensile skill is often taken for granted until it is lost or diminished, as in the case of peripheral nerve injury (PNI). After a peripheral nerve lesion, muscle denervation and sensory loss contribute to prehensile limitations, leading to incoordination and maladaptive strategies. To effectively foster neural recovery and prehension following injury, clinicians should address not only impairments and function but motor control through the provision of specific sensory and motor experiences.

This chapter (1) considers adaptations to injury; (2) reviews the clinical presentation following injury; (3) discusses evaluations to establish a baseline and monitor neural recovery; and (4) reviews rehabilitation tactics used to prevent deformity and enhance recovery and prehensile skill.

Adaptation to Injury

Immediately after PNI the central (CNS) and peripheral nervous systems (PNS) adapt to a reduction in sensory input.[1-3] Neural adaptation to changes in input, or *plasticity*,[4] ranges from axonal degeneration to topographic reorganization.[1,5] The residual effects of PNI depend on the degree of axon and connective tissue involvement (see Chapters 42 and 43). Table 45-1 (online) shows the relationship between injury classification schemes by Seddon[6] and Sunderland.[1,7] An appreciation of postinjury adaptations may aid in the design of effective interventions.

Early Peripheral Changes

Postinjury peripheral changes include the onset of Wallerian degeneration and initiation of neural recovery. Wallerian degeneration involves axonal disintegration and demyelination distal to the lesion site,[8] and phagocytic macrophages interact with Schwann cells to remove debris.[9] With long-standing nerve injury, the endoneurial tubes shrink and collapse due to a reduction in cross-sectional area and the end-organs often degenerate.

Following a PNI, nerve function diminishes in the largest diameter fibers first and later the smallest. Large-diameter fibers (group A and B) are myelinated with a fast conduction rate, and small fibers (C or IV) are unmyelinated with a slower conduction rate.[8] After a nerve lesion, functional loss may proceed in the following sequence: motor, proprioception/vibration, touch, pain, and sudomotor function. Large-diameter fibers carrying motor, proprioceptive, and vibration information may be lost first, yet may be the last to return. Because pain information is primarily carried by the smallest diameter fibers, it is usually one of the last sensations to be lost and the first to return.

Recovery from PNI involves remyelination, collateral sprouting of axons, and axonal regeneration.[9] Regeneration following neurapraxia or axonotmesis begins immediately, whereas a neurotmesis usually requires nerve repair. After a 2- to 3-week latency period, a repaired nerve begins to regenerate. For the nerve to regenerate, the central axon must survive, the environment must support axonal growth, the axon must make timely contact with receptors, and the CNS must integrate signals from the PNS.[9] Axonal regeneration is guided by Schwann cells. In a favorable environment, the axon sprouts a "finger-like" growth cone initiating the process, and the Schwann cells provide a source of neurotrophic factors, which diffuse across the distal to proximal stump.[10] The regrowth rate in adults is 1 to 3 mm a day or more for a nerve laceration and repair[11,12] and about 3 to 4 mm a day after a crush.[12] The timing for axon regrowth after relief from nerve compression is more variable.

Factors that influence nerve recovery include (1) the lesion type (e.g., crush, stretch, laceration); (2) distance from the cell body; (3) age; (4) time since injury; (5) health; and (6) genetic factors.[13] Genetic factors include muscle fiber type, density, motor unit number, height, and weight. Constraints that influence recovery include the ability of the axon to cross the repair site, a slow rate of axon regrowth, and mismatching of sensory and motor fibers. Research examining methods to overcome constraints has included the use of neurotrophic factors, electrical stimulation, and exercise.[10,14-16] These methods are reviewed later in the chapter.

Early Central Changes

Lost or diminished sensory input induces CNS changes, including remodeling of cortical and subcortical structures and alterations at the spinal cord level. Neural reorganization may stem from any one of the following mechanisms:

1. *Removal or unmasking* of inhibitory controls in the affected region.[17,18] For example, changes in excitatory and inhibitory mechanisms in the spinal cord may alter tonic inhibition, causing tactile hypersensitivity.[19]
2. *Migration* of cells that serve other body parts into deafferented cortical regions[3,20]
3. *Strengthening* of existing connections and subthreshold excitatory inputs based on postinjury experience[21-23]
4. *Reorganization of subcortical regions* that project to the cortex such as the basal ganglia, brainstem, or thalamus[17,24]
5. *Neurogenesis and sprouting* of new pathways[25,26]

Prehensile Control

Feedback and Anticipatory Control

Somatosensory feedback and anticipatory control are essential components of grasp and manipulation.[27-30] Current

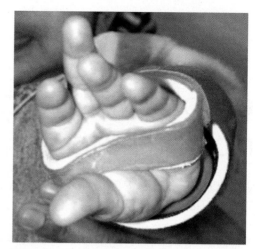

Figure 45-1 Anticipatory grip formation during reach-to-grasp facilitated with support from a dorsal wrist orthosis.

visual information and memories from past sensorimotor experiences are used to preshape the hand (Fig. 45-1) in advance of contact to accommodate object size and shape,[30] aiding the acquisition of stable grasp points.[31] Visual and somatosensory information are also used to anticipate the frictional conditions at the digit–object interface and estimate object weight to adequately grade fingertip forces (grip and load) used to grasp and lift objects.[32,33] If anticipatory control is sufficient, the peak rate of increase in grip (normal or squeeze) and load (tangential or lift) force will be higher for heavier or more slippery objects.[29]

Performance during reach-to-grasp tasks, including the movement path, velocity, and finger width (aperture), and exhibited during grip formation can be examined using kinematic (spatial–temporal) analysis. Kinetic (force) information on fingertip force scaling can be obtained from multiaxial force transducers shown in Figure 45-2A and documented as shown in Figure 45-2B. Kinematic and kinetic analyses allow for close examination of alterations in the spatiotemporal features of the movement and force control as occurs when sensory input is distorted or absent, as in cases of denervation,[27,34] focal hand dystonia,[35] and large-fiber neuropathy.[36]

Previous kinematic and kinetic analyses indicate there is a strong relationship between impaired visual skills or somatosensation and anticipatory control.[27-29,31] Visual or somatosensory deficits may lead to insufficient finger opening, object grasp at incorrect contact points, slips at object contact, temporal delays, and the use of excessive fingertip forces during fine-motor tasks. PNI can impair the sebaceous glands in the fingertips, causing objects to seem more slippery. If somatosensory input is diminished, grip force and movement time may increase to prevent slips and ensure success.[29] To examine the effect of injury on fingertip force scaling, Cole and colleagues[34] induced median nerve compression and then generated sensory nerve action potentials via electric stimulation proximal to the carpal canal. It was not until the compression caused a 50% reduction in sensory nerve action potentials that sensibility began to diminish and subjects began to use greater than 50% increase in grip force to secure objects.

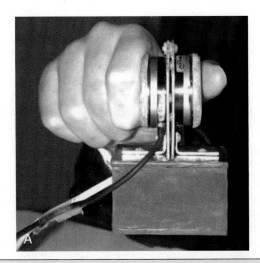

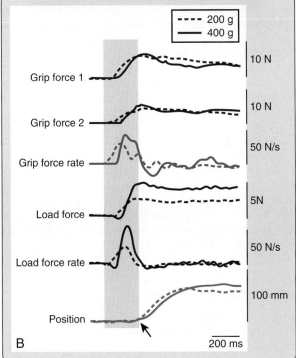

Figure 45-2 A, Grip device equipped with two parallel multiaxial force transducers and a magnetic position sensor (*in box*); **B,** The type of data obtained with this device includes grip force for each digit, grip force rate (first derivative of grip force), load force, load force rate (first derivative of load force), position (object lift-off table), and lift acceleration (second derivative of position—not shown). The arrow on "Position" depicts when the object is lifted off the table. The area shown in grey occurs before the weight of the object is known. Because the grip and load force rates (rate of onset of force) are higher for the heavier object, this subject displayed anticipatory control or advanced planning of fingertip forces.

Secondary to diminished sensation and muscle denervation experienced after PNI, the number of motor units[37] and joint motion available is reduced. Thus, altered sensory and motor function reduces the degrees of freedom or the number of ways the involved hand and arm can move,[38] necessitating the use of alternative prehensile patterns. For example, after a radial nerve injury there is little active wrist and finger–

thumb extension. Thus, it may be difficult to preshape the hand in preparation for object contact. After median nerve injury, thenar muscle denervation may require a shift from precision to power grips or the use of bilateral versus unilateral grip patterns. With a low ulnar nerve injury, a visible Froment's sign (excess thumb interphalangeal [IP] joint flexion during lateral pinch) suggests that the adductor pollicis is affected, resulting in overpowering from the flexor pollicis longus to pinch. Fingertip force generation is significantly affected by median and ulnar nerve injuries, influencing dexterity and handedness. Although activation of intact muscles aids function, coordination is compromised, increasing the effort used, and, therefore, the cost of engaging in prehensile tasks.[39]

Presentation of Specific Nerve Injuries

Radial Nerve Injury

Injury to the radial nerve can stem from humeral shaft fractures (middle and distal third), elbow dislocations, fractures, and compression between the head of the radius and the supinator (radial tunnel syndrome).[13] Nerve compression in the axilla from the incorrect use of crutches or awkward sleeping postures (Saturday night palsy) can also lead to a radial nerve injury. The effect of injury on function depends on the level of the injury (Fig. 45-3). A "wrist drop" is the classic deformity associated with a radial nerve injury characterized by forearm pronation, wrist flexion, thumb flexion and abduction, slight metacarpophalangeal (MCP) joint flexion, and IP joint extension (Fig. 45-4). The individual is unable to extend the wrist and fingers simultaneously or abduct the extended thumb. Depending on the level of the injury, there may be atrophy of the dorsal forearm due to involvement of the finger and thumb extensors and the extensor carpi ulnaris. With higher level injuries there may be atrophy of the extensor muscle mass near the lateral epicondyle due to involvement of the brachioradialis, extensor carpi radialis longus and brevis, or the triceps.

Wrist-Level Injury

The sensory branch of the radial nerve can be injured at the wrist as it resurfaces in the anatomic snuff box. Injury mechanisms may include a radioulnar joint dislocation or nerve compression (wrist-band injury). A lesion at this level only affects sensibility on the dorsal thumb, index, middle, and radial side of the ring finger to the PIP joint (excluding the nail beds), with some variation.

Forearm- or Elbow-Level Injury

Forearm-level injury can result in full or partial denervation of the following muscles: extensor carpi ulnaris (ECU), extensor digitorum communis (EDC), extensor digiti minimi (EDM), abductor pollicis longus (APL), extensor pollicis longus (EPL), extensor pollicis brevis (EPB), and extensor indicis proprius (EIP). Forearm-level injuries can result in

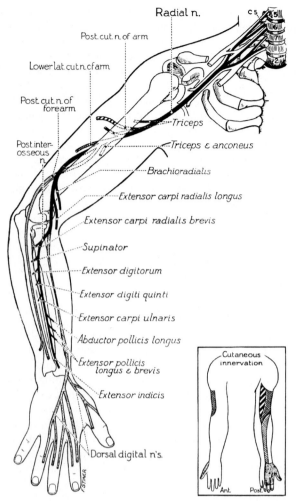

Figure 45-3 The course and distribution of the radial nerve. (From Haymaker W, Woodhall B. *Peripheral Nerve Injuries.* Philadelphia: W.B. Saunders, 1953).

lost or diminished ulnar wrist extension, MCP joint extension of all digits, and thumb abduction or extension. As described for low-level injuries, sensibility through the dorsoradial aspect of the hand is affected.

Elbow-level lesions result in diminished sensibility to the dorsoradial portion of the hand and full or partial denerva-

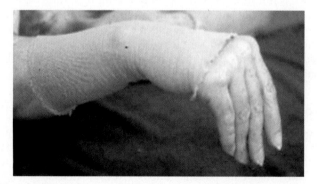

Figure 45-4 Wrist drop secondary to radial nerve injury near the elbow.

tion of the muscles described earlier with the addition of the supinator, extensor carpi radialis longus (ECRL), and extensor carpi radialis brevis (ECRB). With injury at this level, radial wrist extension is lost or weakened, and supination is weakened. Lesions proximal to the elbow also involve the brachioradialis and triceps, resulting in the addition of slightly weakened elbow flexion and lost or weakened elbow extension.

Functional Implications

Lost or diminished sensibility on the dorsoradial aspect of the hand from a wrist-level injury (or higher) has little effect on hand function because the volar surface continues to obtain the sensory input needed for prehension. However, the injured individual should remain vigilant during daily tasks to prevent superficial injury or scalds and burns to the dorsum of the hand. Forearm- or elbow-level lesions limit the ability to turn the hand over and extend the wrist to receive objects. Inadequate wrist stabilization may prevent the formation of stable prehension patterns, such as a spherical grip or radial digital grasp used to open jars or bottles and to perform manipulative tasks such as buttoning. Limited finger and thumb extension will hinder grip formation and object release and may lead to hand asymmetries as found in other populations.[40] To compensate for poor grip formation, the wrist may flex to passively extend the fingers or objects may be transferred to the involved hand by the noninvolved hand. Object release may be accomplished by wrist flexion, shaking objects free, or through use of the noninvolved hand to retrieve them. Reach-to-grasp activities and tasks such as writing or typing are difficult to complete with the wrist in flexion and the fingers and thumb in extension, limiting the use of adequate grip force.

Median Nerve Injury

Injuries to the median nerve can result from lacerations, humeral fractures, elbow dislocations, distal radius fractures, and lunate dislocations into the carpal tunnel.[13] Nerve compression can occur between the two heads of the pronator teres (pronator syndrome), when it branches off as the anterior interosseous nerve and in the carpal tunnel. Functional changes associated with median nerve injury depend on the level of injury (Fig. 45-5). The classic deformity associated with a median nerve injury is the sign of "benediction" with the thumb resting in adduction and the index and long fingers in extension and adduction. With higher-level lesions there may be atrophy of the pronator teres and flexor carpi radialis resulting in loss of volar muscle mass near the medial epicondyles. Thenar muscle atrophy is often visible with long-standing injury (Fig. 45-6).

Wrist-Level Injury

Wrist-level injuries result in full or partial denervation of the opponens pollicis (OP), abductor pollicis brevis (APB), flexor pollicis brevis-superficial head (FPB), and the first and second lumbricals. Thumb flexion, palmar abduction, and

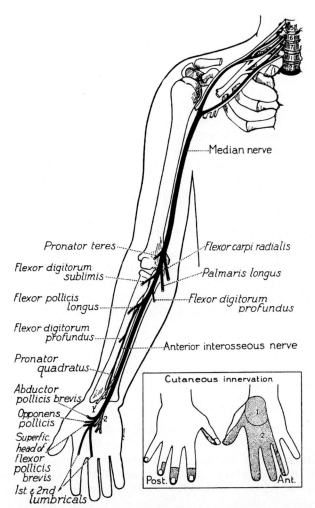

Figure 45-5 The course and distribution of the medial nerve. (From Haymaker W, Woodhall B. *Peripheral Nerve Injuries*. Philadelphia: W.B. Saunders, 1953).

opposition are lost or weakened with wrist-level lesions. Sensibility may be impaired through the volar thumb, index, long, and the radial half of the ring finger and the nail beds. If the injury occurs in the carpal tunnel, sensibility to the thenar eminence is spared because the cutaneous branch travels outside of the carpal tunnel.

Forearm- or Elbow-Level Injury

Forearm- or elbow-level lesions result in full or partial denervation of the muscles previously mentioned with the addition

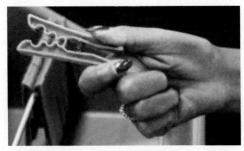

Figure 45-6 Evidence of thenar muscle atrophy.

of the pronator teres (PT), flexor carpi radialis (FCR), flexor digitorum superficialis (FDS), palmaris longus (PL), flexor pollicis longus (FPL), flexor digitorum profundus (FDP) to the index and long fingers, and the pronator quadratus (PQ). Motions lost or weakened include pronation, wrist flexion and radial deviation, thumb IP joint flexion, and flexion of the index and middle fingers at the PIP and DIP joints. MCP joint hyperextension may be observed due to the overpowering activation of the EDC.

Functional Implications

Prehensile skill is compromised after median nerve injury. Lost or diminished finger flexion, thumb flexion, palmar abduction, and opposition impedes grip formation during reach-to-grasp tasks. The ability to stabilize opposing forces between the radial fingers to grasp, and to use the intrinsic muscles for in-hand manipulation, is lost or diminished.[41-43] Insufficient activation of lumbricals I and II prevents finger-to-thumb-pad approximation used for precision grip, resulting in a raking pattern or a weak lateral pinch. Inadequate thumb mobility prevents in-hand manipulation of small objects, thus, compensatory patterns are often used such as two-handed manipulation or stabilizing items against the body. In-hand manipulation used to rotate (turn), translate (move palm to fingertips or fingertips to palm), and shift (move along fingertips) coins, pegs, or a key in one hand is affected. A complete median nerve injury may also result in a 60% loss of lateral pinch strength and 32% loss of power grasp strength.[42]

Lost or diminished sensation in the volar–radial side of the hand impairs somatosensory feedback needed for object recognition, coordination, and grading of movement. If feedback is impaired, excess grip force is often employed to prevent object slippage and drops.[29] Premature fatigue from the use of excess grip force may limit endurance during writing and related tasks as shown in other groups.[44] Reach-to-grasp and pointing movements are less accurate with diminished tactile feedback.[27] Furthermore, insufficient tactile feedback makes it difficult to determine the start and end position in tasks such as typing, text messaging, and calculator use.[45] Median nerve injury significantly limits the ability to complete activities of daily living (ADL), often requiring individuals to change hand dominance if the dominant hand is injured.

Ulnar Nerve Injury

Causes of ulnar nerve injury include direct lacerations and fracture of the medial epicondyle of the humerus or olecranon of the ulna.[13,46] Compression may occur at the cubital or Guyon's canal.[47] The effect of injury on function depends on the individual's age and level of the lesion (Fig. 45-7). High-level lesions in young individuals recover fairly well after repair, whereas adults rarely regain motor function.[48] The classic deformity associated with an ulnar nerve injury is a "partial intrinsic minus" deformity (Fig. 45-8) due to loss of the interossei and lumbricals III and IV with less posturing in the index and long fingers (lumbricals intact). Yet, as

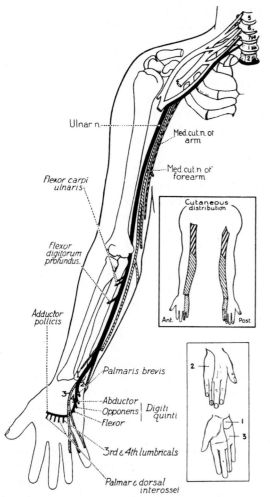

Figure 45-7 *The course and distribution of the ulnar nerve. (From Haymaker W, Woodhall B. Peripheral Nerve Injuries. Philadelphia: W.B. Saunders, 1953).*

reinnervation occurs, the posturing often increases. This deformity is noted for MCP joint hyperextension with PIP joint flexion at the ring and small fingers. With long-standing injury the hypothenar eminence and intrinsics between the IV and V metacarpals may be atrophied. After high-level injuries, there may be medial forearm atrophy.

Wrist-Level Injury

Low-level lesions result in full or partial denervation of: abductor digiti minimi (ADM), flexor digiti minimi (FDM),

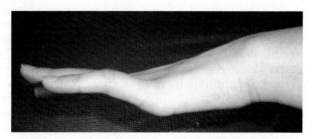

Figure 45-8 *Intrinsic minus posturing with hyperextension at the ulnar metacarpophalangeal joints due to ulnar nerve injury.*

opponens digiti minimi (ODM), III and IV lumbricals, dorsal interossei (DI), palmar interossei (PI), flexor pollicis brevis (deep head) (FPB-deep), and adductor pollicis (AP). Due to partial or full denervation of the intrinsics, finger abduction and adduction, thumb adduction, and opposition of the small finger are lost or weakened. Also, MCP joint flexion at the small and ring finger with simultaneous extension of the IP joints is lost or weakened. Because FDS and FDP function remain intact and the EDC can contract, ulnar-sided "intrinsic minus," or claw, posturing is more pronounced than in individuals with high ulnar nerve lesions.[49] With a wrist-level injury, sensibility is lost or diminished through the volar–ulnar aspect of the palm distally and the small and ulnar half of the ring finger.

Forearm- or Elbow-Level Injury

Lesions at the elbow and above result in full or partial denervation of the muscles listed earlier plus the flexor carpi ulnaris (FCU) and FDP to the ring and small fingers, resulting in lost or weakened ulnar deviation and distal interphalangeal (DIP) joint flexion. Without the FDP and FDS, the "intrinsic minus" position through the ring and small fingers is less severe but noticeable due to contraction of the EDC. Sensibility is now lost or diminished through the dorsal and volar surface of the small and ulnar half of the ring fingers and the ulnar aspect of the proximal palm.

Functional Implications

During many daily tasks the ulnar border of the hand interfaces with a contact surface area. Therefore, lost or diminished sensation through the ulnar side of the hand increases the risk for burns, lacerations, and skin breakdown. To prevent injury, it is vital that the injured individual remains vigilant. Individuals should be advised to wear gloves when exposed to extreme temperature, sharp or rough surfaces, or friction during repetitive physical labor tasks.

The ulnar side of the hand acts as a point of stability for powerful grip and pinch as well as manipulation. Weakness after ulnar nerve injury affects gross grasp needed for opening jars and carrying heavy objects. Lost or weakened intrinsic muscle function restricts active grasp and release and reduces strength.[42] Following an ulnar nerve block, Kozin and colleagues[42] found a mean decrease of 38% gross grasp strength and 77% key pinch strength. Limited key pinch strength makes it difficult to secure fasteners and open doors. Froment's sign is an inefficient substitution for weak key pinch. Posturing into intrinsic minus prevents ulnar digit extension to accommodate large objects during grasping or attempts to catch a football or basketball. Quarterbacks and pitchers with ulnar nerve injuries may have difficulty controlling ball release during throws. Lost or weakened FDP function prevents DIP joint flexion used to secure items against the palm during the translation component (palm-to-fingers or fingers-to-palm movement) of in-hand manipulation.

Intervention

Clinicians have an opportunity to influence prehensile recovery following PNI by conducting sensitive evaluations and

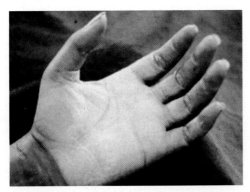

Figure 45-9 *Evidence of trophic changes, which alter skin texture due to sympathetic denervation of the sebaceous glands.*

implementing creative treatment strategies. Individual participation in carefully designed, therapeutic activity after injury may contribute to neural regeneration and reorganization following injury and repair.

Evaluation

As with other hand injuries it is important to consult with the referring physician to discuss how much tension was placed on the nerve repair, the ideal orthotic position and the duration of limb immobilization. Nerve injuries are typically immobilized for a minimum of 3 weeks.

History

After obtaining relevant information from the physician, pertinent medical history and demographics can be obtained from a questionnaire or interview, including the cause and timing of the injury, date of injury, age, type of treatment to date, social/work information, and hand dominance. The nature of current problems, comorbidities, and an assessment of psychosocial factors, ADL status, and vocational or school requirements should also be acquired. A pain assessment using an instrument such as the McGill Pain Questionnaire[50] or the visual analog scale (or pain faces scale for children)[51] should be conducted. The presence of an advancing *Tinel's sign*, induced by tapping on the nerve (to elicit a distal tingling sensation), may be used to gauge current and ongoing progression in regeneration. The physical assessment needs to be customized to the phase of recovery and compared with the noninvolved limb.

Sympathetic Function

Sympathetic function is assessed via observation and palpation and includes an assessment of (1) vasomotor function (e.g., skin color, skin temperature, edema); (2) sudomotor function (sweat); (3) pilomotor function (gooseflesh); and (4) trophic changes (nutrition to skin and nails). Figure 45-9 shows the effect of loss of function in the sebaceous glands of the palm innervated by sympathetic nerve fibers. A quick test of sympathetic function is the wrinkle test, found to have 97% sensitivity and 95% specificity.[52] (See Chapter 11 for more detail.) Absence of sympathetic function is highly

suggestive of absent sensibility because of the high resilience those fibers have to mechanical trauma.[53] Some sympathetic changes are seen immediately, but others are not noticeable until 3 to 6 weeks after nerve injury.

Motor Function

During phase one (immobilization) the motor assessment includes an examination of active (AROM) and passive range of motion (PROM) of *noninvolved* joints. After immobilization (phase two), AROM and PROM of the *involved* joints can be tested as well as prehension patterns through general observation or with tests of hand function such as the Sollerman's Test of Hand Grip,[54] which is a standardized hand function test based on common hand grips and consisting of 20 ADL items (see Chapter 12). To guide testing of muscle function the therapist can follow the predictable sequential pattern of muscle reinnervation and the ability to (1) produce an observable and palpable contraction without joint motion; (2) hold a position, yet not produce the same position; (3) move the involved joint actively; and (4) tolerate resistance.[55]

After the patient has been cleared by the surgeon for strength testing and resistive exercise, there are a few ways to measure strength. The manual muscle test (MMT) is the most widely used and involves a standard 0 to 5 grading scale (absent to normal grades). The action of the muscle being tested is resisted at the distal end of the moving bone while the proximal joint is stabilized. Resistance can be provided isometrically by asking the individual to hold the position or isotonically by resisting throughout the range. Another frequently used tool is the hand-held dynamometer. This device measures the magnitude of force generated versus the amount of resistance tolerated. Although calibrated grip-and-pinch dynamometers measure gross hand strength, hand-held dynamometry tests the strength of individual muscles.[43] During muscle testing it is important to be aware of substitution patterns.[13] Classic substitution patterns for each nerve injury are listed in Table 45-2.

Sensibility

The sequence of return in sensibility is from (1) deep pressure and pinprick, to (2) moving touch, to (3) static light touch, and then to (4) discriminative touch.[13] Initially, localization is poor, and the sensation elicited radiates proximally or distally. Accurate touch localization is one of the last functions to return. Passive sensibility can be tested using the Semmes–Weinstein monofilaments or the Weinstein Enhanced Sensory Test (WEST) for touch–pressure; and the Discriminator for static and moving two-point discrimination. Active sensibility can be tested using Moberg's Picking-Up Test or general tests of tactile gnosis or stereognosis (see Chapter 11 for more details).

Dexterity

Patients with PNIs often require alternative strategies and prehension patterns to perform everyday tasks, increasing the effort while decreasing the movement efficiency.[39] Timed dexterity tests can be used to document baseline performance

Table 45-2 Potential Substitution Patterns for Each Nerve Injury

Radial Nerve	Median Nerve	Ulnar Nerve
Elbow extension assisted via gravity via supination and shoulder external rotation.	Pronation via brachioradialis from supination with gravity assist. Shoulder IR can substitute.	Thumb adduction via medial APB with slight palmar abduciton. Thumb adduction held by APB with slight flexion via FPL (look for APB, EPL, FPL contraction).
Supination via biceps.	Wrist flexion via FCU and APB into ulnar deviation.	Finger abduction via EDC if MCP joint extends. If MCP joint flexion blocked at index and small fingers abduct via EIP and EDM. Test abduction of long finger in MCP neutral.
Wrist extension via tenodesis action of finger flexors. If fingers held extended, then wrist cannot extend.	Finger flexion compromised except action of ulnar FDPs. Finger flexion achieved passively via tenodesis of wrist extensors.	Finger adduction via finger flexors if MCP joint flexion allowed. Prevention: block MCP joint flexion by testing on a flat surface. Watch for index substitution by EIP.
Finger extension via tenodesis action of wrist flexors.	Thumb IP joint flexion achieved via pull of APL from thumb abduction and wrist extension. Test with wrist in neutral and thumb adducted.	MCP joint flexion via lumbricals at index and long. Ring and small MCP joint flexion achieved only with addition of IP joint flexion.
Thumb extension via assist from APB (slip to EPL tendon).	Palmar thumb abduction via APB. Test: thumb moves perpendicular to index to avoid substitution by APL.	IP joint extension weak in index and long fingers. Substitution at ring and small fingers achieved via EDC if MCP joint hyperextension blocked.
	Partial thumb opposition achieved via FPB (deep) and adductor pollicis. Substitution: flexed thumb pulp contacts lateral small finger.	
	MCP joint flexion at index and long fingers via intrinsics.	
	IP joint extension at index and long fingers weak, yet present because interossei are intact.	

APB, abductor pollicis brevis; APL, abductor pollicis longus; EDC, extensor digitorum communis; EDM, extensor digiti minimi; EIP, extensor indicis proprius; FCU, flexor carpi ulnaris; FDP, flexor digitorum profundis; FPB, flexor pollicus brevis; FPL, flexor pollicus longus; IP, interphalangeal; IR, internal rotation; MCP, metacarpophalangeal.

and improvements in fine-motor efficiency. Common dexterity tests (see Chapter 12 for details) include the Nine Hole Peg Test, the Purdue Pegboard Test, and the Jebsen Taylor Hand Function Test.[56] These and other tests can be used to test components of in-hand manipulation. Although normative data are available on most tests, it is worthwhile to also compare performance against the noninvolved hand.

Treatment Methods

Impairments and function are important issues to address following PNI. Yet, methods aimed at motor learning and control can facilitate the transition from poor to smooth coordination, enhancing function. Initially, therapeutic strategies that encourage the use of noninvolved structures or provide supplemental feedback may aid this process. Substituting one form of feedback for another while awaiting peripheral nerve regeneration may preserve central neural function.[57,58] Once regeneration ensues engagement in meaningful but carefully planned tasks as used with focal hand dystonia[59] or central lesions[60] may aid reorganization and lead to better functional recovery.

Management by Phase

Postinjury management can be organized into three phases of recovery: phase one refers to early healing when immobilization is required; phase two is the period of reinnervation when remobilization, sensory reeducation, and active motor control is emphasized; and phase three stresses strengthening

and functional performance. Rehabilitation methods often include orthotic positioning, AROM, biofeedback, neuromuscular electrical stimulation (NMES), and functional tasks.[13] Adjunctive methods include massage, edema management, and sensory reeducation. The goals and common treatment methods for each phase are listed in Table 45-3. Orthotic positioning is reviewed in greater detail in the next section.

Phase One. Following nerve repair, a custom-made immobilization orthosis or cast is used to protect the repair by limiting tension on the repair site for a minimum of 3 weeks. The specific orthosis and position depend on the nerve repaired. Static orthoses provide appropriate biomechanical positioning to prevent overstretching of denervated muscles and deformity of associated structures. Management of pain, edema, and inflammation can be addressed with anti-inflammatory medications and modalities such as ultrasound, phonophoresis, and cryotherapy. Education is often provided to (1) aid in edema reduction via elevation and active movement of noninvolved joints; (2) protect areas of diminished or absent sensation; and (3) review home programs. During this period of immobilization, limitations in performance of ADL are addressed using adapted methods and assistive devices.

Phase Two. After immobilization, place-and-hold techniques and active motion foster muscle activation and movement. Place-and-hold techniques require muscle activation at

Table 45-3 General Goals and Treatment Methods for Each Phase

	Goals	Methods
Phase One	Protect repair site if surgery was performed or rest overused structures and avoid compression or traction of nerve	Static positioning
	Manage edema	Elevation, compression, active movement of noninvolved joints
	Protect areas of diminished or absent sensibility	Education
	Encourage active movement of non-involved joints	AROM exercises and tasks
	Sensory substitution	Use of "sensor glove"
		Mirror visual feedback
Phase Two	Regain AROM	AROM exercises and tasks incorporating involved structures
	Enhance sensorimotor control	Practice grasping and manipulating objects of various shapes, sizes, and textures, complex manipulative tasks
	Sensory reeducation	Desensitization and active somatosensory training
		Use of "sensor glove"
	Enhance function while maintaining appropriate biomechanical positioning at involved and noninvolved joints	Orthotic positioning
		Practice prehensile and ADL tasks with and without orthoses
	Maintain PROM at involved and surrounding joints	PROM exercises, myofascial release, positioning, education
Phase Three	Improve strength	Theraputty, theraband, cuff weights, exercise machines, work simulators, aquatic therapy, biometrics device
	Enhance aerobic conditioning	Aerobic activities (e.g., arm ergometer)
	Return to prior level of function	Work simulation
		Simulation of difficult ADL tasks
	Reevaluate current status regarding: compensatory strategies; capacity for continued improvement and need for surgical intervention	Issue adaptive equipment/orthoses, preoperative conditioning

ADL, activities of daily living; AROM, active range of motion; PROM, passive range of motion.

various lengths and are performed by having the clinician or the individual place the limb in the desired position where it is briefly held. Active motion is initially encouraged through a protected range with gravity eliminated then progressed to full motion against gravity. Aquatic therapy can be beneficial, as the buoyancy of the water can provide assistive AROM. Orthotic positioning is often used to facilitate new movement and function as reinnervation occurs.

To enhance function and neural control in phases two and three, therapeutic activities should focus on motor relearning and adaptive strategies. Traditionally, biofeedback and NMES assist with motor learning and control. Biofeedback provides visual or auditory feedback (or both) when the targeted muscle contracts, aiding relearning of muscle activation or relaxation. NMES augments muscle activation when there is evidence of innervation, but also provides proprioceptive and tactile input to enhance muscle activation and awareness (Fig. 45-10). However, the use of electrical stimulation in full or partially denervated muscle remains controversial.

Multisensory approaches can help maintain cortical representation and allow for faster integration of sensory input on reinnervation. The "sensory glove" introduced by Rosén and Lundborg[57] provides auditory feedback to substitute for tactile input during fine-motor tasks after PNI. The type of auditory stimuli varies depending on the texture of the object being grasped. Mirror visual feedback (MVF),[20,58] which uses a mirror image to provide an illusion of movement in the involved hand, may also be another useful strategy. During MVF the individual is instructed to observe a movement being completed by the noninvolved hand in a mirror image located at midline (involved hand is behind the mirror). Theoretically, the visual system interprets the mirror image

to be movement of the involved hand, thus stimulating mirror neurons in the brain. The goal is to restore volitional control in the affected hand. During the phase of immobilization, the patient simply observes the reflected image and during the phase of reinnervation, the patient attempts to perform the motion observed in the mirror. Based on the reported success relieving phantom limb pain and complex regional pain syndrome,[20] MVF may be successful after PNI[58] and warrants further investigation.

During the design of therapeutic activities it is important to remember that visual information influences anticipatory control during reach to grasp and object manipulation.[32] Engagement with familiar objects and tasks may initially aid motor control. However, as improvement is noted, the introduction of novel objects and tasks may challenge the nervous system to better refine sensorimotor control.[41]

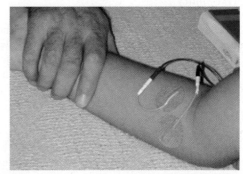

Figure 45-10 Electrode placement for neuromuscular electrical stimulation (NMES) used to facilitate muscle activation in the pronator muscle group.

Phase Three. Once full available AROM is obtained with gravity eliminated and against gravity, strengthening can begin. Resistance can be in the form of theraputty, theraband, free weights, cuff weights, exercise machines, work simulators, and computer games (e.g., Biometrics Device). Aquatic therapy can also be useful since buoyancy of the water can also provide a form of resistance. As in other phases, correct technique should be emphasized to prevent injury.

If an individual plateaus, therapy may shift to consideration of long-term solutions to address residual deficits. Solutions may include the use of devices or orthoses to substitute for absent movement, stability, or strength. If surgical intervention is a consideration, the individual should receive preoperative education and therapy.

Orthotic Positioning

Because of full or partial denervation after injury, individuals are at risk for secondary impairments, such as muscle atrophy, overstretching of the involved muscle–tendon unit, and joint contracture, if care is not properly taken to prevent them.[61] Orthoses can immobilize or mobilize involved structures via static or dynamic components. Orthotic design and wear schedule vary depending on the type, extent, and location of the injury along with the phase of neural recovery. Multiple client factors (e.g., cognition, age) and the desired outcome also influence design. Regardless of recovery phase, patient education is vital to maximize compliance with orthosis care and wear.

Orthosis design after PNI requires attention to detail to ensure that there is sufficient support, reasonable fit, allowance for optimum sensation, ease in donning and doffing, a proper line of pull, and appealing aesthetics.[61] In phase one, orthotic positioning (or casting) aims to (1) protect the nerve repair (or rest the involved nerve), (2) maintain anatomic integrity, and (3) prevent deformity. The method and time period of immobilization depend on the severity of the injury and extent of initial medical care. If surgical repair was performed, the individual is immobilized for a minimum of 3 weeks. PNIs not requiring surgical care should be positioned based on the type and level of injury. Positioning goals in phase two are to (1) maintain passive ROM and (2) enhance function during reinnervation.

Radial Nerve Injury

Phase One. After this injury the fingers and wrist need to be supported to prevent shortening of the flexors and overstretching of the extensors. A volar resting orthosis with the wrist in neutral to partial extension and the MCP joints in extension should be worn nightly. During the day a dorsal wrist cock-up supporting the MCP joints in extension with elastic slings allows for digit movement and leaves the volar surface free for sensory input.

As with other compression injuries, rest is needed to reduce the pain and inflammation that occurs with radial tunnel syndrome. According to Gelberman and colleagues[46] the optimal position for radial nerve decompression is 90 degrees of elbow flexion, forearm midposition or supination, and slight wrist extension. This position of rest can be provided in a long-arm orthosis (Fig. 45-11).

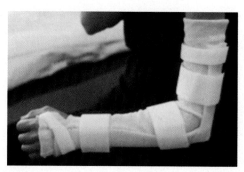

Figure 45-11 Elbow orthosis for use with cubital tunnel syndrome or radial nerve decompression contoured to enhance stability.

Phase Two. At this phase wrist and digit extension often remain absent or weak. A dorsal wrist cock-up orthosis with MCP joint support stabilizes the wrist and MCP joints, allowing for the execution of basic fine-motor skills. Another option is to reestablish a *tenodesis* pattern to improve hand function during reinnervation (Fig. 45-12A). The tenodesis

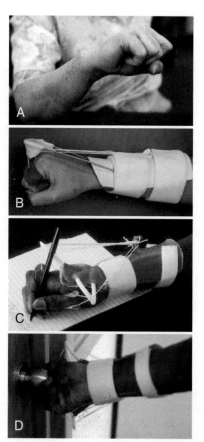

Figure 45-12 A, Use of tenodesis after radial nerve injury to extend the wrist by flexing the fingers. **B,** Tenodesis orthosis: Finger flexion stabilizes wrist in extension (Colditz JC. Splinting for radial nerve palsy. *J Hand Ther* 1987;1(1):18-23). **C, D,** Demonstration of functional use of a modified radial nerve orthosis, which extends beyond the wrist and includes the thumb.

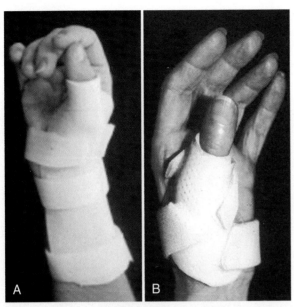

Figure 45-13 A, Wrist-based thumb spica supports wrist and thumb in functional position. **B,** In-hand thumb spica orthosis supports the thumb and allows use of the digits.

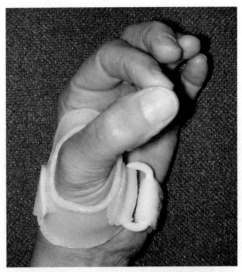

Figure 45-14 Opponens orthosis to position fingers and thumb pulp to pulp.

orthosis uses the intact finger flexors to control wrist extension.[62] Static nylon cord attached to finger slings suspends the proximal phalanges from an outrigger attached to a dorsal forearm base (Fig. 45-12B). Within the orthosis, active finger flexion passively places the wrist in neutral for a power grip, whereas active wrist flexion passively extends the fingers, allowing for object release. The radial nerve orthosis can be varied to include the thumb, expanding the available prehension (Fig. 45-12C, D). Both orthoses foster a power grip and allow use of the impaired hand in ADL. As strength and control improve, other options such as a dynamic Lycra glove or kinesiotaping can be used.

Phase Three. A functional assessment determines if positioning is necessary at this time. If contractures are present, static progressive orthotic positioning may help increase PROM. If an individual has no return, or if recovery of function is insufficient, a referral to a hand surgeon may be warranted to explore surgical options.

Median Nerve Injury

Phase One. To prevent a thumb adduction or webspace contracture, individuals with wrist-level lesions need to wear a night orthosis to maintain passive range in the first webspace. With a high-level lesion, an immobilization orthosis fit in a functional position or a wrist-based thumb spica (Fig. 45-13A) should be worn nightly to maintain length of the intrinsics to the index and middle fingers while supporting the thumb in opposition with the webspace maintained. A short opponens orthosis (Fig. 45-13B) can be worn during the day to provide support to the thumb and allow for use of the digits.

Phase Two. Absent or limited active thumb mobility is the primary impediment to function at this time. A short opponens orthosis that positions the thumb in palmar abduction and opposition (Fig. 45-14) allows thumb-to-fingerpad

contact for a radial–digital or pincer grasp. If thenar atrophy is present, the short opponens orthosis may be too uncomfortable. An option is to form a soft orthosis using a "putty-like" material; securing it with an elastic band (Fig. 45-15) or covering it with a thin plastic orthosis. As strength and motor control improve, other options, such as a Benik Hand Splint or neoprene thumb strap, can provide limited support during motion.

Phase Three. Evaluation of function will determine how to proceed at this time and may include the continued use of orthoses. If the individual has no return, or functional recovery is insufficient, surgical options may need to be explored.

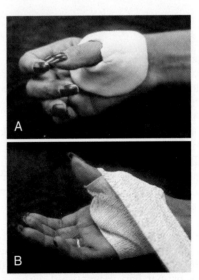

Figure 45-15 A, Alternative opponens orthosis using a "putty-like" material to form a soft orthosis, which can be secured with an elastic band **(B)**.

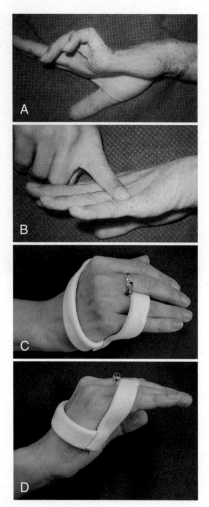

Figure 45-16 Dorsal metacarpophalangeal (MCP) joint block orthosis to prevent intrinsic minus or claw posturing. **A,** Ulnar nerve claw deformity. **B,** By blocking MCP joint hyperextension, redistribution of the action of the extensor digitorum communis to the interphalangeal (IP) joints allows IP joint extension. **C,** Ulnar claw orthosis blocks MCP joint hyperextension. **D,** Active IP joint extension is possible when MCP joint hyperextension is blocked by the orthosis.

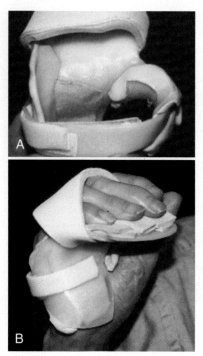

Figure 45-17 A, Orthosis fabricated for long-standing ulnar nerve injury with joint contractures, padded for comfort due to atrophy and excessive bony prominences. **B,** Orthosis in place with MCP joints in flexion and IP joints in extension.

Ulnar Nerve Injury

Phase One. Ulnar nerve injuries not requiring surgical repair should be positioned with a dorsal MCP joint blocking orthosis with the MCP joints in flexion to prevent a fixed claw deformity of the ring and small fingers in the intrinsic minus position (Fig. 45-16). An MCP joint blocking orthosis helps redistribute force from the EDC to the IP joints to promote full IP joint extension. If IP joint contracture is present, the immediate goal is to regain motion with serial casting or positioning. Mild contractures are correctable with a static progressive or dynamic PIP joint extension orthosis.

Phase Two. Once strength and motor control improve, less restrictive orthoses can be used. For example, finger loops or cuffs placed over the ring and small fingers can be attached to a palmar bar or wristband with a static line to minimize intrinsic minus posturing, while allowing greater digit flexion and sensibility.

Phase Three. Assessment of function at this time determines how to proceed and may include continued orthosis wear in cases of long-standing injury (Fig. 45-17). If the individual has no return, or recovery is insufficient, surgical options such as tendon transfers may be explored.

Enhancing Neural Recovery and Prehension

Methods used at the time of nerve repair or afterward to enhance neural recovery include the application of neurotrophic factors, direct electrical stimulation to the repaired nerve, exercise or activity, and sensory reeducation.

Axonal Regeneration After Nerve Repair

Neurotrophic factors are important for regeneration of neurons.[63] Unfortunately, after PNI there is a loss in retrograde transport of neurotrophic factors back to the cell body.[64] This can lead to cell death and halt regeneration. Research suggests that the application of multiple neurotrophic factors (e.g., brain-derived [BDNF] and glial-derived [GDNF]) acting on two different populations of cells may increase survival of damaged neurons and enhance regeneration.[65] Alternatively, the use of human bone marrow stromal cells (MSCs) may enhance peripheral nerve regeneration.[66] MSCs are easily harvested through bone marrow aspiration and differentiate into a wide variety of cells, such as stem cells. Early findings suggest that MSCs grow into thick, robust Schwann cells useful in the production of neurotrophic factors. Although neurotrophic factors have been shown to have a positive effect on nerve regeneration, there currently is no clinical application because of the concerns regarding correct dosage and method of application.[67] Studies explored in animal models may alleviate these issues in the future.

Brushart and colleagues[14,15] used a rat model to determine that intraoperative low-frequency electrical stimulation provided to the nerve 1 hour after repair accelerates the axons' ability to cross the repair site and helps direct them to the appropriate sensory or motor fiber. Electrical stimulation was also found to correlate with an up-regulation of neurotrophic factors in the neurons.[14] In the future it may be feasible and safe to provide electrical stimulation directly to human nerves intraoperatively to enhance success of nerve repair.[68]

Prehension and Sensorimotor Control

Neural regeneration and reorganization are activity-dependent processes[21] induced more favorably in enriched environments.[69] Exercise has proven beneficial for axon regeneration in animals,[16] yet for humans participation in meaningful, and challenging, goal-directed activity that engages attention and motivation may best enhance neural recovery.[21,59] If used prudently, biofeedback and NMES can augment feedback and promote task success.

Even if motor return is good, functional outcome can be poor if hand sensibility is not restored.[70] Sensory retraining is one method of fostering neural reorganization. According to Lundborg,[71] sensory reeducation aims to (1) aid interpretation and promote normalization of distorted hand maps, (2) refine cortical receptive fields to a higher resolution of sensory information, and (3) improve sensory processing. The two phases of sensory retraining are (1) desensitization to address neuropathic pain and (2) sensory reeducation to enhance functional prehension. Please see Chapter 46 for further details on sensory reeducation.

Case Study

MC is a 5-year-old right-hand-dominant male who fell through a glass door and sustained a deep laceration to his right axilla, resulting in a complete transaction of the brachial artery and vein, the ulnar and median nerves, and the medial brachial cutaneous nerve. The structures were all repaired within 4 hours of injury. The biceps muscle was partially lacerated but not repaired. Immediately after surgery, MC was placed in a right shoulder immobilizer for 4 weeks.

Phase One

At 4 weeks after surgery, the hand surgeon determined that MC had complete motor and sensory deficits through the median and ulnar nerve distributions. He was referred to

therapy for fabrication of orthoses, exercises, and education. At the initial visit, his hand was postured in an intrinsic minus position in digits 2 through 5, yet PROM was within normal limits (WNL). Two orthoses were fabricated and issued: (1) a nighttime resting hand orthosis in slight wrist extension, MCP joint flexion, and IP joint extension and (2) a static daytime orthosis to prevent posturing in the intrinsic minus position. The orthoses were fabricated and issued, but due to insurance issues MC was unable to attend therapy at our facility and was referred out to another center. Unfortunately, MC and his family were not compliant with follow-up therapy and orthotic wear. He also missed several postoperative physician visits. Five months after the initial referral (6 months after surgery), MC returned for weekly therapy at our facility with a new insurance policy.

Evaluation

Six months postoperatively, medical and social history were reviewed and an assessment was made of (1) resting posture and available prehension patterns, (2) sensibility, (3) AROM and PROM, (4) strength (Myometer and Jamar dynamometer), (4) dexterity (9-hole peg test, Jebsen Taylor Hand Function Test), (5) ADL skills, and (6) individual and family preferred learning styles.

At rest MC postured his wrist in flexion, MCP joints in slight flexion, and IP joints in flexion. Because of weakness and joint contracture, MC could only exhibit the following patterns: a raking grasp, weak lateral pinch, and a weak scissors grasp between his fingers. During bimanual tasks, MC could not stabilize objects with his right hand, and he relied on both hands to grasp and lift objects. Findings for the initial and final objective assessments are listed in Tables 45-4 through 45-8 (online).

Functional Limitations

MC's primary concerns at this time were his inability to use his right hand to hold toys, assist with dressing, or wipe himself after toileting. He also had difficulty with bimanual tasks such as holding the handlebars on his bike, securing fasteners, and stabilizing a plate and food for cutting. MC had to change his dominance from his right to his left hand due to his limitations.

Factors Affecting Neural Recovery

It was important to consider neural recovery factors when establishing treatment goals with MC and his family and speculating on outcomes. MC's age, health, and timeliness of repair were supportive of good recovery. He was now a 6-year-old male in good general health and had received his nerve repair within 4 hours of injury. He was active and energetic and enjoyed participating in therapeutic activities and had specific functional goals that he wished to address. Constraints to achieving a favorable outcome included the level of his lesion, the involvement of multiple peripheral nerves, and compliance. MC's laceration was at the axilla level, the median and ulnar nerve injuries were severe, and he and his family had a history of noncompliance. His initial delay in acquiring rehabilitation services contributed to joint contracture and suboptimal resting hand posture and may have delayed sensory and motor recovery.

Intervention

For MC it was essential to prioritize goals and treatment and continually reevaluate his progress due to his significant involvement from multiple PNIs. At this phase of treatment MC exhibited significant AROM impairments in his right upper extremity (RUE). The late initiation of his rehabilitation program and his age required modification of the typical treatment goals and strategies listed earlier. His goals for treatment and the strategies used to attain them are shown in Table 45-9 (online). Individual education included a review of therapy goals, precautions, timeline/expectations in recovery, and explanation of functional deficits and the cause.

Phase Two

Due to his age, MC required multimodal individual education, including demonstration, hand-over-hand assistance, verbal, and written or pictorial instructions. To initiate and retrain grasp and release we used MVF. Strategies used to enhance AROM included aquatic tasks using a "water table" for wrist flexion–extension exercises, bilateral dowel exercises, volleyball and baseball with the arm in an "Aircast" to strike the ball, prone scooter board play, play in a tire swing, table hockey using elbow flexion–extension or wrist flexion–extension, and an arm ergometer. To isolate muscle activation we used biofeedback and place-and-hold exercises, which were both successful. We progressed to strengthening via progressive resistive exercises using cuff weights, theraband, theraputty, a biometrics device, and a medicine ball for bilateral games. To enhance sensorimotor control we used the biometrics device to encourage grading of fingertip forces while playing video games. We also encouraged construction of wooden projects (toy boat, car), and participation in manipulative games such as Jenga, Connect Four, Yahtzee, Legos, and Connex. We used virtual reality games and cuff weights to reinforce use of the RUE and to enhance endurance. Sensory reeducation tasks incorporated textured discrimination tiles, stereognosis games, and touch localization with and without vision. Participation in preferred bimanual tasks such as meal preparation and dressing gave MC the opportunity to improve function.

Orthosis type and wear schedule were adapted as progress was made. The long-arm opponens orthosis issued in phase one to provide wrist stability and position the thumb for grasp was used until wrist extension returned. We then issued a short opponens orthosis to position the thumb for grasp combined with kinesiotaping to facilitate active wrist extension. At this time we also issued a figure-of-8 orthosis to prevent intrinsic minus posturing.

Unfortunately, MC's poor sensibility and neuropathic pain (which increased on reinnervation) reduced his willingness to use his RUE for ADL tasks. Sensory reeducation strategies progressed as follows: (1) desensitization, (2) identification of static versus moving touch, (3) touch localization, (4) tactile gnosis, and (5) tactile discrimination.

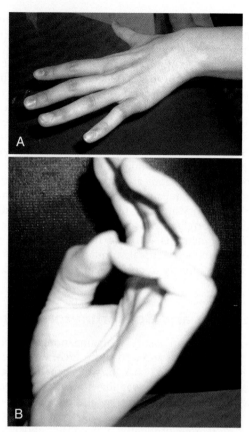

Figure 45-18 Case study: Median and ulnar nerve injury. **A,** Intrinsic minus posturing and muscle atrophy between metacarpals 2 through 5. **B,** Inability to oppose with thumb or small finger after 6 months.

Phase Three

Goals for this phase are listed in Table 45-9 (online). MC primarily focused on strengthening his RUE and improving his prehensile control. After 1 year of therapy, MC displayed maximum therapeutic benefit and was referred to a hand surgeon for consultation regarding surgical options. He continued to display intrinsic minus posturing and had evidence of muscle wasting (Fig. 45-18A). He also was unable to oppose his thumb or small finger (Fig. 45-18B).

At discharge his reevaluation showed progress in most areas as shown in Tables 45-4 through 45-8 (online) including dexterity. Based on his current function and surgical consultation it was determined that he would receive tendon transfers. See Chapter 59 for tendon transfer results.

Summary

Because of the tremendous potential for peripheral nerve regeneration, rehabilitation after compression or traction injuries or after lacerations and repair can be quite rewarding. The key to success is to adhere to precautions initially to rest and protect the nerve, then provide an enriched therapeutic environment as the individual progresses through the phases of recovery. This strategy enhances not only peripheral recovery but central reorganization. Furthermore, if greater emphasis is placed on fostering reorganization and recovery of sensorimotor control, the patient may be able to regain flexible and efficient prehensile skill after nerve injury.

REFERENCES

The complete reference list is available online at www.expertconsult.com.

CHAPTER 46

Sensory Reeducation

BIRGITTA ROSÉN OT, PhD AND GÖRAN LUNDBORG, MD, PhD

THE SENSATIONAL HAND—CONCEPTUAL
  FRAMEWORK
FACTORS INFLUENCING OUTCOME AFTER NERVE
  INJURY AND SENSORY REEDUCATION
CORTICAL REMODELING—RESPONSE TO
  SENSORY INPUT
SENSORY REEDUCATION—PRINCIPLES AND
  PLANNING
SENSORY REEDUCATION IN PHASE 1—SENSORY
  PREPARATION

SENSORY REEDUCATION IN PHASE 2
HOW IS BRAIN ORGANIZATION INFLUENCED BY
  SENSORY REEDUCATION?
ENVIRONMENTAL INFLUENCE ON SENSORY
  REEDUCATION
ASSESSMENT—RESULTS OF SENSORY REEDUCATION
CONCLUSION

CRITICAL POINTS

- After nerve injury the cortical representation of the
  hand becomes disorganized, diminishes, or may
  disappear, a fact that may seriously jeopardize hand
  function.
- The brain is much more plastic than was previously
  believed, possessing a large capacity for cortical
  functional reorganization even at the adult stage.
- The goal of sensory reeducation is to find ways to
  maintain or restore cortical hand representation after
  nerve injury and repair.
- Following repair of major nerve trunks, there is initially
  a period (phase 1) lasting for several months when no
  regenerating fibers have reached the senseless hand,
  followed by phase 2 representing reinnervation of the
  hand.
- It is our belief that sensory reeducation should start
  immediately after nerve repair (phase 1) to preserve the
  cortical hand representation.

Repair of injured nerve trunks in the upper extremity of
adults usually results in incomplete recovery of sensory function in the hand. One explanation for this is that after nerve
injury the cortical representation of the hand becomes disorganized, diminishes, or may disappear, a fact that may seriously jeopardize hand function.[1-4] It is as if the hand "speaks

a new language to the brain." The purpose of sensory reeducation is to facilitate acquisition of the "new language" and
to enhance recovery of sensory function in the hand.

It was long believed that the cortical body map was firmly
established in the adult brain, but according to evolving
concepts the brain is much more plastic than was previously
believed, possessing a large capacity for cortical functional
reorganization even at the adult stage. Rapid reorganizations
occur as a result of changes in activity and sensory inflow.
For example, a decrease of the cortical representation of a
body part is seen as a result of anesthesia, amputation, and
nerve injury. In addition, the brain possesses a cross-modal
and multimodal capacity, implying that one sense can substitute for another.[5-9]

A major goal is thus to find ways to maintain or restore
the cortical hand representation in such situations. Not only
may sensory reeducation be of importance after a nerve
reconstruction, it may be equally important in situations with
only a slight change in the somatosensory cortex to maintain
or restore the cortical somatosensory patterns so as to facilitate the sensorimotor neural networking.

Following repair of major nerve trunks, there is initially
a period (phase 1) lasting for several months when no regenerating fibers have reached the senseless hand, followed by
phase 2, representing reinnervation of the hand.[10] Each of
these phases requires a specific treatment strategy, and it
is our belief that sensory reeducation should start immediately after nerve repair to preserve the cortical hand
representation.

The Sensational Hand— Conceptual Framework

The richness in specific tactile information from the hand, combined with the flexible processing of the brain, has made the human hand a sophisticated instrument with an enormous capacity to perceive, to execute, and to express— simultaneously—in the explorative act of touch.[11,12] A functioning sense of touch creates a base for the use of the hands, and such touch is a vital part of activity—activity that is a basic driving force in humans.

In *Lettre sur les aveugles* ("Letters on the Blind"), from 1749, the French philosopher Diderot discusses the role of learning in the development of normal perception, for example, that "touch gains in power owing to its use."[13] That is briefly what sensory reeducation and sensory relearning is about—"Use it or lose it"—and sensory reeducation is indeed a challenge in the efforts to improve a person's function after a nerve injury.

Jean Ayres described in her *sensory integration theory* the dynamic relationship between behavior and neural processing of input from the senses.[14] The brain must organize input from many sources into meaningful patterns that can be utilized for interaction with the environment and participation in daily-life activities.[14] Such a continuous cross-modal and multimodal networking in the brain[5,15] can be used in sensory relearning. Let other senses help when touch sensibility is weak. For example, touching a fruit can systematically be associated with its taste, smell, and color, creating "a tactile meal."

Four major modalities of somatic sensibility can be defined: touch, proprioception, pain, and temperature sense.[16] A hierarchy of touch functions can also be identified: If detection of touch is present, the next level is discrimination of touch, basic tactile gnosis.[18,19] Localization of touch is also an aspect of discriminative touch, and identification of objects, shapes, and textures with active touching is the third level—a more refined tactile gnosis.[18,20]

Functionality of sensation has been analyzed. An adequate feedback system for control of grip force by the integration of sensory and motor mechanisms and the proprioceptive elements has been investigated in depth,[21,22] and this knowledge is essential for sensory feedback. The superiority of sensibility in a well-coordinated hand is also emphasized, whereby sensibility and memory are discussed as key factors that control our acquired motor programs.[23] Direct recording techniques from the cortical surface of the brain, and modern brain imaging techniques such as positron emission tomography, magnetic resonance imaging (MRI), magnetic encephalography, and transcranial magnetic stimulation have also made it possible to explore issues of tactile processing in the brain, and brain plasticity.[16,17]

Napier described the hand as "an organ of touch which feels round corners and sees in the dark."[24] Sterling Bunnell, the father of hand surgery, described sensation as the "eyes" of the fingers, illustrated by Moberg with the classic *seeing fingertips*, meaning that a hand without sensibility is blind. The expression *functional sensibility* is frequently used in hand surgery literature, as a basic function for *what the hand can do* (i.e., purposeful use of the hand).[25] It is the subtle sensibility that gives the grip "sight," not just to perceive but to understand the touch. Brand and Yancey also pointed out the important functional protective aspect of hand sensibility: "Pain the gift nobody wants."[26] Wynn-Parry and later Dellon and Curtis express this holistic view on the hand and hand sensibility, and the importance of not only motor reeducation but also sensory reeducation programs to improve poor results after nerve injuries.[27,28]

Moberg established the term *tactile gnosis* in his classic articles from 1958 and 1962 as the specific aspect of functional sensibility representing the interplay between peripheral function of the nerve and the interpretation of sensory impressions in the brain. Tactile gnosis enables recognition of qualities and the character of objects without using vision.[25,29,30] Tactile gnosis capacity is specifically addressed in sensory reeducation programs.

The hand is sometimes described as a sense organ strongly linked to the brain and to the personality.[6] This approach has in recent years also gained importance in discussions of surgical techniques to improve poor results after nerve lesions.[31] The emphasis in these discussions is not only on the importance of advanced surgical techniques but also on the rapidly expanding knowledge in neurobiology with several tools to influence injured neurons and to use the inherent plasticity of the neurons in further development of sensory reeducation.

Factors Influencing Outcome after a Nerve Injury and Sensory Reeducation

Nerve injuries may seriously interfere with an individual's capacity to function adequately, and the acquired disability is often dramatic. A hand with limited sensibility is usually a hand with very limited function. There is a high probability of lost work capacity and impaired quality of life for the patient.[32,33] There is often lifelong hand function impairment, pain, dysesthesia, allodynia, and cold intolerance.[34] There is also a substantial economic impact of nerve injuries on the patient as well as on society.[35]

Age

Although the outcome from nerve repair is disappointing in adults, it is well-known that children usually achieve superior functional results without any formal sensory reeducation.[36] The shorter regeneration distance in children and a better regeneration capacity in general contribute to these good outcomes. However, the superior ability of the cortex's central adaptation to the new pattern of afferent impulses presented by misdirected axons also provides an explanation for superior recovery in children. There seems to be a critical age period for recovery of functional hand sensibility, with the best results being seen in those younger than the age of 10 years, followed by rapid decline leveling out after late adolescence. Interestingly, there is a striking analogy between this pattern and the pattern illustrating the scores of immigrants on a grammar test, plotted against the age at which they start to learn a new language.[37] Thus, the critical period for regaining discriminative tactile capacity after nerve repair is analogous to a corresponding critical period for acquisition of a second language, indicating a strong learning component in acquisition of functional sensibility as well.

Timing of Repair, Type of Nerve, Level and Type of Injury

It is agreed that freshly transected nerves should be repaired acutely with no or minimal delay.[38,39] Early repair will substantially reduce the postoperative nerve cell death.[40]

The type of nerve that is injured considerably influences the outcome. If a pure motor nerve is injured, the risk for mismatch between motor axons and sensory axons is eliminated, thus optimizing the accuracy in reinnervation. For pure sensory nerves such as a digital nerve, the situation is analogous.

After nerve transection there is an initial delay followed by sprouting and axonal outgrowth. A nerve outgrowth rate of 1 to 2 mm per day in humans has been suggested. In digital nerve injuries there is only a short distance separating the regenerating axons from their distal targets, while injuries at the upper arm level create different situations with longer time interval to regeneration of the hand. Nerve lesions at wrist level may require 3 to 4 months before the first signs of reinnervation in the hand occur.

A crush or compression lesion always results in better functional outcome than does total severance of a nerve trunk. The initial delay is shorter and the growth of axons proceeds at a faster rate after a crush injury than after a nerve transection. The Schwann cell basal lamina are still in continuity and can thus guide the axons back to their original peripheral targets. The correct peripheral reinnervation of crush injuries is reflected in a perfect restoration of the original cortical representational areas corresponding to the reinnervated body part.[3,41]

Central Nervous System Factors— Cognitive Capacity

The surgeon's ambition is to use repair techniques that bring a maximal number of nerve fibers into correct peripheral cutaneous areas. However, there are at least three strong indications that *central nervous system factors* associated with cortical remodeling represent a major reason for the inferior functional outcome following nerve repair. First, children up to the age of 10 to 12 years usually present excellent recovery of functional sensibility in contrast to adult patients. This critical "age window" for perfect sensory recovery presented by children corresponds well with what is known from other types of learning processes, for instance, the ability to acquire a second language.[37] Second, cognitive functions are important explanatory factors in adults for variations in recovery of tactile discrimination.[42] Third, the peripheral repair technique in nerve lesions has not been found to influence the functional outcome in a clinical randomized study at a 5-year follow-up.[43] Silicone tubular repair, leaving a short distance between the nerve cuts, was compared with the outcome

from routine microsurgical repair in a clinical randomized prospective study. The study included 30 patients with median or ulnar nerve injuries in the distal forearm. Postoperatively, the patients were assessed regularly over a 5-year period with neurophysiologic and clinical assessments. After 5 years there was no significant difference in outcome between the two techniques except that cold intolerance was significantly less severe with the tubular technique. The most significant improvement of perception of touch occurred during the first postoperative year, while improvement of motor function could be observed much later.[44] In the total group there was however an ongoing improvement of functional sensibility throughout the 5 years after repair, although there was no further impairment in nerve conduction velocity or amplitude after the first 2 years.[41] This supports the thesis that central nervous system factors associated with the cortical remodeling after a nerve repair are important, and that efforts to improve the results following nerve repair in the future must address the brain as well as the peripheral nerve.

In addition to the large number of peripheral and central factors, active and conscious use of the hand in activities of daily life, combined with high motivation by the patient, has long been reported to be of great importance for useful return of functional sensibility.[45] Bruyns et al. found that intensive education, high compliance to hand therapy, and an isolated injury predict quicker return to work in patients with median and/or ulnar nerve injuries.[32] A recent meta-analysis showed that age, site, injured nerve, and delayed repair significantly influence the prognosis after nerve repair.[46] Early psychological stress has also been found to influence the outcome in a negative direction.[47]

Cortical Remodeling— Response to Sensory Input

The human hand and the brain have developed into a sophisticated functional unit,[48] and the hand is largely represented in the somatosensory cortex of the brain with arrangements of sharply divided territories receiving impulses from specific areas of the hand. This is reflected in the mapping of the body revealing great variation in tactile discrimination. The fingertips, lips, and the tongue, which occupy large areas, exhibit the highest resolution.[49] However, the plasticity of the brain enables changes in the territories when the prerequisites and demands for sensory input are changed. This is a functional reorganization that is described by several authors.[2-4,50-53]

According to evolving concepts over the last decades, the brain is much more plastic than was formerly believed, possessing a substantial capacity for cortical functional reorganizations also at the adult stage.[4,54] In primate experiments using techniques for direct recording from the brain cortex,[55,56] strong evidence has been presented that there is a capacity for rapid cortical reorganization in the somatosensory cortex of adult primates that may occur for several reasons, such as changed sensory experience and performance of the hand, overuse, amputation, and local anesthesia. The brain can be sculpted by experience, and this dynamic is true for the entire lifetime. The brain's capacity for remodeling is what makes sensory reeducation and sensory relearning possible. In various neuropathies, focal hand dystonia, and during immobilization, a disorganized somatosensory cortex may be one important reason for problems with hand function.

Experience-Dependent Cortical Remodeling

Effects of Increased Sensory Input

Direct recordings from the somatosensory cortex in monkeys demonstrated experience-induced cortical remodeling secondary to increased tactile stimulation of separate fingers.[1,3] Simultaneous tactile stimulation of nearby separate receptive fields of the adult rat paw for a few hours also induces a selective enlargement of the cortical area representing the stimulated skin fields.[57] This phenomenon has been demonstrated in experimental studies involving human subjects.[58-60] Continuous co-activation of separate receptive fields in a fingertip for 2 to 3 hours results in an expansion of the fingertip cortical representation in the S1 area, a phenomenon that is linked to a significant improvement of two-point discrimination.[58-60]

This is interesting from a functional point of view. Tasks requiring increased discriminatory skill relate to an expansion of the cortical projection area corresponding to the fingers involved in the task. You can see the same phenomenon in fingertips subjected to long-term massive tactile stimulation. Patients with blindness using their index fingers for reading in Braille demonstrate an expansion of the finger representation.[61] The string hand of violin players occupies enlarged projection areas in the somatosensory as well as motor cortex of the brain.[51,62] These changes in representation have been demonstrated in other groups of professional musicians in both the somatosensory and auditory domains.[63]

When Increased Sensory Input Becomes a Problem

Stereotypic and repetitive fine motor movements can degrade the sensory representation of the hand in the somatosensory cortex and lead to a loss of normal motor control.[64,65] This can be observed in musicians suffering from overuse syndromes such as functional dystonia (i.e., the inability to control and regulate individual finger movements). In such situations the cortical hand map is distorted and remodeled into a disorganized pattern.[66-68] The physiologic basis is probably repetitive monotonous tactile stimulation and use of the hand over extended time periods. In monkeys, trained to perform monotonous repetitive hand movements involving simultaneous tactile stimulation of various parts of the hand, fusion of the normally well-separated cortical projection sites of individual fingers has been seen.[69] The cortical "hand-glove" becomes a mitten. Reversal of the reorganization changes by use of specific training programs including very specific sensory discriminative tasks have shown good results in dystonia treatment.[66,70,71] Some of this information is available to our readers in Chapter 135.

Effects of Decreased Sensory Input

Diminished or complete arrest of tactile input may result in degradation of cortical representations.[9,72] Hands in persons with cerebral palsy that are contracted into severe flexion postures, devoid of sensory experiences, are associated with a diminished sensory capacity. Surgical procedures to open the hand allow for the possibility of new tactile experiences to wake up such sensibility in disguise.[73] If the lower extremity is immobilized, its representation in the motor cortex decreases, a phenomenon that is reversible with regained mobility.[74] Sensory reeducation may be helpful in this situation of prolonged immobilization.

Nerve Injury and Repair

After a major nerve injury there is a cortical response with an instant and long-standing reorganization of the somatosensory brain cortex. The silent area without sensory input triggers an expansion and invasion from adjacent cortical areas.[3,9,75,76] This is the beginning of a dynamic interplay in the cortical neural networks, which is influenced by several biologic and psychological events during regeneration and reinnervation. These changes, which happen within minutes, are probably based on unmasking of normally occurring, but inhibited synaptic connections. There are reasons to believe that such connections are susceptible to further changes. During this postinjury period before regeneration occurs, the hand is without sensation and there is no sensory input from the areas normally innervated by the injured nerve. In the following sections this period will be named *phase 1*.

The microsurgical nerve repair techniques have been refined to an optimal level; however, there is still a significant disorientation of regenerating axons at the repair site. Therefore, the skin areas of the hand will, to a large extent, not be reinnervated by their *original* axons. The result is additional new changes in the cortical territory where the nerve is normally represented. The original well-organized hand representation is changed to a distorted pattern[75] (Fig. 46-1). The nerve does not recapture all of its original territory. The former specific cortical representation of separate fingers disappears and changes into an overlapping pattern between the fingers.[77] This knowledge is based primarily on primate experiments, but analogous findings have been made also in humans on the basis of functional MRI techniques.[78] The specific cortical territories representing each finger in primate experiments have shown a completely changed pattern. The hand speaks a new distorted language to the brain, requiring a relearning process. This is referred to as *phase 2*, representing reinnervation of the hand. After a nerve injury at the wrist level, phase 2 usually begins 3 to 4 months after nerve repair. The timing for onset of sensory reeducation may be of critical importance. Each of the two phases following a nerve repair requires a specific treatment strategy, and we suggest that sensory reeducation should start immediately after nerve repair to preserve the cortical hand representation.

In summary, there are good reasons to look for factors in the central nervous system, in addition to the cellular and biochemical events, that are associated with degeneration and regeneration in the peripheral nervous system to explain the incomplete sensory recovery after nerve repair. A nerve injury in the upper extremity is followed by profound functional reorganization changes in the brain cortex, mainly due to misdirection of regenerating axons. These central events,

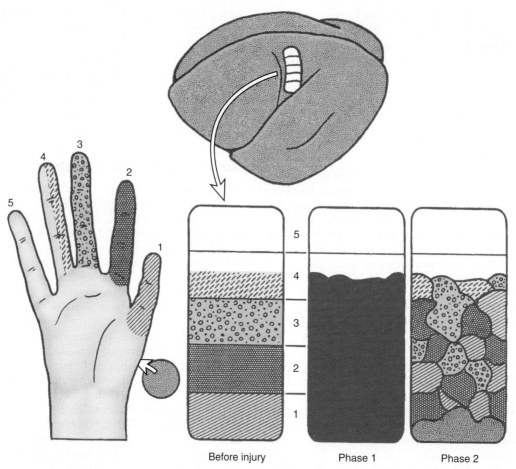

Figure 46-1 A schematic illustration of how the "hand map" in the brain changes after repair of the median nerve. Before injury each finger has its specific area; in phase 1 this area becomes "silent" and becomes occupied by adjacent areas. In phase 2, when the new axons have grown to the skin and to the muscles, the map is again changed, since the axons do not grow in exactly the same paths as before the injury. The map becomes unstructured and is difficult to interpret.

which are an expression of the brain's capacity for rapid plasticity, play a predominant role in the sensory reeducation programs of today. This is a challenging and important area for multidisciplinary clinical development and research in the field of rehabilitation following nerve injuries.

Sensory Reeducation— Principles and Planning

The practice of sensory reeducation has long existed in rehabilitation settings along with motor reeducation but was not recognized as such until Wynn-Parry and Dellon designed the first formal programs.[27,28] The functional improvement seen after training may be based on normalization of the distorted hand map, or it may be due to adaptations in higher brain centers with a capacity to decipher the distorted hand map. Further study is needed to determine which explanation is correct.

Learning is a key word in the rehabilitation process after all injuries. New sensory and motor codes are presented to the brain with which the brain must cope for purposeful sensorimotor interaction and functional use. A relearning process is required to adapt to the new and distorted afferent

sensory input when familiar objects are touched. The mind does not understand the new "sensory code" associated with specific textures and shapes. To facilitate and enhance this process, specific programs for sensory reeducation are routinely used for regaining tactile gnosis. According to these strategies, the brain is reprogrammed on the basis of a relearning process. Sensory reeducation is based on vision guiding touch and on higher cortical functions such as attention and memory during several daily short practice sessions occurring over several weeks or months.[24,27] With active use of the hand, the patient learns to code the integrated passive and active afferent stimuli with slower and fewer conducting nerve fibers than normal.[28,79]

The sensory reeducation training is integrated in the overall rehabilitation program and individualized based on the patient's level of sensory function. As mentioned previously, following repair of major nerve trunks there is initially a period (*phase 1*) lasting for several months when no regenerating fibers have reached the senseless hand, followed by *phase 2* representing reinnervation of the hand.[10] Each of these phases requires a specific treatment strategy.

In phase 1 there is no protective sensibility, and it is important to carefully watch the hand during use to prevent skin injuries. The lack of protective sensation is an important message to communicate to the patient in this early phase. In phase 2 the axons have reached the hand. Hypersensitivity to normal touch is common during this period. If so, desensitization exercises should precede the training sessions. Hyperesthesia and allodynia and its treatment are described elsewhere in Chapters 113 through 116.

Specific, simple, and repetitive sensory relearning exercises of increasing complexity and difficulty should be performed at home by the patient on a daily basis in frequent brief training sessions. Weekly training sessions with the therapist may be scheduled to provide guidance and feedback. Training in a quiet location for high attention is recommended, and active and conscious use of the hand in daily activities combined with high motivation by the patient are important factors. The rehabilitation after a nerve repair is a long process that can take several years, so it takes a lot of patience. The complexity after a nerve injury with interacting phenomena that depend on so many factors is not easy for the patient to understand. Therefore, the information and education of the patient about the injury and the sensory reeducation concept are crucial. If the patient does not understand the training concept, it is very difficult for him or her to be motivated to follow through with the retraining. A written home program should always be given to each patient. The patient should also be encouraged to use the affected hand very consciously in daily activities.

Timing—Onset of Sensory Reeducation

In the sensory reeducation program proposed in this chapter, the training technique is the classical one according to Wynn-Parry and Dellon,[27,79] but focus is on the *timing* of initiation of the training program not only in phase 2 but also in phase 1. The strategy is to activate the cortical area representing the damaged nerve, thereby diminishing the cortical reorganization and maintaining the cortical hand map. Borsook et al.[52] demonstrated that following amputation of the hand, touch of the face, being close to the hand in the cortical body map,[49] gives rise to phantom sensations as soon as 24 hours after injury. Weiss et al. demonstrated plasticity after finger amputation within 10 days after amputation.[80] An analogous phenomenon can also be seen after local anesthetic blocks that temporarily can induce shifts in neuronal receptive fields with cortical reorganization.[81]

The traditional procedure calls for the introduction of sensory reeducation once touch can be perceived in the involved area.[27,79] However, at this point the reorganizing brain presents a random pattern, which may not be possible to reverse. Cheng et al. presented a prospective randomized study on early tactile stimulation after digital nerve repair (3 weeks after surgery) that showed excellent results and significantly better discriminative sensibility in the study group.[82] If the "vacant" cortical area of a denervated hand could be provided relevant information from the hand using visual clues early after repair, it might help to minimize the synaptic reorganization. This may well make the brain better prepared for the relearning program once the nerve has regenerated and reinnervated the peripheral targets.

The design and protocols of the sensory reeducational programs have not changed over the last decades. This is surprising, considering the enormous advances in neuroscience and brain imaging techniques that have increased our understanding of mechanisms underpinning brain plasticity. We therefore have presented new strategies for sensory reeducation that utilize the capacity for cross-modal and multi-modal capacity of the adult brain as well as the remodeling capacity of the brain.

Sensory Reeducation in Phase 1— Sensory Preparation

In phase 1 we focus on maintaining the cortical hand representation by using the brain's capacity for sensory imagery as well as cortical visuo-tactile interaction. Phase 1 lasts until there is measurable sensibility present in the hand that can be assessed with Semmes–Weinstein monofilaments.[83] To be able to start sensory reeducation at this critical early stage without any existing sensibility in the hand, we use the holistic organization of the brain with an extensive capacity for cross- and multimodality. The sensory relearning in this early phase, in combination with mobility training of the hand, is aimed at activating and maintaining the hand map in the brain to make the sensory relearning easier once the axons have regrown. This gives the brain an illusion of sensibility in the hand.

The use of vision to guide the retraining of sensation is the basis for classic sensory reeducation, but there is a continuous interplay among *all* senses. Multisensory neurons that receive more than one type of sensory input may be used to extract information from one sensory modality and use it in another by using polymodal association areas.[5,15,84]

The multimodal capacity of the brain and brain's capacity for adaptation with deprivation of sense can be illustrated in individuals with blindness. When such a person reads Braille or carries out other tactile discrimination tasks, the primary visual cortex is activated together with the somatosensory cortex.[85]

Sensory Imagery

Similarities exist in the cortical functions between perception and imagery.[86] Auditory cortical areas are recruited in the absence of sound during imagining music,[86] the visual cortex is active during visual imagery,[87] and imagination of odors is associated with increased activation in olfactory regions in the brain.[88] Just imagining a movement activates the premotor cortex.[89] The pattern of somatosensory activation during motor imagery is very similar to the pattern observed during a real movement execution.[90] Few observations of *sensory imagery* with involvement of primary sensory cortical areas have been reported. Just thinking about stroking the dorsum of the hand activates the sensory cortex.[91] It is recommended that the patient can try to imagine touch in the hand during phase 1.

Observation of Touch, Reading or Listening to "Sensory" Words, Observing "Sensory Pictures," Mirror Training

Activation of motor neurons that may also serve as mirror neurons in the premotor cortex by the observation of hand

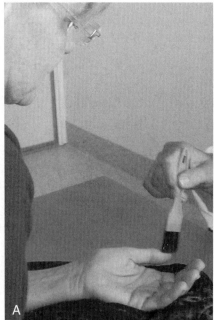

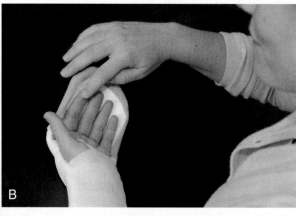

Figure 46-2 By touching the areas in the hand that have no sensibility in combination with concentrated watching, the hand map in the brain is activated. This is repeated several times per day. **A,** Someone else can touch the fingers without sensibility and corresponding fingers on the other hand simultaneously during careful watching. **B,** The patient can touch the fingers lacking sensibility using the corresponding finger area of the other hand, or someone else can do the stimulation.

activity is a well-known phenomenon, which is believed to play a fundamental role in both action and imitation.[92] Mirror neuron areas are also involved in understanding the intention of actions.[93] Reading or listening to *action words* related to hand movements activates hand representational areas in the motor cortex,[94] and hypothetically *reading or listening to "sensory" words or watching "sensory" pictures* would relate to activity in the somatosensory cortex. Other ways to activate the somatosensory cortex include observing a body part being touched. Keysers showed this during *observation of touching* the legs,[95] and we have demonstrated a visuo-tactile cortical interaction during mere observation of tactile stimulation of the hand.[96] It is suggested that the somatosensory cortical areas, SI and SII cortex, are related to the mirror neuron system.[91,97,98] The patient's observation of his or her hand being touched is one component of early sensory training the first day after surgery, which might activate the cortical hand area due to visuo-tactile interaction (Fig. 46-2).

The effect can hypothetically be further enhanced by using mirror training introduced by Ramachandran.[99,100] A mirror is placed transversally in front of the patient with the nerve-injured hand hidden behind the mirror and the healthy hand being reflected in the position of the injured hand. Touching the healthy hand gives the illusion of touching the nerve-injured hand. In these training sessions, a clinical observation is that the patient often gets a perception of the tactile stimuli in the nerve-injured insensate hand by the combined mirror illusion and the true touch of the healthy hand. Exercises normally performed in phase 2, when there is sensibility in the hand, can be used (Fig. 46-3).

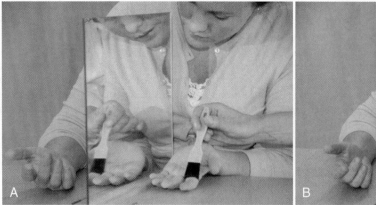

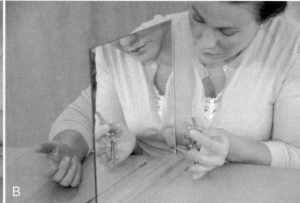

Figure 46-3 Mirror training positioned so the uninjured hand is reflected in the mirror looking like the injured hand. The injured hand is hidden behind the mirror. This creates an illusion that makes the brain think there is activity in the injured hand. **A,** Localization of touch; **B,** training with familiar objects.

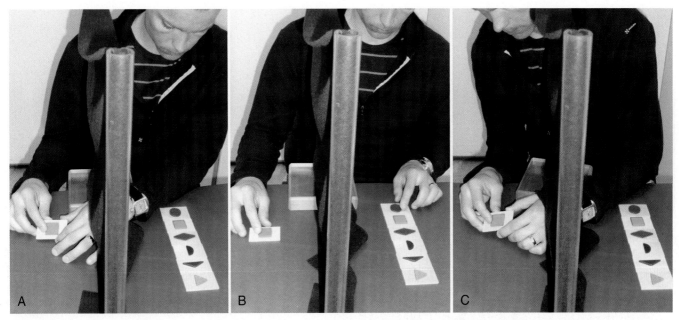

Figure 46-4 *Combining visual and sensory information to teach the brain to understand the "new language" from the right hand. Examples of how the training can be performed with and without vision:* **A**, *Touch a hidden texture, shape, or object, and try to identify it.* **B**, *Touch a copy of the texture, shape, or object with the uninjured hand and the hidden object with the injured hand at the same time, and compare the feeling.* **C**, *Was it correct? If not, or if it was too difficult, touch and watch at the same time and then look in the other direction or close your eyes again.*

Cortical Audio-Tactile Interaction

Another principle is to use another sense such as hearing to substitute for sensibility, thereby utilizing the brain's multi-modal capacity. This method allows early sensory relearning so as to feed the sensory cortex with "relevant" information.[101] Cortical audio-tactile interaction has been recently demonstrated with functional MRI technique.[102]

In a prospective randomized multicenter study, significantly better tactile gnosis compared with controls was observed in persons with median or ulnar nerve repair.[103] These observations were noted within a week after surgery with training in the Sensor Glove (Össur, Iceland) (www. ossur.com), which utilizes audio-tactile interaction.[103] Microphones are mounted dorsally at fingertip levels or in a glove connected to earphones via a miniature stereo processor in the Sensor Glove system. With this system the patient can listen to what the hand feels. Auditory stimuli substitute for absent tactile stimuli. Specific and typical friction sounds are associated with touching of various textures. Exercises with identification of textures and localization were performed several times per day according to the training technique described above.[103]

Whatever method is chosen in phase 1 after the nerve repair, there are good reasons to start sensory relearning much earlier than we do today with the aim of minimizing or inhibiting the reorganization process in the somatosensory cortex induced by the nerve injury. The author's experience is that the method of choice must be individualized. The patient must be comfortable with the exercises and must understand the purpose of such training in phase 1.

Sensory Reeducation in Phase 2

Techniques for Sensory Reeducation

Phase 2 starts when there is measurable sensibility in the palm (minimum Semmes–Weinstein monofilament no. 6.65, 300-g force). When there is some protective sensibility in the fingertips that can be localized correctly, discriminative exercises with identification of shapes, textures, and objects may be initiated. The classic training technique described by Wynn-Parry and Dellon is used. This technique is based on stimulation with varying and increasing difficulty with the eyes open and closed alternately. In this way, another sense (vision) assists the training and improves the deficient sense (sensation)[27,79,104] (Fig. 46-4). Hyperesthesia/allodynia is common in the regeneration phase after a nerve injury, and in such cases desensitization exercises should precede sensory reeducation.

Once the area with diminished sensibility has been established, the first modality to reeducate is the capacity to *localize touch*. Errors in localization of touch after a nerve reconstruction are part of the functional problem in identification of objects without vision. The points stimulated on the skin no longer match with their central projection, and the patient cannot interpret the modified sensation to a meaningful whole (Fig. 46-5). When localization has improved, touching and exploration of items—presenting various sizes, shapes, and textures—is introduced. A variety of tools and specifically designed products can be used for this (Fig. 46-6), but it is recommended also that real and

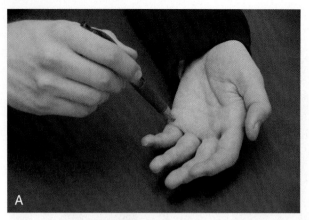

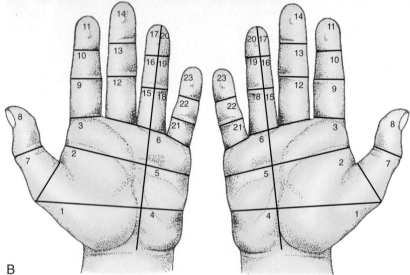

Figure 46-5 To localize touch, the area with diminished sensibility is identified. **A**, The patient is then instructed to touch the skin in one of the areas with a blunt object such as the end of a pen. The object can be pressed or moved hard enough to perceive the touch. The touch can also be compared to an area with normal sensibility. The patient should be instructed to concentrate on *where, what, and how.* Is it in the area where you touch or somewhere else? Is it static or moving touch? Does it feel different from the area with normal sensibility? The touch should be repeated several times, first with eyes open and then with eyes closed until the patient feels that he or she knows where the stimulus is. It is suggested to work on a few areas first until they can be localized correctly. Then, move to adjacent areas. It may also be useful to start to work with areas close to areas with normal sensibility. A good feedback is to get someone else to apply the stimulus to ensure that there is a sensory relearning. **B**, For this purpose the grid can be useful.

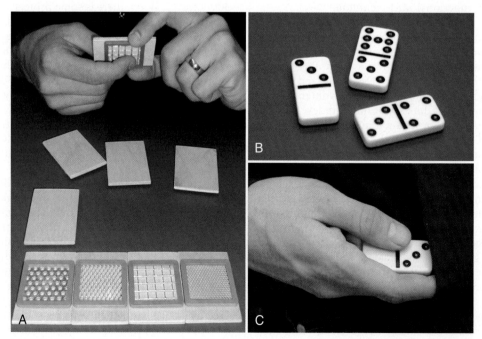

Figure 46-6 Combining identical textures (**A**) and domino brackets of various difficulties (**B**, **C**) for home training.

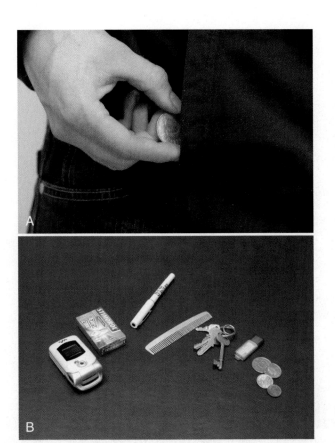

Figure 46-7 A, B, The patient should be encouraged to carry a few familiar objects in the pocket and try to identify them, and think about their shape, texture, weight, and which object is touched. The size of the objects is decided based on tactile gnosis assessment. If, for example, perception threshold in the fingertips is 4 g, and 15-mm objects cannot be identified correctly, the training objects must be simple and bigger.

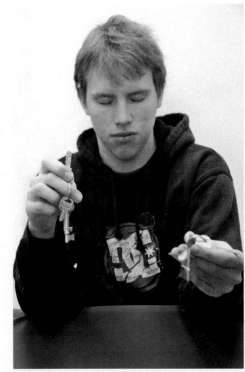

Figure 46-8 Sensory and motor training with emphasis on coordination and identification. Here the patient with eyes closed holds identical keys in right and left (injured) hand, and tries to find a specific key with the left hand.

familiar objects be used (Fig. 46-7). That makes it easier for the patient to incorporate the sensory relearning concept in daily activities, and that is of utmost importance. Exercises that incorporate both sensory and motor training are also highly recommended (Fig. 46-8).

The first sensory reeducation program included timed identification of a series of familiar objects of increasing difficulty.[79] In Dellon's program the training is timed with the regeneration process and return of specific qualities of sensation. The selection of exercises is chosen based on neurophysiologic evidence of cutaneous sensibility. Training is performed depending on when the patient can perceive and identify moving and/or constant touch distally.[27]

Bilateral tactile stimulation, including the injured hand as well as the noninjured hand, might help to influence positively the central substrate for sensory relearning. Sensory input is normally processed to the greatest extent in the contralateral hemisphere, but there is also, to some extent, an ipsilateral activation.[17,105] The whisker representational area in the somatosensory cortex of rats integrates information from both contralateral and ipsilateral whisker pads.[106] In humans there is a transfer of improved tactile performance from a sensory-trained finger to the contralateral hand that has been demonstrated,[107] and it has been shown that practice-related improvements in sensory discrimination can gen-

erate across skin location, hemisphere, and modality.[108] So, there may be good reasons to use both hands in the training process. Use of additional ipsilateral pathways from the non-injured hand may provide correct tactile information to the hemisphere that is contralateral to the injured hand, thereby facilitating the learning process. A conscious sensory relearning in daily activities is very good to use in the bilateral training. Recovering patients should make it a rule to try to feel the structure and shape of everyday objects (Fig. 46-9).

Enhancing the Effects of Sensory Reeducation in Phase 2 Using the Rapid Plasticity of the Brain

It is reasonable to use the brain's capacity for rapid redistribution of cortical resources as a component in the rehabilitation process. That has been well described in the literature in rehabilitation of patients following a stroke. For instance, it has been shown that selective anesthesia of ventral roots of C5–C8 (motor innervation of shoulder and elbow) results in enhanced motor function of the hand (innervation C8–C11).[109] The mechanism is that deafferentation of a specific cortical area (shoulder and elbow representations) allows expansion of adjacent cortical representational areas (the hand). We have recently shown that selective cutaneous deafferentation of the forearm in healthy adults results in improved hand sensation and in expansion of the adjacent cortical hand representation.[110] The rapid improvement in

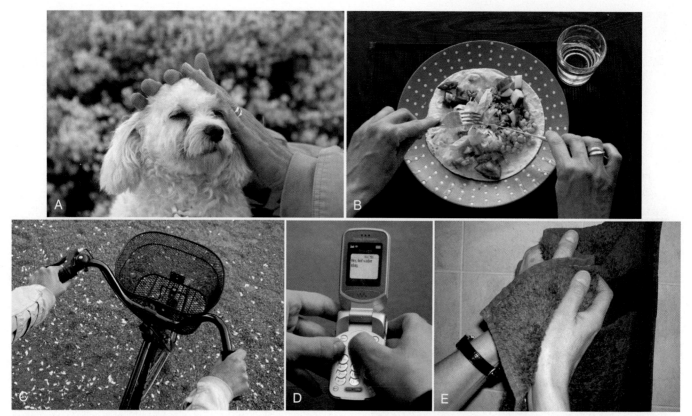

Figure 46-9 A–E, It will help reeducate the sensibility if the patient makes it a rule to try to feel the structure and shape of everyday objects—preferably bilaterally.

sensory functions that may occur within minutes after selective anesthesia is presumably due to unmasking of existing synapses that are normally inhibited. Long-lasting effects may be due to a long-term potentiation of synapses or even formation of new synaptic sites.[111]

So, in addition to traditional sensory reeducation in phase 2, we perform a selective temporary anesthesia of the forearm proximally to the nerve-injured hand during a limited period at a point when the patient has regained some protective sensibility at the fingertip level. This is established with regular follow-ups using a standardized test procedure.[83] The method is used especially in cases with good reinnervation at fingertip level, but poor tactile gnosis.[112] The purpose is to allow expansion of the cortical hand representation. Cutaneous anesthesia of the volar part of the forearm is induced by an anesthetic cream. The treatment is done under careful supervision at the clinic and after prior determination that the patient has no history of adverse reactions to local analgesics. The patient receives EMLA® (lidocaine plus prilocaine; AstraZeneca, Mississauga, ON, Canada), starting with frequent EMLA applications and then with a decreasing number of applications.[112] The treatment is combined with an intense sensory reeducation program with assisted supervised training at the point when the "window" for training is wide open. A double-blind study showed that tactile gnosis (functional sensibility) improved significantly in patients with minimum Semmes–Weinstein monofilament no. 4.31 (1.4-g force) in the fingertips who had received this treatment in combination with intensive sensory reeducation compared with those who received intensive sensory reeducation with a placebo cream applied to their forearms. All patients improved their tactile gnosis, presumably as a result of the intensive sensory reeducation alone, but the EMLA® group was significantly better than the placebo group.[112]

The use of repeated selective temporary anesthesia in sensory training should hypothetically keep a larger cortical area available for the injured body part and, in turn, would increase the brain's ability to interpret the signals from the territory of the injured nerve. This may open a window of opportunity during which it is possible for sensory reeducation to have a better and more long-lasting effect. The optimal frequency for application is yet to be determined in future studies. This is a new and original concept, which may enhance the effect of sensory reeducational programs.

How Is Brain Organization Influenced by Sensory Reeducation?

Little is known about the effects of sensory reeducation on brain organization. One possibility is that sensory training can reverse the disturbed cortical organization toward a normalized pattern. Another possibility is that the cortical hand map is permanently distorted and that the key is an improved processing and perceptual capacity in the sensory networks at a higher cortical level, facilitating interpretation of the distorted hand map. Although young individuals may have a greater capacity for normalization of the cortical hand map following nerve repair as compared with adults, such capacity for normalization of the cortical hand map by training probably does not exist in the mature brain. The topic was studied by Florence et al., investigating the effects of enriched environmental sensory experience on cortical organization on monkeys that had previously undergone nerve repair of the median nerve.[113] One group was subjected to an enriched environmental sensory experience involving presentation of food treats on an artificial grass surface and toys while the control group was allowed only restricted mobility with no such enriched sensory experience. Using direct cortical recording techniques, it was demonstrated that the enriched sensory environment had a significant effect on receptor field size with smaller, normalized, and better located receptive fields likely to provide better resolution. In addition, the cortical hand maps were less distorted in the sensory-enriched animals compared with the sensory-restricted animals. Sensory relearning programs in humans, including an enriched environment, may thus hypothetically explain functional improvement after rehabilitation.

Environmental Influence on Sensory Reeducation

Several factors may influence the results from the sensory reeducational programs in a positive or negative way. For instance, active and conscious use of the hand in daily activities as well as attention during training combined with high motivation by the patient is extremely important. An enriched environment is fundamental to facilitate learning. It has been demonstrated that an enriched environment influences learning by stimulating formation of new synapses. Factors such as a stimulating environment, meaningful activities, and encouragement influence the molding of the brain in a positive direction.[114-116] It has also been demonstrated that passive unattended and repetitive tasks lead to negative changes of the associated territories in the sensory cortex. These observations have been discussed especially as a genesis model for dystonia and repetitive-strain injury problems.[2,65]

Whether music stimulates learning is yet to be definitely demonstrated, but it is argued by several authors that music influences brain activity.[63,117-119] It remains to be investigated if music can enhance sensory relearning and what kind of music would be best suited in such learning. The holistic organization of the brain and the continuous interplay between the brain regions speaks in favor of using all senses very consciously in the sensory relearning process.

Assessment—Results of Sensory Reeducation

Assessment of outcome provides important feedback for the patient and therapist during the rehabilitation period and should be performed in a standardized manner using evidence-based test instruments on a monthly or bimonthly basis. As discussed earlier, much of the recovery can be seen for a long time after the repair; so, after a nerve repair, for example at the wrist level, it can be recommended to follow the patient for at least one year after the injury. The sensory reeducation and relearning is usually a long process, and the patient needs constructive feedback along the way to keep up motivation for a training that has several abstract elements. Good clinical documentation can be a useful tool in this process, and the patient should take an active role in the evaluation of the assessments. This may help him or her to plan the training together with the therapist and to focus on the weak parts in the outcome. An instrument that is sensitive to subtle changes in details of specific functions as well as overall outcome over time is recommended. Several methods have been suggested over the years, and their pros and cons are discussed elsewhere in the literature.[122,123] We suggest use of the "Model for Documentation of Outcome after Nerve Repair," which includes separate domains for sensory, motor, pain–discomfort, and also a "total score."[83,120] Details in function and an overall score can be determined. This model instrument is standardized and is a tool suited for clinical as well as for scientific purposes.[41,121-123] A long-term recovery curve in adults with estimated predicted values for an outcome score after repair of the median or ulnar nerve at the wrist level has been calculated, and can be good feedback during the sensory reeducation process.[124]

Much of the relearning process is probably gained by a conscious use of the hand in daily activities, using vision as a guide for the impaired sensibility. However, to facilitate and enhance this process, specific programs for sensory reeducation should be used as a clinical tool in adult patients for regaining functional sensibility. The therapist's supporting and guiding role during the long and often very trying training period for the patient after a nerve injury must be emphasized.

Conclusion

Improvements of functional sensibility after sensory reeducation have been reported.[79,82,112,125-129] However, the outcome after a nerve repair is often disappointing, especially tactile gnosis in adults. A recent systematic review also shows that very few solid scientific studies have been published investigating the effectiveness of such programs.[129] Little is known about how such programs influence functional cortical organization. Hence, this is an important field for future research and for implementation of an evidence-based clinical routine for the treatment and documentation of recovery after nerve injuries to make clinical research in this field possible.

REFERENCES

The complete reference list is available online at www.expertconsult.com.

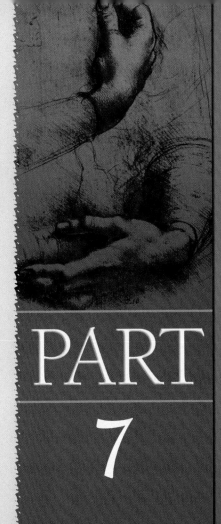

PART
7

Compression
Neuropathies

Basic Science of Nerve Compressions

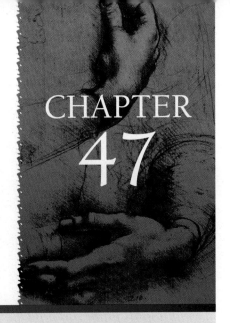

CHAPTER 47

SIDNEY M. JACOBY, MD, MATTHEW D. EICHENBAUM, MD, AND A. LEE OSTERMAN, MD

CRITICAL POINTS

Features of Connective Tissue

- The outermost connective tissues of the nerve, the perineurium, and the epineurium provide diffusion barriers to keep toxins out of the nerve and offer biomechanical support to resist tension and compression of the nerve.
- The Schwann cell is a primary mediator of the neural response to prolonged compression resulting in morphologic changes to the cell and a loss of myelin.

Classification of Nerve Compression

- The accumulation of fluid (edema) within the endoneurial compartment increases endoneurial pressure and decreases blood flow to the nerve. This is the primary pathophysiology of nerve compression.
- Most nerve compression syndromes are type I (neuropraxia) injuries generating mild to moderate sensory symptoms. More severe injuries that include motor impairment are probably type II (axonotmesis).
- Nerve compression at one segment along a nerve pathway may increase vulnerability to nerve compression injury at a site distal or proximal to the segment. It is suspected that axoplasmic transport is disrupted along the pathway.

Critical to the diagnosis and treatment of nerve compression syndromes is a firm understanding of the anatomy, pathophysiology, and presentation of peripheral nerve lesions. Clinicians who treat patients with compressive neuropathies should specifically possess a strong understanding of the peripheral nervous system's response to acute and chronic compression. In addition to clinical acumen, the health-care provider often relies on imaging and electrodiagnostic studies to assist in the diagnosis of peripheral nerve lesions. Once an accurate diagnosis has been established, the health-care team can devise a treatment plan that adequately addresses all potential sources of nerve compression.

Peripheral Nerve Pathway

As spinal nerve roots pass from the cervical spine through intervertebral foramina on their way to becoming peripheral nerves of the upper extremity, there are numerous sites of potential nerve compression. At each site, a potential mismatch exists between space available in the compartment and the contents of the compartment itself. Any decrease in the transectional area of the compartment or any volume increase in the contents of the compartment may result in restricted gliding between the tissues passing through that space.[1] Any increase in intraneural pressure may then similarly impair both the extrinsic and intrinsic blood supply to the nerve

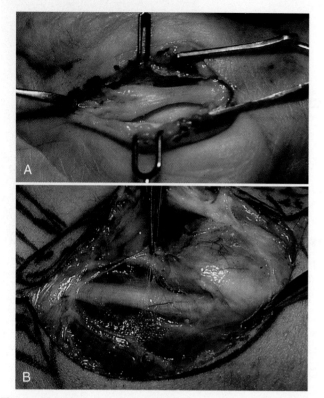

Figure 47-1 A, Intraoperative photograph depicting high-grade compression of the median nerve at the carpal tunnel. Note the pseudoneuroma formation at either end of the hourglass defect (left, distal extent of carpal tunnel; right, proximal origin of carpal tunnel). **B,** Intraoperative photograph depicting compression of the ulnar nerve at the cubital tunnel. The ulnar nerve usually does not show as obvious a narrowing, and pseudoneuroma as seen in median nerve compression. This suggests that ischemia and traction may play a more important role in cubital tunnel symptoms (left, distal extent of cubital tunnel; right, proximal origin of cubital tunnel).

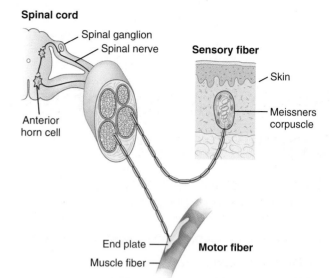

Figure 47-2 Peripheral nerve with its central connections originating in the spinal elements and peripheral connection in the end-organ.

tissue, ultimately resulting in a cascade of biochemical changes that result in functional deficit, pain, or anesthesia in the region that particular nerve supplies. Two of the most common and well-known sites of nerve compression are the carpal and cubital tunnels (Fig. 47-1). Another common site of nerve compression occurs at the radial nerve with the "Saturday night palsy" because one may have a temporarily limited cognitive capacity to alleviate prolonged compression to the upper arm. The severity of clinical symptomatology that results from these classic compressive neuropathies is directly related to the degree of vascular insult, nerve swelling, and ultimately, the cumulative neurologic damage on a cellular level.

Peripheral Nerve Microanatomy

As is true in every facet of surgery and rehabilitation of the hand and upper extremity, a firm understanding of anatomy allows the health-care provider to truly appreciate the severity and implication of the pathologic process. The peripheral nervous system is arranged in such a way that a variety of tissue types function synergistically to relay motor and sensory stimuli to and from the central nervous system (Fig. 47-2).

The main functional unit of the nervous system is the axon (nerve fiber) itself. Axons are themselves further bundled into fascicles, which in turn are organized into nerve trunks surrounded by a tough connective tissue matrix (Fig. 47-3A). Peripheral nerves possess three unique layers of connective tissue sheaths. From the outside inward, these layers are known as the epineurium, perineurium, and endoneurium (Fig. 47-3B). The epineurium is composed of fibroblasts and extracellular matrix consisting mostly of collagen as well as elastic fibers and mast cells.[2] The epineurium provides structural support and biomechanical protection for nerve fascicles, acts as a diffusion barrier, and also contains blood vessels and adipose cells as supportive elements. Moving further inward, each fascicle is surrounded by perineurium, which is a mechanically strong membrane that resists tension and compression forces. It is more organized than the innermost layer, endoneurium, which itself is a sheath of connective tissue cells that surrounds a single axon.[3-6] In addition to the structural integrity the perineurium provides to the nerve fascicle, it acts as a "blood–nerve barrier," regulating and controlling the internal milieu of the nerve fascicles.[7] Any breach or compression of the critical blood–nerve barrier results in the loss of normal homeostasis and ultimately leads to neural dysfunction. Leakage at the level of the endoneurium results in increased intraneural pressure and nerve fiber edema. Breakdown in the blood–nerve barrier results in the accumulation of protein and ingress of lymphocytes, fibroblasts, and macrophages, which ultimately initiates inflammation and eventually scar formation.[8] Nerve fibers are thus surrounded and protected by a sophisticated network of supporting collagen structures that provide mechanical stability, nutrition, and homeostasis that allow the nerve to function normally. Any breach, internal derangement, or exogenous compression or tension will result in neural dysfunction.

Any discussion on the basic anatomy of the peripheral nerve system would be incomplete without reference to Schwann cells, the primary glial or supporting cells of the peripheral nervous system (Fig. 47-4). These cells form the

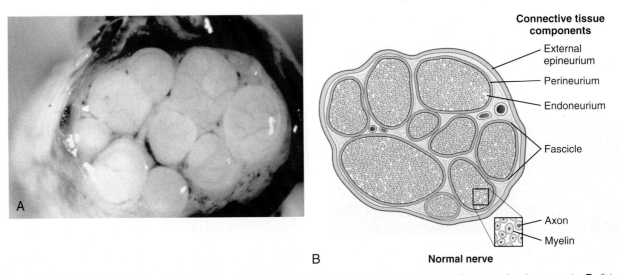

Figure 47-3 A, Magnified view (20×) of a nerve fibers bundled into fascicles and surrounded by a tough connective tissue matrix. **B,** Schematic representation of the connective tissue components of a normal nerve including endoneurium, perineurium, and epineurium. Mesoneurium (not shown) is loose areolar tissue that permits gliding of the nerve; vascular pedicles pass through this layer at different intervals en route to the nerve trunk. Epineurium is the most abundant connective tissue layer, providing a supportive and protective framework for the axon; it has a well-developed vascular plexus that feeds the endoneurial plexus. Perineurium is a thin sheath that surrounds each nerve fascicle and acts as a blood–nerve barrier and provides a bidirectional barrier to diffusion. Endoneurium is a loose collagenous matrix that provides support for underlying nerve fibers.

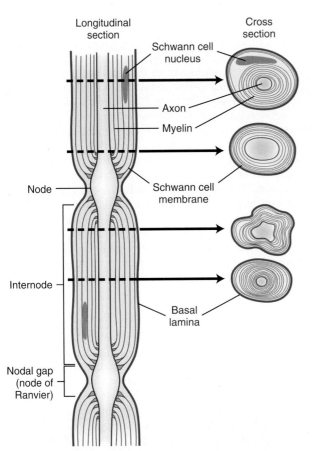

Figure 47-4 Schematic representation of Schwann cells, which form the myelin sheath around axons by wrapping an extension of their plasma membrane around the nerve fiber.

myelin sheath around axons by wrapping an extension of its plasma membrane around the nerve fiber. Continuing investigation into the processes contributing to and treating peripheral nerve damage has identified the myelin-forming Schwann cell as a primary mediator of the neural response to prolonged compression. A classic investigation by Ochoa et al. in the early 1970s provided the first description of the pathoanatomic changes in nerve myelin following nerve compression.[9] Working with an animal model, the authors inflated a pneumatic cuff around the knee of adult female baboons creating a local conduction block in the medial popliteal nerve with subsequent leg and foot weakness. Electron microscope examination of sample nerve fibers from the region underneath the pneumatic cuff revealed a characteristic pattern of myelin disruption consisting of displacement of the node of Ranvier from its normal location. This displacement occurs with paranodal stretching of myelin on one margin of the node and invagination of the paranodal myelin on the other margin. The ruptured membrane essentially cleaves the paranodal myelin from its surrounding Schwann cell, creating an environment in which axonal conduction is disrupted and local demyelination occurs. The significance of Ochoa's investigation was the identification of a nonischemic cause of diminished nerve conduction and localized axonal demyelination in the setting of neural compression.

Basic Nerve Physiology

Normal neural function depends on the propagation of electrical impulses termed *action potentials* from one cell to the next. A complicated, yet coordinated system of mechanoelectrical events must occur for a nerve to function properly.

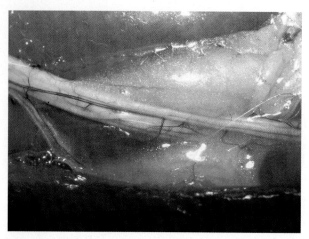

Figure 47-5 The microvascular system of the nerve trunk consisting of extraneural and intraneural blood vessels.

Just as with any other cell, neural cells depend on adequate vascular inflow for optimal function.

The cell bodies of the somatic nervous system reside in the ventral horns (in motor nerves) or dorsal root ganglia (in sensory nerves), and function as the "workhorse" of the neural cell. Axons are the delicate peripheral extensions of the nerve cell body responsible for the propagation of an action potential. Together with surrounding helper cells or Schwann cells, the axons constitute nerve fibers, of which several subtypes exist. Group A nerve fibers denote the largest myelinated somatic afferent and efferent fibers, and have the fastest conduction velocity. Group B nerve fibers contain myelinated autonomic and preganglionic fibers, while group C consists of the thinnest, nonmyelinated visceral and somatic pain fibers, as well as pain fibers belonging to the sympathetic system.[1]

Whatever the specific cell type, all nerves contain a biologic membrane that has a resting potential attributable to the separation of electric charges produced by the semipermeable nature of the membrane.[2] This porous membrane excludes sodium but allows potassium to flow into the cell. An action potential is an "all-or-none" phenomenon in which an excitatory depolarizing event is initiated and a self-propagating signal is delivered from the cell body to the target end-organ. Current travels quickly down the length of the axon but is unable to flow across the myelinated segments of the nerve fiber, instead "jumping" from one internodal segment to the next. Myelinated nerve fibers therefore increase the velocity of propagation as the action potential quickly propagates down the axon jumping from internodal segment to the next, a process termed *saltatory conduction.*

Nutritional supply to nerve fibers is provided by a well-developed microvascular system that perfuses the epineurium, perineurium, and endoneurium. Peripheral nerves have a dual blood supply of intrinsic exchange vessels in the endoneurium and an extrinsic plexus of supply vessels in the epineurial space that crosses the perineurium to anastomose with the intrinsic circulation (Fig. 47-5). A reduction or disruption of nerve blood flow may result in neural ischemia. Extrinsic vessels support smaller regional vessels that further

subdivide to provide nutrition along the length of nerve fibers. When regional vessels approach the nerve trunk, they divide into ascending and descending branches running longitudinally in the epineurial layer. Inside the fascicles, a longitudinal pattern of capillaries run within the endoneurium. As the vessels pass through the innermost part of the perineurium into the endoneurium, they often cross in an oblique manner, making them quite vulnerable to external pressure.[10-15]

Pathophysiology of Nerve Compression

Compared to complete peripheral nerve lesions, compressive neuropathies are unique as the nerve remains in continuity and there is no severance or tearing of the neural elements. The details of nerve degeneration and regeneration as a result of compression loading have been studied extensively over the past 30 years and have yielded a tremendous amount of information regarding the pathophysiology of nerve compression.[16-26] In general, these studies demonstrate that nerve injury will relate to both the degree and duration of compression, with both mechanical and ischemic factors contributing to neurologic dysfunction.[8]

Situations such as trauma or sustained compression will induce the accumulation of edema into the endoneurial space of the nerve trunk.[27] Because of the diffusion barrier created by the perineurium and the lack of lymphatic vessels in the endoneurial space, the fluid may not easily escape. The result is an increase in endoneurial fluid pressure and encroachment of the normal endoneurial microcirculation. Lundborg et al. showed that following 2 to 8 hours of experimental compression-induced ischemia (80 mm Hg) in nerves of rabbits, the endoneurial fluid pressure may increase rapidly and persist for at least 24 hours.[14] Another example of metabolic conduction block is the sensory loss and motor paralysis that can occur after deflating the tourniquet around the upper arm. This type of metabolic block, caused by local arrest of intraneural microcirculation, is immediately reversible when the compression is removed. With extended compression, however, edema within the fascicles can result in increased endoneurial pressure, which could compromise endoneurial capillary flow for hours or days, potentially permanently affecting function of the nerve.[1]

Classification of Nerve Injuries

The success of the peripheral nerve repair process ultimately correlates with the extent and duration of compression. Clinically useful injury-grading systems have been developed that allow correlation of the microscopic changes occurring after nerve injury and patient symptomatology.[28]

Neurapraxia, a type I injury, is the mildest form of injury and simply involves a conduction block. If there is anything to be seen histologically, it will be a segmental area of demyelination. The axon is not injured and therefore does not undergo regeneration. The majority of patients with compression neuropathies fall into this category. A type II injury is termed *axonotmesis* and will involve injury to the axon. Fibrillations would be seen with electromyography, along with a decrease in amplitude on electrodiagnostic testing consistent with loss of axons. This injury has the potential for eventual nerve regeneration. A type III injury is a more severe form of axonotmesis, as some degree of scar tissue forms in the endoneurium. Recovery is therefore less predictable. Patients with severe compression neuropathies fall into the category of type III damage. When the nerve is in continuity but completely blocked with scar tissue and no possibility of recovery, the injury pattern is suggestive of a type IV injury. A type V injury is the complete transection of the nerve. Types IV and V injuries would therefore not apply to compression neuropathy.

Interestingly, some patients with nerve compression such as carpal tunnel syndrome (CTS) have near-normal results on electrodiagnostic studies. Although diagnostic studies may in fact be negative, these patients will sometimes present with severe symptoms lending credibility to the theory of dynamic ischemia to the nerve rather than structural injury to the axon or its surrounding supporting cells.

Biologic Sequelae of Nerve Compression

Numerous methods have been used to induce acute or chronic compression of a peripheral nerve in animal models. For example, tourniquets have been applied around the limbs of rats, rabbits, and primates for varying amounts of time. In baboons, pressures as high as 500 to 1000 mm Hg have been achieved in an effort to induce structural nerve changes.[9,29,30] Because of the difficulty in precisely controlling tourniquet compression, other researchers have applied a miniature inflatable cuff around a mobilized nerve to achieve more consistent compression for several hours.[31,32] These studies have shown that nerve injury is related to the degree and duration of compression, with mechanical and ischemic factors precipitating nerve dysfunction.

Acute Effects (Within Hours)

There have been several well-designed studies of healthy human volunteers in which extraneural pressure in the carpal tunnel was elevated for a maximum of 4 hours while nerve function was simultaneously monitored.[18,28] Pressure was precisely controlled with a clamp that applied an adjustable load to the palm, while the extraneural pressure in the carpal tunnel was measured with a fluid-filled catheter. Nerve function was blocked at 50 mm Hg, whereas some function was lost at 40 mm Hg. In subjects with different blood pressures, the critical extraneural pressure threshold above which nerve function was blocked was 30 mm Hg less than diastolic pressure. Combined with the observation that CTS may manifest with the treatment of hypertension, this finding provides another layer of support for an ischemic mechanism of acute nerve dysfunction.[33]

Short-Term Effects (Within Days)

Human studies on the acute effects of nerve compression have demonstrated a rapid effect of intermediate pressure on nerve function; however, they have not addressed the effect of low extraneural pressure for an extended amount of time. Rydevik, Lundborg, and others have studied the effects of persistent intraneural edema in animals after short-term (order of days) compression at low pressures.[8,23,24] Compression of 8 hours' duration was shown to increase endoneurial pressure to a point that resulted in a reduction of intraneural blood flow. Interestingly, these studies also demonstrated that after low levels of compression for as little as 2 hours, endoneurial fluid pressures increased rapidly and persisted for at least an additional 24 hours after the compression was relieved. These long-lasting effects are probably due to the increased vascular permeability of the epineurial and endoneurial vessels after prolonged compression.

Long-Term Effects (Within Weeks)

To more closely mimic CTS, models of nerve compression have utilized silastic cuffs placed around the rat sciatic nerve and median nerve in primates.[16,19,20,22,34] Not surprisingly, a dose–response relationship between the duration of compression and neural injury was observed. Initial changes showed a breakdown in the blood–nerve barrier, followed by subperineurial edema and fibrosis. Later changes included a localized, and later diffuse, demyelination, and finally Wallerian degeneration.[8]

Histopathology of Nerve Compression

Most nerve compression syndromes are treated with decompression and sometimes transposition, in the case of the ulnar nerve at the elbow. Since nerves are rarely biopsied, most reports on the histopathology of chronic nerve compression (CNC) are limited to cadaver reports or to the few case reports on patients in whom a nerve segment was resected and compared with a nerve at the site proximal or distal to injury.[5,35,36] Material derived from cadaveric studies demonstrate changes consistent with degeneration and regeneration in the unmyelinated nerve fibers at the same time that segmental demyelination is the predominant finding in myelinated fibers.[21,37,38] Increased connective tissue density has also been observed along the median nerve in human cadavers from individuals who died between the ages of 60 and 81.[39] Not surprisingly, the greatest density of connective tissue was found at the level of the wrist crease where the flexion moment is greatest. These findings corroborate the notion that extracellular matrix is deposited in the nerve at sites of bending. Biopsy samples obtained for human case reports revealed thickening of the walls of the microvessels in the endoneurium and perineurium as well as neural edema, thickening, and fibrosis at the site of injury and myelin thinning.

Schwann cell changes, increased vascular permeability, and neurovascularity are just some of the histopathologic

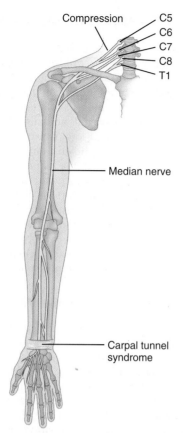

Figure 47-6 *Schematic depicting a proximal compressive lesion at the level of the cervical spine as well as a distal compressive lesion at the carpal tunnel.*

changes associated with CNC. Gupta, in Chapter 42, explores the histopathology of nerve compression with an emphasis on morphologic and physiologic changes of the Schwann cell.

Double-Crush Phenomenon

The controversial concept of a double-crush phenomenon was introduced by Upton and McComas almost 30 years ago.[40] They hypothesized that a proximal level of compression could predispose distal sites to be more sensitive to compression (Fig. 47-6). A clinical correlate would be the case of cervical radiculopathy that predisposes for development of a more peripheral nerve compression. In fact, Upton and McComas noted a high incidence of carpal and cubital tunnel syndrome with associated cervical nerve root injuries. They believed that the summation of compression along the nerve would result in alterations of axoplasmic flow and subsequent pathology. Similarly, the possibility of a distal site of compression causing the more proximal nerve to be susceptible to secondary compression exists and has been termed *reverse double-crush phenomenon*. The prevailing theory in both circumstances is that any compression could induce structural and biochemical changes in the nerve cell bodies and alter axoplasmic transport that could hypothetically render a nerve more vulnerable to developing compressive neuropathy and act as a "crush."[41] This hypothesis may

also apply to systemic conditions such as obesity, rheumatologic or endocrine disorders, and alcoholism, all of which are known to similarly render the nerve more susceptible to the development of a compressive neuropathy.

Chronic Nerve Compression— A Clinical Correlate

CTS is the most common compressive neuropathy and offers a model for compressive nerve injury because the clinical symptoms are very well correlated to defined pathophysiologic events in the nerve.[1] Gelberman et al. carried out studies to identify critical pressure levels for nerve viability in human patients.[42] They monitored the tissue fluid pressure in the carpal canal and found that patients with clinically evident CTS presented with an average carpal pressure of 32 mm Hg, versus 2.5 mm Hg in control subjects. With increasing pressure in the canal to levels of 50 to 60 mm Hg, a complete block of motor and sensory conduction in the median nerve occurred, with sensory function disappearing 10 to 30 minutes before motor function.[13]

Initial symptoms of CTS usually occur at night, as there is no active muscle pump action in the arm, a redistribution of tissue fluid into the arms has taken place, and the wrist often rests in a flexed position during sleep.[1] Ischemia in the median nerve responds by generating impulses perceived by the patient as paresthesias in the median nerve distribution. If symptoms become constant, it is likely that a more advanced pathologic process has developed in the nerve. Patients may experience loss of dexterity, weakness in the median nerve–innervated thenar muscle group, and prolonged, unrelenting paresthesias in the medial three and half digits of the hand. These advanced symptoms represent a more pronounced pathologic process in which some nerve fibers have suffered from a local metabolic disorder caused by edema, whereas other fibers suffer from neuropraxia caused by local myelin thinning and degradation. Surgical decompression may lead to a relief in symptoms based on a metabolic problem, but fibers that suffer from neurapraxia may need more time to recover. With advanced changes consistent with axonotmesis, axons must regenerate if function will ever be restored. Such a recuperative process may take weeks or months, and may be markedly impaired in patients with co-morbidities or advanced age.

Basic Research in Vibration Exposure

Contemporary knowledge of nerve compression syndromes indicates that vibration exposure and the loading of neural structures is one of the strongest factors associated with the development of CTS and other peripheral neuropathies.[8] Pathologic changes indicative of peripheral neuropathy have been demonstrated in multiple experimental and clinical studies of vibration exposure.[43-46] Additionally, both human nerves and animal models exposed to vibration have undergone histologic evaluation and demonstrate findings consistent with compressive-type injuries.[35,47] The use of vibrating tools with a frequency range from a few hertz to several thousand hertz probably causes adverse effects after direct hand exposure beyond a critical temporal threshold. Indeed, a hand–arm vibration syndrome with principally neurosensory derangement has been described after extended exposure to hand-held vibrating tools.[48,49] Other studies have clearly shown a cumulative effect of vibration on peripheral nerve function, with numerous epidemiologic studies demonstrating a strong correlation between vibration exposure and the development of compressive neuropathies, especially CTS.[37,50-52]

Research investigating the effects of vibration exposure on peripheral nerve function has demonstrated results similar to the findings of studies evaluating the pathophysiology of basic nerve compression. A study assessing the effect of cyclically fluctuating extraneural pressure was performed using a rat tibial-nerve model.[53] A pressure that fluctuated between a minimum value of 20 mm Hg and a peak value of 50 mm Hg (2.7 and 6.7 kPa, respectively), with a mean value of 35 mm Hg (4.7 kPa), was directed to the nerve at one cycle per second for 20,000 cycles, a frequency of 1 Hz. The subsequent diminishment in nerve function was similar to that due to static compression by a pressure of 30 mm Hg (4.0 kPa).[23] Although this study primarily demonstrated that the effect of rapidly fluctuating compression on nerve function correlated with the mean pressure, rather than the peak or minimum pressures, it also illustrated that a low-frequency cycled compression of a nerve—in effect, vibration—would cause pathologic changes in peripheral nerve after a short initial exposure.

Animal models have been used to investigate the series of events occurring in peripheral nerves following vibration exposure. Acute vibration of 82 Hz at a magnitude of 0.21 mm Hg for 5 hours daily for up to 5 days resulted in intraneural edema and transient structural degradation in nerve fibers near the vibration inducer.[46,51] In a degradative process similar to that described in compressive peripheral nerve injuries, demyelination occurs initially after injury due to vibration exposure, with axonal degeneration developing as a later finding.[28,43,44]

Similar to direct neural compression, vibration exposure results in increased intraneural edema and increased pressure within the nerve with subsequent reduction in sensory and motor conduction velocities. Continued exposure to vibration has been shown to cause further degradation of neural function as peripheral demyelination occurs, and Schwann cells and fibroblasts proliferate as part of the regenerative response following the injury.[54,55] Peripheral neuropathy occurs as additional vibration exposure results in increased connective tissue, causing perivascular and perineural fibrosis. Finally, axonal injury represents a late stage of vibration-induced neuropathy as chronicity of vibration exposure continues.[56,57]

Clinical Responses to Vibration

A study by Stromberg et al. compared the histological findings of specimens from the dorsal interosseous nerve proximal to the wrist in 10 males exposed to vibration at work to a control group consisting of 10 age-matched cadavers. The authors found that all 10 subjects had pathologic findings consisting of myelin degradation with perineural and interstitial fibrosis, demonstrating that work-related vibration exposure can provoke structural damage in peripheral nerve trunks at the wrist.[49] This conclusion may explain the less successful results for carpal tunnel release in patients with a known history of vibration exposure.[23]

The identification of the hand–arm vibration syndrome (HAVS) has further reinforced the role of vibration exposure in causing peripheral neuropathies.[48,49] Biopsy specimens taken from the fingers of HAVS sufferers have demonstrated three significant pathologic changes: (i) intense artery wall muscular layer thickening with individual muscle cell hypertrophy; (ii) peripheral demyelinating neuropathy with increased numbers of Schwann cells and fibroblasts; and (iii) increased amounts of connective tissue causing perivascular and perineural fibrosis. Because the pathophysiologic characteristics of HAVS include notable vascular and muscular changes in addition to the damage created in the neural elements, any vibrating tool in contact with the hand with a frequency range from a few hertz to several thousand hertz may inflict adverse effects after exposure beyond a critical temporal threshold.[58] Similarly, it has been clearly shown that there is a cumulative effect of vibration on both the vascular and sensorineural components of the HAVS.[20,52] Furthermore, because vibration results in increased peripheral edema and increased intraneural pressure, nerve conduction velocities are reduced. This results in diminished sensory and motor function in the limbs of affected patients. Additional research has demonstrated that vibrotactile receptors in the skin may be susceptible to vibration damage and that loss of function in these receptors may result in profound sensory loss.[48,59]

Effects of Joint Position and Hand-Loading

Multiple studies have evaluated the effect of hand and wrist position on pressures exerted upon neural structures in the upper extremity.[23,60-66] The measurement of extraneural pressure in the carpal tunnel in study subjects with CTS demonstrated that flexion or extension of the wrist increased pressure exerted on the median nerve by between 2 and 10 times.[23,25] Normal subjects revealed a similar response to flexion and extension despite having carpal tunnel extraneural pressures of an absolute lower magnitude. Cadaver studies of the ulnar nerve at the elbow also established a comparable increase in pressure transmitted to the nerve with increasing joint flexion.[60,62] Extraneural pressure monitoring has also been used to study the carpal tunnels of healthy individuals subjected to changes in finger position, wrist flexion and extension, and forearm rotation. Rempel et al. published findings demonstrating minimum carpal tunnel pressures between neutral and full forearm pronation, while greatest values were obtained at the limit of supination.[64] Additional studies of people unaffected by compressive neuropathies have confirmed that carpal tunnel pressure increases to the greatest degree with increasing wrist extension, and to a lesser extent with increasing wrist flexion, forearm supination, and metacarpophalangeal joint flexion.

Similar studies have investigated the pressure on the carpal tunnel in the setting of finger-pinching and grasping maneuvers and tasks.[45,61,63,65-70] Flexor tendon loading has been shown in cadaver models to increase the extraneural pressure within the carpal tunnel.[67,70] Multiple studies of healthy volunteers confirmed an increase in carpal tunnel pressure with holding objects and gripping tasks.[61,63,65,66] Full flexion of the digits into a fist demonstrated the highest associated extraneural pressure in the carpal tunnel in a series by Seradge et al. that investigated the effect of gripping and hand-loading on carpal tunnel pressure.[69] Two additional inquiries into the association between carpal tunnel extraneural pressure and finger position and loading demonstrated that carpal tunnel pressure increases proportionally with increasing fingertip loading.[8,41] Supplementary data revealed that tasks involving pinching the index finger and thumb created measured pressures double that of tasks accomplished by pressing the index finger alone.[45,68]

In sum, the body of research investigating the effect of limb and joint position and functional loading on extraneural pressure provides evidence that protective orthotic fabrication along with activity and occupational modifications alone can ameliorate the clinical findings associated with less severe compressive neuropathies.

Evaluation of Nerve Compression

Developing effective treatment plans for patients with compressive neuropathies depends upon the successful identification and diagnosis of all sites of neural compression. As previously discussed, the concept of the double-crush phenomenon allows for the possibility that neural element compression may occur simultaneously in multiple locations. Accordingly, a complete evaluation must account for the course of an affected nerve from its radicular origin in the spinal cord to its terminal motor and sensory branches at the muscles and dermatomal region it innervates. To this end, physical examination findings, specific nerve provocation tests, and electrodiagnostic studies should be appropriately utilized to create a global picture of potential sites of compression, as well as the most likely etiology. Subsequently, an appropriate treatment plan can be formulated and initiated.

Summary

Nerve compression syndromes of the upper extremity are extremely common and may result in debilitating symptoms. Clinicians should possess a thorough understanding of the anatomy, pathophysiology, and presentation of compressive peripheral nerve lesions so as to best diagnose and treat their patients. An appreciation for the underlying causes of neural entrapment as well as the most common exposures and positions that contribute to neuropathic findings should assist the thoughtful practitioner in successfully identifying compression neuropathies of the upper extremity. The use of provocative testing, sensory examination, and electrodiagnostic assays can help direct appropriate treatment and rehabilitative regimens.

REFERENCES

The complete reference list is available online at www.expertconsult.com.

Carpal Tunnel Syndrome: Surgeon's Management*

PETER C. AMADIO, MD

CRITICAL POINTS

- Carpal tunnel syndrome (CTS) is the most common peripheral neuropathy treated by hand surgeons.
- Most cases of CTS are idiopathic, but the pathology clearly involves increased pressure in the carpal tunnel.
- The association of specific jobs with CTS is controversial.
- Nonsurgical treatments, such as activity modification, orthosis use at night, and steroid injection, can be helpful in milder cases.
- The most effective treatment is surgical decompression, by sectioning of the flexor retinaculum (transverse carpal ligament).
- The evidence supporting one surgical approach over another is mixed; limited exposures may have less pain immediately postoperatively, but also seem to have a higher risk of incomplete release and possibly nerve injury.
- The use of postoperative immobilization or therapy is not supported by high-quality evidence.

Compression of the median nerve at the wrist, or carpal tunnel syndrome (CTS), is the most common upper extremity compressive neuropathy.[1-4] Recent data have indicated that CTS may affect as much as 3% of the population at any one time.[2] Approximately half of these individuals will seek medical attention, and half of those will ultimately be treated with carpal tunnel release, making carpal tunnel surgery the most common hand surgical procedure.[4] It is also one of the most common causes of lost work time in the United States. However, there is little consensus on the most appropriate nonsurgical treatment, the optimal surgical procedure or rehabilitation protocol, or even the most appropriate way to assess outcome. More significantly, in most cases, the etiology remains idiopathic, making preventive strategies entirely conjectural.

History

Although CTS is the most common condition surgically treated by hand surgeons, the term and our current understanding of the condition both date from the last half-century, as documented in several recent reviews.[5-7] The earliest reports of median neuropathy were cases of median nerve entrapment after fracture of the radius. Early treatments included amputation and orthosis use. Although amputation is no longer favored as a treatment for CTS, orthosis use is still employed. Later, excision of prominent palmar callus was tried and, even later, median neurolysis. In 1933, Abbott and Saunders[8] injected dye into cadaver carpal tunnels and noticed increased resistance to dye flow with wrist flexion. On the basis of this study, they condemned the wrist flexion (Cotton-Loder) position, which had been commonly used until that time for the treatment of Colles' fracture. CTS after Colles' fracture remains an important clinical problem.

*This chapter reproduces much of the content published in previous editions of this book, but has been extensively reformatted and updated.

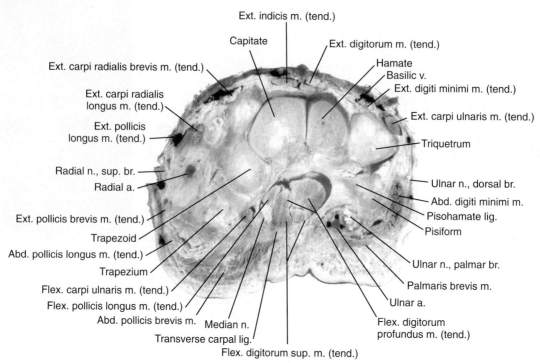

Figure 48-1 Cross-section of the wrist at the carpal tunnel. a., artery; Abd., abductor; br., brevis; Ext., extensor; Flex., flexor; lig., ligament; m., muscle; n., nerve; sup., superficialis; tend., tendon; v., vein.

Although post-traumatic CTS was the first type to be noticed, by the later 1800s, nontraumatic cases were also noted, although their true nature was not known.[5] In 1880, Putnam[9] described 37 patients with nocturnal paresthesias. He noted that "simply letting the arm hang out of the bed or shaking it about … [or the use of] prolonged rubbing would relieve the symptoms."[9] These are, of course, classic symptoms of CTS. Putnam recognized the median nerve as the source of the symptoms, but did not consider compression as an etiology. When compression was considered, the location selected was erroneous, with the brachial plexus being considered the site. Unfortunately for patients with CTS, this hypothesis of brachial plexopathy as an etiology became popular and resulted in a variety of misdirected surgery until the late 1940s.

In 1913, Marie and Foix[10] described an autopsy finding of a large median pseudoneuroma just proximal to the carpal tunnel. They suggested that "perhaps in a case in which the diagnosis is made early enough … transection of the ligament could stop the development of these phenomena." Unfortunately, this advice went unheeded for two decades, until Learmonth[6] described two cases in which he divided the flexor retinaculum to treat a median neuropathy. Subsequently, Phalen et al.[11] popularized the condition and emphasized the frequent intraoperative finding of synovial fibrosis without inflammation.

Anatomy

The carpal tunnel is an inelastic structure. Its floor is composed of the concave arch of the carpal bones. The hook of the hamate, the triquetrum, and the pisiform constitute the ulnar border, whereas the radial aspect includes the trapezium, the scaphoid, and the fascia over the flexor carpi radialis. The roof of the carpal tunnel is made up of the deep forearm fascia, the flexor retinaculum, and the distal aponeurosis of the thenar and hypothenar muscles. The flexor retinaculum extends from the scaphoid tuberosity and the trapezium to attach to the pisiform and the hook of the hamate. The contents of the carpal tunnel consist of the median nerve and nine flexor tendons. The flexor pollicis longus, four flexor digitorum profundus, and four flexor digitorum superficialis tendons pass through the carpal tunnel, with the nerve lying superficially and anteroradially in the tunnel (Fig. 48-1).

At the distal edge of the carpal tunnel, the median nerve most commonly divides into six branches: two common digital nerves, three proper digital nerves, and the recurrent motor branch, which innervates the thenar musculature. The nerve gives off the palmar cutaneous branch proximally and radially, approximately 5 cm proximal to the wrist crease. This branch travels with the main nerve for 1.4 to 2.6 cm and then penetrates the antebrachial fascia between the palmaris longus and flexor carpi radialis. It emerges subcutaneously, usually proximal to the wrist crease, to innervate the palm.

Many variations in the branching pattern and anatomy of the median nerve have been described.[12,13] These include high (i.e., proximal) division, persistence of the median artery, anomalous subretinacular muscle and tendon attachments, and proximal cross-connections with the ulnar nerve, most of which are rare. More commonly seen are proximal incursions of the lumbrical muscles,[14,15] variations in the branching and courses of the recurrent motor branch[16] (Fig. 48-2) and palmar cutaneous branch,[17,18] and distal cross-

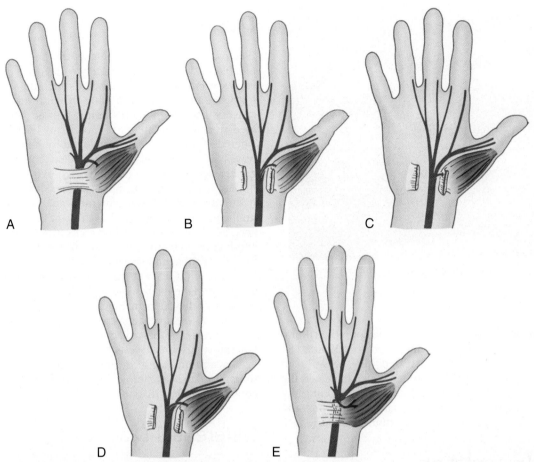

Figure 48-2 Variations in median nerve anatomy in the carpal tunnel. **A,** The most common pattern of the motor branch is extraligamentous and recurrent. **B,** Subligamentous branching of a recurrent median nerve. **C,** Transligamentous course of the recurrent branch of the median nerve. **D,** The motor branch can uncommonly originate from the ulnar border of the median nerve. **E,** The motor branch can lie on top of the flexor retinaculum. (From Green D. *Green's Operative Hand Surgery.* 4th ed. Philadelphia: Churchill Livingstone; 1999.)

connections with the ulnar nerve.[19] As discussed later, an awareness of these variations is essential when performing surgical release of the carpal tunnel.

Pathogenesis

The etiology of CTS is unknown in most cases; however, the pathogenesis appears to be clearly related to increased pressure within the carpal tunnel.[20-25] Experimentally increasing carpal tunnel pressure produces characteristic symptoms of CTS in normal volunteers, and patients with CTS have increased resting CTS pressure, which can rise to as much as 1000 mm Hg with activity, compared with normal levels of 30 to 50 mm Hg with activity, and 10 mm Hg at rest.[26]

Factors Influencing Pressure in the Carpal Canal

In general, any disorder that decreases the cross-sectional area of the carpal tunnel or that produces increased carpal tunnel canal volume content may result in increased pressure in the carpal canal. In the former category, fractures and carpal arthritis are common culprits. In the latter category, and occurring somewhat less frequently, are tumors and

synovitis, increasing the size of the nerve or synovium. Most commonly, however, none of these factors is present, and although there is a statistical association of such conditions as diabetes[27] and certain work activities involving forceful grip and wrist flexion[8-32] with a diagnosis of CTS, a specific cause-and-effect relationship has not been definitively established.

Recent studies have suggested a role for the lumbricals, intermittent space-occupying structures within the carpal tunnel.[15] The lumbrical muscles are distal to the carpal tunnel with the fingers held in extension, but they lie within the carpal canal when the fingers are actively flexed, especially with the wrist flexed. Clinically, this may be important, because sustained contraction of the finger flexors may increase the hydrostatic pressure that the median nerve experiences as a result of crowding in the carpal canal by the lumbricals. As noted in the subsequent chapter on therapy interventions, it may be appropriate to consider the possibility of lumbrical incursion when devising orthotic fabrication strategies.

External Pressure

Intracarpal tunnel pressure may be affected by external pressure to the palm. Cobb and associates.[33] showed that when

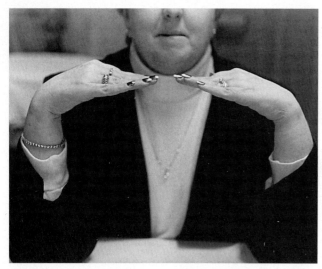

Figure 48-3 Phalen's test.

a 1-kg external force was applied over the flexor retinaculum, the pressure in the carpal canal increased to 103 mm Hg. Force over the thenar area increased the pressure to 75 mm Hg, and force over the hypothenar area increased the pressure to 37 mm Hg.[33] These findings may be clinically significant. Tools, orthoses, and casts can all apply pressure to the palm and thereby elevate carpal tunnel pressure.

Clinical Presentation

The classic clinical presentation of a patient with CTS is paresthesias in the thumb, index finger, and middle finger. Not uncommonly, patients also report a loss of dexterity, particularly with manipulation of small objects, such as coins, needles, or pins. These symptoms are characteristically experienced or exaggerated at night, or with characteristic activities, such as holding a book or newspaper or driving a car, and are worsened by repetitive forceful hand motion. As noted by Putnam[9] 130 years ago, improvement in symptoms after shaking or straightening the affected hand is common.

Clinical findings in CTS include the limitation of paresthesias to the distribution of the distal median nerve (i.e., the tips and palmar aspects of the thumb, index finger, middle finger, and radial half of the ring finger, with sparing of the palm). These symptoms can often be reproduced with pressure over the median nerve, either constantly (Durkan's sign[34]) or by tapping (Tinel's sign), but these signs have only moderate sensitivity and specificity.[35-37] The wrist flexion test, or Phalen's test (Fig. 48-3), is performed by flexing the wrist maximally for 60 seconds to determine whether this produces or exaggerates numbness and tingling in the affected fingers. Although it is commonly performed, this test has limited sensitivity and specificity. Thenar atrophy and loss of sensibility (two-point discrimination or Semmes-Weinstein pressure thresholds) can be observed, indicating more chronic median nerve compression. These findings, when present, are very specific, but they are not sensitive because they are only present in advanced cases.

Diagnostic Tests

Electrodiagnostic testing remains the best-known and most reliable study for confirmation of a diagnosis of CTS. Normal values vary, but general standards include abnormal values for distal motor latency of more than 4.5 msec and for distal sensory latency of more than 3.5 msec.[38] A difference in median and ulnar latency of more than 1.0 msec is also considered significant. Electromyography that shows positive waves or fibrillations in the thenar musculature reflects greater severity and chronicity of nerve injury. Again, this finding is highly specific but is not sensitive because it is less frequently present. A recent meta-analysis of the literature on the use of electrophysiologic testing and its sensitivity and specificity found median nerve electromyography and nerve conduction velocity studies to be valid, reproducible, and highly sensitive and specific.[39]

Ultimately, CTS remains a clinical syndrome, and as many as 15% of patients in some series have clinically evident and surgically relieved median nerve compression in the presence of normal electrodiagnostic results.[40,41] Consequently, in some series, the best diagnostic predictors have not been laboratory or clinical tests but symptom questionnaires and even symptom diagrams. In some cases, response to specific therapies, such as steroid injection, has also been used to confirm a clinical diagnosis of CTS.

Differential Diagnosis

The differential diagnosis of CTS is vast.[42] It may be confused with other peripheral neuropathies, such as pronator syndrome,[42] diabetic neuropathy,[27] or hand–arm vibration syndrome,[43-46] as well as cervical radiculopathy and even central nervous system pathology.[42] It may be distinguished from these other conditions, typically by the distribution of symptoms, which are limited to the median innervated fingers and spare the palm or dorsum of the hand (which are affected by more proximal neuropathies). The finding of split symptoms in the ring finger, with sparing of the ulnar side, is nearly pathognomonic of CTS.

Conservative Management

The efficacy of nonsurgical management of mild CTS has been well documented. Conservative management is generally not an option for moderate to severe CTS, especially in patients who have signs of muscle atrophy or significant sensory impairment. The diagnosis of CTS should be confirmed with clinical testing, and potential proximal compression sites should be ruled out. Conservative management options that have been described for CTS include orthosis use, nonsteroidal anti-inflammatory drugs, injection of the carpal tunnel with a corticosteroid, tendon and nerve gliding exercises, vitamins, iontophoresis, ultrasound, and activity or job site modifications. The following sections describe various conservative treatment options, including those that may warrant further study and consideration based on current research.

Steroid Injection

The purpose of a steroid injection is ostensibly to decrease the mass of the thickened flexor tendon synovium by decreasing the inflammatory process, but this has never been documented, and it is generally agreed that there is little inflammation in most cases of CTS.[47-49] Thus, although steroid injection has been shown to be effective, the mechanism of this effect is unknown. Studies show that injection and orthosis use initially provide relief in approximately 40% to 80% of patients, but by 18 months after injection, this number decreased to 22%.[50-53] There is value in steroid injection, even if symptoms return, in that improvement in symptoms confirms the diagnosis, and a positive response may be indicative of a favorable outcome if surgery is required. However, poor relief after injection does not predict a poor surgical result.[50]

Anti-Inflammatory Drugs and Vitamin B₆ Treatment

Nonsteroidal anti-inflammatory drugs have never been shown to be effective in a scientific study of CTS.[54,55]

In 1976, Ellis et al.[56] proposed that a deficiency in pyridoxine (vitamin B_6) may cause CTS. Although adding vitamin B_6 to the diet is still occasionally advocated in the literature and the press, no controlled, randomized, prospective study has shown vitamin B_6 to be clearly efficacious compared with other conservative treatments for CTS.[52,57-59]

Surgical Management

Indications

Acute CTS requires prompt recognition and early open carpal tunnel release.[22,60,61] Wrist trauma, as well as infections and systemic rheumatologic and hematologic disease, can acutely increase carpal canal pressure, threatening median nerve viability. Thus, when CTS occurs in the context of acute injury, it is important to distinguish neurapraxia secondary to nerve contusion from acute CTS. In such cases, the surgeon should measure carpal tunnel pressure. If it is elevated, then carpal tunnel release should be considered on an urgent basis. If not, the surgeon may elect a period of observation or, depending on the severity of injury, the surgeon could still elect release to inspect the nerve and rule out complete or partial transection or the presence of intraneural hematoma. CTS developing after closed fracture reduction should also prompt exploration because entrapment of the nerve between fracture fragments and even nerve transection have been reported.[62] CTS in the context of presumed or confirmed septic flexor tenosynovitis should also be acutely released to avoid septic necrosis of the nerve.[63]

For idiopathic CTS, a relative indication for surgical release exists when clinical or electrodiagnostic evidence of denervation of the median nerve–innervated muscles is present. In the absence of significant clinical or electrodiagnostic denervation changes, failure to respond with a few weeks of nonsurgical treatment remains a reasonable guideline, as noted by a recent review of the available evidence.[64]

Particularly among patients who must continue in a manual labor occupation, prolonged nonsurgical treatment without symptomatic improvement does not appear to be fruitful.

Procedures

Open Carpal Tunnel Release

For nearly a century, sectioning the flexor retinaculum has been the mainstay of treatment of CTS. Alternatives, such as synovectomy without transection, have had some success, as reported in studies with lower levels of evidence,[65] but the strongest evidence has always supported release of the flexor retinaculum, especially open release. Division of the flexor retinaculum significantly increases the cross-sectional area of the carpal tunnel, with imaging studies showing a mean 24% increase in carpal canal volume.[66] With the relatively high incidence of variations in the location of the median nerve and the ulnar neurovascular structures, open carpal tunnel release remains the preferred procedure of most surgeons for decompression of the median nerve at the wrist. This technique affords full inspection of the transverse carpal ligament and the contents of the carpal canal (Fig. 48-4).

Local, regional, or general anesthesia may be used, but except in the anxious patient, local anesthesia provides adequate local pain relief for uncomplicated release. The use of local anesthetic mixed with epinephrine obviates the need for a tourniquet[67] (another source of intraoperative pain), but may interfere with the surgeon's ability to assess intraoperative nerve vascularity, which some consider a prognostic sign. A rapid return of blood flow on tourniquet release is associated with better outcomes.[68,69] My preference is local infiltration of the tissues with lidocaine, with conscious sedation reserved for patients who request it. Although some have expressed a concern that local anesthetic infiltration can obscure tissue planes, and thus express a preference for axillary or intravenous regional block, I have never found this to be a problem. Unless epinephrine is used, tourniquet control is used to minimize bleeding and improve visibility, although there is no evidence comparing outcomes with and without tourniquet use. When tourniquet use may be relatively contraindicated, such as after axillary node excision or radiation, I do not hesitate to use lidocaine with epinephrine

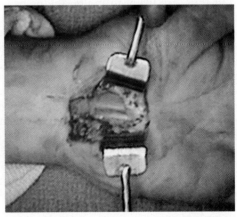

Figure 48-4 Open carpal tunnel release offers a wide exposure.

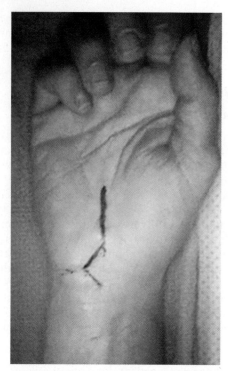

Figure 48-5 Preferred incision for open carpal tunnel release.

(both 1:100,000 and 1:200,000 work well) and forego tourniquet use. If epinephrine is used as an alternative to a tourniquet, it is important to wait several minutes for vasoconstriction to occur before making an incision.

In open release, a palmar incision is made ulnar to the depression between the thenar and hypothenar eminences, more or less in the line of the middle–ring web space, to minimize damage to branches of the palmar cutaneous branches of the median and ulnar nerves. Staying radial to the hook of the hamate minimizes risk to the ulnar neurovascular bundle. The incision is extended from Kaplan's cardinal line along the axis of the third web space proximally (Fig. 48-5). Extension proximal to the wrist crease is not required, but I prefer it, because it is easier to identify the median nerve at this level, release the distal antebrachial fascia, and then dissect from proximal to distal, in the direction of, and thus less likely to injure, the branches of the median nerve, whatever variation they may follow. Others prefer a distal to proximal dissection or even a direct palmar to dorsal approach. There is little evidence to support that any of these variations is better than the others.[64]

In the subcutaneous tissues overlying the flexor retinaculum, an effort should be made to preserve the larger branches of the palmar cutaneous branch of the median nerve, the nerve of Henle,[70] and cutaneous branches of the ulnar nerve. The superficial palmar fascia is divided in line with the skin incision. The underlying flexor retinaculum is divided longitudinally along its ulnar aspect. I prefer to avoid incision into the periosteum of the hamate because periosteal injury may predispose to pillar pain, but again there is no evidence to support this opinion. At the distal end of the incision, the superficial palmar arterial arch is identified in its bed of

adipose tissue and is protected. This represents the distal limit of dissection. After hemostasis is achieved, the wound is irrigated and closed with nonabsorbable suture. Some prefer to close the palmar fascia as well.

Open decompression of the median nerve has stood the test of time, providing reliable symptom relief in patients with a multitude of associated diagnoses. The procedure allows for visualization of all anatomic variations, and if necessary, removal of space-occupying lesions, such as osteophytes or proliferative synovium. A number of high-quality studies and meta-analyses of open carpal tunnel release document patient satisfaction and symptom improvement rates ranging from 86% to 96%.[71-74] Nocturnal pain improves to a greater extent than any other symptom.[75] The resolution of symptoms and functional limitations tends to follow a temporal course, with nocturnal pain, tingling, and subjective numbness that improve within 6 weeks after surgery.[72,75] However, two-point discrimination, if abnormal initially, may remain abnormal. Weakness and functional status improve more gradually. Grip and pinch strength worsen initially and usually return to preoperative levels after approximately 2 or 3 months, with maximum improvement at approximately 10 months. In a series of 44 patients with mean follow-up of 35 months after open carpal tunnel release, Osterman[76] reported a 96% rate of patient satisfaction and symptom improvement, with 84% of patients returning to their preoperative jobs after surgery.

One of the advantages of open release is that technical complications are uncommon. The most common is incomplete release.[77] Wide exposure should minimize the risk of inadvertent nerve or vascular injury. Deep wound infection is also uncommon, although superficial "stitch abscesses" occur. The principal postoperative problem is usually palmar tenderness, so-called pillar pain on either side of the cut retinaculum.[78-83] Interestingly, this pain occurs after all types of carpal tunnel release. One study reported a 41% rate of postoperative allodynia over the thenar and hypothenar eminences at 1 month after surgery, decreasing to 25% at 3 months and 6% at 12 months. Postoperative palmar pain may contribute to delayed return to work, particularly among manual laborers and those receiving worker's compensation.

Pillar pain is localized to the thenar or hypothenar areas and must be distinguished from palmar incisional or scar tenderness. The relevant anatomy appears to be the osseous and muscular attachments of the flexor retinaculum, the origin of the three thenar and three hypothenar muscles. Usually, this pain decreases over time and again appears to be independent of the type of release performed. A more rare complication is flexor tendon bowstringing, which may cause painful snapping of the tendons over the hook of the hamate with grip or, in extreme cases, painful adherence of the median nerve to the palmar subcutaneous tissues. I attempt to identify the potential for this problem intraoperatively by asking the patient to grip strongly after the release is completed; if the tendons and nerve displace out of the tunnel anteriorly, I reconstruct the retinaculum with a distally based flap (Fig. 48-6).[84-86] I also perform this procedure if the patient has a job that requires forceful pinch or grip with the wrist flexed and the work cannot be modified, such as dental hygienists.

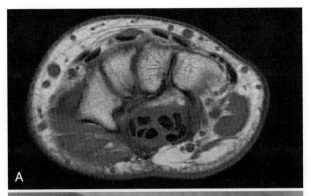

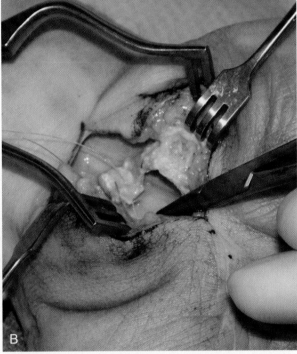

Figure 48-6 Reconstruction of the flexor retinaculum with a distally based rotation flap. **A,** Preoperative magnetic resonance imaging showing bowstringing. **B,** The flap being rotated into place.

For many years, traditional postoperative management after open carpal tunnel release included a period of immobilization ranging from several weeks to a month or more. More recently, early mobilization has been more commonly considered after open release, with a consequent reduction in postoperative morbidity and more rapid return to work. Based on several reports showing no benefit to postoperative immobilization,[87-89] I now allow my patients to begin moving their fingers and wrists immediately after surgery, requesting only that they limit the weight that they lift and that they lift with the forearm supinated, so that the wrist will be extended during lifting. This is discussed in more detail later.

Endoscopic and Mini-Open Carpal Tunnel Release

A variety of less invasive techniques, such as endoscopic and mini-open carpal tunnel release, have been proposed to decrease the morbidity of carpal tunnel release by selectively transecting the flexor retinaculum through small incisions, often placed outside the palm or at least away from the high-contact midpalm of the hand.[71,89-96] Despite these innovations, the incidence of pillar pain, by strict definition, is probably the same, regardless of technique. Proponents of alternative techniques state that less incisional tenderness is present, but most studies suggest that this difference is only significant in the first few weeks after surgery.[72,74,95,97-100] Nonetheless, endoscopic and mini-open procedures do appear to be associated with a few weeks' earlier return of grip and pinch strength and an earlier return to work. These benefits are to some extent outweighed by higher rates of technical complications in most series, with higher rates of incomplete release, median nerve injury, and (something exceedingly unusual with open release) injury to the ulnar neurovascular bundle.[72,101-110] Although many surgeons criticize incisions for open procedures that cross the wrist, all endoscopic release techniques require an incision in the distal forearm. The one-portal releases employ only this proximal incision (Fig. 48-7), whereas the two-portal techniques use this proximal incision and a small distal palmar incision. The one- and two-portal releases use a variety of specially designed devices to release the retinaculum.

Mini-open procedures avoid the distal forearm incisions by using small palmar incisions, usually with special retractors to improve visualization (Fig. 48-8).

Adjunctive Procedures

Although there is little evidence to support their routine use, a variety of adjunctive procedures have been described for use in conjunction with carpal tunnel release. Reconstruction of the flexor retinaculum, synovectomy, and neurolysis have all had their proponents, but current evidence does not support their routine use.[64]

Postoperative Management

The details of postoperative management are discussed in Chapter 49. From the surgeon's perspective, at this point, there is a rough consensus that, regardless of the way that the flexor retinaculum has been cut, activity should begin soon after surgery, As discussed later, return to work should not follow an arbitrary guide, but instead should depend on hand, handedness, patient occupation, and the availability of modified work.

Recurrent or Unrelieved Carpal Tunnel Syndrome

Primary carpal tunnel release is usually successful; nonetheless, the need for reoperation for persistent or recurrent symptoms ranges in studies from 1.7% to 3.1% of cases.[104,111,112] Although most patients improve after reoperation, persistent symptoms to some degree are likely, and failure occurs more frequently than after primary carpal tunnel surgery, especially in the patient who undergoes multiple reoperations.[77] Careful patient selection before reoperation is paramount.

In the evaluation of the patient with recurrent or unrelieved symptoms after carpal tunnel release, consideration

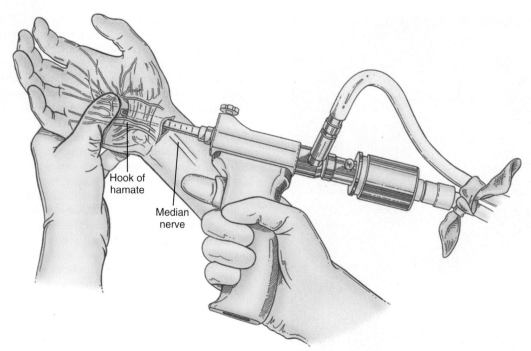

Figure 48-7 Endoscopic one-portal carpal tunnel release is performed through a transverse incision proximal to the volar wrist crease. (Modified from MicroAire Surgical Instruments, Inc. In: Green D: *Green's Operative Hand Surgery.* 4th ed. Philadelphia: Churchill Livingstone;1999.)

must be given to both organic and nonorganic etiologies. A detailed history of current symptoms and preoperative symptoms before the initial carpal tunnel release is mandatory. Multiple examinations may be necessary, with attention paid to the reproducibility of abnormal findings. There is the possibility of an inaccurate original diagnosis of CTS or unrecognized concurrent cervical radiculopathy or pronator syndrome.[42] Patient motivation and the possibility of secondary gain must also be considered. Objective tools, such as the Minnesota Multiphasic Personality Inventory, may be useful in the evaluation of possible nonorganic reasons for persistent or unrelieved symptoms.[113] Electrodiagnostic tests have an important role in this patient group, and unresolved elec-

trodiagnostic abnormalities with clinical findings of median neuropathy after carpal tunnel release warrant a diagnosis of persistent or recurrent CTS.[111,112]

Patients with persistent or early recurrence of symptoms are more likely to have incomplete release of the transverse carpal ligament than those with delayed recurrent symptoms.[112,114,115] The distal portion of the flexor retinaculum extends approximately 1 cm distal to the hook of the hamate and is the portion most commonly missed in cases of incomplete release, particularly with endoscopic techniques.[110] Patients with delayed recurrent symptoms after primary carpal tunnel release are more likely to have intraneural scarring of the median nerve, adherence of the median nerve with traction dysesthesias, regrowth of the flexor retinaculum, or median nerve subluxation from the carpal canal.

Nonsurgical treatment should be attempted before revision of carpal tunnel release. Patients with repetitive, high-demand occupations should have a trial of activity modification. The same demands that may have precipitated the original CTS can contribute to postoperative recurrence. Local steroid injections are appropriate.

The surgical technique of reoperation is similar to that for primary surgery, but usually with a longer incision, so that dissection can begin and end in previously undisturbed tissue planes. It is essential that the median nerve be fully visualized and completely decompressed. It is also important to avoid intraneural dissection, unless a partial laceration is identified and repair or interpositional nerve graft is indicated. In patients with perineural fibrosis, local flaps or vein wrapping can be used to reduce postoperative adhesions.[85,116-123] Risk factors for failure after reoperation include the presence of an active worker's compensation claim, pain in the ulnar nerve distribution, and the absence of abnormality on preoperative electrodiagnostic studies.[77]

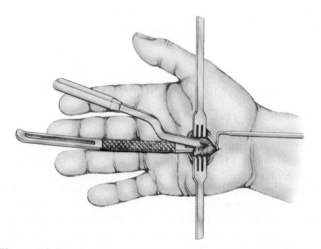

Figure 48-8 Mini-open carpal tunnel release can be performed with a specially designed cutting guide through a small palmar incision. (Courtesy of Kinetikos Medical Inc., San Diego, California.)

Carpal Tunnel Syndrome in Pregnancy

CTS severe enough to warrant treatment rarely occurs during pregnancy (0.34% incidence in a retrospective series of 10,873 pregnant patients[124]), is usually diagnosed during the third trimester, and is associated with generalized edema. The symptoms, most commonly paresthesias, generally respond to conservative treatment or resolve spontaneously postpartum.[124-127] Orthosis use, with or without steroid injections, has been found to be effective for decreasing the uncomfortable symptoms. The health care team treating CTS in the pregnant or lactating woman should coordinate all aspects of the treatment plan with the patient's obstetrician or pediatrician.

In one large series,[124] in 7 of 50 pregnant patients with the diagnosis of CTS, conservative treatment was unsuccessful. These patients underwent surgery in the postpartum period and had resolution of symptoms postoperatively. Some postpartum patients with mild residual hand symptoms as a result of CTS may initially respond to conservative treatment, but years later, symptoms may become severe enough to warrant surgical release. Patients with residual postpartum hand symptoms require long-term follow-up.

Return to Work

The interval between surgery and return to work depends primarily on patient motivation, handedness, the affected side, and specific work requirements.[128] In some cases, insurance status may also play a role, particularly when worker's compensation or litigation is involved. Return to work involving sedentary or light nonrepetitive activity usually occurs within a few days or weeks if the dominant hand is involved, and within a few days if the nondominant hand is affected. Longer return-to-work times can be expected for patients who return to jobs that require repetitive motions of the wrist and digits, forceful gripping, simultaneous wrist and digit flexion, frequent direct impact to the palm, vibration, or heavy manual labor, especially if the dominant hand is affected. These motions and static postures are associated with increased carpal tunnel pressure and may be responsible for symptom recurrence.[21,24,26] Occupations for which return to work may be particularly delayed include dental hygienists[46,129-132] and meat packers.[133-138] Job-specific rehabilitation strategies are discussed in Chapter 49.

Predictors of Outcome

Many studies support the importance of clinical evaluation in the accurate diagnosis of CTS. Patients who can preoperatively identify on a hand symptom diagram an anatomically appropriate pattern of pain and paresthesias are more likely to have a satisfactory outcome after carpal tunnel release.[139] In contrast, the results of electrodiagnostic studies have little predictive value on outcomes after carpal tunnel release.[140] However, among two groups of patients—those with diabetes and the worker's compensation population—those reporting poor results after carpal tunnel release tend to have normal or only minimally abnormal findings on preoperative electrodiagnostic studies.[141-143]

In a prospective study of patients with CTS treated with steroid injections and wrist orthoses, women younger than 40 years were the least likely to have resolution of symptoms. Among operatively treated patients, those with a prolonged (ranging in studies from 3 to 5 years) duration of symptoms before surgery are much less likely to have complete symptom resolution than patients treated more expeditiously.

Economic and psychosocial variables have a well-documented effect on the return to work and the extent of symptom relief for both surgically and nonoperatively managed patients.[73,144-149] Residual symptoms, prolonged absence from work, and the need to change jobs are significantly more common after carpal tunnel release in patients with physically strenuous jobs, especially among worker's compensation recipients. Palmar pain, in particular, contributes to prolonged postoperative recovery. The management of occupation-associated CTS is challenging and mandates close communication and cooperation among the patient, physician, therapist, and employer.

Summary

CTS is the most common peripheral neuropathy treated by hand surgeons. Most cases of CTS are idiopathic, but the pathology clearly involves increased pressure in the carpal tunnel. The association of specific jobs with CTS is controversial. Nonsurgical treatments, such as activity modification, orthosis use at night, and steroid injection, can be helpful in milder cases. The most effective treatment is surgical decompression, by sectioning of the flexor retinaculum (transverse carpal ligament). The evidence supporting one surgical approach over another is mixed; limited exposures may have less pain immediately postoperatively, but also seem to have a higher risk of incomplete release and possibly nerve injury. The use of postoperative immobilization or therapy is not supported by high-quality evidence.

REFERENCES

The complete reference list is available online at www.expertconsult.com.

Therapist's Management of Carpal Tunnel Syndrome: A Practical Approach

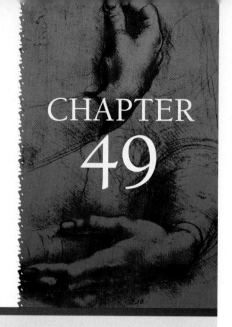

ROSLYN B. EVANS, OTR/L, CHT

CLINICAL EXAMINATION
CONSERVATIVE MANAGEMENT: LITERATURE
   REVIEW AND IMPLICATIONS FOR TREATMENT

POSTOPERATIVE MANAGEMENT
SUMMARY

CRITICAL POINTS

Conservative Treatment

- Complete clinical evaluation for the entire upper extremity
- Decrease carpal tunnel pressure/Improve local neural circulation
- Proper orthosis geometry
  - Wrist position 2 degrees of flexion, 3 degrees of ulnar deviation
  - Lumbrical block if Berger's test is positive or flexor synovitis present
  - Thumb kinetic chain included in neutral in presence of associated carpometacarpal (CMC) joint osteoarthritis
  - Full night resting pan orthosis for exquisite nocturnal pain
- Activity adjustment to minimize effects of posture, tendon load, lumbrical incursion, and flexor synovitis or tendinitis
- Avoid repetitive gripping, pinching, or strengthening
- Refer for electrodiagnostic testing or surgical consult if any atrophy of the opponens muscle, Semmes–Weinstein monofilaments above 3.61 for long finger, constant daytime paresthesia, no improvement in nocturnal pain, or provocative testing after a week of nocturnal orthotic use.
- Therapy inappropriate beyond a few sessions unless other tissues are being treated.

Postoperative Treatment

- Wrist control positioning to decrease incisional tension and to prevent over use

- Proper wound care to promote uneventful healing
- Suture removal at 15 to 17 days after surgery when tensile strength adequate to prevent wound dehiscence
- One-inch Micropore paper tape (3M) to minimize skin–incision line tension for 4 to 6 weeks full time; longitudinal to incision
- Gentle tendon and nerve gliding, allow tissues to strengthen slowly, avoid activity for repetitive grip. No value in testing grip strength
- Modalities only indicated if scar is painful or with flexor inflammation other than functional electrical stimulation to promote flexor tendon glide
- Short-term therapy is usually sufficient, but in some cases not necessary

It is interesting to note that this most common of all treated disorders in the upper extremity[1,2] (which experience teaches that with a *knowledgeable* therapist and *skilled* surgeon is, in most cases, easy to diagnose, operate, and bring to functional recovery) is the subject of so much controversy and research. With this perspective in mind, a practical approach to the therapist's management of carpal tunnel syndrome (CTS) is suggested based on literature review and my clinical experience.

Despite its frequency, many issues concerning this symptom complex are in question.[1,3] Controversy exists in the literature regarding cause,[2,4-12] techniques of evaluation,[13-35] results with conservative care,[36-59] technique of surgery,[1,13,60-72] and the value of postoperative care.[69,73-80]

A passionate debate rages concerning the effect of occupation on CTS and other injuries that may be a result of cumulative-type injuries, with many questions concerning this common and debilitating problem having no clear-cut answer.[2,4,45,81-93]

Several updated reviews of anatomy, pathophysiology, diagnosis with clinical and electrodiagnostic testing, conservative and surgical treatment, and evidence for the same, are suggested for the interested reader.[1,9,13,31,94,95]

The introduction of managed care, with changes in referral patterns to therapy, has increased the number of inappropriate referrals and the number of patients referred with either no diagnosis or incorrect diagnosis by the primary care physician or a physician from another specialty area. This increases the demands for clinical evaluation and treatment skills for therapists. In today's climate, upper extremity therapists must be able to perform a *clinical examination* equal to that of a hand surgeon in order to provide appropriate treatment and suitable recommendations for the patient. In addition the therapist must be able to provide acceptable outcomes[65,96] within treatment parameters set by third-party payers.[96] These pressures can best be met by correct diagnosis and treatment procedures that are based on current medical science.

Conservative mismanagement of CTS by the therapist is most commonly related to the inability to diagnose it or to identify associated problems that have been missed or misdiagnosed, to inappropriate orthosis geometry, and to exercise regimens that *increase* rather than decrease carpal tunnel pressure (CTP).

The *purpose of this chapter* is not to review the obvious or to repeat what is elsewhere in this text, but to focus the attention of the hand clinician and physicians from other specialty areas on the variables that affect intratunnel pressures in the carpal canal, which can be influenced with conservative therapeutic management, and to offer a perspective from clinical experience and literature review on therapeutic interventions that have some or no benefit for this peripheral nerve compression. A few points are made on postoperative management, which may prevent complications and decrease the expense of treatment and lost time from work. Chapter 48 covers surgical management of CTS.[72]

Treatment for CTS includes both conservative and operative interventions, with the goal being to decrease pressure on the median nerve so as to improve neural circulation and decrease symptoms. Conservative options have some support for short-term symptom relief if treated early, but ultimately surgical intervention is necessary for complete resolution of symptoms in most cases.[13,39]

Conservative intervention by the hand therapist might have potential influence on pressures in the carpal tunnel (in cases treated early) by altering postures, tendon load, muscle activity, and external forces, through activity modification and orthotic positioning. Flexor tendon inflammation, one probable cause of CTS,[5,35,98,99] can be decreased with medication, changes in load to the flexor system, and a lumbrical positional orthosis[100] Modalities and nerve gliding as conservative treatments are without strong support and are discussed in the next section.

Clinical Examination

Early and accurate diagnosis is important for providing the correct or appropriate conservative treatment, for identifying the correct surgical candidate, and for minimizing potential disability.[47] The duration of symptoms is a key determinant in estimating the predictive factors of recovery[101] and postsurgical outcomes.[49] Conservative treatment is of most value when instituted in the earliest stages of compression. It is critical to identify and treat this compression syndrome before axonal loss occurs in the median nerve,[102] and equally important to consider the pathophysiologic changes occurring with the different stages of nerve compression when interpreting diagnostic test results and predicting response to conservative management.[31]

My experience is that patients referred to hand therapy by the primary care physician, and even the neurologist, are often misdiagnosed with CTS for complaints of "hand pain," making a complete clinical evaluation of the upper extremity by the therapist critical to the delivery of appropriate care. Symptoms associated with basilar thumb arthritis, flexor tendon inflammation at the A1 pulley or carpal tunnel level, or de Quervain's tendinitis or tendinosis may be the origin of the hand pain. The clinical evaluation should include a directed history to identify any systemic or metabolic problems that could be contributory, assessment of mechanical forces imposed on the extremity in the course of work or avocational activity, a review of symptoms, and treatment to date. The initial interview usually includes asking the patient questions about pain, paresthesias, and motor weakness. Patient complaints of pain, "numbness and tingling" in the median nerve distribution, and complaints of hand swelling[18] are often easy to diagnose after a few provocative tests. Complaints of increased symptoms at night are a good diagnostic predictor for CTS.[101] The initial stages of CTS usually occur at night as revealed by serial overnight recordings of intracarpal tunnel pressure in patients suffering from CTS.[51] Tissue fluid in the arms is redistributed at night when there is no active muscle pump, and both intraneural blood pressure and systemic blood pressure are decreased during sleep.[103] Wrist flexion position during sleep may also contribute to median nerve ischemia.[11,104-106]

Author's Approach

My approach in a busy clinical practice is to follow history taking with a clinical examination beginning with Semmes–Weinstein monofilament testing (Semmes–Weinstein Pressure Aesthesiometer Kit, North Coast Medical, Campbell, CA) to determine light touch and deep pressure thresholds[107-110] of both median and ulnar nerve distribution. Testing is performed both with the upper extremity joints in neutral position (especially the forearm) and also following Phalen's testing,[111] which positions the wrist in flexion for 60 seconds.[14] A quick screen includes Tinel's test[19,112] (percussion over the carpal tunnel), lumbrical incursion, or the Berger test[113,114] (the patient holds a full fist position with the wrist at neutral for 30 to 40 seconds, which creates lumbrical incursion into the carpal canal), Durkan's test[26,115] (external pressure applied over the transverse carpal ligament using a calibrated piston (Gorge Medical, Hood River, Oregon), or more practically, with digital pressure, and observation of soft edema.[18]

Tests specific to CTS are then supplemented with a screen including provocative tests for proximal compression (distal to proximal) in the fibrous bridge between the heads of the flexor digitorum superficialis (FDS), between the humeral and ulnar heads of the pronator teres, beneath the lacertus fibrosis, thoracic outlet, and for C6 through C8 radiculopathy.[108,116,117] The various sites of median nerve compression—brachialis muscle, Struthers' ligament, the bicipital aponeurosis, pronator teres, FDS, the accessory head of the flexor pollicis longus (FPL), and vascular structures—are recently reviewed.[95,118] As previously noted a quick screen is performed for commonly seen associated problems of first CMC arthritis, de Quervain's tendinitis, stenosing tenosynovitis (trigger fingers), wrist or digital tendinitis, epicondylitis, or ulnar nerve compression.

I recommend (for the primary care physician) that a patient be sent for electrodiagnostic studies and surgical consult with symptoms of nocturnal pain, daytime paresthesia, positive provocative tests (Phalen's, Tinel's, Berger's test, or paresthesia with sustained index-to-thumb pinch); middle finger Semmes–Weinstein readings of 3.61 or greater, and of course with any atrophy in the opponens pollicis muscle. These patients' pain may be helped by treatment of associated tenosynovits, changes in activity level, and nocturnal positioning, but need release of the transverse carpal ligament to become asymptomatic.

Clinical Evaluation: Literature Review

Some authors conclude that there is little scientific evidence regarding the reliability and validity for comprehensive upper extremity clinical examination[24] and that sensitivity and specificity vary greatly with comparison subjects within the various studies,[20] but others have demonstrated the value of clinical diagnostic testing for CTS.* However, the existence of a gold standard for the evaluation of CTS is still in question.[28,121]

The American Academy of Orthopaedic Surgeons approved Evidence-Based Clinical Practice Guidelines on May 18, 2007, for the diagnosis of CTS with recommendations for diagnosis including patient history, physical examination (sensory testing, manual muscle testing, provocative testing), discriminatory tests for alternative diagnoses, and electrodiagnostic tests. The guidelines do not include MRI, computerized axial tomography, or pressure-specified sensorimotor devices in the wrist and hand (PSSD).[4]

Through meta-analysis the German Societies of Hand Surgery; Neurosurgery; Neurology; Orthopaedics; Clinical Neurophysiology and Functional Imaging; Plastic, Reconstructive and Aesthetic Surgery; and Surgery for Traumatology recommend similar guidelines for diagnosis, including an accurate history and clinical neurologic examination (including clinical tests) and electrophysiologic investigations (distal motor latency and sensory neurography). They regard radiography, MRI, and high-resolution ultrasonography as optional supplementary investigations.[13]

---

*See references 16–19, 21–23, 25–27, 29–35, 111, 113, 115, 116, 119, and 120.

Szabo and colleagues have concluded that if a patient has (in descending order for sensitivity) a positive Durkan's test, abnormal sensibility with Semmes–Weinstein testing, an abnormal hand diagram (patient mapping of discomfort and quality of their symptoms), and nocturnal pain, the probability of a correct CTS is 0.86. If all four of these conditions are normal, the probability that the patient has CTS is 0.0068. They found that the addition of electrodiagnostic tests did not increase the diagnostic power of the four clinical tests.[26] Their work is supported by others.[25]

MacDermid determined in a systematic review of the properties of clinical tests for CTS that although 60 studies were reviewed in detail, many were of poor quality (mean quality score was 6.6 of 12, with only 15 of 60 obtaining a score of 8 or greater).[30] The most frequently studied test was Phalen's, with an overall estimate of 68% sensitivity and 73% specificity. Next was Tinel's, with estimates of 50% and 77%, and then carpal compression, with estimates of 64% and 83% for sensitivity and specificity, respectively. Two-point discrimination and testing of atrophy or strength of the abductor pollicis brevis proved to be specific but not very sensitive.[30,31]

Berger suggested that provocative testing to produce lumbrical incursion may be as sensitive and specific as Phalen's test for CTS.[113] The test is performed by asking the patient to make a fist with the wrist in the neutral position. The test is positive if pain and paresthesia occur within 30 to 40 seconds. A full fist results in approximately 3 cm of lumbrical muscle incursion into the carpal tunnel and can increase the carpal tunnel contents, possibly contributing to median nerve compression.[114]

Other studies have introduced the complaint of subjective swelling of the affected hand as an important diagnostic and prognostic factor with CTS,[18] and the distal metacarpal compression maneuver as being helpful in diagnosis and orthosis design.[23] Goloborod'ko describes a provocative test in which the examiner uses his or her fingers to simultaneously exert dorsal pressure on the first metacarpal and pisotriquetral complex and volar pressure on the lunate. The test is considered positive if symptoms of CTS are reproduced.[29] The Hand Elevation Test has been found to be 88% sensitive and 98% specific and is recommended in conjunction with other known tests to assist in the diagnosis of CTS.[120] Paresthesias with the first three provocative tests indicate a positive result.

The effect of tenosynovitis as both a contributing cause of CTS,[98] and recurrent CTS,[122] and its effect on commonly used clinical screening tests for CTS[35] emphasizes the importance for the therapist of being able to both diagnose and treat the symptoms of flexor tendon inflammation as opposed to, or in conjunction with, CTS. A recent experimental study speculates that noninflammatory fibrosis of the subsynovial connective tissue is related to CTS and that a change in the subsynovial connective tissue volume or stiffness may be the source of median nerve compression.[98] El Miedany and associates in a study of provocative testing in patients with confirmed forearm symptoms and tenosynovitis found that the sensitivity of Tinel's, Phalen's, reverse Phalen's, and carpal tunnel compression tests was higher for the diagnosis of tenosynovitis than for the diagnosis of CTS (Tinel's, 46% vs. 30%; Phalen's, 92% vs. 47%; reverse Phalen's, 75% vs. 42%; carpal tunnel compression test, 95% vs. 46%). Similarly, higher specificity of these tests was found with tenosynovitis than CTS. They suggested that these tests can be used as an indicator for medical management of the condition of tenosynovitis.[35]

Although opinions and results vary from study to study, most agree that clinical evaluation of CTS has value in itself or as an adjunct to electrodiagnostic testing, and that early diagnosis is critical to good outcomes in the treatment of CTS.[49,50,101,123]

Conservative Management: Literature Review and Implications for Treatment

Even with early detection, the value of conservative treatment has not been proven.[4,13,36-40,42-44,46,52,60,124,125] Many patients experience relief of symptoms with orthotic positioning, local corticosteroid injection, anti-inflammatory medications, and changes in applied forces,† but eventually require surgical decompression of the median nerve.[13,43] The efficacy of surgical decompression over conservative measures has been substantiated by a number of investigators,[1,13,38,39,42,43,49,69,131] and has been demonstrated to be more cost-effective than orthotic positioning.[131]

Clinical research for conservative interventions for CTS include use of local and oral steroids, NSAIDs,[58,128,130,132] positioning with orthoses,[53,56,57,75,104,126,127,133] ultrasound, phonophoresis,[56,128,134] iontophoresis,[128,135] lidocaine patches,[136] exercise therapy,[45,56,137] yoga,[138] manual mobilization,[23,139,140] neural mobilization,[57,125,141-145] vitamin B$_6$,[146] workplace adjustment,[147,148] low-level laser therapy,[149,150] and weight loss.[7,8,151,152]

Increased weight or body mass index (BMI) have been identified as risk factors for CTS. Individuals classified as obese (BMI > 29) are 2.5 times more likely than slender individuals (BMI < 20) to be diagnosed with CTS.[151] Other studies have found statistically significant correlations between BMI and CTS. The importance of aerobic activity and overall fitness should be stressed, especially for those with sedentary occupations and weight problems.

There is increased interest in "neurodynamic maneuvers" or neural mobilization techniques for nonoperative treatment of CTS.[41,52,141-145,153-155] Median nerve excursions have been measured[156-160] and are the basis for clinical exercise regimens that combine cervical, shoulder, elbow, forearm, wrist, and digital motions to effect various degrees of nerve excursion.[142,143] It is postulated that CTP is reduced by combining intermittent active wrist and digital flexion and extension exercises[137] and that differential flexor tendon gliding exercises serve to reduce tenosynovial edema and improve the venous return from the nerve bundles, thus reducing CTP.[52] The physiologic rationale for nervous system mobilization supports the concept that nerve excursion or gliding improves local tissue nutrition by encouraging axonal transport and thus may improve nerve conduction.[30,153] A recent study concludes that forearm supination is the preferred position for passive median nerve gliding exercise because of

large distally oriented nerve gliding, whereas active full digital grip may produce proximally oriented median nerve gliding.[160]

Although some evidence supports the efficacy of nerve gliding exercise,[41] well-respected clinicians in the discipline caution that we should not be "overzealous" with active and passive maneuvers and should be responsive to clinical nerve-related symptoms with exercise that could potentially increase strain to the entrapped nerve.[154,155] Walsh notes that "there is limited evidence reporting favorable outcomes when using neural mobilization to treat specific patient populations, and the appropriate parameters of dosage (i.e., duration, frequency, and amplitude) remain to be confirmed."[154] At this point the efficacy of nerve gliding is not clear.[125,154,155]

Michlovitz has provided us with a general review of available literature[40] and cited the difficulty in making conclusions about the literature regarding success of treatment for CTS "due to variations in outcome measures, severity of CTS, and inconsistencies in duration, dosage, and follow-up time for interventions." Based on literature review she recommended that patients with mild or moderate CTS be provided with a conservative program of positioning the wrist in neutral for nocturnal wear. She suggested that intermittent exercise (nerve gliding exercises), activity modification, and pain-relieving modalities could be helpful in modulating pain and reducing symptoms.[40] Her review is supported by a randomized controlled trial by Baysal and coworkers which supports a combination of orthotic positioning, exercise, and ultrasound therapy in the conservative treatment of CTS.[56]

Meta-analysis of these many studies on conservative treatment yields inconclusive support for these interventions. The lack of clinical heterogeneity was cited as a significant problem, making comparisons and conclusions difficult. Our best available evidence for conservative interventions based on these analyses of literature review follows.

In a systematic review of randomized, controlled trials Gerritsen and colleagues found that diuretics, vitamin B$_6$, nonsteroidal anti-inflammatory drugs, yoga, and laser acupuncture seem to be ineffective in providing short-term symptom relief (varying levels of evidence), but steroid injections seem to be effective (limited evidence). They found conflicting evidence for the efficacy of ultrasound and oral steroids, and limited evidence that ultrasound is effective for long-term relief. Orthotic positioning was found to be less effective than surgery. They concluded that there is little known about the efficacy of most conservative treatment options for CTS.[37]

O'Conner and associates in a meta-analysis of conservative treatments other than steroid injection concluded that current evidence shows significant short-term benefit from oral steroids, positioning, ultrasound, yoga, and carpal bone mobilization. Other nonsurgical treatments did not produce significant benefit. Trials of magnet therapy, laser acupuncture, exercise, or chiropractic care did not demonstrate symptom benefit compared with placebo or control.[55]

Verdugo and colleagues, in a review for the Cochrane Database, found that a significant proportion of people treated medically require surgery, and the risk of reoperation in surgically treated people is low. They concluded that surgical treatment of CTS relieves symptoms significantly better than orthotic positioning.[39]

---

†See references 4, 18, 44, 47, 48, 53, 55, 57, 101, 104, and 126–130.

In a qualitative systematic review of 24 studies, chosen from 2027 articles on conservative management for CTS, Muller and coworkers found grade B evidence (recommendation for an intervention based on evidence that is consistent with two or three randomized controlled studies) to support interventions of orthotic positioning, ultrasound, nerve gliding, carpal bone mobilization, magnetic therapy, and yoga for people with CTS.[41]

Piazzini and associates conducted a meta-analysis for reviews of conservative treatment of CTS from January 1985 to May 2006 and found (1) strong evidence (level 1) on efficacy of local and oral steroids; (2) moderate evidence (level 2) that vitamin B_6 is ineffective and that orthoses are effective, and (3) limited or conflicting evidence (level 3) that NSAIDs, diuretics, yoga, laser, and ultrasound are effective, whereas exercise therapy and botulinum toxin B injection are ineffective.[44]

Evidence-based guidelines from the German Societies of Hand Surgery; Neurosurgery; Neurology; Orthopaedics; Clinical Neurophysiology and Functional Imaging; Plastic, Reconstructive and Aesthetic Surgery; and Surgery for Traumatology determined that among conservative treatment methods, treatment with a nocturnal orthosis and local infiltration of a corticosteroid preparation are effective; that oral steroids, positioning, and ultrasound show only short-term benefit; and that surgical treatment is clearly superior to all conservative methods. They found that open and endoscopic procedures (when the endoscopic surgeon has sufficient experience) are equivalent, and that a routine epineurotomy and interfascicular neurolysis cannot be recommended. They also concluded that early functional treatment postoperatively is important.[13]

A Practical Approach to Reducing Carpal Tunnel Pressure and Associated Symptoms

The goal of all these interventions is to decrease CTP, which will theroretically improve vascular permeability, tissue nutrition, and decrease symptoms. It is therefore important for the hand therapist to understand the effects of therapeutic interventions on CTP to avoid treatments that are ineffective or excessive.

Effect of Posture, Load, and External Pressure on Carpal Tunnel Pressures

A review of experimental work on CTP may offer some insight into reducing these mechanical pressures with positioning, alterations in work or avocational postures, and load applied to the structures that sit within the carpal tunnel. CTPs are affected by changes in the posture of the wrist, fingers, thumb, and forearm; by loads applied to the palmaris longus (PL), flexor digitorum profundus (FDP), FDS, flexor pollicis longus (FPL), and the lumbrical muscles; by externally applied forces to the palm and wrist area; and with exposure to vibration.

Effect of Wrist Posture

We observe clinically that wrist position with CTS is critical and that changes in position by as much as 20 degrees can alter nerve compression symptoms. Prefabricated orthoses with metal bar inserts often increase paresthesias and pain if the wrist is positioned in too much extension. We also observe the effect of extreme or sustained work postures on CTS and tendon inflammation.

The shape of the carpal tunnel changes with wrist posture.[6,162-164] A posture of wrist flexion decreases cross-sectional area in the region of the pisiform and hamate, whereas extension decreases cross-sectional area at the level of the pisiform.[164] The PL, by virtue of its insertion into the palmar aponeurosis (i.e., the distal portion of the flexor retinaculum), may alter the shape of the carpal tunnel as it applies tension to the retinaculum when the wrist is extended.[165]

CTPs depend on tendon load through the carpal tunnel as well as wrist position. Regardless of loading condition, catheter pressures have been found to be higher with wrist extension than with wrist flexion.[166,167] This has been shown previously for wrist postures associated with unloaded conditions.[62,151,168-171] Changes in flexor tendon trajectories due to wrist posture may also increase contact forces on the median nerve, subjecting it to shear pressure.[172]

Keir and Bach[167] explored the hypothesis that the extrinsic finger flexor muscles have the potential to move into the proximal end of the carpal tunnel with wrist extension. Muscle excursions of the FDP and FDS were measured relative to the pisiform during wrist extension in cadaveric specimens. They found that the extrinsic finger flexor muscles have the potential to enter the carpal tunnel during wrist extension, possibly contributing to elevated CTPs during this activity. They conclude that the use of finger flexors when the wrist and fingers are extended should be avoided.[167]

Fung and associates determined in a recent study of wrist posture and motion that frequent flexion, extension, and sustained force of the wrist increase the risk of developing CTS, but that neutral wrist position and repetitive digital motion were not associated with CTS.[105] Keir and colleagues provide guidelines for wrist posture that can be applied to the design of tools and hand-intensive tasks implicating fairly neutral postures. Their investigations defined postures of 26.6 degrees of extension, 37.7 degrees of flexion, radial deviation of 17.8 degrees, and ulnar deviation of 12.1 degrees to keep CTP below the critical 30 mm Hg.[106]

Intratunnel pressures have been measured at 2.5 mm Hg with the wrist in neutral, 31 mm Hg with normal wrist flexion, and 30 mm Hg in maximal wrist extension in normal subjects.[168] Burke and coworkers also found that wrist position had a significant effect on CTP and demonstrated that intratunnel pressures are the lowest with the wrist near neutral, most specifically at 2 degrees of wrist flexion and 3 degrees of ulnar deviation.[133] They recommended this position for wrist control orthotic use. Weiss determined that the average position of the wrist associated with the lowest pressure was 2 ± 9 degrees of extension and 2 ± 6 degrees of ulnar deviation, and recommended an orthosis position similar to that recommended by Burke.[127]

Other investigators support a neutral orthotic position for night only[129] or full-time positioning.[53]

Orthotic positioning has been found to be the most effective if applied within 3 months of symptom onset.[126] Other investigators support the use of short-term nocturnal orthotic use for CTS regardless of the degree of median nerve impairment, demonstrating a reduction in wrist, hand, or finger

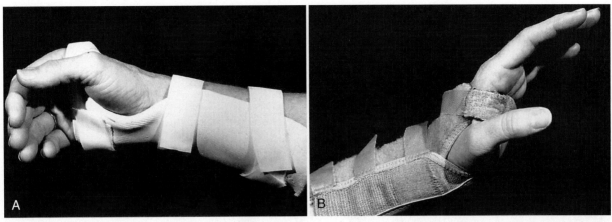

Figure 49-1 A, The proper position for a wrist control orthosis to minimize carpal tunnel pressures is neutral with the wrist postured at 2 degrees of flexion, and 3 degrees of ulnar deviation.[205] **B,** Improper orthosis position may elevate carpal tunnel pressure by 30 to 40 mm Hg.[8,12,206]

discomfort.[104] Symptom relief and neurophysiologic improvement after night-only orthotic wear therapy (in neutral position) has been found to last up to the 6-month follow-up visit by some investigators.[129] Walker and associates in a study comparing full-time to part-time orthotic wear with wrist neutral found that physiologic improvement occurred with full-time wear;[53] however, others have found no significant alterations in intratunnel pressures with or without orthoses.[173]

Clinical Implication. The proper position for a wrist control orthosis is neutral, with the wrist postured at 2 degrees of flexion, and 3 degrees of ulnar deviation (Fig. 49-1A). Prefabricated orthoses that often position the wrist in extension may increase CTP (Fig. 49-1B). A working posture of wrist neutral to slight flexion when digital load is required may minimize intratunnel pressures. Orthoses applied at night with early symptoms are the most effective and are needed for daytime only if it is necessary to control work postures in neutral. Presurgical positioning with orthoses has value if applied early, if tenosynovitis is a coexisting problem, or as pain relief intervention as a precursor to surgery. These orthoses can be remolded for proper fit to wear postoperatively to control tension on the incision and to prevent overuse and associated inflammation.

Repetitive digital motions with work activity may be tolerated with wrist postures of neutral; positions of wrist extension combined with repetitive finger loads should be avoided.[105]

Effect of Finger Position

We observe clinically that limiting finger motion is sometimes required to decrease the symptoms and pain associated with CTS and that in a number of cases wrist control positioning alone does not offer relief of pain. This is especially true in manual laborers with well-developed lumbricals or with anxious and often elderly patients who attempt to improve their symptoms by continually flexing their digits (i.e., the "compulsive gripper"). These same patients find relief of symptoms if the metacarpophalangeal (MCP) joints are positioned in moderate extension, which limits flexor tendon excursion and lumbrical incursion into the carpal tunnel.

With the wrist in neutral, intratunnel pressures are relieved by finger positions that pull the lumbricals up out of the tunnel. Several recent studies examine the dynamic relationship of the lumbrical muscles and the carpal tunnel.[6,114,161,174-178]

Lumbrical incursion into the carpal tunnel that is associated with finger flexion movements increase intratunnel pressures by increasing the contents of the carpal canal.

The four lumbricals take their origin from the FDP tendons as the latter cross the palm.[174,179] Anatomic studies have demonstrated that the lumbrical muscles originate distal to the carpal tunnel with the fingers held in extension, but that all four lumbrical muscles lie within the carpal canal when the fingers are actively flexed.[114,161,174,176] As a composite fist is made, the FDP tendons pull the proximal portion of the lumbricals into the carpal canal.

Lumbrical incursion has been studied in four finger positions.[114] The lumbrical muscle origins were found to be an average of 7.8 mm distal to the carpal tunnel with full finger extension, 14 mm into the tunnel with 50% finger flexion, 25.5 mm with 75% finger flexion, and 30 mm with 100% finger flexion. The lumbrical muscles were distal to the proximal aspect of the hook of the hamate only for the position of full digital extension and 50% finger flexion.[114]

This information is important clinically because the hook of the hamate has been found to be the most constrictive portion of the carpal canal,[165,180] therefore lumbrical incursion to this level could likely have the greatest effect on median nerve compression.[177] Others have demonstrated that the median nerve is compressed and flattened to the greatest degree at the level of the hook of the hamate.[181] So, with finger flexion greater than 50%, this already crowded area becomes even more crowded as the lumbricals move in to take up more space and apply more pressure to the median nerve.

Ham and colleagues have also studied the effect of finger flexion on lumbrical incursion and the median nerve. Successive cross-sectional areas of the carpal tunnel were measured using MRI with the fingers in both full extension and full flexion in 12 healthy volunteers. In this study the presence, amount, shape, and size of the lumbrical muscles influenced the alignment and shape of the median nerve in the carpal tunnel. Other changes that were noted in this

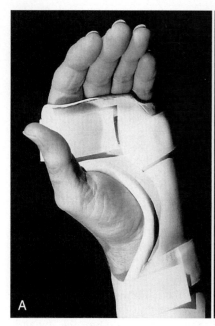
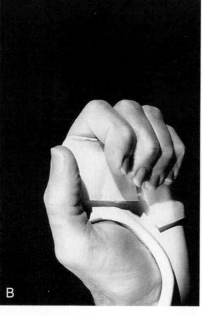

Figure 49-2 A, Patients with well-developed lumbricals, a positive Berger's test, associated flexor or extensor synovitis, or who tend to constantly flex the digits to relieve symptoms should be positioned with the wrist neutral and metacarpophalangeal joints blocked at 20 to 40 degrees of flexion to prevent lumbrical incursion and decrease flexor and extensor excursion. **B,** This orthotic position decreases pressure at the A1 pulley as well as in the carpal tunnel by forcing a hook-fist position, which creates differential excursion between the flexor digitorum profundis and flexor digitorum superficialis tendons.[183,184]

study during finger flexion were fat compression, flattening and displacement of the median nerve in the presence of lumbrical muscles, and pressure from the superficial and deep flexor tendons.[178]

Ditmars and Houin make the point that the lumbricals retract into the carpal tunnel with MCP flexion and actually contract during active interphalangeal (IP) joint extension, causing median nerve compression within the distal end of the tunnel. They state that this mechanism is suggested when the patient complains of intermittent numbness that occurs while writing, holding books, or carrying objects (as with an intrinsic-plus position) for a period of time.[6]

A study on the effects of finger posture on CTP as it relates to wrist position demonstrated that an angle of 45 degrees flexion at the MCP joint may be optimum when designing orthoses or work postures.[182]

Clinical Implication. The clinical implication from review of these studies and from clinical experience is that, in some cases, wrist control positioning alone may be insufficient to decrease intratunnel pressures (or to limit excursion in an inflamed flexor tendon system). A lumbrical block added to the wrist control orthosis that holds the MCP joints at 20 to 40 degrees of flexion decreases finger flexion by 50% and decreases intratunnel pressures.[114,161,176,177] A recent study comparing the effects of a custom fabricated orthosis with the wrist in neutral and MCP joints in neutral to prefabricated wrist cock-up orthoses supports this concept of addressing lumbrical incursion with the addition of a lumbrical block.[57]

In patients with well-developed lumbricals, a positive Berger's test[113,114] or swelling at the volar wrist indicating flexor synovitis or in patients who are "compulsive grippers," the MCP joints should be blocked in moderate extension to decrease the effects of lumbrical incursion (Fig. 49-2). I often fabricate a complete resting pan orthosis including the thumb kinetic chain, and digits in a neutral position for patients with severe nocturnal pain who cannot undergo surgery

immediately or for those with associated triggering digits or with symptomatic basilar thumb arthritis (Fig. 49-3). Limiting flexor tendon excursion in patients with flexor synovitis or hypertrophic synovium[99] is critical to decreasing pain and inflammation and prevents triggering of digits with stenosing tenosynovitis[183,184] often seen in association with CTS by forcing the patient to work the digits in a hook-fist position.

Work postures that require repetitive gripping in patients with CTS should be altered, as should postures that require sustained grip or pinch with an intrinsic-plus position. As noted in the previous section, activity requiring repetitive finger motions is best tolerated with the wrist in neutral. The use of therapy aids that encourage repetitive gripping, such as therapeutic putty or hand grippers, should be avoided as a part of a strengthening program for any hand that is inflamed or edematous as a result of other injury or for

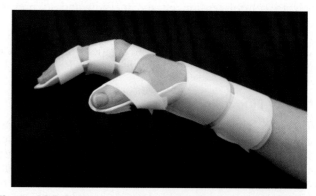

Figure 49-3 Patients with associated thumb carpometacarpal osteoarthritis, flexor tendinitis, or exquisite nocturnal pain find relief with a full resting pan orthosis that includes the thumb kinetic chain in a neutral position, the wrist at 0 degrees, the metacarpophalangeal joints in slight flexion, and the interphalangeal joints neutral. This orthotic position addresses all issues and provides the greatest mechanical relief for carpal tunnel pressure.

patients with the diagnosis of CTS. Repetitive flexion exercise increases intratunnel pressures and can contribute to CTS and trigger fingers.[6,184] A better option is to strengthen the hand with isometric-type exercise or dowel use that allows less than 50% finger flexion. Strengthening should not be a part of a conservative management program for CTS.

Effects of Combined Tendon Load and Posture

Wrist and finger posture combined with load, as with gripping and pinching, have been found to elevate CTPs.[166,173,185,186] Active-resistant flexion of the fingers creates ulnar sliding of the median nerve beneath the flexor retinaculum.[187]

The combined effects of posture and tendon load have been studied in cadaveric wrists.[166] It has been demonstrated that CTPs depend on wrist posture and the loading of tendons passing through the carpal tunnel. CTPs were measured in eight cadaveric wrists under four muscle loading conditions, with the thumb, index, and long finger in a pinch-grip posture measured with both zero load and 1-kg mass to the flexor tendons of the index and long fingers, the PL, and the FPL. This study demonstrated that muscle load elevated pressure in the carpal tunnel above the critical pressure. The effect of muscle loading from greatest to lowest was loading of the PL, the finger flexors, the FPL, and no load. The PL created the highest pressure with the wrist extended and only moderate pressure with the wrist in flexion. The authors speculate that the insertion of the PL into the flexor retinaculum may change the shape of the tunnel when the tendon is under pressure. Loading the finger flexors with the wrist flexed increases median nerve pressure 2.5 times that of loading the flexor tendons in neutral. Tendon load with the wrist in either 45 degrees of extension or flexion increased intratunnel pressure by 30 mm Hg. Loading the FPL in wrist flexion or extension induced pressures no different from zero load conditions, but when the FPL was loaded with the wrist in ulnar deviation, the pressure was twice that of the unloaded state. A forceful grip in ulnar deviation highly compressed the median nerve.[166]

Pressure has been measured within the carpal tunnel during nine functional positions of the hand and wrist,[185] adding support to earlier work by Cobb and colleagues.[177] Intratunnel pressures exceed normal pressures[55,188,189] by more than 200 mm Hg when making a strong fist in normal subjects, and in fact making a fist increased the intratunnel pressure significantly more than variations of either wrist flexion or extension in normal subjects.[185] Power grip was found to elevate intratunnel pressures to 223 mm Hg, isometric flexion of a finger against resistance to 41 mm Hg, wrist flexion to 56 mm Hg pressure, and wrist extension to 77 mm Hg.[185]

Rempel and coworkers examined the relationship between CTP and fingertip force and found that (1) fingertip loading increased CTP for all 10 wrist postures tested, (2) fingertip loading elevated CTPs independent of wrist posture, and (3) relatively small fingertip loads have a large effect on CTP. They concluded that sustained pinch and grasp aggravate median nerve neuropathy at the wrist.[186]

Clinical Implication. These measurements of intracarpal pressures vary some from study to study depending on the method of study, but all demonstrate that CTP changes with posture and load. The implication from these studies is that work postures should avoid the positions of forceful grip, pinching with the wrist ulnarly deviated, strong gripping with the wrist in more than 10 to 15 degrees of flexion, or positions of wrist extension. Isolated fingertip pressures and sustained grasp should be avoided in working situations. Again the case is made for working with the wrist and fingers in a neutral posture. We should be cautious as we ask the patients with other diagnoses (e.g., distal radius fractures or rotator cuff repair) that contribute to inflamed or swollen tissues to exercise with Theraband (which requires sustained hand grip), work simulation tools, work samples, exercise putty, and hand grippers.

The effect of tenosynovitis as both a contributing cause of CTS[98] and recurrent CTS[122] and its effect on commonly used clinical screening tests for CTS[35] emphasizes the importance for the therapist being able to both diagnose and treat the symptoms of flexor tendon inflammation as opposed to, or in conjunction with, CTS. Therapists should be aware that some commonly utilized provocative tests for CTS (Tinel's, Phalen's, reverse Phalen's, and carpal tunnel compression tests) have been found to be better diagnostic tools for tenosynovitis than CTS[35] and can be an indicator for medical management for tenosynovitis.

Effect of Thumb Position

Clinically, we observe that some patients with inflammation at the first CMC joint also experience median nerve symptoms, and that patients, if questioned carefully, point out that median nerve paresthesias worsen with sustained pinch as when holding the newspaper or a pen. The effect of first CMC joint inflammation, the pull of the opponens muscle on the flexor retinaculum, and sustained intrinsic contraction as when holding a heavy book have been implicated as a source of increased intratunnel pressures.[6]

It has been demonstrated that loading the FPL in wrist flexion or extension does not increase intracarpal pressures more than an unloaded state, but FPL load with the wrist ulnarly deviated increases pressures twice that of the unloaded state.[166] Keir and associates allude to the possibility of the thenar muscle applying traction to the flexor retinaculum, much as the PL does, with load to the index finger in opposition.[166]

Clinical Implication. All patients with median nerve symptoms should be evaluated for first CMC joint inflammation or basilar thumb arthritis, and if symptomatic, should be fitted with a short opponens orthosis for daytime (Fig. 49-4A) and a long opponens orthosis for night (Fig. 49-4B), and they should avoid work postures that combine pinch and wrist ulnar deviation. Positioning the thumb kinetic chain requires knowledge of thumb anatomy and kinematics and precision fabrication. Improper positioning within the orthosis contributes to CMC pain. As the orthosis is fabricated the therapist should manually seat the metacarpal in the trapezium, allow for slight flexion of the MCP joint, and ensure that the patient can oppose the thumb P2 to index P3 for function. Patients should avoid repetitive gripping and pinching with work and avocational activities. Adduction forces to the first CMC can be minimized by increasing the size of the writing

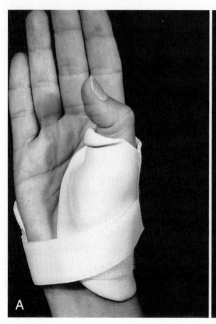
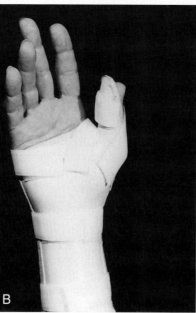

Figure 49-4 A, Carpal tunnel patients with first carpometacarpal (CMC) joint inflammation or painful arthritis should be fitted with a short opponens orthosis for daytime wear. This orthosis prevents CMC dislocation and adduction forces with pinching activities and may decrease joint inflammation and edema where the flexor retinaculum attaches to the trapezium. **B,** Night positioning for these patients should include control for both the wrist and thumb kinetic chain.

pen or pencil, applying arthritic grips to golf clubs, or by increasing grip size on other tools.

Effect of Forearm Position

Rempel and colleagues have demonstrated that CTP is affected by MCP joint motion and forearm positions in a complex way.[190] They measured CTP in 17 normal subjects in relation to pronation and supination position and MCP joint angles. The highest mean pressures (55 mm Hg) were recorded with full supination and with the MCP joints at 90 degrees of flexion. The lowest mean pressures (12 mm Hg) were recorded with 45 degrees of pronation and 45 degrees of MCP flexion. MCP joint angle (90 degrees of flexion) increased CTP to 60% above the minimum, and pronation–supination (90 degrees of supination) to 225% above the minimum.[190]

Clinical Implication. Based on the results of this study, a working position near 45 degrees of pronation and modest flexion for the MCP joint may minimize CTP. If CTP plays a role in the cause of activity-related CTS, then redesigning tools and tasks to minimize CTP will decrease the risk of developing CTS. Isometric forearm strengthening in a neutral position following musculoskeletal injury may be more appropriate in some cases than concentric or eccentric strengthening. This study may cause us to rethink the recommended technique for sensibility testing with the Semmes–Weinstein monofilaments in which the patient's forearm rests supinated while the wrist and digits are supported against a mold of theraputty for testing. This supinated position may increase median nerve pressures not only in the carpal tunnel, but at the flexor–pronator level.

Effect of Externally Applied Pressure

We observe that some therapy techniques designed for strengthening the hand or for stretching connective tissues appear to increase median nerve symptoms.

The application of externally applied forces to the palm in cadaver hands increases CTPs, and the magnitude of that pressure change depends on the location of the applied force.[191] It has been demonstrated that 1 kg of external force increases CTP by 103 mm Hg if applied over the flexor retinaculum, 37 mm Hg over the hypothenar region, and 75 mm Hg over the thenar area adjacent to the distal aspect of the carpal tunnel. The highest pressures are generated by pressure adjacent to the hook of the hamate (mean 136 mm Hg).[191]

Clinical Implication. Perhaps we should take a closer look at the use of hand grippers, some work simulation tools, progressive static positioning that applies force through the thenar or hypothenar regions to increase wrist extension, and the effects of cast pressures on median nerve symptoms, to ensure that our treatments are not contributing to median nerve compression.

Effect of Work Tasks

The international debate about the relationship between CTS and repetitive motion and work is ongoing. Several authors note the adverse effects of speculative causal theories and negative speculative illness concepts as they relate to CTS.[2,93] Derebery reviews the facts and myths surrounding work as a cause of CTS and states that "the concept of work-related CTS has grown to such proportion as to be problematic for society," and that cultural perceptions, expectations, and misconceptions have contributed to support by health care industries of a "largely mythical medical paradigm."[93] Lozano and colleagues recently evaluated 117 articles presenting original data on the cause of CTS in a quantitative analysis of published scientific evidence. They concluded that "current scientific evidence is inadequate to implicate environmental or occupational factors in CTS."[2]

The National Institute for Occupational Safety and Health (NIOSH) concluded, in a multistudy review of over 30 epidemiologic studies that examined workplace factors and their relationship to CTS that, with exposure to a combination of the job factors studied (repetition, force, posture, etc.), the risk for CTS was increased. The highest rates of CTS were found in occupations that required intensive manual exertion (meatpackers, poultry processors, and automobile assembly workers).[82] However, even though job tasks that involve highly repetitive manual acts or specific wrist postures were associated with incidents of CTS, causation was not established. The Occupational Safety and Health Administration has adopted rules and regulations regarding cumulative trauma disorders. Occupational risk factors of repetitive tasks, force, posture, and vibration have been cited.

The current position of the Industrial Injuries and Prevention Committee of the American Society for Surgery of the Hand is that "current medical literature does not provide the information necessary to establish a causal relationship between specific work activities and the development of well-recognized disease entities" such as CTS.[86] This position, as just noted, is recently supported by the meta-analysis by Lozano and colleagues[2] and also in a prospective 17-year study of 471 industrial workers from 1984 to 2002 in which obesity and gender were found to be consistent predictors of CTS, but workplace demands were found to have an uncertain relationship.[92] To add perspective, the Australian court system does not recognize that repetitive strain injury (RSI) exists at all as a physical disorder.[85]

Opposing views can be found. A meta-analysis of the epidemiologic evidence of the relationship between workplace ergonomic factors, such as repetition, force, static muscle loading, and extreme joint position, and the development of muscle, tendon, and nerve entrapment disorders of the neck and upper limbs of exposed workers was conducted by investigators at McMaster University, Hamilton, Ontario, Canada. Their review of 54 relevant studies produced 3 that met inclusion criteria, and 1 of these was found to have major flaws. The reviewers concluded from this analysis that there exists strong evidence of a causal relationship between repetitive, forceful work and the development of musculoskeletal disorders of the tendons and tendon sheaths in the hands and wrists and nerve entrapment of the median nerve at the carpal tunnel.[84]

Examples of work tasks that are thought by some to be high risk are keying on a computer;[192] operating a mouse;[147] the use of excessive strength; incongruous postures and movements of wrist, hand, and elbow; constant pressure on the palm; tearing motions; and the use of gloves.[89] Data from a recent study demonstrate a higher incidence of CTS in the working than the nonworking population and suggest that a substantial proportion of CTS cases diagnosed in lower-grade white-collar and blue-collar workers are attributable to work.[193]

Alterations in work tasks as an effective conservative intervention also do not have strong support, and conflicting studies can be found. Viikari and Silverstein, in a review article on the effect of or role of postural factors, high hand-grip and pinch forces, repetitive hand and wrist movements, external pressure, and vibration in the occurrence of CTS, conclude that there is enough evidence from experimental studies to suggest that both the incidence and severity of CTS could be improved with changes in work patterns, such as

reducing the duration, frequency, or intensity of forceful repetitive work, extreme wrist postures, vibration.[91]

A recently published meta-analysis studying conservative interventions (e.g., exercises, relaxation, physical applications, biofeedback, myofeedback, and workplace adjustments) for adults suffering complaints of the arm, neck, or shoulder (CANS) noted that overall the quality of the studies was poor. They concluded from this review that there is limited evidence for the effectiveness of keyboards with an alternative force-displacement of the keys or an alternative geometry, and limited evidence for the effectiveness of exercises compared with massage, breaks during computer work compared to no breaks, massage as an add-on treatment to manual therapy, and manual therapy as an add-on treatment to exercises.[45]

Clinical Implication. Although causation is debated, and strong evidence to support work task or ergonomic changes in the workplace is lacking, correcting postures to neutral and minimizing stresses to the tendon systems that decrease often-associated tenosynovitis are practical solutions to address CTS until surgery can be undertaken. This can be done with a session of identifying tasks that could cause tendon inflammation (postures, forces, and repetitions associated with activities such as gardening, work-outs, sports, factory or assembly work, and keyboarding). We recognize that we do not have scientific evidence for causation or treatment as it relates to work; however, common sense and experience teaches that rest, and working with neutral postures and decreased duration and intensity can serve to decrease symptoms.

Conclusions for Conservative Management

In summary, conservative intervention for CTS should be minimal, unless associated with other problems such as tenosynovitis, triggering digits, de Quervain's, arthritis, or as sequelae to traumatic injury. As noted previously establishing the clinical diagnosis is critical.

Intratunnel pressures may be relieved with alterations in posture, muscle activity, tendon load, and reduction of external forces. Wrist orthotic positioning is optimal at 0 to 2 degrees of flexion and 3 degrees of ulnar deviation to decrease pressure on the median nerve.[127,133] The MCP joints should be positioned at 20 to 40 degrees of flexion when the lumbrical incursion or full-fist test is positive; if the flexor tendons are inflamed or wrist flexor synovitis is present; if the A1 pulley region is tender or triggering is present with any digit;[184] or for the inadvertent or "compulsive gripper."

Once the patient is positioned, instructed in activity modification, ergonomic changes, and proximal postural changes, he or she should be discharged with a home program and rechecked informally to screen for sensory changes or change in symptoms, unless being treated for additional problems. Outpatient therapy treatment with modalities or exercise regimens is probably not going to prevent the need for surgical intervention, is costly, and uses allowable insurance coverage when it may be needed postoperatively. Median nerve symptoms related to flexor tendon synovitis may well be the most likely scenario for responding to conservative treatment with orthotic positioning, changes in flexor tendon activity, and medications. As noted in the evaluation section, I notify the referring physician that the patient should be evaluated for surgical decompression with symptoms of daytime paresthesia, nocturnal pain that prevents sleep with the orthoses in place, long finger Semmes–Weinstein readings above 3.61, or atrophy in the opponens muscle.

Patients benefit from the proper education and from questioning regarding their understanding of their symptoms to ensure compliance with the home program. Many patients have misinformation from non-peer-reviewed sources. Scangas and associates in a recent study of the disparity between popular and scientific illness concepts of carpal tunnel causation note the significant disparities between popular (Internet) and scientific (*Index Medicus*) theories.[194] Our responsibility, as health professionals, is to ensure that our own knowledge is based on peer-reviewed scientific literature and that our patients are properly educated to avoid the perpetuation of negative speculative illness concepts.

Postoperative Management

The literature confirms that carpal tunnel decompression is effective and the preferred treatment for CTS, but it should be noted that surgical management is not without a small percentage of residual problems.[6,50,66,123,195,196] Postoperative problems have been defined as incomplete relief of pain, poor recovery of sensory and motor function, symptom recurrence, perineural scarring with associated symptoms, scar tenderness, pillar pain, laceration to flexor tendon or nerve, and neuroma in continuity. Other problems can include postoperative wound infection, wound dehiscence from early suture removal, suture abscess, trigger fingers that were not picked up preoperatively and that limit patient's willingness to exercise, PL inflammation, incomplete tendon glide, and complex regional pain syndrome.[6,50,66,123,195,196] These complications exist and are reported by hand surgeons with both open (OCTR) and endoscopic (ECTR) release.[61]

The value of postoperative care is debated.[52,74,75] It has been demonstrated that rehabilitation after surgery facilitates a faster return to work, but has no effect on functional recovery or symptom reoccurrence.[75] Obviously, therapy does not influence a nerve that is still mechanically compressed or the rate of regeneration of a recovering nerve, but patients that have complications of wound problems, painful scar, incomplete flexor tendon glide, stiff joints from associated osteoarthritis, painful first CMC joint arthritis, undiagnosed trigger fingers, an inflamed PL, or pillar pain benefit from supervised therapy.

Many surgeons do not refer patients for therapy following carpal tunnel release (CTR). A recent randomized study failed to show the benefit in a 2-week course of hand therapy after CTR using a short incision and concluded that the cost of supervised therapy for uncomplicated CTR is unjustified.[78] I would agree with this in most cases; however, the key word here is *uncomplicated*, the key point is *short incision*, and it should be noted that these cases were operated on by *experienced hand surgeons*. The therapist who treats patients from a wide referral source knows the benefits of supervised therapy for patients that experience the postoperative problems noted or who tend to overexercise or underexercise.

The value of postoperative positioning also is debated. Finsen and coworkers found no difference in complication rates with regard to scar pain, pillar pain, grip, or pinch in CTR patients positioned versus those not using an orthosis for 4 weeks.[74] Martins and colleagues in a prospective review comparing the effects of wrist immobilization following CTR concluded that patients treated with wrist immobilization in the immediate postoperative period have no advantages when compared with those treated with no immobilization in the end result following CTR.[76] Others support their findings.[73,79,80] My experience is that postoperative positioning with orthoses for a short 2- to 3-week interval following CTR is helpful to control overuse and inflammation and to prevent incisional line wound tension. Orthotic positioning does not appear to contribute to problems with tendon or nerve gliding because patients remove the orthosis for controlled wrist extension and finger exercise.

It is my experience that scar tenderness is the most common postoperative management problem seen following OCTR and that this complication is most often seen with incisions that cross the wrist or when sutures are taken out before the wound has gained adequate tensile strength, producing subsequent dehiscence.

In a study of predictors of return to work following CTR, Katz and colleagues demonstrated that persistent symptoms and scar tenderness most strongly correlated with failure to return to work.[197] Although other demographic predictors were defined in this study, the authors concluded that the work disability at 6 months after CTR is 29% and the principal predictor is clinical outcome of symptom relief and scar tenderness.[197]

Cassidy and coworkers have suggested that there is an anatomic basis for the increased tenderness of incisions that traverse the area from 5 mm proximal to the wrist flexion crease to 10 mm distal to this crease. In a cadaver study of 10 hands, nerve density was measured within the dermis, between the epidermis and superficial fascia, and between the superficial fascia and the transverse carpal ligament to assess whether a variation in nerve density exists in the region of standard CTR. The results of this study indicate that subcutaneous nerve density peaks in the region extending from 5 mm proximal to the wrist crease to 10 mm distal to the wrist crease, averaging twice the number of nerves seen proximally or distally.[64]

Early suture removal following OCTR that results in even minor dehiscence often results in the formation of hypertrophic scar, increased scar tenderness, and lengthened therapy. A point so simple as this, which violates the most basic principles of wound healing, costs the employer and patient time and money and results in poorer outcomes for the physician and therapist.

Scar tenderness can be minimized by incisions that do not cross the wrist,[63,64] detailed attention to wound healing, and by preventing wound site tension with a wrist control orthosis for a short duration of 2 to 3 weeks. The most effective scar management techniques are, in my clinical experience, a carefully planned surgical incision that does not cross the wrist crease, benign wound healing with suture removal around 16 to 17 days after surgery, and wrist control positioning that prevents wound site tension the first few weeks following OCTR. Paper tape (1-inch Micropore paper tape [3M]) applied longitudinally over the incision from 2 weeks to 2 months after surgery helps to prevent hypertrophic scarring by minimizing wound (skin) tension,[198-200] especially for incisions that cross the wrist. Topical silicone occlusive gel sheeting can also be used to pad painful scars and to improve hypertrophic scar;[201,202] however, it has been demonstrated in a bilateral breast reduction model that Micropore paper tape applied to scars actually developed significantly less scar than scars treated with silicone occlusive sheeting (SIL-K) or silicone gel Epiderm.[199]

Occasionally wrist pain is related to inflammation of the PL tendon (positive if the patient experiences pain along the PL tendon with applied manual resistance) associated with CTR. Patients with PL inflammation are tender with deep pressure at the insertion and have pain with resistive wrist flexion or stretch into wrist extension. These patients are treated with orthotic positioning the wrist in 5 degrees of flexion for 3 weeks, avoidance of stretch into extension, and avoidance of flexion loads.

In my clinic we see most postoperative CTR patients 24 hours after surgery for wound care and orthotic positioning. The postoperative dressings are taken down, the hand is cleansed, massaged, re-dressed lightly with a contact layer of xeroform and sterile dressings, and then positioned with a wrist control orthosis in a position of about 25 degrees of extension.

Patients are instructed to begin working on a gentle composite fist for the first few days, progressing to differential tendon gliding exercises,[203,204] and gentle nerve gliding exercises[141-143] by the fourth postoperative day. Specific written instructions to the patient decrease the postoperative problems associated with overexercise, underexercise, overuse, and wound problems associated with moisture or infection especially in the elderly, the diabetic, and the athlete.

Trigger fingers that were not diagnosed prior to CTR can complicate the postoperative course. Pain at the A1 pulley with deep pressure, uneven glide, or frank locking can be addressed by altering flexor tendon excursions at the A1 level.[184] These cases are best positioned with combined wrist control and lumbrical block which positions the MCP joints at about 20 degrees of flexion (see Fig. 49-2A). This position, which forces the patient to work the digits in the hook-fist position, creates maximal differential gliding of 10 to 11 mm of the FDS and FDP[204] and forces the swollen portion of the tendons to glide at different levels through the A1 pulley, thus preventing the painful locking that occurs with a full composite fist.[184] This position also decreases pressures at the A1 pulley, allowing the pulley and tendons to rest, thus decreasing inflammation. Azar and associates, in a study of the dynamic pressures of the flexor tendon pulley system in cadavers, demonstrated that a resting position pressure between the annular pulley and flexor tendon of 0 to 50 mm Hg is increased to 500 to 700 mm Hg with flexion of the fingers into the distal palmar crease.[183] If locking persists with this orthosis design, positioning the distal joint with a one-joint dorsal orthosis that includes the middle and distal phalanx allowing only motion at the PIP joint prevents locking. This orthosis can be hand-based if wrist control positioning is not indicated. Thumb triggers can be positioned with a one-joint dorsal orthosis that includes the proximal and distal phalanx.

In most cases, minimal therapy is needed following CTR, and in some cases no therapy is needed. Postoperative care, as with all hand surgeries, includes standard techniques of edema control, wound care, motion for both uninvolved and involved joints, and early intervention for inflammatory or sympathetic problems. I do not attempt to strengthen patients postoperatively except for light isometric exercises for the intrinsic muscles. Patients are advised to allow the operated hand to slowly strengthen with normal use, to avoid repetitive gripping and pinching exercises (with exercise putty or handgrippers) that may contribute to inflammation at the A1 pulley and that may aggravate the first CMC joint, if joint changes exist, to avoid the use of vibratory tools for 3 months, and to manage the scar with Micropore paper tape for 2 months after surgery. Strategies for return to work include communication with work supervisors regarding minimizing stresses, repetitive motions, ergonomic changes, avoidance of vibratory tools, and the use of padded work gloves in some cases. The point has been made that although there are several opinions regarding effective treatment for CTS, there is very little scientific support for the range of options currently used in practice (surgery, physical therapy, drug therapy, chiropractic treatment, biobehavioral intervention, and occupational medicine).[46]

Summary

Most cases, if followed early, with the precautions noted earlier, do not require much therapy. The greatest contributions made in therapy preoperatively are proper clinical examination of the extremity with recommendations to the primary care physician regarding treatment or referral to a surgeon, proper instruction to the patient for techniques to decrease CTP, and proper orthosis geometry. The most important contribution after surgery is the proper management of wound healing to help prevent scar problems, proper patient instruction about exercise techniques that prevent inflammation and maximize tendon excursion and nerve gliding, and communication with concerned parties on reentry into the workplace.

REFERENCES

The complete reference list is available online at www.expertconsult.com.

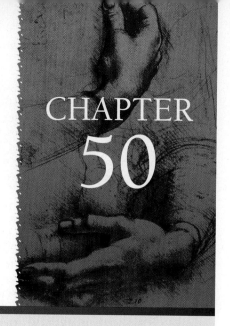

Diagnosis and Surgical Management of Cubital Tunnel Syndrome 📹

MARK S. REKANT, MD

ANATOMY	TREATMENT
PATHOPHYSIOLOGY	POSTOPERATIVE CARE
ETIOLOGY	RESULTS
PHYLOGENIC CONSIDERATIONS	COMPLICATIONS
CLASSIFICATION	OUTCOMES AND PROGNOSIS
DIAGNOSIS	SUMMARY

CRITICAL POINTS

- The ulnar nerve is subject to compression as it pierces the medial intermuscular septum (MIS); at the arcade of Struthers; within the cubital tunnel; and between the humeral and ulnar heads of the flexor carpi ulnaris (FCU).
- Pressure can be imparted to the ulnar nerve about the elbow in three ways: compression, stretch, and friction.
- The capacity of the cubital tunnel is greatest when the elbow is in extension.
- Pressure within the cubital tunnel is increased with elbow flexion and is further increased with contraction of the FCU.
- Patients with intermittent symptoms, no atrophy, and mild electrodiagnostic findings may respond well to nonoperative treatment.
- Surgical management options include endoscopic release, in situ decompression, medial epicondylectomy, and anterior transpositions.
- Postoperative therapy depends on the surgical procedure performed.
- The potential for full motor recovery after surgery is greatly reduced in those patients in whom preoperative symptoms have been present for more than 1 year or who have intrinsic muscle atrophy before surgery.

The term *cubital tunnel syndrome* was defined in 1958 by Feindel and Stratford[1,2] although the ability of the anatomic structures near the elbow joint to exert pressure on the ulnar nerve was known more than a century ago. In 1898, Curtis[3] performed the first published case of management of ulnar neuropathy at the elbow, which consisted of a subcutaneous anterior transposition.

Anatomy

The ulnar nerve is the terminal branch of the medial cord of the brachial plexus containing fibers from C8, T1, and, occasionally, C7. Figure 50-1 illustrates the potential sites of compression of the ulnar nerve in the region of the elbow. At the level of the insertion of the coracobrachialis muscle in the middle third of the arm, the ulnar nerve pierces the MIS, a site of potential compression,[4] to enter the posterior compartment of the arm. Here, the ulnar nerve lies on the anterior aspect of the medial head of the triceps, where it is joined by the superior ulnar collateral artery. The MIS extends from the coracobrachialis muscle proximally, where it is a thin and weak structure, to the medial humeral epicondyle, where it is a thick, distinct structure and lies medial to the brachial artery as far as the middle third of the arm.

Another potential site of compression is the arcade of Struthers.[4] This structure is found in 70% of patients, 8 cm proximal to the medial epicondyle, and extends from the MIS to the medial head of the triceps. The arcade of Struthers is formed by the attachments of the internal brachial ligament (a fascial extension of the coracobrachialis tendon), the fascia and superficial muscular fibers of the medial head of the triceps, and the MIS.

Next, the ulnar nerve passes through the cubital tunnel. The cubital tunnel begins at the condylar groove between the medial epicondyle of the humerus and the olecranon of the ulna. The floor of the cubital tunnel is the elbow capsule and medial collateral ligament of the elbow joint. The roof is

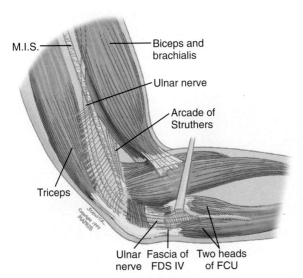

Figure 50-1 Potential sites of compression of the ulnar nerve in the region of the elbow. FCU, flexor carpi ulnaris; FDS, flexor digitorum superficialis; MIS, medial intermuscular septum.

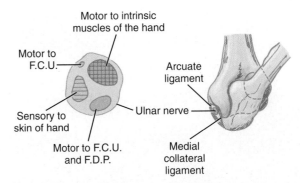

Figure 50-2 Internal topography of the ulnar nerve at the medial epicondyle. FCU, flexor carpi ulnaris; FDP, flexor digitorum profundus.

formed by the deep forearm investing fascia of the FCU and the arcuate ligament of Osborne, also know as the cubital tunnel retinaculum (CTR).[4-7] This retinaculum is a 4 mm wide fibrous band that bridges from the medial epicondyle of the humerus to the medial aspect of the olecranon. Its fibers are oriented perpendicularly to the fibers of the FCU aponeurosis, which blends with its distal margin. The medial epicondyle and olecranon form the walls.

The capacity of the cubital tunnel is greatest when the elbow is in extension because the arcuate ligament is slack. Cadaveric measurements demonstrate that as the elbow moves from extension to flexion the distance between the medial epicondyle and the olecranon increases 5 mm for every 45 degrees of elbow flexion.[8] The shape of the tunnel changes from a round to an oval tunnel, with a 2.5-mm loss of height. The shape change with flexion results in a 55% volume decrease in the epicondylar canal. Once through the cubital tunnel, the ulnar nerve passes between the humeral and ulnar heads of the FCU muscle. Fibrous bands have been described that compress the ulnar nerve distal to the cubital tunnel.

Sunderland[9] described the internal topography of the ulnar nerve at the medial epicondyle (Fig. 50-2). Sensory and intrinsic muscle fibers were found to be located superficially with the motor fibers to the FCU and flexor digitorum profundus deep within the nerve. The central location of these motor fibers provides protection from external forces.

Pathophysiology

Pressure can be applied to the ulnar nerve about the elbow in three ways: compression, stretch, and friction.[7] Small pressures applied to a nerve initially affect the endoneural microcirculation. The nocturnal paresthesias reported by patients stem from the increased tissue pressure and edema that occur during sleep. A critical pressure level has been reported to be 30 mm Hg within the tunnel.[10] Functional loss caused by acute compression is a result of ischemia and not of

mechanical deformation.[10] Pechan and Julis[11] have measured intraneural pressure in the ulnar nerve at the cubital tunnel in cadaver experiments: The pressure was 7 mm Hg with full elbow extension and 11 to 24 mm Hg at 90 degrees of flexion. Werner and colleagues noted that, during elbow flexion, pressure within the tunnel increases sevenfold and can increase more than 20-fold with contraction of the flexor carpi ulnaris.[12]

Experimental studies have demonstrated a progressive thickening of the external and internal epineurium as well as thickening of the perineurium. Persistent paresthesias are related to chronic alterations in the blood flow resulting from intraneural fibrosis.[10,13] The muscle wasting and loss of two-point discrimination found in advanced nerve compression are related to loss of nerve fiber function.

Extraneural compression of longer durations (28 days) has been studied.[14] As with the short-term studies, subperineurial edema may persist even after the removal of the extraneural compression. Inflammatory and fibrin deposits occur within hours, followed by proliferation of endoneurial fibroblasts and capillary endothelial cells. Fibrous tissue from endoneurial fibroblasts proliferates within several days, followed by invasion of mast cells and macrophages into the endoneurial space. Axonal degeneration is noted in nerves subjected to compression for 4 weeks.

Histologic examination of nerves at the site of compression injury reveals proliferation of the endoneurial and perineurial microvasculature, edema in the epineurial space, and fibrotic changes.[3,14,15] Initial changes occur in the nerve–blood barrier, followed by edema and epineurial fibrosis. Thinning of the myelin sheath then occurs at the periphery of the nerve. Axonal degeneration follows prolonged compression (Fig. 50-3). The rate and severity of these changes differ throughout the nerve, possibly because of variations in the amount of connective tissue. These pathologic changes appear to be dose-dependent, based on the duration and force of compression.

Etiology

Potential points of nerve compression or irritation include the arcade of Struthers, MIS cubital tunnel at the level of the medial epicondylar groove, and Osborne's fascia, which is part of the fibrous origin and connects the two heads of the

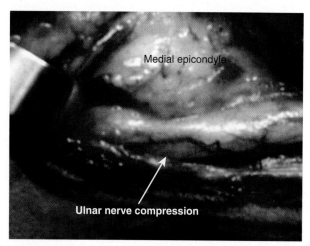

Figure 50-3 Ulnar nerve compression at the level of the medial epicondyle.

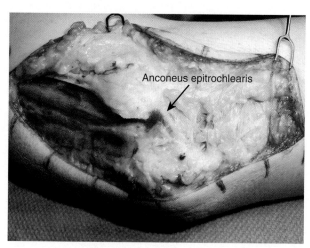

Figure 50-5 Presence of muscle anomaly, the anconeus epitrochlearis.

FCU (Fig. 50-4). Additional causes include subluxation of the ulnar nerve over the medial epicondyle,[16] cubitus valgus, bony spurs, hypertrophied synovium, muscle anomalies,[17-20] ganglia, and direct trauma.

Laxity of the fibroaponeurotic band can result in subluxation or dislocation of the ulnar nerve from the epicondylar groove. This occurs during elbow flexion. Asymptomatic hypermobility of the nerve is found in approximately 16% of the population and is often bilateral.[16]

One muscle anomaly, the anconeus epitrochlearis (Fig. 50-5) was identified as occurring in 3.2% of symptomatic patients treated surgically.[18] The anconeus epitrochlearis muscle was first described by Wood[20] in 1868 and later by LeDouble[19] in 1897 in their works about anomalous muscles in humans. The presence of this muscle is frequently associated with a prominence of the medial head of the triceps; that is, the ulnar nerve is completely covered by the triceps up to the medial humeral epicondyle, at the level of the ulnar canal, and near the olecranon notch. This configuration peculiarity exacerbates the clinical syndrome and the consequent surgical difficulties. In 1986, Dellon[17] demonstrated the presence

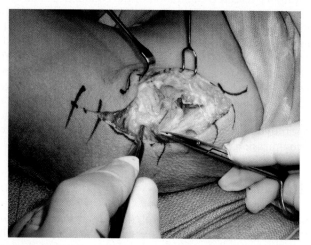

Figure 50-4 Fascia overlying the flexor carpi ulnaris is a potential site of nerve compression or irritation.

of the anconeus epitrochlearis in 11% of 64 cadaver dissections and of the ulnar nerve beneath the medial head of the triceps in 24% of the dissections. Clinical history of intense muscular activity (in work or sports) in young patients with cubital tunnel syndrome without other risk factors may sometimes be present.

Axial MRI is used to identify the anconeus epitrochlearis muscle extending from the medial epicondyle to the medial aspect of the olecranon and permits measurement of the diameter and recognition of the size and shape of the muscle. Coronal and sagittal slices allow for the identification of muscle position and the measurement in craniocaudal length. Short-time inversion recovery images reveal the features of muscle edema, if present. The relationships among the ulnar nerve, the muscle, and the adjacent soft tissue may be demonstrated with the use of MRI.[21]

Phylogenic Considerations

During ulnar nerve dissections of nonhuman primates, Dellon[17] demonstrated that in nonanthropoid apes such as the baboon, the ulnar nerve is within the triceps and the anconeus epitrochlearis muscle is present. In anthropoid apes, the ulnar nerve is more superficial, covered by a thin sheet of triceps medial head fibers blending into the MIS, the anconeus epitrochlearis muscle is present, and Osborne's band is not well developed.[17,22] During evolution, the medial head of the triceps regressed in humans, leaving a thin layer of fascia from the medial head of the triceps to the MIS, with the ulnar nerve lying below this thin film of fascia. The anconeus epitrochlearis muscle became so thin that the fibrous band described by Osborne may be identified as the remnant of the muscle.[17,23] Comparative anatomy studies such as the treatise of Padoa[22] clarified that the anconeus epitrochlearis muscle and the prominent medial head of the triceps strengthened elbow adduction and extension for brachiation in climbing. In humans, this function is not required; thus, the anconeus epitrochlearis became a potential compressive agent, as did the prominence of the medial head of the triceps.

Classification

McGowan[24] provided the following classification system:
- Grade I—Mild lesions with paresthesias in the ulnar nerve distribution and a feeling of clumsiness in the affected hand; no wasting or weakness of the intrinsic muscles
- Grade II—Intermediate lesions with weak interossei and muscle wasting
- Grade III—Severe lesions with paralysis of the interossei and a marked weakness of the hand

Wadsworth[7,25] classified the cubital tunnel syndrome on an etiologic basis: (1) acute and subacute external compression and (2) chronic internal compression caused by a space-occupying lesions or lateral shift of the ulna (injury of the capitelar physis in childhood).

Childress[16] studied 2000 ulnar nerves in 1000 normal subjects and found an incidence of 16% with subluxation of the ulnar nerve from the humeral epicondylar groove during elbow flexion. Two types of subluxation were defined: (1) the nerve moves onto the tip of the epicondyle when the elbow is flexed to or beyond 90 degrees, and (2) the nerve passes completely across and anterior to the epicondyle when the elbow is completely flexed. Approximately 75% of ulnar nerves with recurring subluxation are the first type.[16]

Diagnosis

Patients with cubital tunnel syndrome often complain of sharp or aching pain on the medial aspect of the elbow, which may radiate proximally or distally.[14,26] These patients also typically report numbness and tingling radiating into their little finger and ulnar half of the ring finger. Additional complaints may include weakness with grip and small finger usage. Symptoms vary from a vague discomfort to hypersensitivity, which is initially intermittent in nature and gradually becomes more severe and constant. Many patients report an exacerbation of their symptoms during sleep, especially with elbow flexion. Patients with longstanding neuropathy note loss of grip and pinch strength as well as loss of fine dexterity. Lastly, those with prolonged compression present with intrinsic muscle wasting, clawing, and abduction of the little finger.

Physical examination findings include a positive percussion test (Tinel's test) over the ulnar nerve at the elbow, abnormal mobility of the ulnar nerve at the medial epicondyle, or a positive cubital tunnel compression or elbow flexion test with increased symptoms with the elbow maximally flexed. The elbow flexion test, if positive, causes reproduction or exacerbation of pain or parasthesias (or both). Evaluation should also include muscle and sensory testing, including vibratory perception and light touch with Semmes–Weinstein monofilaments. See Chapters 6, 11, and 52 for further discussion of clinical testing procedures.

Electrodiagnostic testing may further aid in diagnosis and treatment. The loss of evoked sensory potential is a very sensitive indicator of altered conduction.[27] Ulnar nerve compression gives rise to reduced electrical velocities across the elbow of less than 50 m/sec. Electromyographic (EMG) studies may show denervation potentials in the ulnar-innervated muscles and are consistent with cubital tunnel syndrome when nerve conduction velocity is less than 41 m/sec.[28]

Roentgenographic studies should be done to determine the degree of cubitus valgus or assess bony lesions that can potentially compromise the cubital tunnel.

More recently, ultrasound imaging of the ulnar nerve at the elbow has been used to help confirm the diagnosis of ulnar nerve entrapment.[29] Ultrasound is the most commonly used imaging modality because it is inexpensive, provides high resolution, is readily available, and allows for dynamic imaging during elbow flexion. Most studies suggest that the key ultrasonographic finding is enlargement of the ulnar nerve at the site of entrapment.[30-32] As with previous studies,[30-32] the ulnar nerve was enlarged in those with entrapment compared with controls.

Treatment

Nonoperative Management

Nonoperative management includes patient education, activity modification, local heat and ultrasound,[33] and night orthotic positioning. See Chapter 52 for a detailed discussion of nonoperative management. The patient with intermittent symptoms, no atrophy, and mild electrodiagnostic findings may respond well to nonsurgical treatment. Should symptoms become unremitting and increasingly symptomatic, ulnar neuropathy at the elbow, either idiopathic or secondary to identified trauma, can be treated surgically.

Surgical Management

Surgical options include endoscopic release, in situ decompression, medial epicondylectomy, and anterior transpositions. All surgical options grant decompression of the ulnar nerve about the elbow's cubital tunnel.

Endoscopic Release

The endoscopic approach to in situ decompression of the ulnar nerve is not new. Tsai and coworkers[34] used an endoscopic technique for cubital tunnel syndrome as early as 1992. Excellent results, as defined by the Bishop rating system, were obtained in 61% of patients and good results in 33% of patients.[21] The effectiveness and safety of endoscopic cubital tunnel release was also confirmed by studies using cadaver specimens.[35,36]

The procedure has resulted in early postoperative relief of symptoms and good patient satisfaction. All patients improved symptomatically within a week of surgery. Good and excellent long-term outcomes were observed in 92% of patients, with an average follow-up interval of 16 months. As in other studies,[35,37] the best results were obtained in the group of patients with mild and moderate preoperative symptoms. In addition to avoiding potential injury to the medial antebrachial cutaneous nerves, potential problems involving scarring, recurrence, and elbow contracture also can be avoided with an endoscopic release.

In Situ Decompression

In situ decompression involves a relatively small incision with release of the overlying arcuate ligament or aponeurotic roof. This procedure has many similarities to release of the transverse carpal ligament at the wrist performed during carpal tunnel release. Wilson and Krout[38] reported on 16 consecutive patients (17 elbows) treated with simple decompression. They reported eight excellent, five good, and four fair outcomes, as well as one revision. The authors concluded that the ulnar nerve could be restored to normal by simple decompression. Miller and Hummel[39] reported on 12 patients with progressively worsening parasthesias, moderate to severe weakness, and EMG changes who were treated with simple decompression. Six of seven patients had improvement of pain, 9 of 12 had improvement in parasthesias, and 11 of 12 showed improvement on EMG studies. One ulnar nerve required transposition.

The authors concluded that the best outcome of simple decompression is obtained in the patient with mild weakness, recent onset of symptoms, and mild abnormality of sensory action potentials. The advantages of simple ulnar nerve decompression include simplicity of incision, decreased incisional soreness, and quicker recovery with minimal disturbance of the blood supply, use of local anesthesia, and lack of postoperative immobilization. The disadvantages of in situ decompression include potentially inadequate decompression, potentially higher recurrence rate, ulnar nerve subluxation, and failure to address all potential pathology in the patient with advanced motor and sensory loss and abnormal bony anatomy (i.e., cubitus valgus).

Medial Epicondylectomy

In 1959, King and Morgan[40] reported their technique, in which a 12- to 15-cm incision is made over the medial epicondyle. The medial antebrachial cutaneous nerve is identified and protected. The ulnar nerve is identified, released, and protected in a similar fashion as with simple decompressions. The humeral medial epicondyle is exposed with sharp subperiosteal dissection and with elevation of the common origin of the flexor–pronator muscles. The origin of the medial collateral ligament and ulnar nerve posteriorly are protected throughout the procedure. The exposed epicondyle is removed with a bony osteotome, taking care to avoid the joint and the origin of the ulnar collateral ligament. The osteotomy surface is finely rasped and contoured with a bony rongeur and rasp. The flexor–pronator muscle flap is reattached to the redundant periosteal flaps, providing a smooth gliding surface for the decompressed ulnar nerve. Hemostasis is ensured with deflation of the tourniquet prior to closure. Removal of the medial epicondyle affords decompression of the cubital tunnel by removing one side of the condylar groove, or so-called tunnel.[3,41-44] This permits the ulnar nerve to be under minimal tension during flexion and extension of the elbow without need for formal anterior transposition.

Craven and Green[45] studied 30 patients who reported symptoms of cubital tunnel syndrome lasting for an average of 10.8 months. These patients were treated with medial epicondylectomy. Twenty-eight of 30 patients had complete pain relief as well as improvement in conduction velocity from an average of 33 m/sec to 54 m/sec with no recorded flexor–pronator weakness. The authors recommended this technique for cubital tunnel syndrome in the patient with abnormal nerve conduction velocity across the elbow. Heithoff and associates[46] reviewed 43 patients with chronic ulnar neuropathy who were treated with medial epicondylectomy. At an average follow-up of 2.3 years, 8 patients had excellent, 23 had good, 9 had fair, and 3 had poor results. The poor results were related to failure of the neuropathy to improve over time. No problems were reported related to osteotomy site tenderness, elbow instability, flexor–pronator weakness, or increase in ulnar nerve vulnerability. The authors concluded that medial epicondylectomy is a satisfactory means of decompression.

In a primate study, Ogata and colleagues[47] demonstrated that anterior transposition is associated with significant decrease in blood flow for several days. No decrease in blood flow was reported with simple release or epicondylectomy. Advantages of medial epicondylectomy include the relative simplicity of the procedure and, because medial epicondylectomy requires less dissection than ulnar nerve transposition, a lower risk of ulnar nerve injury. This technique has the added advantage of also treating persistent medial epicondylitis and ongoing symptomatic epicondylar nonunion. This technique provides a more thorough decompression of the ulnar nerve than does an in situ decompression without a formal anterior transposition. The disadvantages of a medial epicondylectomy are greater initial patient discomfort postoperatively from the bone tenderness as well as potential for collateral ligament injury (elbow instability) from too judicious bone removal from the medial epicondyle, wrist flexor–pronator muscle weakness, and heterotopic bone formation.

Anterior Transpositions

The third option for surgical relief for ongoing ulnar neuropathy at the elbow is anterior transposition. Three types of anterior transposition have been proven to be effective: subcutaneous, intramuscular, and submuscular. All three techniques have their advantages and disadvantages. All three techniques involve fully mobilizing the ulnar nerve from the cubital tunnel with transposition to the anterior aspect of the elbow.

The surgical approach is a posteromedial curvilinear incision extending from 7 cm distal to the medial epicondyle to 8 to 10 cm proximal (Fig. 50-6). Care should be taken to identify and preserve branches of the medial antebrachial cutaneous nerves (Fig. 50-7) that may travel athwart the incision. This exposure enables direct visualization to release the fascial bands overlying the flexor–pronator muscles, the aponeurotic roof to the potential proximal entrapment of the ulnar nerve in the arcade of Struthers.

As the nomenclature implies, subcutaneous transposition involves placing the transposed nerve below the skin and subcutaneous fat. Curtis is reported[15,17] to have described this technique in 1898, which has become increasingly popular in modern times. In fact, given the relative ease of fully decompressing all potential points of ulnar nerve irritation and compression with minimal patient morbidity, this is the author's typical procedure of choice (Fig. 50-8). Eaton and colleagues[15] described a fasciodermal sling to support the transposed ulnar nerve. These authors concluded that

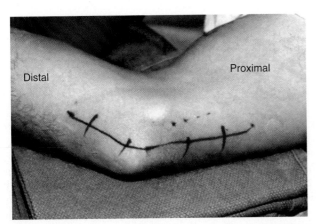

Figure 50-6 The surgical approach for an anterior transposition is a posteromedial curvilinear incision extending from 7 cm distal to the medial epicondyle to 8 to 10 cm proximal.

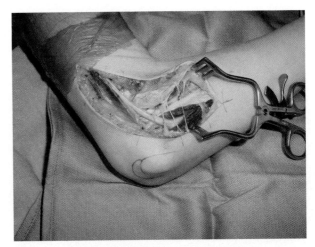

Figure 50-8 Subcutaneous transposition.

subcutaneous transposition using an epineural sling is an effective minimally invasive option for managing ulnar neuropathy. Subcutaneous ulnar nerve transposition is technically easier to perform than either submuscular or intramuscular transposition. However, its disadvantages include, especially in the thin patient, the vulnerability of the nerve to repeated trauma because of its position in the subcutaneous tissue.

The alternative options involve placement of the nerve deeper—either in the muscle of the flexor–pronator mass or below it. Submuscular transposition was popularized and well described by Learmonth.[48] The flexor–pronator muscle mass is incised from its origin about the medial epicondyle (Fig. 50-9) and repaired in a lengthened fashion after the ulnar nerve is transposed below the muscle (Fig. 50-10). This technique is potentially advantageous because the ulnar nerve is protected amid a vascular muscle bed. The procedure has been modified by performing an osteotomy of the medial epicondyle with the attached flexor–pronator muscles and then reattaching the epicondyle with screw fixation.[49,50]

The advantages of anterior submuscular transposition include release of all potential compression sites and protec-

tion of the nerve in a less vulnerable position beneath the flexor–pronator origin. The disadvantages include longer postoperative immobilization, possible weakness of the flexor–pronator mass, and a more technically demanding procedure.

Anterior transpositions have the advantage of moving the ulnar nerve from an unsuitable scarred area to a more favorable one. In addition, the nerve is effectively lengthened a few centimeters which, in effect, decreases overall tension of the nerve with elbow motion. The disadvantage to anterior transposition is a larger incision with increased healing time, particularly with submuscular transposition as there is need for muscle tendon healing. Another potential risk is devascularization of the nerve when it is moved from its natural bed.

Postoperative Care

Depending on the type of surgical procedure performed, postoperative dressing consists of a bulky soft dressing with

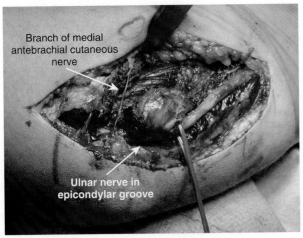

Figure 50-7 Care should be taken to identify and preserve branches of the medial antebrachial cutaneous nerves.

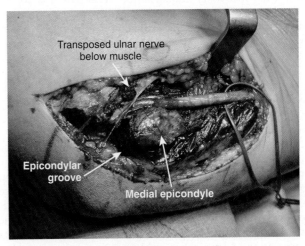

Figure 50-9 In a submuscular transposition the flexor–pronator muscle mass is incised from its origin about the medial epicondyle.

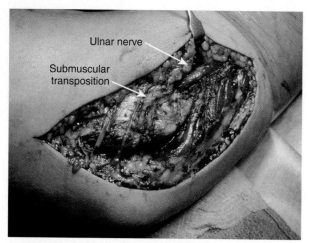

Ulnar nerve

Submuscular transposition

Figure 50-10 The ulnar nerve is transposed below the muscle, and the flexor–pronator muscle is repaired in a lengthened fashion.

an elastic bandage for an in situ decompression to usage of a long-arm posterior plaster orthosis with the elbow in 90 degrees of flexion for 1 to 2 weeks for a medial epicondylectomy or subcutaneous transposition. Submuscular transposition requires immobilization for 3 to 4 weeks to allow for muscle tendon repair with gradual resumption of elbow extension.

Results

Treatments by in situ decompression, medial epicondylectomy, and anterior transpositions of all three methods have all demonstrated predictable, satisfactory results. Pain is usually relieved, and other sensory symptoms show consistent improvement. The improvement of the evoked sensory potential correlates well with the improvement in clinical symptoms.[27] However, weakness tends to persist, and intrinsic muscular atrophy is the least likely to improve.[18,27,41,51] There is little prognostic difference between successful surgical procedures, but a guarded prognosis always should be given with secondary transposition. The potential for full motor recovery after surgery is greatly reduced in those patients in whom preoperative symptoms have been present for more than 1 year or who have intrinsic muscle atrophy before surgery.

Complications

Potential complications from surgery aside from infection include postoperative stiffness, persistent soreness, nerve injury, and recurrent compression. Irritation or laceration of the posterior branches of the medial antebrachial cutaneous nerves from dissection or retraction may result in a transient or permanent loss of sensation or hypersensitivity about the medial aspect of the elbow. A postoperative flexion contracture can occur, most commonly following a submuscular transposition. Ulnar nerve subluxation may occur subsequent to a simple release or decompression, with the

potential for instability following detachment of the medial collateral ligament during a medial epicondylectomy or submuscular transposition.

Outcomes and Prognosis

In general, all described procedures yielded good-to-excellent results in 85% to 90% of patients.[8,24,27,49] There is currently no consensus on the optimal operative treatment. The debate about it is highly dogmatic, with surgeons claiming excellent results for each of the treatment options. The choice of operative treatment is largely based on the surgeon's preference and experience. Several recent articles demonstrate findings indicating success with limited or simple decompression.[52,53]

Heithoff and associates[46] reviewed 12 clinical studies involving 350 patients in which a medial epicondylectomy was performed. Results were satisfactory in 72% to 94% of patients. Kaempffe and Farbach[54] reviewed 27 patients with partial medial epicondylectomies over an average of 13 months. Subjective improvement was noted in 93% of the cases.

In a meta-analysis by Zlowodzki and coworkers,[53] comparing ulnar nerve transposition with simple decompression for the treatment of ulnar nerve compression in patients without a prior traumatic injury or surgery involving the affected elbow, no significant differences were seen in postoperative motor nerve-conduction velocities or clinical scores. This systematic review of nonrandomized studies showed simple ulnar nerve decompression to have the best results[53]; however, the authors pointed out a potential selection bias: patients with less severe symptoms were treated more frequently with simple decompression, whereas patients with higher-grade compression syndromes were treated more often with transposition.[53]

In a prospective randomized study, Nabhan and associates[52] compared simple decompression with anterior subcutaneous transposition in 66 patients with cubital tunnel syndrome. Thirty-two patients underwent simple decompression, and 34 underwent anterior subcutaneous transposition. No significant difference in pain, motor and sensory deficits, or nerve conduction-velocity studies were found between the two groups at 3- to 9-month follow-up. The authors recommended simple decompression of the ulnar nerve. Biggs and Curtis[55] reported on 23 in situ neurolysis and 21 submuscular transpositions. The results were equally effective, but three deep wound infections developed in the transposition group. The authors concluded that in situ release is equally effective and offers fewer complications.

Bartels and colleagues[56] reported on 75 simple decompressions and 77 anterior subcutaneous transpositions in a prospective randomized trial. The authors found no difference in clinical outcome between the two groups. The complication rate was 9.6% in the simple decompression group and 31.1% in the transposition group. The authors concluded that simple decompression was easier to perform because of reduced soft tissue dissection and the absence of muscle detachment. Additionally, simple decompression was associated with fewer complications, even in the presence of subluxation.

An earlier meta-analysis by Bartels and coworkers[57] of the literature from 1970 to 1997 revealed that simple decompression resulted in the best outcome; subcutaneous and submuscular transpositions the worst outcomes. Heithoff[58] reviewed 14 clinical studies in which a simple decompression was performed. Results were satisfactory in 75% to 92% of the patients.

Summary

Cubital tunnel syndrome is the second most common nerve compression in the upper extremity and the most prevalent at the elbow. Patients with mild symptoms may respond to nonsurgical treatment as described in Chapter 52. However, patients with unremitting pain, paresthesias, and potential motor weakness require surgical decompression at the point of compression. There are many surgical options, each with their own pros and cons. Clinical presentation most often guides surgical options along with the surgeon's experience and postoperative rehabilitation is surgery-dependent. Outcomes are generally good and are likely to be optimal if the duration of symptoms is less than 1 year.

REFERENCES

The complete reference list is available online at www.expertconsult.com.

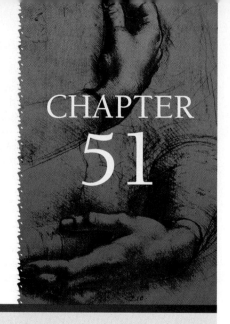

Other Nerve Compression Syndromes of the Wrist and Elbow 🎥

JOSHUA M. ABZUG, MD, GREGG MARTYAK, MD, AND
RANDALL W. CULP, MD, FACS

RADIAL TUNNEL SYNDROME
RADIAL SENSORY NERVE COMPRESSION
ANTERIOR INTEROSSEOUS NERVE/PRONATOR
  SYNDROME

ULNAR TUNNEL SYNDROME
SUMMARY

CRITICAL POINTS

- The clinical features of radial nerve compression and irritation at the wrist require careful examination to rule out the more common conditions of tennis elbow and de Quervain's tenosynovitis at the wrist.
- Proximal median nerve compression is less common than carpal tunnel syndrome (CTS), rarely requires surgical intervention, and can be differentiated from CTS as it is not likely to cause nocturnal pain.
- Surgical decompression of the ulnar tunnel is the most common treatment since the primary cause is space-occupying lesions.
- The clinical features of these nerve compressions correlate well with sensory and motor changes common to the involved nerve. Electrodiagnosis is less helpful with the radial tunnel and pronator syndrome conditions than for the more common nerve compressions such as carpal and cubital tunnel syndromes.

Radial Tunnel Syndrome

Radial tunnel syndrome was first described as a distinct clinical entity in 1956 when Michele and Krueger[1] described the "radial pronator syndrome." They presented a pain syndrome distinct from lateral epicondylitis and proposed an anatomic basis for compression of the posterior interosseous nerve (PIN) that could cause refractory lateral elbow pain. In a summary of the 1960 Annual Meeting of the British Medical Association, Capener became the first to report operative release of the supinator for refractory tennis elbow.[2] In 1972, Roles and Maudsley[3] coined the term *radial tunnel syndrome*

and proposed that entrapment of the PIN could cause lateral elbow and forearm pain.

Anatomy

The anatomy of the radial nerve and its branches about the elbow is variable. A theoretical space,[4] the radial tunnel originates near the level of the radiocapitellar joint where the nerve lies on the capsule of the radiocapitellar joint.[3] The medial border of the tunnel is formed by the brachialis muscle proximally and the biceps tendon more distally. The roof and lateral border of the tunnel begin as the brachioradialis and extensor carpi radialis longus (ECRL) muscles, and more distally are represented by the deep surface of the extensor carpi radialis brevis (ECRB). The radial tunnel was originally described as terminating at the entrance of the nerve into the proximal border of the supinator; other investigators[3] have suggested that the radial tunnel continues to the distal border of the supinator. Five potential areas of entrapment have been described (Box 51-1 and Fig. 51-1).

At the level of the elbow, the nerve is covered by fibrofatty connective tissue. Thickened bands of fascia from the capsule course around the nerve and anchor the surrounding musculature to the elbow capsule. The first potential area of compression of the radial nerve or its branches can occur here.[3,5] The roof of the tunnel begins as a collection of fascial interconnections between the brachialis and the brachioradialis. The structures of the roof continue distally, the biceps tendon becomes the medial border of the tunnel, and the proximal portion of the ECRB becomes the lateral border of the tunnel. At this level, the deep surface of the ECRB may contain thickened fibrous bands from its tendinous origin[5] and contribute to the second possible area of compression of the nerve.

The third potential area of compression is a group of vessels with an intimate association with the radial nerve and

Box 51-1 Potential Areas of Compression

Thickened fascial tissue superficial to radiocapitellar joint
Fibrous origin of ECRB or fibrous bands within the ECRB
Radial recurrent vessels–leash of Henry
Proximal border of supinator—arcade of Frohse
Disal edge of supinator

ECRB, extensor carpi radialis brevis.

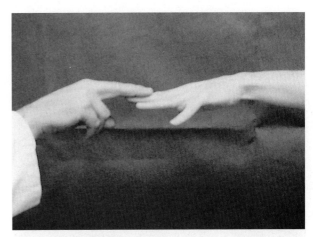

Figure 51-2 *Resisted middle finger extension.*

its branches.[3] These vessels have been referred to as *leash of Henry* and usually are branches of the proximal radial artery. They course laterally across the biceps tendon and proximally into the radial tunnel. These branches may impinge on the nerve throughout the proximal portion of the radial tunnel.[6]

At the proximal border of the supinator, the radial nerve has divided into its superficial branch and its deep branch, the PIN. The PIN continues, penetrating the supinator muscle on the proximal radius. As it penetrates, a fibrous band on the leading edge of the supinator, the *arcade of Frohse,* may impinge on the nerve.[7] This represents the most common region where the PIN is compressed. In a series of 90 patients, 83 had distinct compression at this site.[8] The arcade arises as a semicircular structure from the tip of the lateral epicondyle and the medial aspect of the lateral epicondyle. Anatomic variations in the composition of these origins have been reported by Spinner.[7] The lateral origin of the arcade is always firm and tendinous in nature, whereas the medial half of the arcade is firm and tendinous in 30% of specimens. In his 1979 report, Werner[8] described the arcade as fibrous in 78 of 90 cases. In addition, Prasartritha[9] reported that the arcade was tendinous in 57% of dissections performed on 30 Thai cadavers. The nerve then continues distally within the

supinator muscle and emerges as its distal aspect, giving branches to the superficial extensors. The final potential area of compression of the PIN is the distal border of the supinator muscle.[9,10] Fibrous or tendinous bands present in this region of the supinator were reported to occur in 65% of dissections performed on 30 Thai cadavers.[9]

Clinical Features

The patient with radial tunnel syndrome usually complains of pain in the dorsal forearm. It is localized to the mobile wad musculature: the ECRL, ECRB, and brachioradialis (BR), and over the course of the radial nerve in the proximal forearm. The pain is usually 4 to 5 cm distal to the lateral epicondyle and may radiate proximally and distally over the forearm. The pain is characterized as a deep burning or aching, worse after activity involving forearm pronation and wrist flexion.[6] Rest pain and night pain are also features of radial tunnel syndrome.[8,11-13] Sensory complaints and muscular weakness have been reported but are not characteristic of the syndrome.[14,15]

Characteristic physical examination findings have been described. The first is resisted extension of the long finger with the elbow in full extension, forearm in pronation, and the wrist in neutral (Fig. 51-2). The test is positive when pain is produced in the ECRB or BR over the course of the radial nerve. The second provocative maneuver is resisted supination of the forearm, with the elbow in extension (Fig. 51-3). This maneuver is painful when patients with radial tunnel syndrome have compression of the PIN at the arcade of Frohse.[16] A third characteristic finding with palpation is a point of maximal tenderness within the extensor musculature 4 to 5 cm distal to the lateral epicondyle (Fig. 51-4).[11,16]

The differential diagnosis of radial tunnel syndrome includes intra-articular elbow pathology, PIN compression, cervical radiculopathy, lateral epicondylitis, and other entities (Box 51-2). An important distinction is between radial tunnel syndrome and lateral epicondylitis. These two entities have been reported to coexist in 5% of patients.[8] Differentiation between the two syndromes can be difficult because of the overlap in symptoms and difficulty with physical examination. The areas of maximal tenderness are separated by several centimeters at best. Classically, the pain in lateral

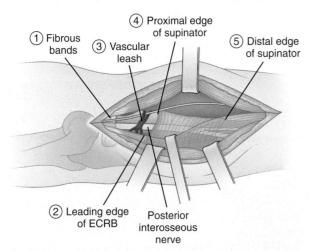

Figure 51-1 *Five compression sites of the posterior interosseous nerve. ECRB, extensor carpi radialis brevis. (From Steichen JB. Radial tunnel compression sites. In: Gelberman RH, ed. Operative Nerve Repair and Reconstruction, Philadelphia: JB Lippincott, 1991.)*

① Fibrous bands
② Leading edge of ECRB
③ Vascular leash
④ Proximal edge of supinator
⑤ Distal edge of supinator
Posterior interosseous nerve

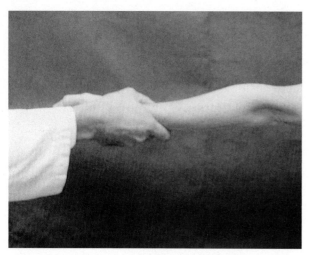

Figure 51-3 Resisted supination.

epicondylitis occurs at or just distal to the lateral epicondyle over the ECRB portion of the common extensor origin (Fig. 51-5).[17] The pain in radial tunnel syndrome is located between 4 and 5 cm distal to the epicondyle within the extensor musculature, either laterally between the BR and ECRB muscles or medially between the mobile wad and the brachialis muscle (Fig. 51-4).[18] Provocative tests for radial tunnel syndrome as listed earlier can be, but usually are not, positive in lateral epicondylitis.[6] Passive stretch of the ECRB muscle and common extensor muscle origin are more likely to be painful in lateral epicondylitis. Passive stretch of the common extensor origin can be performed by extending the elbow and flexing the wrist and fingers.[19] Also, lateral elbow pain is increased with resisted wrist extension in patients with lateral epicondylitis, but not for radial tunnel syndrome.

Diagnostic injection can also be performed to help in the diagnosis of radial tunnel syndrome and to differentiate it from lateral epicondylitis. An injection between the brachialis and BR within the radial tunnel has been reported to help confirm the diagnosis of radial tunnel syndrome.[15] To help confirm the diagnosis, the injection should produce some degree of motor block and transient relief of symptoms.[15] In patients with possible coexistent radial tunnel

and lateral epicondylitis, an injection over the lateral epicondyle common extensor origin that results in incomplete relief of pain favors the diagnosis of radial tunnel syndrome.

PIN compression is differentiated from radial tunnel syndrome by the presence of motor abnormalities. These abnormalities can range from partial weakness to complete loss of function and may be preceded by pain over the course of the radial and posterior interosseous nerves. Radiocapitellar pathology can be differentiated from radial tunnel syndrome with a history of antecedent trauma or chronic overuse syndrome, MRI or plain radiography, and mechanical abnormalities on physical examination.

Electrophysiologic Diagnosis

The presence of abnormalities on electrophysiologic examination of patients with a clinical diagnosis of radial tunnel syndrome remains controversial. Many believe that radial tunnel syndrome may be present despite normal electrophysiologic studies. Abnormalities have been reported by multiple investigators, but there is no consensus on what abnormalities are uniformly present or diagnostic. In their initial report, Roles and Maudsley[3] reported increased motor latencies in 8 of 10 patients. Electromyographic (EMG) abnormalities have been reported in the presence of normal nerve conduction velocities (NCVs) by Jebsen and Engber.[20] Lister[6] and Ritts[15] and their associates have also reported EMG abnormalities.

In 1980, Rosen and Werner[21] reported on 28 patients with a clinical diagnosis of radial tunnel syndrome. They

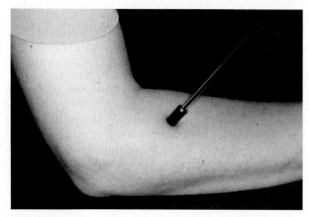

Figure 51-4 Point of maximal tenderness in radial tunnel syndrome.

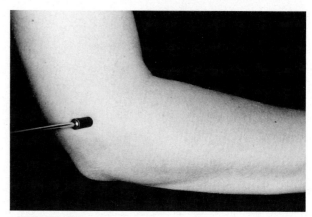

Figure 51-5 Point of maximal tenderness in lateral epicondylitis.

performed preoperative and postoperative testing, which included motor conduction velocity at rest, motor conduction velocity with active supination, and EMGs. They found no differences in motor conduction velocity at rest between controls and study subjects, nor did they find any differences between sides on subjects. They did demonstrate significant differences in NCV with active supination, as well as EMG differences between controls and subjects. They concluded that a dynamic compression of the PIN at the level of the supinator can produce lateral elbow pain and local tenderness where the nerve passes through the supinator.

In 1991, Verhaar and Spaans[22] concluded that the signs and symptoms present in patients with radial tunnel syndrome are not caused by compression of the PIN. They based their report on 16 patients with radial tunnel syndrome who underwent EMGs and NCVs, as well as NCV testing while performing resisted supination. They reported no EMG abnormality in any of the patients. They reported one patient with an increased motor latency, which returned to normal on follow-up examination without operative treatment.

In 1998, Kupfer and colleagues[23] reported a series of 25 patients who underwent preoperative and postoperative electrodiagnostic examination. They recorded radial nerve motor latency with the forearm in neutral, passive supination, and passive pronation. They demonstrated that an increased latency can occur in all three positions. Statistically significant increases in latency were demonstrated with respect to the control group. They also demonstrated a statistically significant decrease in motor latency postoperatively. They concluded that the differential motor latency of the radial nerve was a sensitive diagnostic factor in patients with radial tunnel syndrome.

Operative Treatment

Operative treatment of radial tunnel syndrome is indicated after failure of nonoperative management (see Chapter 52). Before surgery is considered, all other potential causes for pain should be ruled out. Coexistent lateral epicondylitis and intra-articular pathology of the radiocapitellar joint should be identified and treated if possible. There are four common approaches to surgical decompression of the radial nerve and its branches. Pertinent features of each approach are presented.

Anterior (Modified) Henry Approach

In the anterior (modified) Henry approach,[24] a curvilinear incision is made beginning approximately 5 cm proximal to the lateral epicondyle and extending distally along the anterior portion of the brachioradialis muscle. The incision is then carried obliquely across the elbow flexion crease near the medial border of the BR muscle. Proximally, the fascia is divided between the biceps/brachialis and the BR. Distally, the fascia is opened medial to the BR.

Next, the interval between the brachialis and BR is developed, and the radial nerve is identified. The BR is retracted gently with the radial nerve, and the interval with radial nerve is developed distally. At the level of the lateral epicondyle, the superficial branch of the radial nerve is identified and protected. Moving from proximal to distal, the nerve is mobilized by freeing it from the capsule of the radiocapitellar joint and any constricting fascial bands. The ECRB is then lifted off the nerve, and its deep origin divided if it contains any potentially compressing fibrous bands. Next, the branches of the recurrent radial artery are identified and ligated. The PIN is dissected free, and the proximal border of the supinator muscle, the arcade of Frohse, is identified and carefully divided. Moving distally, the supinator muscle is divided, and the PIN is dissected out as it proceeds through the supinator. Care is taken to preserve any branches of the nerve to the supinator. At the distal border of the supinator, branches of the nerve may take acute angles to innervate the superficial extensor muscles, and caution is warranted. The PIN should be freed from any fibrous bands in the distal portion of the supinator.

Posterior Approach of Thompson

In Thompson's posterior approach,[25] a curvilinear incision is made from several centimeters proximal to the lateral epicondyle on the supracondylar ridge, anterior to the lateral epicondyle, and distally to the ulnar side of Lister's tubercle. The interval between ECRB and the extensor digitorum communis (EDC) is identified, and the fascia is incised. If difficulty is encountered in entering this interval, distal palpation of the abductor pollicis longus (APL) and extensor pollicis brevis can be used to identify the plane between the ECRB and the EDC, and the dissection is carried from distal to proximal, mobilizing the ECRB and EDC to reveal the supinator muscle covering the proximal radius.

At this point, the PIN can be identified proximally or distally in the supinator muscle. From proximal to distal, the origin of the ECRB and ECRL are detached from the lateral epicondyle and retracted. The PIN is identified at the proximal border of the supinator, and the arcade of Frohse is identified. The dissection of the PIN and release from potential sites of compression proceed as previously described.

Another approach is to identify the PIN distally and trace it proximally through the supinator muscle. The dissection is then carried proximally, the leash of Henry is identified, and muscular branches are ligated. The PIN or the proper radial nerve is dissected free from fascial and muscular adhesions on the joint capsule up to the level of the lateral epicondyle.

Transmuscular Brachioradialis-Splitting Approach

Multiple skin incisions have been described for the transmuscular brachioradialis-splitting approach.[5] Straight longitudinal,[3] S-shaped curvilinear,[26] and transverse incisions have been recommended.[5] The subcutaneous tissue is divided, and the lateral antebrachial cutaneous nerve identified and protected if present. The BR is identified by palpation, and the fascia covering it is split longitudinally. With use of blunt dissection, the BR is divided by the surgeon while two retractors are used to maintain the interval created. The dissection proceeds until a layer of fat is visualized. The dorsal sensory branch of the radial nerve is identified in the fat, and beneath that the PIN and the proximal border of the supinator muscle are identified. After the branches of the radial nerve are identified, the exposure is extended by further distal and proximal splitting of the BR. Potential compressing structures can now be identified and released from proximal to distal within the window of the BR muscle.

Approach Through the Brachioradialis/Extensor Carpi Radialis Longus Interval

A lazy S-shaped incision is made over the BR-ECRL interval.[27] The subcutaneous tissues are divided, and the interval between the BR and ECRL is identified. Care is taken to identify and protect the lateral antebrachial cutaneous nerve. The interval between the BR and ECRL is developed from their origins on the lateral epicondyle to the middle of the supinator. The dorsal sensory branch of the radial nerve is identified and traced proximally. The PIN is identified. Proximal dissection also reveals motor branches from the radial or PIN to the ECRB. Retraction of the ECRL and ECRB laterally allows for exposure of the distal border of the supinator muscle and release of the remainder of the supinator muscle.

Surgical Decision Making

The operative approach used should be individualized and depends on the expected location of pathology and the surgeon's experience. Advantages and disadvantages for each procedure are summarized in Table 51-1 (online).

Results of Surgical Treatment

Initial reports of operative treatment for radial tunnel syndrome were favorable, but recent reports have been less favorable. See Table 51-2 (online) for a summary of relevant reported studies.

Complications of Surgical Treatment

Postoperative problems resulting from surgical decompression of the radial tunnel vary. Hypertrophic scarring requiring steroid injection and even excision or Z-plasty has been reported[6,12,14] as symptoms due to ECRB scarring has been identified during revision surgery.[6] Superficial radial neurapraxia has also been reported by multiple authors and usually resolves without complication.[12-14] Complete PIN palsy has been reported[12] and resolved with conservative treatment. The development of complex regional pain syndrome, also known as reflex sympathetic dystrophy, has also been reported but is not common.[6,20] Treatment with stellate ganglion blocks and hand therapy resulted in resolution. With strict adherence to operative technique, other complications, including infection, hematoma, and elbow stiffness, are rare.

Radial Sensory Nerve Compression

Anatomy

In 1932, Wartenberg described five cases of compression of the superficial branch of the radial nerve as a mononeuritis termed *cheiralgia paresthetica,* which is commonly referred to today as Wartenberg's syndrome.[28] Entrapment of the sensory branch of the radial nerve was actually first reported in 1926 by Matzdorff.[29]

The radial nerve is a branch off the posterior cord of the brachial plexus and comprises the anterior divisions of nerve roots C5, 6, 7, and 8. Once the nerve is formed, it courses anterior to the subscapularis, teres major, and latissimus dorsi muscles before passing deep to the long head of the triceps. Subsequently, the radial nerve passes through the posterior space and then goes between the medial and lateral heads of the triceps to lie in close approximation to the posterior shaft of the humerus.

On the humeral shaft, the nerve lies in the spiral groove and proceeds distally through the lateral intermuscular septum to run directly over the annular ligament at the level of the radial head. Distal to the lateral epicondyle of the distal humerus, the radial nerve divides into the superifical radial nerve and the posterior interosseous nerve.

The superficial branch of the radial nerve, the dorsal radial sensory nerve (DRSN), initially lies deep to the brachioradialis muscle. Subsequently, it passes between the BR and the ECRL muscles to emerge from under the lateral border of the BR muscle. At this point, the nerve runs in the subcutaneous tissue to provide sensation to the radial aspect of the dorsum of the hand. In 3% to 10% of individuals, the DRSN pierces the tendon of the BR to become subcutaneous. Another anatomic variation described is the presence of a split BR tendon with exiting of the DRSN between the two slips of tendon. Turkof and coworkers demonstrated this anomaly to be present in 3.3% of 150 dissected arms.[30]

The DRSN terminates in three branches: a dorsal branch, a palmar branch, and a branch that becomes the dorsoulnar and dorsoradial digital nerve of the index and long fingers. The dorsal branch innervates the cutaneous area of the dorsal ulnar aspect of the thumb and the dorsal radial aspect of the index finger, whereas the palmar branch innervates the cutaneous area of the dorsal radial aspect of the thumb.

Compression of the DRSN has been shown to occur at two potential sites. The first is where the DRSN emerges between the tendons of the BR and the ECRL. Pronation of the forearm causes these tendons to come together and compress the nerve. Repetitive pronation and supination may cause compression at this site secondary to the creation of a scissoring effect. The scissoring effect occurs because these tendons are free to adjust their position with these movements, however, the DRSN is tethered by fascial attachments and ultimately scar tissue.[31] The other potential site of compression is where the DRSN runs in the subcutaneous tissue in the distal forearm.[31] Compression occurs at this site secondary to the lack of excursion the nerve requires during repetitive wrist flexion and ulnar deviation.[31]

Clinical Examination

Patients with radial sensory nerve entrapment, Wartenberg's syndrome, typically present with complaints of pain and a burning sensation over the dorsoradial aspect of the forearm and wrist. These symptoms are often exacerbated by palmar flexion and ulnar deviation of the wrist. In addition, rapid, repeated pronation and supination of the forearm has been shown to exacerbate symptoms.[31] These activities may include the use of a screwdriver, using a typewriter, computer keyboard, or prolonged use of a pen for writing. Patients may also complain of grip strength weakness, occurring secondary to pain.[31] Symptoms may manifest due to a tight wristwatch[28,29,32,33] or use of handcuffs.[34] Other causal factors may include diabetes,[28] repeated exposure to severe cold,[28] trauma,[28,32,35] and lipomas.[36]

Physical examination for radial sensory nerve entrapment can be performed by way of provocative maneuvers. Tinel's sign over the radial aspect of the midforearm is usually positive in nerve entrapement.[16] The clinician can also perform the so-called false-positive Finkelstein's test. The test is positive if pain is produced with flexion of the thumb and ulnar deviation at the wrist.[37]

It is important for the clinician to recognize the potential for other factors causing similar symptomology. De Quervain's tenosynovitis must be considered when evaluating for compression of the radial sensory nerve. Pick reported that the diagnosis of this entity is based on the presence of local swelling, point tenderness over the first dorsal compartment, and a positive Finkelstein's test.[38] A Finkelstein's test is performed by palmar flexion and ulnar deviation of the wrist as well as adduction of the thumb. The test is considered positive when these maneuvers elicit pain over the dorsal radial forearm. This can be differentiated from the earlier described false-positive Finkelstein's test seen in radial sensory nerve entrapment, since the false-positive Finkelstein's test is independent of thumb position.[18] Another differentiation is that patients with de Quervain's tenosynovitis should have a normal sensory exam in the distribution of the DRSN.

The cutaneous distribution of the lateral antebrachial cutaneous nerve has been shown to overlap with the cutaneous distribution of the radial sensory nerve in 75% of patients.[39] The lateral antebrachial cutaneous nerve can easily be injured during release of the first dorsal extensor compartment. Neuroma-like symptoms around the incision can be related to either the lateral antebrachial cutaneous nerve or the radial sensory nerve. Injury to these nerves can be differentiated by performing a nerve block.[16] This procedure is performed by injecting local anesthetic superficial to the fascia in the proximal third of the forearm to block the lateral antebrachial cutaneous nerve. If the lateral antebrachial cutaneous nerve is the cause of the patient's complaints, the symptoms should be relieved temporarily. If the symptoms persist, the sensory branch of the radial nerve can be injected where it emerges between the BR and ECRL tendons.[31]

Cervical disk disease causing radiculopathy must be investigated; therefore, a thorough physical examination including assessment for cervical spine pathology should be performed.

Electrophysiologic Evaluation

The utilization of electrophysiologic tests for the diagnosis of radial sensory nerve compression has demonstrated usefulness in the literature. Dellon and Mackinnon found that 16 of 19 examinations demonstrated a focal conduction block or localized site of radial sensory nerve entrapment.[31]

Nonoperative Treatment

Management of DRSN compression is attempted nonoperatively before surgical intervention is undertaken. Therapist's management is covered in Chapter 52. In addition to therapy, a local corticosteroid injection can be performed in the area of entrapment between the tendons of the BR and ECRL.

Operative Treatment

Operative treatment of radial sensory nerve entrapment is performed to free the nerve from any potential sites of compression. A volar approach is recommended to avoid making an incision directly over the course of the nerve, which may involve the nerve in postoperative scar.[16] The fascia along the course of the nerve is freed distally and proximally for a total of approximately 10 cm, thus allowing the nerve more excursion during wrist flexion and ulnar deviation. It is important to be careful not to damage any of the crossing branches of the lateral antebrachial cutaneous nerve. In addition, the radial sensory nerve should be decompressed in the area between the tendons of the BR and ECRL tendons to prevent any scissoring effects. This can be performed by resecting a portion of the BR tendon.[40] If the nerve emerges between two slips of BR tendon, the dorsal slip, which is usually thinner, should be resected.[41] The wound is then thoroughly irrigated and closed. A bulky dressing is applied and the wrist in placed in neutral.

Dellon and Mackinnon demonstrated 85% good or excellent results with operative intervention.[42]

Rehabilitation

The patient is seen in follow-up 3 to 5 days after surgery. The dressings are removed, and the patient is encouraged to begin active range-of-motion exercises of the fingers, wrist, and elbow. Physical or occupational therapy (or both) is prescribed for desensitization of the radial sensory nerve distribution. Heavy lifting should be avoided for approximately 4 weeks. Full activity and return to work without restrictions can be expected by 6 to 8 weeks after surgery. See Chapter 52 for a full discussion of postoperative rehabilitation.

Anterior Interosseous Nerve/ Pronator Syndrome

Anatomy

Median nerve compression in the proximal forearm was originally described in 1951 by Seyffarth, who coined the term *pronator syndrome* to describe the symptomology of aching pain in the forearm and wrist as well as paresthesias in the median nerve distribution.[43] The median nerve is formed by the convergence of the medial and lateral cords and comprises the anterior divisions of nerve roots C5, 6, 7, 8, and T1. Once the nerve is formed, it travels along the medial aspect of the arm medial to the brachial artery, without giving off any branches, until it reaches the area of the pronator teres muscle. The branches that arise in this area sequentially innervate the pronator teres, flexor carpi radialis, palmaris longus, and the flexor digitorum superficialis (FDS).

The median nerve passes deep to the lacertus fibrosis before passing between the two heads of the pronator teres muscle, the humeral head, and the ulnar head. The nerve subsequently continues between the FDS and profundus. Just proximal to the wrist, the nerve becomes more superficial, traveling between the tendons of the FDS and flexor carpi radialis. The median nerve then lies immediately deep to the palmaris longus tendon just before entering the carpal tunnel at the distal skin crease of the wrist.

The anterior interosseous nerve (AIN) is a major branch of the median nerve, which arises 5 to 8 cm distal to the medial epicondyle, just distal to the proximal border of the ulnar head of the pronator teres.[44] The AIN continues distally with the median nerve, lying anteriorly on the interosseous membrane, to supply motor branches to the flexor pollicis longus, flexor digitorum profundus of the index and long fingers, and the pronator quadratus, where it terminates.

Multiple sites of compression have been described in the literature as potential causes for pronator syndrome. The most proximal site of compression is beneath the ligament of Struthers secondary to a supracondylar process on the distal humerus.[45-47] As the nerve travels distally, the next potential site of compression is where it passes deep to the lacertus fibrosis.[45,48-54] More distal, the nerve courses between the two heads of the pronator teres muscle. At this juncture, the nerve can be compressed by fibrous bands between the muscle heads, a fibrous arch across the ulnar head, or from a tendinous ulnar head.[45,48-52,55] Beaton and Anson noted that the nerve passed between both heads of the pronator muscle in 82.5% of 240 arms. The nerve passed below a solitary humeral head in 8.8% of the arms and below both heads in 6.3% of the arms. The nerve pierced the humeral head in 2.5% of the arms.[56] In addition, vascular leashes that cross the nerve may be potential sites of compression.[49,50] Finally, the median nerve may be compressed in the proximal forearm by an arch formed by the FDS muscle.[45,48-52,55]

Another diagnosis that can occur secondary to compression is AIN syndrome, which was first described in 1952 by Kiloh and Nevin.[57] This entity causes a pure motor deficit since the AIN, as described earlier, is purely a motor branch of the median nerve. Potential sites of compression of this nerve include the humeral head of the pronator teres, the FDS as it courses with the median nerve through the arch of this muscle, an accessory head of the flexor pollicis longus (Gantzer's muscle), a tendinous origin of the palmaris profundus, and an accessory lacertus fibrosis.[44]

Clinical Examination

Pronator syndrome typically presents with patients complaining of pain in the volar aspect of their proximal forearm. Activities such as repetitive pronation and supination aggravate the symptoms. Additional complaints of patients include paresthesias in the thumb, index, and long fingers, as well as numbness in the palm in the distribution of the palmar cutaneous branch of the median nerve. These symptoms can be differentiated from CTS due to the lack of nocturnal symptoms.[57-60]

Physical assessment for pronator syndrome can be performed by trying to elicit pain when creating tension on potential anatomic sites of compression. The first maneuver involves trying to reproduce symptoms by assessing resisted forearm pronation, with the forearm in neutral, as the elbow is gradually extended. Symptoms that correlate with this maneuver indicate compression at the pronator teres muscle. In addition, one can attempt to elicit pain with resisted elbow flexion at 120 to 130 degrees with the forearm in the supinated position.[59] This maneuver correlates with compression occurring at the lacertus fibrosis. The clinician can also attempt to elicit symptoms by resisting flexion of the proximal interphalangeal joint of the long finger. Positive correlation of symptoms with this maneuver demonstrates compression at the FDS.[58] Lastly, the pronator compression test can be performed to aid in accurate diagnosis of pronator syndrome. This test is performed by having the examiner place pressure over the area of the pronator teres on both upper extremities. A positive test occurs when there are paresthesias in the median nerve distribution of the involved extremity, occurring within 30 seconds, and no paresthesias in the uninvolved extremity.

Patients with AIN syndrome also complain of pain in the proximal volar forearm, and their symptoms are aggravated with repetitive forearm motion.[57,59] In addition, patients may complain of difficulty with fine-motor movements, such as writing or picking up small objects. This is caused by weakness in the muscles innervated by the AIN. These muscles include the pronator quadratus, the flexor pollicis longus, and the flexor digitorum profundus of the index. It is important to note that patients with AIN syndrome do not complain of paresthesias. Physical examination assessment of AIN syndrome includes manual muscle testing of the muscles innervated by the AIN and observation of pinch.

The clinician must recognize the potential for other factors causing similar complaints. A thorough physical examination including assessment for cervical spine pathology should be performed. Potential causative factors can include cervical radiculopathy, brachial plexopathy, and thoracic outlet syndrome. In addition, CTS must be considered as a potential diagnosis. Therefore, Phalen's test and Tinel's sign for the median nerve at the level of the wrist should be performed. CTS has a significant correlation with nocturnal symptoms, whereas pronator syndrome does not.

The double-crush syndrome can cause a symptomatic compression neuropathy secondary to multiple sites of compression along the course of a single nerve. Neural function can become impaired secondary to single axons, compressed at one site, rendering the nerve more susceptible to damage at another site.[61]

Electrophysiologic Evaluation

Electrophysiologic testing for the diagnosis of pronator syndrome has been somewhat controversial in the literature.[48,58,59] Studies have demonstrated that the use of nerve conduction studies have not been a sensitive indicator of median nerve entrapment in the proximal forearm and elbow.[59,62] One reason for this is that Tetro and Pichora have demonstrated that CTS may cause slowing of median NCV for a variable distance proximal to the wrist.[59] Hartz and colleagues also demonstrated in their study that localization of the abnormality found in electrophysiologic testing was only rarely possible.[50] However, more reliable results have been demonstrated with EMG studies.[48,62] The most beneficial aspect of electrophysiologic testing may be in ruling out CTS as a potential confounder when diagnosing other compression lesions of the median nerve.[58,59]

Nonoperative Treatment

Haussmann and Patel have shown that half of patients diagnosed with pronator syndrome recover within 4 months.[57] The first step in managing pronator or AIN syndrome is to have the patient avoid any aggravating activities. These activities, as mentioned earlier, are often related to repetitive pronation–supination or forceful grip activities, such as weight-lifting and tennis. The patient may also benefit from resting the extremity for approximately 2 weeks in a posterior elbow orthosis with the elbow in 90 degrees of flexion and the forearm in neutral rotation. A full discussion of the therapist's management for pronator or AIN syndrome follows in Chapter 52. Cortisone injections into the area of the pronator teres have been suggested when other options have been unsuccessful.[58,59]

Operative Treatment

Operative treatment has been recommended only after conservative measures have failed to provide relief after 8 to 12 weeks. It is imperative that decompression of the median nerve occurs at all possible sites of compression.[58] Therefore, the surgical technique is the same for both pronator syndrome and AIN syndrome.

Mackinnon has described the following technique. The patient is placed supine on an operating room table with the affected extremity placed on a hand table. A tourniquet is applied. The incision is described as a lazy S that begins in the antecubital fossa and progresses distally for about 10 cm. Dissection is carried out through the soft tissue, taking care to preserve cutaneous sensory branches of the nerve. The lacertus fibrosis is identified and divided. This eliminates the first potential site of compression. Following that, the tendon of the ulnar head of the pronator teres is identified in the distal extent of the incision. This tendon is extended utilizing step-lengthening, thus releasing compression off the median nerve at the level of the pronator teres. The median nerve is followed distally to identify the insertion of the ulnar head of the pronator teres. The tendinous portion of the ulnar head of the pronator teres is excised. The arch of the tendinous portion of the FDS is identified and divided, thus releasing the next potential site of compression.

Once these structures have been released, the surgeon can follow the median nerve proximally with a finger to evaluate for the presence of a ligament of Struthers. If the ligament is present, the skin incision can be extended proximally above the elbow crease. The ligament can be identified and divided if present.

The wound is then thoroughly irrigated, and the subcutaneous tissues and skin are closed. A bulky dressing is placed with a posterior orthosis. The elbow should be slightly flexed and the wrist in the neutral position.[40] Tetro and Pichora have shown that most studies report 85% to 90% good to excellent outcomes following surgical decompression.[59]

Rehabilitation

The patient is seen in follow-up 3 to 5 days after surgery. The orthosis and dressings are removed, and the patient is

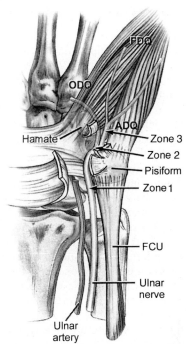

Figure 51-6 The three zones of Guyon's canal. The volar carpal ligament has been reflected to reveal zone 1, which contains both the motor and sensory fascicles of the ulnar nerve. Zone 2 is made up of motor fibers and dives deep to the hypothenar musculature to curve radially around the hamate book. Zone 3 is made up of the sensory branch and is superfical to the musculature and follows the main trunk of the ulnar artery. (From Berger RA, Weiss A-PC, eds. *Hand Surgery*. Philadelphia; Lippincott Williams & Wilkins, 2003.)

encouraged to begin active range-of-motion exercises of the fingers, wrist, and elbow. During the first 2 weeks, an orthosis or sling may be used at night for patient comfort to prevent full elbow extension. The patient should continue exercises in an attempt to regain full elbow extension and forearm supination. Full activity and return to work without restrictions can be expected by 6 to 8 weeks after surgery.

Ulnar Tunnel Syndrome

Anatomy

Several authors have described the three anatomic zones of the ulnar tunnel or Guyon's canal.[63-65] Zone 1 contains motor and sensory branches of the ulnar nerve and is bordered by the flexor digitorum profundus and transverse carpal ligament dorsally, the FCU tendon and pisiform ulnarly, and the volar carpal ligament radially and volarly. Zone 2 contains the motor branch only and if compressed produces motor changes only. The borders in this zone are the palmaris brevis muscle dorsally, opponens digiti minimi, pisohamate and pisometacarpal ligaments volarly, abductor digiti minimi ulnarly, and transverse carpal ligament and flexor digiti minimi radially. Zone 3 contains only the sensory branch, and its borders include the palmaris brevis muscle dorsally, hypothenar fascia volarly, abductor digiti minimi ulnarly, and the long flexor tendons radially (Fig. 51-6). Zone 1 injuries occur more frequently than injuries in the other zones.[63,64]

Clinical Features and Examination

Space-occupying lesions such as ganglions, benign tumors including lipomas, and anomalous muscles are primary contributors to ulnar tunnel syndrome.[65] Other causes include trauma from hamate fractures and persistent or prolonged compression of the hypothenar eminence from using the hand as a "hammer,"[65] pneumatic tool use,[66] and resting on handlebars of a bicycle.[67,68] Dupuytren's disease, rheumatoid arthritis, burns, and scleroderma may also contribute space-occupying lesions.[65,69,70]

Sensory symptoms such as pain and paresthesias are typically worse at night and exacerbated by prolonged wrist flexion or extension. The sensory changes occur only in the volar aspect of the ulnar nerve sensory distribution in the ring and small digits, thereby distinguishing ulnar tunnel syndrome from cubital tunnel syndrome. Patients often report exquisite tenderness over the hook of the hamate. Prolonged compression of the motor nerve fibers in zones 1 and 2 may result in intrinsic muscle weakness, especially of the interossei, ulnar lumbricals, and the adductor pollicis. The hypothenar muscles may be spared with zone 2 injuries. Prolonged compression may result in a typical ulnar claw deformity of the hand.[65]

The patient's history regarding the mechanism of injury to the ulnar nerve guides the clinical examination, especially if co-morbidities are present that might increase the index of suspicion for a space-occupying lesion if no specific incident or trauma is reported. Standard radiographs should include standard lateral and anteroposterior views as well as a carpal tunnel view. CT and MRI may help differentiate fractures and determine the nature of space-occupying lesions. Electrodiagnostic tools aid diagnosis and may localize the zone of injury. Testing across the elbow should be included to rule out cubital tunnel syndrome.[65]

Treatment

Surgical decompression is indicated and considered the mainstay of treatment in patients with space-occupying lesions and some fractures. Nonoperative management is discussed in detail in Chapter 52, and it may be necessary for those patients who do not respond to typical medical treatment with NSAIDs, a resting wrist orthosis, and ergonomic modifications, and who do not present with a space-occupying lesion or fracture.[65]

Summary

Careful history and physical examination, as well as appropriate diagnostic studies, are mandatory in the diagnosis of nerve compressions of the wrist and elbow. Other pathologic conditions that cause similar signs and symptoms must be ruled out. After diagnosis, nonoperative treatment modalities should be exhausted before surgical intervention. The selection of an operative approach should be made individually, based on the suggested area of compression, the presence of other existing pathology, and the surgeon's experience. All potential areas of compression should be identified and explored. Surgical intervention is followed by a course of rehabilitation and a home program of exercises specific to the nerve that has been decompressed and the procedure performed.

REFERENCES

The complete reference list is available online at www.expertconsult.com.

Therapist's Management of Other Nerve Compressions About the Elbow and Wrist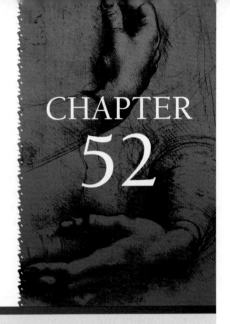

ANN PORRETTO-LOEHRKE, PT, DPT, CHT, COMT AND
ELIZABETH SOIKA, PT, DPT, CHT

CRITICAL POINTS

Principles of Conservative Management

- Muscle length and myofascial mobility
- Neural mobilization
- Orthoses and protection
- Activity modification

Concepts of Neural Mobilization

- **F**ix the adjacent joint
- **L**imit the range of motion (ROM)
- **O**scillate proximal or distal (or both) to level of compression
- **S**low, rhythmic motion
- **S**ymptom free

Principles of Postoperative Management

- Protected ROM
- Neural mobilization
- Scar management
- Sensory desensitization
- Activity modification

For the upper extremity specialist, identifying and treating nerve compression syndromes about the elbow, forearm, and wrist can be both challenging and frustrating. Unless referred by a highly skilled physician, these patients present to therapy with such vague prescriptions as "elbow pain—please evaluate and treat." Often, these conditions are classified as repetitive stress injuries (RSI) in patients who are involved in occupational or recreational activities that have precipitated or exacerbated their symptoms over time. This chapter covers conservative and postoperative management of cubital tunnel syndrome at the elbow, radial tunnel as well as pronator

syndrome at the forearm, and Wartenberg's and ulnar tunnel (also known as Guyon's canal) syndromes at the wrist.

History

The patient's history is one of the most critical elements of the examination and provides useful information for formulating a plan of care. When taking a patient's history, it is important to ask the following six questions: Who? What? Where? When? Why? To What Extent?

Who? The patient's age, gender, past medical history, and social history can provide essential clues for the therapist. Was there a recent trauma, such as a motor vehicle accident, that caused the onset of symptoms? Was there a history of a childhood fracture that may have caused compensation patterns that are now contributing to the patient's problem? Other medical conditions such as diabetes mellitus and hypothyroidism can predispose patients to peripheral nerve compression syndromes.[1,2]

What? What are the patient's primary complaints? Does the patient describe symptoms of burning, numbness and tingling, pain, or weakness? How long have the symptoms been present? Were they of sudden onset or more gradual? Is there a specific activity or motion that provokes or exacerbates the patient's symptoms?

Where? Where are the symptoms located? Are they localized to one specific region, or do they tend to travel? This can assist the therapist in identifying a localized nerve entrapment versus more vague complaints that may be indicative of a proximal component.

When? When do the symptoms occur? Are they provoked with a specific activity or do they have a delayed onset? Responses to these questions provide clues about the chronicity of the problem. In the work environment, does the patient's job involve repetitive elbow flexion and extension while standing on a production line? At night, does the patient have a tendency to sleep in a fetal position with elbows maintained in flexion?

Why? Has the patient experienced these symptoms in the past, or is this a new onset? What caused the patient to seek out treatment for this problem? What is the patient now unable to do? Often, patients with more chronic issues describe a history of mild pain or paresthesias that slowly progresses to the point of limiting function. This is the stage at which most patients seek treatment.

To what extent? Are the symptoms merely bothersome or are they limiting the patient's ability to perform specific work-related tasks or fulfill social roles such as caring for a child? Answers to this question enable the clinician to determine the degree of irritability present at the nerve compression site. Are the patient's symptoms considered highly irritable or mildly irritable? Does the patient take anti-inflammatory or other medications to perform daily tasks?

Responses to these six questions give the therapist a clinical picture of the patient's condition that help guide the examination process and ultimately determine how to proceed with conservative treatment.

To ensure the best possible outcome, it is critical to perform a proximal screen to rule out cervical involvement and thoracic outlet syndrome (TOS). This can be performed in a relatively quick, systematic fashion. An upper quarter screening exam, described in Chapter 10, involves examining cervical spine and upper extremity motion for limitations and pain. The screening exam also checks the cervical myotomes and dermatomes for overt neurologic "red flags." Spurling's maneuver, also described in Chapter 10, is also helpful for ruling out cervical nerve root conditions resulting from foraminal encroachment. A positive test indicates involvement of the cervical spine in producing the patient's distal upper extremity complaints.

The elevated arm stress test (EAST) (also known as the *Roos test*) and Cyriax release test (CRT) can be utilized to rule out symptoms originating from the thoracic outlet region. The EAST involves asking the patient to place the shoulders at 90 degrees of abduction and elbows at 90 degrees of flexion (Fig. 52-1). The patient then performs rhythmic hand grasping and releasing for 3 minutes, or until distal symptoms are provoked.[3] The CRT, originally described by Dr. James Cyriax, is performed by elevating, or "unloading," the upper extremities by performing passive scapular elevation.[4] This is best accomplished by having the patient sitting in a comfortable position with arms supported on a tabletop or pillows. The therapist stands behind the patient and passively elevates the scapulae by supporting the patient's elbows and forearms as in Figure 52-2. This position is held for 3 minutes or until symptoms are reproduced. As with the EAST, a positive test results in reproduction of the patient's distal complaints. The sensitivity and specificity of the EAST and CRT have not been reported to date. It is important that therapists consider the entire cluster of signs and symptoms observed during the physical examination and not rely on just the results of a few special tests to make their therapy diagnosis.

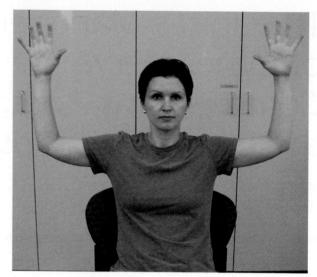

Figure 52-1 Elevated arm stress test.

In some instances a patient may present with positive provocative signs with both localized testing as well as with cervical or TOS testing. In these cases, it is important to address both the proximal and distal issues as part of the treatment program to ensure optimal outcomes. A study by Smith and colleagues found a significantly greater number of cyclists with clinical signs and symptoms of ulnar neuropathy also presented with positive clinical tests indicative of TOS, suggesting a double-crush phenomenon.[5] Forty-three percent of these subjects tested positive with the CRT and 32% positive with the EAST.

Following completion of the proximal screen, the therapist can perform specific provocative tests for each distal nerve compression syndrome. These are discussed in detail later in the chapter.

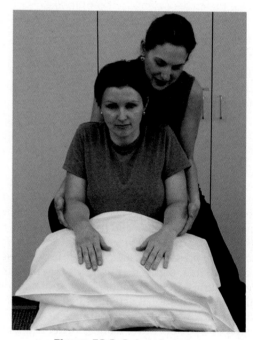

Figure 52-2 Cyriax release test.

Basic Principles of Conservative Management

The therapist needs to consider four main principles when initiating treatment for peripheral nerve compressions. These concepts are introduced in this section, but are explained in more detail under each syndrome. The four principles, shown in the first section of the critical points list at the beginning of the chapter, include addressing muscle length and myofascial mobility, neural mobilization, orthoses and protection, and activity modification.

Muscle Length and Myofascial Mobility

The development of peripheral nerve compression is often the product of a cycle of overuse, inflammation, nerve irritation, and muscle guarding. Over time, muscles and their adjacent fascia can become hypomobile, leading to increased stress on the peripheral nerves during activities. Localized manual treatment techniques, such as myofascial release or slow, prolonged stretch, can be beneficial for these patients. To avoid ischemia resulting from increased neural tension, the peripheral nerve must be placed on slack both proximal and distal to the area being treated. This is critical for patients whose nerves are in a highly irritable stage. To place a peripheral nerve on slack proximally, instruct the patient to perform active scapular elevation combined with tipping the head to the involved side (i.e., ipsilateral cervical side-bending). Slackening the distal portion of the nerve depends on which nerve entrapment syndrome is being addressed. Other treatment techniques, such as use of Kinesio tape, can improve myofascial mobility. Thermal modalities such as moist heat and continuous ultrasound may also be beneficial in facilitating blood flow to the involved area prior to and during muscle stretching.

Neural Mobilization

The second principle of conservative management can be addressed early in rehabilitation while improving myofascial mobility. The goal of neural mobilization is twofold: improving both extraneural (i.e., epineurium in relation to its surrounding soft tissues) and intraneural (i.e., axonal flow and intrafascicular motion) mobility.[6,7] The principles of neural mobilization are based on the anatomic and biomechanical properties of peripheral nerves and their response to stress and strain. Chapter 118 provides a detailed review of the literature on nerve mobilization for examination and treatment of the peripheral nervous system.

The biggest mistake therapists make with neural mobilization techniques is doing too much too fast. It is important for the treating therapist to possess a basic understanding of the biomechanical properties of peripheral nerves when initiating a neural mobilization program. Strain is defined as the change in nerve length induced by a longitudinal tensile stress. This is referred to as percent elongation.[8] Gliding of the nerve relative to its surrounding nerve bed is called excursion.[9] The goal of neural mobilization is to maximize the excursion of the nerve while minimizing the strain. Stretching a nerve more than 8% beyond its resting length causes venous congestion and inhibits blood flow; therefore, it is critical to avoid placing strain on the nerve with mobilization techniques.[10] Rather than tensioning the nerve, the authors prefer to glide, or "floss," the nerve. The flossing motion is similar to flossing teeth—the entire nerve segment moves proximally, then distally. "Neural flossing" can provide excellent neural mobilization while avoiding tension on the nerve.

Butler describes "sliding techniques," which involve elongation of the nerve bed at one joint while reducing the length of the nerve bed at an adjacent joint.[6] This method promotes larger longitudinal excursion of the nerve while minimizing the strain. Coppieters and Butler confirmed the clinical assumption that sliding techniques result in a substantially larger excursion of the nerve than traditional tensioning techniques.[11] The nerve segment closest to the moving joint undergoes the greatest amount of strain.[12] When performing neural mobilization for a specific nerve compression syndrome, it is important to avoid active ROM at the joint closest to the involved site in a highly irritable stage. For example, performing a neural mobilization technique for a patient with cubital tunnel syndrome involves maintaining the elbow in a static position while placing the nerve on slack proximally and performing gentle ROM with the wrist and digits. Nerve stiffness is greater when a nerve is elongated more quickly; therefore, it is important that nerve mobilization techniques be performed in a slow, rhythmic fashion to avoid excess strain.[13] Slow, rhythmic neural gliding techniques, with the therapist taking care to avoid stretch on the nerve, are especially beneficial for patients with highly irritable nerve compression syndromes.

If a patient has been immobilized in a cast or orthosis, the nerve becomes less tolerant to strain. To avoid adverse neural tension, a therapist must be cognizant of this when initiating neural mobilization. Symptoms of this may include pain, paresthesias, and protective reflexes.[13]

The mnemonic **FLOSS** sums up the general concepts of neural mobilization that ensure safe and effective treatment. FLOSS is described throughout this chapter with each nerve compression syndrome.

Fix the adjacent joint
Limit the ROM
Oscillate proximal or distal (or both) to level of compression
Slow, rhythmic motion
Symptom free

Orthoses and Protection

The third component provides a means of diminishing neural tension to create a healing environment. Orthoses are generally used to abate acute symptoms or symptoms that are observed at rest and increased with activity. Orthoses and the use of Kinesio tape can be beneficial in preventing patients from inadvertently performing aggravating motions both day and night. With motor involvement, use of orthoses can improve patient function.

Activity Modification

The fourth principle involves patient education in avoiding motions and positions that create stress on the peripheral nerve. Repetitive loading can result in physiologic and structural alterations in the nerve.[13] This principle accounts for both how the patient moves (i.e., posture and neuromuscular control) and ergonomics with home and work-related tasks. Helping the patient to understand how movements and positions provoke symptoms often helps to alleviate nerve irritation with daily activities. Posture and muscular recruitment patterns greatly affect how a patient regularly uses the involved arm. Simple suggestions about keyboard height or use of a headset, for instance, can have a profound effect on curbing the cycle of overuse.

With all distal upper extremity nerve compression syndromes, it is important to consider the patient's entire body habitus, especially during activities that provoke symptoms. Poor recruitment of large muscle groups, such as the abdominals and scapular stabilizers, leads to heavy reliance on the small distal musculature of the forearm and wrist. How many patients with cubital tunnel syndrome find themselves leaning on their involved elbow while working at the computer? Neuromuscular reeducation to improve core stability promotes optimal scapular positioning while effectively unloading the involved structure, allowing for rest and healing during daily activities. At the shoulder girdle, strengthening scapular stabilizers and rotator cuff muscles minimizes distal compensation patterns. Use of a figure-of-8 or clavicle strap is also beneficial, especially in the early stages of rehabilitation (Fig. 52-3).

Basic Principles of Postoperative Management

The principles of postoperative management, described in the third part of the critical points list at the beginning of the chapter, include performing protected ROM and use of orthoses if needed, neural mobilization, scar management, sensory desensitization, and activity modification.

Protected Range of Motion

Initiate gentle motion within a range that avoids placing stress on the structure that was released or repaired. For example, a patient with a radial tunnel release may need to avoid end-range forearm pronation early in the rehabilitative process to prevent tension at the surgical site or the nerve. Protected ROM applies to some, but not all, postoperative programs. ROM considerations for each procedure are covered in detail later in the chapter. The use of orthoses can be beneficial for protection of the repaired structures or minimization of neural tension. A long arm orthosis may be utilized for a patient with a submuscular ulnar nerve transposition for protection of the flexor–pronator group that was cut during the procedure. Specific use of orthoses are discussed with postoperative management.

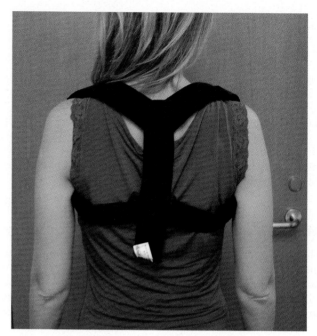

Figure 52-3 Figure-of-8 strap.

Neural Mobilization

Restoring neural mobility can minimize adherence from scar tissue formation at the release site, while facilitating mobilization of the perineural fascia proximal and distal to the original site of entrapment. When initiating neural mobilization after surgery, it is critical for the therapist to understand the pathway of the peripheral nerve. An "in situ" ulnar nerve decompression maintains the ulnar nerve in the cubital tunnel behind the medial epicondyle, whereas an ulnar nerve transposition reroutes the nerve to the anterior aspect of the elbow. Reviewing the patient's surgical report can give the treating therapist a clear picture of the nerve pathway, allowing for optimal treatment.

Scar Management

This involves performing superficial and deep scar tissue mobilization over the closed incision to optimize differential gliding between the scar and surrounding soft tissue. Following removal of stitches and closure of the suture line, the patient is instructed in scar tissue mobilization. It is important to avoid sliding over the skin, but rather maintaining firm contact to move the deeper tissue beneath the scar line. Use of silicone gel sheeting (SGS) provides pressure to the healing scar to further enhance scar remodeling (Fig. 52-4). For patients who do not elect to use SGS (due to insurance limitations and out-of-pocket costs), the authors have found Kinesio tape to be a cost-effective and beneficial method of improving scar tissue mobility. Paper tape may be another low-cost alternative. Its use is described in Chapter 49.

Sensory Desensitization

The fourth principle may be used variably with postoperative management. A sensory desensitization program is almost

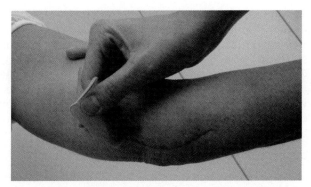

Figure 52-4 Silicone gel sheeting applied to a patient with a subcutaneous ulnar nerve transposition.

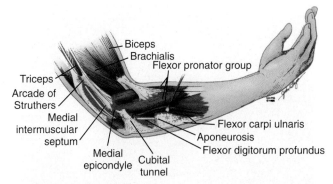

Figure 52-5 Anatomy of the ulnar nerve at the elbow, which demonstrates the five potential sites of nerve compression. (Copyright © The Mayo Foundation. From Amadio PC. Anatomical basis for a technique of ulnar nerve transposition. *Surg Radiol Anat.* 1986;8:155-161.)

always indicated with a radial tunnel release; however, it may not be needed for a patient after a pronator release. Hypersensitivity to external stimuli such as light touch, deep pressure, and vibration can affect quality of life and impair function; therefore, it is important to begin an early, regimented desensitization program as soon as signs or symptoms are identified. This is accomplished by exposing the hypersensitive area to a tolerable stimulus, working from the periphery toward the most sensitive area. A stimulus is deemed tolerable if it approaches the threshold of hypersensitivity but produces minimal discomfort. The patient works from a fine texture such as cotton toward coarser textures like burlap as the area accommodates to the stimulus. Readers are referred to the companion Web site for the Desensitization and Reeducation chapter by Lois Barber from the third edition.

Activity Modification

Just as with conservative treatment, activity modification can play an important role in preventing recurrence of peripheral nerve compression following surgical release. Consideration of the patient's trunk and scapular stability as well as ergonomics optimizes a patient's postsurgical outcome.

Specific Nerve Compression Syndromes

Cubital Tunnel Syndrome

The ulnar nerve courses along the posteriomedial aspect of the humerus and then along the medial elbow within the bony canal formed by the medial epicondyle and olecranon. It then exits beneath the arcuate ligament and enters the forearm between the two heads of the flexor carpi ulnaris (FCU) muscle. Ulnar nerve compression can potentially occur at the arcade of Struthers, a portion of fascia that connects the intermuscular septum and triceps, and within the cubital tunnel itself. The roof of the cubital tunnel consists of the arcuate ligament and the floor consists of the medial collateral ligament (Fig. 52-5). Elbow flexion tightens the roof and the floor of the cubital tunnel, placing increased pressure on the ulnar nerve.[14] Cubital tunnel syndrome is the

second most common nerve compression syndrome in the upper extremity.[15]

When taking the patient's history, complaints of paresthesias or dysesthesias can help in discerning the level of ulnar nerve compression. Complaints of paresthesias on both the volar and dorsal aspects of the ulnar half of the ring finger and entire small finger are indicative of a compression at the level of the cubital tunnel. Conversely, compression of the ulnar nerve at the level of the wrist (i.e., ulnar tunnel, or Guyon's canal) produces paresthesias on the volar aspects of the ulnar ring and small fingers only. When questioning the patient, it is important to consider elbow postures during daily activities and sleep. Does the patient maintain the elbow in a flexed position while on the phone throughout the day? Is there a tendency to rest on the affected elbow while watching TV or driving? Sleeping in the fetal position with terminal elbow flexion can also contribute to ulnar nerve irritation. In advanced cases of cubital tunnel syndrome, patients may present with intrinsic muscle wasting with significant grip and pinch deficits, or complaints of hand clumsiness.

When evaluating a patient with suggested cubital tunnel, it is important to perform a quick screen to rule out TOS, as the ulnar nerve is most often affected. Once the patient is cleared of proximal involvement, localized testing can begin. Observation of the patient's hand posture may reveal first dorsal interosseous atrophy or mild clawing on the ring or small fingers (or both) in advanced cases. Clawing is less pronounced with involvement at the cubital tunnel, versus distally at the ulnar tunnel, as the ulnar-innervated flexor digitorum profundus (FDP) muscles to the ring and small fingers are affected along with the intrinsic muscles. With involvement of the nerve at the ulnar tunnel, the FDP muscles remain intact, which leads to more profound clawing resulting from the imbalance between the intrinsic and extrinsic muscles. With weakness of the intrinsics, the patient may also present with a positive Wartenberg's sign, indicating lack of ability to adduct the small finger.

Hands-on testing of the elbow begins with the elbow flexion test, one of the most sensitive and specific tests for identifying ulnar nerve compression at the cubital tunnel.[7] Prior to performing this test, it is important to observe if the patient's ulnar nerve subluxes anteriorly to the elbow when performing active elbow flexion and extension. This can

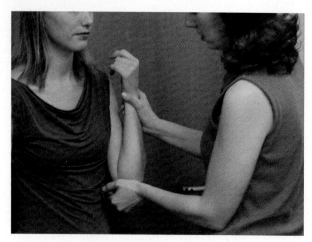

Figure 52-6 Elbow flexion test.

often be palpated at the medial epicondyle and produces an audible "snap." If the ulnar nerve does not sublux, the elbow flexion test can be performed. The authors prefer to maintain the shoulder in a neutral position, versus flexion, to avoid placing tension on the brachial plexus beneath the pectoralis minor muscle. Once the ulnar nerve is identified in the cubital tunnel, manual pressure is applied in the groove as the elbow is placed in terminal flexion with the forearm supported in supination. Care must be taken to maintain the wrist in neutral because flexion can promote compression of the ulnar nerve at the wrist. The test position is held for 60 seconds while the therapist monitors for reproduction of the patient's ulnar nerve symptoms (Fig. 52-6).

Observation of the patient's alignment with elbow flexion is also important because patients with cubital valgus demonstrate higher susceptibility to the development of cubital tunnel syndrome due to tightening of the retinaculum over the ulnar nerve in this position.[16,17]

This is caused by the olecranon process of the ulna moving toward the lateral epicondyle of the humerus during elbow flexion, thereby creating a smaller container for the ulnar nerve within the cubital tunnel. This can be observed with active range-of-motion (AROM) testing or during the elbow flexion test.

Typically, resisted testing does not reproduce symptoms of cubital tunnel syndrome; however, in a small population, resisted elbow extension can reproduce ulnar nerve symptoms. This is due to an anomalous muscle called the anconeus epitrochlearis. Amadio and Beckenbaugh reported that this muscle, which attaches at the medial epicondyle and the olecranon process, occurs in approximately 10% of patients undergoing surgery for cubital tunnel syndrome.[18] Contraction of this muscle places direct compression on the ulnar nerve within the cubital tunnel. Patients who perform repetitive forceful elbow flexion and extension activities may be more at risk for the development of cubital tunnel syndrome due to these biomechanical characteristics.

Strength testing for more involved patients may reveal deficits with lateral pinch and grip. A patient with weakness of the first dorsal interosseous, deep head of flexor pollicis brevis (FPB) and adductor pollicis (AP) muscles demonstrates compensation using the flexor pollicis longus (FPL) muscle with hyperflexion of the thumb interphalangeal (IP)

joint during lateral pinch (positive Froment's sign). The patient may also present with hyperextension at the metacarpophalangeal (MCP) joint (positive Jeanne's sign). Sensory testing can also be performed to differentiate between cubital tunnel and ulnar tunnel syndrome; that is, sensibility deficits of the dorsal ulnar aspect of the hand are present with cubital tunnel but not with ulnar tunnel compression. Details on sensibility testing procedures are provided in Chapter 11.

Conservative Management

Conservative treatment of cubital tunnel syndrome involves use of the four principles described in the first portion of the critical points list at the beginning of the chapter.

Restoring Muscle Length and Myofascial Mobility. The path of the ulnar nerve lies beneath the FCU muscle. Overuse of the flexor–pronator group can contribute to muscle stiffness and loss of myofascial mobility, which can produce stress on the ulnar nerve. Performing myofascial techniques involving slow, prolonged stretch[19] as well as the patient's performing gentle stretching may lessen the pressure placed on the ulnar nerve as it exits the cubital tunnel. It is critical to "unload" or place the proximal portion of the ulnar nerve on slack while gently stretching the flexor–pronator muscles. This can be achieved by having the patient perform ipsilateral cervical sidebending and scapular elevation. With the forearm in supination, the patient grasps the opposite hand to gently stretch the wrist into extension, while maintaining the elbow in terminal extension (Fig. 52-7). Kinesio tape placed with the elbow in terminal flexion can also be beneficial for improving myofascial mobility of the ceiling of the cubital tunnel (Fig. 52-8, online).

Neural Mobilization. When performing nerve gliding techniques for cubital tunnel syndrome, it is important to avoid tensioning the nerve. The elbow itself stays in a static position, while movement is provided by the surrounding joints. Since the ulnar nerve is stretched most with terminal elbow flexion, the elbow should be placed in extension with full forearm supination. The patient's opposite hand assists with alternating wrist, ring, and small finger flexion and extension while maintaining active scapular elevation and ipsilateral cervical side-bending to place the ulnar nerve on slack proximally. This is performed in a slow, rhythmic fashion to avoid pain, paresthesias, or dysesthesias along the ulnar nerve distribution. For example, a patient with left cubital tunnel syndrome performs an ulnar nerve gliding technique by elevating, or "shrugging," the left shoulder while tipping his head to the left as he performs active-assistive wrist and ring and small finger flexion and extension. The patient's left elbow remains in extension with the forearm in supination throughout the nerve gliding sequence. The following FLOSS template is utilized for the neural mobilization techniques discussed with each section of the chapter.

- *Fix the adjacent joint*: For the highly irritable nerve, the elbow remains in extension or slight flexion. When the nerve is mildly irritable, the elbow can be moved through midrange with the nerve on slack proximally.
- *Limit the ROM*: Avoid adverse neural tension by limiting terminal elbow flexion.[12]

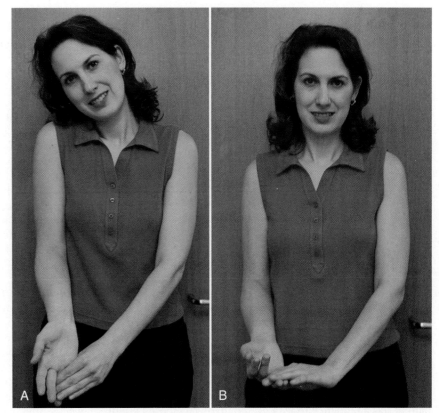

Figure 52-7 Neural mobilization for cubital tunnel syndrome (*highly irritable stage*). **A,** Step 1: Patient performs ipsilateral scapular elevation and cervical sidebending as the wrist and ring and small fingers are extended. The forearm remains in supination and elbow in extension. **B,** Step 2: The scapula and cervical spine are returned to neutral as the wrist and ring and small fingers are brought into slight flexion. This is performed in a slow, rhythmic fashion.

- *Oscillate distal or proximal (or both) to the level of compression*:
  Highly Irritable Stage: The scapula elevates as the wrist and ring and small fingers are extended. The elbow remains in extension with the forearm in supination during the mobilization. As the scapula returns to neutral, the wrist and digits are brought into slight flexion.
  Mildly Irritable Stage: With the nerve on slack proximally, the patient performs midrange elbow flexion to 60 degrees combined with alternating wrist and digit flexion and extension.
- *Slow, rhythmic motion*: Perform at the pace of one repetition every 1 to 2 seconds to maximize excursion and minimize strain on the nerve.
- *Symptom free*: Avoid pain, paresthesias, and reflexive muscle guarding.
Please refer to video on the companion Web site for details.

Orthoses and Protection. A prefabricated or custom-made elbow flexion block is a standard method of conservative treatment for cubital tunnel syndrome. Although shoulder abduction increases tension on the ulnar nerve,[12] orthotic positioning is focused at the elbow and the patient is instructed to sleep with the arms at the sides. Often, it is helpful to have the patient use a pillow beneath the elbow to support the shoulder in a neutral, more adducted position. In the authors' opinion, prefabricated elbow orthoses are more comfortable and better tolerated by patients than custom thermoplastic orthoses. Apfel and Sigafoos compared the ROM constraints by four different prefabricated orthoses

and a "homemade" version of an elbow flexion block using a folded towel around the elbow with tape.[20] They found that the Pil-O-Splint with stay, Hely & Weber splint, and the folded towel were all effective in preventing elbow flexion beyond 100 to 110 degrees, which causes the most pressure at the cubital tunnel (Fig. 52-9).

During daily tasks, a Heelbo pad, which is a sleeve with a gel pad that can be placed over the medial aspect of the elbow, is helpful for minimizing concentrated stress at the cubital tunnel (Fig. 52-10). Caution must be taken to ensure the sleeve does not increase compression circumferentially around the patient's arm, as these sleeves sometimes tend to fit tightly. Use of stretched Kinesio tape, applied with the

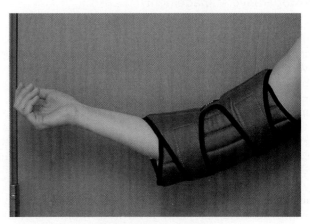

Figure 52-9 Pil-O-Splint.

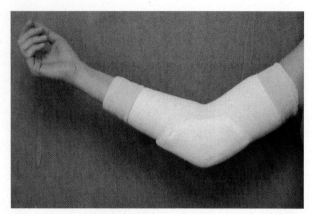

Figure 52-10 Heelbo pad.

elbow in terminal flexion, can also be helpful in limiting a patient's tendency to flex the elbow with daily activities. For advanced cases of cubital tunnel syndrome resulting in a claw deformity, a hand-based custom anticlaw orthosis can be used (Fig. 52-11, online).

Activity Modification. Educating the patient about avoiding terminal or near-terminal elbow flexion is a critical element of conservative treatment. This is especially important if the patient has a tendency to lean on the involved elbow. Patient education involving abdominal bracing assists in recruiting the trunk and scapular stabilizers to minimize the tendency for the patient to rest with his or her involved elbow in a flexed position. Sometimes an external support, such as a figure-of-8 strap, can help the patient maintain good scapular alignment, especially if the patient is unable to tolerate supporting his or her arms on armrests. Use of a tray on which to rest the forearms while typing on a keyboard prevents pressure at the cubital tunnel and minimizes stress on the ulnar nerve. For patients who use the phone for the majority of their workday, use of a headset or wireless earpiece can prevent the need for maintaining the elbow in flexion for extended periods. Sleeping in a fetal position can place increased stress on the ulnar nerve at the cubital tunnel. Patient education to avoid this position as well as use of orthoses may also be beneficial.

Postoperative Management

In Situ Ulnar Nerve Decompression. This procedure involves releasing the fascial roof of the cubital tunnel to decompress the ulnar nerve. These patients tend not to have postoperative therapy unless they have pain or hypersensitivity that limits the return to function. Typically, patients have no ROM restrictions and are able to achieve full elbow and forearm motion on their own. Since the ulnar nerve remains situated in the cubital tunnel, the neural mobilization described in the conservative treatment section is utilized. Scar tissue mobilization techniques and sensory desensitization are employed, if indicated.

Subcutaneous Ulnar Nerve Transposition. This procedure involves removing the ulnar nerve from within the cubital tunnel and transferring it anterior to the elbow beneath the skin and subcutaneous fat. The patient comes in for the first postoperative therapy visit within 2 weeks after the procedure. A long arm orthosis is not required, but may be used with patients who present with significant discomfort or need protection when returning to one-handed work. With this procedure, there are no ROM restrictions postoperatively; however, it may take up to 4 to 6 weeks for the patient to feel comfortable performing full elbow extension. Neural mobilization techniques can begin at the initial therapy session; however, the technique is modified to accommodate the new pathway of the ulnar nerve across the anterior aspect of the elbow. Instead of maintaining the elbow in slight flexion, the elbow is now statically placed in 60 to 90 degrees of flexion. The mobilization technique remains the same with regard to distal and proximal motions. Scar tissue mobilization techniques and sensory desensitization are utilized as well. At 3 to 4 weeks after surgery, a strengthening program can begin.

Submuscular Ulnar Nerve Transposition. This procedure involves removing the ulnar nerve from within the cubital tunnel and placing it anterior to the elbow beneath the flexor–pronator muscle mass. Because the flexor–pronator group must be detached and reattached to allow the ulnar nerve to slide beneath, a custom orthosis is utilized postoperatively for protection. A long arm orthosis is fabricated for the patient at the first postoperative visit, usually 2 or 3 weeks after surgery, placing the elbow near 90 degrees of flexion with the forearm in neutral to slight pronation and slight wrist flexion (Fig. 52-12, online). AROM to the elbow, forearm, and wrist are initiated, instructing the patient to maintain slight forearm pronation and wrist flexion to minimize tension on the flexor–pronator muscle group. (ed. note: In some clinical settings earlier postoperative therapy may begin 2 weeks after surgery with ROM exercises restricted to passive only to avoid stress on the flexor pronator origin. Passive exercises are performed within a comfortable range avoiding aggressive end range stretching. At 4 weeks, AROM may begin.) The patient removes the custom orthosis five to six times per day to perform AROM. Neural mobilization techniques, similar to those described in the Subcutaneous Ulnar Nerve Transposition section, can begin at this time. The long arm orthosis is worn for the first 6 weeks postoperatively between exercises and at night. Often, a light compressive sleeve is needed to minimize localized edema at the elbow to reduce further joint stiffness. At 6 weeks after surgery, passive range of motion (PROM) can be initiated and the custom orthosis discontinued. It is important to ensure that the patient does not develop an elbow flexion contracture, as this is not uncommon. If a patient develops a contracture of more than 20 degrees, a static extension orthosis may be used at night. At 8 weeks after surgery, a strengthening program is initiated. Scar management, sensory desensitization, and activity modification are employed as part of the postoperative rehabilitation.

Ulnar Tunnel Syndrome

Ulnar tunnel syndrome (UTS) involves compression of the ulnar nerve at the level of the volar wrist and hand. There are three potential sites of entrapment[8]: (1) just proximal to or within Guyon's canal, which results in both sensory and motor involvement[18]; (2) between the abductor digiti minimi and flexor digiti minimi muscles near the hook of the hamate, which results in motor involvement only and; (3) at the distal end of Guyon's canal, in which the sensory branch alone is involved.[21] The main causes of UTS include ganglion cysts, ulnar artery thrombosis, and ulnar-sided wrist fractures or dislocations.[22] Anomalous muscles, such as the accessory abductor digiti minimi or flexor digiti minimi brevis, can also play a role.[23] Repetitive trauma, such as bicycling while resting the hypothenar eminence on the handlebars or long-distance truck driving resting on a steering wheel, can also contribute to this compression syndrome.

Conservative Management

Restoring muscle length and myofascial mobility: This impairment is not typical with UTS.

Neural mobilization: Utilizing the principle of FLOSS, the following can be performed:

- *Fix the adjacent joint:* The wrist remains in a neutral position.
- *Limit the ROM:* Avoid end-range wrist extension.[12]
- *Oscillate distal or proximal (or both) to the level of compression:* With the nerve on slack proximally and elbow in an extended position with wrist in neutral, the patient performs midrange ring and small finger extension and flexion. With mild irritability, midrange wrist extension can be added to the mobilization in combination with digit extension.
- *Slow, rhythmic motion:* Perform at the pace of one repetition every 1 to 2 seconds to maximize excursion and minimize strain on the nerve.
- *Symptom free:* Avoid pain, paresthesias, and reflexive muscle guarding.

Please refer to video on the companion Web site for details.

Orthoses and Protection. Padded gloves or gel pads can assist with distributing pressure at the hypothenar eminence. Late-stage UTS with motor involvement can result in profound clawing of the ring and small fingers due to the muscle imbalance of the intact FDP muscle and weakened intrinsics. A custom anticlaw orthosis can improve function with grasping and holding objects.

Activity Modification. Patient education in avoiding weight-bearing or pressure on the hypothenar eminence with wrist extension is most beneficial. Avoiding using the hand as a hammer and minimizing exposure to vibration (as with grasping a steering wheel) can limit deleterious effects on the nerve. With typing, a split keyboard can help prevent excessive ulnar deviation and wrist extension and minimize ulnar nerve tension in this region.

Postoperative Management

Ulnar Tunnel Release. This procedure involves decompressing the ulnar nerve along the entrapment points described earlier. These patients tend not to have postoperative therapy unless pain or hypersensitivity limits return to function. Typically, patients have no ROM restrictions and are able to

achieve full wrist motion on their own. The neural mobilization described in the conservative management section is used. Scar tissue techniques and sensory desensitization are employed, if necessary.

Radial Tunnel Syndrome

Near the level of the humeroradial joint (HRJ) of the elbow, the radial nerve divides into the posterior interosseous nerve (PIN) and the superficial terminal branch of the radial nerve (dorsal radial sensory nerve). This bifurcation may occur within the area spanning 3 cm proximal and distal to the HRJ; therefore, radial nerve compression about the elbow can affect the radial nerve proper or the PIN (or both). The radial tunnel is approximately 5 cm in length, extending between the HRJ and the supinator muscle. The HRJ capsule and the deep head of the supinator constitute the floor of the tunnel. The biceps and brachialis tendons define the medial border of the tunnel, and the extensor carpi radialis longus (ECRL), brevis (ECRB), and brachioradialis (BR) muscle bellies border the tunnel laterally. The superficial branch of the radial nerve exits the tunnel on the superficial surface of the supinator. Conversely, the PIN travels deep to the superficial head of the supinator through the fibrous supinator arch known as the arcade of Frohse. The nerve continues distally between the two heads of the supinator muscle.[24]

Radial nerve or PIN compression can be caused by HRJ degeneration, radial head fractures, tumors, and ganglion cysts.[25] The nerve may be compressed within the arcade of Frohse, between the superficial and deep heads of the supinator, between the septum of the ECRB and EDC, or by vascular leashes from the recurrent radial artery. Iatrogenic causes of radial tunnel syndrome (RTS) or PIN syndrome may include counterforce bracing for lateral epicondylitis or placement of strapping during orthotic fitting.

RTS and PIN syndrome, although of similar cause, manifest very differently in the clinical setting. The PIN is a motor nerve innervating the supinator, wrist extensors, and digital extensors; therefore, PIN syndrome is characterized by weakness in these muscle groups.[26] The radial nerve innervates the ECRL proximal to PIN bifurcation, thus radial wrist extension is spared with PIN palsy.[24] Generalized pain at the dorsal forearm, with point tenderness approximately 4 cm distal to the lateral epicondyle is the classic presentation on RTS. Palpable tenderness directly over the lateral epicondyle is more suggestive of tendinopathy than nerve irritation.[24] RTS is estimated to coexist in 5% of individuals with lateral epicondylitis.[27]

Occupational risk factors that contribute to RTS include use of pinching tools, repetitive force exertion of greater than 1 kg (>10 times per hour), working in elbow extension, and maintaining forearm in pronation or supination during work tasks.[28] Symptom exacerbation with use, particularly repetitive forearm rotation, as well as nocturnal pain is commonly associated with RTS.[29]

Dorsal forearm pain may result from impairments at the level of the cervical spine, thoracic outlet region, shoulder, or elbow. If RTS is suggested, it is imperative to rule out proximal issues by performing the screenings discussed previously in this chapter. Particularly similar in presentation to RTS is lateral epicondylitis, and provocative maneuvers to

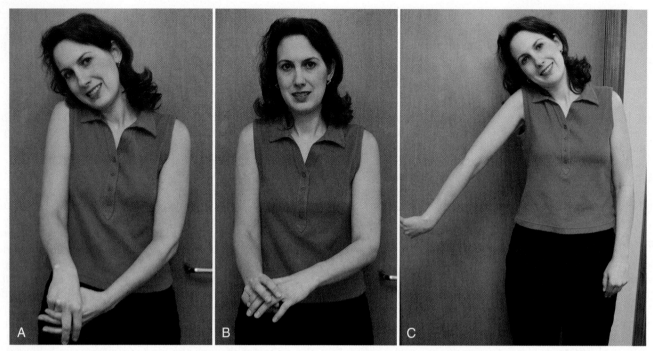

Figure 52-15 Neural mobilization for radial tunnel syndrome. **A,** *Highly irritable stage.* Step 1: Maintaining the index and middle finger metacarpophalangeal joints in extension and the forearm in pronation, the patient performs ipsilateral scapular elevation and cervical sidebending combined with midrange wrist flexion. **B,** *Highly irritable stage.* Step 2: The wrist is brought back into extension as the scapula and cervical spine return to neutral. This is performed in a slow, rhythmic fashion. **C,** *Mildly irritable stage.* With the nerve on slack proximally, midrange elbow extension with combined forearm pronation, wrist flexion, and ulnar deviation (verbal cue: "Like a turtle scooping sand at the beach") with return to start position. This is performed in a slow, rhythmic fashion.

"tease out" the pain-generating structure are outlined in this section.

The following provocative maneuvers may reproduce pain with both RTS and lateral epicondylitis; however, the location of the pain provides the differential diagnosis. Generalized pain at the dorsal forearm, with point tenderness approximately 4 cm distal to the lateral epicondyle, is characteristic of RTS, and palpable tenderness directly over the lateral epicondyle is diagnostic for lateral epicondylitis.

- Resisted middle finger MCP extension (Fig. 52-13, online)
- Resisted forearm supination (Fig. 52-14, online)
- Resisted wrist extension
- Upper limb neurodynamic test with radial nerve bias (combined scapular depression, shoulder abduction, elbow extension, forearm pronation, wrist flexion with ulnar deviation, and thumb adduction)[6]

Although RTS and lateral epicondylitis may occur in concert with one another, treatment focuses on the area of highest irritability with provocative testing.

Conservative Management

The principles of conservative management are much like other nerve compression syndromes discussed within this chapter.

Restoring Muscle Length and Myofascial Mobility. Restore the length of the supinator and ECRB muscles via myofascial techniques and gentle stretching. The patient performs active scapular elevation with ipsilateral cervical sidebending

during the soft tissue techniques to place the nerve on slack proximally.

Neural Mobilization.
Figure 52-15.
- *Fix the adjacent joint*: For the highly irritable nerve, the elbow and forearm remain stable at 90 degrees elbow flexion and forearm pronation during the mobilization. When the nerve is mildly irritable, all joints can be moved through midrange with the nerve on slack proximally.
- *Limit the ROM*: Avoid adverse neural tension by limiting combined wrist flexion, elbow extension, and forearm pronation.[30]
- *Oscillate distal or proximal (or both) to the level of compression*:
  Highly Irritable Stage: Maintaining the index and middle finger MCP joints in extension and the forearm in pronation, the patient performs ipsilateral scapular elevation and cervical sidebending combined with midrange wrist flexion. The wrist is then brought back into extension as the scapula and cervical spine return to neutral.
  Mildly Irritable Stage: With the nerve on slack proximally, midrange elbow extension with combined forearm pronation, wrist flexion and ulnar deviation (verbal cue: "Like a turtle scooping sand at the beach") with return to start position.
- *Slow, rhythmic motion*: Perform at the pace of one repetition every 1 to 2 seconds to maximize excursion and minimize strain on the nerve.

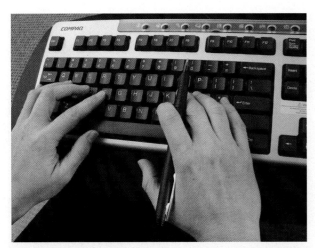

Figure 52-17 Ergonomic consideration: Unloading the radial nerve by holding a pen while keyboarding.

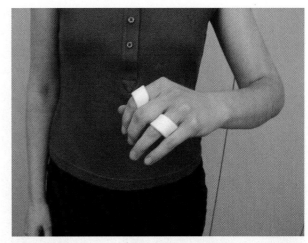

Figure 52-18 Ergonomic consideration: A yoke orthosis, used traditionally for extensor tendon rehabilitation, can be beneficial in supporting the middle finger metacarpophalangeal joint in extension during activities to unload the radial nerve.

- *Symptom free*: Avoid pain, paresthesias, and reflexive muscle guarding.

Please refer to video on the companion Web site for details.

Orthoses and Protection.
- In the highly irritable stage, use of a wrist hand orthosis (WHO) in slight wrist extension may decrease tension at the involved site.
- Kinesio tape: The authors have found taping beneficial for unloading the wrist extensor muscle mass and facilitating supination. This can be used regardless of the stage of irritability (Fig. 52-16, online).

Activity Modification.
- Ergonomic equipment consideration: Split keyboard, vertical or pencil-shaped mouse, use of tools with a pistol grip.
- Activities or positions to avoid: Repetitive forearm rotation, wrist flexion–extension, elbow extension, and prolonged static pinch and grip; avoid use of a counterforce strap.
- Behavior modification with daily tasks: Hold steering wheel at 9 and 3 o'clock, push shopping cart and lawnmower in a forearm neutral position, place pencil or pen under index finger during extensive computer work to hyperextend the MCP joint and place the radial nerve on slack (Fig. 52-17), consider wearing a yoke orthosis to place the MCP joint of the index or middle fingers (or both) in extension to unload the radial nerve (Fig. 52-18).
- Scapular and core stabilization: Consideration of figure-of-8 strap for postural retraining.

Postoperative Management

Surgical decompression often includes release of the ligament of Frohse and the superficial head of the supinator muscle.[31] AROM to the elbow, forearm, and wrist are initiated 3 to 5 days after surgery. Care must be taken to avoid combined elbow extension, forearm pronation, and wrist flexion, as this position places excessive tension on the radial nerve and surrounding soft tissues. An orthosis is not routinely indicated after this procedure, as gentle motion is encouraged to prevent neural adhesions and minimize scar adherence. However, a removable wrist extension orthosis may be used for comfort and protection while the patient is engaged in necessary activities of daily living and work in the early postoperative period. On review of the surgical report, the therapist can initiate neural mobilization based on the FLOSS principles outlined in the conservative management section. Activity modification follows conservative principles as well. Scar management and sensory desensitization are very important components of postoperative care, as the authors see a prevalence of hypersensitivity associated with this procedure. At 3 weeks after surgery, strengthening of the wrist and hand muscles may be initiated, with progression to the elbow and forearm at 6 weeks.[32]

Posterior Interosseous Nerve Syndrome

Whether the patient is seen for conservative management or postsurgically, the therapist's role is to facilitate improved fine-motor function through use of adaptive equipment and orthoses. Consideration for use of a dynamic wrist and digital MCP extension orthosis can facilitate function while the patient awaits motor return. Scar tissue management, edema control, and pain management techniques may be employed following postsurgical PIN release. In addition, patient education on avoidance of repetitive gripping and forearm rotation tasks minimizes tension and compression on the nerve. Therapists may educate patients on the rate of motor recovery after nerve injury, understanding this may take longer than 6 months (see Chapter 45).

Wartenberg's Syndrome

Wartenberg's syndrome is a painful condition involving the superficial branch of the radial nerve, also referred to as the dorsal radial sensory nerve (DRSN). The nerve becomes tensioned and compressed between the BR and ECRL muscles

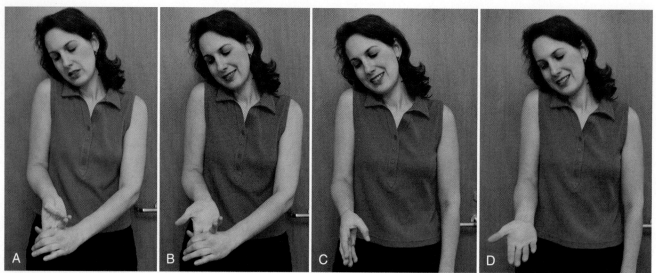

Figure 52-19 Wartenberg's syndrome. **A,** *Highly irritable stage.* Step 1: Place the forearm passively in supination with the index and middle finger metacarpophalangeal joints supported in passive extension, and perform midrange active thumb opposition. **B,** *Highly irritable stage.* Step 2: The forearm and fingers remain in position as the patient performs midrange active thumb retroposition. This is performed in a slow, rhythmic fashion. **C,** *Mildly irritable stage.* Step 1: With the nerve on slack proximally, the patient performs midrange forearm pronation with active thumb opposition. **D,** *Mildly irritable stage.* Step 2: The patient performs midrange forearm supination in concert with active thumb retroposition. This is performed in a slow, rhythmic fashion.

depending on the position of the forearm and wrist. With forearm pronation, the ECRL tendon crosses under the BR tendon and in a scissor-like fashion compresses the DRSN. In supination the DRSN lies between the BR and ECRL tendons without compression.

The nerve becomes tensioned with forearm pronation, wrist flexion, and ulnar deviation. Repetitive activities involving the transition between forearm pronation and supination with combined wrist flexion and extension can illicit inflammation and pain at the junction between BR and ECRL muscles.

Positive provocative tests for Wartenberg's syndrome include the following:

- Positive Tinel's sign located at the intersection between the BR and ECRL muscles, located 4 cm proximal to Lister's tubercle
- Resisted wrist extension with radial deviation, tested with forearm supination
- Passive wrist flexion with ulnar deviation, tested with forearm pronation

Wartenberg's syndrome is sometimes seen in conjunction with de Quervain's tenosynovitis.[33,34] To differentiate the two, perform the Finkelstein's test with the forearm in neutral, then repeat with full pronation. A more painful test in pronation is indicative of Wartenberg's syndrome because of the greater degree of DRSN compression in pronation. Isolated first dorsal compartment tenosynovitis produces the same amount of pain regardless of the forearm position.

Conservative Management

Restoring Muscle Length and Myofascial Mobility. Because the DRSN becomes scissored between the BR and ECRL muscles, improving the myofascial mobility of these muscles and the entire dorsal compartment of the forearm as a whole

is beneficial. Care must be taken to avoid tensioning the DRSN when performing stretching or myofascial techniques. This can be accomplished by placing the radial nerve on slack proximally. During myofascial techniques, it is also beneficial to place the nerve on slack distally by placing the fingers and wrist in extension. This position allows the therapist to perform gentle localized stretching or myofascial release without exacerbating the patient's symptoms.

Neural Mobilization.
Figure 52-19.

- *Fix the adjacent joint*: For the highly irritable nerve, the forearm remains stable in a supinated position. When the nerve is mildly irritable, all joints can be moved through midrange with the nerve on slack proximally.
- *Limit the ROM*: Avoid adverse neural tension by limiting combined wrist flexion and ulnar deviation with forearm pronation and thumb opposition.[35]
- *Oscillate distal or proximal (or both) to the level of compression*:

  Highly Irritable Stage: Place the forearm passively in supination and perform gentle, midrange active thumb opposition and retroposition with the index and middle finger MCP joints supported in passive extension.

  Mildly Irritable Stage: With the nerve on slack proximally, midrange forearm pronation is incorporated with active thumb opposition, while supination is performed in concert with active thumb retroposition.
- *Slow, rhythmic motion*: Perform at the pace of one repetition every 1 to 2 seconds to maximize excursion and minimize strain on the nerve.
- *Symptom free*: Avoid pain, paresthesias, and reflexive muscle guarding.

Please refer to video on the companion Web site for details.

Orthoses and Protection.

- Highly irritable stage: A volar-based orthosis maintaining the wrist in extension and thumb retroposition minimizes tension on the DRSN.
- The authors have also found Kinesio tape applied along the dorsoradial wrist to be beneficial in reducing pain and discomfort associated with Wartenberg's syndrome (Fig. 52-20, online).

Activity Modification.

- *Ergonomic equipment considerations*: Split keyboard, vertical mouse, use of large-diameter tools and writing instruments, use of pen between index and middle fingers to unload radial nerve with forearm pronation activities (see Fig. 52-17).
- *Avoidance of activities* combining wrist flexion–extension and forearm rotation: Tennis; mowing the lawn; packing boxes or working on an assembly line; avoid wearing bracelets or a tight-fitting watch around the wrist; avoid wearing long sleeves or gloves during the exacerbated stage.
- *Behavior modification with daily tasks*: Pushing grocery cart with a forearm neutral position; holding steering wheel at 9 and 3 o'clock positions.

Pronator Syndrome

The median nerve is vulnerable to compression or tethering at the level of the elbow and proximal forearm. The term *pronator syndrome* (PS) has become a catch-all diagnosis for median nerve compression syndromes about the elbow and forearm, regardless of the anatomic structure causing the compression. The path of the median nerve around the elbow, although varying among individuals, includes four potential sites of compression. Beginning proximally, the median nerve may be compressed at the *ligament of Struthers*, with attachments extending from the supracondylar process of the humerus to the medial epicondyle.[36] This ligament is considered an anomalous variation at the elbow because it is only present in 0.7% to 2.7% of individuals.[37] When present, this ligament may contain and compress the median nerve and brachial artery.

The second site of potential compression about the elbow is the *lacertus fibrosus*, or *bicipital aponeurosis*, a fibrous band of tissue extending between the distal biceps tendon and the flexor–pronator mass. At the level of the antecubital fossa, the median nerve and brachial artery travel under the lacertus fibrosus.[37] Sudden, forceful elbow flexion against substantial resistance can result in complete or partial disruption of the distal biceps tendon as well as tethering of the median nerve at the lacertus fibrosus.[38] Furthermore, this nerve may be compromised during repetitive elbow flexion and extension activities.[36]

On entering the forearm, the median nerve most commonly travels between the superficial and deep heads of the pronator teres (PT) muscle, the third potential nerve compression site. Repetitive or resisted forearm rotation activities may contribute to nerve compression at this level. Finally, as the median nerve continues distally toward the wrist, its path lies deep to the fibrous flexor digitorum superficialis (FDS) arch, approximately 6.5 cm below the level of the humeral epicondyles. This is the fourth potential site of compression.[36]

The incidence of PS is considered rare, but it affects women four times more often than men. It is most prevalent in the fifth decade of life.[37] Individuals with PS most commonly present with the chief complaint of pain at the proximal volar forearm that is exacerbated by repetitive forearm rotation or elbow motion. Their occupation may require heavy grasping or twisting, such as carpentry work, which can repetitively compress the median nerve at the PT, superficialis arch, or lacertus fibrosus. In addition to forearm pain, individuals may report paresthesias in the thumb, index, middle, and radial half of the ring fingers. A distinguishing characteristic of PS is sensory symptoms into the palm of the hand over the thenar eminence, consistent with innervation of the palmar cutaneous branch of the median nerve.[37] Compression of the median nerve at the level of the carpal tunnel does not result in paresthesias in the palm of the hand because the compression occurs distal to this sensory branch. Another feature of PS that distinguishes it from carpal tunnel syndrome is the absence of noctural paresthesias.[37] Perceived weakness and fatigue are also characteristic symptoms of PS.[36]

A thorough understanding of the anatomic course of the median nerve provides rationale for PS testing. Lee and LeStayo describe three provocative tests to localize compression of the median nerve at various points along its path[37]:

- *Resisted forearm pronation with elbow extension*: The first test is performed with patient's forearm in the neutral position. The examiner resists forearm pronation as the elbow is gradually extended. A positive test reproduces the patient's symptoms and is indicative of median nerve compression at the PT.
- *Resisted elbow flexion*: The second test reproduces pain and paresthesias if the median nerve is compressed at the level of the lacertus fibrosus. The examiner performs resisted elbow flexion with the patient's elbow flexed from 120 to 130 degrees and the forearm in full supination.
- *Resisted proximal interphalangeal flexion at the middle finger*: If this results in symptom reproduction, the likely point of compression is the superficialis arch.

Another clinical test that may aid in the diagnosis of PS is the pronator compression test.[39] The examiner exerts pressure over the PT muscle bellies, bilaterally, for 30 seconds. A positive test results in median nerve paresthesias in the involved extremity. With chronic PS (>4 months), Semmes–Weinstein sensory testing at the hand and Tinel's sign at the proximal forearm may be positive.[36]

Conservative Management

The principles of conservative management of PS are much like those for other nerve compression syndromes discussed within this chapter.

Restoring Muscle Length and Myofascial Mobility. Based on the examination findings, soft tissue techniques address the involved structure: biceps brachii with lacertus fibrosus, PT, or FDS muscles. A myofascial technique for addressing the biceps brachii may include slow, prolonged stretch to the distal biceps tendon with the elbow in extension and the

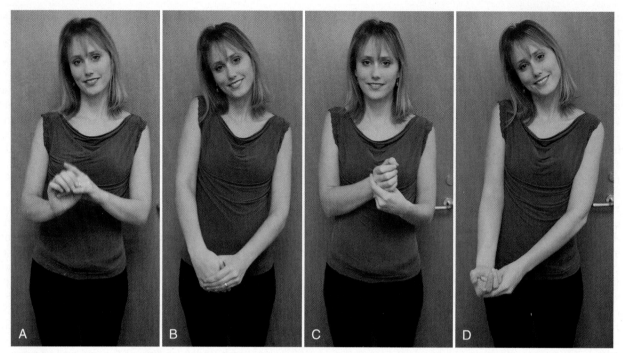

Figure 52-21 Pronator syndrome. **A,** *Highly irritable stage.* Step 1: The forearm is stabilized in neutral to slight pronation, and oscillation is performed with slight elbow extension combined with wrist flexion. **B,** *Highly irritable stage.* Step 2: The patient then performs slight elbow flexion combined with partial wrist extension. This is performed in a slow, rhythmic fashion. **C,** *Mildly irritable stage.* Step 1: Start with the elbow flexed to 90 degrees, forearm neutral, and slight wrist extension. **D,** *Mildly irritable stage.* Step 2: Perform scapular elevation combined with slight elbow extension, forearm supination, and slight wrist flexion ("giving a low five"). This is performed in a slow, rhythmic fashion.

forearm in pronation. Care must be taken to avoid excessive neural tension when performing soft tissue specific techniques. The patient performs active scapular elevation with ipsilateral cervical sidebending during the soft tissue techniques to place the nerve on slack.

Neural Mobilization.
Figure 52-21.
- *Fix the adjacent joint*: For compression at the lacertus fibrosus, the elbow and forearm are stabilized due to the biceps involvement in both elbow flexion and forearm supination. Conversely, if the level of compression is between the two heads of the PT muscle or the arch of the FDS muscle, the forearm remains stable.
- *Limit the ROM*: Avoid adverse neural tension on the median nerve by limiting full wrist extension and forearm supination, especially in a synergistic fashion.[35]
- *Oscillate distal or proximal (or both) to the level of compression*:
  1. Lacertus Fibrosus
     Highly Irritable Stage: The elbow stabilized at 90 degrees with forearm in neutral; oscillation is performed with scapular elevation combined with partial wrist extension followed by scapular depression with wrist flexion.
     Mildly Irritable Stage: During this mobilization, slight elbow extension combined with forearm supination and wrist extension are performed with the nerve on slack proximally.
  2. Pronator Teres
     Highly Irritable Stage: The forearm is stabilized in neutral to slight pronation; oscillation is

performed with slight elbow extension combined with wrist flexion followed by slight elbow flexion combined with partial wrist extension.
     Mildly Irritable Stage: Beginning with the elbow flexed to 90 degrees, forearm neutral, and wrist in slight extension, the scapula is elevated combined with slight elbow extension, forearm supination, and slight wrist flexion.
  3. FDS Arch
     Highly Irritable Stage: With the forearm stabilized in supination, oscillation is performed with slight elbow flexion combined with partial wrist, index finger, and middle finger extension followed by slight elbow extension with wrist and digit flexion.
     Mildly Irritable Stage: Same mobilization as for the highly irritable stage, but move through a slightly larger arc of motion.
- *Slow, rhythmic motion*: Perform at the pace of one repetition every 1 to 2 seconds to maximize excursion and minimize strain on the nerve.
- *Symptom free*: Avoid pain, paresthesias, and reflexive muscle guarding.
Please refer to video on the companion Web site for details.

Orthoses and Protection.
- For a highly irritable nerve compression, Lee and LeStayo recommend use of a posterior elbow gutter orthosis at 90 degrees elbow flexion and forearm neutral for 2 weeks, removing for gentle ROM only. Gentle midrange neural mobilization techniques can be performed within the orthosis.[37]

- Kinesio tape: The authors have found this taping method beneficial for unloading the flexor–pronator mass (Fig. 52-22, online).

Activity Modification.

- *Ergonomic equipment considerations*: Adjustable split keyboard to minimize pronation during typing, vertical or pencil-shaped mouse to avoid pronation, use of tools with a pistol grip.
- *Activities or positions to avoid*: Repetitious forearm rotation or elbow flexion and extension.
- *Behavior modification with daily tasks*: Hold steering wheel at 9 and 3 o'clock positions; push shopping cart and lawnmower in a forearm-neutral position.
- *Scapular and core stabilization*: Consider a figure-of-8 strap for postural retraining.

Postoperative Management

A surgical release for PS often involves decompression of the median nerve at the ligament of Struthers, bicipital aponeurosis, fibrous bands of the PT muscle, and dissection of the FDS arch. If the PT muscle is released during the procedure, it is reattached and must be protected during the postoperative phase.[36,40]

- *Protected ROM*: Avoid end-range forearm supination.
- *Orthoses and protection*: Koo and Szabo recommend plaster orthosis at 90 degrees elbow flexion, 45 degrees forearm pronation, and slight wrist flexion until stitch removal.[36]
- *Neural mobilization*: On review of the surgery report, the therapist can initiate neural mobilization based on the FLOSS principles discussed under conservative management.
- *Scar management* and *sensory desensitization*: Due to the extensive "lazy S" incision traversing 10 cm proximal to elbow crease and distally to the midforearm, scar management is very important with these patients.[36] Deep scar tissue mobilization and SGS are critical components in the rehabilitation process. These patients typically demonstrate fewer hypersensitivity issues than those patients with radial tunnel releases.
- *Activity modification and postoperative precautions*: If the PT muscle is released and reattached, avoiding active pronation and full passive supination during the early phases of rehabilitation protects this structure. In these cases, an orthosis preventing forearm rotation is employed. Koo and Szabo avoid resistance activities until 6 to 8 weeks after surgery.[36]

Anterior Interosseous Nerve Syndrome

The anterior interosseous nerve (AIN), a main branch of the median nerve, supplies motor function to the FPL, FDP of the index and middle fingers, and pronator quadratus muscles. Potential sites of AIN compression include the deep head of the PT muscle, an accessory lacertus fibrosus, fibrous arch of the FDS, or an anomalous or accessory slip of the FPL muscle in the forearm (Gantzer's muscle). Tumors, thrombosed vessels, and fractures may contribute to AIN compression.[36] Casey and Moed reported four cases of AIN syndrome over a 3-year period resulting from constrictive postoperative dressings.[41]

The incidence of AINS is rare, accounting for less than 1% of upper extremity nerve compression neuropathies.[36] Patients may report vague pain in the proximal forearm that increases with activity. Activities, such as writing, manipulating buttons and zippers, and picking up small objects, that require tip pinch may be reported as functional limitations. These individuals may report a history of trauma or repetitious activity that precedes the onset of pain and motor loss. Spontaneous motor deficits of the FDP and FPL muscles bilaterally after vaccination or viral illness may indicate Parsonage–Turner syndrome.[36] A thorough history can help a therapist rule out proximal involvement leading to the motor loss that mimics AINS.

Postural analysis of the hand during tip-pinch activity reveals extension of the index finger distal interphalangeal and thumb interphalangeal joints with compensatory hyperflexion of the index finger proximal interphalangeal and thumb MCP joints. Isolated active flexion of the FPL, index finger, or middle finger FDP muscles may be absent or weak.

Conservative Management and Postoperative Management

Whether the patient is seen for conservative management or postsurgical rehabilitation, the therapist's role is to facilitate improved fine-motor function through use of adaptive equipment or orthoses. The use of zipper pulls and large-diameter pens may be beneficial. Silver ring or oval-8 orthoses may assist with tip pinch by stabilizing the IP joints in flexion at the thumb and index finger. Scar tissue management, edema control, and pain management techniques may be employed after surgical AIN release. In addition, patient education in avoidance of repetitive gripping and forearm rotation tasks minimizes tension and compression on the AIN. Therapists may educate patients on the rate of motor recovery after nerve injury, understanding this may take longer than 6 months.

Summary

Evaluation and treatment of upper extremity nerve compressions about the elbow, forearm, and wrist can be approached with a systematic method. Taking into account the individual patient's history and home and work situations enables the shaping of the treatment goals and plan. Restoring soft tissue and neural mobility, in addition to protection and activity modification, create the framework for conservative management. Early intervention can assist with reducing repetitive stress on the involved structures and optimize therapeutic outcomes. For postoperative care, applying these same principles leads to timely restoration of function.

REFERENCES

The complete reference list is available online at www.expertconsult.com.

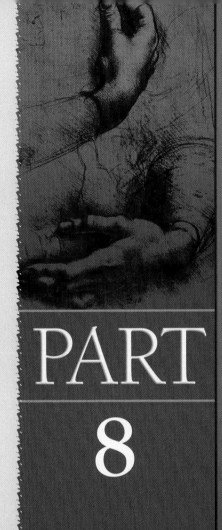

PART

8

Proximal Nerve
Conditions

CHAPTER 53

Cervical Radiculopathy

MITCHELL K. FREEDMAN, DO, MADHURI DHOLAKIA, MD,
DENNIS W. IVILL, MD, ALAN S. HILIBRAND, MD, AND
ZACH BROYER, MD

CRITICAL POINTS

- The peak age range for cervical radiculopathy is 50 to 54 years.
- Between 50% and 75% of patients experience recurrent cervical pain within 1 to 5 years.
- Poor prognostic indicators for neck pain in the workplace include age, previous musculoskeletal pain, high quantitative job demands, low social support at work, low physical capacity, job insecurity, poor work posture, and sedentary repetitive and precision work.
- The diagnosis of cervical radiculopathy must be made on the basis of history and physical examination in combination with appropriate imaging studies.
- Magnetic resonance imaging is the study of choice to confirm the diagnosis of cervical radiculopathy.
- Nonsteroidal anti-inflammatory drugs, acetaminophen, muscle relaxants, opioids, and anticonvulsants can be used to treat radiculopathy.
- Physical therapy, acupuncture, traction, and transcutaneous electrical nerve stimulation units can be used to treat cervical radiculopathy.
- Cervical interlaminar and transforaminal epidural steroid injections may provide improvement in radicular symptoms.
- The goals of operative treatment include relief of arm pain and facilitation of neurologic recovery via elimination of compressive pathology.

Cervical radiculopathy occurs less frequently and at an older age than lumbar radiculopathy. Between 5% and 36% of all radiculopathies are from the cervical spine.[1] Radhakrishnan et al.[2] reported that the peak age range for cervical radiculopathy is 50 to 54 years, where there is an incidence rate of 202 per 100,000 people. The overall incidence rate is 83.2 per 100,000 (107.3/100,000 males and 63.5/100,000 females). A history of physical exertion or trauma was present before onset of pain in 14.8% of cases. A confirmed disk protrusion was seen in 21.9% of cases, and spondylosis, disk protrusion, or both were seen in 68.4% of patients with radiculopathy. The prevalence of cervical radiculopathy by level is as follows: 70% at C7, 9% to 25% at C6, 4% to 10% at C8, and 2% at C5.[2]

Incidence and Prevalence

Kondo et al.[3] found the combined incidence of symptomatic herniations and protrusions to be 5.5 per 100,000 people, with occurrence in men being 6.5 per 100,000 compared with 4.6 per 100,000 in women. The incidence in both sexes was highest at 45 to 54 years, followed closely by the incidence at 35 to 44 years. The most common disk involved was C5-C6 followed by C4-C5 and then C6-C7.[3] Kelsey et al.[4] reported that the C5-C6 and C6-C7 levels were involved in 75% of patients, based on review of myelograms and radiographs.

Risk Factors

Risk factors for neck pain in the adult population include smoking and exposure to tobacco and poor psychological health.[5] The prognosis was better in younger patients as well as in patients with greater optimism, less need to socialize, and patients in which coping involves self-assurance. Poor psychological health, anger, frustration, and worrying were associated with a poor prognosis. Between 50% and 75% of patients experienced recurrent pain within 1 to 5 years.[6] In the working population, risk factors for neck pain include age, previous musculoskeletal pain, high quantitative job demands, low social support at work, low physical capacity, job insecurity, poor work posture, and sedentary, repetitive, and precision work. Headaches, emotional problems, smoking, ethnicity, and poor job satisfaction may be associated with neck pain.[7] Women are more likely to suffer neck pain than men. General exercise and white collar employment were positive prognostic factors, whereas a poorer prognosis was associated with workers who had little influence over their work situation, blue collar workers, those with prior neck pain, and those with prior sick leave. Between 60% and 80% of workers reported recurrent pain within 1 year.[8]

Definition and Causes

Cervical radiculopathy is a disease of the cervical nerve roots that results in pain that radiates into one or both upper extremities. It occurs as a result of compression or inflammation (radiculitis) of the nerve root. Compressive causes of radiculopathy include cervical disk herniation, cervical spondylosis, synovial cysts, fractures that cause compression of the nerve root, trauma with nerve root avulsion, intraspinal tumors, osseous malignancies or metastasis, meningeal cysts, arteriovenous fistulas, and vertebral artery compression. Radiculitis may also occur as a result of herpes zoster or with diabetic and autoimmune etiologies. It may even be idiopathic.

Differential Diagnosis

The differential diagnosis of radiculopathy includes brachial plexopathy and mononeuropathies, including the long thoracic, suprascapular, and axillary nerves. Acute onset of pain suggests the differential diagnosis of neuralgic amyotrophy (Parsonage-Turner syndrome). Distal nerves, such as the ulnar, median, and radial nerves, can cause distal pain and paresthesias that can simulate radiculopathies. Mechanical problems involving the shoulder and wrist must be considered as well. Rotator cuff dysfunction or medial and lateral epicondylitis are in the differential diagnosis of the etiology of pain in the extremity and can also develop as a result of muscular imbalances secondary to cervical radiculopathy. Cervical and thoracic myofascial pain, discogenic disease, and facet dysfunction may cause pain to radiate into the upper extremity as well, especially from the lower cervical spine.

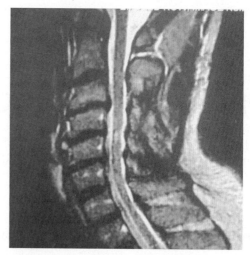

Figure 53-1 Cervical magnetic resonance imaging with sagittal view of T2 image showing signal change secondary to myelopathy resulting from cervical stenosis.

Cervical myelopathy (Fig. 53-1) can be caused by trauma with fractures or dislocations, cervical herniated nucleus pulposus, spondylosis with stenosis, tumor, arteriovenous malformations and dural arteriovenous fistulas, syringomyelia, subacute combined degeneration (vitamin B_{12} deficiency), infection (epidural abscess; tabes dorsalis, a late form of syphilis; lymes, human immunodeficiency virus–related myelopathy), and hereditary paraparesis.[9] The differential diagnosis must include other reasons for upper motor neuron dysfunction, including brain syndromes (stroke, encephalomyelitis, tumor), anterior horn syndrome, and multiple sclerosis.

History

The history includes any incidents or repetitive activities that may precipitate the painful syndrome. The patient should draw a picture of the location of the pain or specifically point to the areas where pain occurs as well as the pattern of paresthesias. The semantics of medicine are such that patients may describe pain in the shoulder and really mean the trapezius or shoulder blade, or even the cervical spine. Thus, it is important to identify the areas involved in a graphic manner. Inquire specifically about activities that exacerbate symptoms in the cervical spine, shoulder, or arm. Paresthesias in the area of the shoulder and lateral elbow are reminiscent of problems with the C4 and C5 nerve roots, respectively. The thumb is classically C6, the middle finger is C7, the small finger is C8, the medial elbow is T1, and the axilla is T2.[10] Diffuse upper extremity paresthesias raise concerns about brachial plexopathy. Weakness in the lower extremities or bowel or bladder retention or incontinence raise concerns about cervical myelopathy.

A full medical history must be taken to evaluate the patient for visceral problems that may contribute to the pain or may impair aspects of treatment. Causes of visceral pain that may result in pain in the area of the shoulder and shoulder blade include cardiac disease (myocardial infarction/ischemia, aortic aneurysm, pulmonary pathology (malignancy, pneumonia, and pulmonary embolism), and gastrointestinal disorders (peptic ulcer disease, cholecystitis, pancreatitis). Previous medications, exercise therapies, modalities, and injection treatments must be reviewed as well as the response to each of these treatments. A full functional and social history must be reviewed to look for activities that may be contributing to maintaining the pain syndrome or are limited secondary to the pain syndrome.

Physical Examination

Physical examination begins with watching the patient walk into the room, when possible, to see whether there is a spastic gait. The patient should disrobe sufficiently so that the muscle bulk of the upper back and upper extremities can be observed. Atrophy may be seen by comparing one side of the body with the other side. Scapular winging should be evaluated by looking at the patient while the patient is standing still and with provocative testing. Winging with scapular protraction correlates with serratus anterior weakness secondary to a long thoracic nerve lesion. The upper, middle, and lower trapezius must also be examined for weakness to determine the integrity of the spinal accessory nerve. Palpation of the cervical paraspinal musculature and trapezius is performed to look for tender points and trigger points. Range of motion in the cervical spine must be evaluated for flexion, extension, rotation, and side bending to each side. Spurling's test requires the patient to extend the neck and rotate and side bend the neck as the examiner applies downward pressure to the top of the head. Findings are consistent with cervical radiculopathy when pain radiates into the limb that is ipsilateral to the side of rotation. Tong et al.[11,12] used electrodiagnosis to establish a sensitivity of 30% and a specificity of 93%.

Imaging Studies

If pain is reproduced in the shoulder with range-of-motion screening, the shoulder should be examined for subacromial impingement syndrome and rotator cuff dysfunction. The elbow should be examined for regional nerve compression syndromes, such as cubital or radial tunnel or tendinopathies of the common extensor tendon (tennis elbow) or common flexor tendon (medial epicondylitis). The chapters on shoulder and elbow examination and specific clinical conditions provide further information to assist with comprehensive examination and differential diagnosis. Motor testing, sensation, and deep tendon reflexes are evaluated in the upper and lower extremities. If the patient has brisk reflexes or lower extremity spasticity, clonus, or a Babinski's sign, then upper motor neuron pathology is a consideration. When upper motor neuron pathology is suspected, the cranial nerves must be evaluated to ensure that the pathology is not cephalad to the cervical spine. If there is bowel or bladder incontinence, then sensation of the genitalia and rectum to pinprick must be evaluated. Voluntary rectal contraction and rectal tone are

evaluated. In upper motor neuron pathology, there may be rectal weakness with an increase in tone (after spinal shock has resolved). Bulbocavernosus and anocutaneous reflexes are brisk in upper motor neuron pathology.

Myotome testing should be performed of the elbow flexors (biceps/brachialis, C5), wrist extensors (extensor carpi radialis, C6), elbow extensors (triceps, C7), finger flexors to the middle finger (flexor digitorum profundus, C8), and small finger abductor (abductor digiti minimi, T1). The deep tendon reflexes evaluated include biceps (C5), brachioradialis (C6), and triceps (C7). Dermatomal sensory testing with a light touch or pinprick is performed. Dermatomal distribution is as follows: C2, occipital protuberance; C3, supraclavicular fossa; C4, over the acromion; C5, lateral epicondyle; C6, extensor surface of the thumb; C7, extensor surface of the middle metacarpophalangeal joint; C8, extensor surface of the fifth metacarpophalangeal joint; and T1, over the medial epicondyle.[10] Chapter 10 provides a comprehensive review of the upper quarter screen described in this chapter.

Pulses in the upper extremities should always be evaluated, especially the radial pulses and carotid artery pulses. Blood pressure should be checked in one and possibly both arms for diagnostic and therapeutic purposes. Medications that may be used to treat radiculopathy may have cardiovascular side effects, and the baseline blood pressure must be known before initiation of treatment with muscle relaxants as well as nonsteroidal anti-inflammatory drugs (NSAIDs).

Cervical spine plain films are of limited use in the diagnosis of radiculopathy. They show age-related degenerative changes, alignment, congenital abnormalities, and gross fractures. Flexion and extension films can show dynamic instability. However, the presence of cervical degenerative changes alone is not diagnostic of pain because these changes are frequently seen in asymptomatic patients.[13]

Magnetic resonance imaging (MRI) is the study of choice for cervical radiculopathy. It can accurately evaluate neural structures and the intervertebral disks painlessly, noninvasively, and without radiation exposure. The spinal cord can be evaluated for intrinsic damage, including edema, blood, tumor, and syrinx. MRI can also help to differentiate between a soft and a hard disk, which may add information about the acuity of disk herniation (Figs. 53-2 and 53-3A and B). In a retrospective review of 34 surgical patients, Brown et al.[14] found that MRI predicted 88% of lesions versus 81% for computed tomography (CT) myelography and 50% for CT scan.

CT myelography is invasive and is not as sensitive as MRI in viewing the spinal cord or intervertebral disk. However, in cases where there is instrumentation, or if MRI is contraindicated (e.g., pacemakers, metallic implants, spinal cord stimulators), then CT myelography is an alternative. A plain CT scan provides excellent visualization of the bony elements and is used to detect nonunion of fusions and acute fractures. It may be used to look for disk herniations if MRI is contraindicated and myelography is deemed too invasive.

These studies do not provide a definitive diagnosis without a clinical context. The results must be matched with the history and physical findings, and potentially with complementary studies to make a diagnosis. CT scan findings can be abnormal in asymptomatic patients.[15] Myelograms show disk abnormalities in 21% of asymptomatic patients.[16] Boden

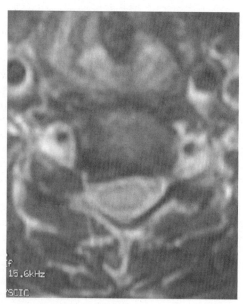

Figure 53-2 Sagittal image of osteophytic cervical disc herniation at C5-C6.

et al.[17] found abnormalities in MRI scans of 19% of asymptomatic patients. Abnormalities were found in 14% of patients younger than 40 years and 28% of patients who were older than 40 years.

Electromyography and nerve conduction is a physiologic test that evaluates the peripheral nervous system. It is used not only to evaluate for radiculopathy but also for plexopathy, individual peripheral nerve lesions, and myopathy. The electromyography and nerve conduction findings may not become abnormal for 10 days to 6 weeks postinjury. The sensitivity of needle electromyography and nerve conduction in cervical radiculopathy is 61% to 67% compared with the gold standards of clinical evaluation, myelogram, and intraoperative impression.[18] Radiculopathy is confirmed by showing spontaneous activity in two or more muscles innervated by the same root level but different peripheral nerve roots. Muscles innervated by root levels above and below the involved levels should be normal.[1] In the lumbar spine, abnormal paraspinal musculature alone does not diagnose radiculopathy and can be abnormal in up to 30% of asymptomatic patients older than 40 years.[19] Chapter 15 provides detailed information on electrophysiologic evaluation of the upper quarter.

Cervical facet syndrome may be the cause of pain in the cervical spine as well as the head and proximal upper extremity. Diagnosis of cervical facet (zygapophyseal joint) dysfunction is made by diagnostic injection into the zygapophyseal joint directly or by diagnostic block of the medial branch of the dorsal rami above and below the symptomatic joint. Referral patterns of facet joints were mapped by Dwyer et al.[20,21] History and physical examination as well as degenerative changes found on anatomic images do not provide a diagnosis. A single uncontrolled diagnostic injection carries a 27% false-positive rate.[22] The patient must have 50% to 80% relief with provocative pain maneuvers on at least two occasions to make a definitive diagnosis. Comparative injections include placebo versus local anesthetic or short-acting versus long-acting anesthetic.[23]

Cervical selective nerve root injections may be used for diagnosis as well. They should be used as an adjunct to the history, physical examination, and previously mentioned diagnostic studies, and not in isolation. The diagnostic injection may help to determine whether a given nerve root is involved in cases where: (1) the pain radiation is not classic for a given root; (2) there are multiple anatomic abnormalities that could result in cervical radiculopathy; or (3) there is a distal pain generator, such as a median or ulnar nerve

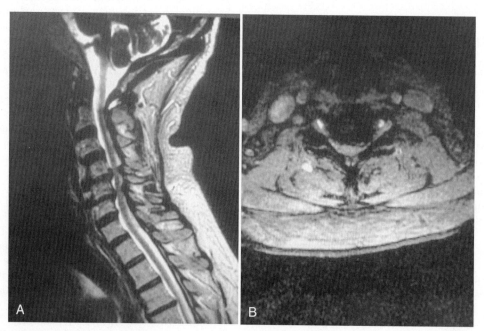

Figure 53-3 A, T2 image of sagittal view of cervical stenosis. **B,** T2 image of axial view of cervical stenosis.

lesion, that may be causing confusion as to the etiology of the symptoms. Anesthetic joint injection of the shoulder or elbow may also be a useful adjunct to determine whether other mechanical problems can be contributing to the pain syndrome instead of or in addition to radiculopathy.[24] In the lumbar spine, false-positive responses have been noted. Placebo and blocking afferents from mechanical structures and peripheral nerve generators may be a part of the reason for false-positive responses.[25]

Drug Treatment

The primary treatment medication categories used for cervical radiculopathy include NSAIDs, muscle relaxants, opioid analgesics, oral corticosteroids, topical agents, antidepressants, anticonvulsants, and acetaminophen. For most cervical conditions, NSAIDs are the first-line intervention. NSAIDs have anti-inflammatory, analgesic, and antipyretic effects. Reducing inflammation is important in treating cervical radiculopathy. NSAIDs achieve their anti-inflammatory effects at high dosages and reduce pain at low dosages. The choice of NSAID must be individualized. If an individual NSAID is not effective, the patient may respond to an NSAID from another class. However, major risk factors include gastrointestinal side effects, renal and hepatic failure, and cardiovascular disease. The results of studies with COX-2 inhibitors are contradictory with regard to gastrointestinal safety profiles.[26,27]

Oral corticosteroids may be useful in the treatment of cervical radiculopathy. They are generally well tolerated, effective, and safe. There have been no documented cases of avascular necrosis when the total prednisone dose or equivalent stayed below 550 mg.[28]

Peloso et al.[29] reviewed the effects of medication on primary outcomes in adults with mechanical neck disorders and whiplash. Although 36 trials were reviewed, a limited number of medications were studied. These included oral NSAIDs and analgesics, psychotropics, corticosteroid injections, local anesthetics, and botulinum toxin A injections. The benefits of muscle relaxants, analgesics, and NSAIDs were questionable. Results showed that botulinum toxin A is no better than saline injections at reducing pain and disability. Chronic neck pain showed some benefit with local anesthetics, and patients with chronic neck pain and associated arm symptoms benefited from epidural injections of a corticosteroid plus a local anesthetic agent. If given within 8 hours of an injury, corticosteroid injections appear to reduce the pain of whiplash.[29]

Muscle relaxants fall into two main categories, antispasmodics and antispasticity medications. Muscle relaxants are not more effective than NSAIDs and have more side effects.[30,31] Their sedative side effects may help patients with pain to rest better when they are used at night.

Opioid analgesics are an option, but should only be used for a time-limited course. Physicians who prescribe opioids must incorporate government-mandated documentation and should use opioid contracts and screen for high-risk patients with a history of substance abuse or substance-seeking behavior. Because of the potential of these drugs for physical dependence, other options should be considered.[32]

Topical agents, including a lidocaine 5% patch and NSAID-containing patches, are attractive to patients who wish to avoid systemic side effects. Common patient complaints include cost, adhesive allergy, and movement of the patch. Compounded topical agents may be beneficial, but there is little evidence-based research to support their off-label use.

Antidepressants have been used successfully to decrease radicular pain and improve restorative sleep. Although selective serotonin reuptake inhibitors lack many of the side effects of tricyclic antidepressants, their efficacy in relieving neck pain compared with tricyclic antidepressants is not known. Dual-action reuptake inhibitors (serotonin and norepinephrine) may offer an advantage over single-action agents because of their effects on norepinephrine. Currently, there are no studies to support this conclusion.[33]

Anticonvulsants, such as gabapentin, are increasingly being used to treat radicular pain. They have been shown to be safe and effective for other types of neuropathic pain conditions. There are no randomized, placebo-controlled, crossover studies that support monotherapy or combined therapy for radicular pain.

Therapy

The primary goals of treatment of cervical radiculopathy are reduction of pain, restoration of strength and function, and prevention of recurrence.[34] Physical therapy is, in most cases, among the recommended first-line treatments. The evidence that physical therapy is of benefit in cervical radiculopathy derives mainly from case series, case reports, and anecdotal experience, because there are few randomized controlled trials addressing this subject in the literature. Therapy should be initiated as soon as possible after symptom onset because patients with acute (<1 month) cervical pain and radiculopathy have been shown to have significantly greater functional improvement after physical therapy intervention than patients with chronic (>6 months) symptoms.[35]

A physical therapy program is generally performed two to three times a week for approximately 4 weeks and may consist of any or all of the following interventions: isometric neck exercises, postural exercises, mechanical traction, cervical manipulation, and the use of modalities such as a cervical collar or transcutaneous electrical nerve stimulation (TENS). Isometric neck exercises are performed early in the course of treatment, when movement of the neck is painful.[36] As pain diminishes, stretching exercises are added to the therapy program to restore neck range of motion. Stretching and strengthening exercises target the cervical paraspinal, shoulder girdle, scapular stabilizing, and lumbar muscles. In a small case series, Cleland et al.[37] found that 10 patients showed significant improvement in pain and function after a physical therapy program that consisted of cervical traction or mobilization and strengthening exercises of the neck flexors and scapulothoracic muscles. In their review of 88 randomized controlled trials, Gross et al.[38] found moderate evidence that various types of neck stretching and strengthening exercises were beneficial for patients with mechanical neck disorders and whiplash-associated neck pain.

Modalities such as heat and ice, electrical stimulation, and use of a cervical collar are employed in the acute phase of disease to reduce pain. No consensus exists regarding the use of soft cervical collars in cervical radiculopathy. Soft collars have been shown in several studies to be of no benefit or less benefit than active therapies and rest.[39] Collars may provide some comfort during sleep or activity during the acute stage of disease, but their use should be limited to no more than 2 to 3 weeks[36] to prevent the development of weakness of the cervical paraspinal musculature.

TENS is a modality that delivers electrical current to the painful area via surface electrodes. TENS is postulated to reduce pain by modulating sensory afferent signals to the substantia gelatinosa (gate-control theory) as well as causing the release of endogenous endorphins.[40] There is conflicting evidence regarding the usefulness of electrotherapies in the treatment of neck pain. A small number of studies have shown TENS to be useful in reducing pain and restoring mobility in patients with acute nonradiating neck pain.[36] In contrast, a Cochrane review found no definite evidence supporting the use of electrotherapies in the treatment of acute neck pain.[41] Precautions and contraindications for electrotherapy should be considered before treatment and are discussed in detail in Chapter 117. Gross et al.[38] and Hurwitz et al.[39] reported that patients with acute cervical pain as a result of whiplash injury or mechanical neck disorder who were treated with phosphatidylethanolamine N-methyltransferase were found to have less pain and analgesic use compared with a placebo group.

Traction is one of the most commonly used modalities in the treatment of cervical radiculopathy, although little literature supports its effectiveness. In physiologic studies, cervical traction using 25 pounds of force has been shown to cause spinal elongation of 2 to 20 mm.[42] Intermittent cervical traction with the neck in 30 degrees of flexion has been shown to cause up to a 21% increase in anterior intervertebral space.[43] A small study comparing patients with unilateral C7 radiculopathy treated with either modalities and exercise alone or intermittent mechanical traction and modalities and exercise found that grip strength was significantly greater after five treatment sessions in the group receiving traction. This difference in grip strength had disappeared, however, after 10 treatment sessions,[44] suggesting that the beneficial effects of traction may be immediate and temporary. The increase in posterior cervical intervertebral space seen after traction has been noted to be temporary, returning to baseline 20 minutes after treatment cessation.[45] Gross et al.[38] found moderate evidence that intermittent cervical traction was of short-term (<3 months) benefit for neck and radicular pain compared with control or placebo.

Mechanical cervical traction may be applied via a motorized device or via a free-weight and pulley system. Traction is created using a head or chin sling attached to a system that provides pull in a cranial direction. When initiating traction therapy, a weight of 5 to 10 pounds is recommended, followed by a gradual increase in weight to a maximum of 50 pounds.[42] A treatment duration of 15 to 25 minutes, if tolerated by the patient, is generally recommended.[42] Home traction units may be ineffective or may cause increased pain if not used properly and with supervision.[36,42] Traction should not be applied with the neck in extension, because of the risk of increased pain, vertebrobasilar insufficiency, or spinal instability.[42] In addition, cervical traction is contraindicated in patients of advanced age or those with ligamentous instability, diskitis, osteomyelitis, vertebral or spinal cord tumor, osteoporosis, uncontrolled hypertension, clinical suspicion of myelopathy, severe anxiety, history suggestive of vertebrobasilar insufficiency, rheumatoid arthritis, midline herniated nucleus pulposus, or acute torticollis.[42]

Manual cervical traction is performed by a physical therapist, usually in conjunction with other spinal manipulation techniques. Low-velocity manipulation, often referred to as cervical mobilization, consists of gentle pressure applied in the available range of cervical flexion, extension, lateral bending, and rotation.[36] Gross et al.[38] found strong evidence that multimodal treatment programs including both exercise and mobilization or manipulation reduced pain and improved function in patients with neck and radicular pain. However, manipulation alone was found to be ineffective in reducing pain. High-velocity manipulations of the cervical spine, often performed by chiropractors or physicians trained in osteopathic manipulation, should be used with caution because such treatment is associated with a small (1/10,000–6/100,000) but serious risk of adverse events, such as stroke, weakness, or paralysis. The risk of these adverse events may be increased in patients with cervical stenosis or vascular disease. Other, more common potential neurologic complications of high-velocity cervical manipulation include headache, fainting, dizziness, lightheadedness, paresthesias in the upper limbs, or transient (6–72 hours) increase in pain.[42,46] Systemic anticoagulation, uncontrolled diabetes, atherosclerosis, suspicion of vertebrobasilar insufficiency, osteoporosis, ligamentous laxity, spondyloarthropathies, and acute disk herniation are all contraindications to high-velocity manipulation.[40]

A physical therapy program for cervical radiculopathy also includes patient education or "neck school," instruction in proper body mechanics, and ergonomic assessment. Neck school consists of instruction, often in small groups of 4 to 10 patients, on topics such as neck anatomy and stress reduction techniques.[36] Neck school may be helpful in preventing recurrences of cervical radiculopathy, but has been found to be ineffective in reducing pain.[38]

Regarding body mechanics, patients with cervical radiculopathy should avoid positions that increase load on the cervical intervertebral disks, such as neck forward flexion and rotation or prolonged neck extension, and should take care that the arms and shoulders are supported when patients are seated.[46] An ergonomic evaluation ensures that the patient's positioning in the workplace, especially when a computer is used, is not exacerbating the symptoms.

Finally, the patient should be reevaluated at frequent intervals throughout the course of physical therapy. If, after 4 to 6 weeks, the patient and therapist do not note improvement in symptoms, the physical therapy program should be discontinued and consideration should be given to other treatment modalities, such as medications or injection procedures. If the therapy program does result in improvement in symptoms, the patient should be instructed in a self-directed home exercise regimen. See Chapter 55 for a detailed review of the therapist's management of upper-quarter neuropathies.

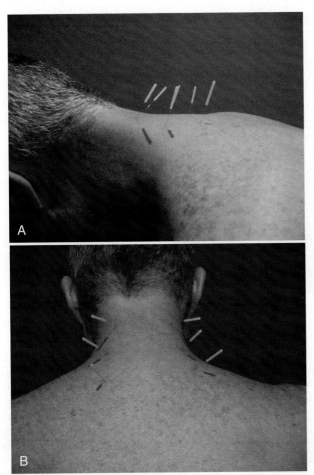

Figure 53-4 Posterior **(A)** and lateral views **(B)** of cervical acupuncture.

Acupuncture

Acupuncture (from the Latin *Acus*, "needle," and *pungere*, "prick") refers to an ancient technique of inserting and manipulating hairlike filiform needles into points on the body with the aim of preventing or treating illnesses[47] (Fig. 53-4A and B); Acupuncture may include stimulation via manual, electrical, thermal (burning of the moxa herb, or moxibustion), or laser techniques.[48] Western science believes that acupuncture analgesia is achieved by stimulation of the peripheral nervous system, autonomic nervous system regulation, anti-inflammation, and direct needling. According to Pomeranz and Berman,[49] acupuncture analgesia occurs by stimulation of small-diameter nerves in muscles that trigger the release of endorphins and monoamines in the spinal cord, midbrain, and hypothalamic–pituitary complex. Acupuncture needle placement and the type of stimulation achieve different effects through this three-level system. Needles placed close to the site of pain maximize spinal circuitry stimulation, providing a more intense analgesic effect because all three centers are used, whereas needling at sites anatomically distant from the painful area activates only the midbrain and hypothalamic–pituitary system. Usually, a combination of the two sites is used to maximize the effect.[50]

Although the practice is accepted by many patients, the effectiveness of acupuncture for cervical radiculopathy remains controversial in the medical community. Acupuncture reduces neck pain and produces statistically, but not clinically, significant effects compared with placebo.[51] Two recent reviews of acupuncture for neck pain showed mixed results. White and Ernst[52] found that an equal number of trials offered positive and negative outcomes. Smith et al.[53] concluded that there is no convincing evidence of the analgesic efficacy of acupuncture in chronic neck or back pain.

A typical initial treatment trial consists of three to four visits over 2 weeks. If there is evidence of objective functional improvement, a total of up to 8 to 12 visits over 4 to 6 weeks is recommended.[54] Acupuncture treatment is safe. Serious injuries are rare when treatment is provided by licensed practitioners. White et al.[55] and MacPherson et al.[56] found no serious events in a 2001 study of 66,000 acupuncture treatments in the United Kingdom. Ernst et al.[57] found that the most common adverse effects were minor bleeding after needle removal, hematoma, and dizziness.

Cervical Injection

In the cervical spine, injections into the epidural space are performed with either an interlaminar or a transforaminal approach. Because of the anatomy of the cervical spine and the important structures in the vicinity, injections must be done under fluoroscopy to assure safe and effective placement.

Interlaminar injections require entering the posterior epidural space. This space narrows at the more cephalad levels. At C7, the space is 1.5 to 2.0 mm, and at higher levels, it decreases to 1.0 mm. Pathology can decrease these dimensions even further. Therefore, the commonly injected sites are the C6-C7 and C7-T1 levels, with maximum space and safety at C7-T1.[58]

Transforaminal epidural steroid injections can be performed at the specific level of the radiculopathy (Fig. 53-5).

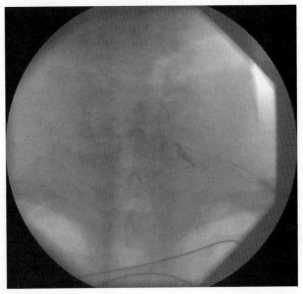

Figure 53-5 Anteroposterior fluoroscopic view of cervical transforaminal epidural steroid injection.

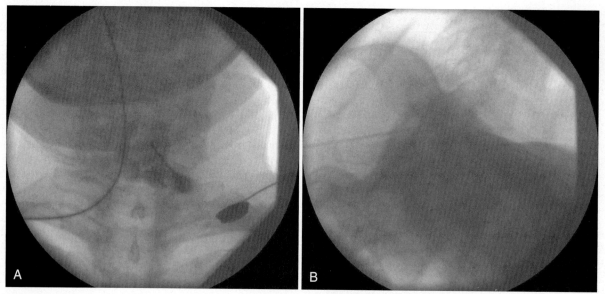

Figure 53-6 A, Anteroposterior fluoroscopic image of cervical translaminar epidural steroid injection. **B,** Lateral fluoroscopic image of cervical transforaminal epidural steroid injection.

In selective nerve root block, a steroid is not injected because the only purpose is to anesthetize a specific nerve root to determine whether that particular nerve root is the pain generator. If the pain resolves, then the anesthetized nerve can be assumed to be the cause of pain. When a therapeutic block is performed, steroids are injected, with or without lidocaine, to decrease inflammation.[59]

There are no randomized studies that support the idea that cervical epidurals are beneficial for axial pain. Cervical interlaminar injections showed efficacy for radiculopathy in two randomized studies (Fig. 53-6A and B). Stav et al.[60] showed that cervical epidural injections were significantly more effective than trigger points at 1 week and 1 year. Cervical interlaminar injections were effective in 76% of patients with radiculopathy at 1 week and in 68% at 1 year. Trigger point injections were effective in 36% at 1 week and in only 12% at 1 year.[60] In another randomized trial, Castagnera et al.[61] showed a 71% improvement in patients at 1 month, followed by a 79% improvement rate at 3-, 6-, and 12-month intervals with cervical interlaminar injections.

Cervical transforaminal injections have been shown to result in improvement in radicular symptoms in nonrandomized studies. Kolstad et al.[62] performed a prospective study in which patients who were scheduled for cervical surgery were injected twice. At 6 weeks and at 4 months, there was a significant decrease in pain, with 5 of the 21 patients canceling surgery. Lin et al.[63] retrospectively showed improvement in 70 patients who underwent cervical epidural injections for radiculopathy. Sixty-three percent of the patients had improvement of symptoms, obviating the need for surgery, at an average of 13 months of follow-up. Cyteval et al.[64] achieved good pain relief in 60% of patients undergoing cervical transforaminal injection without rebound at the 6-month point. Bush and Hillier[65] prospectively showed that patients had good pain relief 7 months after injection.

Cervical interlaminar and transforaminal epidural injections have few serious complications. However, severe morbidity can occur when there is a complication. Waldman[66]

reported three vasovagal syncopal reactions, one superficial infection, and two dural punctures in a series of 790 patients who received cervical epidural steroid injections. Dural puncture was reported in 0.5% to 5.0% of patients undergoing epidural injections. This can lead to resultant postural headaches. The headache increases with standing and sitting, and is alleviated in the supine position. Nausea, vomiting, and photophobia may also occur.[67]

Serious complications of cervical epidural injections have been noted, including abscess and infection.[68] Also, if improper technique is used, then the needle may be directed through the dura into the spinal cord, resulting in traumatic spinal cord injury and possibly syrinx formation, with resultant central cord syndrome.[69]

Serious negative outcomes have also occurred with cervical transforaminal epidural injections. An anonymous survey of physicians in the American Pain Society reported 78 complications, including 16 vertebrobasilar brain infarcts, 12 cervical spinal cord infarcts, and 2 combined brain and spinal cord infarcts. There were 13 fatalities, and 5 of the fatalities were of an unspecified etiology. Complications may not be reported because of existing or pending litigation.[70]

Surgical Treatment

Over the last 50 years, surgical treatment of cervical radiculopathy has been shown to be more successful than the treatment of almost any other spinal disorder. The goals of operative treatment of cervical radiculopathy include relief of arm pain and facilitation of neurologic recovery via elimination of the compressive pathology (i.e., herniated disk, compressive osteophyte, or abnormal motion). Achievement of these goals has been reported in the vast majority of patients treated with a variety of surgical approaches and techniques. Nevertheless, these procedures are generally reserved for individuals who have already undergone unsuccessful nonoperative intervention.

In most patients with cervical radiculopathy, nonoperative treatment results in improvement in arm pain and resumption of normal activities.[71] The natural history of untreated cervical radiculopathy is one of improvement in approximately two thirds of individuals.[72] Consequently, surgical intervention in patients with radiculopathy should generally await the completion of appropriate nonoperative intervention. There are a few notable exceptions to this rule. The first exception is the small group of patients who have disabling weakness of an anti-gravity muscle group that is critical to the patient's daily functional activity, such as the patient who presents acutely with three fifths strength in the right biceps because of a foraminal herniated nucleus pulposus on the right side at C4-C5. Such a scenario may seriously limit the patient's ability to perform daily activities, such as raising the hand to the head to shave, brush the teeth, or comb the hair. A similar scenario in which patients may forego nonoperative treatment and proceed to surgical intervention would be the mechanic or surgeon who has dominant hand intrinsic muscle weakness that makes it difficult to perform work-related tasks. A third, more ambiguous indication for surgical intervention is "intractable pain." Generally, these patients cannot obtain sufficient relief of radicular symptoms despite conservative treatment.

A more common but much more difficult decision-making process for surgery arises in the setting of the patient who presents with complaints of radiculopathy but has evidence of significant spinal cord compression on MRI or CT myelography. Between 5% and 10% of the general population has some degree of cervical spinal cord compression by MRI, yet less than 1% of the general population has cervical myelopathy.[73] Patients with radicular symptoms and concurrent cord compression on MRI may forego nonoperative treatment when they are symptomatic as a result of myelopathy and are experiencing difficulty with coordination, dexterity, balance, or walking. The natural history of untreated cervical myelopathy is not benign.[74] Patients may be asymptomatic but show physical findings indicative of spinal cord compression, including Hoffman's sign or hyperreflexia. The neurologic status of these patients should be monitored periodically. In these patients, decision making is limited by the lack of evidence suggesting the likelihood of progression to symptomatic myelopathy. We generally counsel these patients about their condition and encourage an attempt at nonoperative treatment. However, if the radicular component persists, a stronger recommendation is made to pursue surgical intervention than in the patient without cord compression.

Once the decision is made to proceed with operative intervention, consideration must be given to the optimal surgical approach. Successful relief of radicular pain has been reported with posterior and anterior approaches in more than 90% of patients. The posterior approach requires fashioning an opening or "foraminotomy" just lateral to the spinal canal at the takeoff of the cervical nerve root from the spinal cord. This approach facilitates direct decompression of the nerve when there is a herniated disk that compresses the nerve root in the neural foramen. The posterior approach to radiculopathy relieved pain in more than 90% of affected patients.[75,76]

The anterior approach is more commonly chosen to treat this pathology.[77] There are broader indications for the anterior approach, including compressive pathology, which may be foraminal or directly anterior to the spinal cord. In addition, anterior surgery generally involves "stabilization" of the pathologic motion segment via interbody fusion or placement of an artificial disk. The anterior approach is also preferred for patients who have significant mechanical neck pain, advanced arthritic changes, or a spondylolisthesis (Fig. 53-7A and B).

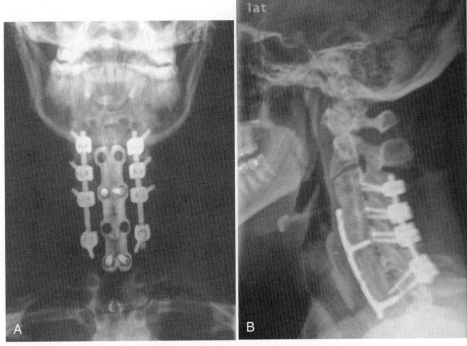

Figure 53-7 Anteroposterior **(A)** and lateral **(B)** x-rays after C3-C7 anterior and posterior fusion.

The classic description of long-term outcomes of pain relief and neurologic improvement was published by Bohlman[78]; the authors reported relief of arm pain and neurologic recovery in more than 90% of patients at an average follow-up of 5 years. More recent data from the recent U.S. Food and Drug Administration–supervised trials of cervical disk replacement support the results of Bohlman[78] with patient-generated outcomes data.[79,80]

There has been little direct comparison between anterior and posterior surgical approaches to the treatment of cervical radiculopathy. A prospective study was performed by Herkowitz et al.[81] in which 44 patients with cervical radiculopathy were randomized to undergo anterior or posterior surgery. With an average follow-up of 4.5 years, successful pain relief was observed in 94% of patients undergoing anterior surgery compared with 75% of patients undergoing posterior surgery.

Complication rates with these operations are low, but can be devastating. In a study of nearly 500 patients undergoing cervical spine surgery for radiculopathy or myelopathy, the incidence of postoperative paresis or paralysis was 0.2%. Other rare but life-threatening complications that occur in approximately 1 per 1000 patients include vertebral artery and esophageal injuries. A complication common to both approaches is an inadequate decompression resulting in little, if any, symptomatic improvement in the postoperative period. There are no reliable data on the incidence of this complication, but based on reported outcomes, it may be assumed to be less than 10%. With the posterior approach, there is approximately a 1% risk of infection and a potential for iatrogenic instability leading to recurrent symptoms if more than 50% of the facet joint is sacrificed in performing the decompression. With the anterior approach, there is a risk of pseudarthrosis, generally less than 10%, which may manifest as recurrent pain after a pain-free interval of 3 to 6 months after surgery. Dysphagia and dysphonia are also common after anterior surgery, although most of these symptoms resolve within 6 weeks of surgery.[82]

In summary, surgical treatment of cervical radiculopathy improves on the natural history of cervical radiculopathy and has a greater likelihood of success than nonoperative treatment. However, surgery exposes patients to greater risks than nonoperative intervention and is therefore generally offered to patients only after unsuccessful nonoperative treatment. In the future, prospective studies comparing outcomes of surgical and nonsurgical treatment of surgical radiculopathy may better define the most appropriate role for surgical intervention in treating this disorder.

Summary

The examination and management of cervical radiculopathy can be challenging to both physicians and therapists because of the extensive differential diagnosis involved as a result of referred pain into the upper extremity. There are many treatment options available to patients to alleviate pain and paresthesia. A trial of conservative treatment with physical therapy is warranted. If no improvement is observed, then other interventions, such as acupuncture, epidural injections, and surgery, may be considered. Early management is crucial to avoid the development of abnormal pain processing and syndromes.

REFERENCES

The complete reference list is available online at www.expertconsult.com.

Thoracic Outlet Syndrome

54

A. LEE OSTERMAN, MD AND CHRIS LINCOSKI, MD

ANATOMY
HISTORY
CLASSIFICATION
DIAGNOSIS
PHYSICAL EXAMINATION

DIAGNOSTIC STUDIES
ELECTRODIAGNOSTIC TESTING
TREATMENT
RESULTS
RECURRENT THORACIC OUTLET SYNDROME

CRITICAL POINTS

- Thoracic outlet syndrome is a controversial entity.
- Diagnosis requires a thorough examination and is primarily clinical.
- Three main presentations exist: Neurogenic, arterial, and venous.
- Most cases can be managed non-operatively.
- Surgical decompression of the thoracic outlet space can be helpful in recalcitrant cases.

There are few clinical entities in hand surgery and therapy that are more controversial and create as confusing a clinical picture as thoracic outlet syndrome (TOS). TOS is defined as compression of the neurovascular structures in the thoracic outlet.[1] An incomplete understanding of the anatomy and the lack of objective physical findings contribute to the confusion and controversy surrounding TOS. This entity remains the most difficult upper extremity compressive neuropathy to manage, given its elusive diagnosis and lack of consistent response to treatment. This chapter briefly reviews the history of this controversial entity and the relevant anatomy and discusses the current standards of diagnosis and recommended surgical treatment. The next chapter (Chapter 55) discusses the role of physical therapy for the treatment of TOS.

Anatomy

The thoracic outlet is the region from the intervertebral foramina to the coracoid process and contains the brachial plexus, subclavian artery, and vein[2] (Fig. 54-1). There are three distinct anatomic areas where compression can occur: the interscalene triangle (or scalene interval), the costoclavicular space, and the subcoracoid space. Any condition, such as congenital variations, space-occupying lesions, inflammation, or fibrosis secondary to trauma, can narrow these spaces, resulting in compression neuropathy of the brachial plexus or arterial or venous compression.

The interscalene triangle is bordered anteriorly by the anterior scalene muscle, posteriorly by the middle scalene muscle, and inferiorly by the clavicle (Fig. 54-2). The brachial plexus and subclavian artery pass through this space, and the subclavian vein passes anterior to it. The scalene muscles act as secondary respiratory muscles by causing elevation of the first rib during deep inspiration. Use of these muscles can cause neurovascular compression because of their intimate relationship with the brachial plexus and subclavian artery that pass between the anterior and middle scalene muscles. Abnormalities of the scalene muscles have been reported with overlapping insertions and variable fusions of the anterior and middle scalenes[3] (Fig. 54-3). The scalenus minimus is an anomalous muscle originating from the transverse process of the C6-C7 vertebrae and inserting on the first rib and pleural fascia. It courses between the subclavian artery and lower brachial plexus. This anomalous muscle can narrow the scalene interval, resulting in neurovascular compression. It has been reported in 30% to 50% of cases of TOS.[3]

The costoclavicular space or triangle is bordered anteriorly by the clavicle, costocoracoid ligament, and subclavius muscle; posteromedially by the first rib; and posterolaterally by the scapula[4,5] (Fig. 54-4). Compression of the subclavian vessel and brachial plexus can result from several causes: fracture callus or hematoma of the first rib or medial clavicle,

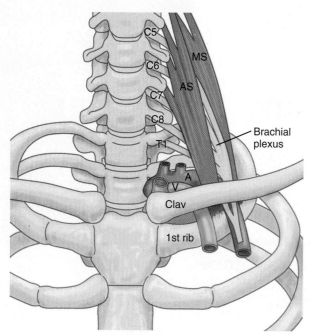

Figure 54-1 The thoracic outlet is a normal space defined by the borders of the scalene muscles and the first rib. The subclavian vein is anterior to the anterior scalene, but beneath the clavicle (Clav). A, subclavian artery; AS, anterior scalene; MS, middle scalene; V, subclavian vein.

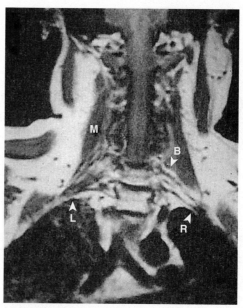

Figure 54-3 Magnetic resonance imaging of the brachial plexus showing a normal plexus without abnormal masses. B, brachial plexus; L, lung apex; M, scalene muscle; R, first rib.

poor posture with drooping shoulders, or congenital narrowing or abnormalities. Hypertrophy of the subclavius can result in compression of the subclavian vein, causing Paget–Schroetter syndrome.[6] The costoclavicular ligament is also implicated in compression of the subclavian vein.[7]

The subcoracoid space is the least common site for entrapment of the three potential areas of compression.[4] The neurovascular bundle runs inferior to the coracoid and below the pectoralis minor, which inserts on the coracoid process. The pectoralis minor can impinge on the neurovascular bundle in hyperabduction of the extremity. Arm abduction stretches the neurovascular bundle around the coracoid and also tenses the pectoralis minor, which causes further compres-

sion. Wright[8] coined the term *hyperabduction syndrome* and described Wright's hyperabduction test. He noted this in short, stocky men who repetitively extend their arms above their heads. Hyperabduction of the arm also moves the clavicle posteriorly and superiorly, narrowing the costoclavicular space.

Cervical ribs are one of the structures most commonly associated with TOS. Cervical ribs are present in 0.2%–0.6% of individuals and bilateral in 50% to 80%.[4] They may be completely formed, but are more often incomplete and have

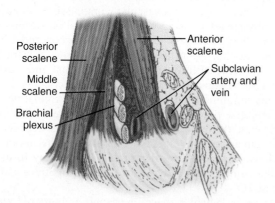

Figure 54-2 The interscalene triangle is bordered anteriorly by the anterior scalene muscle, posteriorly by the middle scalene, and inferiorly by the clavicle. The brachial plexus and subclavian artery pass through this space, and the subclavian vein passes anterior. The scalene muscles act as secondary respiratory muscles by causing elevation of the first rib during deep inspiration.

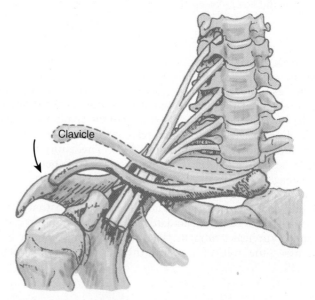

Figure 54-4 The costoclavicular space or triangle is bordered anteriorly by the clavicle, costocoracoid ligament, and subclavius muscle, posteromedially by the first rib, and posterolaterally by the scapula. The space is dynamic and as we move our shoulder forward the clavicle rotates (*arrow*) and the space narrows.

a fibrous band or anlage connecting the bony tip of the cervical rib to the first rib. Wright[8] and Roos[7,9] described nine types of fascial bands causing neurovascular compression. These fibrous bands frequently attach to the tip of a cervical rib, the transverse process of C7, or the first rib, and are commonly implicated in arterial compression. They can also result in compression of the brachial plexus, causing neurologic symptoms.[10]

First rib anomalies can further narrow the thoracic outlet. These anomalies can include fusion of a cervical rib to the first rib, fusion of the first rib to the second rib, and abnormally positioned or bifid ribs. Fracture of the first rib can result in callus, which can cause compression of the neurovascular structures.

History

The history of TOS is rich with contributions from legendary surgeons: Galen, Vesalius, Halstead, Ochsner, DeBakey, and Adson. The history of TOS begins with Galen and Vesalius, with the recognition of cervical ribs. The diagnosis of cervical rib syndrome is first attributed to Willshire[11] in 1860. Surgical rib resection was first reported by Coote[12] in 1861 for cervical rib compression. First rib resection was originally reported by Murphy in 1910.[13]

Later, a shift in thinking about the pathogenesis of TOS occurred. Adson and Coffey[14] reported on compression of the neurovascular structures by the scalene musculature. They recommended a new procedure, anterior scalenotomy, and removal of any abnormal tendinous insertions.[14] He subsequently described Adson's sign (discussed later). Ochsner et al.[15] reported on scalene muscle abnormalities and coined the term *scalenus anticus syndrome* in 1935. Scalenotomy subsequently became the most popular procedure for TOS. Scalenotomy fell out of favor after a recurrence rate of 60% was noted,[16] and attention was focused on identifying other etiologic factors. Compression between the first rib and clavicle was implicated, with Falconer and Weddell[17] introducing the term *costoclavicular compression syndrome* in 1943.

Gradually, attention became less focused on the scalene musculature and more on the contribution of the first rib. Roos[9] described a transaxillary approach to first rib resection in 1966. He reported a 93% improvement rate, and this subsequently became the preferred procedure for TOS. Roos focused the attention of surgeons back onto the brachial plexus compression rather than on the vascular compression and described many congenital bands causing TOS.[7,8] Atasoy[18] combined Adson's work implicating the scalene interval as a site of compression and the work of Roos implicating the first rib. In 1996, Atasoy[18] reported combined transaxillary cervical rib resection and transcervical scalenectomy for complete decompression of the thoracic outlet.

The great number of surgeons who have contributed to this diagnostic entity, first focusing on vascular compression and later on neurologic compression, has led to a variety of nomenclature associated with TOS. This variety of nomenclature underscores the difficulty with diagnosis and its varied presentation. The greater entity of TOS has been called cervical rib syndrome, scalene anticus syndrome, subcoracoid–pectoralis minor syndrome, costoclavicular syndrome,

first thoracic rib syndrome, scalenus medius syndrome, Paget–Schroetter syndrome, rucksack palsy, droopy shoulder syndrome, and hyperabduction syndrome. In this chapter, the encompassing term *thoracic outlet syndrome*, as proposed by Peet et al.,[19] is used.

Classification

Wilbourn[20] classified TOS into two main types, vascular and neurogenic (Box 54-1). The vascular type is much less common and represents fewer than 5% of TOS procedures performed. Vascular TOS is further subdivided into two subtypes, arterial TOS and venous TOS. Given the different subtypes, TOS can have a varied presentation. Compression of the subclavian vein and compression of the subclavian artery represent venous and arterial TOS, respectively, whereas compression of the brachial plexus results in neurogenic TOS. It is estimated that the brachial plexus is the most commonly compressed structure (90%), followed by the subclavian vein (6% to 7%) and subclavian artery (3% to 4%).[4,21] The vascular subtypes exhibit objective signs and symptoms of diagnosis, whereas the neurogenic types often do not. Thus, much controversy surrounding TOS relates to the neurogenic type.

Arterial Thoracic Outlet Syndrome

Arterial TOS is the least common type, representing fewer than 1% of cases in a series of more than 2500 cases reported by Sanders et al.[22] Arterial TOS can be acute, chronic, or acute-on-chronic. Acute TOS is rapidly clinically evident and can result in limb-threatening ischemia. Signs and symptoms include pain, pallor, pulselessness, and paresthesias. Chronic or acute-on-chronic arterial TOS frequently presents with thromboembolic complications. Chronic arterial compression leads to intimal damage, arterial stenosis, thrombus formation, thromboembolic complications, and aneurysm formation. This is frequently diagnosed late. A history of unilateral Raynaud's disease should raise suspicion for a missed diagnosis of chronic arterial TOS. Likewise, a patient with neurologic compression as a result of TOS syndrome should be examined for signs of microembolic disease, including claudication, fingertip ulcerations, and cold intolerance. Arterial TOS is almost always caused by a bony anomaly causing compression.[20] Almost all patients have

---

> **Box 54-1 Classification of Thoracic Outlet Syndrome**
>
> **VASCULAR**
> Arterial thoracic outlet syndrome
> Venous thoracic outlet syndrome
>
> **NEUROGENIC**
> True neurogenic thoracic outlet syndrome
> Disputed neurogenic thoracic outlet syndrome

either a well-developed cervical rib or another bony anomaly causing compression.[23,24] Dense fascial bands originating from a cervical rib or an elongated transverse process of C7 have specifically been implicated.[25] Additionally, a malunion of the clavicle or first rib may cause arterial compression.[20] These may result in compression of the subclavian artery, with positional changes seen with Adson's test and Wright's hyperabduction maneuver. The subclavian artery may be palpable superior to the clavicle, and a bruit may be present. If arterial TOS is encountered, a chest radiograph should be performed to evaluate for cervical rib or other bony anomaly. The diagnosis of vascular TOS can be evaluated initially by noninvasive tests, such as duplex imaging, and confirmed with angiography. The treatment of acute arterial TOS is with urgent embolectomy. Treatment of chronic arterial TOS is with surgical decompression with arterial repair or reconstruction.[20]

Venous Thoracic Outlet Syndrome

Venous TOS is occlusion of the subclavian vein in the thoracic outlet. It is more common than arterial TOS, but much less common than neurogenic TOS. It represents only 2% to 3% of all cases of TOS. As with arterial TOS, venous TOS can be acute or chronic. Acute venous TOS can occur because of a thrombus or can occur suddenly after sudden maximal arm use, termed *effort thrombosis* or *Paget–Schroetter syndrome*. This typically occurs in muscular young men after strenuous exercise, and is believed to be caused by impingement from the costoclavicular ligament. This may also occur with overhand athletes because of abduction of the arm, causing compression and occlusion of the subclavian vein.[26] Acute occlusion results in a sudden painful swelling of the arm, whereas chronic occlusion presents more insidiously with swelling or cyanosis. The best test for diagnosis is dynamic venography.[27] If findings on static venography are normal, the arm may be abducted to 180 degrees, showing pathologic compression in this position. Subclavian venous thrombosis most often occurs as a result of secondary causes, such as an underlying clotting abnormality or subclavian catheters. Extrinsic compression of the subclavian vein can also occur because of a tumor. Primary compression of the subclavian vein usually occurs in the costoclavicular space.[27] Treatment involves removing the clot with thrombolysis and subsequent correction of the underlying abnormality.[27,28] If compression is caused by a congenitally tight costoclavicular space, this can be treated with surgical decompression by transaxillary first rib resection.

Neurogenic Thoracic Outlet Syndrome

Neurogenic TOS is by far the most common type, as classified by Wilbourn.[20] The most common etiology of neurogenic TOS is neck trauma in an individual with anatomic predisposition to narrowing at the thoracic outlet.[29] Hyperextension neck injuries result in scarring of the scalene muscles. Ochsner[15] described hypertrophy, degeneration, and fibrosis of the anterior scalene muscles. This is believed to result in neurologic compression. The second most common etiology of neurogenic TOS is repetitive stress injuries. Poor posture is also believed to play a role.

Wilbourn[30] subclassified neurogenic TOS into "true" neurogenic and "disputed" neurogenic types. True neurogenic TOS is exceedingly rare and shows objective signs of nerve compression, usually of the lower brachial plexus. Objective signs and symptoms include paresthesias in the lower plexus distribution, intrinsic wasting, decreased grip strength, and hypothenar atrophy. Patients typically have minimal pain, but do have objective findings of neurologic compression. True neurogenic TOS is almost always associated with a bony anomaly, such as a cervical rib causing nerve compression.[30] Paresthesias are the most common presenting symptom and occur in up to 95% of individuals.[31] Paresthesias most characteristically involve the medial forearm and the fourth and fifth digits.

Symptoms of disputed neurogenic TOS are more vague and can include shoulder pain, extremity weakness, headache, neck and scapular muscle spasm, arm dysesthesias, and paresthesias. Because of the preponderance of lower plexus involvement, paresthesias more commonly affect the medial forearm and fourth and fifth digits; however, they can also be vague, involving the entire arm. This vague presentation is characteristic of the disputed neurogenic type rather than the true neurogenic type. Patients may complain of a "dead arm" sensation, where the entire arm may "go to sleep." Patients may also note weakness and fatigue of the extremity, especially in the intrinsic musculature. Symptoms can be worsened with overhead activity and placing the arm in a hyperabducted position. Disputed neurogenic TOS may also cause vague vascular symptoms, such as swelling, cyanosis, and a cool hand.

Diagnosis

Because of the varied presentation of compression at the thoracic outlet, the diagnosis of TOS can be difficult. Additionally, the vast majority of patients with neurogenic TOS have the disputed type without objective findings or positive electrodiagnostic test results, making this diagnosis particularly challenging. The diagnosis is primarily clinical, with ancillary studies performed to rule out other diagnoses. Approximately 98% of symptoms are neurologic. It commonly presents between 20 and 40 years.[1] The incidence in women is three times that in men. The reasons for this are unclear, possibly related to an increased incidence of bony and soft tissue anomalies in the neck.[32] Interestingly, it is more common in patients with private health insurance and is rarely diagnosed in the Medicaid or worker's compensation population.[33] The incidence is increasing in the United States, but it is less prevalent in other countries, such as the United Kingdom.

TOS may occur simultaneously with carpal tunnel syndrome, cubital tunnel syndrome, or other compressive neuropathies, as a double-crush phenomenon. Proximal compression of the brachial plexus can result in increased susceptibility to compression in the carpal tunnel and cubital tunnel. Conversely, a reverse double-crush scenario is possible, with distal compression resulting in increased susceptibility to proximal compression because of altered proximal axoplasmic flow. Wood and Biondi[34] reported double-crush phenomena in 42% of cases of TOS. The most common double-crush associated with TOS was carpal tunnel syndrome, affecting 41 of 165 patients. Carpal tunnel is believed to occur in 20% to 45% of cases of TOS, and cubital tunnel syndrome is believed to occur in approximately 10% of cases.[35] These syndromes need to be excluded for the diagnosis of TOS to be made.

Initial workup should include a thorough and comprehensive physical examination, provocative tests, and diagnostic studies, such as cervical spine radiographs, chest radiographs, electrodiagnostic testing, and somatosensory evoked potentials (SSEPs).

Physical Examination

Because the diagnosis of TOS is frequently clinically based, with lack of objective confirmatory tests, the physical examination should be comprehensive. The physical examination should begin with the patient unclothed above the shoulders. The patient's shoulder posture should be noted and the arms inspected for swelling. Tenderness in the neck, shoulder girdle, and clavicular fossa as well as Tinel's sign, scapular winging, and muscle spasm should be noted. A thorough physical examination of the upper extremity should be performed, including detailed muscle strength and sensation using Semmes–Weinstein monofilaments. Provocative tests should be conducted to rule out other conditions, such as carpal tunnel syndrome, cubital tunnel syndrome, cervical radiculopathy, tendonitis, and rotator cuff tears, starting distal and proceeding proximally. Only then should provocative tests for TOS be performed.

Adson's Test

Adson's test (or Adson's maneuver) is performed by placing the arm at the side and having the patient hyperextend the neck, turn the face toward the affected side, and take a deep breath, as originally described by Adson and Coffey[14] (Fig. 54-5A and B). The physician stands behind the patient and monitors for loss of radial pulse and reproduction of paresthesias. Inspiration tightens the accessory respiratory muscles, the scalenes, narrowing the scalene interval and causing compression of the brachial plexus and subclavian artery. A positive test result is classically described as obliteration of the radial pulse with inspiration. However, test results can be positive in normal, asymptomatic individuals, limiting the diagnostic value of the test.[14] Sanders and Hammond[27] believe that it has no clinical value for the diagnosis of TOS. Reproduction of the patient's symptoms should also be noted.

Wright's Hyperabduction Test

The arm is externally rotated and abducted to 180 degrees, with the elbow flexed 90 degrees, as the patient inhales deeply (Fig. 54-6). A positive test result shows a decrease in the pulse as the maneuver is performed. In Wright's[36] original description, a position of hyperabduction during sleep was noted to cause arm paresthesias. MacKinnon[37] modified the test by having the elbow extended, minimizing cubital tunnel compression. Some would consider reproduction of

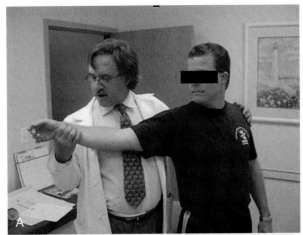

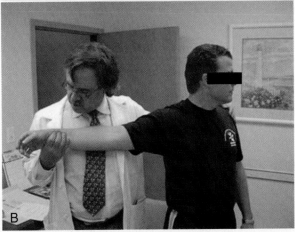

Figure 54-5 A, Adson's test is performed by having the patient place the arm at the side, hyperextend the neck, turn the face toward the affected side, and take a deep breath, as originally described by Adson. **B,** A reverse Adson's test can follow the standard test by having the patient turn the head in the opposite direction. The examiner should look for pulse obliteration and reproduction of symptoms. Many patients can normally have a pulse diminution without symptoms.

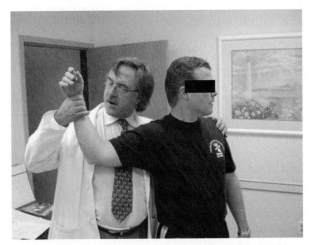

Figure 54-6 Wright's hyperabduction test. The arm is externally rotated and abducted to 180 degrees, with the elbow flexed 90 degrees, as the patient inhales deeply. A positive result shows a decrease in the pulse as the maneuver is performed.

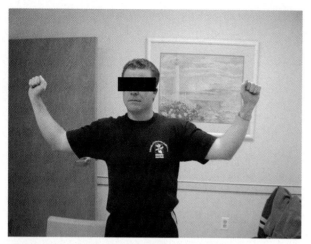

Figure 54-7 The Roos' test or elevated arm stress test. The arms are held in a position of 90 degrees of abduction and externally rotated ("stick-up position"). The patient then opens and closes the hands slowly for a period of 3 minutes. Reproduction of symptoms in the entire extremity or rapid fatigue of the extremity constitutes a positive result.

symptoms as a positive test result.[14] Hyperabduction causes compression in the subcoracoid region by the pectoralis minor muscle.

Roos' Test

Roos' test is also called the elevated arm stress test (Fig. 54-7). The arms are held in a position of 90 degrees of abduction and externally rotated ("stick-up position"). The patient then opens and closes the hands slowly for a period of 3 minutes. Reproduction of symptoms in the entire extremity or rapid fatigue of the extremity constitutes a positive test result. Patients with TOS typically cannot complete this test. Many authors[1,2,38] described this as the most reliable test for TOS. The test is of the most diagnostic benefit when symptoms occur rapidly after elevation of the arm.[21] One study showed reproduction of symptoms in 94% of patients with neurogenic TOS.[19] We believe that this maneuver can reproduce symptoms of other pathologies, including carpal tunnel syndrome, cubital tunnel syndrome, and rotator cuff syndrome, and the results should be interpreted with caution.

Hunter's Test (Brachial Plexus Tension Test)

This test involves reproduction of the patient's symptoms by placing particular portions of the brachial plexus under maximal tension. Tension of the lower plexus is performed by placing the arm at 90 degrees of abduction, with the elbow extended, the wrist extended, and the palm upward. Maximal stretch of the lower trunk will result in pain and paresthesias in the medial forearm and fourth and fifth digits. Whitenack et al.[25] also described different positions that result in maximal stretch of the upper and middle plexus.

Halsted Maneuver

The Halsted maneuver is also referred to as the military brace test or costoclavicular test. The patient moves the shoulders

inferiorly and medially, protruding the chest, as in a military posture. This test narrows the thoracic outlet. Further narrowing can be accomplished by having the examiner apply downward traction to the arm, causing compression of the clavicle on the thoracic outlet.

Upper Limb Tension Test of Elvey

The upper limb tension test is performed in three positions. Position 1 is abduction of both arms to 90 degrees with the elbow extended. Position 2 is position 1 plus dorsiflexion of the wrists. Position 3 is positions 1 and 2 plus tilting of the head to the contralateral side. A positive test result is indicated by pain and paresthesias radiating down the arm, with the strongest evidence of TOS indicated by a positive response in position 1. A recent study showed this to be a positive physical finding in 98% of a series of 50 patients with TOS.[19]

A study of the false-positive rate with provocative physical examination testing in healthy subjects showed that outcomes of pulse alteration or paresthesias were unreliable.[39] When a positive outcome was defined as pain, Adson's test, the Halstead maneuver, and the supraclavicular pressure test (pressure over the supraclavicular fossa at the medial scalene muscle for 30 seconds) had reasonably low false-positive results. A positive outcome defined as discontinuation of the elevated arm stress test because of pain, or pain in the arm after multiple maneuvers, also had a low false-positive rate.[40] Others have also suggested low specificity of the diagnostic physical examination maneuvers discussed earlier.

Diagnostic Studies

Initial diagnostic studies for the evaluation of TOS are cervical spine radiographs, chest radiographs, electrodiagnostic testing, and SSEPs. There are tests that are useful for the diagnosis of vascular TOS and true neurogenic TOS; however, there are no "gold standard" diagnostic studies to confirm neurogenic TOS. The initial diagnostic studies are performed in disputed neurogenic TOS to rule out other entities. Cervical spine films evaluate for cervical disk disease, degenerative joint disease, or neural foramina narrowing, all of which can mimic TOS. Cervical spine films and chest radiographs should be evaluated for the presence of cervical ribs, an elongated C7 transverse process, and structural anomalies of the first rib and clavicle, which are commonly present in true neurogenic TOS (Fig. 54-8). The C7 transverse process is elongated if it projects lateral to the plane of the T1 transverse process on the anteroposterior view. The apical lung segment should be evaluated on a chest radiograph to exclude a tumor. Pancoast tumor must be included in the differential diagnosis of a patient with paresthesias in the C8-T1 distribution.

If vascular compression is suspected, noninvasive tests, such as duplex ultrasonography, pulse volume recordings, and plethysmography, can be used. If vascular compression is not suspected, these tests do not need to be included in the routine evaluation of neurogenic TOS. Vascular TOS can be further evaluated, with angiography and venography representing the "gold standard" for arterial and venous TOS, respectively (Fig. 54-9). There are reports of the use of

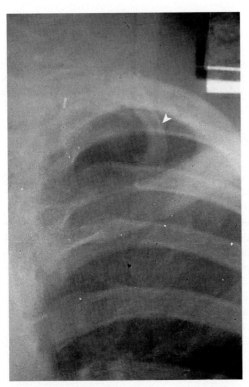

Figure 54-8 Routine chest x-ray showing a cervical rib (*arrow*).

Electrodiagnostic Testing

Although patients with disputed neurogenic TOS have negative findings on electrodiagnostic testing, electromyography (EMG) and nerve conduction velocity (NCV) remain an important part of the initial evaluation of suspected TOS. EMG and NCV are performed to rule out sites of distal compression and evaluate for possible double-crush syndrome. Because there are no gold standard tests for disputed neurogenic TOS, it is important to rule out other pathology, such as carpal tunnel syndrome and cubital tunnel syndrome, which can present with similar symptoms. This can be done with EMG and NCV. Routine electrodiagnostic tests are not useful to confirm the presence of disputed neurogenic TOS.[45] However, they have utility for the diagnosis of true neurogenic TOS. True neurogenic TOS shows reduction of the amplitude of ulnar and median compound nerve action potentials and a decreased or absent medial antebrachial cutaneous (MABC) sensory nerve action potential (SNAP). EMG in this setting can be helpful for the diagnosis of true neurogenic TOS.[46] The advantage of electrodiagnostic testing is that, if the findings are positive, they can provide objective data for diagnosis. In patients with objective physical signs of nerve compression, such as intrinsic wasting, EMG and NCV show chronic denervation, reduced amplitude and prolongation of ulnar SSEP latency, delay in F wave latency, changes in median nerve motor action potential and ulnar nerve SNAP, and decreased MABC SNAP amplitude. A report of MABC SNAP in 16 patients showed decreased MABC SNAP amplitude in neurogenic TOS with lower plexus involvement, suggesting its possible use as an early diagnostic tool.[47] Similarly, for suspected upper plexus lesions, the lateral antebrachial cutaneous nerve amplitude can be tested.[48]

SSEPs are a measure of the electrical conduction of a distal sensation through the brachial plexus, nerve roots, spinal cord, and central nervous system. Several studies suggest that SSEPs are useful in the diagnosis of TOS in patients with objective signs of muscle wasting and weakness, and are not useful in patients with only subjective signs of TOS.[49-51] They can be helpful in true neurogenic TOS, but there is no consensus in the literature as to their utility in disputed

magnetic resonance angiography for the diagnosis of arterial TOS; however, evidence-based studies of CT angiography have recently been described, and this may become the imaging modality of choice.[41]

The best use for MRI is to exclude the diagnosis of cervical spine pathology rather than for the diagnosis of TOS. There are some case reports of MRI being used to identify compression of the brachial plexus[42,43]; however, currently, MRI is not the standard of care for the diagnosis of TOS. A recent blinded study that was performed to evaluate positional change in patients with TOS showed that MRA done in a provocative position, such as the Halsted maneuver, is more valuable in the diagnosis of TOS[44] (Fig. 54-10).

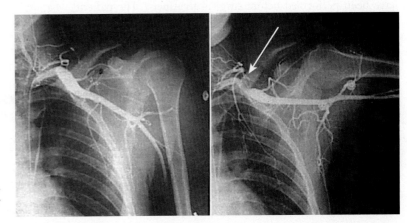

Figure 54-9 Stress angiography showing narrowing of dye flow at the thoracic outlet (*arrow*) in the abducted externally rotated arm position.

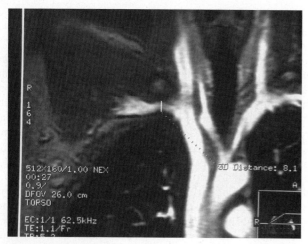

Figure 54-10 Magnetic resonance angiography showing occlusion of contrast at the thoracic outlet level.

neurogenic TOS. Komanetsky et al.[52] reported 21 patients with TOS who were examined with SSEP monitoring. There was no significant difference in brachial plexus conduction time (interpeak latencies) between the TOS group and the control group. However, significant differences were noted with arm positioning, specifically, abduction and external rotation, suggesting that SSEPs are not helpful in the diagnosis of disputed TOS.[52]

Treatment

The first-line treatment is physical therapy. Most cases of TOS can be managed effectively with a therapy program, including a comprehensive program of postural modification, nerve gliding exercises, education, and strengthening.[53] This therapy is discussed in the following chapter. The remainder of this chapter discusses surgical treatment.

Indications for surgery are straightforward for true neurogenic and vascular TOS. Patients with arterial compression or signs of arterial insufficiency should undergo urgent decompression, typically through a combined approach.[54] Indications for surgery in true neurogenic TOS include intrinsic wasting, frequently accompanied by objective EMG and NCV evidence of nerve compression.[55] Indications for disputed neurogenic classification are less clear. At a minimum, an extensive course of physical therapy should have been performed before surgical treatment. The patient should be evaluated for sites of distal compression and treated if necessary before contemplation of surgical treatment for TOS. MacKinnon and Patterson's[54] indications for surgery are failure of 3 months of supervised therapy and double-crush with failure of surgical management of the distal compression. However, others have developed differing surgical indications for disputed neurogenic TOS. Urschel[55] believed that it was mandatory to have prolongation of ulnar and median NCV across the thoracic outlet in addition to failure of conservative treatment before considering surgery.

There are two general surgical approaches to TOS. The first involves anterior scalenectomy, with or without brachial plexus neurolysis. The second involves removal of the first rib. In all cases, abnormal anatomy that may be causing compression should be addressed, such as a cervical rib or fibrous attachments to a cervical rib. Removal of the first rib can be accomplished through either a transaxillary approach or a supraclavicular approach. Each technique has proponents, and results are similar.[56] There is no consensus as to the best surgical approach or procedure for TOS.

Transaxillary Rib Resection

Transaxillary rib resection was first performed in 1966 by Roos,[56] who popularized this approach. Proponents believe that it is a safer approach because dissection is not near the brachial plexus and axillary vessels. It also avoids the complication of long thoracic and phrenic nerve injuries, and produces a more acceptable cosmetic result (Fig. 54-11A to C). Disadvantages of this approach include poor visualization of the posterior aspect of the first rib and lack of access to the brachial plexus (which frequently lies medial to the first rib) and congenital bands or cervical ribs. Formal exploration of the upper brachial plexus cannot be done through this approach. The entire rib should be resected. Poor visualization of the posterior aspect of the first rib can result in a long residual first rib stump. Rib stump length is believed to play a role in recurrent TOS.[57,58]

Supraclavicular Rib Resection

The supraclavicular approach allows wider exposure of the brachial plexus and more direct access to the cervical ribs or fibrous bands causing compression. If anomalous first ribs or fibrous bands are present, they should be removed. This can be best accomplished through the supraclavicular approach. This approach also allows easier access to the brachial plexus and scalenes for scalenectomy and upper plexus neurolysis and is the approach favored by many neurosurgeons.[59] The disadvantage of the supraclavicular approach is a higher incidence of thoracic duct and phrenic nerve injuries. Phrenic nerve paralysis has been reported in up to 7% of cases.[60]

An incision parallel to the clavicle is made approximately 2 cm above the clavicle and beginning 1 cm lateral to the midline (Fig. 54-12A and B). Supraclavicular nerves are identified, the platysma is incised, and the anterior scalene muscle is identified. The phrenic nerve is identified adjacent to the anterior scalene. The anterior scalene muscle is then divided at its insertion on the first rib. Neurolysis of the brachial plexus and middle scalenectomy can then be performed. This exposure can be used for isolated scalenectomy and brachial plexus neurolysis without first rib resection. If the first rib is to be removed, it can be done easily through this approach.

Anterior Scalenectomy and Brachial Plexus Neurolysis

Anterior scalenotomy was described by Adson and Coffey in 1927.[14] This remained a popular operative treatment method until Clagett[61] reported a high failure rate with this procedure and recommended first rib resection instead. Anterior scalenectomy is reported to have a higher success rate than anterior scalenotomy, which does not involve

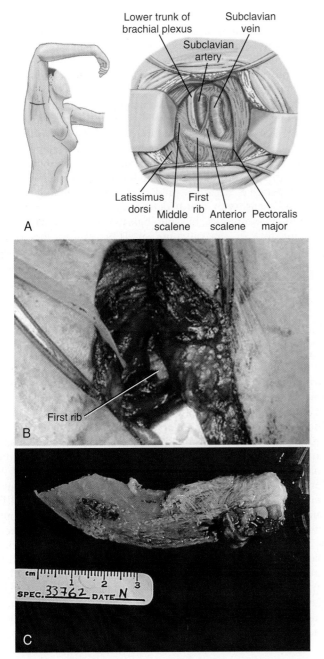

Figure 54-11 A, Diagram of the transaxillary approach. **B,** Visualization of the first rib. **C,** Excised first rib.

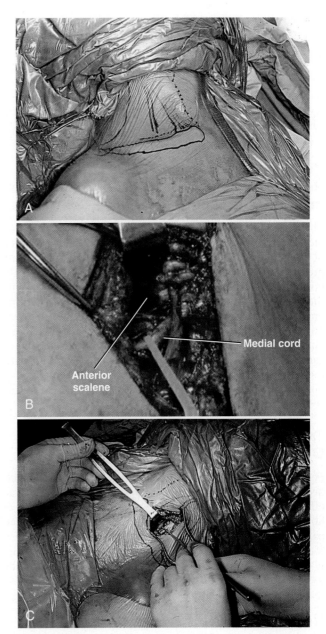

Figure 54-12 A, Supraclavicular approach allowing direct access to the brachial plexus and scalene. **B,** View of the plexus emerging behind the anterior scalene. **C,** After resection of the scalene, the artery and liberated plexus are evident.

removal of the anterior scalene muscle.[62] Anterior scalenectomy removes offending structures compressing the brachial plexus more effectively than scalenotomy alone. Also, middle scalenectomy can be performed easily, resulting in more complete decompression than scalenotomy alone. The reported failure rate of anterior scalenectomy alone is 12%.[62] Today, this procedure is most commonly used in conjunction with brachial plexus neurolysis. Combined neurolysis reportedly improves results.[63] It can also be performed as a combined approach with first rib resection and anterior scalenectomy.

Anterior scalenectomy involves a 5-cm incision superior and parallel to the clavicle. Dissection is carried through the platysma muscle. Then the clavicular head of the sterno-cleidomastoid is transected. The anterior scalene muscle is then identified. Structures at risk during this dissection include the thoracic duct and phrenic nerve. The anterior scalene muscle is then transected and removed in its entirety. Portions of the middle scalene muscle can also be removed if this muscle contributes to impingement of the brachial plexus. The complication rate is reported to be less than 2%, and includes brachial plexus injury, hemothorax, pneumothorax, phrenic nerve injury, lymphocele, and chylothorax.[48] Anterior scalenectomy can be performed with less morbidity than first rib resection.

Wehbé and Whitaker[64] described epineurectomy, which is excision of the epineurium and circumferential dissection of the affected nerves, with release of any offending structures. This involves a supraclavicular approach, with anterior scalenectomy, followed by extensive dissection of the brachial plexus and removal of the epineurium and any compressing structures. Wehbé and Whitaker[64] reported a 90% rate of alleviation of symptoms and a 10% recurrence rate.[50] Others recommend brachial plexus neurolysis only for revision surgery or in post-traumatic cases in which there is suspected scarring.

Combined Approach: Transaxillary Resection of the First Rib and Anterior and Middle Scalenectomy

This technique has been popularized by Atasoy, who recommended a combined approach for complete decompression of the thoracic outlet. First rib resection effectively decompresses the lower plexus, and scalenectomy decompresses the upper plexus. The first rib resection is performed first, with the rationale being that scalenectomy is easier to perform once the distal insertions of the anterior and middle scalene muscles are released from the first rib. Results of this combined procedure show the lowest recurrence rate among various series of different operations for TOS.[60,65] To date, there are no randomized prospective trials involving a combined approach. This technique is also advocated for unsuccessful TOS surgery or recurrent TOS.

Treatment of Vascular Thoracic Outlet Syndrome

For patients with arterial compression, urgent surgical decompression is performed, followed by removal of an offending compressive structure, such as a cervical rib or fibrous bands. A combined approach is recommended. For patients with venous compression, thrombolysis is performed, followed by first rib resection. Percutaneous angioplasty can be performed at the same time as first rib resection to correct any residual subclavian vein stenosis.[66]

Results

The results of most series show improvement in symptoms. Most patients show improvement after surgical treatment. However, a known percentage of patients do not improve with surgery in most series, and a small percentage of these patients had significant disability. Results are difficult to interpret because of the lack of a consensus about the diagnosis of TOS, lack of defined surgical indications, and lack of randomized prospective trials. Good to excellent results have been reported in 70% to 90% of patients in most reported studies.[60,61,67] Leffert and Perlmutter[68] reported 282 transaxillary first rib resections and noted an 85% improvement in pain. He also noted a high incidence of complications, with a 31% rate of intraoperative pneumothorax. A review of 11 patients treated with brachial plexus neurolysis and scalenectomy without first rib resection showed that 82% had good outcomes, with return to normal everyday activity and either complete or significant relief of symptoms. The authors' conclusion was that microsurgical decompression through a supraclavicular approach without first rib resection is an effective treatment for TOS.[69] A series of 770 supraclavicular rib resections showed 59% excellent results and 27% good results, with a low incidence of complications.[70] Results with scalenectomy with first rib resection have not been conclusively proven to be better than those with anterior and middle scalenectomy alone.[71,72] It is believed that removal of the first rib does not result in improvement; rather, improvement occurs because of the scalenectomy that is required to access the rib. Thus, some authors no longer perform first rib resection and instead perform anterior and middle scalenectomy alone.[73] Because there are few randomized comparative studies, there is no consensus as to the best surgical approach.

Preoperative negative predictive factors include acute ischemia, sensory or motor deficit, and poorly systematized neurologic symptoms.[74] Psychological factors also play a significant role in the outcome of TOS surgery. Predictive factors associated with persistent disability include a history of major depression, unmarried status, and having less than a high school education.[75]

Recurrent Thoracic Outlet Syndrome

True recurrent TOS occurs after a symptom-free interval following surgical intervention. If there was no improvement or symptom-free interval after surgery, the possibility of an incorrect diagnosis, secondary gain, or technical errors in surgery should be entertained. Technical errors include inadequate first rib removal, failure to remove a cervical rib, and inadvertent removal of the second rib instead of the first.[76] A long residual first rib stump has been correlated with recurrent TOS.[77] True recurrence assumes a correct diagnosis with successful treatment. Surgical decompression is reliable, but results tend to deteriorate over time.[78] True recurrence is usually caused by scar tissue surrounding the brachial plexus or caused by a residual first rib stump causing further impingement. In revision surgery, the supraclavicular approach is most commonly used because it provides excellent exposure to the brachial plexus for neurolysis. The complication rate associated with revision surgery is higher, and the success rate is lower.[79]

Summary

TOS is compression of the neurovascular structures in the thoracic outlet. This condition is one of the most challenging upper extremity compressive neuropathies to manage, given the difficulty in diagnosis and lack of consistent response to treatment. The foundation of effective management is a thorough understanding of the anatomy of the thoracic outlet, the types and clinical presentation of TOS, and the physical examination procedures, diagnostic studies, and electrodiagnostic testing used. A course of therapy should always be tried as the first line of treatment before surgical intervention.

REFERENCES

The complete reference list is available online at www.expertconsult.com.

Therapist's Management of Upper Quarter Neuropathies

MARK T. WALSH, PT, DPT, MS, CHT, ATC

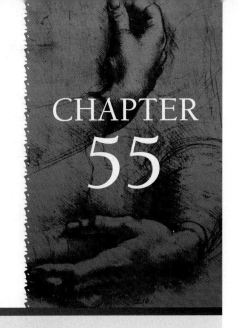

MAJOR TYPES
ANATOMIC RELATIONSHIPS IN BRACHIAL PLEXUS
  NEUROPATHIES
INCIDENCE OF BRACHIAL PLEXOPATHY
DIAGNOSIS AND CLASSIFICATION

THERAPIST'S MANAGEMENT
THERAPY INTERVENTION
CASE EXAMPLE
SUMMARY

CRITICAL POINTS

- There are two major types for the therapist to consider, compressive and entrapment.
- Appropriate therapist classification of patients into one of two types is imperative to providing appropriate treatment.
- Therapist management requires a comprehensive evaluation to determine the level and tissue involvement.
- Therapy is guided by patient classification and three phases of intervention: control, restorative and rehabilitative.

This chapter focuses on painful conditions in the upper extremity related to the brachial plexus, otherwise known as brachial plexus neuropathies (BPN). Other peripheral neuropathies of the involved upper extremity and cervical spine pathology can complicate the diagnosis. The existence of one type of BPN is referred to as *thoracic outlet syndrome* (TOS) and remains controversial.[1,2] As this pain syndrome becomes more ingrained within the central nervous system, accompanying alterations in the neural biomechanics of the brachial plexus and peripheral nerves occur, making diagnosis and treatment more difficult. It is the intent of this chapter to communicate a clearer understanding of brachial plexopathy and its varied manifestations, allowing the clinician to develop a logical sequence of evaluation, assessment, and treatment.

Major Types

Compressive Brachial Plexus Neuropathies

Two major types of brachial plexopathy are discussed. The first, compressive brachial plexus neuropathy (CBPN), is classically described as TOS. This implies that compression on the neurovascular structures is occurring as they pass through the thoracic inlet as a result of a reduction in the diameter of this potential space. The mechanism for this compression could be anatomic anomalies,[3-5] muscular hypertrophy or adaptive shortening of surrounding fascia, or space-occupying lesions.[5] Postural dysfunction is a major component of both types of brachial plexopathies.[6,7] Alterations in posture, especially longstanding ones, may result in the narrowing of spaces necessary for the neurovascular structures to freely traverse the thoracic inlet. Longstanding forward head posture can potentially create space limitations in shape and size secondary to adaptive shortening of tissues of the scalene triangle, costoclavicular, or axillary interval.

Brachial Plexus Entrapment Syndrome

The second type of brachial plexopathy, brachial plexus entrapment syndrome (BPES), is less understood. The term may often be used synonymously with the diagnosis of neurogenic TOS (NTOS). More recently this has been referred to as cervical brachial pain syndrome (CBPS). A result of a traction injury to the brachial plexus,[8,9] whiplash injuries,[10] or other compressive neuropathies in the upper extremity,[11-14] BPES impairs neural tissue mobility and tolerance to tension as a result of intraneural or extraneural fibrosis from direct trauma,[15] local pathology within the cervical or thoracic spine,[10,16] or longstanding compression or overuse. This limitation in the nerve's adaptability or compliance is referred to as *adverse neural tension* (ANT),[17,18] or, more recently, neural tension dysfunction (NTD).[19] As a result of NTD movement of the patient's involved extremity beyond the limits of the nervous system's compliance creates abnormal tension in the peripheral nervous system (traction) further exacerbating the patient's symptoms.

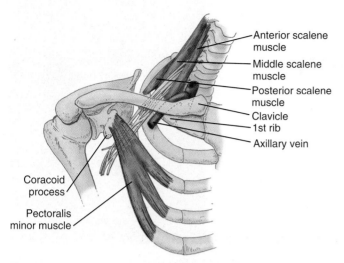

Figure 55-1 Illustration of the anatomic relationships of the thoracic inlet. (From Pratt N. *Clinical Musculoskeletal Anatomy.* Philadelphia: JB Lippincott, 1991.)

Anatomic Relationships in Brachial Plexus Neuropathies

Several anatomic relationships are important to the therapist's evaluation and management of BPN. The first relationship is at the level of the cervical spine between the exiting nerve roots of the brachial plexus and the prevertebral fascia.[20] The trunks of the brachial plexus enter the thoracic inlet through the scalene triangle. An important distinguishing feature at this level is the relationship of the subclavian artery as it accompanies the trunks of the brachial plexus through the scalene triangle. In comparison, the subclavian vein enters the thoracic inlet anterior to the scalene triangle. Clinically this may explain why patients present with neurogenic and classic arterial symptoms without venous symptoms (Fig. 55-1).

Moving laterally, the neurovascular bundles converge and traverse the costoclavicular interval, inferior to the clavicle and superior to the first rib. Continuing laterally, the neurovascular bundle enters the upper extremity through the axilla. At the costoclavicular interval, the patient may present with neurologic symptoms related to the anterior and posterior divisions of the brachial plexus. At the axilla the symptoms may follow a cord distribution. Figure 55-1 further illustrates these relationships. Clinically, each of these could present with differing neurologic complaints and pain distribution. The final relationship to consider is muscular. Machleder and colleagues[21] and Sanders and coworkers[22] described histologic changes of the scalene muscles in patients presenting with a diagnosis of BPN. These changes include increased type I collagen and type II muscle fiber atrophy within the scalene muscles. These histologic changes support the theory that longstanding cervicobrachial pain may be an underlying cause and pathology for BPN. The increased percentage of connective tissue within the scalene muscles compared with normal muscle tissue may indicate a "stiffening" of the scalene triangle, resulting in a decrease in compliance of these muscles, placing the neurovascular structures at greater risk.

Potential Anatomic Spaces (Intervals) of Involvement

There are three potential spaces for CBPN or the development of BPES within the thoracic inlet. The first and most medial space is the interscalene triangle located within the boundaries of the posterior cervical triangle. The presence of a prefixed or postfixed brachial plexus along with other anatomic anomalies may add to poor neurovascular mobility and tension attenuation. Injury to the shoulder girdle or repetitive trauma may lead to symptoms and pathology. As previously discussed, the second potential space is the costoclavicular interval. The third potential space moving laterally is the axillary interval. In this area of the anterior structures, the deltopectoral fascia, pectoralis minor, and coracoid have all been implicated as potential sources of compression of the neurovascular structures.[23]

Incidence of Brachial Plexopathy

BPN occurs more often in women, usually between the fourth and the sixth decades of life.[24] Brachial plexopathies have also been associated with a history of cervical,[10] thoracic,[25] or shoulder trauma[16,26]; arthritis[16]; bad posture; and repetitive motion disorders.[27] Brachial plexopathies can include symptoms that are related to the venous, arterial, neurologic, or autonomic systems.[28] The symptoms associated with multiple system involvement are often extremely variable, making the diagnosis of CBPN or BPES predominantly a clinical diagnosis made by a process of exclusion rather than specific objective signs or diagnostic tests. Therefore careful and meticulous evaluation and hypothesis formulation are necessary to identify the potential causes of the multiple problems that may coexist in many of these patients.

Diagnosis and Classification

Diagnosis

The diagnosis and classification of these patients continues to remain controversial. Arguments have been put forth to support and refute the existence of brachial plexopathy, especially those labeled as TOS.[1,2] The classification and diagnosis of brachial plexopathy centers on four types, based on symptoms: vascular–arterial, vascular–venous, true (specific) neurogenic, and false (nonspecific) neurogenic TOS.[29] The problem is that the term *TOS* is often used as a diagnosis for other neuropathologies that include the brachial plexus. This confused diagnostic scheme makes it difficult for the treating clinician to develop an appropriate treatment strategy. Either way, brachial plexopathy needs to be considered as upper quarter neuropathic pain. This requires the therapist to have a clear understanding of pain. The reader is referred to Chapter 113 for further information on pain mechanisms and Chapter 114 for additional information on pain assessment and management.

Cuetter and Bartoszek[29] classified thoracic outlet and brachial plexopathy into four categories. They identified two vascular components, arterial and venous, and believed that these were undisputed because diagnostic tests are available to confirm occlusion or changes of either vascular system. In addition, specific clinical examination techniques, discussed later in this chapter, may further support the presence of vascular involvement. The remaining two classification categories are neurogenic. Sanders and associates also identified three types: arterial, venous, and neurogenic.[30] These have been identified as true (nondisputed) or false (disputed) NTOS.[31,32] Four criteria for true NTOS are (1) the presence of a cervical rib on radiograph, (2) intrinsic wasting of the hand, (3) sensory changes, and (4) pain or paresthesia over the lower trunk distribution implicating lower trunk involvement.[31,32] LeForestier and colleagues[31] also included a fifth criterion: positive electrodiagnostic findings. However NTOS may also exhibit symptoms related to the upper plexus.[33] Approximately 5% of neurovasculopathies within the thoracic inlet are true neurogenic or vascular.[32,34] The remaining 95% are classified as false NTOS[32,34] and may be more appropriately classified as BPES as will be discussed later. Within this classification, false NTOS symptoms are identical to those found in true NTOS; however, these cases lack the four criteria. Ribbe and coworkers[35] developed a TOS index of signs and symptoms in an attempt to establish clear criteria for the diagnosis of TOS. The index included positive symptoms provoked by arm elevation, paresthesia over the ulnar nerve or lower trunk distribution, tenderness of the brachial plexus over the supraclavicular fossa, and a positive Roos' test. The lack of a standardized classification system clouds the identification or diagnosis of BPN and hinders the development of a logical treatment approach.

Proposed Therapist's Classification

Compressive Brachial Plexus Neuropathy, or Thoracic Outlet Syndrome

As a result of this lack of consensus, I found it necessary to develop a clinical classification dividing brachial plexopathies into two major types. The contrast between these two types is found in Table 55-1. The first type of brachial plexopathy is classic TOS or which I classify as CBPN, a compressive vasculopathy or neuropathy of the brachial plexus. Classic TOS, as described in the literature, has six identifiable components. (1) Posture appears to play a role in the patient's symptoms. (2) The onset of discomfort is usually described as insidious with transient symptoms. (3) These symptoms are usually associated with extremity position, posture, or particular motions described by the patient such as overhead work or extended periods of static upper extremity positioning. (4) After the offending posture or activity is corrected, symptoms usually subside. These same symptoms may be transiently provoked during treatment. (5) The TOS provocative tests, discussed later, may be more reliable in identifying the potential anatomic interval of compression. (6) Finally, most of these patients present with minimal resting pain, minimal sleep disturbance, low pain scores (verbal reporting or visual analog pain scales), rapid recovery when symptoms are provoked, less mechanical tissue sensitivity to

Table 55-1 *Therapist's Clinical Classification Criteria*

	TOS (CBPN)	BPES
Posture	Offending posture = ↑ Symptoms	Antitension postures = ↓ Symptoms
Onset	Insidious	Trauma-related (cervical/shoulder)
		Repetitive strain injury (RSI)
Irritability	Low	High
Symptoms	Transient often posture/activity	Continuous (features of neuropathic-dependent pain)
Special Tests	↑ Number positive tests = ↑ Sensitivity	Poor sensitivity—diffuse symptoms
	Adson's	Scalene triangle
	Wright's	Axillary interval
	Halsted's	Retroclavicular space
Neurodynamic Tests	Low symptom response	High symptom response
	Mild limitation of motion	Significant limitation of motion
Treatment: Soft/Neural Tissue Mobilization	Transient symptom provocation	Protracted symptom provocation

CBPN, compressive brachial plexus neuropathy; BPES, brachial plexus entrapment syndrome; TOS, thoracic outlet syndrome.

physical examination, with rapid resolution of symptoms once the offending clinical examination is terminated, and the knowledge needed to relieve their symptoms, indicating *low tissue irritability*.

Brachial Plexus Entrapment Syndrome

The second type of brachial plexopathy is brachial plexus entrapment syndrome (BPES), often associated with trauma[8,9] that involves either a traction injury directly or indirectly to the brachial plexus, or local soft tissue inflammation resulting in a compromise of adequate blood flow to the brachial plexus or intraneural or extraneural fibrosis. This fibrosis compromises brachial plexus neural excursion and its ability to attenuate tensile forces placed across the plexus from upper limb or combined cervical motion. These patients typically report delayed onset of their intractable pain that can occur several days, weeks, or months after their injury.[36] It is theorized that the delay in onset of the symptoms is explained by the normal course of biologic healing and the development of neuropathic pain. Mature scar formation eventually compresses the neurovascular structures or limits brachial plexus mobility, creating neural tension dysfunction. Under these conditions, upper quarter motion results in repetitive traction to the neural tissues and development of symptoms. In these patients, the reliability of the TOS provocative tests for determining the interval of involvement is poor and may easily provoke symptoms by placing traction on the neural or surrounding tissues, creating a false positive result. Treatment that might be used for the classic TOS patient may provoke symptoms in patients with BPES at the time of treatment, or the response may be delayed by several hours to a day. Often these patients report a significant increase in symptoms at the next follow-up appointment. Finally, the tissue response in patients with BPES tends to be much more *irritable*. Symptoms are easily provoked with minimal movement of the upper quarter, and patients often report spontaneous bursts of pain and other features of neuropathic pain. The reader is referred to Chapters 113 and 118 for further discussions on neurogenic pain. In addition, additional concomitant dysfunction, such as myofascial trigger points, shoulder pathology, or cervicothoracic spine involvement, may accompany the brachial plexus symptoms.

This theory of differentiating TOS from BPES was explored by Jordan and associates in the development of a Cervical Brachial Symptom Questionnaire.[14] They identified several factors that predicted responsiveness to treatment in a group of 85 patients treated for TOS and compared the TOS treatment-responsive group ($N = 59$) and nonresponsive group ($N = 26$). The authors identified this latter group as suffering from treatment-resistant cervical brachial pain syndrome (CBPS). The results indicated the TOS treatment-responsive group was less likely to have comorbidities, fewer surgeries, fewer widespread sensory symptoms, and was less likely to have weakness extending beyond the lower trunk distribution. In comparison, the CBPS group had sensory and strength complaints extending beyond the lower trunk distribution, greater history of non-TOS-related surgeries, and greater comorbidities, such as complex regional pain syndrome and fibromyalgia.[14]

Differential Therapy Diagnosis

In addition to classifying these cases, it is also essential for the therapist to consider differential diagnoses of other potential conditions that may mimic the symptoms associated with brachial plexopathy. Major ones are listed in Box 55-1. Myofascial trigger points, as indicated by Travell and Simons,[37] can mimic the distribution of brachial plexopathy involvement. Table 55-2 contains common myofascial trigger points that may mimic brachial plexopathy symptomatology.[37] Glenohumeral joint pathology or dysfunction may also provoke symptoms that are similar in nature to the brachial plexopathies referred to as the dead arm syndrome.[38] As reported by Upton and McComas[39] and others,[39-41] the presence of double- or multiple-crush syndromes may also disguise the involvement of the brachial plexus. Eurroll and Hurst,[42] MacKinnon,[43] and Seror[44] reported that these associated double crushes could include carpal tunnel syndrome, ulnar nerve involvement, or anterior interosseus syndrome.[45] The presence of these disorders and others may help explain treatment failure. Therapists must also consider visceral

Box 55-1 Therapist Differential Diagnosis

Cervical dysfunction/pathology
Glenohumeral joint pathology
Myofascial trigger points
Visceral pathology
Multiple/double crush

Table 55-2 Common Myofascial Trigger Points

Muscle	Area of Referral
Trapezius	Face and interscapular region
Scalene	Posterolateral arm/radial three digits
Supraspinatus	Lateral arm/forearm
Infraspinatus	Lateral arm/forearm and radial half of hand
Latissimus dorsi	Posteromedial arm, forearm, and ulnar half to hand
Pectoralis	Anterior shoulder, medial arm, and ulnar two digits
Subscapularis	Posteromedial arm and wrist
Serratus	Medial arm, forearm, and ulnar half of hand/digits

causes such as an apical lung tumor encroaching on the brachial plexus or coronary pathology.

Therapist's Management

Examination

History

To classify an upper quarter compression neuropathy, a careful and thorough examination is essential. This examination starts with a detailed inquiry about the mechanism of the problem and the specific distribution and qualitative attributes of the patient's symptoms. As previously discussed, the distribution of symptoms can vary greatly. The history also provides insightful information about particular positions, postures, or activities that relieve, accentuate, or aggravate the symptoms. This helps the therapist determine the tissue or anatomic space involved. Figure 55-2 is an example of the presentation of symptoms related to the upper and lower trunks of the brachial plexus. The neurogenic symptoms are classically distributed over the lower trunk[46,47] but may also include the upper trunk,[47] middle trunk,[5,47,48] and cords of the brachial plexus.[23] With upper trunk plexopathies (C5-C6 distribution), the pain may tend to be more proximal in nature. This proximal pain may be distributed over the anterior and lateral aspect of the cervical region, portions of

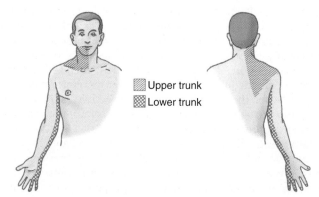

Figure 55-2 *Illustration of the distribution of symptoms that may involve the upper trunk or lower trunk of the brachial plexus.*

the face, and the scapular and interscapular region of the involved side.[49] Distal paresthesia and pain may be distributed over what appears to be the median or ulnar nerve distribution (or both) or the C5-C6 dermatomal region. In contrast, lower trunk (C8-T1) plexopathy symptoms of pain and paresthesia are distributed mostly distal. The paresthesia may be located over the medial aspect of the arm, the forearm, and the ulnar aspect of the hand, appearing to be ulnar nerve-related. If involvement of the brachial plexus occurs at a more lateral position, such as the division or cord level, the variability of the symptom distribution may be even more pronounced. The use of a body diagram to represent symptom distribution may provide further insight, to which the Cervical Brachial Symptom Questionnaire previously alluded.[14]

Taking the patient history also includes investigating past injuries or medical problems to determine prior upper quarter trauma or symptoms (e.g., a previous motor vehicle accident with cervical spine injury,[10] or blunt trauma directly over the superior aspect of the shoulder and upper trapezius region). Prior injury might suggest preexisting mobility problems of the plexus. The medical history also provides valuable information about contributory medical conditions such as diabetes mellitus, hyperthyroidism or hypothyroidism, arthritis, or other systemic neurologic disease. It is also important to note the length of time the symptoms have been present. There is a tendency for secondary tissue dysfunctions to develop the longer the symptoms have persisted; knowing the duration of symptoms assists in developing an accurate prognosis. In general, symptoms that are more diffuse[14] or have persisted for a longer period require extended therapy and are less likely to completely resolve.[50] Specific questioning about occupational or avocational activities that could compromise the neurovascular structures within the thoracic inlet is also essential.

Symptoms

Neurogenic Symptoms. Information regarding symptom distribution and previous history leads to more specific questions about the qualitative nature of the symptoms. Symptoms with neurogenic features involve the motor, sensory, or autonomic nervous system, such as specific muscle performance deficits, alterations in sensibility, and vasomotor instability. These may be intertwined in the pain as associated sensory disturbances of paresthesia and numbness over the same distribution. Accompanying these early neurologic symptoms may be autonomic nervous system complaints such as hyperhidrosis and burning pain over the same distribution. Raskin and coworkers[51] and others[28] reported that headache was present in 26 of 30 patients diagnosed with TOS. Validation of the diagnosis was based on relief of symptoms after first rib resection. Utilizing an isokinetic testing technique, Ozcakar and associates[52] were able to confirm and quantify the weakness and fatigue often reported by the patients.

Late neurogenic symptoms can include complaints of pain; sensory changes; and paresthesia distributed over the posterior lateral cervical region, anterior shoulder, and posterior lateral aspects of the humerus.[1,46,47] More evident intrinsic muscular weakness of the hand with lower trunk involvement, reflex changes, and actual sensory loss[6] may be present. These sensory changes may also manifest with pencil

Box 55-2	Common Symptomatology of Brachial Plexus Neuropathies

Headache ipsilateral side
Neck pain
Shoulder/arm pain: Intermittent (TOS) or neuropathic features (BPES)
Shoulder/arm paresthesia: Intermittent (TOS) or continuous (BPES)
Arm/hand fatigue (arterial)
Arm heaviness (venous)
Pain/paresthesia with lifting/carrying: Brachial plexus traction
Pain/paresthesia with overhead activities
Tinel's sign over the brachial plexus: Neural hyperalgesia

BPES, brachial plexus entrapment syndrome; TOS, thoracic outlet syndrome.
    Compiled from Ide J, Kataoka Y, Kamago M, et al. Compression and stretching of the brachial plexus in thoracic outlet syndrome: Correlation between neuroradiographic findings and symptoms and signs produced by provocation manoeuvres. *J Hand Surg.* 2003;28-B:218–223; and from Ozcakar L, Inanici F, Kaymak B, et al. Quantification of the weakness and fatigue in thoracic outlet syndrome with isokinetic measurements. *Brit J Sports Med.* 2005;39:178–181.

pointing of the digits for the involved nerve distribution. The most common complaints are listed in Box 55-2.

Vascular Symptoms. Venous symptoms include reports of distal edema, especially after activity and pain described as a dull ache over a nonspecific distribution. The patient may also report a sensation of heaviness in the involved extremity.[46,47] With more significant venous involvement, cyanosis may also be present. Arterial symptoms can include descriptions of fatigue, ischemia-like pain, coldness in the distal part of the extremity, and Raynaud's phenomenon.[46,47] The complaint of ischemic pain may be diffuse or specific to a localized area over the distal extremity. Although rarely seen, late arterial signs could include distal thrombosis or embolization with ischemia changes.[53] Clinical signs of vascular involvement include loss or a decrease in the quality of distal pulses when performing provocative stress tests; vascular involvement may also be detected with an arteriogram.

Diagnostic Tests

Diagnostic tests can also be of assistance. Radiographs may indicate the presence of a cervical rib, other bony conditions, or a prominent C7 transverse process, which may suggest the presence of a rudimentary fibrous band that has the potential of occupying space in the scalene triangle. Arteriograms may indicate a possible blockage of subclavian or axillary vessels. The use of somatosensory evoked potentials,[51,54] nerve conduction velocities of the medial antebrachial cutaneous nerve, and electromyography studies are also helpful.[31,54,55] All of these tests may provide additional information about the location and degree of the neuropathology and can *rule out* the presence of double- or multiple-crush syndromes.

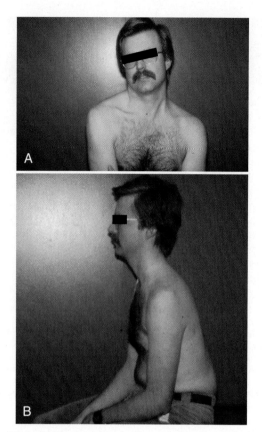

Figure 55-3 Photograph of common cervical posture seen in patients with brachial plexus neuropathy. **A,** Frontal plane. **B,** Sagittal plane. Note how examining in one plane only may not give the therapist the complete picture.

The use of imaging techniques has been found to be more predictive when combined with the provocative testing positions. Gillard and colleagues confirmed vascular changes when visualized with sonography in 48 patients diagnosed with TOS, utilizing MRI in 29 patients and 12 healthy individuals as controls.[56] Demirbag and associates determined there was a significant difference in MRI findings in the patient group when comparing neutral to provocative test positions and a significant difference in the positional change values in MRI between the groups.[57] Although further studies are needed to demonstrate imaging's usefulness, these studies show promise in bringing more objectivity to the diagnosis of CBPN (TOS).

Observation

While obtaining the history from the patient, the therapist should observe the patient's standing and sitting postures. The therapist should look for any cervical asymmetry, thoracic kyphotic changes, or accessory breathing patterns. Examples of cervical postures are demonstrated in Figure 55-3. As is evident from these photos, observing the posture strictly in the sagittal plane may result in incorrect or insufficient information. Figure 55-3B demonstrates the classic forward-head and rounded-shoulder posture in the sagittal plane, with a flattened upper thoracic kyphosis commonly seen in CBPN. In the frontal plane (Fig. 55-3A) cervical asymmetry is evident with rotation and lateral flexion of the

cervical spine toward the affected side, accompanied by increased upper trapezius muscle tone. Through this observation alone, the therapist is able to hypothesize the patient's level of irritability. This posture demonstrates the patient's effort to decrease the tension on the brachial plexus by elevating the scapula via contraction of the upper trapezius and levator scapulae and rotating and laterally flexing the cervical spine toward the involved side. The therapist must also inspect for the presence edema in the supraclavicular fossa and any atrophy and trophic, temperature, or color changes in the extremity. The position of the upper extremity should also be noted to determine whether the patient is using distal joints to reduce neural tension by maintaining the elbow in flexion, the forearm in neutral, and the wrist and digits in flexion.[58,59] These components may exist separately or in combination, and each may vary in the amount it contributes to the patient's position and pain.

Upper Quarter Screening

Details of the upper quarter screen are presented in Chapter 10, but in regard to upper quarter neuropathies, the cervical spine's active range of motion (ROM) is assessed to determine limitations in motion and the presence of mechanical spine pain, which may be provoking the patient's pain. Special tests, including Spurling's test for foraminal encroachment[60] and the vertebral artery test, are executed to determine nerve root or vascular involvement.[61] Myotome scanning and reflex testing provide further information on neural conduction. Tinel's test in the supraclavicular fossa, in the axilla, and along the peripheral nerves allows identification of neural hyperalgesia or other peripheral nerve pathology in the upper extremity. Ide and associates reported that in 111 patients diagnosed with combined compression and stretch TOS, 103 patients had a positive Tinel's sign over the supraclavicular fossa.[62] Finally, the supraclavicular fossa and axilla should be auscultated for the presence of a bruit.

Careful sensory evaluation is undertaken using vibrometry and monofilament cutaneous pressure sensation testing. These threshold tests are reported to be more sensitive than other forms of sensibility testing for early detection of peripheral neuropathies.[7,63] Sensory evaluation should be carried out to investigate: (1) dermatomal distribution, to rule out possible cervical root involvement; (2) peripheral nerve distribution, to rule out the possible local peripheral nerve compressive neuropathies; and (3) sensory disturbance related to the brachial plexus and its divisions. On completion of the general upper quarter screen, assessment for active motion dysfunction is undertaken. This process is explained in Chapter 118. The purpose of active dysfunction testing is to determine whether imparting tension on the peripheral nervous system in various locations alters active motion of the cervical spine or upper extremity. The presence of active motion dysfunction assists the therapist in identifying the nervous system's role in the presenting complaints.

Provocative (Special) Tests

Specific provocative tests, described later in this chapter, are carried out only after the therapist has taken an adequate history and completed an upper quarter screening to develop an initial hypothesis about the level of irritability. These provocative positions can potentially place adverse tension on the peripheral nervous system or brachial plexus, exacerbating the patient's symptoms and creating false positive results. These special tests were originally designed to determine the integrity of the vascular system and the brachial plexus.

Numerous authors have questioned the specificity, sensitivity, and reliability of these tests. Most of these studies examined asymptomatic subjects as to the frequency of positive tests defined as diminished or lost pulse. None of these studies compared normal subjects with a patient population or considered provocation of symptoms. Falconer and Weddell[64] examined the specificity and sensitivity of the costoclavicular maneuver in four case studies—three vascular and one neurogenic—that had a positive costoclavicular maneuver. They confirmed the involvement of the costoclavicular interval surgically. In 100 normal subjects, 50 males and 50 females 19 to 47 years of age, the costoclavicular maneuver was positive for pulse changes in 25 males and 29 females. In 50% of the males and 60% of the females, either a positive Adson's or costoclavicular maneuver was obtained.[64] In contrast, Adson[65] found 9 males and 11 females had a decrease or obliteration of pulse performing his provocative maneuver. In 1980, Gergoudis and Barnes investigated the reliability and validity of the provocative maneuvers. The authors used photoplethysmography to measure the changes in vascular status that occurred with Adson's, costoclavicular, and Wright's test in 130 normal subjects. They determined that 60% had an abnormal finding with at least one test, 27% with two tests, and less than 7% had an abnormal finding when all three tests were performed.[66] It should be noted that the provocation of any kind of symptoms from a neurogenic standpoint was not measured. In 1987, Warrens and Heaton examined the validity of these provocative maneuvers by determining the frequency of false positive results and the role of photoplethysmography. In 64 normal volunteers, they found 17% were reporting some symptoms. They determined that complete obliteration of the pulse occurred in 58% of the population with at least one test, and 30% had bilateral findings. The incidence of positive findings was 27% for the costoclavicular maneuver, 15% for Adson's test, and 14% for Wright's test. Using photoplethysmography, at least one test was positive in 39% of the subjects. In only 2% of the population were all three tests positive.[67]

In determining the prevalence of a positive elevated arm stress test (EAST) or Wright's maneuver, Costigan and Wilbourn used two groups: 24 normal subjects and 65 patients diagnosed with carpal tunnel syndrome (CTS). They determined that the EAST was positive for 92% of the CTS patients and 74% of the controls.[68] Novak and coworkers reported that in 65 of 115 patients with possible TOS, the EAST was positive in 94% of the 65 patients and in 100% of the 65 patients with confirmed TOS when direct pressure over the supraclavicular region was combined with the EAST. A positive result was symptom production, but not necessarily the exact symptoms reported by the patient.[27] In 1995, Rayan and Jensen studied the prevalence of a positive response for three provocative maneuvers in a typical patient population of 100. The subjects were divided into two groups: those younger than 40 and those older than 40. They reported that 87 of 100 subjects had at least one positive test for vascular signs and that 41 of 100 had at least one positive test

for a neurogenic response.[69] Plewa and Delinger examined 50 healthy subjects and reported changes in pulse in 11% for both Adson's and costoclavicular maneuver, 62% for Wright's test, and 21% for supraclavicular pressure. Provocation of symptoms (pain or paresthesia) was positive for 11% with Adson's maneuver, 15% with costoclavicular maneuver, and 36% with Wright's test. They concluded that as the number of positive maneuvers increased in each subject, the specificity improved because only six subjects had all three tests positive.[70] In 1999, Toomingas and colleagues examined the position of abduction/external rotation among male industrial and office workers. They determined the positive prevalence value was 24% of the population in 1987 and 15% in 1992. Distal symptoms were positive in 12% to 20% of the population, whereas proximal symptoms were present in 5% to 6%. It was their opinion that the symptoms of numbness in the hands had the highest specificity and sensitivity associated with decreased sensitivity to touch.[71]

Most recently the accuracy of the special tests has been examined using MRI and ultrasonography. Demirbag and associates, using MRI, measured various space size and anatomic relationships of the thoracic inlet and confirmed that the provocative tests of Adson, hyperabduction (Wright), and Halsted (costoclavicular) resulted in significant alteration of these measurements in a group of 29 patients. There was also a significant difference noted between the patient group and the control group of 12 for the Halsted and hyperabduction test.[57] Gillard and associates reported mean sensitivity and specificity values of 72% and 53%, respectively, for the three primary tests alluded to earlier using ultrasonography. They also determined that combining more than one test improved sensitivity.[56] Finally Ide and coworkers, using neuroradiographic techniques to examine 150 patients diagnosed with compressive, mixed compressive/stretch, and stretch TOS, determined that the "stretch test" (axial distraction of the upper extremity in neutral) and 90 degrees of abduction/external rotation position (Wright) resulted in greater sensitivity for the compression and mixed compression/stretch group of patients.[62]

Provocative Test Application Techniques

The original proponents of provocative tests used them to delineate the location of compression of the neurovascular structures in the thoracic inlet. In the case of Adson, the proposed test implicated compromise at the scalene triangle. This test, described by Adson and Coffey in 1927,[3] involves cervical rotation and extension to the tested side with the upper extremities supported in the patient's lap. This is followed by a deep inspirational breath, which is held for 30 seconds while the examiner palpates for changes in the radial pulse. Obliteration or diminution of the pulse is a positive test. As discussed previously, the importance of the pulse remains in question.[66] Of equal or greater importance is symptom provocation reported by the patient.[6] The clinician is also reminded that this position may stress the contralateral scalene triangle and indirectly provoke symptoms.

The stress hyperabduction test (Wright's test) described by Wright[23] in 1945 implicates the axillary interval. This test is performed in two steps as the patient sits comfortably positioned with the cervical spine in neutral. The arm is passively positioned in 90 degrees of adduction and 90 degrees

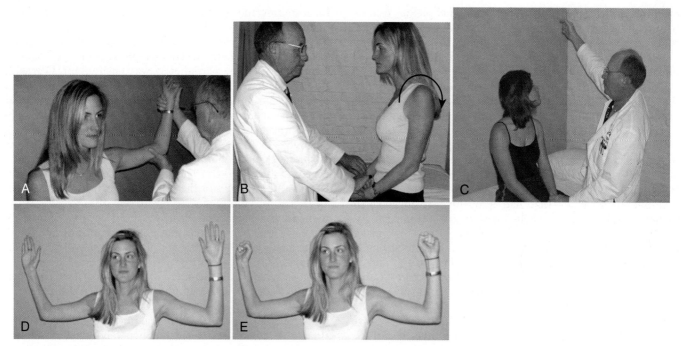

Figure 55-4 The four commonly applied tests for thoracic outlet syndrome: **A,** Wright's. **B,** Costoclavicular. **C,** Adson's. **D, E,** Roos'. The breath is held only for the Adson's test.

of external rotation for up to 1 minute while the clinician monitors the patient's symptoms and the quality of the radial pulse. The maneuver may implicate the subclavian vessels and plexus as it is stressed across the coracoid pectoralis loop. A positive test is loss of pulse and implicates the axillary interval. When this test was performed on 150 normal young adults, 83.3% had obliteration of their radial pulse on the right and 82% on the left.[23]

Halsted[4] initially described, and Falconer and Weddell further researched and described the costoclavicular maneuver or military brace position for stressing the costoclavicular interval.[64] This test is performed with the patient in the sitting position while the clinician helps position the patient into scapular protraction, elevation, retraction, and depression. The patient holds this position for 30 seconds. The patient's arms remain comfortably supported on the thighs while the examiner simultaneously monitors for any pulse changes. The test is positive when radial pulse changes occur or symptoms are provoked.

In 1966, Roos and Owens[47] described a provocative maneuver that uses exercise stress and positioning. No specific anatomic interval is tested. The patient sits in a neutral position, humerus abducted to 90 degrees, full external rotation, and elbows flexed to 90 degrees. The patient then performs repetitive finger flexion and extension that can be continued for up to 3 minutes. The examiner monitors for any evidence of dropping of the extremities, indicating possible fatigue and arterial compromise. The therapist also observes the color of the distal extremity, comparing left to right. According to Roos, this test stresses all three intervals and places the arterial, venous, and nervous system in tension. The test is considered positive when the patient is unable to maintain the elevation for 3 minutes because of fatigue or pain. Examples of these four maneuvers are depicted in Figure 55-4.

Smith,[72] Lindgren,[73,74] Elvey,[8] and Butler and Gifford[75] hypothesized three additional tests to stress the neurovascular structures through the thoracic inlet. Smith described the stress hyperextension position,[72] which potentially implicates all three intervals and is nonspecific for vascular or neural involvement. A positive test is a change in pulse and provocation of symptoms. In 1992, Lindgren and colleagues[74] described the cervical rotation/lateral flexion test, designed to assess the elevated position of the first rib in patients presenting with brachialgia (TOS). They examined the reproducibility of this test by comparing it with the cineradiography for first rib position. In 23 symptomatic patients, the test was positive for restricted cervical motion. First described by Elvey[8] and refined by Butler and Gifford,[75,76] the upper limb tension test systematically places the neurovascular structures of the upper extremities into segmental tension. A positive response is indicated by the provocation of symptoms and motion limitations. The test should be performed on the noninvolved side first to determine each patient's normal response. See Chapter 118 for further definitions and an explanation of the correct application of this test.

Tissue Mobility and Palpation

The pectoralis minor and the deltopectoral fascia should be observed for tightness with the patient in a supine position, noting shoulder height and symmetry in the frontal plane. The therapist can also examine for pectoralis minor tightness. Standing at the patient's side facing the patient's head, the therapist places his or her inside hand on the inferior angle of the thoracic cavity and then passively forward flexes the shoulder on the same side. The therapist palpates the inferior costal angle to determine whether any anterior and superior movement occurs. This movement is the result of pectoralis minor tightness as the coracoid process translates

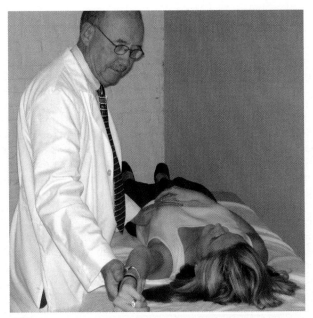

Figure 55-5 Photograph of testing for pectoralis minor tightness. If the pectoralis is tight, the costal inferior angle will translate anteriorly into the examiner's palpating hand.

superiorly and posteriorly and is illustrated in Figure 55-5. An alternative method to evaluate pectoralis minor tightness is to measure the relative difference in resting height from the surface of the plinth to the acromioclavicular joint, comparing the involved and uninvolved side when observing the patient from the head in the supine position. An examination for active myofascial trigger points as described by Travell and Simons[37] is performed to ascertain whether the pain or symptoms are related to the myofascial trigger points mimicking brachial plexus pathology. The most common myofascial trigger points capable of this are listed in Table 55-2. Finally, examination should be undertaken for any evidence of sternoclavicular joint tenderness or muscle spasm of the cervical and shoulder girdle region. This is done to differentiate tissue involvement of the cervical region and upper quarter, which may help support or refute the hypothesis of BPN.

Therapy Intervention

Effectiveness of Conservative Management: Compressive Brachial Plexus Neuropathy (Thoracic Outlet Syndrome)

The therapist is likely to encounter different opinions about the role of conservative care for the management of TOS or BPES. Much of the discrepancy that surrounds the implementation of conservative care is related to controversies regarding the existence of this entity and the criteria used to verify the diagnosis. Peet and coworkers[77] reported one of the first descriptions for conservative management for TOS in 1956. Treatment techniques for the 55 patients in their study included moist heat, massage, shoulder elevator strengthening, pectoralis strengthening, and postural correction exercises. They reported improvement in 70.9% of the patients; 20 patients improved in 3 to 28 days, and 13 patients improved in 4 to 12 weeks. In 1968, Urschel and associates, using a conservative approach of moist heat, active motion, shoulder elevation strengthening, and cervical traction, reported their treatment was "effective" for 50% of the 120 patients in the study. Treatment duration varied from 3 months to several years.[78] In 1974, Dale and Lewis described a conservative treatment program consisting of shoulder girdle strengthening and medication. They stated that 63% of the 150 extremities "did well."[79] McGough and colleagues studied a large population of 1300 patients. Treatment consisted of shoulder girdle strengthening, postural correction, moist heat, massage, and medication; only 9.4% required surgery. The average treatment time was 7.2 months, ranging from 2 months to 2 years.[80] Woods described a treatment program including medication, exercise, and transcutaneous electrical nerve stimulation (TENS). Of the 109 patients in the study, 50% obtained relief within 9 months mean treatment time; TENS was found effective in 40 of the 109 patients.[81] The major weaknesses with each of these studies were a lack of consistent criteria for the diagnosis and that only descriptive outcomes were reported.

In 1979, Smith described a treatment protocol composed of orthopedic manual techniques to increase flexibility of the thoracic inlet, flexibility exercises, and behavioral and postural modification. A significant decrease in symptoms was obtained in 75% of the 20 patients. The mean treatment time was 10 visits, with a range of 1 to 14.[72] In 1984, Walsh recreated this treatment approach using inclusion criteria of insidious onset of symptoms, no history of trauma, and two or more of the provocative maneuvers positive for pulse changes and symptom provocation. Symptoms were predominantly transient paresthesia and pain. Asymptomatic relief was obtained in 68.5% of 16 patients involving 19 extremities; 10.5% reported moderate relief, 5.2% reported temporary relief, and 15.8% reported no relief. Surgery was performed in three of the six patients with moderate or no relief. There was one reoccurrence that was relieved after 14 additional visits.[82]

Other conservative approaches have been tested. Ingesson and coworkers described a physiotherapeutic method of treatment for CBPN (TOS). Treatment included general and specific components. General components were patient education, avoidance of provocative postures and activities, and ergonomic intervention. Specific components were relaxation for involved muscles; breathing exercises and training; stretching of shortened muscles; postural training, including coordination for anterior and posterior postural muscles; specific mobilization of the cervical and thoracic spine; and a home exercise program. A "positive effect" was achieved in 50% of the patients (63 of 125); 45 of the remaining 62 patients required surgery.[83] In 1990, Sucher presented four case studies in which patients were treated with myofascial release techniques as the primary tactic. In all four cases symptoms were "markedly improved." The particular techniques were not described in detail. However, it appears that contract–relax, spray and stretch, and vigorous stretching of involved musculature or surrounding fascia were discussed.[84]

In 1995, Novak and associates reported on 42 patients treated conservatively for TOS. Treatment included education about pathophysiology, avoidance of offending positions, and postural awareness. Therapy treatment incorporated postural correction, pain control, stretching and therapeutic exercise, aerobic conditioning, and a home exercise program. Symptomatic improvement was obtained in 25 patients, 10 were unchanged, and 7 worsened. Poor overall outcome was related to obesity, worker's compensation, and concomitant double-crush injury (carpal or cubital tunnel syndrome). Arm and hand pain was significantly improved in patients who did not have these concomitant problems.[85] In 1997, Lindgren reported on 139 patients treated with a therapeutic model of scapula ROM, upper cervical spine-normalizing exercises (chin tucks while standing against the wall), resisted cervical forward flexion, rotation and extension to normalize first rib function, and stretching the anterior cervical spine and levator muscles. At the time of discharge from the hospital, 88.1% of the patients were satisfied with the outcome and improved impairment.[73]

Cramer described a reconditioning program for athletes to decrease the rate of recurrence of injury-induced brachial plexus neuropraxia. The program included 4 weeks of conservative management and 8 weeks of progressive reconditioning consisting of cervical strengthening three times per week and cervical mobilization and modified shoulder strengthening two times per week. No specific patient data were presented to support this approach.[86]

Effectiveness of Conservative Management: Brachial Plexus Entrapment Syndrome

Numerous other authors have also described conservative approaches. The concept of adverse neural tension (ANT),[18,75] or neural tension dysfunction (NTD),[19] provides additional causes and treatment approaches to be considered in the treatment of BPN patients. The recent concept of ANT or NTD is what led me to the development of the classification system of CBPN and BPES. Several authors have examined the effect of treatment of BPES (cervical brachial pain syndrome). Allison and coworkers in a single-blind, randomized controlled trial of 30 patients and a control group compared the effects of two different manual therapy techniques: cervical and neural mobilization versus indirect manual techniques of articular structures of the glenohumeral joint and thoracic spine. They reported improved pain intensity, pain quality scores, and functional disability levels in the manual therapy groups. The neural mobilization group also had significantly lowered visual analog scale (VAS).[11] In 2003 Coppieters and associates published their findings comparing two intervention groups: cervical contralateral lateral glide mobilization versus therapeutic ultrasound in 20 patients with neurogenic CBPS. They reported a significant reduction in pain perception, a decrease in shoulder girdle elevation (superior scapulae elevation), and increased ROM (elbow extension) with the upper limb neural tension test in the manual therapy group.[13] In a quasiexperimental study of 50 patients, Hanif and colleagues treated NTOS patients with a combination of strengthening exercises of the paraspinal and scapular muscles along with stretching of the scalene,

sternocleidomastoid, and pectoralis muscles, performed once a day, 4 days a week, for 6 months. Thirty-one of the patients had a full or marked recovery, 16 partial improvement, and 6 no change or worse.[87] Landry and associates compared the long-term functional outcomes in patients with NTOS treated surgically and conservatively. The conservative intervention was physical therapy; however, no specific interventions were described. The patients undergoing surgery missed more work; however, there was no significant difference in number of subjects that returned to work, symptom severity, or change in symptomatic status since onset. They concluded that first rib resection did not improve functional status.[88]

Variability in the duration of the various conservative treatment strategies relates to the lack of diagnostic criteria and specific treatment approaches. Guidelines for treatment duration are based on patient symptom response and the therapist's physical examination. In general, (1) the longer the duration of symptoms, the longer conservative care may be necessary; (2) multiple-system involvement such as glenohumeral joint pathology, myofascial trigger points, or double-crush syndromes may necessitate longer-term conservative measures; (3) conservative care may take longer for the patient with BPES than for those that have the classically described TOS (CBPN); (4) social, medical, emotional and occupational factors play an important role in the patient's response to conservative care; and (5) the presence of multiple- or double-crush syndrome may require treatment to address the cervical spine, distal pathology, and BPN.

Treatment Considerations

General: Three Phases of Treatment

Multisystem involvement is often present in patients diagnosed with TOS and BPES. Treatment programs are developed from information obtained from the evaluation and assessment. There is no recipe or cookbook approach for treating these patients, especially when their conditions are highly complex. Whether the problem is CBPN (TOS) or BPES, the purpose of the control phase of treatment is to decrease and control the patient's symptoms. In the more complex cases, it may be useful to formulate a problem list for each identified impairment or tissue dysfunction. This list may include bursitis or specific tendinitis of the shoulder; adhesive capsulitis; active myofascial trigger points; mechanical, cervical, or thoracic spine pain; double or multiple crushes; and other soft tissue conditions. The therapist must keep in mind that a double- or multiple-crush syndrome involvement may necessitate treatment for a more distal peripheral neuropathy.[24,39,42] The problem list should be prioritized based on the overall goal of the control phase. Therefore the brachial plexus component of the patient's symptomatology may in fact be the last issue addressed in the intervention plan. Initially, attempting to manage the brachial plexus component may only exacerbate the patient's symptoms and result in failure. Also imperative in this phase is identifying activities, positions, and treatments that exacerbate or relieve the patient's symptoms. The therapist's understanding of the level of tissue irritability and methods of relief is essential for progressing to restorative phase.

The restorative phase of conservative management commences only after control and comfort have been achieved. The patient should have a minimal level of resting pain and no sleep disturbance. During this phase, treatment of tissues that create impairments such as limited motion or provoke the symptoms directly related to the compression or entrapment of the brachial plexus and its accompanying neurovascular structures may be initiated. Treatment may transiently exacerbate the patient's complaints; however, this should not last beyond the treatment session. To ensure that it does not, the therapist must have command of the methods necessary to regain symptom control. Postural awareness and correction are also being initiated during this phase.

The final phase, the rehabilitative phase, involves conditioning and strengthening the muscles necessary to maintain postural correction, rehabilitate weakened muscles in the extremity, and increase activity tolerance and endurance. Postural correction is carried over into activities of daily living and occupational situations that may lead to NTD situations. Functional and occupational activities are addressed via patient education and ergonomic intervention.

Control Phase.

Patient Education and Behavior Modification. In general, the treatment approach for classic CBPN (TOS) and the more complex case of BPES can be combined based on the primary goal of symptom control and relief. Although the duration of treatment varies greatly for each of the two conditions, the BPES patient is likely to require more time. Control-phase treatment centers on behavior modification, postural correction and awareness, and the development of a diaphragmatic breathing pattern. Behavior modification addresses factors contributing to symptoms, quality of life, and occupational or avocational activities. Behavior modification may include instructing the patient in appropriate positioning of the upper extremity at rest to avoid placing tension across the brachial plexus and accompanying vascular structures. Passive shoulder elevation corrects the depressive traction component on the brachial plexus and has been beneficial in decreasing symptoms. Positioning suggestions include using the opposite, noninvolved extremity to support the involved extremity in the brachial plexus slack position, as demonstrated in Figure 55-6, or resting the affected extremity on the armrest of a chair or a pillow on the lap. While standing, the patient can obtain additional relief from tension by placing her hand in a coat pocket or by supporting it on her belt. Resting the affected arm on the armrest of a chair or pillow for 30 minutes before bedtime may also aid in decreasing symptoms before sleeping. Obtaining adequate rest after strenuous activities is important for relaxation of any muscular components involved. It is beneficial during the initial phases of treatment to have the patient refrain from engaging in strenuous aerobic activities, which may create exertional breathing. This increases accessory muscle activity and potentially compromises the neurovascular structures throughout the thoracic inlet.

Activities that aggravate the patient's symptoms are identified during history taking. Many times, the patient is unaware of similar activities that include the same exacerbating movements. The patient should be educated to avoid all activities and motions that exacerbate symptoms during the initial

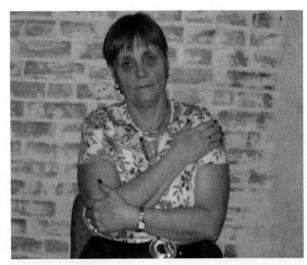

Figure 55-6 Brachial plexus slack position; note the posture of the head and cervical spine favoring the involved side.

phase of treatment. This educational process continues throughout the entire course of care. The patient should avoid any pressure over the thoracic inlet. Additional padding that increases the surface area can diminish pressure from automobile shoulder-restraint straps. Women should wear a strapless bra or use additional padding to increase the strap surface area. Finally, the patient should avoid carrying heavy objects, including handbags, with the affected extremity. These activities increase shoulder depression and traction on the neurovascular structures.

Proper sleep positioning is often important to obtaining symptom control and avoiding sleep disturbance. Sleep positions should place the affected upper extremity in a position that minimizes tension on the brachial plexus and its neurovascular structures, the cervical spine, and distal peripheral nerve tissues. Examples of sleep positions are demonstrated in Figure 55-7. The position should maintain the spine in neutral and support the upper extremity, avoiding tension on the neurovascular structures in the thoracic inlet. Finding a helpful sleep position may require nothing more than changing the side of the bed the patient sleeps on.

Postural Education. The postural educational process should be integrated into daily activities and occupational situations. Eliminating offending resting postures such as the forward-head and rounded-shoulder posture or upper extremity over head positions during work is an important component of this education. Modifications in the workplace may be necessary to achieve these goals. It is important to respect a longstanding offending posture and the accompanying tissue adaptations that result from it. Therefore reestablishment of a balanced posture and stability of the upper quarter during use requires patience. Postural awareness and correction is only taken seriously by the patient when the therapist presents these concepts appropriately. It is necessary to spend time at each treatment session discussing and working on posture and breathing. A proper balance of stretching and strengthening exercises is necessary to permit postural correction. Overcorrecting to an established "textbook" posture often leads to further exacerbation of symptoms. Because most of these patients are 40 years of age or

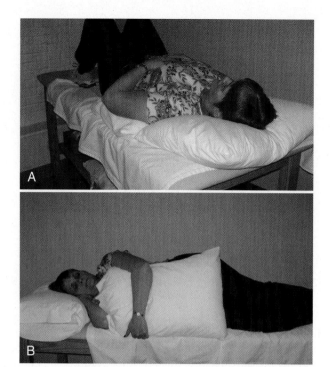

Figure 55-7 Examples of sleep positions. **A,** Supine. **B,** Side-lying.

older, these posture abnormalities result in longstanding adaptive tissue changes. These soft tissue adaptations occur within the fascia, muscle, articular structures, and neurovascular structures. Postural correction should also take into account the nervous system to avoid additional adverse neural tension on the plexus and its accompanying nerve roots and peripheral nerves. It may also be helpful to involve family members in the postural correction process and teach them to recognize abnormal breathing patterns to increase patient awareness. A low-impact, tolerable aerobic exercise program to encourage large segmental and muscle group activity is implemented during this stage as well. As reported by Novak and colleagues,[85] many of these patients have body weight issues and compromised fitness status.

Proper Breathing Patterns. Altered breathing patterns at rest and during activity are common in patients with BPN. Accessory breathing patterns using the scalene, intercostal, and pectoralis minor muscles often occur when patients are focused and statically postured. All of these structures affect the path of the neurovascular structures as they progress laterally through the thoracic inlet. This accessory breathing pattern is identified by shallow breaths with increased cephalic excursion and a decrease in circumferential expansion of the thoracic cavity. This same breathing pattern may be evident during activities such as playing an instrument, working at a computer, reading, or writing. Patient education and instruction about these aberrant breathing patterns is essential in developing a diaphragmatic breathing pattern. Diaphragmatic breathing requires instruction by the therapist to help the patient reestablish the diaphragm as the major muscle responsible for breathing. Diaphragmatic breathing allows for accessory muscle relaxation and improved excursion of the thoracic cavity. Patient command of this is beneficial when progressing into the latter phases

of treatment that incorporate diaphragmatic breathing into manual treatment techniques and the home program.

Additional Considerations. Treatment of BPES patients involves two additional considerations. It is imperative the therapist recognize the level of neuropathic pain involved and identify the extent to which each of the five clinical pain patterns described by Gifford and Butler[89] is involved: (1) peripheral nociceptive, (2) peripheral neurogenic, (3) central nervous system-related, (4) sympathetic nervous system-related, and (5) affective–motivational. Although one or two of these may dominate the patient's complaints, all five may be present, further complicating the problem. Through identification of these different pain patterns, a more direct treatment approach is established and the prognosis is improved. Patients with predominant central nervous system, sympathetic nervous system, or affective–motivational pain patterns are more difficult to treat, and their outcomes are often less successful. Often, it is necessary for a therapist to accept that complete resolution of a patient's symptoms is unrealistic. The goal in this particular group of patients may be to improve the quality of the patient's life by controlling symptoms and obtaining greater pain-free environmental ROM, thus allowing the patient to use the upper extremity in a more functional and comfortable manner.

During this time, identified secondary problems may be treated directly, for example, addressing active myofascial trigger points that are referring symptoms, providing pain modulation through modalities and exercise, or treating double- or multiple-crush situations. It is also appropriate to implement large-amplitude motions using all extremities through a low-impact aerobic program or using general nerve mobilization techniques via the spine and lower extremities. See Chapter 118 for further information and direction.

Restorative Phase. The primary purpose of the restorative phase of treatment is to "restore" or reverse soft tissue dysfunction identified during the evaluation. This phase of treatment is initiated only after comfort and symptom control have been achieved. In classic compressive TOS, soft tissue mobilization described by Smith[72] may be instituted. The goals of these manual techniques are to improve flexibility of the associated tissues, restore normal tissue resting lengths, and assist in restoring normal posture. Addressing these problems may increase the size of the potential compression intervals and minimize neurovascular compression.[84,90] Soft tissue mobilization includes addressing joint and soft tissue mobility of the acromioclavicular and sternoclavicular joints and scapulothoracic articulation as necessary. In addition, it is appropriate to improve first rib position,[73] mobility, and cervical spine function. These techniques also address adaptively shortened muscles such as the pectoralis group and the scalene muscles via deep massage and stretch while avoiding brachial plexus tension. Brachial plexus gliding or peripheral nerve mobilization may be instituted. Examples of these techniques are demonstrated in Figure 55-8.

It is beyond the scope of this chapter to discuss the specifics of peripheral nerve mobilization. See Chapter 118 for additional information. In general, the purpose of peripheral nerve mobilization is to restore normal neurophysiology and neurobiomechanics, thereby improving neural compliance and excursion.[50] It is theorized that alleviating intraneural

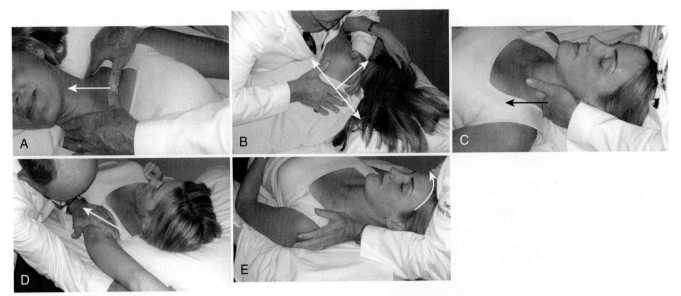

Figure 55-8 Manual techniques that can be used to improve the flexibility of the thoracic inlet. **A,** Sternoclavicular joint. **B,** Scapular-thoracic articulation. **C,** First rib. **D,** Pectoralis minor tightness. **E,** Scalene stretch.

and extraneural compression results in improved vascular function and axoplasmic flow.[75,76] This is accomplished by using components of the upper and lower limb tension tests to restore neural mobility. However, therapists are advised to obtain further information regarding these techniques and their appropriate use before proceeding with peripheral nerve mobilization techniques. Use of these techniques, especially during the early portions of the first two phases, without symptom control could significantly exacerbate the patient's symptoms.

A home exercise program is instituted during the restorative phase treatment. Originally described by Peet and coworkers[77] and subsequently modified by numerous other authors, the home program aims to improve the flexibility of the entire thoracic inlet region and its accompanying neurovascular structures. The following examples are not intended to be all-inclusive; other exercises may be more appropriate for a particular patient. Scalene stretching is preferably done in a supine position to minimize cervical muscle activity while maximizing stretch. Cervical protraction and retraction or "axial extension" exercises[50] can help eliminate the forward-head and rounded-shoulder posture and reestablish proprioceptive input for proper cervical spine positioning. The therapist is reminded to correct any occipital rotation and restore lumbar posture. Incorporating diaphragmatic breathing into the exercise program assists the patient in habituating appropriate breathing patterns and is a gentle way of adding restorative forces to the involved tissues and indirectly mobilizing the brachial plexus.[91] Diaphragmatic breathing can be combined with scalene, deltopectoral fascia, and pectoralis minor stretching. For example the patient performs shoulder forward flexion to a subthreshold position of symptom onset, and then uses diaphragmatic breathing to stretch the pectoralis minor by using the diminishing circumference of the lower thoracic cavity on exhalation to stretch the pectoralis minor. Pectoralis stretching can also be accomplished with a corner stretch or while the patient stands with

arms elevated at 90 degrees in a doorway. Scapulothoracic flexibility exercises can be performed to improve soft tissue and brachial plexus flexibility and scapular motor control. In addition, scapulothoracic stabilization techniques such as quadruped positioning or using a therapeutic ball may help restore optimal scapulothoracic motor control. Cervical spine flexibility may be improved with active ROM, contract–relax, and a host of other techniques. Appropriate nerve gliding exercises may be instituted in conjunction with these techniques or as separate exercises. Examples of some home exercises are demonstrated in Figure 55-9.

In patients classified with BPES these exercises may need to be modified to avoid placing tension on the neurovascular plexus and its accompanying peripheral nerves. Treatment for previously identified secondary problems continues. During this stage, the therapist must be mindful of any active motion dysfunction resulting from neurogenic involvement to avoid the end-ranges of motion, which may lead to adverse tension and exacerbation of pain. If symptom control has been achieved, specific nerve gliding techniques for the brachial plexus may be instituted. Because of the longstanding nature of the problems faced by this patient population, a home program is imperative and may be more important than specific hands-on techniques performed in the clinic. It is only over an extended period that the adaptive tissue changes can be corrected and balances between the soft tissues and the neurovascular structures can be restored. At no time during this phase should any treatment or home exercise program provoke more than mild transient symptoms. As previously alluded to, most of these patients present with neuropathic pain, and aggressive handling or too rapid a progression in therapy may provoke their initial level of tissue irritability.

Rehabilitative Phase.

Compressive Brachial Plexus Neuropathy. The primary strategies of this phase for patients with compressive BPN are

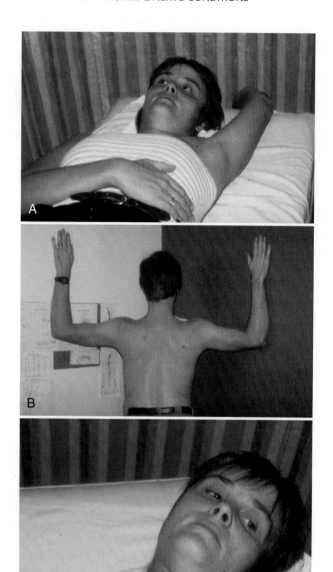

Figure 55-9 A, Diaphragmatic breathing combined with humeral forward flexion for pectoralis tightness. **B,** Corner stretching for pectoralis group and deltopectoral fascia tightness. **C,** Scalene stretching.

intended to increase overall aerobic capacity and fitness, improve postural muscle imbalances, and institute workplace modifications, while continuing to emphasize posture awareness and breathing. In addition, a balanced nutritional program is encouraged to assist overweight patients; excess weight is a problem because obesity has been associated with TOS.[85] Strengthening of postural muscles and incorporating scapular motor control continues to support the emphasis on postural awareness. It is sometimes unrealistic to expect that a longstanding postural fault or habit can be totally overcome through these techniques. It is realistic to expect the patient to reverse the offending posture as often as possible throughout the day. Rehabilitation exercises should also address work conditioning, be work task specific, and include modifications that help avoid inappropriate stresses across the brachial plexus region. In conjunction with this, the

continued application of posture and diaphragmatic breathing in the workplace should be addressed. The patient's awareness of these latter two components often begins to fail, resulting in continuance or recurrence of symptoms. Finally, during the rehabilitative phase of treatment for CBPN, continuous reassessment of patients' subjective, objective, functional, and vocational status should be performed to address any final issues before discharge.

Brachial Plexus Entrapment Syndrome. These same strategies may also be instituted in patients with BPES. The return to, or institution of, any strengthening exercises involving the upper extremities should be approached with caution to avoid exacerbation or recurrence of the patient's symptoms by placing inappropriate tension on the nervous system. In addition, specific nerve mobilization techniques for localized and secondary involvement of the peripheral nervous system should be implemented and previous nerve mobilization techniques continued as needed. This may require periodic visits to the clinic to appropriately modify or progress the exercise prescription. It is also important during this phase for the therapist to reevaluate expectations of recovery for the patient. It has been my unfortunate experience on several occasions, on achieving a 60% to 70% improvement, that further attempts to improve upper extremity conditioning resulted in exacerbation of the patient's initial complaints. This necessitated a return to the initial phase of treatment to regain control before progressing again through the remaining two stages. The goals and expected outcome established by the therapist and patient may have to be tempered by the reality that 100% alleviation of symptoms may not be possible. Therefore educating patients about acceptable levels of activity tolerance and the positions that exacerbate their symptoms becomes extremely important in allowing continued daily activities and occupational tasks.

Case Example

The following case example may help exemplify the treatment approach for brachial plexus neuropathy patients:

A 29-year-old woman was involved in a motor vehicle accident 18 months before she was referred to our clinic with the diagnosis of "brachial plexus neuropathy." Three physicians and two physical therapists provided previous treatment without any significant improvement. Previous therapy included palliative modalities and a rigorous conditioning program. Despite this intervention, her symptoms progressively worsened. Objectively, the patient presented with three active myofascial trigger points, restricted cervical spine motion, glenohumeral joint limitations, and evidence of brachial plexus neural tension dysfunction. The patient also had positive active and passive motion dysfunction (neurodynamic testing) of the involved extremity, indicating NTD.

Control-phase treatment was directed toward the patient's myofascial trigger points and employed appropriate techniques to deactivate the trigger points and interventions to eliminate brachial neurovascular tension and compression. This was achieved by placing the patient in the brachial plexus slack position (see Fig. 55-6). From this position, localized stretching of the involved trigger points was

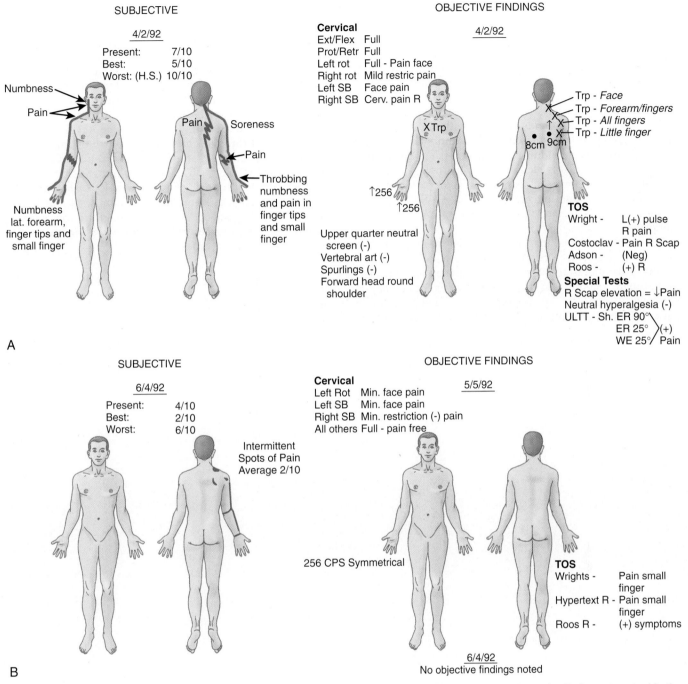

Figure 55-10 Actual patient diagrams of pretreatment and post-treatment findings for the patient in the case example. **A,** Pretreatment subjective pain diagram. **B,** Post-treatment subjective pain diagram.

performed, minimizing stimulation of the sensitized peripheral nervous system. Restricted cervical ROM was managed with an active ROM program and manual mobilization techniques. At this point, the BPN components of her problem were not specifically addressed.

Progression into the restorative phase was initiated once the active myofascial trigger points were deactivated; cervical spine motion improved, and symptoms were controlled. Interventions now included soft tissue mobilization and peripheral nerve mobilization (gliding). These techniques

continued until the patient no longer demonstrated evidence of ANT signs, negative provocative TOS maneuvers, inactive myofascial trigger points, and symmetrical cervical motion. Although complete subjective relief was not attained, the patient returned to work and functional activities she had been avoiding before treatment. During the rehabilitative phase she was instructed in additional postural strengthening exercises. Postural and breathing awareness and symptom avoidance education continued. Figure 55-10 contrasts the pretreatment and post-treatment findings for this patient.

Summary

The treatment of patients with upper quarter (brachial plexus) neuropathy, especially those presenting with long-term neuropathic pain, can be a complex and challenging problem for the occupational or physical therapist. Literature supports the use of conservative care as the preferred initial approach with these patients suffering with CBPN or BPES. Many of these patients present with additional secondary system complaints, including active myofascial trigger points, primary or secondary glenohumeral pathology, cervical pathology, and more distal peripheral neuropathies in the form of double or multiple crush. For this reason, treatment of these patients is rarely straightforward and is usually complex.

Treatment requires that the therapist understand the pathologic mechanism contributing to the patient's complaints. This understanding, which is obtained only through a thorough examination performed by the therapist, is extremely important in appropriately classifying these patients' conditions into one of two types: CBPN or BPES.

Treatment should initially address the issues of comfort and symptom control. Gradual progression through the three phases of treatment requires that the therapist be alert to the patient's symptom responses throughout the course of care. The therapist must also appreciate that tissue maladaptations occur over a number of years, especially when there was a strong postural and concomitant repetitive nature to their symptoms. In these particular cases, treatment requires patience and understanding that this is an ongoing process, best addressed through compliance with the home exercise prescription, postural awareness, and correction of abnormal breathing patterns. Finally, treatment progression requires the therapist to proceed in a very gentle, systematic, and controlled manner with minimal symptom response. Proper education of the patient for behavior modification, exercise compliance, symptom control, and postural awareness is requisite for optimal outcomes.

REFERENCES

The complete reference list is available online at www.expertconsult.com.

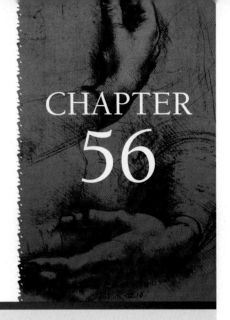

CHAPTER 56

Traumatic Brachial Plexus Injuries

LANA KANG, MD AND SCOTT WOLFE, MD

ANATOMY AND CLASSIFICATION

PHYSICAL EXAMINATION

IMAGING STUDIES

ELECTRODIAGNOSTIC TESTS

PROGNOSIS

SURGICAL INTERVENTION

REHABILITATION

OUTCOMES

SUMMARY

CRITICAL POINTS

Indications for Surgical Intervention

Absolute:
- Open, contaminated wounds
- Iatrogenic injuries, or
- Associated vascular injuries

Relative:
- Closed avulsion injuries (ideally within 3 to 6 weeks after injury)
- Closed traction/stretch injuries (ideally within 3 to 6 months if no improvement)

Priorities
- Address life-threatening conditions
- Classify and isolate the level and pattern of injury
- Initiate early management, multidisciplinary approach

Pearls
- Use multiple diagnostic tools including a thorough physical examination, imaging, and electrodiagnostic testing
- Plan to perform intraoperative electrodiagnostic assessment

Pitfalls
- Inadequate preoperative identification of intact versus damaged nerves
- Lack of a back-up plan at the time of surgery
- Insufficient discussion of expectations with the patient and family members

Healing Timelines and Progression of Therapy
- Prepare the patient and family for years of ongoing treatment and need for rehabilitation and monitoring
- Anticipate individual variability

Adult traumatic brachial plexus injuries (TBPI) can be devastating, frequently occurring during life-threatening events, such as falls from heights, penetrating wounds, physical assault, or motor vehicle accidents. In our current society of high-speed travel and high-risk sports activities, it is not surprising that these injuries are increasing in incidence.[1-3] Although TBPI can be fraught with serious physical and psychosocial deficits, timely management with a multidisciplinary approach can optimize functional restoration for these patients.

The true incidence of TBPI is unknown but is believed to be steadily rising throughout the world.[2,3] These injuries typically afflict male patients aged 15 to 25.[4] Based on evaluation of 1068 patients over an 18-year period, Narakas[4] reported that 70% of TBPI result from motor vehicle accidents, and 70% of these involve motorcycles or bicycles; in turn, 70% of these cyclists have other major injuries.

TBPI are classified according to the mechanism, level, and pattern of injury. The two major mechanisms of injury are closed blunt trauma or penetrating open trauma. Closed trauma exceeds penetrating trauma and includes traction or compression injuries, with traction accounting for 95% of cases.[5] Traction mechanisms can result in avulsion, rupture, or stretch injury to the nerves. With the head and neck violently moved away from the shoulder, a mechanism of traction is believed to result in upper trunk and C5–C6 root injury; with the arm in an overhead position, it is believed to result in lower trunk and C8–T1 injury.

Root avulsion injuries can be further subclassified into peripheral or central avulsions based on the mechanism that produced them. Peripheral avulsions are the result of traction forces that overcome the fibrous attachments of the rootlets, which are stronger at the C5 and C6 levels than the C7 through T1 level.[6,7] Central avulsions occur less commonly and result from longitudinal or bending forces on the spinal cord that avulse the root but do not result in translation of the root outside the epidural sleeve.[2,8]

Anatomy and Classification

Levels of injury are described based on the anatomy of the plexus moving in a cranial to caudal direction: (1) the root, (2) the trunk, (3) the division, (4) the cord, and (5) the peripheral nerves (Fig. 56-1).

Injuries that occur at the level of the root are localized relative to the dorsal root ganglion (DRG). Preganglionic (or supraganglionic) injuries are located proximal to the DRG, whereas postganglionic (or infraganglionic) injuries occur distal to the DRG. The exact site of the lesion relative to the DRG has clinical implications for sensorimotor functional

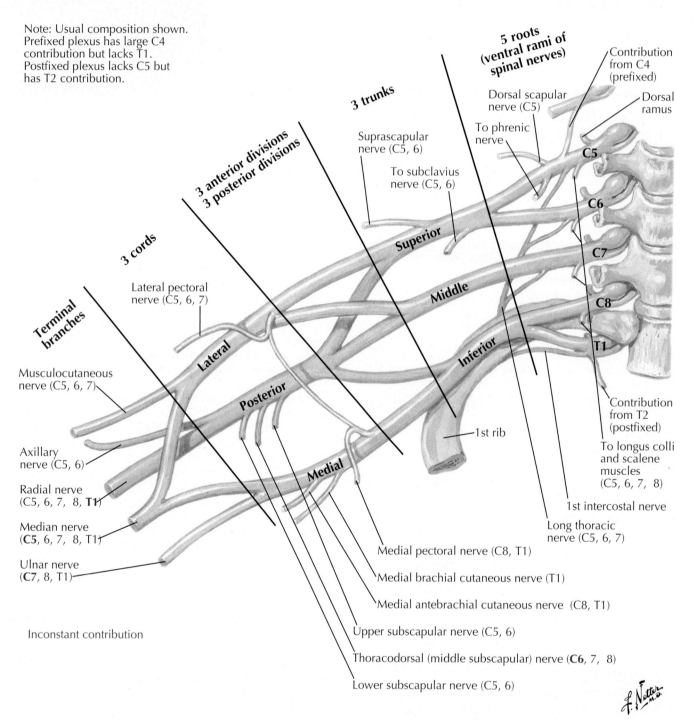

Note: Usual composition shown. Prefixed plexus has large C4 contribution but lacks T1. Postfixed plexus lacks C5 but has T2 contribution.

5 roots (ventral rami of spinal nerves)

3 trunks

3 anterior divisions
3 posterior divisions

3 cords

Terminal branches

Contribution from C4 (prefixed)

Dorsal scapular nerve (C5)

Dorsal ramus

To phrenic nerve

Suprascapular nerve (C5, 6)

To subclavius nerve (C5, 6)

Lateral pectoral nerve (C5, 6, 7)

Superior

Middle

Inferior

Lateral

Posterior

Medial

C5

C6

C7

C8

T1

Musculocutaneous nerve (C5, 6, 7)

Axillary nerve (C5, 6)

Radial nerve (C5, 6, 7, 8, **T1**)

Median nerve (**C5**, 6, 7, 8, T1)

Ulnar nerve (**C7**, 8, T1)

1st rib

Contribution from T2 (postfixed)

To longus colli and scalene muscles (C5, 6, 7, 8)

1st intercostal nerve

Long thoracic nerve (C5, 6, 7)

Medial pectoral nerve (C8, T1)

Medial brachial cutaneous nerve (T1)

Medial antebrachial cutaneous nerve (C8, T1)

Upper subscapular nerve (C5, 6)

Inconstant contribution

Thoracodorsal (middle subscapular) nerve (**C6**, 7, 8)

Lower subscapular nerve (C5, 6)

Figure 56-1 Anatomy of the brachial plexus. The brachial plexus has five major segments: roots, trunks, divisions, cords, and branches. The clavicle overlies the divisions. The roots and trunks compose the supraclavicular plexus, and the cords and branches compose the infraclavicular plexus. (Netter illustration from www.netterimages.com. © Elsevier Inc. All rights reserved.)

deficits, physical examination findings, electrodiagnostic test results, and treatment options. Motor loss is found in both pre- and postganglionic injuries. In preganglionic injuries, the root has been avulsed from the cord, thus disrupting those motor fibers and motor unit potentials (MUPs) that arise from the corresponding anterior horn cells. As the sensory cell bodies reside in the dorsal root ganglion, sensory axons and their corresponding sensory nerve action potentials (SNAPs) are preserved in root avulsion injuries despite complete anesthesia in the corresponding dermatome. This finding is distinct from postganglionic injuries and pathognomonic for root avulsion injury. Postganglionic injuries may have a similar motor and sensory clinical exam, but have electrodiagnostic abnormalities in both MUPs and SNAPs. Although encouraging research has been done in animal models for reimplantation of avulsed rootlets directly into the spinal cord,[9,10] such efforts in humans have not demonstrated successful recovery of function. Thus, preganglionic injuries are treated with procedures such as nerve or muscle transfer, rather than with reimplantation or nerve grafting.

A classification system based on pattern of injury is useful for describing a combination of both mechanisms and levels of injury. These patterns of injury are also associated with a frequency of occurrence. The two major categories are supraclavicular and infraclavicular. Injuries that occur in the supraclavicular region constitute 70% to 75% of TBPI and involve global damage to the plexus in 50% of these cases. Upper trunk (C5–C7) injury constitutes 35% and isolated C8–T1 injuries 3% of these supraclavicular injuries. In five-level injuries that involve all major roots of the brachial plexus (C5 through T1), 60% consist of a combination of ruptures of the upper cervical roots and avulsions of the lower cervical roots.[11,12]

Infraclavicular injuries occur with a frequency of 25% to 33% and involve the cords or the peripheral nerves.[12-15] These injuries are more commonly incomplete and are associated with shoulder girdle fracture–dislocations, clavicle fractures, and scapulothoracic dissociations.[12-15] Thirty percent involve single or multilevel cord injuries, and 25% involve isolated peripheral nerve injuries.[12-15] In 5% to 25% of infraclavicular injuries there is an associated axillary arterial injury.[12-15]

As will be described later in the chapter, understanding the pattern of injury is helpful for determining the prognosis for recovery and the appropriate treatment.

Physical Examination

The musculoskeletal examination of patients with TBPI is a critical part of the evaluation process. A systematic motor and sensory examination allows one to map the location of injury with some precision, which is then used to guide diagnostic evaluation and choice of treatment. The physical examination is also helpful in determining the prognosis for recovery. A thorough physical exam is necessary in patients with subacute or chronic injuries to determine the potential nerve, muscle, and tendon donors available for nerve transfer, free-muscle grafts, or tendon transfer.

In patients with major life-threatening injuries, a detailed examination of the brachial plexus and peripheral nervous system may not be possible in the acute context. The ideal

Table 56-1   Manual Muscular Testing Scale[11,12]

Grade	Muscle Strength
M0	No contraction
M1	Flicker or trace of contraction
M2	Active movement with gravity eliminated
M3	Active movement against gravity
M4	Active movement against gravity and resistance
M5	Normal power

setting for the physical exam involves a patient who is alert, responsive, and cooperative. The basic principles of the musculoskeletal exam apply. It begins with inspection and observation of upper extremity posturing, joint contractures, and muscle atrophy. Active and passive joint range of motion is measured. Manual muscular strength is graded from 0 to 5 using the Medical Research Council grading scale[16,17] and recorded in tabular form (Table 56-1) to help determine the myotomal pattern of injury and to document baseline muscle function for future comparison.

Specific signs are helpful in determining a preganglionic pattern of injury. One example is the constellation of findings associated with Horner's syndrome. This syndrome occurs with loss of sympathetic ganglionic function after avulsion of the T1 nerve root and is recognized by meiosis (papillary constriction), enophthalmos (inset orbit), ptosis (drooping of the eyelid), and anhydrosis (dry eye) that together indicate disruption of the sympathetic outflow from and to the head and neck from the sympathetic ganglion at the T1 level. Patients with high-energy preganglionic injuries frequently have extensive abrasions, swelling or ecchymosis in the supraclavicular region, as well as a head tilt away from the injured side (indicating injury to the sternocleidomastoid). Severe, burning neuralgic pain usually accompanies preganglionic traction injuries. Postganglionic injuries usually can be differentiated by a positive Tinel's sign over the site of presumed injury, absence of neurogenic pain, and within days, the shiny, atrophic and dry skin of the involved dermatome(s), characteristic of loss of sympathetic input to the affected part.

Systematic testing of individual nerves and their motor function is based on the anatomy of the brachial plexus and its peripheral branches. Injury to neighboring spinal levels, including C3 to C4 and T2, as well as anatomic alterations in plexus anatomy can confuse the pattern of injury. Variability in the spinal level constitution of the plexus is not uncommon and should be considered when mapping out the pattern of injury. This variability may take the form of a "pre-fixed" plexus when the C4 nerve root contributes to the plexus and when the plexus comprises roots from C4 through C8. A "postfixed" plexus occurs less frequently and occurs when the T2 nerve root contributes to the plexus and when the plexus comprises the C6 through T2 roots.[12] Complete high-energy injuries of the plexus may involve injury to the spinal accessory nerve as well, and documentation of this injury is critical for determining subsequent treatment options.

The examination is begun with the patient's torso exposed, or with a patient gown tied so the neck, shoulders, arms, and scapulae are visible. Strength and mobility of the trapezius, sternocleidomastoid, rhomboids, and serratus anterior are assessed sequentially and against manual resistance, by asking the patient to shrug the shoulders, turn the head from side to side, approximate the scapulae in the midline, and push against a wall with both outstretched arms, to the best of their ability. The trapezius and sternocleidomastoid muscles are innervated by the 11th cranial nerve (spinal accessory nerve), the serratus anterior muscle is innervated by the long thoracic nerve (T5–T7A), and the rhomboid muscles are innervated by the dorsal scapular nerve.[4,5] Denervation of the rhomboids or serratus connotes a very proximal rupture or avulsion of the upper trunk, given that their respective peripheral nerve innervations arise from the upper roots of the plexus. Although loss of the serratus anterior muscles is the most common cause of classic scapular "winging," dysfunction of the trapezius also results in alteration of scapular motion, winging, and loss of normal mechanics of humeral elevation on the glenoid. The suprascapular muscles (supraspinatus and infraspinatus) are innervated by the suprascapular nerve (C5–C6), which is the first and only branch off the upper trunk; loss of function is demonstrated by atrophy and palsy of abduction and external rotation of the shoulder.

The patient is next asked to face the examiner, and both heads of the pectoralis major muscle (clavicular and sternal) are palpated during attempted and resisted flexion and adduction of the humerus to assess the integrity of the lateral (C5–C7) and medial pectoral nerves (C8–T1). The latissimus dorsi is innervated by the thoracodorsal nerve (C6–C8) and makes up the posterior fold of the axilla; it can be tested by having a seated patient arise by pushing up on the arms of a chair. The subscapular muscles (subscapularis and teres major) are innervated by the upper and lower subscapular nerves (C5–C6), respectively, and can be tested with the "lift-off test." In this test, the standing patient is asked to place the dorsum of the hand on the ipsilateral buttock and then lift the hand off the back against the resistance of the examiner.

The axillary nerve (C5) is tested during resisted abduction of the shoulder, observing and palpating all three components of the deltoid. Additional terminal branches of the plexus are tested with elbow flexion (musculocutaneous nerve [C5–C7]); elbow, wrist, and digital extension (radial nerve [C6–C8 with inconstant contributions from C5 and T1]); wrist and digital flexion (median [C6–T1] and ulnar nerves [C8–T1]); and intrinsic hand and thumb motion (median and ulnar nerves). Each muscle of the forearm and hand should be methodically tested and recorded because detection of partial injuries can be critical prognostic information.

Sensory examination can be difficult, especially in an anxious patient or those with multiple trauma with secondary fractures or soft tissue injuries. Nevertheless, the quality of sensory dysfunction should be tested to the best of the examiner's ability. Light touch and pinprick testing is sufficient to demonstrate the integrity of peripheral nerves; two-point discrimination can be useful for partial or recovering nerves later on. Because of the redundancy and variation in dermatomal innervation, discriminatory sensory testing between the dermatomal levels is less reliable than it is for the autonomous zones; nevertheless, identification of a dermatomal pattern of dysfunction helps to localize a root level of injury. Sympathetic loss should be identified with abnormal dryness, cooler temperatures, and discoloration of the skin. Tinel's sign should be tested and is elicited along any injured peripheral nerve by percussion over the nerve. An advancing Tinel's sign on serial examinations indicates a recovering lesion and has good prognostic implications.

Catastrophic vascular injury occurs in 11% to 55% of plexus injuries and is recognized by loss of vascular perfusion and pulses to the injured extremity.[11,13,18-20] These injuries include rupture of the subclavian–axillary artery in 10% of supraclavicular and in over 20% of infraclavicular lesions and rupture or thrombosis of the axillary artery in infraclavicular injuries.[11] Closed injuries of the shoulder girdle, such as shoulder dislocation, may be accompanied by vascular occlusion in up to 64% of cases[21] and are rare but not insignificantly associated with fractures of the proximal humerus.[22,23] Prompt diagnosis and urgent treatment are critical in these circumstances.

More subtle vascular lesions can be detected with special tests for thoracic outlet syndrome.[24] In addition to the presence of bruits, thrills, or abnormal distal pulses, dysfunction of the subclavian artery is tested with Adson's test. This test is positive if there is loss of the ipsilateral radial pulse while turning the patient's head to the ipsilateral side, slightly elevating the chin, and having the patient perform pulmonary inspiration to elevate the first rib. Wright's test and Roos' stress test are two additional methods that point to the diagnosis of thoracic outlet syndrome. Wright's test is performed by assessing the ipsilateral radial pulse while hyperabducting and externally rotating the patient's arm. This test is considered positive if the pulse diminishes or symptoms are reproduced.[25] Roos' stress test is performed by having the patient positioned with both elbows flexed 90 degrees and level with the shoulders, which are abducted and externally rotated, and then having the patient repetitively open and close the ipsilateral hand for several minutes. Reproduction of symptoms or a sensation of heaviness or fatigue in the shoulder is considered a positive test result[25] (Fig. 56-2).

Imaging Studies

Initial trauma examination includes standard radiographic imaging of the cervical spine and chest. Risk of injury to the brachial plexus increases in the presence of associated cervical spine fracture or dislocation, transverse process fracture, clavicle and superior rib fracture, and shoulder fracture or dislocation. Shoulder girdle injuries should be assessed with dedicated anteroposterior and axillary views. Damage to the neighboring phrenic nerve can complicate preganglionic injuries of the upper rootlets and is diagnosed with an elevated hemidiaphragm detected on a plain chest film. Arteriography or magnetic resonance angiography should be

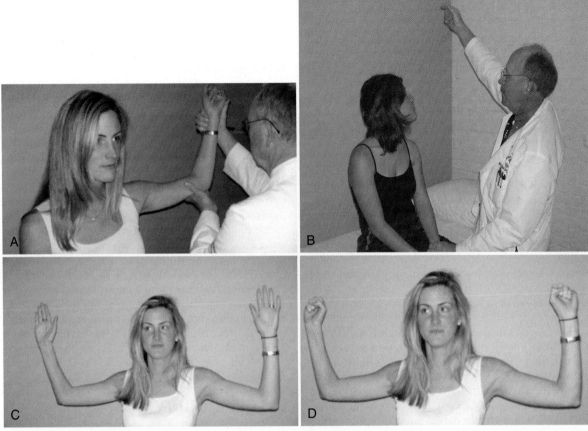

Figure 56-2 Commonly used tests for thoracic outlet syndrome. **A,** Wright's. **B,** Adson's. **C, D,** Roos'. (Photos courtesy of Mark T. Walsh, DPT, MS, CHT.)

performed when injury to the arch or subclavian vessels is suggested.

Advanced imaging of the cervical cord is performed using CT myelography or MRI. CT myelography is still considered the gold standard for determining the level of root injury.[26] It allows assessment for the development of pseudomeningoceles that develop when dural sheaths heal after root avulsion. The CT myelogram is preferably performed 3 to 4 weeks from injury. This is the time needed to allow resolution of the blood clots that form after acute nerve root avulsions that potentially impede the flow of dye and thus block detection of the pseudomeningocele (Fig. 56-3).

At some tertiary centers, MRI is performed in conjunction with CT myelography. Technological improvements have made MRIs of high quality that permit examination of the varying degrees of bony and soft tissue injury, inflammation, and scarring. MRI potentially allows identification of neuromas, hematomas, abscesses, seromas, and other occult sources of compression or injury to the plexus. MRI is attractive because it is less invasive than myelography, is not time-dependent, is becoming increasingly available, and can evaluate lesions of the plexus distal to the spinal cord and nerve roots. However, no study is perfect, and MRI is less

accurate for detecting root avulsions than CT myelography, except for the C8 and T1 levels, which can be more difficult to assess due to the obliquity of the spinal nerves at this level.[27-29] Thus, a combination of imaging modalities is probably more accurate and frequently necessary.[2,14]

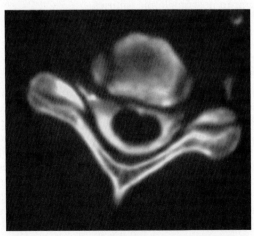

Figure 56-3 CT myelogram performed 3 to 4 weeks after injury outlining the branching of the roots from the spinal cord.

Electrodiagnostic Tests

Electrodiagnostic evaluation is vital to the examination and preoperative planning of TBPI. The information derived from these studies provides a different perspective to the understanding of the pattern, extent, and severity of a TBPI. In this regard it is complimentary to other forms of information. It can provide both corroborative and unforeseen data, localize a lesion, and provide prognostic information about the quality and extent of axonal injury.

Electrodiagnostic testing consists of electromyelography (EMG) and nerve conduction studies. The former tests the electrical activity of a muscle, and the latter tests the conductive electrical capacity of a nerve. Together they can provide a baseline assessment and are ideally performed 3 to 4 weeks after the injury, to allow Wallerian degeneration of denervated axons to occur. Potential recovery and regeneration can be followed by serial examination every 6 weeks in the acute injury period. Chapter 15 provides detailed information on electrodiagnostic testing.

EMG is performed by needle examination of muscles at rest and with activity. EMG can detect denervation injury as early as 10 to 14 days in the proximal muscles and 3 to 6 weeks in the distal muscles. Muscle denervation is revealed as fibrillation activity of muscles. The presence of many fibrillation potentials at rest with no motor unit potentials (MUPs) with poor voluntary muscle contraction indicates severe denervation; the presence of MUPs and only a few fibrillation potentials at rest is indicative of a partial injury. Differentiation of preganglionic from postganglionic injuries can be achieved by examination of the paraspinal and peripheral muscles innervated by nerves that arise from the level of the roots.

Nerve conduction studies assess both motor and sensory nerve activity. Injury is reflected by a decrease in the amplitude of compound muscle action potentials (CMAPs). As stated previously, preganglionic injury and postganglionic injury can also be differentiated by characteristic patterns of SNAPs. Because the sensory nerve cell body lies just outside the DRG, SNAPs are preserved in preganglionic injuries in the setting of complete anesthesia in the affected dermatome; this is a pathognomonic sign for root avulsion injury. SNAPs are absent in postganglionic injuries.

Prognosis

The decision for surgical intervention is based on a number of factors that must be individualized to the patient's injuries. These include the patient's medical condition in acute trauma situations and ability to withstand surgery, age, and co-morbidities. In general, younger patients have enhanced potential for nerve recovery and are treated more aggressively in both acute and chronic situations. It was once suggested that patients older than 50 years are not candidates for surgery, but satisfactory results in older patients have been reported in several studies, particularly with new and innovative nerve transfer procedures.[18,24,30]

Another important prognostic factor is the extent and level of injury. Supraclavicular injuries have less chance of spontaneous recovery than infraclavicular injuries.[12,15] Root avulsions and root ruptures are seen more commonly in supraclavicular injuries and have little chance for recovery without surgical intervention. Individual peripheral nerves can be tethered in their course toward their target organ, which places them at risk for segmental axonal injury, at a second site downstream from a proximal injury. This is particularly true for the axillary nerve within the quadrangular space, the suprascapular nerve at the suprascapular notch,[12] and the musculoskeletal nerve at the coracobrachialis arch. The potential for segmental injury mandates surgical exploration in suggested cases. In general, infraclavicular injuries are less susceptible to nerve disruption because they occur farther away from an "anchorage" point.[12,15] A general rule is that surgery is not indicated acutely in closed infraclavicular injuries.

Complete peripheral nerve injuries that result from iatrogenic causes, such as cervical or axillary lymph node dissection, rib resection, and during orthopedic shoulder procedures, are best treated with diagnosis and operative repair or transfer within 3 months of injury. In contrast, TBPIs that result from low-energy gunshot wounds are the result of neurapraxic injury and have a good chance of spontaneous healing and are generally observed for 3 to 6 months for signs of improvement.

Surgical Intervention

The timing of surgery is perhaps one of the most critical factors in surgical management. Indications for acute exploration are sharp lacerations, open crush injuries, and concomitant vascular injury. In cases of open trauma with contaminated devitalized tissue, nerve ends should be identified and tagged for later repair after initial debridement, bony stabilization, and repair of arterial injuries. Early exploration is also indicated within 1 to 2 weeks in unequivocal cases of complete C5 through T1 avulsion injuries.[15]

Delayed exploration refers to surgery performed longer than 3 months after injury. It is recommended for complete injuries with no recovery at 12 weeks and for injuries that show no clinical improvement in proximal muscle function despite evidence of distal muscle recovery. Nerve reconstruction on adults with a TBPI that is older than 9 months after injury is less predictable, although improvement has been reported in cases up to and beyond 12 months after injury,[18,24,31,32] particularly with the increased use of nerve transfer procedures.

Prioritization of surgical goals needs to be outlined for the patient and the surgical team. In general, most brachial plexus surgeons agree that elbow flexion is the most important function to restore. Next is active shoulder control, including abduction, external rotation, and scapular stabilization. Triceps function is next in order of significance and has greater success of return of function after surgical treatment than for distal radial nerve function. Restoration of functional motor recovery of muscles below the elbow is a laudable goal, but generally unlikely to succeed with standard nerve reconstruction at the plexus level, given the distance from nerve repair to target muscle. Newer transfer techniques in the forearm, when permissible, show excellent early promise.[33] Finally, sensory median nerve function has been shown to be desirable for significant relief of pain associated with multilevel injuries.[34]

Surgical options include nerve repair, neurolysis, nerve grafting, nerve transfer, and free-muscle grafts. Direct nerve repair is done in the acute setting, especially for sharp lacerations; in closed injuries primary repair is limited by the degree of tension on the repair from early scar formation and contracture. Neurolysis is rarely performed alone except in cases of scar entrapment associated with unrelenting pain. Intraoperative nerve recordings should be performed before and after neurolysis to demonstrate improvement in nerve conduction following neurolysis.[12,35]

Intraoperative electrodiagnostic evaluation is routinely used during all methods of surgical intervention for brachial plexus. The exact form and technique of testing varies with the nature of the injury and the planned technique. Somatosensory-evoked potentials (SSEPs) are one intraoperative electrodiagnostic tool used to demonstrate continuity between the central and the peripheral nervous system via a dorsal root.[2] The actual state of the ventral root is not tested directly but is instead inferred from the state of the sensory nerve rootlets, as suggested by the integrity of a few hundred intact fibers. SSEPs are absent in postganglionic or combined pre- and postganglionic lesions. In comparison, motor-evoked potentials (MEPs) involve transcranial electrical stimulation[2,36] to assess the integrity of the motor pathway via the ventral root. Intraoperative MEPs are not useful for cases of complete distal lesions because of the obligatory time needed for regeneration into distal muscles; they are, however, useful for cases of partial lesions because the size of the lesion is proportional to the number of functioning axons.

Another form of intraoperative electrodiagnostic testing involves the use of a hand-held nerve stimulator. Often, these readily available instruments can be used to quickly identify functioning and nonfunctioning nerves, both before and after neurolysis. Mackinnon and Kline have shown hand-held nerve stimulators to be vital for a variety of novel nerve transfer techniques (as will be described later). A portable device (Varistim III; Medtronic, Jacksonville, FL) is used to confirm the function of donor nerves and to identify expendable fascicles such as those that innervate the flexor carpi radialis, flexor digitorum superficialis, or palmaris longus of the median nerve and the flexor carpi ulnaris of the ulnar nerve.[37-39] The selected donor fascicle is neurolysed and mobilized. To optimize specificity of stimulation the ground needle of the stimulator is placed close to the neurolysed portion of the donor nerve. Sufficient residual nerve functions should be verified by electrical stimulation of the remainder of the donor nerve before transfer.

Nerve grafting may be performed in cases of well-defined ruptures and neuromas and is most successful in defects of less than 10 cm.[30,32,39-41] Intraoperatively, there must be good viability of the remaining fascicles after neuroma resection. This is assessed by direct visualization under the operative microscope and confirmed with frozen section of the transacted nerve end. Ideally, good fascicular and axonal demarcation is preserved on the proximal side, with relatively little perifascicular fibrosis. Intact SSEPs help to confirm the integrity of the proximal stump; however, they contain no motor neuronal information. The sural nerve is the most common donor graft and is able to provide up to 40 cm of length. Other potential donors include the brachial and antebrachial cutaneous nerves, which have the advantage of being generally obtainable within the same operative field. Less commonly used donors include the radial sensory and, rarely, the ulnar nerve (vascularized or not).[42] Nerve grafts are generally reversed in polarity (to avoid the chance that regenerating axons will travel down an exiting branch) and stacked in predetermined lengths (cable grafts) to span a defect. Fibrin glue is often used to tack the stacked cable grafts together at each end, using a technique pioneered by Narakas[43] (Fig. 56-4). Shorter defects (<10 cm) do better than longer ones,[41] and grafts for proximal function do better than those for distal function because of the increased distance for regenerative nerve conduction to reach the desired target.

Novel options in nerve transfer, or neurotization, have revolutionized the treatment of adult brachial plexus surgery over the past decade.[33,44-48] Nerve transfer is a surgical option for acute, delayed, and even selected chronic cases. The technique usually involves transfer of an intact nerve to a denervated nerve, but, rarely, a functioning nerve can be transplanted directly into muscle, when no distal nerve stump remains.[49] In the case of intraplexal nerve transfer, fascicles of functioning peripheral nerves are harvested and transferred to the distal segment of a denervated nerve, close to the denervated muscle end plates. Examples include

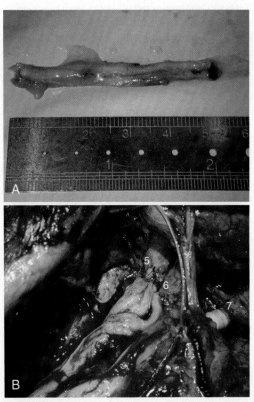

Figure 56-4 A, Nerve graft preparation using 5-cm cables of sural nerve and fibrin glue. **B,** Multiple cable grafts inserted from C5 through C7 roots.

transfer of medial pectoral or ulnar fascicles to the musculo-cutaneous nerve[45,48] and the transfer of the long head triceps nerve branch to the axillary nerve.[47] In extraplexal nerve transfer, a nearby motor nerve from outside the brachial plexus (e.g., the spinal accessory nerve, intercostal nerve, or phrenic nerve) is transferred to a denervated peripheral nerve of the brachial plexus (e.g., suprascapular nerve, musculocutaneous nerve, or axillary nerve). The choice of these procedures depends on the availability of undamaged extraplexal nerves.

Oberlin's procedure is an example of an intraplexal transfer aimed at restoring biceps function.[46,48] It involves transfer of one or more ulnar nerve fascicles to the nerve of the biceps. A 15-cm incision is made along the medial arm beginning at the pectoralis muscle and coursing distally along the neurovascular bundle. The biceps fascia is opened and the musculocutaneous nerve identified. The motor branches to both heads of the biceps are identified approximately 12 cm distal to the acromion and stimulated to ensure complete denervation; the branches are traced proximally where they usually coalesce into a single motor branch from the parent musculocutaneous nerve, and then divided sharply for transfer to the ulnar nerve. The ulnar nerve is identified by external neurolysis, and the epineurium is opened. Several fascicles of the ulnar nerve are chosen 3 to 4 cm distal to the level of the musculocutaneous branch to the biceps and stimulated with a portable nerve stimulator. A single large fascicle can usually be identified to produce maximal contraction of the flexor carpi ulnaris without significant contraction of the ulnar intrinsic muscles. This fascicle (or fascicles) is divided far enough distally to transfer directly to the motor branch(es) of the musculocutaneous nerve (Fig. 56-5).

When restoration of deltoid function is indicated, the radial nerve branch to the long, lateral, or medial heads of the triceps has been shown to be a promising intraplexal option to improve shoulder abduction.[47,50] This innovative technique involves the use of a single triceps branch transferred directly to the motor branch of the axillary nerve.[47] A posterior incision 15 cm long over the sulcus between the lateral and long heads of the triceps is made, and the radial nerve is identified deep between the long head and the lateral head of the triceps. Branches are elevated and stimulated to confirm branching to medial, long, and lateral heads. The axillary nerve is located in the quadrangular space and traced to identify the branch of the teres minor, posterior deltoid,

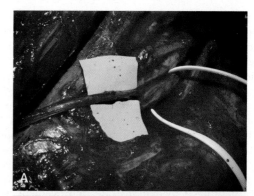
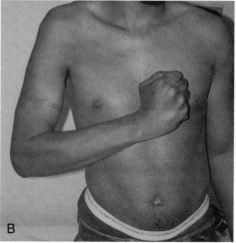

Figure 56-5 A, Oberlin's microtransfer of a single fascicle of the ulnar nerve (*white vessel loupes*) to the motor branch of the biceps. **B,** Recovery of biceps function at 6 months.

anterior branch to the skin, and the branch to the anterior and middle deltoid. It has been reported that the deep (medial) head branch is longer and a more robust axonal contribution for axillary reinnervation[44]; with this in mind, a branch to one head of the triceps deemed suitable during surgical dissection is divided distally and reflected to directly approximate the motor branch of the axillary nerve. If a size discrepancy exists, a nerve conduit can be used for better approximation and grouping of the fascicles (Fig. 56-6).

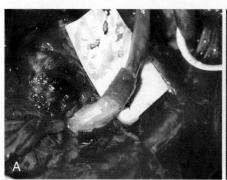
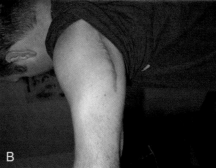
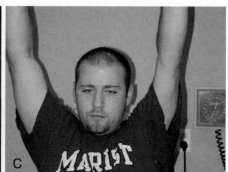

Figure 56-6 A, Nerve transfer from the long head of the triceps to the axillary motor branch with nerve conduit for C5 to C6 avulsion injury in a 20-year-old football player. **B,** Twelve-month hypertrophy of the deltoid. **C,** Overhead elevation at 12 months.

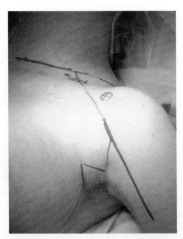

Figure 56-7 Standard incisions for brachial plexus surgery. The supraclavicular exposure is performed through a "necklace" incision placed 1 cm above and parallel to the clavicle. The incision is lengthened across the clavicle and medial to the coracoid process for direct exposure of the infraclavicular plexus. Intraplexal nerve transfers can be performed by lengthening the skin incision down the medial surface of the arm. Intercostal nerve transfers are performed with a zigzag extension of the incision across the axilla along the fifth and sixth ribs below the breast.

Other traditional transfers used early in the field of nerve transfer surgery made use of extraplexal sources that include the spinal accessory to the suprascapular nerve or to the musculocutaneous nerve, the phrenic nerve to the axillary nerve, the contralateral C7 nerve to the median nerve (usually in cases of complete or multilevel plexopathy with limited donor options), and the intercostal nerves to several potential peripheral nerve recipients (musculocutaneous, long thoracic, axillary, radial, and median nerves).

The spinal accessory nerve is a pure motor nerve that innervates the sternocleidomastoid and trapezius muscles. Its proximity to the suprascapular nerve allows direct microapproximation without a need for a graft. Exposure is performed using a 15-cm necklace incision situated 1 cm above and parallel to the clavicle[24,44,51] (Fig. 56-7). Division of the platysma allows supraclavicular nerve identification and preservation. The spinal accessory nerve is identified just deep to the superolateral margin of the trapezius near the clavicle and traced distally to its bifurcation. Nerve stimulation and contractility of the trapezius confirms viability of the spinal accessory nerve. The distal portion of the spinal accessory nerve is divided sharply and the end coapted to that of the recipient suprascapular nerve.

The phrenic nerve is another traditional nerve donor that has been transferred to the suprascapular nerve without grafting, achieving grade 3 muscle recovery within 8 months[18,52]; however, phrenic nerve harvest has the potential of compromising diaphragmatic and pulmonary function and is often contraindicated in patients who have had chest trauma.

Another traditional extraplexal source of satisfactory donors is the intercostal nerves as described in 1988 by Narakas and Hentz.[53] The intercostal nerves are harvested via a thoracic exposure and subperiosteal dissection along the inferior surface of the ribs. Their vulnerable location in the setting of high-energy trauma can preclude ease of availability as from chest tube placement or from abundant callus

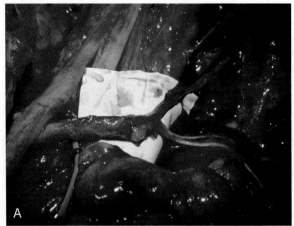

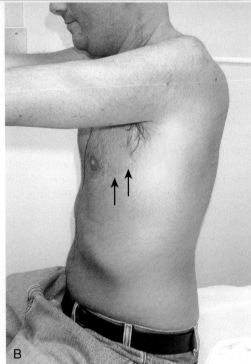

Figure 56-8 A, Three intercostal nerves glued together with fibrin glue and microcoapted to the axillary nerve without an intercalated nerve graft. **B,** Five years after ICN transfers (*arrows*) to axillary and musculocutaneous nerves for C5 through C7 avulsion injury.

associated with rib fractures. Another disadvantage is that these nerves are a mixed motor and sensory nerve with a limited number of available axons, necessitating transfer of multiple nerves to any particular recipient nerve. Improved results with intraplexal nerve transfers with the pectoral, ulnar, radial, or median nerves have allowed reserved use of intercostal nerves for elbow or shoulder reinnervation when other available donor nerves are unavailable. Nevertheless, the surgical technique should remain accessible to the surgeon. The procedure starts with a long curvilinear incision that starts proximal in the axilla and continues inferiorly along the midthoracic line beneath the ipsilateral nipple that corresponds to the inferior margin of the fifth rib (Fig. 56-8). The pectoralis major muscle is reflected medially and superiorly, and slips of the serratus are bluntly divided to expose each rib. Electrocautery is used to open the periosteal sleeve, and a curved elevator is used to dissect the periosteum from the internal surface of the rib. Sharp dissection through the periosteum identifies the intercostal nerve and intimately associated artery; extreme care should be taken to avoid perforating the pleura, which lies immediately deep to the nerves. The nerves are stimulated to identify the motor branch and traced to the anterior nipple line. Both motor and sensory portions are tagged for later direct approximation to motor and sensory (usually median) nerve recipients.

Although transfers to the more distal musculocutaneous nerve and axillary nerves have been described, both require use of an interpositional nerve graft.[53] Nerve transfers to the shoulder and elbow have been shown to be significantly more effective when performed without an intercalated nerve graft.[54]

Newer nerve transfer techniques are evolving. These include double nerve transfers performed for both elbow flexion and shoulder abduction.[55] For elbow flexion, the technique includes transfer of both the ulnar and medial nerves to the biceps and brachialis branches of the musculocutaneous nerve, respectively. For shoulder abduction this has been accomplished by dual nerve transfers to restore strength of supraspinatus, infraspinatus, and deltoid muscles.[24,55]

Restoration of function below the elbow remains a challenge. Intrinsic muscle function and wrist or digital flexion cannot readily be restored by nerve transfers. Neurotization of the median nerve to obtain sensation and finger flexion is a potential surgical alternative, as is staged double-functioning free-muscle transplantation.[56-58] Additional discussion on nerve transfers is available in Chapter 61.

Free-muscle transfers are an alternative option for complete TBPI or when donor nerves are unavailable.[3,59] It involves transplantation to a new location of a muscle and its neurovascular pedicle with microvascular anastomosis between the donor and recipient nerves and vessels. A number of muscles are available for transfer, including the gracilis, the latissimis dorsi, and the rectus femoris, which are powered by the anterior division of the obturator nerve, the thoracodorsal nerve, and the femoral nerve, respectively. Its use for restoration of elbow flexion is generally reserved for chronic injuries or when the native biceps and brachialis have been severely injured by direct trauma (Fig. 56-9). Intercostal nerves are often used to innervate the transferred muscle, and its vascular pedicle anastomosed to a branch of the subclavian artery. The gracilis muscle is frequently used for its proximally based neurovascular pedicle that allows for earlier reinnervation and for its long tendon length that enables reconstruction of hand and wrist function in addition to the primary goal of elbow flexion.[3]

Rehabilitation

Therapy should be initiated soon after injury. Formal attention to maintaining motion is needed to minimize contracture formation and to stimulate activity in muscles with any potential recovery that is frequently subclinical. For all known isolated nerve injuries, appropriate orthoses should be fabricated to counteract the corresponding muscle

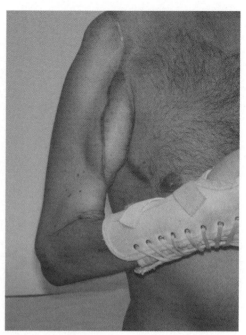

Figure 56-9 Clinical photograph 5 years after free-gracilis transfer for chronic complete plexus palsy. Intercostal nerves were used to motor the gracilis muscle.

weakness. Especially if surgery is anticipated, results from operative intervention depend on intact and preexisting joint motion.

Postsurgical rehabilitation is a team effort that is closely coordinated between surgeon and therapist. Immediate postoperative therapy usually entails a period of immobilization to allow for soft tissue healing and the resolution of edema. Ideally, microvascular anastomoses are tension-free to enable passive range of motion in all directions. When this is not attainable, clearly outlined and time-dependent therapy guidelines are communicated to all managing teams.

Patients and family members must be prepared for the prolonged time to recovery and the required investment to dedicated therapy. This includes regularly scheduled therapy sessions and periodic 3- to 4-month interval follow-up visits that last anywhere from 2 to 5 years after surgery to monitor full recovery.

Outcomes

The risks and benefits of surgical treatment should be clearly discussed with the patient so that expectations do not exceed the limits of the best possible outcome. Prognosis is highly dependent on the pattern of injury: complete C4 through T1 ruptures are the most severe and least amenable to reconstruction, C5 through T1 avulsion injuries are amenable to restoration of shoulder and elbow function with limited distal functional recovery, and proximal injuries with lower trunk sparing have the best prognosis with surgical intervention.[29]

Peer-reviewed literature confirms that experience with a variety of nerve transfers continues to improve and evolve. Functional milestones after intercostal transfer to the musculocutaneous nerve include the elicitation of chest pain by squeezing of the biceps muscle at approximately 3 months postoperatively, visible biceps contraction (M1) during deep inspiration at 6 months, and antigravity elbow flexion within 18 months of surgery.[60] This has been confirmed with a meta-analysis by Merrell and colleagues of 1088 nerve transfers, which showed 72% of intercostal to musculocutaneous nerve transfers exhibiting M > 3 and 37% M > 4 biceps function.[54] Some series have reported up to 65% antigravity elbow flexion within 12 months, and that voluntary biceps control was no longer dependent on the respiratory cycle by 3 years after surgery.[52]

As stated previously, despite the encouraging results with intercostal nerve transfer, greater functional success has been achieved more recently by transferring intact branches of the ulnar or median nerve directly to the motor branches of the biceps or brachialis. Early results with these novel transfers demonstrated 75% to 100% of patients achieved antigravity (M3) biceps strength or better (see Fig. 56-5B), and recent results show between 75% and 94% M4 strength.[46,48,61,62] Oberlin's transfers have had success rates with between 94% and 100% achieving M3 biceps function.[48,61,62] The meta-analysis by Merrell and colleagues also revealed that over 70% of cases achieve M > 3 elbow flexion.[54] In 2005, Mackinnon and coworkers reported M4 or better strength of elbow flexion in six patients in her series with dual transfers for elbow flexion, with clinical reinnervation noted at a mean of 5.5 months.[45]

Novel transfers for shoulder abduction show similar promise. Leechavengvongs reported excellent results in five of seven cases using the long head branch of the radial nerve branch to axillary nerve, with a mean shoulder abduction of 124 degrees by 28 months.[47] Most authors today would agree that a powerful combination of transfers for shoulder abduction includes the spinal accessory to the suprascapular nerve and a triceps branch to axillary nerve. The same meta-analysis by Merrell and colleagues also showed that dual transfers to restore shoulder function (to suprascapular and axillary nerves) yielded significantly improved results compared with single-nerve transfer, and over 70% achieved M3 shoulder abduction when the intercostal and spinal accessory nerves were the donors.[54] Successful transfers to the supra-

scapular nerve (92%) outnumbered those to the axillary nerve (69%).[54] Chuang recently reported 60 degrees of abduction in patients with root avulsions and 90 degrees or more in patients with upper root avulsions, using a combination of nerve transfers for shoulder abduction.[63] In a series of 577 spinal accessory nerve transfers, Songcharoen described 80% motor recovery (M > 3) with transfer to suprascapular nerve, obtaining 60 degrees of shoulder abduction and 45 degrees of shoulder flexion. In the same series, spinal accessory transfer to axillary only achieved 60% success; the poorer results may be attributed to the longer reinnervation distance and the requisite need for interpositional nerve grafts.[52]

There is little outcome data on nerve transfers for restoration of function distal to the elbow. A series of 111 transfers of the contralateral C7 nerve root to the medial nerve yielded 30% M3 and 20% M2 function. Despite the discouraging motor results, 83% obtained protective sensory recovery after this procedure.[52]

Summary

Understanding the pattern of injury is key to determining the prognosis for recovery and the appropriate treatment. A thorough physical examination combined with imaging techniques and electrodiagnostic evaluation guide the surgical options for patients with TBPI. Surgical options include nerve repair, neurolysis, nerve grafting, nerve transfer, and free-muscle grafts. The risks and benefits of surgical treatment should be clearly discussed with the patient so that expectations do not exceed the limits of the best possible outcome since prognosis is highly dependent on the pattern of injury. Patients and their families must understand that compliance with rehabilitation is essential to achieving an optimal outcome and that medical follow-up will be needed for up to 5 years.

REFERENCES

The complete reference list is available online at www.expertconsult.com.

CHAPTER 57

Common Nerve Injuries About the Shoulder 🎥

JOHN M. BEDNAR, MD AND RAYMOND K. WURAPA, MD

DIAGNOSIS AND MANAGEMENT
SUMMARY

CRITICAL POINTS

- Treatment of these nerve injuries requires a thorough examination of the shoulder complex and electrophysiologic testing to identify the location and extent of nerve injury.
- Therapy plays a primary role in both surgical and nonoperative management of common shoulder injuries.
- Treatment plans for therapy should address scapular dysfunction and prevention of a frozen shoulder.

Diagnosis and Management

The shoulder is a complex joint with complicated kinematics that rely on muscle function and balance for mobility and stability. Nerve injury that affects the function of these muscles will significantly alter this balance. Shoulder problems overall are common. Nerve injuries about the shoulder are relatively uncommon but are a commonly undiagnosed cause of shoulder dysfunction. The presenting signs or symptoms may be attributed to a structural problem (e.g., rotator cuff tear, shoulder instability) but will not improve with standard treatment for these conditions. The symptoms of local abnormalities of the shoulder may also present distally in the arm and forearm, complicating diagnosis.

The spectrum of nerve injuries involving the shoulder includes both acute and chronic conditions. These problems coexist with other more common injuries. Nerve injuries may be primary, from pathology arising within the nerve, or secondary, from other ongoing processes within the shoulder resulting in compression or traction neuropathy. Injury to the neurologic system can arise at many anatomic locations,

including cervical roots, brachial plexus, and peripheral nerves innervating the shoulder. Cervical spine pathology can lead to nerve injury at the root or spinal cord level. Existing systemic conditions (e.g., multiple sclerosis, malignancy, enthesopathies) may also make diagnosis difficult. For all these reasons, nerve injuries about the shoulder are often difficult to diagnose and manage.

The injury level and/or primary nerve pathology can be localized from the results of a detailed history and physical examination. Other diagnostic modalities, including electromyography (EMG), nerve conduction studies, spinal cord or cortical evoked potentials, magnetic resonance imaging (MRI), myelography, and computed tomography, are useful in confirming the clinical diagnosis and help guide treatment.

The goal of management is early correct diagnosis. Only after the correct diagnosis is made can appropriate treatment be instituted to avoid atrophy and/or contracture and to restore stability and mobility to the shoulder.

Anatomy

The neurologic elements of the upper extremity originate from the cervical portion of the spinal cord. The upper extremity receives contributions from cervical roots C5, C6, C7, and C8 and thoracic root T1. The brachial plexus is formed by the junctions of the ventral rami of these five roots. Occasionally, there may be contributions from C4 and less commonly from T2. The five cervical roots unite just above the clavicle, forming three trunks: the upper, consisting of roots C5 and C6; the middle trunk, consisting of root C7; and the lower trunk, consisting of roots C8 and T1 (Fig. 57-1). Just below the clavicle, each trunk divides into an anterior and posterior division. The anterior division of the upper and middle trunks forms the lateral cord. The anterior division of the lower trunk forms the medial cord, and the posterior divisions from the upper, middle, and lower trunks form the posterior cord. Note that the cords surround the subclavian artery and are named by their position relative to the artery. The lateral cord branches include the lateral pectoral nerve, musculocutaneous nerve, and median nerve. The

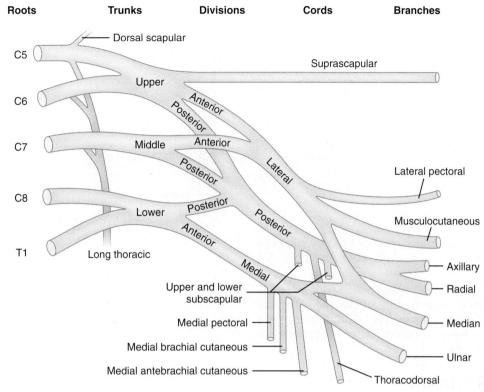

| Roots | Trunks | Divisions | Cords | Branches |

Figure 57-1 Brachial plexus anatomy.

medial cord branches include the medial pectoral nerve, medial brachial and antebrachial cutaneous nerves, and median and ulnar nerves. The posterior cord branches include the upper and lower subscapular nerves, the thoracodorsal, axillary, and radial nerves.

Other branches arise more proximally either from the cords, trunks, or roots to supply the shoulder girdle musculature. The dorsal scapular nerve, supplying the rhomboid muscles, arises directly from the C5 nerve root. The suprascapular nerve, supplying the supraspinatus and infraspinatus muscles, is a branch arising from the upper trunk. The long thoracic nerve, supplying the serratus anterior muscle, arises from contributions of the C5, C6, and C7 nerve roots (Table 57-1).

Types of Nerve Injury

Nerve injury can occur by laceration, traction, or compression. Laceration occurs by direct trauma through penetrating injury or as a result of a fracture or its treatment. Traction is a common mechanism that occurs with blunt trauma. A shoulder dislocation can result in a traction injury to the brachial plexus. A fall onto the shoulder with lateral deviation of the neck will result in a traction injury to the upper trunk of the brachial plexus. An injury with traction on the arm pulled in abduction will place traction on the lower plexus. Compression occurs either from a perineural scar or fracture callus in a post-trauma case or from an extrinsic lesion such as a ganglion or tumor.

The mechanism of injury is determined from the patient history. The degree of injury for each mechanism is determined by physical examination and electrophysiologic testing. The degree of nerve injury is characterized as one of three types based on the classification of Seddon[37] and Sunderland.[39,40]

Neurapraxia: A minimal nerve injury characterized by a temporary, fully reversible nerve conduction block, with good prognosis

Axonotmesis: A moderate nerve injury characterized by a disruption of the axons and myelin sheath with the epineurium left intact to guide regeneration; has a fair prognosis

Table 57-1 Branches of the Brachial Plexus

Peripheral Nerve	Origin
Long thoracic	C5, C6, C7—from roots
Dorsal scapular	C5—from root
Suprascapular	C5, C6—from upper trunk
Upper subscapular	C5—posterior cord
Lower subscapular	C5, C6—posterior cord
Thoracodorsal	C7, C8—posterior cord
Lateral pectoral	C5, C6, C7—lateral cord
Medial pectoral	C8, T1—medial cord
Medial brachial cutaneous	C8, T1—medial cord
Medial antebrachial cutaneous	C8, T1—medial cord
Axillary	C5, C6—posterior cord
Radial	C6, C7, C8—posterior cord
Median	C5 through T1—medial and lateral cords
Musculocutaneous	C5, C6—lateral cord
Ulnar	C8, T1—medial cord

Table 57-2 Nerves Commonly Injured about the Shoulder

Peripheral Nerve	Muscle Innervated
Long thoracic	Serratus anterior
Suprascapular	Supraspinatus
	Infraspinatus
Musculocutaneous	Coracobrachialis
	Biceps
	Brachialis
Axillary	Deltoid
	Teres minor
Spinal accessory	Trapezius

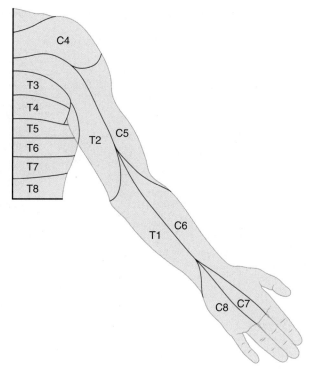

Figure 57-2 Upper extremity dermatome chart.

Neurotmesis: A severe injury characterized by complete destruction of the nerve with poor prognosis for regeneration

Another nerve injury classification system with more categories of nerve injury is described by Sunderland.[39] The rate of nerve regeneration is about 1 inch per month, which must be considered when assessing nerves recovering various distances to muscles or skin.[26]

Physical Examination

Examination for nerve injuries should be a part of every routine physical examination. The patient should be carefully observed with the trunk and upper extremities disrobed so that the normal side can be compared with the symptomatic side. Subtle areas of atrophy, deformity, discoloration, or swelling should be noted. The active and passive range of motion of the neck, shoulders, elbows, wrists, and hands should be measured and these joints tested for stability. The motor evaluation is one of the most important components of the neurologic examination. Each of the muscles of the shoulder should be tested, including those that move and stabilize the scapula. A comprehensive motor assessment can often define the site of a neurologic lesion. The nerve innervation of the muscles of the shoulder is outlined in Table 57-2.

The strength of each muscle should be recorded using the muscle grading system of Sunderland[40] (Table 57-3). Sensory deficits can occur in either a dermatomal (nerve root) distribution (Fig. 57-2) or along the distribution of peripheral nerves. If spinal cord lesions are suspected, a detailed evaluation of all sensory functions (pain, hot/cold, vibration, and position sense) is mandatory.

Table 57-3 Muscle Grading System

Grade	Findings
5 Normal	Able to withstand full resistance
4 Good	Able to withstand some resistance
3 Fair	Move against gravity—no resistance
2 Poor	Move with gravity eliminated
1 Trace	Muscle contraction without movement
0 Zero	No muscle contraction

Diagnostic Tests

Electrophysiologic examination remains the most commonly performed test for evaluation of neurologic injury. This test has two components: an electromyogram and a nerve conduction velocity (NCV) study. The combination of NCV and EMG allow localization of the nerve injury, assess the age and degree of injury, and provide evidence of nerve recovery. Chapter 15 provides detailed information on this diagnostic tool, but it is briefly reviewed in this chapter.

EMG is performed by placing a recording needle into the muscle being studied and observing the nature of the electrical activity in the muscle. A normal muscle is electrically silent at rest and produces a well-defined single-peaked recording when the muscle is contracted voluntarily (motor unit potential [MUP]). A nerve with an acute injury with denervation will produce spontaneous electrical signals at rest recorded as fibrillation potentials or positive sharp waves. The MUP will be altered or nonexistent, depending on the degree of axonal injury. These electrical changes in an acute injury do not become detectable by EMG until 3 weeks after injury. As regeneration occurs, the fibrillation potentials disappear. Intact motor nerves sprout to innervate denervated motor units, producing a polyphasic MUP with multiple peaks. The presence of polyphasic potentials indicate that the nerve injury is more than 3 months old.

EMG can detect the effects of denervation caused by a lower motor lesion. EMG cannot define the location of the lesion between the spinal cord and muscle, unless multiple muscles are individually tested to map the location of the nerve injury. EMG can determine whether the pathologic process involves more than one peripheral nerve. It can also identify whether the observed pathology is part of a generalized peripheral neuropathy or chronic myopathy (e.g., muscular dystrophy).

The NCV is a direct measurement of nerve conduction through the extremity. Myelin is the insulating material for the nerve axons. As myelin is lost as a result of compression or injury, the conduction across the injured segment will decrease. This test helps to define areas of compression or injury along a peripheral nerve. These measurements are obtained by direct stimulation of a nerve proximally in the extremity and measurement of the time required for impulse conduction to a point in the nerve more distal in the extremity. The measurement is recorded in meters per second. Abnormal values (decreased conduction velocity) are determined by comparison with the uninvolved extremity or published normal standards.[21] Nerve conduction can also be measured by stimulating the nerve at a fixed distance from an anatomic landmark and tracking (from a distal muscle) the time from stimulation to recording of a MUP. This measurement is a *motor latency* and is recorded in milliseconds. A *sensory latency* is measured by stimulating the fingertip and recording from the nerve at a fixed distance proximally. These measurements, if prolonged, imply abnormal nerve conduction in the anatomic region being studied.

Spinal Accessory Nerve

The spinal accessory nerve is the 11th cranial nerve and the primary motor nerve to the trapezius and sternocleidomastoid muscles. It is susceptible to injury because of its superficial course through the subcutaneous tissues on the floor of the posterior cervical triangle. This anatomic structure is bound by the trapezius, sternocleidomastoid, and clavicle (Fig. 57-3). Injury occurs from blunt trauma directly to the nerve, traction injury to the nerve from a force depressing

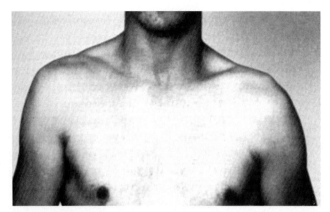

Figure 57-4 Atrophy of the left trapezius muscle secondary to spinal accessory nerve injury.

the shoulder while the head is forced in the opposite direction,[45] or iatrogenic injury from surgical procedures in the posterior cervical triangle, most commonly cervical node biopsy. Injury to the spinal accessory nerve results in paralysis of the trapezius muscle.

Spinal accessory palsy presents as a dull ache or pain, with drooping of the shoulder and noticeable weakness in arm elevation and abduction (Fig. 57-4). Atrophy of the trapezius muscle is present. The sternocleidomastoid muscle may also be atrophied and nonfunctional if the injury is proximal. The patient is unable to shrug the affected shoulder. Winging of the scapula can be seen when viewed from behind because of the lack of the suspensory action of the trapezius.

When the injury is caused by blunt trauma or traction, initial treatment is conservative, with sling immobilization and a therapy regimen to prevent a frozen shoulder and to strengthen the trapezius and surrounding muscles.

These patients may present to therapy with a diagnosis of shoulder impingement. The impingement is secondary to drooping of the shoulder from the spinal accessory palsy and unrelated to acromioclavicular joint pathology. It is difficult to compensate for the lack of trapezius function simply by strengthening adjacent muscles, and the impingement symptoms fail to improve with traditional therapy prescribed for classic impingement syndrome.

The deficit in closed nerve injuries may persist for 3 to 12 months. If no electrophysiologic evidence of regeneration is present by 6 months, the trapezius palsy can be considered permanent.[36]

When the injury is iatrogenic or caused by open trauma, neurolysis and nerve repair are most successful when performed within 6 months of injury.[16] If surgical exploration reveals a nerve transection, nerve repair is performed by either direct repair or nerve grafting if a tension-free repair cannot be performed. If a neuroma-in-continuity is found at surgical exploration, intraoperative nerve conduction studies are performed to determine whether neurolysis alone is effective or whether resection with primary repair is needed. A recovery period of about 1 year is required to assess the results of surgical intervention.

Kim et al.[22] reported on the surgical outcomes of 111 spinal accessory nerve injuries. The most frequent injury mechanism was iatrogenic (103) with 82 of these patients

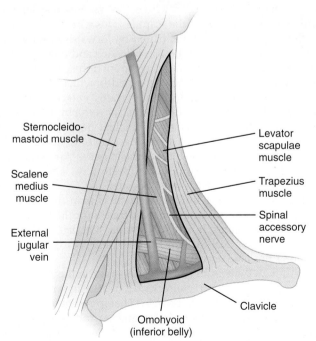

Sternocleido-
mastoid muscle

Scalene
medius
muscle

External
jugular
vein

Levator
scapulae
muscle

Trapezius
muscle

Spinal
accessory
nerve

Clavicle

Omohyoid
(inferior belly)

Figure 57-3 Spinal accessory nerve location in posterior cervical triangle.

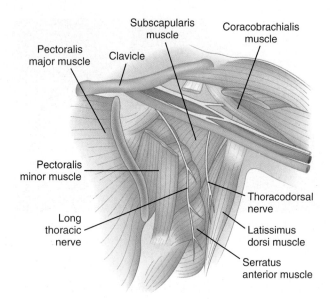

Figure 57-5 Anatomy of the long thoracic nerve.

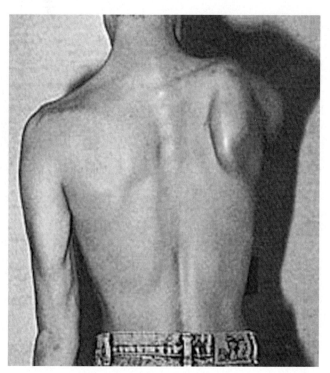

Figure 57-6 Scapular winging resulting from long thoracic nerve injury.

having a lymph node biopsy as the index procedure. Eight were caused by stretch injury and three by traumatic laceration. Nineteen patients at operative exploration were found to have the nerve in continuity. They were treated with neurolysis when intraoperative electrical stimulation demonstrated conduction along the nerve. When the nerve was found to have been lacerated, 26 patients were treated by end-to-end repair and 58 patients were treated by nerve graft. The average graft length was 1.5 inches. Of the patients treated by neurolysis, 95% regained grade 4 or higher trapezius muscle strength. Of the patients treated by suture repair or nerve graft, 77% regained grade 3 or higher strength.

If trapezial function does not return, reconstructive procedures are performed. For isolated, complete, permanent trapezial injuries, muscle transfers are recommended.[2,25,42] The Eden-Lange procedure[36] involves transfer of the levator scapulae muscle to the acromion and transfer of the rhomboid muscle to the infraspinatus fossa of the scapula. Romero and Gerber[36] reported a series of 12 patients treated with the Eden-Lange procedure with a mean follow-up of 32 years. Nine were classified as excellent, two were fair, and one was poor. Pain was adequately controlled in 11 patients. Overhead activity was restored in nine patients. The patient with a poor outcome had a concomitant long thoracic nerve palsy.

Scapular suspension or scapulothoracic fusion are preferred[8,26] in patients with neuromuscular disorders and multiple nerve injuries involving the parascapular muscles.

Long Thoracic Nerve

The long thoracic nerve originates from the ventral rami of C5, C6, and C7 and travels beneath the brachial plexus and clavicle over the first rib.[4] The nerve then courses along the lateral aspect of the chest wall to innervate the serratus anterior muscle (Fig. 57-5). Because of its superficial course and length, this nerve is susceptible to damage from blows to the shoulder or chest wall or from prolonged traction on the shoulder.

The serratus anterior stabilizes the scapula on the posterior thoracic wall, providing a firm point for muscles originating from the scapula to move the arm. In addition, the serratus anterior, together with the trapezius and levator scapulae, acts to upwardly rotate the scapula, allowing greater glenohumeral elevation.

The clinical presentation includes a dull ache or pain around the shoulder, winging of the scapula, and decreased active shoulder motion.[10,20] Often, the patient may present with painless winging of the scapula. This winging deformity of the scapula is most accentuated by forward pushing on a wall (Fig. 57-6) or when the arm is loaded and then elevated. More severe pain usually indicates more diffuse involvement of regional muscles and an associated brachial plexus neuropathy.[18] An idiopathic form of serratus anterior paralysis has been described, termed *neuralgic amyotrophy*, which consists of a syndrome of paralytic brachial neuritis that occasionally may affect only the long thoracic nerve.[32] The differential diagnosis for long thoracic nerve paralysis must include polymyositis, muscular dystrophy, and cervical spondylosis, all of which must be ruled out.

Electrophysiologic studies are invaluable in the diagnosis and prognosis of this injury. EMG determines the location of nerve involvement. It will determine whether the injury involves the cervical roots or brachial plexus or is isolated to the long thoracic nerve.

Although there is no consensus as to the appropriate treatment of this condition, conservative treatment with rest and therapy is a common approach. Therapy should strive to strengthen the serratus anterior and surrounding muscles and maintain the range of motion of the shoulder. These patients may also present to therapy with an incorrect diagnosis of shoulder impingement, secondary to the winging deformity of the shoulder from long thoracic palsy. The winged scapula rotates forward, decreasing the space between the acromium and greater tuberosity and resulting in rotator cuff impingement.

The overall prognosis for serratus anterior paralysis is good, with progressive recovery occurring up to 2 years after the injury.[14] A serratus palsy can be judged permanent[26] if no clinical or electrical evidence of recovery is seen by 12 months after injury.

A number of surgical options are available for persistent deficits:

1. Neurolysis.[9] Nath[28] reported 50 patients treated by neurolysis of the supraclavicular portion of the long thoracic nerve. The average follow-up was 25.7 months. Neurolysis improved scapular winging in 49 (98%) of the 50 cases. Pain reduction was good or excellent in 43 (86%) of the cases.
2. Muscle transfer.[6,27] Perlmutter and Leffert[33] reported the results of 16 patients treated with pectoralis major tendon transfer to the scapula. Eight patients were asymptomatic with normal function, five had intermittent mild discomfort, and one had frequent mild pain with no scapular winging. Two patients failed after a traumatic event.
3. Scapulothoracic arthrodesis. Stabilization of the scapula to the chest wall is an option for pain relief but with significant loss of shoulder motion.[17]

Suprascapular Nerve

The suprascapular nerve originates from the upper trunk of the brachial plexus, with contributions from the fifth and sixth cervical roots. The nerve courses through the posterior cervical triangle, passing under the body of the omohyoid muscle and anterior border of the trapezius muscle. The nerve passes through the suprascapular notch, covered by the transverse scapular ligament, to innervate the supraspinatus muscle. At this point, it also gives off sensory fibers to the capsular ligamentous structures of the shoulder and acromioclavicular joint. The suprascapular nerve continues around the lateral border of the spine of the scapula, through the spinoglenoid notch, to innervate the infraspinatus muscle (Fig. 57-7).

Most injuries involve entrapment of the suprascapular nerve at the suprascapular notch by the transverse scapular ligament before it innervates the supraspinatus muscle.[7,15] An injury here would produce symptoms of both supraspinatus and infraspinatus weakness. Another common area of entrapment is at the spinoglenoid notch. Because the supraspinatus has already been innervated, an injury here produces only infraspinatus weakness.

Injury to the suprascapular nerve is most commonly caused by direct shoulder trauma, including fracture or dislocation,[46] but can also occur from a traction injury.[12] The clinical presentation includes a dull ache or pain along the posterior aspect of the scapula. Weakness of abduction and external rotation of the arm[38] is found on physical examination. Atrophy of the supraspinatus or infraspinatus muscles is found in more advanced cases (Fig. 57-8).

The differential diagnosis should include rotator cuff tears, cervical radiculopathy, myopathy, and brachial plexus

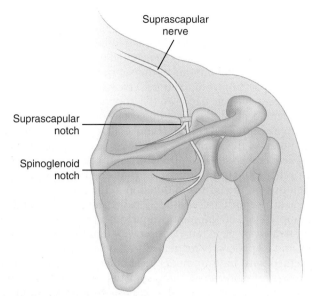

Figure 57-7 Anatomy of the suprascapular nerve.

neuropathy. Patients often initially receive a diagnosis of a rotator cuff injury and undergo a workup for this diagnosis. However, the diagnosis of suprascapular nerve entrapment should be suspected if the MRI study shows a structurally intact rotator cuff with selective atrophy of the supraspinatus and infraspinatus muscles. EMG and NCV studies can confirm the clinical impression of suprascapular nerve entrapment and determine the location at either the suprascapular or spinoglenoid notch. MRI is performed to look for a ganglion arising from the glenohumeral joint compressing the nerve.

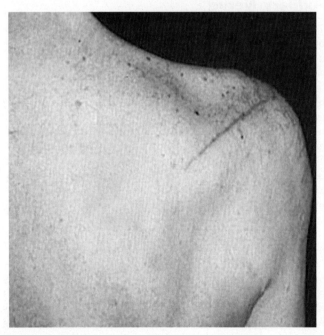

Figure 57-8 Atrophy of the supraspinatus and infraspinatus muscles resulting from suprascapular nerve injury.

Initial treatment is conservative, consisting of rest, anti-inflammatory agents, and therapy to strengthen the involved and surrounding muscles while maintaining shoulder motion. Surgical decompression may be required if an anatomic lesion is identified.[41] Explorations of the suprascapular nerve have revealed hypertrophy of the transverse scapular ligament and compression of the nerve at the suprascapular notch and spinoglenoid notch.[13,35] Ganglion cysts are a common cause of compression of the suprascapular nerve at the spinoglenoid notch of the scapula.[19,29,43] The clinical response to surgical decompression varies from no improvement to complete pain relief with full restoration of muscle bulk and power, depending on the form and duration of the causal lesion.[15,44] Kim et al.[23] reported a series of 42 patients treated by surgical decompression of the suprascapular nerve. Three patients were treated by ganglion excision with good return of function, and 39 patients were treated with neurolysis. Thirty-one presented with mild to moderate shoulder pain and muscle weakness. Preoperative supraspinatus and infraspinatus muscle function was grade 0 to 2. Postoperative supraspinatus muscle function improved to grade 4 or better in 28 (90%) of the patients. Infraspinatus muscle function improved to better than grade 3 in 10 (23%) of patients. Eight patients presented with severe pain and grade 3 muscle strength. Postoperatively, 7 (88%) of the patients in this group reported improvement in pain. All patients had muscle strength that remained the same or improved to grade 4.

Patients with severe, longstanding atrophy and denervation potentials on EMG have a poor prognosis for recovery with surgical decompression. Because the supraspinatus stabilizes the humeral head in the glenoid during arm elevation and the infraspinatus provides 90% of the external rotation power of the shoulder, residual weakness will limit activities of daily living and often preclude return to competitive sports.[30]

Axillary Nerve

The axillary nerve is a branch from the posterior cord of the brachial plexus receiving its nerve fibers from the C5 and C6 nerve roots. The nerve courses laterally and inferiorly, anterior to the subscapularis muscle, passing along the medioinferior aspect of the shoulder joint, around the neck of the humerus into the quadrilateral space. The quadrilateral space is on the posterior aspect of the shoulder, bordered by the teres minor superiorly, teres major inferiorly, humeral shaft laterally, and the long head of the triceps muscle medially. The axillary nerve then passes around the posterior and lateral portion of the proximal humerus, divides into anterior and posterior branches, and innervates the deltoid and teres minor muscles. A sensory cutaneous branch of the nerve supplies the lateral aspect of the upper arm.

Injury to the axillary nerve is usually a result of a proximal humerus fracture, shoulder dislocation, or direct trauma.[1,3] Iatrogenic injury to the nerve can result from any operative procedure involving the inferior aspect of the shoulder capsule, by either compression from a retractor or direct injury during the capsular release. The axillary nerve runs horizontally 5 cm inferior to the acromion; a deltoid-splitting procedure that exceeds this 5 cm will injure the nerve and denervate the anterior deltoid muscle. The high frequency of

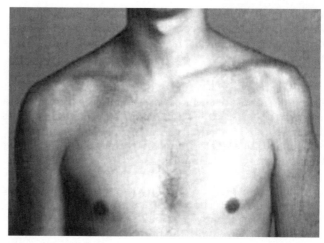

Figure 57-9 Deltoid atrophy caused by isolated axillary nerve injury.

involvement of this nerve with shoulder injuries is explained by its anatomic location, making it more susceptible to stretch or tension.

The clinical presentation can vary considerably, including poorly localized anterior shoulder pain, deltoid atrophy with weakness in arm elevation and abduction, and numbness along the lateral aspect of the upper arm (Fig. 57-9). Abduction weakness may not be clinically apparent because of effective substitution by the supraspinatus muscle. When an axillary nerve injury is diagnosed, the remaining branches of the posterior cord must be evaluated to determine the location of the nerve lesion. This requires examination of the muscles innervated by the thoracodorsal nerve (latissimus dorsi muscle) and radial nerve (wrist and finger extensor muscles). Electrophysiologic testing is helpful in determining the location and extent of the axillary nerve injury.

If a partial injury exists, treatment consists of rest and therapy. Therapy should focus on strengthening of the shoulder muscles, specifically the deltoid and teres minor muscles, and maintaining shoulder range of motion. Because of the short course of this nerve, some degree of recovery should be observed within 3 to 4 months. If no recovery is evident after this period, neurolysis or nerve grafting produces a good outcome.[11,34] Kline and Kim[24] reported a series of 56 isolated axillary nerve palsies of which 90% had nerve lesions in continuity and were treated with operative exploration. If nerve action potentials were recorded crossing the zone of injury, neurolysis was performed. If no conduction was evident, the lesion was resected and nerve grafted. The neurolysis group attained a mean grade of 4 muscle recovery. The nerve graft group attained a mean grade of 3.7 muscle recovery.

Quadrilateral space syndrome involves compression of the posterior humeral circumflex artery and axillary nerve[5] as they pass through the quadrilateral space. It manifests with axillary nerve deficits, as discussed earlier, and a diminished radial pulse with the arm positioned in abduction, elevation, and external rotation (provocative maneuver). This diagnosis can be confirmed by arteriography while performing the provocative maneuver. Once this problem is diagnosed, surgical decompression is usually necessary to relieve symptoms. Cahill and Palmer[5] reported a series of 18 patients treated with surgical decompression of the quadrilateral space. Eight patients reported complete relief of symptoms, eight reported improvement of symptoms, and two patients showed no improvement.

Musculocutaneous Nerve

The musculocutaneous nerve is a terminal branch of the lateral cord, receiving contributions from the C5 and C6 roots. It supplies the coracobrachialis, brachialis, and biceps muscles; innervates the elbow joint; and becomes the lateral antebrachial cutaneous nerve in the forearm. Isolated musculocutaneous nerve injury is uncommon. It usually occurs in association with shoulder trauma. Injury may occur iatrogenically during shoulder operative procedures (e.g., creating an anterior portal for shoulder arthroscopy). A "safe zone" has been described intraoperatively because the nerve is usually noted to cross obliquely to enter the brachioradialis muscle 5 cm below the coracoid process. However, this interval of safety may be diminished by abduction of the arm and with anatomic variation. Iatrogenic injury can also occur from arm traction during an operative procedure.

Clinical presentation of a musculocutaneous nerve injury includes weakness of elbow flexion, especially with the forearm fully supinated, and sensory loss over the lateral volar forearm. Unless it is known with certainty that the nerve is divided, patients with immediate postoperative musculocutaneous nerve deficits are treated nonoperatively with therapy for the first 3 weeks. Therapy should involve strengthening the shoulder muscles, focusing on the involved coracobrachialis, brachialis, and biceps muscles, and maintaining shoulder motion. Three weeks after surgery, electrophysiologic studies can be performed to further assess the state of the nerve. Signs of nerve recovery should be evident within 3 months of injury. If no recovery is noted by 3 to 6 months, surgical exploration and repair are recommended. Osborne et al.[31] reported a series of 85 patients with repair of traumatic lesions of the musculocutaneous nerve. There were 57 patients with good results, 17 patients with fair results, and 11 patients with poor results. The type of injury was the most important factor in determining the result. Twelve of 13 patients with clean, sharp lacerations had good results compared with 30 of 48 patients with closed traction lesions who had good results. The results were better when repaired within 14 days of the injury and when the nerve grafts were less than 10 cm long. The results were worse in the presence of a bony or arterial injury.

Summary

Nerve injuries about the shoulder are uncommon but are a commonly undiagnosed cause of shoulder dysfunction. Injuries to the nerve coexist with other more common shoulder problems. The goal of management is early diagnosis by careful physical examination and electrophysiologic studies.

The correct diagnosis must be made to guide treatment to restore stability and mobility to the shoulder. Therapy relies heavily on the appropriate management of scapular dysfunction, which is thoroughly discussed in Chapter 93.

REFERENCES

The complete reference list is available online at www.expertconsult.com.

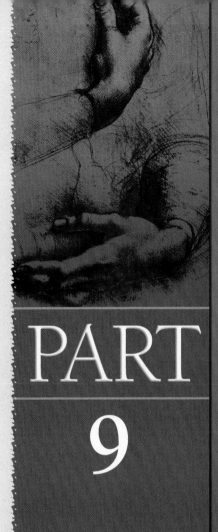

PART

9

Surgical Reconstruction for Nerve Injuries

Tendon Transfers for Upper Extremity Peripheral Nerve Injuries 📹

JOSHUA A. RATNER, MD AND SCOTT H. KOZIN, MD

RADIAL NERVE
MEDIAN NERVE
ULNAR NERVE

COMBINED MEDIAN AND ULNAR NERVE PALSIES
SUMMARY

CRITICAL POINTS

- Potential donors for transfer are those muscles with
  1. Adequate power to motor the recipient tendon
  2. Similar tendon excursion to the recipient
  3. Function synergistic or "in phase" with the recipient
- Transfers for radial nerve palsy restore wrist extension, metacarpophalangeal (MCP) joint extension, and thumb extension.
- Transfers for median nerve palsy restore thumb opposition and interphalangeal (IP) joint flexion.
- Transfers for ulnar nerve palsy restore thumb adduction, MCP joint flexion, IP joint extension, and index digit abduction.
- Timing of surgery depends on the achievement of tissue equilibrium.
- Clinical success requires a multidisciplinary approach to patient care.

Functional deficits resulting from peripheral nerve injuries vary with the particular nerve involved, the location of the lesion, and the extent of concomitant injuries to bone and soft tissue structures. Tendon transfer surgery to restore fundamental wrist and hand function is made possible by the redundancy that exists among the actions of our upper extremity musculature. The development of a surgical plan for tendon transfers involves identifying those muscles that are denervated, evaluating the patient's functional deficits, and considering which muscles are available for transfer. Potential donors for transfer are those muscles with adequate power to motor the recipient tendon, similar tendon excursion to the recipient, and those with function synergistic or "in phase" with the recipient (i.e., wrist extension and finger flexion, thumb adduction and wrist flexion, finger extension

and thumb abduction). Certainly, existing function should not be sacrificed by the harvest of a muscle–tendon unit.

Timing of surgery depends on the achievement of tissue equilibrium. Resolution of wound healing, union of fractures, and mobilization of stiff joints are prerequisites for a well-functioning tendon transfer. Clinical success requires a multidisciplinary approach to patient care including contributions by physicians, nurses, therapists, and electrodiagnosticians. A description of rehabilitation strategies for tendon transfers after peripheral nerve injury can be found in Chapter 59.

Radial Nerve

Anatomy

The radial nerve is a branch of the posterior cord of the brachial plexus. The first few branches of the radial nerve innervate the triceps.[1] Coursing through the posterior compartment of the arm, the nerve lies immediately adjacent to the posterior humerus for a distance of more than 6 cm.[6] Piercing the lateral intramuscular septum, the radial nerve enters the anterior compartment of the arm approximately 10 cm proximal to the lateral epicondyle. The nerve's relationship to both the humerus and the stout fibers of the lateral intramuscular septum place it at particular risk in this region for traumatic and iatrogenic injury. Once in the anterior compartment, the radial nerve lies between the brachioradialis (BR) and the brachialis and continues in this interval distally, giving off motor branches to both the BR and extensor carpi radialis longus (ECRL) (Fig. 58-1). Before entering the forearm through the two heads of the supinator, the radial nerve bifurcates into a sensory branch, dorsal radial sensory nerve (DRSN), and a primarily motor branch, the posterior interosseous nerve (PIN). The extensor carpi radialis brevis

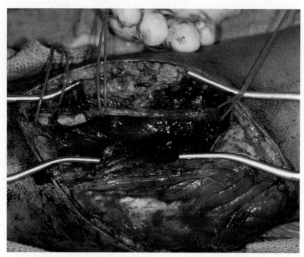

Figure 58-1 In the anterior compartment, the radial nerve lies between the brachioradialis and the brachialis muscles. (Courtesy of Shriners Hospital for Children, Philadelphia.)

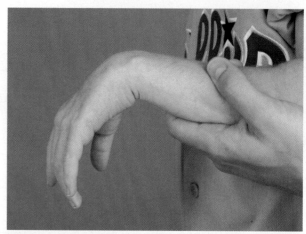

Figure 58-3 A 7-year-old child status post left humerus fracture with high radial nerve palsy and wrist drop. (Courtesy of Shriners Hospital for Children, Philadelphia.)

(ECRB) is variably innervated by either the radial nerve or the PIN (in the majority of cases). The PIN travels through the proximal dorsal forearm innervating the extensor digitorum communis (EDC), extensor carpi ulnaris (ECU), extensor digiti quinti (EDQ), abductor pollicis longus (APL), extensor pollicis longus (EPL), extensor pollicis brevis (EPB), and extensor indicis proprius (EIP) before terminating as a sensory nerve to the carpus, lying deep to the tendons of the fourth dorsal extensor compartment.

Physical Examination

The most proximal muscle innervated by the radial nerve is the triceps, and in the majority of cases of a peripheral nerve injury, its function as an elbow extensor is preserved. As illustrated in Figure 58-2, a radial nerve lesion proximal to the elbow results in loss of function of all the wrist extensor

muscles (ECRL, ECRB, and ECU), yielding a wrist drop (Fig. 58-3). Loss of wrist extension results in the inability to generate power grip, which can easily be tested using a dynamometer. EDC function is tested by asking the patient to simultaneously extend the MCP joints of the index through small digits (Fig. 58-4). EIP and extensor digiti minimi function is evaluated by asking the patient to extend the index and small finger MCP joints in isolation. EPL function is assessed by asking the patient to extend all joints of the thumb at the same time. Extensor pollicis brevis (EPB) function is assessed by having the patient extend the thumb MCP joint while keeping the interphalangeal (IP) joint flexed.

In contrast to a high radial nerve palsy (also known as palsy of the radial nerve proper), a lesion distal to the elbow will involve only those muscles innervated by the PIN (see Fig. 58-2). Clinically, examination of the patient with low radial nerve palsy demonstrates wrist radial deviation during active extension because of maintenance of ECRL function and loss of ECU function.

After initial evaluation and diagnosis of radial nerve palsy, it is recommended that the patient be fitted for a radial nerve orthosis. Traditional outrigger orthoses or newer lower

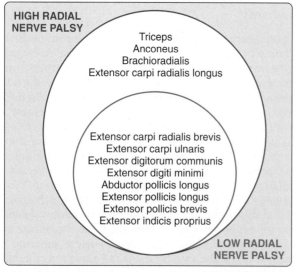

Figure 58-2 A radial nerve lesion proximal to the elbow results in loss of function of all the wrist extensors (extensor carpi radialis longus, extensor carpi radialis brevis, and extensor carpi ulnar), yielding a wrist drop.

HIGH RADIAL NERVE PALSY

Triceps
Anconeus
Brachioradialis
Extensor carpi radialis longus

Extensor carpi radialis brevis
Extensor carpi ulnaris
Extensor digitorum communis
Extensor digiti minimi
Abductor pollicis longus
Extensor pollicis longus
Extensor pollicis brevis
Extensor indicis proprius

LOW RADIAL NERVE PALSY

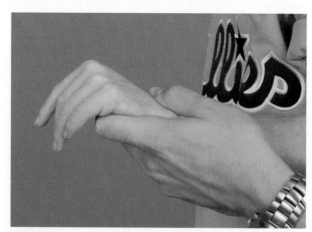

Figure 58-4 Passive extension of the wrist and attempted active finger extension produces no metacarpophalangeal joint extension. (Courtesy of Shriners Hospital for Children, Philadelphia.)

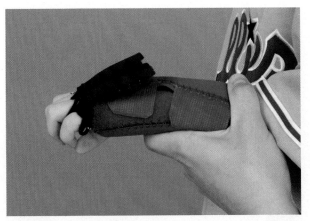

Figure 58-5 Low-profile neoprene orthosis to support wrist in extension and provide metacarpophalangeal joint extension with straps fastened with Velcro. (Courtesy of Shriners Hospital for Children, Philadelphia.)

Table 58-1 Seddon's Classification of Nerve Injury

Type	Definition	Outcome
Neurapraxia	Interruption of nerve conduction; some segmental demyelination; axon continuity intact	Reversible
Axonotmesis	Axon continuity disrupted; neural tube intact	Wallerian degeneration; incomplete recovery
Neurotmesis	Complete disruption of nerve continuity; loss of axons and neural tubes	No spontaneous recovery; surgery required

Adapted from Seddon HJ. *Surgical Disorders of Peripheral Nerve Injuries.* 2nd ed. Edinburgh, Churchill-Livingstone, 1972.

profile orthoses along with an appropriate home exercise program prevent the development of wrist and MCP joint contractures and can considerably enhance function (Figs. 58-5 and 58-6). The reader is referred to Chapter 45 for more detail regarding orthotic fabrication for the nerve-injured hand. During subsequent visits, serial physical examinations of a patient with radial nerve palsy is an important tool for monitoring recovery, guiding treatment, and managing patient expectations.

Despite the limited functional consequence of a loss of BR activity after a radial nerve injury, evaluation of this muscle for signs of reinnervation is extremely important in the weeks and months after injury. Because the BR is the first muscle innervated by the radial nerve in the anterior compartment of the arm, reinnervation of the BR implies nerve conduction distal to the site of the lesion. Once motor function of the brachioradialis is restored, it is likely that wrist and MCP joint extension will soon follow.

Timing of Tendon Transfers

The preferred timing of tendon transfers for a radial nerve palsy falls into one of two categories: early transfers done to

act as an "internal orthosis" or later transfers to restore function when recovery is deemed unlikely. Early transfers are performed within weeks of nerve injury and usually consist of a single tendon transfer for wrist extension. This transfer for wrist extension allows power grip by placing the finger and thumb flexors at a biomechanical advantage. Release of finger opening is accomplished by wrist flexion and the associated tenodesis effect of the long finger extensor tendons. The preferred timing of late transfers varies widely among authors, with intervals ranging between 6 and 18 months.

The expected time to recovery of any peripheral nerve lesion can be calculated based on the work of Seddon (Table 58-1).[2] Neurapraxias tend to recover within 3 to 4 weeks after injury as remyelination occurs promptly. In contrast, an axonotmesis injury involves Wallerian degeneration and implies incomplete and slow regeneration. Assuming a rate of nerve regrowth of 1 mm/day, the expected time to clinically detect return of function can be estimated based on the distance between the nerve lesion and the site of innervation of the BR. Therefore, it is reasonable to expect that a radial nerve lesion occurring at the mid-shaft of the humerus would take at least 6 months to recover. Delaying tendon transfers until that time seems reasonable to allow sufficient time for nerve recovery. During this time, a radial nerve orthosis will enhance function and should be prescribed.

Radial Nerve Tendon Transfers

In an isolated high radial nerve injury, muscle–tendon units innervated by the median and ulnar nerve are possible donors. Given the preserved function of both the wrist flexors (i.e., flexor carpi radialis [FCR] and flexor carpi ulnaris [FCU]) and both pronators (pronator teres [PT] and pronator quadratus), there are several available options. Classic transfers for radial nerve palsy include the Brand,[3] Jones,[4] and modified Boyes[5,6] transfers. Among these transfers is the common use of the PT to ECRB and the palmaris longus (PL) to EPL. The preferred choice of a motor to reanimate the EDC varies with each author. In low radial nerve palsy, a transfer for wrist extension is not required because ECRL function is preserved.

Although each of the three sets of transfers have been used by the authors, the preferred transfers for radial nerve palsy

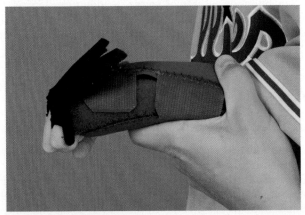

Figure 58-6 Active finger flexion is able to overcome the tension in the straps, which promotes functional use of the hand. (Courtesy of Shriners Hospital for Children, Philadelphia.)

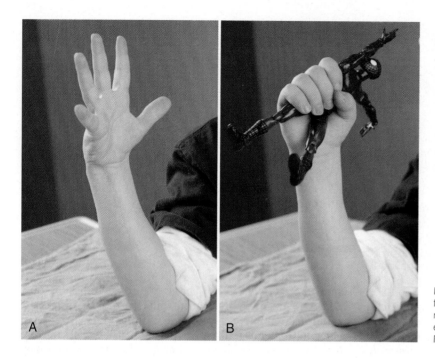

Figure 58-9 *A 5-year-old boy status post tendon transfers for radial nerve deficit.* **A,** *Adequate thumb and finger release with mild wrist flexion.* **B,** *Full grasp with wrist in extension. (Courtesy of Shriners Hospital for Children, Philadelphia.)*

are the PT to ECRB, PL to the rerouted EPL, and FCR to EDC. The rationale for this last choice is the preservation of the FCU, which is an important contributor to power tasks, such as wielding a hammer.[7] Preservation of this ulnar-sided flexor also helps to balance the radial deviation caused by the tendon transfers to the ECRB. This is particularly important in the case of low radial nerve palsy with an intact ECRL. Harvest of the FCU is also more time-consuming compared with the FCR. The FCU has muscle and fascial attachments along the entire ulna that must be freed to maximize its excursion. If the FCR is chosen for the EDC motor, a single utilitarian curvilinear radial-sided incision can be used to perform all the transfers.

In our experience, transfer of the flexor digitorum superficialis (FDS), either through the interosseous membrane or around the ulnar border of the forearm to the EDC, is more prone to fail. Difficulties with rehabilitation to activate this "out-of-phase" transfer (i.e., learning to fire a finger flexor as an extensor) and the development of adhesions after interosseous transfer are common.

Surgical Technique in Brief

The FCR and PL are readily accessible beneath the full-thickness volar forearm flap. Branches of the radial sensory nerve and the radial artery are identified and protected. Dorsal dissection allows exposure of the PT tendon, located beneath the BR musculotendinous junction deep to the emerging radial sensory nerve.[8] The PT tendon is harvested with a strip of periosteum to augment its coaptation to the ECRB tendon (Fig. 58-7, online). Further elevation of the dorsal skin flap exposes the ECRB, EPL, and EDC within the second, third, and fourth dorsal compartments, respectively. The PL is released from its insertion into the palmar fascia and mobilized toward the freed EPL tendon. The EPL must be transposed from the third compartment toward the PL.

This transposition provides better thumb extension and eliminates the thumb adduction vector of the EPL.

Tendon transfers of the thumb and finger extensors are performed before transfers about the wrist. This sequence allows the surgeon to judge sufficient tension using wrist motion. The EPL tendon is woven into the PL, and the FCR is woven into the EDC using a tendon braider (Fig. 58-8, online). Tension is adjusted until wrist flexion of 30 degrees produces adequate thumb and finger extension via tenodesis and wrist extension allows passive finger flexion into the palm. Once digital extension transfers are completed, the PT is woven into the ECRB. Tension is adjusted until a 30-degree extension resting posture of the wrist is achieved. All Pulvertaft tendon passes are secured with braided, nonabsorbable suture. Once skin flaps are closed, the extremity is positioned with the wrist in 30 degrees of extension, the MCP joints in full extension, and the thumb abducted with the IP joint in extension.

Rehabilitation of radial nerve tendon transfers is the subject of the next chapter. In general, tendon transfers for radial nerve palsy lead to improved ability to pick up and release objects (Fig. 58-9).

Median Nerve

Anatomy

The median nerve arises from the lateral and medial cords of the brachial plexus and has contributions from the C5, C6, C7, C8, and T1 spinal nerve roots. The median nerve travels distally into the arm lateral to the brachial artery and medial to the biceps brachii. In the mid to distal one third of the arm, the median nerve crosses anterior to the brachial artery and comes to lie medially to the artery as it approaches

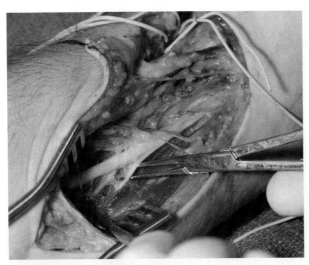

Figure 58-10 In the proximal forearm, the median nerve provides motor branches to innervate the pronator teres, palmaris longus, flexor digitorum superficialis, and flexor carpi radialis (see Fig. 58-9). (Courtesy of Shriners Hospital for Children, Philadelphia).

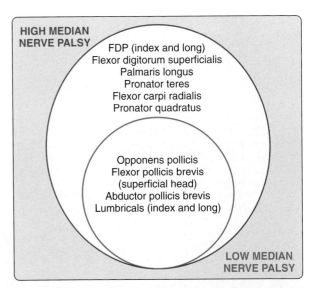

Figure 58-12 Low median nerve injury primarily affects thumb opposition and sensibility. FDP, flexor digitorum profundus.

the antecubital fossa, where it lies deep to the lacertus fibrosus.

The median nerve enters the forearm between the two heads of the PT. In the proximal forearm, motor branches arise to innervate the flexor–pronator musculature including the PT, PL, FDS, and FCR (Fig. 58-10). The anterior interosseous nerve (AIN) originates from the median nerve between 5 and 8 cm distal to the medial epicondyle and provides motor branches to the index and long flexor digitorum profundus (FDP) tendons, the flexor pollicis longus (FPL), and the pronator quadratus. Like the PIN, the terminal branch of the AIN is a carpal sensory branch.

After giving rise to the AIN, the median nerve continues distally between the FDS and FDP before becoming more superficial several centimeters proximal to the wrist crease. The palmar cutaneous branch of the median nerve arises 5 to 7 cm proximal to the wrist crease. Continuing distally, the median nerve enters the carpal tunnel and eventually divides into the recurrent motor branch and three common digital nerves to provide sensation to the palmar surface of the thumb and index, long, and radial half of the ring fingers. Motor branch anatomy has been thoroughly studied.[9] In approximately one half of subjects, the motor branch originates at the distal edge of the transverse carpal ligament and travels proximally and radially in a recurrent fashion to innervate the thenar musculature. Transligamentous and subligamentous variations have also been described.

Given the frequency of surgical procedures performed at the carpal tunnel and the incidence of nonaccidental lacerations to the volar wrist, low median nerve injuries are more prevalent than high median nerve injuries.

Physical Examination

The presentation of a patient with a median nerve injury will vary with the level of the lesion. High median nerve injury will result in a loss of thumb IP flexion, FDP (index and long) function, pronation of the forearm, and loss of thumb

opposition (Fig. 58-11, online). Simple examination findings include the inability to make an "OK" sign, which requires thumb IP and index distal IP flexion. Loss of sensation in the median innervated digits is also present. Low median nerve injury primarily affects thumb opposition and sensibility (Fig. 58-12). The physical examination must test for palmar abduction to isolate abductor pollicis brevis function (Fig. 58-13). Thumb opposition must be carefully assessed and compared with the uninjured side (Fig. 58-14). Opposition is a combination of palmar abduction, MCP joint flexion, and thumb pronation. After a median nerve injury, MCP joint flexion is preserved via function of the flexor pollicis brevis,

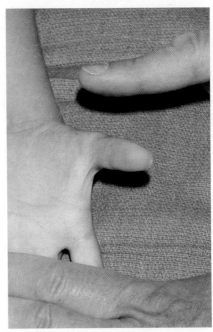

Figure 58-13 Test for palmar abduction to isolate abductor pollicis brevis function. (Courtesy of Shriners Hospital for Children, Philadelphia.)

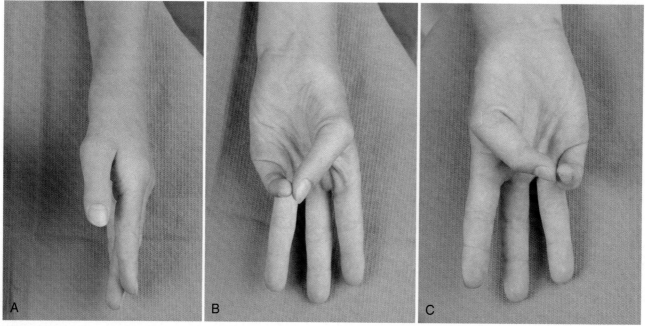

Figure 58-14 An 8-year-old child with absent left thumb opposition. **A,** Lateral view demonstrates absent thenar muscles. **B,** Attempted thumb opposition yields only metacarpophalangeal joint flexion. **C,** Normal right thumb opposition. (Courtesy of Shriners Hospital for Children, Philadelphia.)

which is dually innervated by the median and ulnar nerves. However, true opposition is not possible because palmar abduction and pronation are absent.

Because of the proximity of the median nerve to the ulnar nerve and brachial artery in the arm, a high lesion warrants a detailed assessment of ulnar nerve function and hand vascularity (Fig. 58-15).

Timing of Transfers

Tendon transfers for median nerve injuries are performed when recovery, whether spontaneous or after nerve repair, is no longer expected. Prerequisites for successful transfers that were previously mentioned should be met, especially tissue equilibrium.

Tendon Transfers for Low Median Nerve Palsy: Thumb Opposition Transfers (Opponensplasties)

The loss of thumb opposition results in a considerable impairment of hand function. Bunnell[10] described an opponensplasty that passed a tendon through a constructed pulley at the level of the pisiform, across the palm and to the dorsal ulnar aspect of the thumb metacarpal. This technique provided superior opposition, a motion inclusive of palmar abduction, flexion, and pronation of the thumb.

Numerous variations of the originally described technique have been used to restore opposition of the thumb, using various muscles innervated by the ulnar or radial nerve. Donor muscle–tendon units have included the FDS of the long or ring finger (not available in high median nerve palsy), EIP, EPL, ECU, ECRL, EDQ, PL, and abductor digiti quinti.[11]

Our preferred technique for restoration of opposition in isolated low median nerve palsy is the ring finger FDS opponensplasty (Fig. 58-16, online).

Surgical Technique in Brief

An oblique standard incision is made over the ring finger A1 pulley. The pulley is incised longitudinally, and the FDS

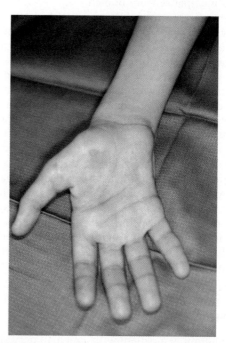

Figure 58-15 A 15-year-old boy with Charcot–Marie–Tooth disease and loss of intrinsic musculature within the hand secondary to median and ulnar nerve involvement. (Courtesy of Shriners Hospital for Children, Philadelphia.)

tendon is isolated and separated from the FDP tendon. The ring finger is flexed, and the FDS tendon is divided transversely just proximal to its bifurcation. The tails of the FDS tendon are left behind to adhere to the floor of the tendon sheath and prevent proximal IP (PIP) joint hyperextension.

At this point, a pulley for the ring finger FDS tendon is constructed. An oblique incision is made at the volar ulnar distal forearm in the region of the FCU tendon insertion into the pisiform. The FCU and the ring finger FDS tendons are exposed, and the ulnar neurovascular structures are protected. The radial half of the FCU tendon is divided transversely approximately 4 cm proximal to its insertion on the pisiform. The radial half of the tendon is separated longitudinally from the ulnar half, creating a distally based strip of tendon graft. The tendon graft is looped distally and passed through the distal portion of the FCU near the pisiform insertion and secured with nonabsorbable sutures (Fig. 58-17, online). The ring finger FDS tendon is pulled through the carpal tunnel into the proximal wound. The ring finger FDS tendon is passed through the FCU loop (Fig. 58-18, online). A subcutaneous tunnel is created between the pisiform and a radial incision along the thumb MCP joint. The donor tendon is routed through the pulley and into the radial thumb incision (Fig. 58-19, online).

Several options for attachment of the tendon transfer have been described with more dorsal insertions, enhancing pronation, and more radial attachments, yielding greater abduction[12,13] (Fig. 58-20, online). The exact position for insertion depends on the needs of the patient and his or her thumb, determined before surgery.

Regardless of the chosen insertion site, correct tensioning is imperative to achieve an optimal result. Tensioning is set using tenodesis, such that maximal thumb opposition is present with passive wrist extension and adequate thumb extension is noted with passive wrist flexion. After skin closure, the thumb is immobilized in opposition and the wrist in slight flexion to remove any tension from the tendon transfer.

Additional Transfers for High Median Nerve Palsy

In addition to restoration of thumb opposition, high median nerve palsy requires reanimation of the FPL and FDP (index and long) tendons. The BR is the preferred donor for thumb IP flexion and is transferred to the FPL (Fig. 58-21). Index and long finger IP flexion is restored by side-to-side transfers of the ring and small finger FDP tendons—innervated by the ulnar nerve—to the index and long FDP tendons. Loss of pronation can be overcome by rerouting the biceps around the radius, which convert the biceps from a supinator to a pronator.

Ulnar Nerve

Anatomy

The ulnar nerve is composed of fibers from the C8 and T1 spinal nerves and is the largest branch from the medial cord of the brachial plexus. Within the proximal arm, the ulnar nerve lies medial to the axillary artery and subsequently the

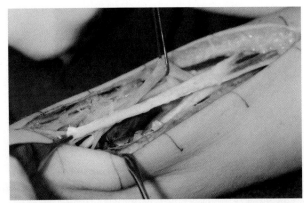

Figure 58-21 Brachioradialis transferred to the flexor pollicis longus for thumb interphalangeal joint flexion. (Courtesy of Shriners Hospital for Children, Philadelphia.)

brachial artery. The ulnar nerve pierces the intermuscular septum 8 cm proximal to the medial epicondyle and courses from the anterior to the posterior compartment of the arm. At the level of the elbow, the ulnar nerve travels through the cubital tunnel posterior to the medial epicondyle and between the two heads of the FCU before entering the forearm (Fig. 58-22). In the forearm, the ulnar nerve provides innervation to the FCU and FDP (ring and small fingers). Within the mid-forearm, the ulnar nerve travels between the FCU and the FDP, continuing toward the wrist, where it lies deep and radial to the FCU tendon.

The ulnar nerve enters the palm through Guyon's canal, dividing into deep and superficial branches. The superficial palmar branch provides sensory branches to the ulnar-sided digits and motor innervations to the palmaris brevis. The deep branch innervates the hypothenar muscles (abductor digiti minimi, flexor digiti minimi, opponens digiti minimi), adductor pollicis, dorsal and palmer interrossei, third and fourth lumbricals, and flexor pollicis brevis (deep head). The terminal branch of the deep motor branch ends in the innervation of the first dorsal interosseous muscle.

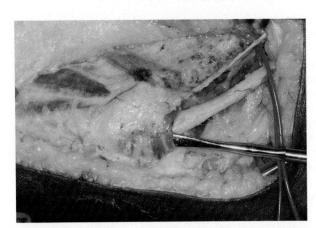

Figure 58-22 The ulnar nerve travels through the cubital tunnel posterior to the medial epicondyle and between the two heads of the flexor carpi ulnaris before entering the forearm. (Courtesy of Shriners Hospital for Children, Philadelphia.)

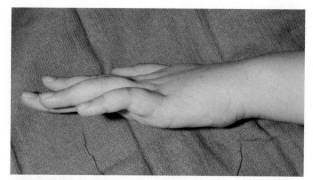

Figure 58-23 *Low ulnar palsy results in clawing of the ring and small digits. (Courtesy of Shriners Hospital for Children, Philadelphia.)*

Physical Examination

The most notable physical finding in low ulnar nerve palsy is the "claw" posture of the ring and small fingers caused by intrinsic paralysis (Fig. 58-23). The index and long fingers do not claw because their lumbrical function is preserved via median nerve innervation. Accordingly, clawing of all digits represents an insult to both the median and ulnar nerves. Abduction of the small finger because of the loss of the palmar interossei providing adduction force and the unopposed abduction moment of the EDQ (radial nerve innervation) may be seen (Wartenberg's sign) (Fig. 58-24, online). Froment's sign is the recruitment of the FPL during lateral pinch, resulting in thumb IP flexion caused by the loss of the powerful adductor pollicis (Fig. 58-25, online). Loss of intrinsic function and coordination will lead to the inability to cross the fingers (Fig. 58-26, online). Loss of intrinsic function in the hand also results in the inability to coordinate MCP joint flexion with IP flexion and results in "roll-up flexion" (Fig. 58-27, online). This hampers encircling larger objects and object acquisition. Sensory loss over the small finger and ulnar border of the ring finger is also found. High ulnar nerve palsy includes the loss of the FCU and the FDP to the ring and small fingers. Because of the resultant loss of ring and small finger IP joint flexion, true clawing is not seen (Fig. 58-28).

Timing of Tendon Transfers

Tendon transfers for ulnar nerve injuries are performed when recovery, whether spontaneous or after nerve repair surgery, is no longer expected. Similar prerequisites described for successful tendon transfer with radial and median palsies must be present. In the interim, hand therapy to preserve passive range of motion is paramount. In addition, fabrication of a lumbrical bar orthosis that prevents MCP joint hyperextension will improve function and prevent volar plate attenuation of the ring and small MCP joints. The reader is referred to Chapter 45 for more detail. Failure to prescribe this orthosis will result in a MCP joint extension contracture and reciprocal attenuation of the central slip, which substantially complicates reconstruction.

Low Ulnar Nerve Tendon Transfers

The goals of tendon transfers for ulnar nerve palsy include restoration of thumb adduction and index abduction for key

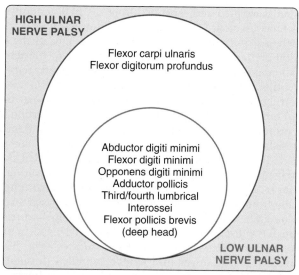

Figure 58-28 *High ulnar nerve palsy includes the loss of the flexor carpi ulnaris and the flexor digitorum profundus in the ring and small fingers. Because of the resultant loss of ring and small finger interphalangeal joint flexion, true clawing is not seen. (Courtesy of Shriners Hospital for Children, Philadelphia.)*

pinch as well as restoration of intrinsic function with MCP joint flexion (with IP extension when necessary).

Tendon Transfers for Intrinsic Function (Intrinsicplasty)

Several techniques to improve intrinsic minus hand function are available that use extrinsic muscles of the wrist and fingers as donor tendons. Two of the more commonly performed operations include transfer of a wrist motor with tendon graft extensions (four-tail graft)[14] and transfer of the FDS (Stiles-Bunnell transfer).[15] Both procedures rebalance the hand and improve asynchronous finger motion and clawing.

In preparing for tendon transfer surgery for ulnar nerve palsy, a decision must be made regarding the need to include IP joint extension as part of the reconstructive strategy. Bouvier's test provides valuable information concerning the need to restore IP joint extension. The test is performed by blocking extension of the MCP joints and asking the patient to extend the IP joints. The ability to extend the IP joints with the MCP joints flexed uses the extrinsic extensors and is deemed a positive Bouvier's test result. In this scenario, the primary goal of the transfer is to provide MCP joint flexion with the insertion of the transfer into the proximal phalanx. A negative Bouvier's test result indicates that the extrinsic extensors cannot extend the IP joints and adding IP extension function with the transfer is necessary. This requires transfer into the lateral bands of the extensor apparatus.

FDS Transfer

This procedure uses the FDS as the donor motor–tendon unit with the goals of rebalancing the hand, correcting the claw deformities, and improving synchronous motion. No increase in strength is anticipated. The FDS from either the index or middle finger is released and split. The two tendon tails or slips are transferred through the lumbrical canals of the ring and small fingers and inserted most commonly into the lateral bands of the finger extensor mechanisms. The tendon slips are usually of adequate length and rarely require tendon graft extensions when harvested at the level of the proximal IP joint. Several variations of this technique have been described, including subdividing the long finger FDS into four slips for transfer to all four fingers, attachment of the tendon slips to the flexor tendon sheaths, and attachment of the tendon slips to the proximal phalanges through bone tunnels.

Surgical Technique in Brief

The finger FDS tendon(s) are harvested at the PIP joint or in the palm using traction to ensure adequate length (Fig. 58-29, online). Both slips are released, sharply dividing distal to Camper's chiasm. The superficialis tendon(s) are withdrawn into the proximal wound, and the longitudinal split in the tendon is extended proximally to create two slips of equal caliber.

Skin incisions are made at the dorsoradial bases of the ring and small fingers. The lateral band projecting to each extensor mechanism is identified. Both transferred tendon slips must follow an unimpeded course through the hand, dorsal to the common digital arteries and nerves and palmar to the transverse metacarpal ligaments (Fig. 58-30, online). A tendon passer is used to create this path and draw each tendon slip separately to the target finger.

Correct tensioning is achieved with the wrist positioned in extension and the finger MCP joints in maximum flexion, taking up approximately 50% of the excursion of the donor tendons. After repair, the wrist is brought through a range of motion, demonstrating tenodesis of all finger MCP joints with the wrist flexed (Fig. 58-31, online). Full passive finger MCP joint extension should be possible with the wrist in extension. The wrist is immobilized postoperatively in approximately 45 degrees of extension with the MCP joints flexed 60 degrees and the IP joints fully extended.

Tendon Transfer for Thumb Adduction (Adductorplasty)

Restoration of lateral pinch by adductorplasty has been described using various techniques. The most commonly performed procedures include the ECRB and FDS transfers. BR, ECRL, EIP, and EDQ have also been described. The choice of donor tendon to be used for adductorplasty may alter or be altered by the donor chosen for the intrinsicplasty.

Surgical Technique in Brief: ECRB Thumb Adductorplasty

A series of transverse incisions is made over the dorsoradial border of the extensor retinaculum. The insertion of the ECRB is released sharply from the base of the third metacarpal, and the tendon is withdrawn from beneath the extensor retinaculum (Fig. 58-32, online). A 2- to 3-cm transverse incision is made over the proximal aspect of the second intermetacarpal space, and the fascia overlying the second dorsal interosseous muscle is incised. A subcutaneous tunnel

is created between the dorsal wrist and hand wounds. A 2- to 3-cm curvilinear incision is then made along the dorsoulnar border of the thumb MCP joint, and the insertion of the adductor pollicis tendon is exposed.

To increase the length of the ECRB tendon, an ipsilateral palmaris longus tendon can be harvested through two or three small transverse incisions or with the aid of a tendon stripper. Other sources of autogenous tendon graft may be used (e.g., plantaris, long toe extensor). Alternatively, the ECRB tendon can be lengthened by longitudinally splitting the tendon in half, leaving the distal 2 cm of tendon intact (Fig. 58-33, online). One limb is sectioned proximally from the musculotendinous junction and brought distally to increase the length of the tendon. A curved clamp is passed through the second intermetacarpal space volar to the metacarpal and directed toward the thumb MCP joint in the interval between the adductor pollicis and first dorsal interosseous muscles (Fig. 58-34, online).

One end of the tendon or tendon graft is sutured to the adductor pollicis tendon at its bony insertion into the phalanx. The other end of the graft is then withdrawn through the second intermetacarpal space. The graft is then passed through the subcutaneous tunnel to the proximal wrist incision, dorsal to the extensor retinaculum. With the wrist in neutral alignment and the thumb held tightly against the volar radial border of the index finger, the graft is woven into the previously released ECRB tendon, taking up 50% to 80% of the donor tendon's excursion. In cases using the ECRB split, similar tensioning is performed. With the wrist placed in flexion, the thumb should adduct firmly against the index metacarpal, recreating lateral pinch. With the wrist extended, the thumb should be easily abducted away from the palm. The wrist is positioned in 45 degrees of extension with the thumb in palmar abduction.

Restoration of Index Finger Abduction

Along with thumb adduction, index finger abduction is the second component for generating forceful key pinch. Restoration of first dorsal interosseous function by transferring an accessory slip of the abductor pollicis longus or by using the EIP tendon is effective. Loss of the ulnar deviation moment provided by the EIP of the index finger, however, can result in an unacceptable overly abducted posture of the index finger. We do not routinely restore index finger abduction because patients are generally satisfied with restoration of thumb adduction alone for lateral pinch.

Additional Tendon Transfers for High Ulnar Nerve Palsy

Transfer of the ulnar innervated ring and small FDP tendons to the median innervated FDP index and long tendons will restore IP joint flexion to the ring and small fingers.

Combined Median and Ulnar Nerve Palsies

Combined low ulnar and low median nerve palsy is the most common combined palsy, followed by high ulnar and high

Table 58-2 Combined High Median and Ulnar Palsy Tendon Transfers

Functional Deficit	Available Donor	Comments
Thumb adduction	ECRL to adductor pollicis	Third MC used as pulley
	BR to adductor pollicis	Third MC used as pulley
	EIP to adductor pollicis	Third MC used as pulley
Thumb IP flexion	BR to FPL	
	FPL tenodesis	Passive only
Index abduction for pinch	APL to first DI	With thumb MCP joint arthrodesis
	EPB to first DI	With thumb MCP joint arthrodesis
	PL to first DI	With thumb MCP joint arthrodesis
Finger flexion	ECRL to FDP	
Intrinsic paralysis	ECU intrinsicplasty	With tendon grafts

APL, abductor pollicis longus; BR, brachioradialis; DI, dorsal interosseous; ECRL, extensor carpi radialis longus; ECU, extensor carpi ulnaris; EIP, extensor indicis longus; EPB, extensor pollicis longus; FDP, flexor digitorum profundus; FPL, flexor pollicis longus; MC, metacarpal; MCP, metacarpophalangeal; PL, palmaris longus.

median. Combined median and ulnar palsies are particularly disabling, not only because of the numerous motor deficits, but also because of the loss of sensibility on the volar surface of all digits.

Because of the limited number of available donors, particularly in high combined palsies, prioritizing patient needs is required. Table 58-2 summarizes the more commonly performed transfers for combined ulnar and median nerve palsies.

Summary

By performing tendon transfers, the devastating effects of a permanent peripheral nerve lesion can be lessened. Vital functions such as pinch, grasp, object acquisition, and object release can be restored in the injured limb. Although a return to preinjury function is not likely, impairment can be minimized with well-planned and well-executed transfers.

Variables influencing outcomes are numerous and include co-morbid conditions, surgical precision, avoidance of complications, patient compliance, and access to skilled rehabilitation professionals.

REFERENCES

The complete reference list is available online at www.expertconsult.com.

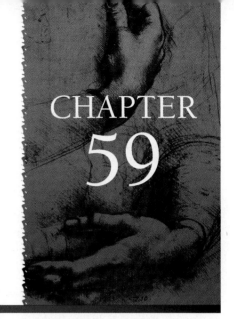

Therapist's Management of Tendon Transfers 🎥

SUSAN V. DUFF, EdD, PT, OTR/L, CHT AND
DEBORAH HUMPL, OTR/L

PREOPERATIVE CARE
POSTOPERATIVE PROGRAMMING
CASE STUDY: PART II (SEE PART I, CHAPTER 45)
SUMMARY

CRITICAL POINTS

- A team approach is critical to effectively address preoperative issues and enhance postoperative success.
- Preoperative factors considered by the team include (1) psychosocial issues, (2) status of neural recovery, (3) musculoskeletal readiness, (4) degree of sensibility, (5) motor learning aptitude, and (6) functional requirements.
- Preoperative therapy may be required to maintain or increase the strength of the muscle(s) proposed for transfer, to maximize preoperative passive range of motion and correct joint contractures, and to provide education regarding anticipated postoperative restrictions and requirements.
- Therapy after surgery has three phases: (1) immobilization, (2) activation of the transfer, and (3) strengthening/return to function.
- The use of custom-fabricated orthoses is an important part of the therapy program after tendon transfers.
  1. The specifics of the surgical procedure as well as the patient's clinical presentation will dictate the exact positioning requirement of the orthosis.
  2. In general, the orthosis is fabricated with the joints affected by the transfer positioned to protect the resting tension of the transfer.
  3. Familiarity with the specific surgical procedure, healing characteristics, and positioning requirements are essential in the fabrication and ongoing monitoring and modification of an upper extremity orthosis. An experienced certified hand therapist is uniquely qualified to fabricate the orthoses required.

Once neural recovery from peripheral nerve injury has plateaued, tendon transfers offer a means to enhance prehension and related function. Yet, the decision to perform tendon transfers requires a great deal of consideration preoperatively to ensure a successful outcome.

This chapter (1) outlines preoperative considerations, (2) reviews evaluations used to establish a baseline and monitor progress, and (3) considers postoperative rehabilitation methods used to foster prehensile skill after tendon transfer(s).

Preoperative Care

Tendon transfers done immediately after a traumatic injury as a salvage procedure require quick decision making by the surgeon, patient, and family. However, if tendon transfers are to be done after rehabilitation from peripheral nerve injury is complete, then a preoperative team assessment is often used to direct preoperative intervention strategies in preparation for the transfer procedure and to aid decision making regarding surgical procedures to be performed.

Benefits of a Team Assessment

A team approach can effectively address preoperative issues and enhance postoperative success. The ideal team would consist of a hand surgeon, physician assistant or nurse practitioner, hand therapist (occupational or physical therapist), electrodiagnostician, social worker, the client, and his or her family. The client's primary therapist is also an important team member because he or she is usually the most familiar with the client's condition. Ideally, details on current function and preoperative goals will be exchanged among team members.

Preoperative Evaluation

Preoperative factors considered by the team include (1) psychosocial issues, (2) status of neural recovery, (3) musculoskeletal readiness, (4) degree of sensibility, and (5) motor learning aptitude.

Psychosocial Issues

Success with postoperative rehabilitation depends on issues such as cognition, past and current abilities/interests, client roles, motivation, and compliance. Pertinent information can be obtained from the primary therapist, family/client interview, and observations of nonverbal behavior.[1] Cognitive screening should be done with young children and individuals with impairments that may affect tendon transfer training. The use of the Disability of the Arm, Shoulder, and Hand Questionnaire[2] or a graphic display of the client's roles and responsibilities may supply useful information. A record of participation in therapy and carryover with home programs can help gauge future motivation and compliance.

Poor compliance can diminish the success of tendon transfer surgery and may stem from

1. *Denial.* Many individuals believe that the situation will resolve itself or determine that because the other limb is working well, they really "don't need to improve."
2. *Frustration.* The client and his or her family may have made many sacrifices to attend therapy and perform exercises without sufficient gratification of nerve recovery.
3. *Lack of trust in the therapy program.* The client may not believe in the rehabilitation process or have confidence in the team members because of outcome or other issues.
4. *Finances.* Therapy visits can be very costly when time, insurance copays, and travel expenses are also an issue.
5. *Time.* Other roles as a family member, job holder, and maintainer of the household may occupy the client's day and limit the availability to participate or attend therapy sessions.

If the underlying reasons for poor compliance can be resolved, the chance for success may improve.

Status of Neural Recovery

Before tendon transfers, the team should ensure that the opportunity for reinnervation has passed and that recovery has plateaued. For example, repeated assessment of muscle strength, sensibility, and dexterity should reveal gradual slowing in progress or lack of progress over the past few months. To verify current ability, the contribution of stabilization techniques used to augment movement and function (e.g., orthotic stabilization or neuromuscular electrical stimulation [NMES]) can be compared with the client's individual effort (see Chapter 45) (Fig. 59-1). Findings from electrodiagnostic tests such as electromyography or nerve conduction studies can further verify that recovery has plateaued, and provide support that the client is ready for surgical intervention.

Musculoskeletal Readiness

Range of Motion. Ideally, full passive and active range of motion (ROM) should be present in the involved extremity before surgery, particularly at the associated joint(s). The involved side should be compared with the noninvolved side with a goniometer. Active ROM should also be assessed during functional tasks because the quality of the motion may differ from what is displayed during goniometry.

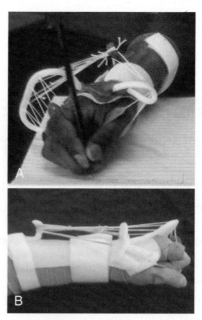

Figure 59-1 Two versions of a modified splint for a radial nerve injury without and with dynamic components. Both support the wrist and MCP joints to allow the client to write or grasp effectively.

Muscle Strength. A strength assessment helps determine which muscles are strong enough to transfer. Although muscle physiologic cross-sectional area is proportional to maximum muscle strength, it is not easily measured.[3] Therefore, strength is often documented with manual muscle testing or hand-held dynamometry (e.g., M500 Myometer; Jtech Medical Industries, Salt Lake City, UT) (Fig. 59-2). Traditionally, a muscle must be graded as 4/5 on a standard 0 to 5 manual muscle testing scale[4] and have sufficient excursion in the new position to be considered for transfer. Proximal muscle weakness and incoordination can reduce muscle power, resulting in substitution patterns that the therapist should be cognizant of (see Table 45-2). Grip and pinch

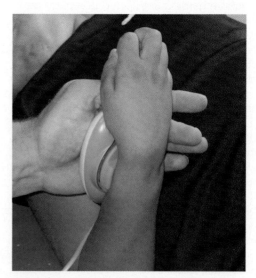

Figure 59-2 Hand-held dynamometer with digital readout used to examine muscle strength.

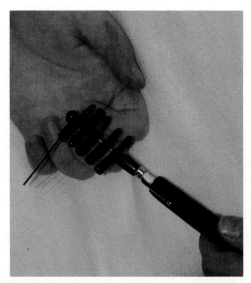

Figure 59-3 Weinstein Enhanced Sensibility Test used to examine pressure sensibility.

dynamometers help determine prehensile strength.[5] However, there are no established recommendations associated with dynamometry and tendon transfers.

Assessments of Dexterity/Function. Measurement of coordination, skill, and function using standardized tests can validate the client's need for tendon transfers and document preoperative performance. Table 59-1 (online) provides a list and descriptions of useful dexterity and functional tests. (See Chapter 12 for a detailed description of functional tests.)

Degree of Sensibility

Because it plays an important role in object manipulation,[6,7] an accurate assessment of passive and active sensibility should be made. Touch pressure and discrimination are two forms of passive sensibility. The touch-pressure threshold is commonly tested with Semmes–Weinstein monofilaments[8,9] or the Weinstein Enhanced Sensibility Test, as shown in Figure 59-3.[10] Discrimination can be assessed with static/moving two-point discrimination using the Disk-Criminator.[11,12] An alternative is the Pressure-Specifying Sensory Device,[13] which was designed to determine the amount of pressure required to perceive one or two metal prongs. Active sensibility or stereognosis can be tested with the Moberg's Picking-Up Test[14,15] or the Byl-Cheney-Boczai Sensory Discriminator Test.[16] The clinician is advised to follow the nerve distribution and assess both limbs for comparison during sensibility testing.

Motor Learning Aptitude

Activation of the muscle–tendon unit after transfer requires learning new control strategies. Preoperative motor learning ability can be measured behaviorally at four levels: acquisition, retention (consistency), transfer (flexibility), and efficiency.[17,18] Initial practice or performance of a new task involves acquisition of a skill or a control aspect of a skill. Retention or consistency is evident when a skill or some aspect of a skill can be demonstrated after a short or long time delay. Transfer or flexibility involves the ability to execute a similar skill or slight variation (e.g., altered force or timing) after a time delay. Finally, efficiency refers to the ability to minimize energy expenditure during task performance such as during the execution of fine motor activities. The ideal test would measure all four levels.

Motor learning aptitude should be assessed with the non-involved versus the involved limb. Acquisition can be assessed by observing performance of a novel task. For example, a client could be asked to quickly place 10 small objects in a set sequence into a container (acquisition). At the next therapy session, retention could be measured by having the client repeat placement of the objects in the same order without coaching. As a transfer task, the client could be asked to place the objects in reverse order without previous review. Finally, efficiency could be measured by timing performance.

Preoperative Therapy

When a client does not yet meet the surgical criteria, he or she may be referred back to therapy to further improve ROM and strength. For instance, muscle wasting or contractures may have developed during the primary healing phase. It is possible that the therapeutic regimen was insufficient or compliance with the recommended protocol was poor, detracting from the outcome. These issues should be resolved before proceeding with tendon transfer surgery.

Methods to Enhance Preoperative Passive ROM

Joint contractures often interfere with successful outcome from tendon transfers. Thus, it is imperative that maximum passive ROM be achieved in the involved joints preoperatively, which can be done with static progressive orthoses or serial casting.

Serial casting can be quite effective at resolving distal contractures. It provides quick improvement in ROM by incorporating a low-load sustained stretch to shortened tissue(s).[19,20] Its use ensures client compliance because the cast cannot be easily removed. Unfortunately, prolonged cast wear may interfere with client roles, alter skin integrity, and temporarily weaken muscles needed for transfer. In those situations, a static progressive orthosis would be best (Fig. 59-4).

Structures susceptible to contracture vary depending on the nerve injured. After a radial nerve injury, due to the loss of finger extension, extrinsic finger flexor muscle–tendon unit shortening may occur and this will limit combined wrist and finger extension. In this case, a forearm to finger tip serial cast or orthosis positioned at the end range of finger and wrist extension may be warranted. The orthosis can be serially adjusted to result in gradual lengthening of the shortened finger flexors and allow increased combined extension of the wrist and fingers. After a median nerve injury, the webspace between the thumb and index finger is vulnerable to an adduction contracture. A thumb webspacer orthosis or serial cast with stabilization of the metacarpophalangeal (MCP) joints of the thumb and index may help to maximize thumb abduction or extension. After an ulnar nerve injury, chronic

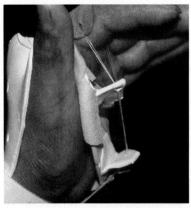

Figure 59-4 *Static progressive orthosis to provide a low-load sustained stretch to the metacarpophalangeal joint.*

intrinsic minus or claw posturing can lead to MCP joint hyperextension and interphalangeal (IP) joint flexion contractures. In this instance, orthoses or serial casts for MCP flexion and IP joint extension are an effective way to increase passive ROM at both joints (Fig. 59-5).

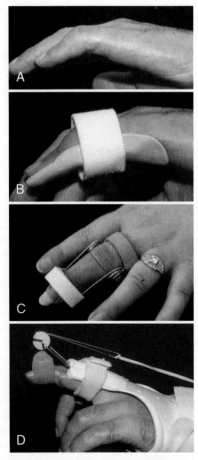

Figure 59-5 A, *Proximal interphalangeal (PIP) joint contracture.* **B,** *Static three-point extension orthosis to increase extension.* **C,** *Spring wire PIP extension orthosis.* **D,** *Dynamic PIP extension orthosis.*

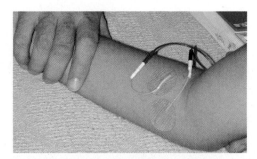

Figure 59-6 *Neuromuscular electrical nerve stimulation to condition the pronator teres muscle before tendon transfer in its new role as a wrist extensor.*

Strengthening Before Transfer

Before surgery, methods to maintain or increase strength of the muscle(s) proposed for transfer should be encouraged. Biofeedback is effective in cueing individuals with various disabling conditions to activate muscles with more strength and vigor.[21] NMES has also been used to augment muscle contraction in potential transfer muscles, as shown in Figure 59-6.[22] Aquatic therapy or whirlpool provides a gravity-reduced environment useful for strengthening muscle without stress and strain. Once muscle activation is sufficient, resistance can be provided in the form of free weights, cuff weights, Thera-Band (The Hygienic Corporation, Akron, OH), theraputty, exercise machines, work simulators, and computer games (e.g., Biometrics device; Biometrics Ltd., Ladysmith, VA). If prehension patterns are limited, cuff weights can provide resistance without requiring grasp of a free weight.

Postoperative Programming

Education

Postoperative guidelines should be reviewed before and after surgery to clarify expectations. Guidelines may include information regarding orthoses, therapy frequency, precautions, and activity limitations. The commitment required to achieve success from surgery should be emphasized, including the therapy timeline and the value of compliance with home exercise programs. These discussions may prompt the client to plan life events such as sports participation around the surgery schedule. Postoperative success and motivation can be enhanced by establishing realistic functional outcomes. A social worker can aid in planning for medical costs or travel to ensure postoperative therapy participation. Referral to another client who has undergone tendon transfers may enhance understanding of the experience.

Postoperative Treatment by Phase

Treatment after surgery consists of three phases: (1) immobilization, (2) activation of the transfer, and (3) strengthening/return to previous function (see Table 59-2 for goals at each phase).

Phase 1: Immobilization

After tendon transfer the limb is usually immobilized in a bulky dressing with a plaster shell at first and then a cast or

Table 59-2 *General Goal and Treatment Methods for Each Phase*

Phase	Goals	Methods
1	Protect repair site	Cast, then change to static orthosis in position that minimizes tension on the tendon transfer
	Manage edema	Elevation, compression, active movement of noninvolved joints
	Protect areas of diminished or absent sensibility	Education
	Encourage active movement of noninvolved joints	Active ROM exercises and tasks
2	Regain active ROM	Active ROM exercises and tasks incorporating involved structures
	Activation of tendon transfer	Use former function of the transferred tendon and the new function simultaneously; perform desired motion with contralateral limb first, then both limbs together; use of place-and-hold techniques; work in gravity-eliminated plane at first
	Enhance sensorimotor control	Practice grasping and manipulating objects of various shapes, sizes, and textures; complex manipulative tasks
	Sensory reeducation	Desensitization and active somatosensory training; use of "sensor glove"
	Enhance function while maintaining appropriate biomechanical positioning at involved & noninvolved joints	Custom orthoses; practice prehensile and ADL tasks with and without orthoses
	Maintain passive ROM at involved and surrounding joints	Passive ROM exercises, myofascial release
3	Improve strength	Theraputty, Thera-Band, cuff weights, exercise machines, work simulators aquatic therapy, Biometrics device
	Enhance aerobic conditioning	Aerobic activities (e.g., arm ergometer)
	Return to previous level of function	Work simulation; simulation of difficult ADL tasks
	Reevaluate current status regarding; compensatory strategies; capacity for continued improvement and need for surgical intervention	Issue adaptive equipment/splints, preoperative conditioning

ADL, activities of daily living; ROM, range of motion.

custom-fabricated thermoplastic orthosis fabricated by a hand therapist for 3 to 5 weeks. Limited evidence has been published exploring the application of early motion after tendon transfers. In a clinical study[23] of 20 patients after transfer of the extensor indicis proprius to the extensor pollicis longus to restore thumb extension, patients were treated with either immobilization or early dynamic motion (dynamic thumb extension with active, limited range flexion). The authors found that the dynamic motion group had better results after 4 weeks, but hand function was similar in both groups after 6 and 8 weeks. Patients treated with early dynamic motion recovered their hand function more rapidly than the immobilized patients, shortening total rehabilitation time and making dynamic motion treatment cost-effective. In a similar study, Rath[24] reported that immediate postoperative active mobilization reduced rehabilitation time by an average of 19 days after opposition tendon transfer compared with immobilization. An earlier return to activities of daily living was a further benefit to patients.

A more recent study by Giessler et al.[25] compared early free active motion with early dynamic motion with extension orthoses. Both regimens (dynamic vs. early active) achieved comparable clinical results.

Nevertheless, a period of immobilization is the more typical practice after tendon transfers and is particularly recommended for the younger or less compliant patient.

Orthotic Fabrication. After cast removal, the client is usually referred to therapy for fabrication of an orthosis to continue to protect the integrity of the transfer. The specifics of the surgical procedure as well as the patient's clinical presentation will dictate the exact positioning requirements. In general, the orthosis is fabricated with the joints affected by the transfer positioned to protect the resting tension of the transfer. For example, after a transfer of the flexor digitorum superficialis (FDS) tendon of the ring finger to the thumb to restore opposition, a wrist-based thumb spica orthosis may be used to position the wrist in 10 to 20 degrees of flexion with thumb opposition. If a swan-neck deformity with PIP joint hyperextension develops in the ring finger, a static three-point hyperextension block orthosis may be warranted to limit PIP joint hyperextension. A protective orthosis should be removed only for exercise and bathing.

Edema Control. Immediately postoperatively, limb elevation prevents distal accumulation of fluid. Exercise proximal to the surgical site also prevents edema formation and may reduce the incidence of secondary joint stiffness. Compressive garments should be used as needed.

Soft-Tissue Mobility. Postoperative treatment includes interventions to prevent adhesions, increase tendon excursion, and enhance mobility at the surgical and donor sites. This can be accomplished in a few ways. One is through massage during activation of the transfer or separately, performed at least twice daily. If needed, vibration can be used to reduce pain before massage.[26] Another method to improve soft tissue mobility and minimize hypertrophic scarring is with the use of a silicone gel sheet, which acts through a process of skin hydration.[27] Use of an elasticized tubular bandage sleeve (Tubigrip) over the gel insert can keep it in place and increase the compression on the scar while contributing to edema control.

Home Program. During the immobilization phase, the primary goal is to protect the transfer. This is accomplished with casting and orthoses. Other goals such as edema control, active ROM of noninvolved joints, and soft tissue mobility can be reinforced at home.

Phase 2: Activation of the Transfer

Mobilization of the transfer requires learning to activate the muscle–tendon unit in a new role. To recruit the transfer, the client is encouraged to move into the former and new role simultaneously. For example, if the pronator teres is transferred to a new role as a wrist extensor, the transfer can be recruited by pronating the forearm and extending the wrist at the same time (Fig. 59-7A). It may be easier to initiate isolated motion such as wrist extension in a gravity eliminated plane (Fig. 59-7B). If he or she is unable to recruit the transfer in a gravity-eliminated plane, it may be easier to first try to place the limb in the new position passively and then ask the client to hold it (place-and-hold technique). Another strategy is to perform the desired motion with the noninvolved limb first and then attempt to move the involved limb actively or move both limbs simultaneously.

The client may feel that it is necessary to move vigorously and force movement of the transfer; however, he or she must be educated to move slowly and perform short sessions of exercise to prevent fatigue of the transferred muscle. A recommended strategy is for the client to activate the transfer through 10 repetitions and then rest while attending to scar massage, edema control, and passive ROM. This sequence could be repeated three times in the session, and the orthosis reapplied at the end of the session.

Below are examples of common transfers used for the radial, median, and ulnar nerve palsies (Table 59-3) along with methods to activate select transfers.

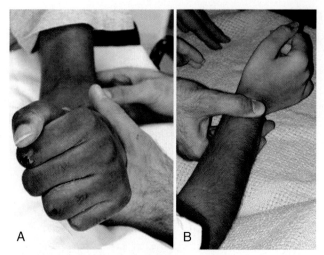

A   B

Figure 59-7 *Initiation of active motion after pronator teres transfer for wrist extension.* **A,** *Attempted wrist extension in combination with forearm pronation.* **B,** *Isolated wrist extension in gravity-eliminated plane.*

Radial Nerve Tendon Transfers. These transfers are often performed to augment wrist or finger/thumb extension after an injury at the forearm/elbow level. The pronator teres is often used to improve wrist extension. If the client has difficulty activating the transfer, the limb may be positioned with the forearm in approximately 20 degrees pronation, while the therapist provides counterpressure and the client attempts further active pronation. Resisted pronation should stimulate the transferred muscle to activate wrist extension (see Fig. 59-7A). To augment digit extension, the flexor carpi ulnaris may be transferred to the extensor digitorum communis (EDC). During therapy, the client may be encouraged

Table 59-3 Common Tendon Transfers

Level	Function	Transfer	Early Precautions
Radial nerve	Wrist extension	Pronator teres to extensor carpi radialis longus and brevis	Avoid simultaneous wrist and digital flexion to prevent overstretching of the transfer
	Finger extension	Flexor carpi ulnaris of flexor carpi radialis to extensor digitorum communis	
	Thumb extension	Palmaris longus of flexor digitorum superficialis to extensor pollicis longus	
Median nerve	Opposition	Flexor digitorum superficialis, palmaris longus, or extensor digiti minim	Avoid simultaneous wrist, thumb, and finger extension
	Thumb IP flexion (high lesions); DIP flexion of index (high lesions)	Brachioradialis to flexor pollicis longus; flexor digitorum profundus of the long, ring, and small fingers to the flexor digitorum profundus of the index finger	
Ulnar nerve	Correct claw (control MCP joint hyperextension)	Flexor digitorum superficialis, extensor indicis proprius, extensor digiti minimi to intrinsic	Avoid full MCP joint extension; avoid simultaneous finger, thumb, and wrist extension
	Thumb adduction	Flexor digitorum superficialis or extensor carpi radialis longus to adductor pollicis	
	Index abduction	Abductor pollicis longus, extensor carpi radialis longus, or extensor indicis proprius to first dorsal interossei	
	DIP flexion of the long, ring, and small fingers (high lesions)	Side-to-side tenodesis of flexor digitorum profundus of index finger	

DIP, distal interphalangeal; IP, interphalangeal; MCP, metacarpophalangeal.

to flex the wrist to neutral (from an extended position) while attempting to extend the MCP joints. Forceful wrist flexion past neutral is not encouraged because this may promote more tenodesis compared with active movement of the transfer. The client would then follow the same rest and exercise sequence as mentioned earlier.

Median Nerve Tendon Transfers. The most common median nerve transfer done after a wrist-level injury is an opponensplasty. To achieve this, the FDS tendon of the ring finger may be transferred to a thenar muscle such as the opponens pollicis or abductor pollicis brevis to enhance thumb opposition. During therapy, activation of the transferred FDS tendon may be encouraged if ring finger MCP flexion is blocked during attempted opposition. This may be further facilitated by active assistance of the thumb into opposition manually or through the assistance of an orthosis to position the thumb in opposition for light activity (Fig. 59-8).

Another transfer for higher level injuries is transfer of the brachioradialis to the flexor pollicis longus. Initially, activation of the transfer may take place in elbow flexion/forearm neutral to activate the brachioradialis in its former role as an elbow flexor. Once the client is able to activate the transfer, repetitive practice in the new role ensues (Fig. 59-9).

Ulnar Nerve Tendon Transfers. Transfers after a wrist or forearm/elbow-level ulnar nerve injury are typically done to reduce posturing in the intrinsic minus or claw position. A common procedure in this case is the Zancolli lasso procedure in which the FDS to the ring and small fingers is detached from its insertion and wrapped around the second annular ligament near the volar aspect of the MCP joint(s), which acts as a pulley. The effect of the transfer is to limit the action of the EDC at the MCP joint by preventing MCP joint hyperextension. The action of the EDC is then transmitted distally, allowing PIP and distal IP (DIP) joint extension, eliminating the claw deformity. To activate this transfer, the client is encouraged to flex and extend the MCP joints in very small ranges (between 20 and 30 degrees from full MCP

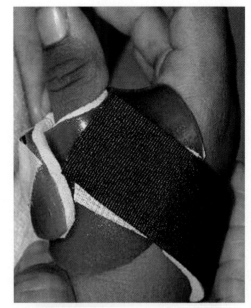

Figure 59-8 Thumb opposition orthosis.

flexion resting posture), with special attention to avoid full MCP extension, which would stretch out and defeat the transfer. Initially, a wrist-based orthosis positioning the MCP joints in flexion and the IP joints in extension may be used. As treatment progresses, the patient may progress to a hand-based orthosis, as shown in Figure 59-10.

Augmenting Muscle Activation. There are various options available to enhance activation of the transferred muscle including mirror visual feedback, therapeutic whirlpool, and vibration.[28,29] Mirror visual feedback requires movement of the noninvolved limb in front of a mirror, which provides visual and proprioceptive feedback while the involved limb rests behind the back of the mirror. This process has been shown to engage mirror neurons in the contralateral

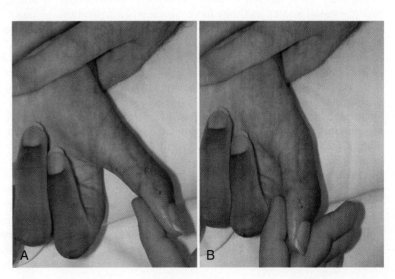

Figure 59-9 Training thumb flexion after transfer of the brachioradialis to the flexor pollicis longus.

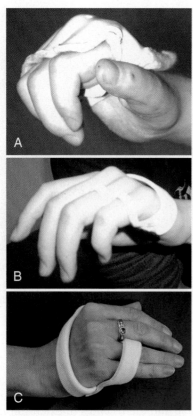

Figure 59-10 Hand-based orthoses to block hyperextension of the metacarpophalangeal joints digits 2 through 5 **(A)** and digits 4 and 5 **(B, C)**.

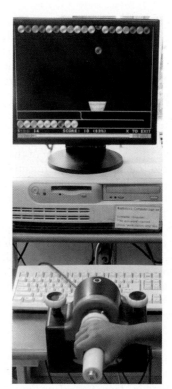

Figure 59-11 Strengthening through engagement in computer-based devices such as the Biometrics Exercise Kit.

hemisphere, which may aid in the initiation of movement in the involved limb.[30] Another option is to place both limbs in a low agitation whirlpool or therapeutic pool, which provides buoyancy and assists active motion. Another useful method is to apply vibration to the muscle–tendon unit to foster muscle activation.[28]

Biofeedback and NMES. Activation of the transfer may be difficult to obtain initially because there may not be any observeable joint motion at first. Therapeutic devices that provide visual and/or auditory biofeedback when activation of the transfer is attempted may aid this process. If biofeedback is not successful at enhancing activation, NMES may be required. Units as simple as a hand-held device such as the M500 Myotrac can be used.

If the transferred muscle cannot be held isometrically during place-and-hold techniques or if the client cannot be encouraged to move into the new position, NMES may help activate the muscle. NMES parameters are customized to the client's age, need, and tolerance. After full ROM with gravity eliminated can be achieved, gravity-resisted motion may be used and then progressed to resisted motion.

Home Program. During the activation phase, an orthosis is often worn during the day but is removed three to five times daily for exercise and practice of specific tasks. Soft tissue mobility techniques and edema control should also be reinforced at home.

Phase 3: Strength and Function

By the eighth week postoperatively, if the client can activate the transfer without assistance, he or she is ready for strengthening and functional task practice. During this phase, nighttime wear of an orthosis may continue for positioning only, or it may be discontinued.

Strengthening. Resistive grip, pinch, and upper limb exercises may be initiated. One form of resistive training that is useful is the Biometrics Exercise Kit (Biometrics Ltd., Ladysmith, VA). This device allows the client to activate or strengthen the transferred muscle through progressive resistance using varied prehension patterns while being visually engaged in a game on a computer screen (Fig. 59-11).

Task Practice. Participation in functional activities should be encouraged in this phase in preparation for return to full activities of daily living and work/school/leisure activities. For example, after a brachioradialis to flexor pollicis longus transfer, thumb flexion/adduction can be used to hold a pen during handwriting (Fig. 59-12). Two components associated with successful intervention are the type of practice used in treatment and the form of feedback provided by the clinician. Part of a task or the whole task can be practiced. Practice may also be organized in a blocked, random, or serial (combination) fashion. Research in typical adults supports the use of blocked practice during acquisition; however, random or serial practice seems to better support retention and skill transfer.[31] Other studies report that blocked practice may lead to a better outcome in clinical populations.[32-34]

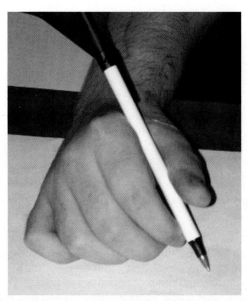

Figure 59-12 *Practicing handwriting after transfer of the brachioradialis to the flexor pollicis longus to enhance thumb flexion/adduction.*

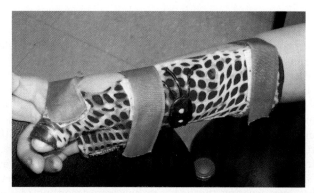

Figure 59-13 Case: wrist-based thumb spica orthosis issued to M.C. 4 weeks after tendon transfers.

Feedback. How frequently and what type of feedback should be provided? Intermittent feedback has been shown to be more helpful for skill acquisition than continuous feedback.[35] Thus, if knowledge of results on errors is provided in a bandwidth or when the error exceeds a tolerance limit, motor learning is facilitated.[36] Informational feedback is more conducive to learning than just positive reinforcement such as "that was good" or "nice job."[18] For example, you may state "your wrist muscles seem stronger than last week, you were able to hold your wrist up for 10 seconds." Furthermore, intermittent feedback is more conducive to learning than concurrent or constant feedback.[37,35]

Home Program. During this phase, activities to strengthen the transfer should be done. The key to success is practice; therefore, a specific practice schedule should be recommended.

Case Study: Part II (See Part I, Chapter 45)

M.C. is a lively 7-year-old boy who sustained a combined high median, radial, and ulnar nerve injury of his right dominant extremity. He received therapy in our outpatient facility for 1 year to monitor nerve recovery, provide sensory reeducation, and improve active ROM and strength. His family had a history of poor compliance with therapeutic regimens and therapy visits; however, they remained quite invested in his anticipated recovery. M.C. revisited the surgeon for a yearly follow-up examination, who recommended tendon transfers to augment wrist and thumb function. M.C. was referred back to therapy for preoperative evaluation of passive ROM, strength, sensibility, and dexterity (Jebsen Taylor Hand Function Test and the 9-Hole Peg Test). One week later, M.C. went to the operating room and had the pronator teres

tendon dissected from the radial shaft and transferred to the extensor carpi radialis brevis. The right index extensor indicis tendon was transferred to the abductor pollicis brevis to aid thumb opposition.

Phase 1: Immobilization

M.C. was immobilized in a long arm cast for 5 weeks as follows: 90 degrees of elbow flexion with forearm neutral, 30 degrees of wrist extension, and 30 degrees of thumb palmar abduction. At 2 weeks postoperatively, he was recast in the same position. At 4 weeks postoperatively, the cast was removed and M.C. was referred back to therapy for fabrication of a resting orthosis, which placed him in 30 degrees of wrist extension, 30 degrees of thumb palmar abduction, 30 degrees of MCP flexion, and 5 degrees of PIP and DIP flexion. The night orthosis was designed to protect the transfers and the muscle donor sites and preserve the arches of the hand because he lacked intrinsic muscle control before surgery. He was also issued a thumb spica orthosis for day wear (Fig. 59-13). M.C. had a history of poor compliance with orthosis wear. Therefore, his family was educated in detail regarding the importance of orthosis wear and home exercise compliance to maximize the results of the surgery.

Phase 2: Activation of the Transfer

The goals of the first session were as follows: (1) enhance soft tissue mobility, (2) increase passive ROM, (3) reduce pain, and (4) activate the transfers (Table 59-4, online). Treatment began with forearm and thumb scar massage to his forearm and thumb scars and passive ROM. M.C. was able to passively stretch into 50 degrees of wrist extension and 60 degrees of thumb abduction. He had a pain level of 6/10 on the Wong-Baker FACES Pain Rating Scale with passive ROM. To address pain during treatment, frequent breaks were taken and snacks provided. To activate the transfer, M.C.'s arm was positioned on the therapy table in 90 degrees of elbow flexion and forearm neutral. With guidance, he was instructed to pronate the forearm to elicit wrist extension. M.C. was then instructed to straighten his index finger while trying to move the thumb away from the palm into abduction. With these strategies combined, M.C. was able to exhibit 25 degrees of active wrist extension and 10 degrees of palmar abduction. Interestingly, overflow from activation of simultaneous movements from his uninvolved extremity seemed to enhance wrist extension and thumb abduction. The sequence of scar massage and passive and active ROM exercises were repeated three times in the session.

Because of M.C.'s family's past issues with compliance, it was even more important for them to have specific guidelines to follow. M.C. and his family were thoroughly instructed to perform the same sequence of activities at home five times per day and issued a detailed written home program with orthosis wear details, exercises, and scar massage. M.C. was seen 5 days after the initial session, and the orthosis was visibly dirty with an intense odor. This was a good sign that M.C. was wearing the orthosis; however, according to the family, M.C. did not take off the orthosis once over the 5-day period, despite all the education provided on the first visit. Therefore, the family was again reeducated on the importance of following the whole regimen at home.

For the next week, M.C. practiced eliciting wrist extension and palmar abduction in a gravity-eliminated plane. During therapy, table hockey games were played using light objects such as cotton balls, foam blocks, and peg dowels. The objects were to be moved across the table using only the dorsum of his hand with gravity-eliminated wrist extension. Biofeedback was also used to improve strength of the transfer, especially into opposition because this motion was more difficult for M.C. to visualize. In addition, M.C. only had 60 degrees of available MCP joint flexion at the time, so the thumb was not able to approximate the PIP joint efficiently. M.C. quickly progressed to gravity-resisted wrist extension 1-½ weeks after cast removal. Active wrist extension against gravity was 10 degrees and palmar abduction was approximately 2 degrees.

The family reported that alternating between wear of the the night and day orthoses was challenging, so the night orthosis was discontinued. Thus, M.C. was only required to wear the thumb spica orthosis for day and night wear. Therapy activities were shifted to include placement and removal of objects from vertical incline surfaces such as loose fitting pegboards, water-cling foam blocks, and a vertical coin slot. M.C. was also instructed to grasp and release ping pong balls using a tenodesis grasp from a surface at shoulder height to engage the entire arm. M.C. used the Biometrics unit with a ROM arc of 0 to 25 degrees of nonresistive active ROM to exercise the wrist into extension. After 2 weeks, M.C. was only required to wear his orthosis for rough play activities and at night.

Phase 3: Strength and Function

By week 8, M.C. began to verbalize the excitement of holding a bike handle, tying shoes, and grasping a mini football because these were activities that he had enjoyed previously, but was unable to perform for more than a year after the initial injury. M.C.'s index finger exhibited 80 degrees of MCP flexion, so he was able to elicit an inferior pincer grasp. However, efficiency of the pinch was inhibited by DIP hyperextension. Kinesiotaping was used to position the DIP joint into 5 degrees of flexion to block DIP hyperextension and provide stability for thumb to index finger opposition. Strengthening activities at this phase included the use of a Thera-Band, theraputty, the Theraband Power Web

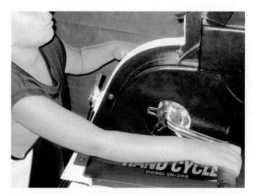

Figure 59-14 Case: conditioning using the arm ergometer.

Exerciser, and graded clothes pins for resisted pinch. Other modalities included the Biometrics unit (for resisted gross grasp, wrist extension, and key pinch tasks), a nut-and-bolt assembly board, and practice securing fasteners such as shirt buttons and shoe laces. These prehensile tasks had frustrated M.C. in the period just after the nerve injury. Sensory reeducation activities were added including texture wands and use of the Dynagel unit (an aqueous gel medium tank that has general thermal and cold properties for resistive exercise and proprioceptive feedback). Coordination activities were introduced such as shifting playing cards, in-hand coin manipulation, and timed grasp and release of various sized pegs and dowels.

By 3 months postoperatively, M.C. was practicing more proximal strengthening activities such as wall push ups, Thera-Band chest presses, and graded ball tosses onto a rebounder. We also added conditioning activities such as the arm ergometer (Fig. 59-14). At 3 months postoperatively, he was progressing nicely in terms of dexterity and function. At 6 months postoperatively, M.C. had improved functional strength for wrist extension, thumb opposition, and key pinch (Fig. 59-15). The family also reported that he was back to performing some of his preinjury activities. At 6 months postoperatively, he had continued to make gains in dexterity and function. Tables 59-5 through 59-9, online, depict clinical findings at 3 and 6 months postoperatively. After a

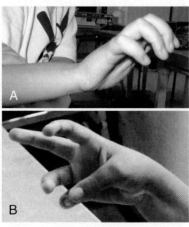

Figure 59-15 Case: M.C. at 6 months postoperatively. **A,** Wrist extension. **B,** Thumb opposition.

successful postoperative treatment program, he was seen less frequently and finally discharged with a home program and followed only in the hand clinic.

Summary

If tendon transfers are an option after a client has plateaued after a peripheral nerve injury, the potential outcome must be fully explored by the hand team and the family because the preparation, surgery, and rehabilitation are lengthy and demanding. The preoperative phase requires a thorough examination with baseline objective tests and maintenance or achievement of maximum passive ROM at associated joints and maximum strength of the muscle(s) to be transferred. The postoperative and rehabilitation phase must include carefully positioned orthoses to protect the transfer, intense muscle reeducation procedures, and effective practice schedules to improve active ROM, strength, and prehension patterns in the involved limb. With diligence and creative programming, the functional benefit of tendon transfers may be achieved, enhancing function in everyday activities.

REFERENCES

The complete reference list is available online at www.expertconsult.com.

Brachial Plexus Palsy Reconstruction: Tendon Transfers, Osteotomies, Capsular Release, and Arthrodesis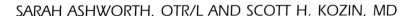

SARAH ASHWORTH, OTR/L AND SCOTT H. KOZIN, MD

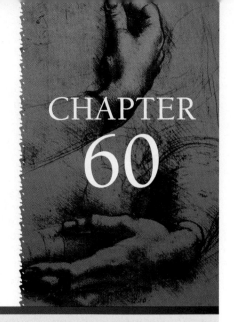

CRITICAL POINTS

- The mainstay for brachial plexus reconstruction consists of tendon transfers about the shoulder, elbow, wrist, and hand.
- Joint releases can be performed for contractures about the shoulder and elbow.
- Corrective osteotomy to reposition the limb and arthrodesis to stabilize flail joints are additional techniques employed in brachial plexus reconstruction.
- The physical examination should include the entire extremity, from shoulder girdle to hand, and must assess the muscle strength, sensory status, and joint motion.
- The range of active motion, muscle strength, and any limitations in passive motion are critical elements during formulation of a treatment strategy.
- The formulation of a list of what's in, what's out, what's available, and what's needed is the basis for the decision-making process.

Children and adults are victims of brachial plexus injuries, which can occur from a variety of causes. The principal etiology is traction across the brachial plexus that results in differential strain across the roots or trunks (Box 60-1).[1,2] The upper and middle trunks course from superior to inferior and possess a slight baseline tension. This anatomic arrangement predisposes the upper brachial plexus to traction injury when compared with the inferior trunk, which traverses over the first rib and is relatively relaxed.[1] Traction can be applied via multiple mechanisms, such as a football injury, a motorcycle accident, or during the childbirth process. Any mechanism that increases the distance between the head/neck and

shoulder results in stretching across the plexus. The degree and extent of damage is related to the vector, amount, and duration of force. Greater force will result in injury to more roots of the brachial plexus.

In addition to traction, there are less common causes of brachial plexus injury, including penetrating trauma, infection, and compressive neuropathy. These etiologies represent a direct insult to the brachial plexus, and their distribution is more variable depending upon the trajectory of the bullet or knife, site of infection, or location of compression. For example, viral infection (also known as Parsonage–Turner syndrome) commonly affects the long thoracic nerve and presents with scapular winging, while brachial plexus compression (also known as thoracic outlet syndrome) usually involves the lower cord and presents with signs and symptoms of ulnar nerve dysfunction.[1,3]

Regardless of the age of the patient and etiology of the brachial plexus injury, similar treatment principles are applied to reconstructive surgery. This chapter focuses on brachial plexus injuries that have incompletely recovered from injury and/or surgery, or are not amenable to nerve reconstruction.

The mainstays for management are tendon transfers about the shoulder, elbow, wrist, and hand. Joint releases can be performed for contractures about the shoulder and elbow. Corrective osteotomy to reposition the limb and arthrodesis to stabilize flail joints are additional techniques employed in brachial plexus reconstruction.

Classification

Brachial plexus injuries can be classified according to the level of involvement (Table 60-1). Upper plexus lesions are most common and involve the fifth and sixth cervical roots

Box 60-1 Etiology of Brachial Plexus Injuries

Trauma
  Nonpenetrating (traction)
  Penetrating (knife, gunshot wound)
Nerve entrapment
  Thoracic outlet syndrome
Infection
  Viral plexopathy (Parsonage–Turner syndrome)
Radiation
  Fibrosis
  Malignant degeneration after radiation
Tumors
  Primary (schwannomas or neurofibromas)
  Secondary (pulmonary apices)
Neuropathies
Iatrogenic
  Axillary or scalene anesthesia
  Surgical biopsy
  Intraoperative positioning
  Median sternotomy
  Inadvertent traction

Table 60-1 *Patterns of Brachial Plexus Injuries*

Pattern	Roots Involve	Primary Deficiency
Upper brachial plexus (Erb-Duchenne)	C5 and C6	Shoulder abduction and external rotation
Extended upper brachial plexus	C5, C6, and C7	Above plus elbow flexion elbow and digital extension
Lower brachial plexus (Dejerine-Klumpke)	C8 and T1	Hand intrinsic muscles Finger flexors
Total brachial plexus lesion	C5, C6, C7, C8, and T1	Entire plexus
Peripheral brachial plexus lesion	–	Variable

a brachial plexus tabulation sheet is an efficient way to record manual muscle strength and prevent inadvertent omission of important data. Muscle strength is graded from 0 to 5, enhanced by the use of a minus modifier to denote incomplete range. The sensibility of the extremity is assessed by standard measures including light touch and two-point discrimination.

Children are more difficult to examine than adults because of their limited attention span, poor ability to follow commands, and lack of cooperation. Extreme patience and repeated examinations are often required to obtain an adequate evaluation. The examination cannot be hurried, and interactive play is utilized to assess the functional use of the extremity. A variety of toys, props, and games are used to accomplish this task (Fig. 60-1). Standardized assessments including the active movement scale, Toronto scale, and modified Mallet classification (Figs. 60-2 and 60-3) can be

or upper trunk. These injuries are referred to as either an Erb-Duchenne or Erb's palsy.[1,4] An extended Erb's palsy also involves the seventh cervical root or middle trunk and is fairly common. Isolated lower plexus lesions are uncommon and referred to as a Klumpke's palsy.[5] The most severe injury is a disruption of the entire plexus—known as a global injury.

Patient Evaluation

The initial examination includes the history, physical examination, and imaging studies. The history should include the details of the initial injury with a focus on the amount and extent of the trauma incurred. The use of the extremity after the initial injury and subsequent return of function are important facts. The treatment rendered subsequent to the injury and its effect on extremity function also constitute essential information. Associated systemic and local injuries that occurred are factors to consider while planning the reconstructive surgery. For example, evaluation of an infant with an obstetric brachial plexus injury should include details about the mother's labor, inquiry into shoulder dystocia, and questions about associated injuries (i.e., fractures of the clavicle or Horner's syndrome).

The physical examination should include the entire extremity, from shoulder girdle to hand. The neck should also be assessed for restriction of motion and pain. The examination must assess the muscle strength, sensory status, and joint motion. The range of active motion, muscle strength, and any limitations in passive motion are critical elements during formulation of a treatment strategy. A uniform grading system for muscle strength and documentation is mandatory when evaluating a patient for surgical reconstruction. Using

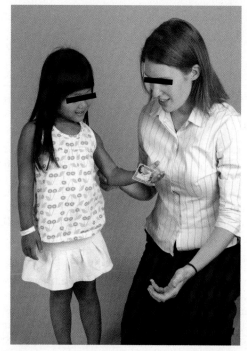

Figure 60-1 A variety of toys, props, and games are used to examine children. (Courtesy of Shriners Hospital for Children, Philadelphia.)

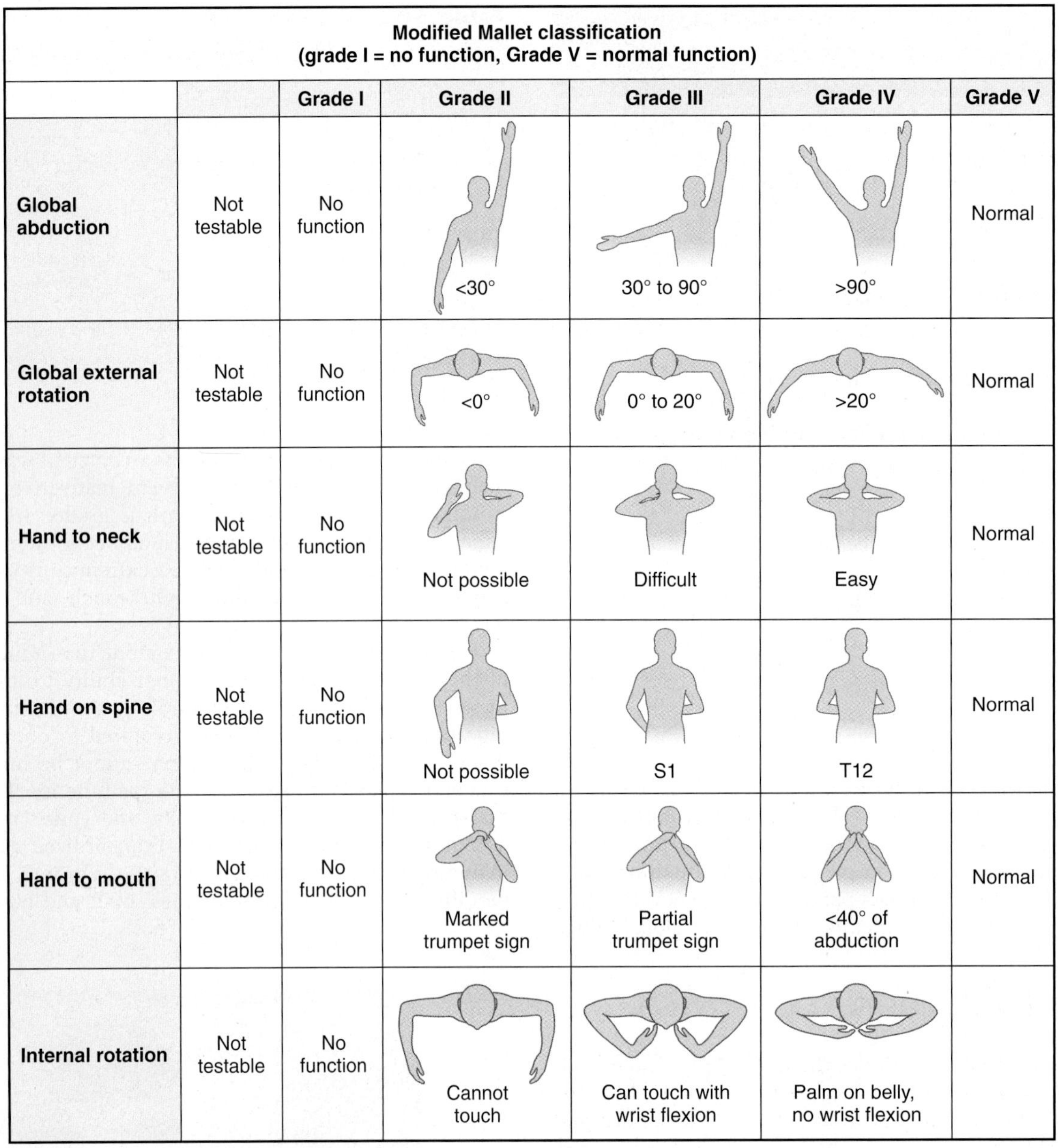

Modified Mallet classification (grade I = no function, Grade V = normal function)						
	Grade I	Grade II	Grade III	Grade IV	Grade V
Global abduction	Not testable	No function	<30°	30° to 90°	>90°	Normal
Global external rotation	Not testable	No function	<0°	0° to 20°	>20°	Normal
Hand to neck	Not testable	No function	Not possible	Difficult	Easy	Normal
Hand on spine	Not testable	No function	Not possible	S1	T12	Normal
Hand to mouth	Not testable	No function	Marked trumpet sign	Partial trumpet sign	<40° of abduction	Normal
Internal rotation	Not testable	No function	Cannot touch	Can touch with wrist flexion	Palm on belly, no wrist flexion	

Figure 60-2 Modified Mallet Classification with additional internal rotational score. Grade I, no function; grade V, normal function.

quickly learned and administered for reliable assessment of younger children.[6] Inclusion of hand-to-belly measurement allows for greater sensitivity to changes of internal rotation of the shoulder. Sensibility can be tested in children using the O'Riain's wrinkle test, stereognosis testing, or subjectively through observation of hand use.[7] Two-point discrimination is unreliable until about 9 years of age.[8] The sophistication of the evaluation modality varies with the age, development, and intellect of the child.

A functional assessment via a questionnaire and examination is a fundamental component in the formulation of a treatment plan. The ability to perform activities of daily living and the techniques used to perform such tasks require evaluation. For example, a patient with deficient finger extension often uses passive wrist flexion and tenodesis of the extensor digitorum communis to extend the fingers for release of

objects. The proposed surgical plan must either avoid limiting wrist flexion (e.g., wrist fusion) or restore active finger extension at the time of arthrodesis. A consideration of the patient's expectations is another important element of the preoperative evaluation. Realistic goals will prevent disappointment and foster a better relationship with the patient.

A baseline outcome measurement is also part of the initial patient workup and preoperative evaluation. Currently, the exact outcome tool that is appropriate for brachial plexus injuries remains unclear, and outcome measurements in children are notoriously difficult. Nonetheless, a critical evaluation of the results after brachial plexus injury and/or surgery is necessary to improve future care of these patients. This task requires faithful documentation of the preoperative state and postoperative change from both subjective and objective standpoints. Adults should at least complete the RAND SF-36

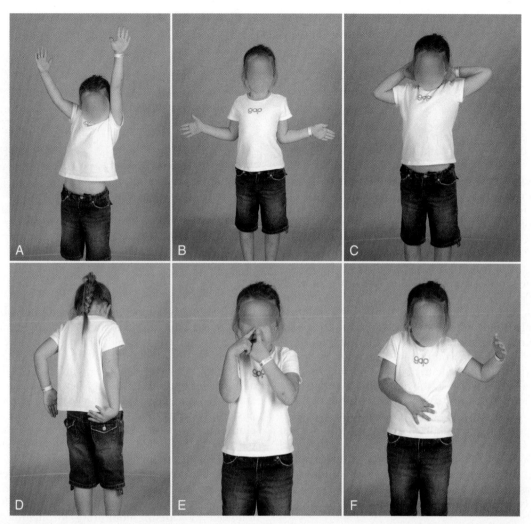

Figure 60-3 A three-year-old child assessed using Mallet measures following arthroscopic capsular release. **A**, Global abduction (grade IV). **B**, Global external rotation (grade IV). **C**, Hand to neck (grade IV). **D**, Hand to spine (grade II). **E**, Hand to mouth (grade IV). **F**, Internal rotation (grade III). (Courtesy of Shriners Hospital for Children, Philadelphia.)

questionnaire before surgical intervention.[9,10] The Mallet classification has been shown to be a reliable instrument for assessing shoulder function in children with brachial plexus birth palsies.[11-13] The Canadian Occupational Performance Measure (COPM) is an applicable outcome tool for both children (can interview caregivers) and adults.[14] The COPM measures changes in client-perceived performance and satisfaction of self-identified goals. For each goal, performance and satisfaction are rated using a 10-point Likert scale, wherein 1 is negative (cannot perform, not satisfied) and 10 is positive (performs very well, very satisfied). This outcome tool also encourages discussion of realistic expectations of intervention to prevent disappointment and ensure that both the patient and the caregivers are fully educated about the potential of any treatment.

Ancillary Studies

Ancillary studies can be helpful at the time of patient examination and during the formulation of a treatment plan. Radiographs of the injured extremity are used to assess for previous

fractures and to evaluate bony development in children. Limitation of passive motion should not always be assumed to be secondary to soft-tissue contracture, and radiographs are required. For the shoulder, anteroposterior and axillary views are adequate in the adolescent or adult patient. However, children who are skeletally immature may require advanced imaging modalities (e.g., magnetic resonance imaging [MRI]) to truly depict the contour of the glenohumeral joint.[15-18] We prefer MRI, as this modality provides the most accurate image of the pediatric glenohumeral joint with precise depiction of the articular cartilage, humeral head position, and glenoid configuration.

Electrodiagnostic tests can provide some useful information about nerve and muscle recovery when the physician is contemplating early nerve repair and/or reconstruction.[19,20] However, electromyography is not quantitative with respect to muscle strength and does not substitute for an astute physical examination coupled with manual muscle testing. Reinnervated muscle will demonstrate an abnormal electromyographic signal, such as increased amplitude and polyphasic waveforms. These findings indicate inherent weakness and altered contractile properties, which often preclude use of that muscle as a suitable donor. However, electrodiagnostic tests have limited value during the formulation of secondary reconstructions.

Shoulder

The shoulder is frequently impaired after a brachial plexus injury, because most of its prime movers are innervated by the upper plexus. The rotator cuff confluence is innervated by C5 and C6 and acts to move the glenohumeral joint and depress humeral head motion during movement, which maintains the concentric relationship between the humeral head and glenoid. This function and precise synchrony between the rotator cuff and deltoid muscles is distorted after brachial plexus injury and impaired by incomplete nerve regeneration. Loss of abduction (deltoid and supraspinous muscles) and a deficit in external rotation (infraspinous muscle) are the most common problems, especially in residual brachial plexus birth palsy (Fig. 60-4). Internal rotation is usually less affected, since multiple muscles (pectoralis major, latissimus dorsi, and subscapularis) possess the ability to provide internal rotation. This resultant imbalance can cause an internal rotation contracture over time, which is especially prevalent in the pediatric population after brachial plexus birth palsy. Therefore, at the time of initial evaluation of an infant after brachial plexus birth palsy, parents or other caregivers are instructed in passive external rotation exercises. The scapula must be stabilized to isolate glenohumeral joint rotation (Fig. 60-5). These passive maneuvers are performed at each diaper change, and the status of the glenohumeral joint is carefully monitored. Early detection of a diminished passive external rotation with manual scapular stabilization requires a referral for formal therapy aimed at

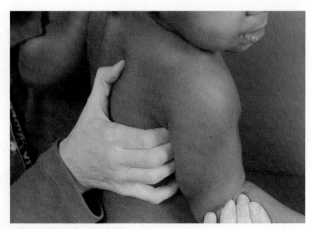

Figure 60-5 Stabilization of the scapulothoracic joint is necessary to isolate the glenohumeral joint during external rotation exercises. (Courtesy of Shriners Hospital for Children, Philadelphia.)

glenohumeral rotation. An established internal rotation contracture (i.e., no external rotation) that does not respond to therapy requires surgical release.[15,21] Failure to maintain external rotation will cause altered development of the glenohumeral joint with an irregularly shaped humeral head and corresponding deficient glenoid cavity (Fig. 60-6). Surgery is recommended when the humeral head is posteriorly subluxed and the glenoid is deformed.[12,17] The clinical test is passive external rotation with the scapula stabilized and the shoulder adducted. Negative range of motion (ROM) implies subluxation and warrants MRI. Release of the anterior joint capsule can be combined with tendon transfer to restore active external rotation.[22-25] In young children (under 3 years of age), isolated release is often preferred, followed by careful monitoring for neurologic return of external rotation.

With respect to internal rotation, it is important to understand the role the subscapularis plays in end-range internal rotation. Weakness from the brachial plexus injury or following surgical release or lengthening to improve external rotation can result in limited ability to bring the hand to the trunk/waist (Fig. 60-3F).[15,21] Baseline assessment of internal rotation ROM and end-range strength is important to predict and minimize postoperative midline function limitations. Weak internal rotation requires early incorporation of active midline activities following surgery.

Elbow

The elbow is frequently impaired after brachial plexus injuries—especially elbow flexion secondary to loss of the biceps and brachialis muscles. Inability to flex the elbow is a considerable impairment, since hand-to-mouth function is impossible. In patients with global injuries and minimal hand function, the affected arm uses elbow function as a support to carry objects along the forearm. The inability to flex the elbow further impairs the function of the limb. For these reasons, restoration of the functional arc of elbow motion (30 to 130 degrees) carries a high priority during brachial plexus reconstruction.[23]

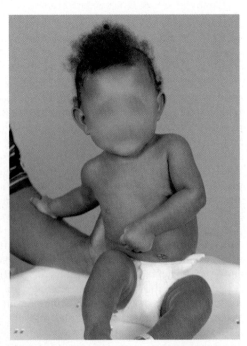

Figure 60-4 Six-month-old child with left brachial plexus birth palsy and deficient shoulder abduction and external rotation. (Courtesy of Shriners Hospital for Children, Philadelphia.)

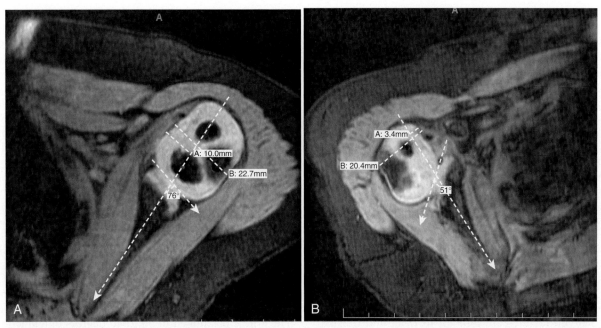

Figure 60-6 Four-year-old female with right brachial plexus palsy. **A**, Normal left shoulder (percent of humeral head anterior, or PHHA = 44%, version = −14 degrees). **B**, Abnormal right shoulder with pseudoglenoid (PHHA = 16.7%, version = −39 degrees). (Courtesy of Shriners Hospital for Children, Philadelphia.)

Forearm

Forearm rotation is often limited following brachial plexus palsies. The forearm joint is motored between muscles that provide supination and pronation. Supination is primarily an upper trunk (C5 and C6) function via the biceps and supinator muscles. In contrast, pronation is a middle and lower trunk function via the pronator teres (C7) and pronator quadratus (C8 and T1). An individual may lack supination, pronation, or both depending on the extent of injury. Although supination is important for specific tasks such as accepting change, eating, and personal hygiene, these activities are unilateral and can be completed effectively with the unaffected arm. Pronation deficiency leads to difficulty with many more bimanual tasks such as keyboarding, writing, and tabletop activities. The decision to restore forearm movement requires careful considerations of the function limitations and potential for gains and losses.[26,27] Contraindications for improving pronation include weak or absent wrist extension, insensate hand, and/or minimal finger movement. Without adequate wrist extension and finger strength, a pronated forearm limits the function of the hand as a stable carrying surface. The pronated hand becomes less functional as compared with the supinated position. An insensate hand uses vision as the afferent signal, and rotation of an insensate hand into pronation increases the risk for injury owing to the inability to visualize the palmar surface of the hand.

Wrist and Hand

Wrist and hand impairment varies with the damage to the middle and lower plexus. Upper brachial plexus lesions have a minimal effect on hand use, while global plexus injuries can severely hamper hand function. A definitive treatment algorithm for the wrist and hand is more difficult to formulate because of the variable clinical presentation. A detailed functional examination and manual muscle testing are the foundation for the development of a treatment paradigm. The formulation of a list of what's in, what's out, what's available, and what's needed is the basis for the decision-making process. Individualized treatment is required, and many of the principles of radial, median, and ulnar nerve transfers are applied. The principles and techniques of these tendon transfers are covered in Chapters 58 and 59.

Conservative Versus Surgical Intervention

Conservative management is beneficial for preventing muscle tightness and subsequent joint contracture when further neurologic recovery is anticipated. Therapy interventions are also helpful to minimize joint contracture and strengthen muscles. Interventions may include active and passive ROM, strengthening, splinting, kinesiotaping, electrical stimulation, muscle and/or sensory reeducation, and adaptive functional training. Surgical intervention is indicated when joint instability or deformity is present or when no further neurologic recovery is expected and functional deficits remain problematic for the patient.

Approach to Reconstruction Options

Contracture Release

The shoulder is prone to develop an internal rotation contracture, especially following brachial plexus birth palsy.

Incomplete recovery after brachial plexus birth palsy often results in decreased movement and muscle imbalance about the shoulder, as rotator cuff and deltoid innervation is incomplete. The internal rotators overpower the external rotators, which results in an internal rotation contracture. This constant position of internal rotation leads to early glenohumeral joint deformity by 6 months of age and advanced deformity by 2 years, which is characterized by increasing glenoid retroversion and posterior humeral head subluxation (glenohumeral dysplasia).[15] Children with an established internal rotation contracture and glenohumeral joint deformity are unlikely to regain optimum shoulder function without intervention.[15,21]

In patients with recovery of biceps and brachialis function, the elbow is prone to develop an elbow flexion contracture. The exact etiology is unclear but seems to be related to the reinnervation process.[28] The contracture is more severe in children without triceps function. Therapy is often beneficial, especially if implemented early in the process. Orthotic positioning and serial casting are useful in reducing flexion contractures. Botulinum toxin can be added in recalcitrant cases. Established contractures are difficult to treat, and capsular release has mediocre results, with the inherent risk of losing pivotal elbow flexion. Therefore, an elbow release is rarely performed in patients with brachial plexus palsies.

Open Release of Internal Rotation Contracture

An anterior approach between the deltoid and pectoralis muscles is performed. If the pectoralis muscle is tight, a musculocutaneous lengthening can be performed. The subscapularis muscle is isolated and released from the underlying anterior capsule. If the contracture is resolved, then the joint arthrotomy is unnecessary. Persistent contracture is usually associated with underlying joint deformity and may require capsular release. The arm is positioned in 45 degrees of abduction and 40 to 50 degrees of external rotation, which is maintained by a shoulder spica cast.

This procedure can also be performed via an axillary incision and release of the subscapularis muscle from its scapular origin, which allows the entire muscle to slide. A similar immobilization and postoperative management is employed. Release of the internal rotation contracture can also be combined with tendon transfer to restore external rotation at the same time or as a staged procedure after supple passive motion has been restored.

Arthroscopic Release of Internal Rotation Contracture

Arthroscopy is performed via an anterior and posterior portal.[1,15] An electrocautery is introduced through the anterior portal. The thickened superior glenohumeral ligament, the middle glenohumeral ligament, and the upper one-half to two-thirds of the subscapularis are released. The upper, intra-articular portion of the subscapularis tendon is then released. As the release continues inferiorly, the tendinous portion of the subscapularis transitions into a more muscular portion. At this point, the release becomes isolated to the capsule, with preservation of the inferior and lateral

muscular portions of the subscapularis. The electrocautery is removed and exchanged for an arthroscopic punch. The inferior glenohumeral ligament is then released to a point slightly posterior to the midportion of the axillary pouch. The axillary nerve is protected. The arthroscopic equipment is removed from the joint. The glenohumeral joint is manipulated into external rotation, both with the arm at the side and with the arm at 90 degrees of elevation. Marked improvement in external rotation is noted, often with a palpable clunk associated with glenohumeral joint reduction. Failure to achieve joint reduction or passive external rotation of less than 45 degrees with the arm in adduction requires additional arthroscopic release of the axillary pouch and the tight subscapularis.

In children with concomitant tendon transfers, the latissimus dorsi and teres major tendons are transferred to the superior-posterior rotator cuff and humerus following arthroscopic release. The child is placed in a shoulder spica cast with the glenohumeral joint positioned in 45 to 60 degrees of external rotation. The amount of abduction varies according to whether or not tendon transfers were performed. The arm is positioned in 30 to 40 degrees of abduction after isolated release and 100 to 120 degrees of abduction after release combined with tendon transfer. The child continues to wear a cast for 3 weeks after isolated release and 4 to 5 weeks after tendon transfer.

The postoperative cast immobilization is continued for 3 to 4 weeks. An orthosis is fabricated that replicates the position while in a cast (Fig. 60-7). The orthosis consists of a trunk portion and a posterior elbow splint with elbow flexion. The arm portion is securely attached to the trunk piece with the prescribed abduction and external rotation. During the first 1 to 2 weeks the orthosis is removed for bathing, therapy, and supervised play. Orthosis weaning is influenced by the presence of shoulder stiffness, active movement, and the patient's activity level. The orthosis is worn at night for 12 weeks after surgery. Restrictions include avoiding passive internal rotation and resistive activities.

Active ROM exercises are begun, focusing on external rotation and shoulder elevation. In children this is best achieved through play activities. Compensatory movements, such as trunk extension, should be limited by gentle manual stabilization or cueing. Early active internal rotation is

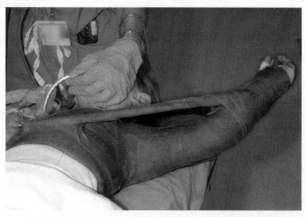

Figure 60-7 Postoperative cast status following arthroscopic release and tendon transfers. An orthosis is fabricated that replicates the position when in cast. (Courtesy of Shriners Hospital for Children, Philadelphia.)

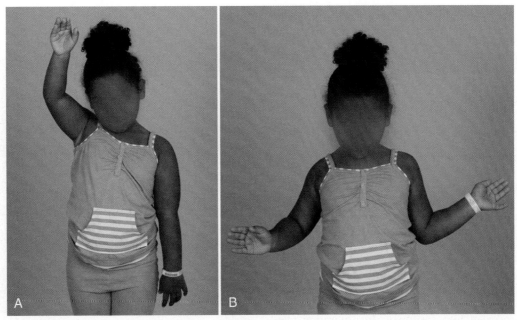

Figure 60-8 Four-year-old female status following right arthroscopic anterior release showing improved shoulder function. **A**, Abduction (Mallet grade IV). **B**, External rotation (Mallet grade IV). (Courtesy of Shriners Hospital for Children, Philadelphia.)

incorporated into treatment to limit midline dysfunction. Passive external rotation with scapular stabilization is initiated and performed several times per day to maintain improved position of the shoulder, and should be incorporated into the home program. Scar massage is initiated as soon as the incisions heal and should be performed four to five times per day. Caregiver education is a large component of early treatment to encourage carryover at home. Frequent practice of stretching, scar massage, and stabilizing techniques during therapy sessions increases confidence and compliance with the home program. This is especially true with young children who may be resistant to some of these interventions. Distraction activities are also beneficial to children with limited tolerance of certain activities.

In children with glenoid dysplasia, open or arthroscopic reduction has been shown to improve joint configuration with reduction of the humeral head and improved glenoid version (i.e., the angle the glenoid center line makes with the plane of the scapula).[21,27] Positive changes are observed both on MRI and with clinical measurements. Improvements in active shoulder ROM primarily occur with abduction and external rotation (Fig. 60-8). Limitations with internal rotation have been noted after subscapularis lengthening, which can be reduced by minimizing the amount of lengthening completed at the time of surgery. Importantly, superior outcomes are associated with better preoperative clinical and MRI status. This indicates that early recognition of glenohumeral dysplasia and timely intervention will result in better shoulder motion and improved joint alignment.

Tendon Transfers

The formulation of a treatment plan requires careful consideration of the above-noted factors, including the patient, joint motion, sensibility, manual muscle testing, and expectations. As mentioned above, the treatment paradigm requires consideration of four general categories: What's in, what's out, what's available, and what's needed. Each category has certain inclusion criteria that require elucidation. The "what's in" collection lists all muscles that are detected by manual muscle testing along with their respective grades. The "what's out" category records all muscles not detected by manual muscle testing. The "what's available" register includes all muscles that have a manual muscle test grade equal to a 4 or 5. Muscles graded 3 or less are not suitable for transfers, since strength tends to diminish by one grade after transfer. Therefore, muscles capable of complete range but unable to except any resistance are listed as a grade 3. Transfer of these muscles would result in a grade 2 strength, which would be able to perform only gravity-eliminated motion and not enhance function. The "what's available" list must also consider the availability and expendability of the muscle. A prerequisite to transfer is that the function of a donor muscle must be preserved after transfer for it to be considered expendable. For example, a grade 4 extensor carpi radialis longus muscle is a viable donor as long as the extensor carpi brevis muscle is intact. Once a list of available muscles has been formulated, then the surgeon contemplates the possibility of achieving "what's needed" with transfer of these tendon(s).

The final surgical decision must also take into account the inherent excursion of the muscle and technical considerations. The *excursion* is the distance a muscle can contract and is proportional to the length of the individual muscle fibers. Tendon transfers should attempt to match the donor and recipient muscle excursions to allow full ROM following transfer. The surgeon must also consider the rehabilitation strategy following tendon transfer and consult with the therapist.

Following tendon transfer surgery, there are four main phases: immobilization, mobilization, light strengthening–functional training, and strengthening. Intervention during the immobilization phase focuses on edema and pain management, and on ROM of uninvolved joints. This phase typically lasts 3 to 4 weeks depending on the type of tendon transfer, the quality of the tendons, and the strength of the suture.

The mobilization phase begins when the cast is removed and lasts until 6 to 8 weeks following surgery. Therapy is initiated with the fabrication of a protective orthosis that maintains a tension-free position of the tendon transfer. Resistive activities and active/passive movements that apply tension to the transfer are avoided. Treatment begins with muscle reeducation of the tendon transfer. Cues to attempt previous action of the transferred muscle in a protected position are useful for muscle reeducation.[29] Tapping and vibration can also facilitate recruitment. Biofeedback is a valuable modality for patients exhibiting difficulty with consistent recruitment of tendon transfers. Once consistent recruitment has been achieved with active ROM, functional activities should be incorporated into treatment. Incorporating play activities for children or identified functional activities can make sessions more meaningful to the patient. Scar management including scar massage and possible use of silicon gel sheets should be initiated as soon as incisional scars are healed.[30]

The therapist should continually examine the patient for possible complications. A sudden or gradual lag in end-range movement may indicate weakness, deep scar formation, attenuation, or rupture of the tendon transfer. When weakness or scar formation is suspected, active assisted ROM or place-and-hold exercises can help build strength and promote tendon gliding. If limitations continue, neuromuscular electrical stimulation may be beneficial to encourage gliding and strengthening. Neuromuscular electrical stimulation should not be initiated until it has been cleared by the surgeon, typically after 6 weeks following the procedure. In cases of suspected attenuation or rupture, the patient must be immediately examined by the surgeon. Mild attenuation may improve with healing and adaptive shortening of the muscle–tendon unit over time. However, substantial attenuation and/or rupture requires revision surgery to improve functional outcomes.[29]

During the light-strengthening phase, the orthosis is worn only for sleep and for protection during highly resistive activities. Strengthening is initiated with light theraband or weights. The therapist must continue to monitor for complications. Muscle fatigue and undesired compensatory movement patterns should be avoided during the initiation of strengthening exercises. Passive motions that apply tension to the tendon transfer are avoided. Once the patient has been cleared from restrictions, usually at 12 weeks after surgery, orthoses are discontinued and strengthening is progressively increased as tolerated.

Latissimus Dorsi and Teres Major Transfer

The child is positioned in the lateral decubitus position on the operating room table. An incision is made across the

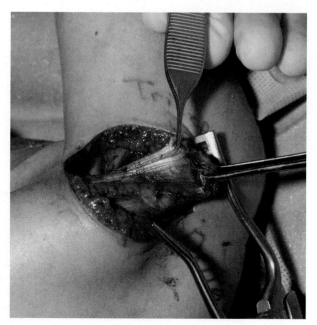

Figure 60-9 Latissimus dorsi and teres major tendons transferred over triceps to posterior rotator cuff. (Courtesy of Shriners Hospital for Children, Philadelphia.)

axilla from the latissimus tendon insertion toward the posterior acromion. The latissimus dorsi and teres tendons are released from their insertions. The latissimus dorsi and teres tendons are transferred over the long head of the triceps to the posterior rotator cuff (Fig. 60-9). The tendons are inserted into the bone just above the infraspinous insertion. The wound is closed with absorbable suture. The arm is positioned in 30 to 40 degrees of external rotation and 120 degrees of abduction, with a spica cast. Casting is continued for 4 to 5 weeks after tendon transfer.[1,15]

Other Shoulder Tendon Transfers

Other tendon transfers about the shoulder for residual brachial plexus palsy involve restoration of glenohumeral abduction. Donor muscles used include the trapezius, levator scapulae, and bipolar latissimus dorsi. The trapezius is transferred with a portion of the acromion to the decorticated posterolateral humerus. The levator scapulae is elongated with a fascial graft to reach the tendon of the supraspinous. The latissimus is transferred on a pedicle similar to the bipolar technique for flexorplasty. Experience with these transfers is not extensive, and expected abduction is limited to only 30 to 60 degrees.[1] In persistent cases of shoulder instability or subluxation, arthrodesis is preferred in adult plexopathies.

Postoperative Management

After 4 weeks of immobilization an orthosis is fabricated to replicate the cast, with the arm abducted and externally rotated (Fig. 60-10). The orthosis is worn for sleep and weaned during the day for therapy, bathing, and supervised play. For patients who quickly demonstrate fatigue with the transfer and have difficulty maintaining their active range,

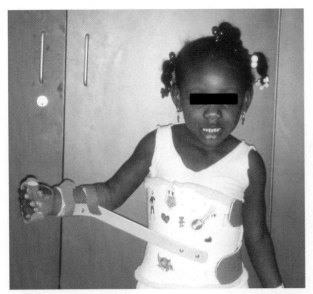

Figure 60-10 After 4 weeks of immobilization, an orthosis is fabricated to replicate the cast with the arm externally rotated after arthroscopic release. (Courtesy of Shriners Hospital for Children, Philadelphia.)

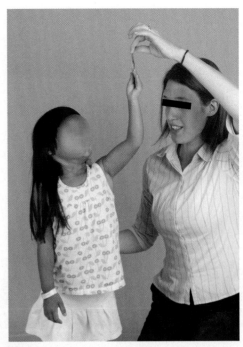

Figure 60-11 When working with children, the therapist must be creative in choosing and setting up activities to engage the patient into the desired movements. (Courtesy of Shriners Hospital for Children, Philadelphia.)

the orthosis may be worn more often during the day to allow for rest between exercises. On the other hand, patients who appear stiff or hesitant to move their arm out of abduction and external rotation may need more time out of the orthosis to allow for relaxation and thus avoid the development of contractures. The orthosis is used at night until 12 weeks after surgery. Restrictions during the mobilization and light-strengthening phases include avoiding passive internal rotation and shoulder adduction. Resistive and weight-bearing activities are also avoided.

Therapeutic intervention focuses on recruitment of the tendon transfer, and active and passive shoulder abduction and external rotation. When working with children, the therapist must be creative in choosing and instituting activities to engage the patient into the desired movements (Fig. 60-11). For example, a painting activity set up on a vertical surface can be used to facilitate both external rotation and shoulder elevation. Consider changing the position of the patient for those with difficulty fully abducting against gravity. Working in the supine position allows for successful active movement in a gravity-eliminated plane. Early active internal rotation and adduction is initiated when cleared to limit difficulty with midline tasks and scapulohumeral abduction contractures.

Latissimus dorsi and teres major tendon transfers can significantly improve shoulder function in patients with brachial plexus palsy. In patients with unbalanced forces around the shoulder, early tendon transfers can stop the progression of glenohumeral joint deformity. On MRI examination, tendon transfers have not been shown to be effective in correcting existing glenohumeral joint deformity.[6] Combining arthroscopic glenohumeral release with tendon transfers has been successful in correcting the alignment of the glenohumeral joint and augmenting active shoulder movement when further nerve recovery is not expected (Fig. 60-12).[15]

Tendon Transfers for Elbow Flexion

The assessment of potential muscles for transfer is performed via inventory of available donors. There are multiple donor muscles described for elbow flexorplasty, including the latissimus dorsi, pectoralis major, triceps, and flexor-pronator muscles.[31-37] The latissimus dorsi or pectoralis major muscle can be transferred by detachment of its humeral insertion and transfer into the biceps tendon using an intervening graft (unipolar transfer). Another option is to release both the origin and insertion sites and transfer the entire muscle into the anterior compartment of the arm (bipolar transfer). The bipolar technique reattaches the muscle origin to the coracoid process or acromion and the insertion into the biceps tendon.[34,37] A bipolar transfer of the latissimus dorsi or pectoralis major muscle is preferred to a unipolar transfer because the bipolar method provides a better "line of pull" and superior restoration of muscle fiber length.

When multiple donor muscles are available, the latissimus dorsi is our preferred donor for elbow flexorplasty. This muscle is expendable, possesses adequate strength, and provides sufficient excursion for elbow flexion.[37] The pectoralis major muscle is another workable donor for elbow flexorplasty, although the cosmetic concerns limit its use.[34] The triceps muscle has similar inherent properties with reference to muscle fiber length and excursion when compared with the biceps muscle. However, loss of active extension is a disadvantage and limits the use of the triceps-to-biceps transfer. In fact, triceps muscle transfer is contraindicated in patients who require forceful elbow extension for upper extremity weight bearing for mobility, such as wheelchair propulsion or crutch ambulation.[38] The transfer or proximal

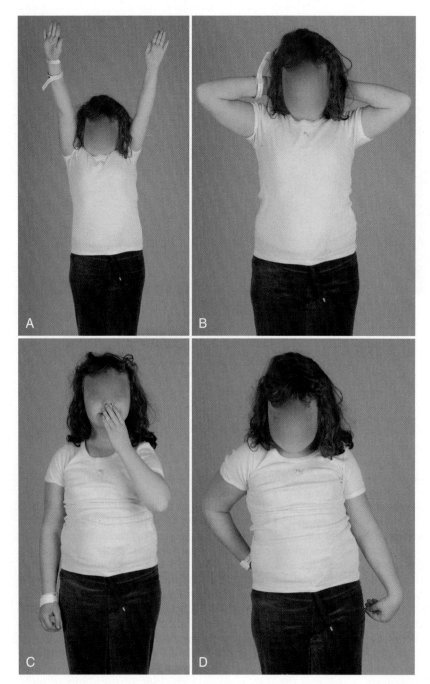

Figure 60-12 Six-year-old female following left arthroscopic anterior release and tendon transfers demonstrating Mallet parameters for shoulder function. **A**, Abduction (grade IV to 170 degrees). **B**, Hand to neck (grade IV from grade II preoperative). **C**, Hand to mouth (grade IV from grade III preoperative). **D**, Hand to spine (grade II with no change from preoperative). (Courtesy of Shriners Hospital for Children, Philadelphia.)

advancement of the flexor-pronator muscle group, known as the Steindler procedure, is less commonly used for restoration of elbow flexion. This technique has the disadvantage of limited motion and strength following transfer and the unwanted pronation that occurs with attempted elbow flexion.

Latissimus Dorsi Transfer (Bipolar Technique)

The patient is placed in a lateral position for harvest of the latissimus dorsi muscle and rotated into the supine position during transfer of the muscle into the anterior arm. A longitudinal incision is made from the posterior axillary fold to the inferior aspect of the latissimus dorsi muscle. The entire muscle is mobilized, including a strip of thoracodorsal fascia and the tendinous insertion into the humerus (Fig. 60-13). The thoracodorsal nerve and vascular pedicle are isolated and protected. An anterior deltopectoral approach is performed to create a passageway for the bipolar transfer. The latissimus dorsi muscle is passed from posterior to anterior with the tendinous insertion proximal and the fascial origin distal.[1]

The latissimus dorsi muscle is passed into the arm through a subcutaneous tunnel. The tendon of origin is secured to the clavicle or acromion via drill holes and the thoracodorsal fascia woven into the biceps tendon, which can be reinforced by fascia lata graft. The transfer is placed in enough tension to create a 30-degree tenodesis effect (i.e., tension in the

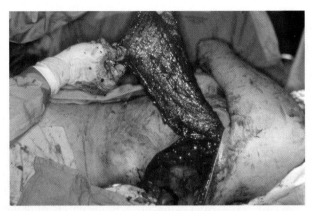

Figure 60-13 Bipolar latissimus dorsi muscle harvested from flank for elbow flexorplasty. (Courtesy of Shriners Hospital for Children, Philadelphia.)

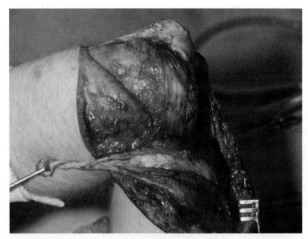

Figure 60-15 Triceps-to-biceps transfer to restore elbow flexion. (Courtesy of Shriners Hospital for Children, Philadelphia.)

transfer prevents the last 30 degrees of elbow extension). The wounds are closed with drains placed in the posterior wound. A long arm orthosis that maintains 100 to 110 degrees of flexion and a Velpeau's dressing is applied.

Pectoralis Major Transfer (Bipolar Technique)

The pectoralis muscle is harvested via an incision that runs longitudinally along the medial border of the sternum and curves laterally inferior to the clavicle (Fig. 60-14).[39] The sternocostal origin is released with a strip of rectus abdominis fascia. The clavicular origin is freed while the underlying neurovascular pedicle (medial and lateral pectoral nerves and arteries) is identified and preserved. The pectoralis major tendon of insertion into the humerus is released in preparation for transfer.

The entire pectoralis muscle is mobilized into the arm and passed through a subcutaneous tunnel. The insertion site is oriented proximal and the sternocostal origin distal. The tendon of origin is secured to the clavicle or acromion and the rectus fascia woven into the biceps tendon, which can be reinforced by fascia lata graft. The transfer is placed in enough tension to create a 30-degree tenodesis effect (i.e., tension in the transfer prevents the last 30 degrees of elbow extension). The wounds are closed, and a long arm orthosis that main-

tains 100 to 110 degrees of flexion with the arm secured to the thorax (Velpeau's dressing) is applied.

Triceps Transfer

The patient's distal half of the triceps is exposed via a posterior incision. The triceps tendon is elevated from the olecranon and elongated with a strip of periosteum. The radial nerve is identified and protected as it passes around the humerus from posterior to anterior. The biceps tendon is exposed using a zigzag or transverse antecubital incision. The triceps tendon is passed laterally through a subcutaneous tunnel and secured to the biceps tendon (Fig. 60-15). The transfer is placed in enough tension to create a 30-degree tenodesis effect (i.e., tension in the transfer prevents the last 30 degrees of elbow extension). The wounds are closed, and a long arm orthosis that maintains 100 to 110 degrees of flexion with the arm secured to the thorax (Velpeau's dressing) is applied.[1]

Flexor–Pronator Transfer (Steindler Procedure)

A medial incision is performed beginning in the arm, across the elbow, and extending into the forearm. The flexor--pronator muscle group is isolated at its origin from the medial epicondyle. The ulnar nerve is identified within the cubital tunnel and carefully protected. The median nerve is also isolated as it passes through the pronator muscle. The flexor–pronator muscle group is elevated with a piece of medial epicondyle in preparation for transfer (Fig. 60-16).

The entire muscle group is transferred in a proximal and anterior direction to increase their ability to flex the elbow. The muscles are secured to the humerus via a screw placed across the piece of transferred bone and into the humerus. This creates an immediate tenodesis effect, and the arm is positioned in an arm orthosis that maintains 100 to 110 degrees of flexion.[40]

Postoperative Management

Regardless of the muscle transfer for elbow flexion, the initial postoperative regimen is similar. The arm is placed in either an orthosis or a cast in flexion for 4 to 6 weeks' time depending on the status and effectiveness of the proximal and distal transfer sites.[41] At the time of cast removal, a posterior long

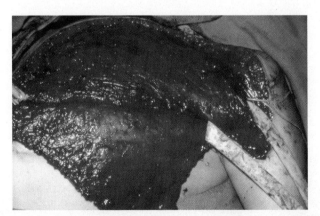

Figure 60-14 Bipolar pectoralis major transfer harvested from chest wall for elbow flexorplasty. (Courtesy of Shriners Hospital for Children, Philadelphia.)

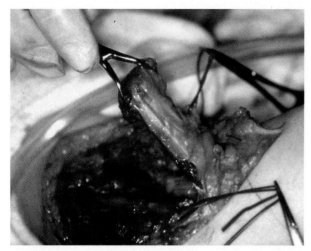

Figure 60-16 *The flexor–pronator muscle group is elevated with a piece of medial epicondyle in preparation for transfer. (Courtesy of Shriners Hospital for Children, Philadelphia.)*

arm orthosis is fabricated with the elbow flexed at approximately 110 degrees. The orthosis is primarily worn at night. The patient is also fitted with an adjustable elbow hinge brace that allows for locking flexion and extension ROM. Initially the extension hinge is locked to 110 degrees, allowing further flexion and blocking extension beyond this point. During the early part of the mobilization phase, treatment focuses on muscle reeducation and scar management.

Muscle reeducation begins with active contraction and isolation of the transfer. To initiate recruitment, the therapist cues the patient to perform the transferred muscles' previous action. Close supervision and careful positioning of the arm in a gravity-eliminated plane are necessary to prevent elbow extension. With a Steindler procedure, the arm should be supported on a table with the elbow flexed to 110 degrees to allow elbow flexion with gravity eliminated. Support is provided to the patient's wrist and forearm, and the patient is cued to contract the flexor–pronator musculature. The therapist should palpate and visually observe contraction of the flexor–pronator muscles for contraction. Biofeedback allows for visual and auditory feedback when activation has occurred to further teach the patient how to isolate activation. This can be especially helpful when antagonistic muscles are transferred.

Once activation is consistent, functional tabletop activities should be included in the program to reestablish desired movement patterns. When the patient can consistently recruit the tendon transfer, the ROM can be progressed 15 degrees each week. After achieving a 30-degree arc of motion (90 to 120 degrees), light resistive activities are initiated. This consists of against-gravity active ROM, hand-to-mouth activities, and more challenging tabletop activities. At approximately 10 weeks with sufficient tendon excursion, patients may begin formal strengthening. Passive elbow extension is not allowed for 3 months. Tendon transfers may actually function better in patients who lack full extension. The slight elbow flexion contractures ease the initiation of active elbow flexion. The goal for end-range extension is typically 20 to 30 degrees.[42] The day orthosis is discontinued after the patient achieves active elbow flexion against gravity from 90 degrees to end-range. Night wear of the orthosis continues until 12 weeks from surgery.

The results following with elbow flexorplasties are positive with three fifths to full muscle strength and enough active flexion for activities of daily living.[41,42] Patients report functional gains in unilateral and bimanual activities. Mild elbow flexion contractures are common following these procedures. In general, bipolar flexorplasties provide more ROM than do unipolar transfers (Fig. 60-17). Steindler flexorplasties produce only about 90 to 100 degrees of elbow flexion (Fig. 60-18).

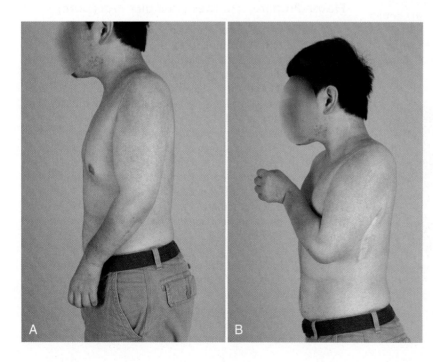

Figure 60-17 *A 12-year-old male following bipolar latissimus dorsi flexorplasty.* **A,** *Elbow extension with slight contracture.* **B,** *Active elbow flexion. (Courtesy of Shriners Hospital for Children, Philadelphia.)*

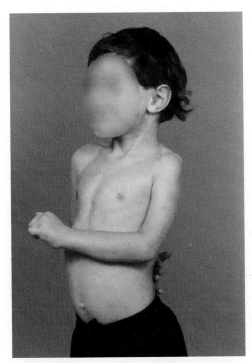

Figure 60-18 An 8-year-old male following Steindler flexorplasty with 90 degrees of elbow flexion. (Courtesy of Shriners Hospital for Children, Philadelphia.)

Tendon Transfer for Elbow Extension

A deficiency in elbow extension can result from brachial plexus injury that involves the middle portion of the plexus. Surgical reconstruction is less commonly performed, because elbow flexion is a greater priority and elbow extension can be accomplished by gravity.[43] In certain cases, elbow flexion is adequate and the lack of elbow extension is disabling. Deficient elbow extension will decrease the patient's available workspace, especially during reaching activities, limit the ability to perform overhead tasks, and impair transfers in wheelchair users.

Evaluation for elbow extension transfer requires an inventory of the available muscles. Options include the latissimus dorsi muscle transferred using a bipolar technique or the biceps-to-triceps transfer, which is commonly used in tetraplegia. Active brachialis and supinator muscles are prerequisites to biceps transfer to maintain elbow flexion and forearm supination. The evaluation of their integrity requires a careful physical examination of elbow flexion and forearm supination strength.[29] The brachialis and supinator muscles can be palpated independent of the biceps muscle. Effortless forearm supination without resistance induces supinator function that can be palpated along the proximal radius. Similarly, powerless elbow flexion incites palpable brachialis contraction along the anterior humerus. Equivocal cases require additional evaluation to ensure adequate supinator and brachialis muscle activity.[44] We prefer injection of the biceps muscle with a local anesthetic to induce temporary paralysis and allow independent assessment of brachialis and supinator function.

Latissimus Dorsi Transfer (Bipolar Technique)

The patient is placed in a lateral position for harvest of the latissimus dorsi muscle. A longitudinal incision is made from the posterior axillary fold to the inferior aspect of the latissimus dorsi muscle. The entire muscle is mobilized including a strip of thoracodorsal fascia and the tendinous insertion into the humerus. The thoracodorsal nerve and vascular pedicle are isolated and protected.

The latissimus dorsi muscle tendon of origin is secured to the clavicle or acromion via drill holes. The remaining muscle is passed through a subcutaneous tunnel and the thoracodorsal fascia woven into the triceps tendon, which can be reinforced by fascia lata graft. The transfer is sutured in place with the arm positioned in full extension. The wounds are closed and the arm placed in a long arm orthosis in complete extension.

Biceps Transfer

The biceps tendon is routed around the medial side of the humerus, either over or under the ulnar nerve. The musculocutaneous nerve is identified just lateral to the biceps tendon and is protected throughout the procedure. The lacertus fibrosis is incised, and the biceps tendon is traced into the forearm toward its insertion into the radial tuberosity. The biceps tendon is released and transferred around the medial aspect of the arm (Fig. 60-19).

A third 7-cm posterior incision is made over the distal third of the triceps and curved around the olecranon. The triceps is sharply split over the tip of the olecranon, and the biceps tendon is passed obliquely through the medial portion of the triceps tendon and attached to the olecranon (Fig. 60-20). The limb is maintained in full extension, and the subcutaneous tissue and skin closed with nonabsorbable

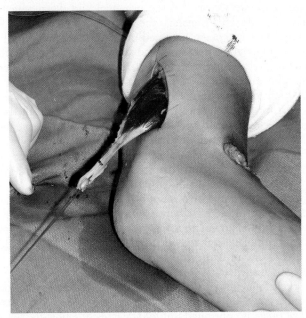

Figure 60-19 Biceps tendon transfer for elbow extension. The biceps tendon is released from the radial tuberosity and transferred around the medial aspect of the arm. (Courtesy of Shriners Hospital for Children, Philadelphia.)

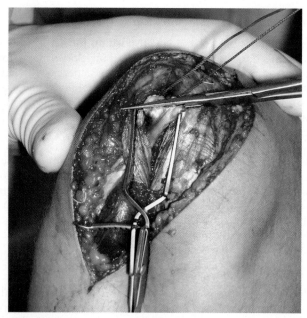

Figure 60-20 Biceps tendon transfer for elbow extension. The biceps tendon is passed obliquely through a split in the triceps tendon and attached to the olecranon. (Courtesy of Shriners Hospital for Children, Philadelphia.)

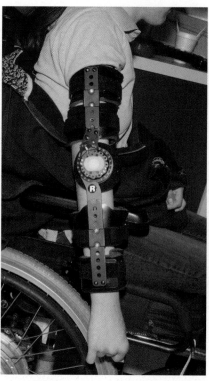

Figure 60-21 A dial-hinge brace (e.g., Bledsoe Brace Systems, Prairie, Texas) is used to monitor amount of allowable flexion. (Courtesy of Shriners Hospital for Children, Philadelphia.)

sutures. The tourniquet is deflated, and dressings and a well-padded long arm cast are applied in the operating room.[29]

Postoperative Management

Regardless of the muscle transfer for elbow extension, the initial postoperative regimen is similar. The arm is placed in an orthosis or cast for 3 to 6 weeks' time depending on the status and effectiveness of the proximal and distal transfer sites. For biceps transfer, shoulder elevation above 90 degrees and extension past neutral are not allowed until 6 weeks after surgery. During the immobilization phase the patient and caregivers are educated on edema management techniques.[29]

An elbow extension orthosis in full extension is then fabricated for nighttime use. A dial-hinge brace (e.g., Bledsoe Brace Systems, Prairie, Texas) is fitted for daytime use and acts as a flexion block at 15 degrees (Fig. 60-21). The brace is adjusted each week to allow an additional 15 degrees of flexion. The brace is not advanced if an extension lag develops. Tendon transfer firing is started in an antigravity plane. The medially routed biceps can be palpated along the medial humerus during active elbow extension. Verbal prompting of active elbow flexion and forearm supination facilitate motor learning. Biofeedback may be used in patients who have difficulty with initiating the transfer or if co-contraction of antagonist muscles is occurring.

Functional activities of daily living are incorporated into the therapy as elbow flexion increases each week. The dial-hinge brace is continued until 90 degrees of elbow flexion is achieved without an extension lag. A nighttime extension orthosis is maintained until 12 weeks. Strengthening is started 3 months after surgery.

Results

Biceps-to-triceps tendon transfer has been shown to effectively produce antigravity elbow extension (Fig. 60-22). In our series of nine patients, eight achieved three fifths or greater elbow extension following tendon transfer. All patients experienced greater reachable workspace and were satisfied with their results.[29]

Forearm

Biceps Rerouting

Biceps rerouting[38] is the preferred technique at our facility for supple supination deformities of the forearm to improve the position. A Z-incision is designed with a horizontal limb across the antecubital fossa (Fig. 60-23). The biceps tendon is traced to its insertion into the radial tuberosity, and a Z-plasty of the biceps tendon is performed along its entire length to ensure sufficient tendon length for passage around the radius (Fig. 60-24). The distal Z-plasty is left attached to the insertion site, and the proximal Z-plasty is left attached to the muscle belly.

The distal attachment is carefully rerouted around the radius through the interosseous space to create a pronation force (Fig. 60-25). The elbow is placed in 90 degrees of flexion and the forearm in pronation. The rerouted distal tendon is repaired back to the proximal tendon that is still attached to the biceps muscle (Fig. 60-26). A long arm cast is applied with the elbow in 90 degrees of flexion and the forearm in pronation for 5 weeks.

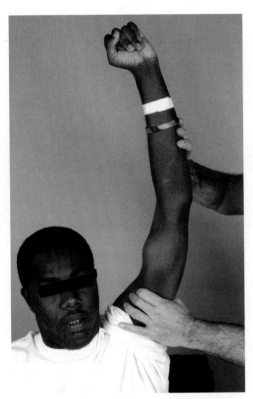

Figure 60-22 A 16-year-old male following biceps-to-triceps tendon transfer with strong antigravity elbow extension. (Courtesy of Shriners Hospital for Children, Philadelphia.)

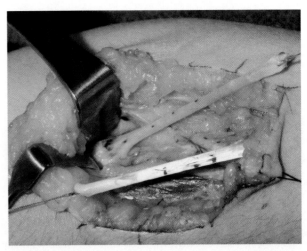

Figure 60-24 Biceps tendon rerouting for forearm deformity. Z-plasty of the biceps tendon along its entire length to ensure sufficient tendon length for passage around the radius. (Courtesy of Shriners Hospital for Children, Philadelphia.)

only 8 weeks after surgery and discontinued at 12 weeks. During the mobilization phase, passive elbow extension and supination are avoided. Light strengthening activities for elbow flexion and pronation can be introduced 8 weeks postoperatively.[26,27]

Frequently, minimal therapy is needed after surgery. During early mobilization the focus is on active ROM, including gentle elbow extension and supination. The forearm will naturally pronate with elbow flexion. Scar management is initiated as soon as the incisional scars are closed. Self-care and other light functional activities that promote pronation should be introduced, such as keyboarding. These are all completed as part of the home program.

The improved pronated position of the forearm enhances the patient's use of the hand for many activities of daily living (Fig. 60-28). A loss of supination ROM is expected and should be discussed before surgery.[27]

After 5 weeks of immobilization, the cast is removed and rehabilitation is started. A long arm orthosis is fabricated with the elbow in a resting position with the forearm pronated and the wrist in neutral or slightly extended position (Fig. 60-27). An alternative to this is a long forearm-based orthosis that prevents supination but allows elbow motion. The orthosis is removed for bathing and home program during the first week. The orthosis is weaned to night use

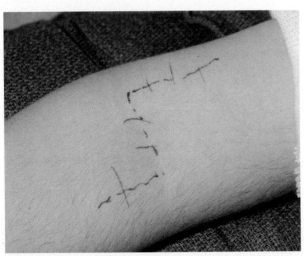

Figure 60-23 Biceps tendon rerouting for forearm deformity. A Z-incision is designed with a horizontal limb across the antecubital fossa. (Courtesy of Shriners Hospital for Children, Philadelphia.)

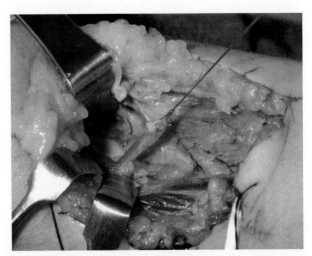

Figure 60-25 The distal biceps tendon is rerouted around the radius through the interosseous space to create a pronation force. (Courtesy of Shriners Hospital for Children, Philadelphia.)

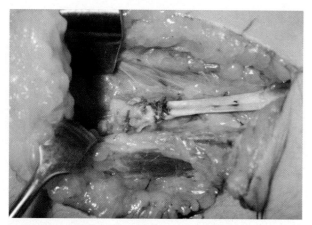

Figure 60-26 The rerouted distal tendon is repaired back to the proximal tendon that is still attached to the biceps muscle. (Courtesy of Shriners Hospital for Children, Philadelphia.)

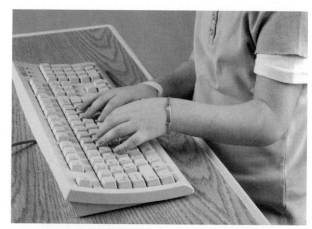

Figure 60-28 Improved pronated position of the left forearm facilitates keyboard usage. (Courtesy of Shriners Hospital for Children, Philadelphia.)

Osteotomies

Humeral Osteotomies

A humeral osteotomy can greatly improve an individual's function. For patients with an internal rotation contracture and advanced glenohumeral joint deformity, changing the resting position of the arm can greatly improve activities requiring external rotation. Likewise, patients who have external rotation without internal rotation for midline tasks, such as fastening buttons or zippers on pants, would benefit from humeral osteotomy. The preoperative examination must include a careful measurement of the patient's active arc of motion, the functional goals, and must consider the amount of movement that must be preserved to maintain current functional status. Simulation of both internal and external rotation activities, such as hair washing and fastening pants with passive assistance, allows the therapist to measure how much motion is required for the individual to complete each task (Fig. 60-29). The assessment must compare active arc of motion and consider the available

compensatory movements, such as wrist flexion to achieve hand-to-belly movement, before giving a final recommendation regarding amount of correction.

We prefer a medial arm incision along the medial intermuscular septum to hide the scar. The interval between the anterior and posterior arm musculature is developed, and the medial intermuscular septum is identified. The ulnar nerve lies just posterior to the septum, and the median nerve and brachial artery are anterior. The periosteum is incised, and reverse retractors are carefully placed anterior and posterior to the humerus.

The length of the humeral shaft necessary for osteotomy and plate fixation is exposed. The size of the plate depends upon the size of the humerus. Usually, a 2.7- or 3.5-mm plate is selected with six or seven holes. The desired amount of external rotation is determined before surgery, and a Kirschner wire is drilled in an oblique angle to simulate the amount of correction. A fine-bladed saw is selected and a transverse osteotomy performed perpendicular to the bone (Fig. 60-30). The humerus is externally rotated, and the osteotomy is reduced. The plate and screws are applied in

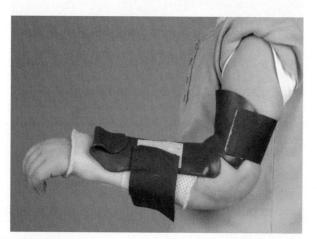

Figure 60-27 Two-piece supracondylar orthosis following immobilization phase after biceps rerouting. (Courtesy of Shriners Hospital for Children, Philadelphia.)

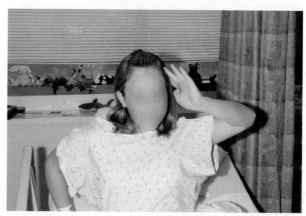

Figure 60-29 A 14-year-old with internal rotation contracture and inability to touch her ear or back of her neck. (Courtesy of Shriners Hospital for Children, Philadelphia.)

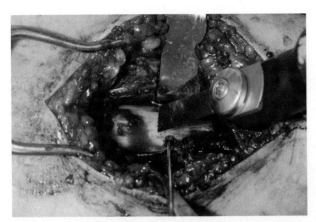

Figure 60-30 A Kirschner wire is drilled in an oblique angle to simulate the amount of correction, and a fine-bladed saw is used for osteotomy. (Courtesy of Shriners Hospital for Children, Philadelphia.)

standard fashion (Fig. 60-31). Wound closure is straightforward using absorbable sutures. The limb is wrapped in a bulky dressing from the hand to the axilla. No orthosis is utilized, although ample dressing is applied to "immobilize" the limb. The elbow is positioned in 90 degrees of flexion.[45] The fingers are left free for early motion. The arm is placed into a sling when the child is walking. The dressings are removed 2 weeks after surgery and radiographs taken to ensure bony alignment.

Based on healing and patient activity level, immobilization lasts for 2 to 6 weeks. Following dressing removal, a humeral fracture brace is fabricated to protect the healing bone (Fig. 60-32). The brace is worn at all times except during bathing until adequate healing is noted. Resistive activities and passive ROM are avoided until the bone healing is complete. Minimal therapy is required. The patient is educated on a home program of active ROM and scar management. Exercises to promote new movements such as hand to ear or neck (external rotation osteotomy) or hand to trunk (internal rotation osteotomy) are included. A few sessions may be necessary for the patient to adapt to the arm in the new position and maximize the functional potential.

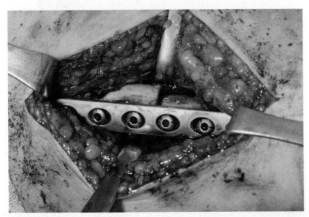

Figure 60-31 The humerus is externally rotated, the osteotomy is reduced, and the plate and screws are applied. (Courtesy of Shriners Hospital for Children, Philadelphia.)

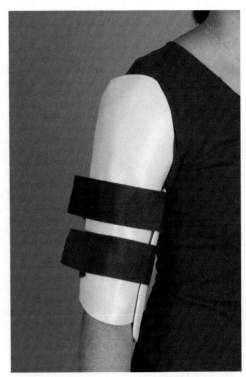

Figure 60-32 Humeral fracture brace to protect the osteotomy and to allow elbow motion. (Courtesy of Shriners Hospital for Children, Philadelphia.)

Humeral osteotomy does not improve overall glenohumeral motion but does enhance upper extremity function by allowing the arc of shoulder rotation to be in a more functional range.[24,31] This allows the hand to be placed in a better position to accomplish certain activities of daily living that require external rotation, such as washing hair, placing the hand on the neck, eating, and throwing a ball (Fig. 60-33). Mallet parameters improve for the desired goals, although some reciprocal loss of motion is expected.

Osteotomy of the Radius and Ulna

Mild rigid supination deformities can be treated with osteotomy of the radius or ulna.[27] However, severe supination deformities require osteotomy of the radius to maximize correction (Fig. 60-34). A separate incision is used for each osteotomy. Fixation is accomplished with a six- or eight-hole 2.4-mm titanium low-contact dynamic compression plate (Synthes USA, Paoli, Pennsylvania) (Fig. 60-35).

The proximal ulna is approached between the flexor carpi ulnaris and extensor carpi ulnaris muscles. The distal third of the radius is approached via a dorsal or radial approach between the extensor carpi radialis brevis and extensor pollicis longus tendons or between the brachioradialis and extensor carpi radialis longus tendons, respectively. Osteotomies of the radius and ulna are performed with a thin blade and sagittal saw under continuous irrigation to prevent heat necrosis (Fig. 60-36). The ulna plate is applied after the ulna is rotated into maximum pronation (Fig. 60-37). A similar technique is used across the osteotomy of the radius.

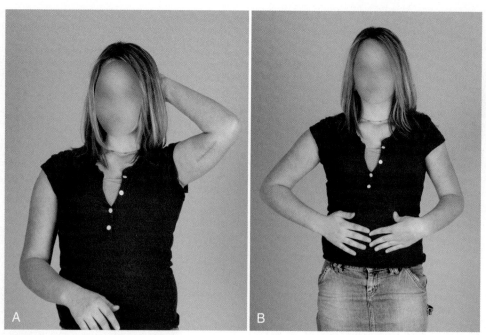

Figure 60-33 The 14-year-old shown in Figure 60-29 after external rotation osteotomy. **A**, Improved hand to ear and neck. **B**, Mild loss on internal rotation with wrist flexion required to place hand on navel. (Courtesy of Shriners Hospital for Children, Philadelphia.)

The forearm rotation is measured at the distal radioulnar joint (bi-styloid axis) using the elbow epicondylar axis as a guide. Inadequate pronation requires readjustment of the osteotomy sites until sufficient pronation is obtained. The subcutaneous tissue and skin are closed in routine fashion. A plaster orthosis is applied for 2 weeks instead of a cast, and the child is monitored overnight for neurovascular problems.

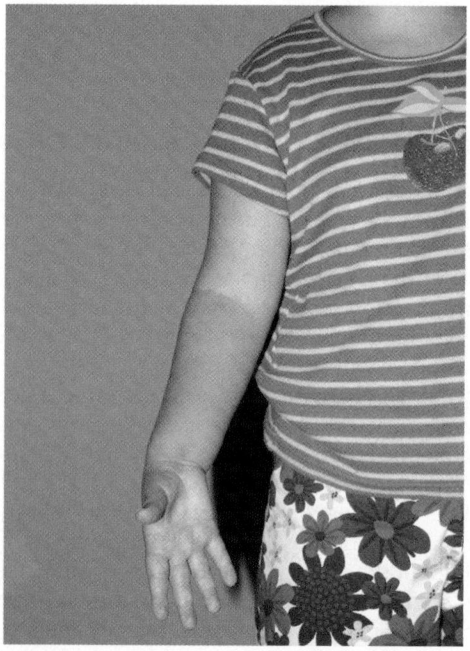

Based on healing and patient activity level, immobilization lasts for 4 to 6 weeks. Upon dressing removal a long forearm-based orthosis is fabricated to prevent rotation and protect the healing osteotomy. The orthosis should not limit elbow ROM. Clamshell or circumferential orthoses offer additional

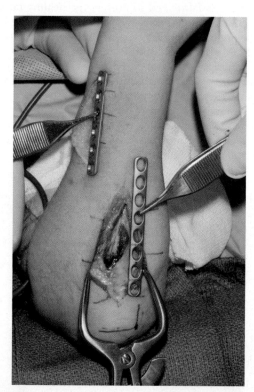

Figure 60-34 An 8-year-old female with residual brachial plexus birth palsy and fixed supination deformity. (Courtesy of Shriners Hospital for Children, Philadelphia.)

Figure 60-35 A separate incision is used for each osteotomy, and bony fixation is accomplished with a six- or eight-hole 2.4-mm titanium low-contact dynamic compression plate. (Courtesy of Shriners Hospital for Children, Philadelphia.)

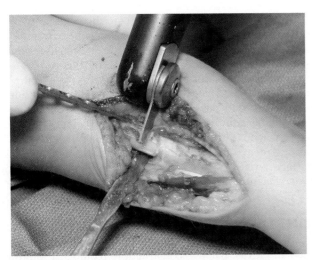

Figure 60-36 Osteotomy of the radius with a thin blade. (Courtesy of Shriners Hospital for Children, Philadelphia.)

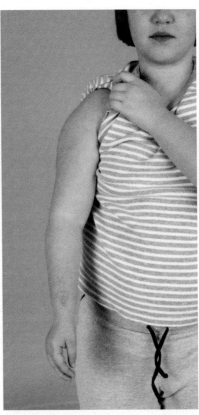

Figure 60-38 Improved forearm position of child shown in Figure 60-34 following osteotomy of the radius and ulna. (Courtesy of Shriners Hospital for Children, Philadelphia.)

support in highly active patients, especially young children. The splint is worn at all times except during bathing, therapy, and the supervised home program until adequate healing is noted. Minimal therapy is often required. The patient is educated on a home program of active ROM and scar management. If the patient's arm was fixed in supination before surgery, active wrist and digital extension exercises should be included in the regimen. Functional activities are incorporated into the home program to reeducate the patient to use the hand in the new position. Light functional activities should be initiated at first visit. The patient may need guidance to compensate for forearm rotation with shoulder and elbow movements.[26]

Osteotomy of the radius or ulna reliably corrects mild fixed-supination deformities. Osteotomy of the radius and ulna can achieve up to 100 degrees of correction.[46] The improved forearm position translates into better ability to perform activities of daily living that require pronation, such as keyboarding and desktop tasks (Fig. 60-38). Complications are related to bony union and inadequate correction. Careful preoperative assessment and postoperative protection will minimize these complications.

Shoulder Arthrodesis

In some cases there is extensive loss of the muscles about the shoulder girdle without available donors for transfer. Persistent shoulder instability and recalcitrant pain can prohibit use of the elbow and hand. In these cases, arthrodesis is the only option to restore stability, eliminate pain, and provide a stable platform for extremity reconstruction and function.[47,48] Minimal therapy is needed with focus on active ROM of the scapula muscles, strengthening of muscles distal to the shoulder, and adaptive techniques to accommodate for limited shoulder motion.[49,50]

Shoulder arthrodesis relies on the scapulothoracic muscles for motion and predictably corrects painful glenohumeral

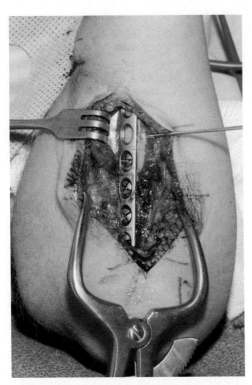

Figure 60-37 The ulna plate is applied after the ulna has been rotated into maximum pronation. (Courtesy of Shriners Hospital for Children, Philadelphia.)

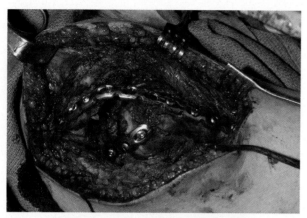

Figure 60-39 Right shoulder fusion with rigid internal fixation using plates and screws. (Courtesy of Shriners Hospital for Children, Philadelphia.)

subluxation. Absent scapular control is a contraindication for shoulder arthrodesis. The optimal position for fusion is controversial but should allow hand-to-mouth function with active elbow flexion. The preferred position is 30 degrees of abduction, 30 degrees of internal rotation, and 30 degrees of forward flexion. Numerous operative techniques have been described to achieve union. Rigid internal fixation is preferred, with plates and screws across the scapular spine and onto the lateral humerus (Fig. 60-39). Postoperative immobilization varies from an abduction pillow to a shoulder spica, depending on the quality of the bone and rigidity of the fixation. Shoulder arthrodesis reliably corrects painful

subluxation and provides stability to the extremity. This proximal stability will allow better use of the extremity via scapulothoracic motion and allow further restoration of distal function using additional tendon transfers.

Shoulder arthrodesis can enhance function in a limb with an unstable shoulder. Pain related to inferior subluxation of the humeral head can be effectively managed by arthrodesis. With a stable and fused proximal shoulder joint, patients are able to reach within their workspace, manipulate objects by grasping them with the hand and/or a brachiothoracic grasp, and incorporate the affected extremity in bimanual activities more efficiently.[49]

Summary

Brachial plexus palsy reconstruction requires a thorough examination of the upper quarter to determine what structures are in, which ones are not, what is available for reconstruction, and what is needed for function. Once the functional goals have been determined for the patient, the surgeon can identify the surgeries that will provide an optimal outcome. The surgeon and therapist must communicate the goals of the reconstructive procedures and develop the optimal postoperative plan of care to help the patient regain function and actively participate in activities of daily living, school, work, and avocational activities.

REFERENCES

The complete reference list is available online at www.expertconsult.com.

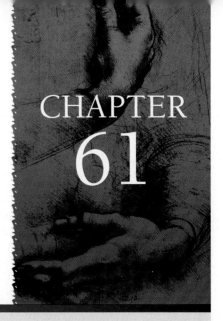

Nerve Transfers

THOMAS H. TUNG, MD

PRINCIPLES OF NERVE TRANSFER
INDICATIONS AND TIMING OF NERVE TRANSFERS
ANATOMY
PATIENT EVALUATION

MOTOR AND SENSORY TRANSFERS FOR ISOLATED
NERVE INJURIES
MOTOR AND SENSORY REEDUCATION
SUMMARY

CRITICAL POINTS

Donor Nerve

- Near target muscle
- Expendable
- Pure motor fibers
- As large a number of motor axons as possible
- Synergistic to target muscle

Transfer

- Tension free transfer through full range of motion
- Divide "donor distal" and "recipient proximal" to allow tension free nerve approximation
- If redundancy exists, trim recipient nerve to minimize distance from regenerating donor axons to target muscle motor endplates

Postop

- Appropriate therapy for motor re-education

Nerve injuries in the upper extremity frequently cause permanent disability with devastating consequences on daily living and the ability to work. Direct primary repair of a nerve transaction is advocated if possible and appropriate for the mechanism of injury. Large nerve gaps, proximal injuries with crush, transaction-, and avulsion-type injuries prohibit direct repair and require secondary nerve reconstruction after acute management and stabilization. Until the last century, the results of nerve repair in the extremity and especially of the brachial plexus were viewed with pessimism. In the latter half of the 20th century, advances in peripheral nerve surgery, including improvements in nerve repair and grafting techniques, and improved knowledge of internal topography, injury pattern, and regenerative ability of the peripheral nerve have contributed to better outcomes.

The level, mechanism, and severity of the injury determine the course of management and the timing of surgical procedures. Factors such as muscle atrophy after denervation and degeneration of the neuromuscular junction limit the opportunity for nerve reconstruction and adversely influence the outcome. If nerve fibers do not successfully reinnervate the target muscle within approximately 1 to 1.5 years of injury, the motor end plates disappear, the muscle architecture is destroyed, and muscle fibers are eventually replaced by fat with time. Therefore, "time is muscle," and with complex injury patterns it is imperative to closely follow the examination and results of diagnostic tests to make a clear diagnosis in a timely fashion such that reinnervation can occur before it is too late.

Advances in nerve repair and in the understanding of the internal topography of the nerve have contributed to the development of nerve transfers. Nerve-to-nerve transfers offer a superior alternative for functional restoration in isolated or multiple-nerve injuries when early reinnervation of the target end-organ is necessary, such as in proximal injuries or in delayed treatment. Expendable sensory or motor axons close to the end-organ allow for earlier regeneration and preclude the need for nerve grafts. Nerve transfers have traditionally been advocated for otherwise unsalvageable root avulsion injuries of the brachial plexus in which reconstruction with nerve grafts is suboptimal or not possible.[1] Nerve graft reconstruction of such proximal injuries requires regeneration over long distances before reaching target end-organs, frequently resulting in suboptimal functional recovery. The patient population with brachial plexus injury provided the stimulus for the application of novel reconstructive options that would offer faster reinnervation of muscles to minimize atrophy and degeneration of the motor end plate. Consequently, nerve transfers became a routine part of the early surgical management of upper brachial plexus injuries with very good outcomes. The experience with tendon transfers and an understanding of the principles of motor reeducation set the stage for the use of nerve transfers as an alternative to muscle or tendon transfers. The advantages typically include shorter operative time, shorter duration of morbidity and recovery, and faster target muscle reinnervation with less atrophy and motor end-plate fibrosis.

This writer has progressively applied this technique to more distal and isolated nerve injuries in the forearm and hand with encouraging results. As our understanding of the innervation patterns of muscles and the internal topography of peripheral nerves increases, our application of nerve transfers has become more widespread in the management of a range of peripheral nerve injuries, including those with more distal and isolated nerve trauma and those for which tendon transfers are conventionally recommended. My practice has evolved toward a broader application of distal nerve transfers to minimize operative time, morbidity, and recovery and to more quickly reinnervate target organs to optimize the functional outcome.

Principles of Nerve Transfer

Nerve transfers involve repair of the proximal aspect of a functioning motor nerve to the distal aspect of a nonfunctioning motor nerve of the target muscle. While many of the principles for nerve transfers are common to tendon transfers, there are unique considerations as well. Redundant and expendable nerve fascicles or branches of the donor nerve are utilized to minimize morbidity and the possibility of downgrading function. As with tendon transfers, a donor nerve that supplies muscles synergistic to the target muscle is preferred to facilitate postoperative therapy and motor reeducation. While a nerve supplying a nonsynergistic, or even antagonistic, muscle group may be used, the rehabilitation in such cases is more difficult and less intuitive, and functional recovery may be less optimal. Biomechanical considerations of muscle type and amplitude, vector, and tension that affect strength of a transferred muscle,[2,3] do not apply, since muscles reinnervated by nerve transfers maintain their anatomic location and attachments. Other advantages of a nerve transfer include (1) the capacity to restore sensibility in addition to motor function, (2) the possibility of restoring multiple muscle groups with a single nerve transfer, and (3) the avoidance of dissection and scarring of the muscle bed that may limit excursion and strength. If known, the donor nerve should have a similar number of nerve fibers as the recipient nerve. Intraplexal transfers may also be more effective than those that use extraplexal nerve donors,[4] generally because of proximity to the target muscles. The most critical factor for the success of a nerve transfer is the quality of the donor motor nerve in terms of axon count.

As with any peripheral nerve surgery, nerve transfer for restoration of motor function demands a timely approach. If nerve fibers do not reach the motor end plate within, ideally, 1 year of injury, the muscle will not work. Thus, an additional advantage of nerve transfer surgeries is that the transfer does not need to be performed in the zone of injury but should be done close to the recipient nerve motor end plate. This in essence shifts a proximal-level nerve injury to a dis-

tal-level injury and avoids dissection in the original area of injury, which may have significant scarring—thus facilitating operative dissection.[5] Sensory reinnervation, on the other hand, can be performed at any time after injury. At the end of this section, specific operations and options for delayed restoration of motor function, with free-functioning muscle transfers, will be discussed.

Nerve transfers may also be used as an alternative to nerve grafting or primary repair in certain cases because of the ability to convert a proximal high-level nerve injury to a low-level nerve injury. For example, a high radial nerve injury may be treated by transfer of redundant median nerve branches [to the flexor digitorum superficialis (FDS) and palmaris longus (PL)] to distal radial nerve branches to reinnervate the extensor carpi radialis brevis (ECRB) and the muscles innervated by the posterior interosseus nerve. The transfer is performed at the proximal forearm, allowing more timely restoration of wrist and finger extension.[6] Proximal ulnar nerve injuries also benefit from distal transfer. The anterior interosseus nerve (just proximal to the pronator quadratus) is transferred to the deep motor branch of the ulnar nerve to restore intrinsic hand function.[7-9] Another very specific nerve transfer procedure may be used for restoration of pronation.[10] A redundant branch to the FDS may be used. In this case, nerve transfer is quite important as there are limited tendon transfer–based alternatives.[11] The donor nerves are selected based on the proximity to the neuromuscular junction of the target muscle to minimize the reinnervation time, and the repair is done without tension. Nerve grafts are used if necessary; however, a primary repair is preferable, and is the routine. Internal neurolysis allows for dissection of donor and recipient fascicles from the main nerve to enable an end-to-end repair whenever possible.[12,13] We often perform distal-nerve transfers simultaneous with proximal-nerve graft reconstruction to avoid the formation of a painful proximal neuroma.

Indications and Timing of Nerve Transfers

The surgical indications for nerve transfers continue to evolve as new donor sources for motor and sensory restoration are proposed and evaluated. Because of the excellent results that can be obtained from nerve transfer, we advocate its use in almost any case where regeneration distance and time to reinnervation can be significantly reduced to improve outcome, and to avoid surgery under hostile tissue conditions, especially where other critical structures have already been reconstructed such as vascular injuries. We prefer to use a nerve transfer in managing the following conditions:

1. Brachial plexus injuries where only very proximal or no nerve is available for grafting
2. High proximal injuries that require a long distance for regeneration
3. Avoidance of scarred areas in critical locations with potential for injury to critical structures
4. Major limb trauma with segmental loss of nerve tissue

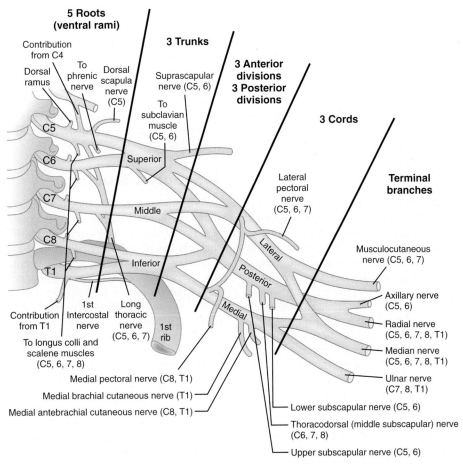

**5 Roots
(ventral rami)**

Contribution from C4

Dorsal ramus

To phrenic nerve

Dorsal scapula nerve (C5)

C5

C6

C7

C8

T1

Superior

Middle

Inferior

Contribution from T1

1st Intercostal nerve

Long thoracic nerve (C5, 6, 7)

1st rib

To longus colli and scalene muscles (C5, 6, 7, 8)

Medial pectoral nerve (C8, T1)

Medial brachial cutaneous nerve (T1)

Medial antebrachial cutaneous nerve (C8, T1)

3 Trunks

Suprascapular nerve (C5, 6)

To subclavian muscle (C5, 6)

**3 Anterior divisions
3 Posterior divisions**

3 Cords

Lateral pectoral nerve (C5, 6, 7)

Lateral

Posterior

Medial

Terminal branches

Musculocutaneous nerve (C5, 6, 7)

Axillary nerve (C5, 6)

Radial nerve (C5, 6, 7, 8, T1)

Median nerve (C5, 6, 7, 8, T1)

Ulnar nerve (C7, 8, T1)

Lower subscapular nerve (C5, 6)

Thoracodorsal (middle subscapular) nerve (C6, 7, 8)

Upper subscapular nerve (C5, 6)

Figure 61-1 Schematic illustration of brachial plexus.

5. As an alternative to nerve grafting when time from injury to reconstruction is prolonged
6. Partial nerve injuries with a defined functional loss
7. Spinal cord root avulsion injuries
8. Nerve injuries wherein the level of injury is uncertain, such as with idiopathic neuritides or radiation trauma and nerve injuries with multiple levels of injury

Recovery of motor function depends on a critical number of motor axons reaching the target muscle and reinnervating muscle fibers within a critical time period. Reinnervation of denervated muscles is generally not possible after 12 to 18 months in adults because of degeneration of the motor end plate. Axonal regeneration occurs at a rate of 1 inch per month or 1 to 1.5 mm/day.[14] The use of distal-nerve transfers can significantly prolong the "window" of opportunity following injury for surgical intervention. A distal-nerve transfer within centimeters of the neuromuscular junction of the target muscle will still have the potential for successful reinnervation even if performed late (8 to 10 months) after the injury.

Anatomy

The use of nerve transfers requires an intimate knowledge of anatomic details of peripheral neuroanatomy. The major nerves of interest derive from the brachial plexus. A few other nerves are mentioned primarily for their use as donor nerves in nerve transfer procedures.

The brachial plexus is the bridge from the spinal cord nerve roots to the terminal nerve branches that innervate the upper extremity (Fig. 61-1). The cervical fifth through eighth (C5–C8) and thoracic first (T1) nerve roots (with variable inclusion of the fourth cervical and second thoracic roots) form the three trunks. The upper (C5 and C6), middle (C7), and lower (C8 and T1) trunks then each divide into an anterior and posterior division. These six divisions then form three cords, with the three posterior divisions becoming the posterior cord, the two anterior upper divisions forming the lateral cord, and the remaining anterior division forming the medial cord. The cords then divide into the terminal nerve branches. The lateral cord goes to the musculocutaneous and median nerves. The posterior cord goes to the axillary and radial nerves. The medial cord goes to the ulnar and median nerves. Note that the median nerve receives components both from the lateral and medial cords.

Specific nerves originate at each segment, with the exception of the divisions, and the pattern of functional deficit will provide clues as to the location and level of injury. Injuries that result in isolated motor or sensory defects are either very proximal or distal. For example, a pure motor injury may indicate a central or motor root lesion or injury to a terminal motor nerve branch such as the anterior interosseous nerve (AIN). A pure sensory nerve injury may involve dorsal root ganglion level injury or injury to a terminal sensory nerve branch such as the lateral antebrachial cutaneous nerve. Mixed patterns of motor and sensory loss indicate an injury in the middle, for example, to the radial nerve. Further examination of function along that nerve helps pinpoint the exact level of injury. For example, if triceps function is maintained but distal wrist and finger extension is lost, the level of radial nerve injury is distal to the takeoff of the nerve branches to the triceps muscle. On the other hand, if a root level injury is suspected, it is important to determine if the injury is very proximal with associated root avulsions. Loss of function of the rhomboids, serratus anterior, or diaphragm hints at a very proximal level of nerve injury. This is because the nerves to these muscles—dorsal scapular, long thoracic, and phrenic, respectively—all originate quite close to the spinal cord. An associated Horner's syndrome, due to damage to the sympathetic ganglia, also suggests a proximal level of nerve injury. Diagnosis of a proximal or root avulsion injury can significantly change management strategies, because simple repair or interpositional grafting will not be possible.[15]

Other nerves that are relevant for the upper extremity peripheral nerve surgeon include ones used in nerve transfer procedures such as the spinal accessory, intercostal, and phrenic nerves. These are usually not involved in brachial plexus or more distal upper extremity nerve injuries and can serve as relatively expendable donor material. Other nerves of interest are used for interpositional nerve grafting in cases wherein direct end-to-end repair is impossible. Historically, expendable graft material (with the respective length of graft each provides) has been harvested from sensory nerves such as the sural (30–40 cm) and medial (20 cm), and lateral (5–8 cm) antebrachial cutaneous nerves.[16]

Patient Evaluation

History and physical examination are important in the assessment and management of peripheral nerve problems. The extent of injury and any spontaneous recovery should be carefully assessed. Critical information includes the mechanism and time of injury, associated concomitant injuries, and, when considering nerve transfers, the availability of motor nerve branches as potential donor nerves.

As with any functional reconstructive procedure, active and passive range of motion at each joint and function of specific muscles should be assessed and optimized. In chronic injuries, passive range of motion may be limited by joint contracture, which should be treated first by physical or occupational therapy. Motor function may be graded using the standard British Medical Research Council scale. Beginning proximally, strength of shoulder abduction and internal and external rotation are measured. Assess elbow flexion and extension with direct palpation of biceps and brachioradialis musculotendinous units. Forearm pronation, supination, wrist extension, flexion, and radial and ulnar deviation are graded. Hand function, including both intrinsic and extrinsic function, is assessed.[17] An examination of sensation by light touch, evaluation of two-point discrimination, and the ten test also will help to pinpoint the level of injury.

The ten test compares sensation in the normal and abnormal areas. As both a normal and abnormal area are touched, the patient is asked to grade the sensation compared to normal or 10 out of 10 sensation. The abnormal area is given a score on a scale from 0, no sensation, to 10, normal sensation.[18,19] This can be helpful, especially in children as they are often able to at least differentiate between normal and abnormal when the two sides are compared. Putative donor nerves for nerve or tendon transfer should be carefully assessed individually.

Diagnostic Studies

Imaging tests can be used to determine associated injuries that may change treatment options as well as demonstrate severity of the primary nerve injury. Plain films of any areas that are suspected of being injured should be performed immediately. For motor vehicle trauma patients these routinely include cervical spine and chest films. For patients with brachial plexus injury, rib fractures on the affected side preclude later use of intercostal nerves for nerve transfer. An elevated hemidiaphragm may indicate a phrenic nerve injury, which would prohibit use of the affected phrenic nerve. An upper extremity angiogram delineates associated vascular injury. Direct assessment of the upper extremity nerve lesion by imaging modalities is still relatively crude. A pseudomeningocele visible on CT myelogram suggests nerve root avulsion.[20] Because the pseudomeningocele may not be visible initially, this test should be done at 3 to 4 weeks postinjury. MRI can also be helpful to show changes such as neuroma formation and serves as a noninvasive method for diagnosis of root avulsion, although CT myelogram remains the gold standard.[21,22] A normal-appearing CT myelogram or MRI scan does not obviate the need for operative intervention, however.

Nerve conduction studies may be used to assess action potentials across putative lesion sites. If the action potential is preserved, neurolysis alone may be sufficient; lack of a potential is usually fairly definitive evidence that some intervention is required to restore function. Some groups also use sensory evoked potentials for brachial plexus injuries to see if lesions are pre- or postganglionic.[17,23] This also helps in determining whether proximal exploration and grafting will be of any use at all (preganglionic lesions indicate nerve root avulsion, which is not amenable to this). We rely less on electrodiagnostic tests to identify postganglionic lesions that allow proximal exploration with excision of neuroma and grafting because of our preference for distally based nerve transfer procedures and the often suboptimal outcomes associated with the reconstruction of proximal lesions and long nerve grafts.

Electromyography may show changes indicating recovery in muscles, but the level of recovery may not be clinically sufficient. Therefore, electromyography is most useful when used to serially track function and, especially early on, may justify some watchful waiting. Overall, electromyography is best used as an adjunct to document spontaneous reinnervation as demonstrated by the presence of motor unit potentials.[24] If there is evidence of progressive reinnervation, in a timely fashion after injury, then operative intervention may be unnecessary.

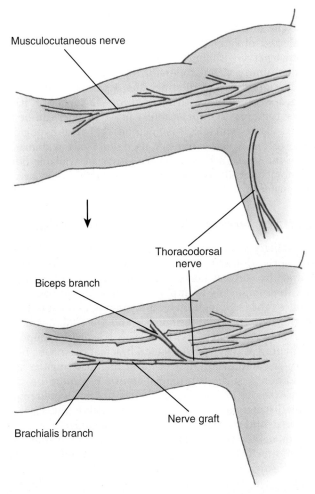

Figure 61-2 Transfer of thoracodorsal nerve to the musculocutaneous nerve.

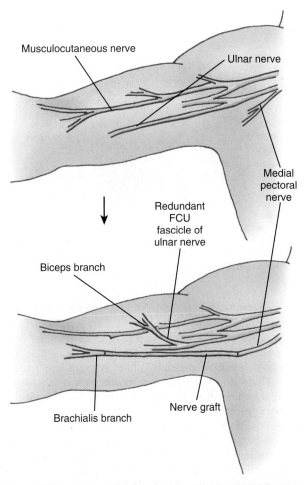

Figure 61-3 Modified Oberlin procedure with transfer of flexor carpi ulnaris (FCU) fascicle of ulnar nerve to the biceps branch of the musculocutaneous nerve and medial pectoral nerve branches to the brachialis branch using a nerve graft.

Motor and Sensory Transfers for Isolated Nerve Injuries

Musculocutaneous Nerve— Elbow Flexion

The restoration of elbow flexion is the top reconstructive priority in the patient with brachial plexus injury. Donor muscles used for the restoration of elbow flexion include the pectoralis major, latissimus dorsi, triceps, and the Steindler flexorplasty using the flexor–pronator musculature. Similarly, the nerves that supply these muscles can be used to reinnervate the biceps brachii and brachialis muscles (Fig. 61-2).[25] Historically, the first donor nerves used were either several intercostal nerves with or without interposition nerve grafts or the spinal accessory nerve transferred to the musculocutaneous nerve. In a meta-analysis of the English literature, Merrell et al. found the use of the spinal accessory nerve to be superior to the intercostal nerves for restoration of any function; however, in patients with grade 4 biceps strength, the intercostal nerves were more reliable for transfer to restore strength.[26] In 1993, we described our results with use of medial pectoral nerve branches transferred to the

musculocutaneous nerve.[27] This transfer moved the level of the repair more distal than previous reconstructions to allow faster reinnervation, and bypassed the coracobrachialis branch to allow more motor axons to reach the biceps and brachialis muscles. In addition, the lateral antebrachial cutaneous nerve was transposed proximally to neurotize the biceps muscle to redirect motor fibers that had regenerated into the lateral antebrachial cutaneous back to the target muscle.

In 1994, Oberlin et al. described a more distal repair by coapting a fascicle of the ulnar nerve in the upper arm directly into the biceps branch of the musculocutaneous nerve.[28] Leechavengvongs et al.[29] and Sungpet et al.[30] later reported excellent results from this transfer in 32 and 36 cases, respectively, with rapid motor recovery of the biceps muscle between M3 and M4 strength with no functional donor morbidity. Given that the brachialis muscle is a stronger elbow flexor than the biceps brachii muscle, we have modified Oberlin's procedure to reinnervate both the biceps and the brachialis branches of the musculocutaneous nerve so as to maximize elbow flexion strength (Fig. 61-3).[31,32]

While the best option to restore elbow flexion will depend on donor nerve availability, our preference is to transfer redundant motor fascicles of the ulnar nerve and the median

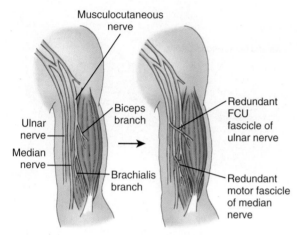

Figure 61-4 Transfer of fascicles of ulnar and median nerves to the biceps and brachialis branches of the musculocutaneous nerve. FCU, flexor carpi ulnaris.

nerve to both the biceps and the brachialis branches of the musculocutaneous nerve (Fig. 61-4).[33] Either donor fascicle may be coapted to either recipient nerve branch. Recent studies have shown that fibers of a distinct fascicular group are located adjacent to each other, even in the proximal limb.[34] There are, however, significant plexus interconnections at the midarm level, and the fascicle length and diameter vary considerably.[35,36] An intraoperative decision is made based on the ability to neurolyse and approximate the nerves to each other, as well as match comparable size of the nerve fascicular diameter. When the median or ulnar nerves cannot be used, other successful nerve transfer donors include the medial pectoral, thoracodorsal, or intercostal nerves.

Suprascapular Nerve—Shoulder Abduction and External Rotation

Reinnervation of the suprascapular nerve is second in importance only to restoration of elbow flexion in the paralyzed upper extremity. A patient able to externally rotate the shoulder not only has better shoulder control but can flex the elbow through a more functional range. The suprascapular nerve originates from the upper trunk and passes across the posterior triangle of the neck through the scapular notch to innervate the supraspinatus and infraspinatus muscles. These muscles initiate abduction and external rotation, and stabilize the humeral head in the glenoid fossa. Muscle transfers used to reconstruct their function have historically included the trapezius muscle, latissimus dorsi, teres major, long head of the biceps, and the posterior deltoid muscle.[25,37] Described donor nerves for transfer to the suprascapular nerve include the distal portion of the accessory nerve, the thoracodorsal nerve, intercostal nerves, and medial pectoral nerves. A nerve graft may be used for reconstruction from a healthy C5–C6 root if available. Successful reinnervation is anticipated, as the distance from the donor nerve root or upper trunk to the target motor end plates is not prohibitive. The distal portion of the spinal accessory nerve after it has given off branches to the upper trapezius is an excellent source of donor motor axons.[12] As the trapezius rotates the scapula with shoulder abduction, the accessory nerve is a

synergistic donor and facilitates the postoperative rehabilitation. The distal end of the spinal accessory can usually be transferred directly to the proximal portion of the suprascapular nerve with an end-to-end repair (Fig. 61-5).

To minimize scapular winging that may be associated with denervation of part of the trapezius, a partial neurectomy in the accessory nerve with an end-to-side repair or partial accessory nerve–to–suprascapular nerve transfer can be performed. This principle is similar to the hemi-hypoglossal nerve–to–facial nerve transfer used for facial reanimation. When the spinal accessory nerve is not an available donor, the thoracodorsal[13] or medial pectoral nerves[38] can be used for transfer.

Axillary Nerve—Shoulder Abduction

The axillary nerve arises from the posterior cord, passes posteriorly through the quadrangular space, and travels around the surgical neck of the humerus, dividing into at least three branches to supply the teres minor and deltoid muscles. The larger deltoid branch innervates the middle and anterior deltoid, while the smaller and most inferior branch innervates the posterior deltoid with a sensory component terminating as the superior lateral brachial cutaneous nerve. Injury or compression may occur at the quadrangular space in addition to a more proximal injury. If a more proximal injury exists, as in a brachial plexus injury that would require a long distance for regeneration, then a nerve transfer is our preferred option. Donor nerves have included the medial pectoral nerves, triceps branch of the radial nerve, intercostal nerves, spinal accessory nerve, and the thoracodorsal nerves for reconstruction of the axillary nerve.[26,39]

Our preferred reconstruction of deltoid muscle function is to transfer the branch(es) of the radial nerve to the long head of the triceps muscle to the deltoid branch of the axillary nerve using a posterior shoulder approach (Fig. 61-6).[40] The radial nerve usually gives off two to three redundant branches to the long head of the triceps. These branches are selected rather than those to the lateral or deep head because of their proximity to the axillary nerve and their favorable size. The transfer is performed to both motor branches supplying the deltoid while the cutaneous branch and nerve to the teres minor are excluded from the reconstruction. Occasionally, the superior lateral brachial cutaneous nerve divides from the posterior deltoid motor branch proximal to the muscle, but more often will pierce the deltoid along with the motor branches. The cutaneous branch is usually the most inferior branch of the axillary nerve, but it can be difficult to differentiate this from the motor branches entering the deltoid. A "tug-test" can be used to identify the sensory branch by placing gentle traction on the nerve, and observing for evidence of skin movement in the area of innervation. Traction on the cutaneous branch will cause some movement of the skin overlying the deltoid muscle, whereas traction on the motor branches will not.

Radial Nerve—Wrist and Finger Extension

Radial nerve injuries are typically reconstructed with direct nerve repair, nerve grafts, or tendon transfers. In selected

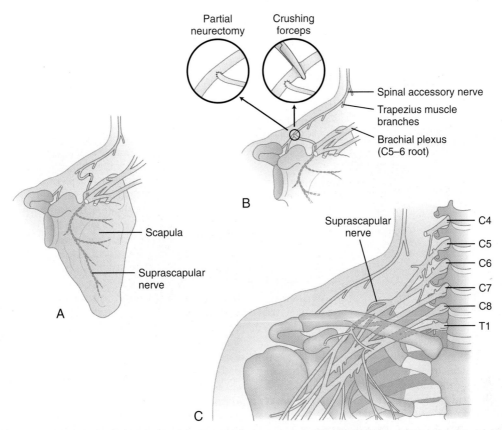

Figure 61-5 Transfer of distal accessory nerve to the suprascapular nerve in a direct end-to-end fashion or as an end-to-side transfer including a partial injury to the accessory nerve to stimulate axonal sprouting.

patients we have used nerve transfers to reconstruct radial nerve function (Fig. 61-7). At the proximal and midforearm, the branches of the median nerve are well described and consistent. Both the radial and median nerves can be readily exposed through a single longitudinal proximal volar forearm incision. A step-lengthening of the pronator teres tendon will facilitate the exposure of the more distal motor branches of the median nerve and especially the AIN. Redundant or expendable nerve branches to the FDS, flexor carpi radialis (FCR), or palmaris longus (PL) may be transferred to the

ECRB branch of the radial and posterior interosseous nerves (PINs).[41] We use the PL and the FDS or FCR branches to the PIN and the ECRB branch, respectively (see Fig. 61-7). The strongest donor (FCR) should be transferred to the ECRB to maximize wrist extension for optimal function. In addition, to restore sensation, the radial sensory branch can be coapted end-to-side to the median nerve at a location distal enough to prevent tension to the transfer. The flexor carpi ulnaris branch of the ulnar nerve provides another donor option; however, this requires a second incision.[42]

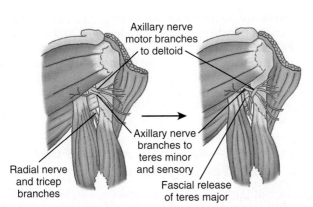

Figure 61-6 Direct transfer of a triceps branch of the radial nerve to the motor component of the axillary nerve through a posterior shoulder approach.

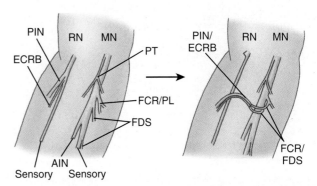

Figure 61-7 Transfer of the palmaris longus (PL) or flexor carpi radialis (FCR) and redundant flexor digitorum superficialis (FDS) branches of the median nerve (MN) to the extensor carpi radialis brevis (ECRB) and the posterior interosseous nerve (PIN) branches of the radial nerve (RN) for restoration of wrist and finger extension through a single proximal forearm exposure.

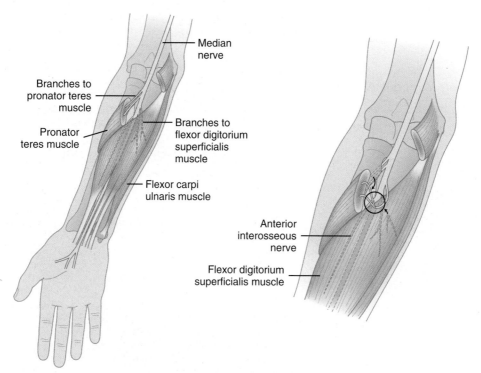

Figure 61-8 Transfer of redundant flexor digitorum superficialis branch of the median nerve to pronator teres branches of median nerve to restore pronation.

Median Nerve—Forearm Pronation, Thumb Opposition, and Finger Flexion

We have used motor nerve transfers reliably to restore pronation, thenar function, and flexor pollicis longus (FPL) function. If loss of pronation exists as an isolated deficit, a redundant or expendable branch from the ulnar or median nerve itself may be used to reinnervate the pronator teres.[43] The branches (usually two) to the pronator are found proximally at the level of the antecubital fossa. Nerve stimulation is used to identify the multiple branches of the median nerve. There are usually two or more branches to the FDS, and one or two can be transferred directly to the branches of the

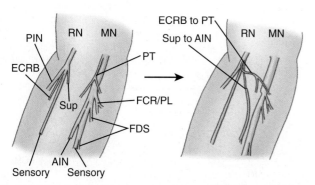

Figure 61-9 Transfer of the expendable extensor carpi radialis brevis (ECRB) and supinator branches of the radial nerve to the pronator and anterior interosseous nerve (AIN) branches of the median nerve for the restoration of pronation and critical digit and thumb function. FCR, flexor carpi radialis; FDS, flexor digitorum superficialis; MN, median nerve; PIN, posterior interosseous nerve; PL, palmaris longus; PT, pronator teres; RN, radial nerve; Sup, supinator.

pronator teres muscle by direct repair (Fig. 61-8). The PL if present or FCR branches may also be used. If the median nerve is not available to provide donor motor axons, then a redundant branch to the FCU from the ulnar nerve can be used.

In the case of combined ulnar and median nerve palsy with intact shoulder and elbow function, such as in C8 T1 avulsions, we have transferred the brachioradialis branch of the radial nerve to the proximal AIN with either a medial antebrachial cutaneous or medial brachial cutaneous nerve graft to restore finger flexion. Our current preference is to use expendable branches of the radial nerve such as the ECRB and the supinator branch to reinnervate the pronator and AIN branches of the median nerve (Fig. 61-9). This can be performed through a single proximal volar forearm exposure used for the median-to-radial nerve transfers described previously.

Thumb opposition can be effectively corrected with standard tendon transfers; however, the terminal AIN at the wrist can be used to reinnervate the motor branch of the median nerve with a short nerve graft. In the case of an isolated palsy of the FPL, another expendable motor branch of the median nerve, such as that to the PL, FDS, or FCR, can be used as donor axons for transfer to the FPL branch.

Ulnar Nerve—Intrinsic Muscle Function and Ulnar Sensory Loss

Recovery of intrinsic muscle function is uncommon following a high ulnar nerve injury, even with early repair,[43,44] and reconstruction with tendon transfers often yields less than satisfactory results.[25] Because the distance required for

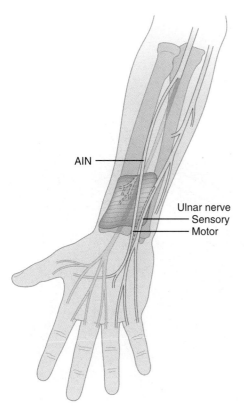

Figure 61-10 To restore ulnar motor function in the hand, the distal branch of the anterior interosseous nerve (AIN) to the pronator quadratus is transferred to the deep motor branch of the ulnar nerve.

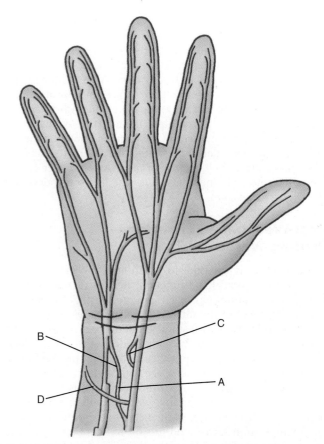

Figure 61-11 For ulnar sensation, the third-webspace fascicle of the median nerve (A) can be transferred to the sensory component of the ulnar nerve (B) at the distal forearm after neurolysis and fascicular dissection. The distal stump of the third-webspace fascicle (C) and the less critical dorsal cutaneous branch of the ulnar nerve (D) can be sutured end-to-side to the median nerve for protective sensation without additional donor morbidity.

regeneration is prohibitively long, the purpose of the nerve transfer in this setting is to convert the high ulnar nerve injury to a low ulnar nerve injury to significantly decrease the length of regeneration required. Patients with ulnar nerve palsy may also have significant pinch and grip weakness as well as clawing of the ulnar digits. If the median nerve is available as a donor nerve, the terminal AIN at the wrist can be transferred to the deep motor branch of the ulnar nerve (Fig. 61-10).[45,46] The disadvantage of this transfer is that it does not provide a synergistic donor and there is limited restoration of ulnar hand function. However, improvement is sufficient to prevent clawing and improve pinch strength, and tendon transfers have not been necessary[46] except for one patient who required a secondary tendon transfer for a persistent small-finger abduction deformity (Wartenberg's sign).[47] Clawing and finger flexion strength may be further improved by tenodesis of the flexor digitorum profundis tendons of the ring and small fingers side to side to the flexor digitorum profundis tendons of the index and long fingers.

Several options are available to restore ulnar nerve sensation. Unlike motor nerve transfers, there is no limit from the time of injury during which reconstruction must be performed to restore sensation. Traditionally an end-to-end transfer of the median nerve branch to the third webspace in the palm to the common ulnar sensory branch in the palm will divert sensation to the ulnar border of the hand. Alternatively, an end-to-side transfer of the ulnar sensory branch to the side of the third-webspace branch of the median nerve is possible, but recovery of sensation may be more limited. Another end-to-side option is to transfer both the sensory component of the ulnar nerve and its dorsal cutaneous branch to the median nerve in the distal forearm (Fig. 61-11). When an end-to-side transfer is performed, the perineurotomy is performed to produce limited and recoverable demyelination of the donor nerve that will increase sprouting without the need for a neurotomy.[48]

The fascicular transfer technique can also be used to reconstruct ulnar nerve sensation. The third webspace can also be used as a donor branch to restore more critical border digit sensation as a sensory fascicular transfer in the distal forearm (see Fig. 61-11). This is our preferred method when using the nerve branch to the third webspace as the donor nerve as in a high ulnar nerve injury or upper brachial plexus palsy. The internal topography of both the median and ulnar nerves at the wrist and forearm is well-defined and consistent. The motor and sensory components of each nerve are readily identified and dissected; in particular, the fascicle to the third webspace can be neurolysed for more than half the length of the forearm proximal to the wrist. However, the sensory fascicles of the ulnar nerve to the fourth webspace and to the ulnar border of the small finger have not in our experience been easily separated at this level. Consequently, our preference is to transfer the digital nerve branches in the palm when using the fourth-webspace branch as donor nerve, and fascicular transfer at the distal forearm when reconstructing ulnar nerve sensation, using the whole sensory component as the recipient nerve. As with all nerve transfers, the donor fascicle is divided as distally as possible and the recipient fascicle divided as proximally as possible, to maximize length and minimize tension at the repair site. Advantages of the fascicular transfer technique include the avoidance of scars on the contact surfaces of the palm and potential injury to the palmar vascular arches, and the ability to combine other procedures such as the terminal AIN transfer to the deep ulnar motor branch or side-to-side flexor tenodesis via a single wrist incision.

First-Webspace Sensation— Median Nerve

Proprioception is essential to pinch and fine motor movement and to overall hand function. Reconstruction of first-webspace sensation has been reported using expendable sensory branches of the ulnar and radial nerves as donors.[31] The main priority is to restore sensation particularly to the ulnar side of the thumb and radial side of the index finger. In some cases, as in an upper trunk brachial plexus injury, sensation to the third webspace will remain intact. The common digital nerve to the third webspace is transferred directly to the nerve to the first webspace in an end-to-end fashion. The distal stumps of the nerve to the third webspace can then be transferred end-to-side to the branch to the fourth webspace to recover some protective sensation to the donor nerves. Also, the common digital nerve to the second webspace can be transferred readily to the ulnar digital nerve to the small finger in the palm or as a fascicular transfer at the wrist.

In the case of a complete median nerve palsy, the common digital branch of the ulnar nerve to the fourth webspace, the dorsal sensory branch of the ulnar nerve, and the sensory radial nerve can all serve as donors.[31,49] As in any case, the repair to the first webspace is performed in an end-to-end fashion to maximize sensory recovery (Fig. 61-12).[50,51] The remaining common digital branches of the median nerve can then be sutured end-to-side to the ulnar or radial nerves for protective sensation. We have no preferred transfer for all instances, as the potential combinations are many, and the optimal transfer depends on the nerve injury, donor nerve availability, and patient preference.

Motor and Sensory Reeducation

The long-term focus of rehabilitation is on motor and/or sensory reeducation. As in tendon transfers, the patient must learn and be able to coordinate new pathways for target muscle activation. Following nerve transfer, the cortical command required to initiate target muscle contraction differs from what was previously needed. The patient "relearns" motor control of the reinnervated target muscle by activating the nerve to the donor muscle, which now stimulates the reinnervated muscle.[43] This concept is similar to the reeducation needed following tendon transfers. In addition, the ability to restore sensation can only improve recovery but

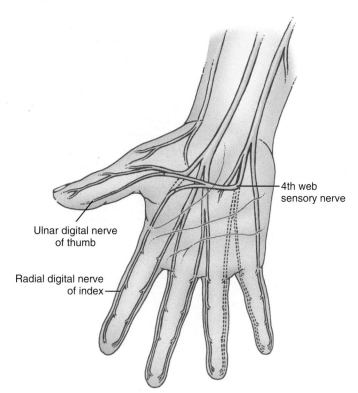

Figure 61-12 To restore critical median nerve sensation, the fourth-webspace branch of the ulnar nerve is transferred in an end-to-end manner to the median nerve branch to the first webspace.

Labels: 4th web sensory nerve; Ulnar digital nerve of thumb; Radial digital nerve of index

does not guarantee optimal function. Sensory reeducation begins when the patient begins to perceive input stimulus from the reinnervated territory. Cortical remapping occurs from continued sensory input from the newly innervated areas.

Summary

Significant advances in peripheral nerve surgery have been made in the last century. The introduction of microsurgical techniques has transformed peripheral nerve surgery into a sophisticated specialty with procedures that produce consistent results. The combined experience from brachial plexus surgery, muscle and tendon transfers, and motor and sensory reeducation has facilitated the evolution of nerve transfer techniques as a reliable surgical option for the treatment of nerve injuries. In the last decade, reconstruction of upper plexus injuries in our institution has progressed from the use of long-nerve grafts to elegant distal-nerve transfers. Our use of distal-nerve transfers far removed from the zone of injury allows us to restore function and sensibility with shorter operative time, through smaller incisions, with less morbidity, and to achieve comparable or better functional results than conventional approaches.

REFERENCES

The complete reference list is available online at www.expertconsult.com.

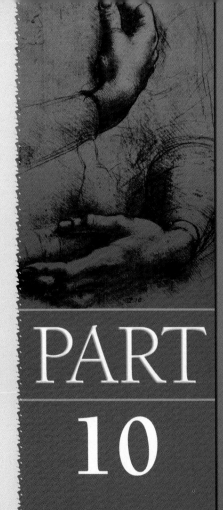

PART 10

Vascular and Lymphatic Disorders

Vascular Disorders of the Upper Extremity

DAVID HAY, MD, JOHN S. TARAS, MD, AND JEFFREY YAO, MD

VASCULAR ANATOMY
DIAGNOSTIC WORKUP
COMMON VASCULAR DISORDERS OF THE UPPER
   EXTREMITY
HAND SURGERY IN PARTICULAR POPULATIONS
SUMMARY

- Routine hand surgery has been found to have minimal risk in patients with previous axillary lymph node dissection or radical mastectomy.
- The risk of interrupting oral anticoagulation regimens for routine outpatient hand surgery probably outweighs the benefit of perioperative surgical risk reduction.

CRITICAL POINTS

- Understanding anatomy is key to understanding vascular injuries and disorders of the upper extremity.
- Thorough, systematic history and physical examination of the upper extremity is essential for the diagnosis of both acute and chronic conditions.
- Multiple specialized diagnostic and imaging tests are available to detail vascular conditions of the upper extremity.
- Traumatic injury to the upper extremity may be limb-threatening, and emergent surgical exploration is indicated if distal ischemia is present.
- Clinicians must have a high index of suspicion for compartment syndrome in the acutely painful, swollen extremity. Clinical diagnosis and emergent fasciotomy are essential to prevent permanent disability.
- Most cannulation and intravascular injection injuries may be treated with supportive measures provided that blood flow to the extremity is not compromised.
- Hypothenar hammer syndrome is seen almost exclusively in patients with repetitive vibratory trauma and/or history of smoking. The majority of patients will find relief with the cessation of these activities and initiation of oral vasodilator therapy.
- Vasospastic disease is most commonly idiopathic or associated with systemic sclerosis. Close coordination with a rheumatologist will allow the patient to enjoy the benefit of recent breakthroughs in treatment of this complex problem.
- Hemangiomas, vascular malformations, and peripheral aneurysmal disease deserve symptomatic treatment, which may include surgical excision in particular cases.

Vascular disorders of the upper extremity make up only approximately 5% of all vascular disease.[1] The relative infrequency of these disorders is contrasted by the potential range of presentation. The clinical picture may range from life-threatening hemorrhage in the emergency department, to subtle symptoms of pain with activity, color changes, or a mass presenting in clinic. Additionally, vascular disorders are often misdiagnosed. It is not unusual for a patient to consult several physicians over the course of 6 to 12 months before his or her problem is recognized and correctly diagnosed.

Vascular Anatomy

Arterial System

The brachial artery is the major inflow vessel to the forearm and hand. It arises from the axillary artery at the lower border of the teres major muscle.[2] At the level of the antecubital fossa, it dives below the lacertus fibrosus and divides into the two principal vessels of the forearm—the radial and ulnar arteries. Before this division, the profunda brachii artery anastomoses proximally with the posterior humeral circumflex beneath the deltoid, and distally with the recurrent branches of the radial and interosseous arteries. At the elbow, the superficial and inferior ulnar collateral arteries anastomose with the recurrent branch of the ulnar artery. Despite this extensive collateral network, interruption or thrombosis of the brachial artery is associated with acute ischemia of the distal limb in approximately 10% of cases (Fig. 62-1).[3]

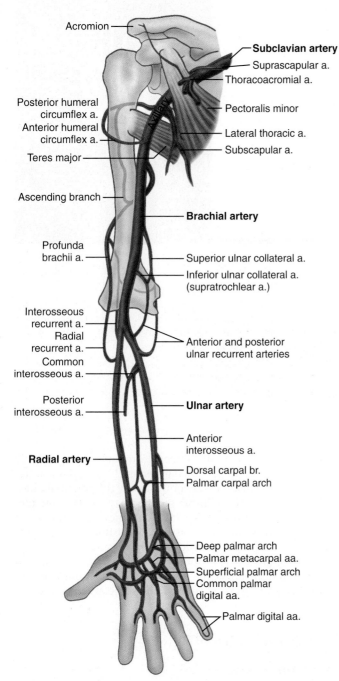

Acromion

Subclavian artery

Suprascapular a.

Thoracoacromial a.

Pectoralis minor

Posterior humeral circumflex a.
Anterior humeral circumflex a.

Teres major

Lateral thoracic a.

Subscapular a.

Ascending branch

Brachial artery

Profunda brachii a.

Superior ulnar collateral a.

Inferior ulnar collateral a. (supratrochlear a.)

Interosseous recurrent a.
Radial recurrent a.
Common interosseous a.

Anterior and posterior ulnar recurrent arteries

Posterior interosseous a.

Ulnar artery

Radial artery

Anterior interosseous a.

Dorsal carpal br.
Palmar carpal arch

Deep palmar arch
Palmar metacarpal aa.
Superficial palmar arch
Common palmar digital aa.

Palmar digital aa.

Figure 62-1 *The vascular anatomy of the upper extremity.*

In the forearm, the radial and ulnar arteries take divergent paths to the wrist. The radial artery remains relatively superficial beneath the brachioradialis muscle in association with the sensory branch of the radial nerve. Its major branch is the radial recurrent artery. Distally, it passes superficially, just lateral to the flexor carpi radialis tendon. At the level of the wrist, it subdivides into a smaller superficial palmar branch, which passes volarly through the thenar musculature and joins the superficial palmar arch. The larger branch passes to the dorsum of the wrist through the anatomic snuffbox and head of the first dorsal interosseous muscle. It then dives deeply to form the major contribution to the deep palmar arch.

The ulnar artery takes a deeper course to the hand. This vessel passes deep to the pronator teres and flexor digitorum superficialis before passing medially to lie deep to the flexor carpi ulnaris muscle and tendon in the distal forearm. It enters the hand via Guyon's canal medial to the ulnar nerve. The ulnar artery provides approximately 60% of the supply to the hand, the majority of which is through the superficial palmar arch. One of its branches at the level of the pisiform contributes to the deep palmar arch.

The ulnar artery has two important branches in the forearm. The ulnar recurrent artery anastomoses with the ulnar collateral branches of the brachial artery. The common interosseous artery arises in the proximal forearm and divides to form the anterior and posterior interosseous arteries. These two vessels travel distally along with the anterior and posterior interosseous nerves. The most distal volar carpal arch is the deep palmar arch.

The majority of blood flow to the hand is supplied by the palmar arches. The superficial arch, which lies distal to the deep arch at the same level as the abducted thumb tip, is in close proximity to the transverse carpal ligament and may be injured during carpal tunnel release. This arch is "complete" in 78.5% of specimens, either by the ulnar artery alone (37%) or from an anastomosis of the ulnar with the radial or interosseous artery (41.5%). An incomplete arch occurs when vessels other than the ulnar artery provide total flow to one or more digits. The thumb is the most common autonomous digit in hands with incomplete arches.[4] According to Coleman and Anson,[4] the deep palmar arch is less variable; they found complete arches in 98% of their specimens, but a more recent study by Ikeda et al.[5] found this pattern in only 77%.

The superficial palmar arch gives off the common digital vessels, which divide to form the proper digital arteries to the fingers. The deep arch gives rise to the princeps pollicis artery, which provides the majority of flow to the thumb via an ulnar volar vessel; this vessel is the one that is most frequently repaired in thumb revascularization. The branches of the deep arch—the deep palmar metacarpal arteries—terminate in the common palmar metacarpal arteries and supply the metacarpophalangeal joint and the interosseous musculature. The dorsal circulation to the hand is often overlooked, but it too provides alternative flow to the digits. Vessels that contribute to the dorsal circulation arise from dorsal branches of the radial and ulnar arteries as well as from the digital dorsal carpal arch. Blood flow to the digits comes predominantly through the common and proper digital arteries branching from the superficial palmar arch.[6] These vessels, which lie in close proximity to the digital nerves, form a ladder-like branching pattern that supplies the bones, joints, and flexor tendons. A corresponding but smaller dorsal network is the vascular supply to the extensor tendons. The digital arteries are larger on the ulnar side of the thumb, index, and long fingers, averaging 1.8 mm at the base of the proximal phalanges and 0.95 mm in the distal phalanges.[7]

There are many variations of the arterial anatomy of the forearm and hand. These anomalies have no particular significance in the normal state, but they may affect the diagnostic picture after injury and alter classic surgical anatomy. Significant variations occur in up to one-third of specimens. For example, the radial artery may originate proximal to the antecubital fossa in 15% of the population.[8] This vessel may be cannulated accidentally during venipuncture or lacerated during a surgical approach to the elbow and distal humerus. A vessel often confused with the radial artery is the superficial brachial artery, which divides distally into the radial and ulnar arteries, whereas the proper brachial artery supplies the distal interosseous artery.[9] A superficial brachial artery exists in 2% of specimens. Finally, a persistent median artery makes a contribution to the palmar arch in 15% of specimens.[10]

Venous System

Venous anatomy is best understood by proceeding from distal to proximal, in the direction of flow. Identifiable veins have been found distal to the nail fold in the lateral and volar positions.[11] These vessels are generally small, measuring 0.5 to 0.8 mm in diameter.[12] The first identifiable dorsal vessel is the terminal vein just proximal to the nail fold. The dorsal system is somewhat larger than the volar system, and these are the vessels used in replantation. These two systems are connected via oblique anastomotic veins. Dorsal and volar veins in the hand drain into the superficial cephalic and basilic veins as well as the deep venae comitantes of the radial and ulnar arteries. The radial and ulnar veins drain into the deep brachial vein, which combines with the basilic vein to form the axillary vein. The cephalic vein does not enter the deep system until just proximal to the clavicle, and it provides collateral circulation when the deep circulation is disrupted. The venous system of the upper extremity has more extensive variations than does the arterial system. However, these vessels usually are not significant unless proximal obstruction of the central venous system causes dilation of the superficial vessels.

Lymphatic System

The lymphatic system is often overlooked in studies of vascular anatomy and does not become clinically important unless obstruction causes swelling and edema of the extremity. Generally, the lymphatic drainage of the hand runs parallel to the superficial venous anatomy and arterial structures of the arm.[13] These two systems join at the level of the axillary lymph nodes, which become engorged and painful when the hand is infected.

Nervous System

Knowledge of the sympathetic nervous system completes one's understanding of the vascular anatomy. Fibers from the lower cervical and upper thoracic ganglia pass into the peripheral nervous system mainly by way of the median and ulnar nerves. However, all nerves that cross the wrist contribute sympathetic fibers to the hand and digits. These fibers control vessel constriction and dilation in response to physiologic stimuli such as cold or stress. They also may participate in pathologic processes such as complex regional pain syndrome (CRPS) and Raynaud's phenomenon.

Diagnostic Workup

History and Physical Examination

Most vascular disorders of the upper extremity may be diagnosed with an appropriate history and physical examination. The examination must be tailored to the clinical situation. An acute, life-threatening arterial injury with pulsatile bleeding is easily recognized. However, even in an emergent situation, assessment of the distal peripheral pulses and the patient's vascular status is mandatory. A brief but comprehensive neurologic examination distal to the traumatic injuries will reveal deficits that require exploration of nearby nerves at the time of vascular repair.

A more detailed history and physical examination are needed when evaluating an individual with nonacute symptoms. Questions and diagnostic tests are involved that are not part of the routine examination of a hand surgery patient. For this reason, the examiner is advised to use a comprehensive and organized data worksheet, which will ensure a complete evaluation as well as aid in diagnosis.

The most common presenting complaints in patients with vascular disorders are pain, color changes, cold intolerance, and skin changes. It is important to determine whether the symptoms are unilateral or bilateral. In addition, the patient's age, handedness, occupation, and work history should be noted.[14]

Pain is present in two thirds of patients with upper extremity vascular disease. Callow[15] notes that sudden arterial occlusion causes pain that is severe and abrupt in onset, but vasospasm may produce only mild paresthesias and marked pallor. Pain with exertion that is relieved by rest is most indicative of an obstructive arterial problem. In contrast, pain at rest may indicate severe arterial insufficiency, although it also could be symptomatic of a neurologic, bony, or other pathologic condition.

Color changes may be part of the "triple response" or Raynaud's phenomenon. Ischemic pallor usually is followed by cyanotic coloring, and a reactive erythema marks the return of flow. Cyanotic coloring also may occur in long-standing venous obstruction or insufficiency. Cold intolerance may manifest as a heightened sensitivity to cold climates, the winter months, or even the refrigerated sections of the grocery store. The patient may complain of mild to severe pain that is relieved when the extremity is warmed. Digital stiffness after exposure to cold also may indicate vascular disease. Thus, it is important to obtain a history of the patient's response to cold exposure. Skin complaints include changes in nail shape (clubbing) or quality (pitting). Skin atrophy often occurs in patients with scleroderma and may result in ulcerations either at the tips of the digits or over the extensor surfaces of the interphalangeal joints.

The examiner should establish whether the patient has a history of limb trauma, swelling, a mass, associated lower extremity symptoms, or nonspecific symptoms of numbness and paresthesias. Significant medical conditions such as diabetes, renal failure, inflammatory arthritis, or collagen-vascular disease should be noted, because they may be associated with vascular problems. Cigarette smoking, alcohol intake, and illicit injection of recreational drugs also may have a bearing on the patient's condition. Often, the patient will be too embarrassed or unwilling to respond to inquiries about lifestyle choices that may explain otherwise puzzling symptoms. The patient should be assured that the information will not be used to prosecute him or her and that it is vital in reaching the correct diagnosis and choosing the appropriate treatment. Finally, questions about family history often will reveal that relatives have experienced similar symptoms, especially when Raynaud's phenomenon is suspected. Additional history may be obtained during the physical examination.

Physical examination for suspected vascular disease should follow the general principles of inspection, palpation, auscultation, and special testing. Again, the patient with acute ischemia may require a comprehensive but abbreviated examination before emergency radiologic or surgical procedures are performed. Chronic symptoms allow an examination that is more complete and detailed.

The complete vascular examination should be performed in a warm room to prevent inadvertent vasospasm, and the patient should wear a gown that allows access to both upper extremities. The examination should be performed on both extremities, even if the symptoms are unilateral. Gross inspection will demonstrate skin texture changes as well as frank ulcerations and tissue necrosis. Color changes consistent with cyanosis may indicate chronic venous insufficiency, and dilated distal veins in an edematous extremity may indicate proximal obstruction. Cold stimulation may trigger the color changes of Raynaud's phenomenon. The axillary, brachial, radial, and ulnar pulses should be palpated throughout the entire extremity. The carotid pulse may be affected in proximal arterial disease. Masses are palpated for thrills, pulsations, or tenderness. Auscultation of vessels and masses may demonstrate bruits.

One important and simple test to perform is the Allen's test. First described by Allen[16] in 1929, this test has many variations. It involves simultaneous compression of the ulnar and radial arteries while the hand is exsanguinated by opening and closing the fist. Pressure over the radial artery is released, and the return of flow to the palm and digits is observed. Compression of the ulnar artery is then released, and further changes are noted. The test is then repeated, releasing pressure on the ulnar artery first (Fig. 62-2). The test is considered abnormal when reflow to all or part of the hand takes more than 7 seconds; this indicates inadequate flow secondary to obstruction or vascular anomaly. Allen's test of the digital arteries may be useful in evaluating digital vessel flow, in which case palpation can be supplemented with various objective methods such as laser Doppler flowmetry (LDF) and pressure manometry to measure return of flow.[17]

During the initial evaluation, physical examination of the extremity should be supplemented by segmental pressure measurements and Doppler studies. Proximal obstruction may be detected by the use of a simple blood pressure cuff. Systolic blood pressure is measured in both arms at the antecubital level. A side-to-side difference of more than 15 mm Hg or a ratio of less than 0.96 is considered abnormal and indicates obstruction proximally.[18] Cuffs may be placed on the upper arm, forearm, and digits to identify obstruction as low as the palmar arch.

Perhaps the most useful supplement to the physical examination is Doppler ultrasonography[19] (Fig. 62-3). A high-

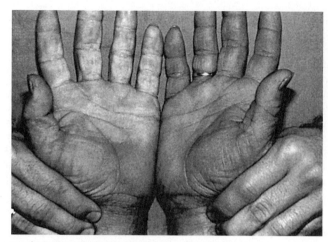

Figure 62-2 When the Allen's test was performed in this patient with artery thrombosis, the hand remained pale when compression on the ulnar artery was released.

frequency ultrasonic probe (10 MHz for upper extremity testing) emits sound waves that are reflected off the patient's blood. The movement of fluid and cells causes a change in the frequency of the transmitted signal known as the Doppler effect. After the reflected signal is processed, it is projected as an audible signal or visible waveform. To administer the examination, special conducting gel is applied to the skin followed by the probe, which is positioned at a 45- to 60-degree angle and manipulated until the strongest signal is obtained. Normal arterial signals consist of a triphasic sound: a high-pitched peak during systole, a fall in pitch during diastole, and then a short increase in pitch before the next systole. Venous sounds are lower in pitch and vary with respirations. Abnormal signals have characteristic audible and waveform changes and can be used to identify the location and nature of the problem. For example, a stenotic arterial segment has relatively fast flow with a resultant high-pitched Doppler signal. The Doppler also may be used to map the location of normal or variant arterial anatomy before surgery and as an adjunct to the Allen's test in patients in whom pulses are difficult to palpate.

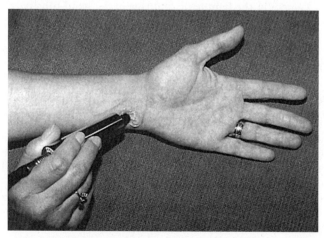

Figure 62-3 Doppler examination allows quick and accurate mapping of the major arteries.

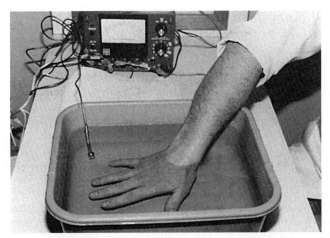

Figure 62-4 Cold stress testing is useful in evaluating patients with vasospastic disorders.

Specialized Vascular Testing

Noninvasive testing in the vascular laboratory is the most significant development in the screening and evaluation of patients with vascular disorders. Initially developed to evaluate lower extremity problems, the vascular laboratory has been applied only recently to disorders of the upper extremity.

One of the most common tests performed in the vascular laboratory is segmental pressure monitoring. As mentioned previously, segmental pressures may be obtained at the level of the arm, forearm, or digit. Serial measurements are obtained quickly with serial pressure cuffs, and accurate ratios are then calculated to screen for obstructive disease.[20] It is also possible to recalculate segmental pressures after exercise stress testing; this may reveal subclinical obstructive disease that causes symptoms only after activity.

Digital plethysmography, or pulse volume recording (PVR), uses a strain gauge or photo sensor that measures changes in the volume of the digit with each pulse. Normally, this change is expressed as a linear tracing that defines the relative difference in volume between pulse waves. Normal tracings show a sharp systolic upslope followed by a dip that has been termed the *dicrotic notch*, and then the sequence is terminated with a less sharp downslope.[21] In the tracing of an obstructed pulse, the normal upsweep is delayed and has a less acute slope; the peak is often rounded, and the downslope is longer and away from the baseline. PVRs may be obtained under stress conditions.

PVR has been shown to correlate well with arteriographic findings.[22,23] It does not localize lesions or provide absolute values that enable comparison of results between patients. Thus, it may be most useful as a screening tool or for monitoring a patient to evaluate the results of treatment. Most studies agree that PVR should be used in conjunction with other noninvasive modalities.

Cold stress testing was developed by Koman et al.[24] to evaluate the upper extremity in patients who suffer from cold intolerance or possible vasospasm (Fig. 62-4). In this test, skin temperature probes that have been placed on each digit are monitored before, during, and after brief exposure to a cold stress, usually an ice-water bath. The baseline measurements provide an index of resting blood flow, and the temperature change after exposure is a measurement of the vascular response to the stress. The temperature curve after the stress is withdrawn reflects the return of blood flow. Patients with a vasospastic disorder may demonstrate lower baseline temperatures, more dramatic temperature decreases after exposure, and prolonged recovery periods. Cold stress testing after sympathetic blockade has been used to predict the outcome of surgical sympathectomy for relief of vasospasm.[25]

LDF[26] and digital nail fold capillaroscopy[27] are among other noninvasive techniques that are being developed to evaluate distal digital blood flow. Both modalities attempt to provide objective diagnosis and prognosis of vasospastic diseases, and to differentiate primary Raynaud's phenomenon from systemic sclerosis and other vasospastic diseases. LDF is based on the detection and analysis of scattered light to assess microscopic blood flow. Different wavelengths of light can be emitted to refine depth of penetration and improve accuracy. However, its precision complicates its application, since different readings from the same finger from slightly different positions can have markedly different measurements. Its full potential has not yet been realized, and current research is refining the technique to take advantage of its inherent strengths.[28] Capillaroscopy uses microscopic digital imaging of the nail fold to elucidate the flow, individual capillary diameter, and regional capillary structure. Investigations have shown structural abnormalities characteristic of systemic sclerosis that are not present in primary Raynaud's phenomenon. Additionally, it may demonstrate real-time acute changes associated with Raynaud's phenomenon as well as long-term changes in the capillary bed associated with long-term disease progression.[29] These and other techniques continue to evolve and improve our ability to understand the microvascular changes associated with vasospastic phenomena. Collaboration with institutional imaging and research groups may provide benefit to both patient care and to the refinement of these techniques.

Diagnostic Imaging

The radiographic evaluation of patients with suspected vascular problems includes plain films and arteriography.[30] New modalities such as radionuclide imaging,[31] duplex ultrasonography,[32] and MRI[33] also are used and represent some noninvasive alternatives to angiography.

All evaluations of vascular problems should include plain film radiographs of the hand (Fig. 62-5). In cases of suspected vascular compression in the neck, films of the cervical spine also are obtained. Radiographs of all masses should be obtained and assessed for the presence of calcifications, which often accompany vascular tumors. Radiographs also will delineate the extent of bony involvement before resection of invasive arteriovenous malformations.

Until recently, contrast studies have been the primary radiographic means of evaluating vascular disorders of the upper extremity. Most often, angiography is performed via cannulation of the femoral artery. The catheter is threaded retrograde to the level of the subclavian or axillary artery, depending on the desired level of study. Contrast material—

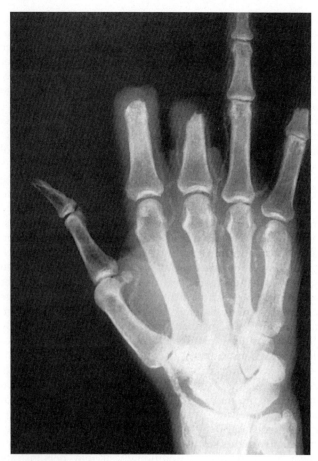

Figure 62-5 Radiograph demonstrating calcification of the arterial system in a patient receiving renal dialysis. The patient developed gangrene in several digits secondary to inadequate perfusion.

usually an iodine-containing radiopaque liquid—is injected proximally, and serial radiographs of the extremity are then taken. This technique allows complete evaluation of the vascular tree (Fig. 62-6A). Digital subtraction arteriography is a newer technique that eliminates background tissues to enhance visualization of the vessels. Venography is performed after catheterization of a peripheral vessel to the superior vena cava.

Angiography is a very sensitive and specific means of detecting most vascular disorders of the upper extremity. Atherosclerotic, embolic, aneurysmal, and inflammatory diseases are well visualized with this modality. Traumatic injuries, including lacerations and intimal damage, also may be detected by angiography. Feeder vessels in arteriovenous malformations may be localized for surgical excision. Angiography also has been used to establish the vascular supply to injured and donor tissue when a free-tissue transfer (Fig. 62-6B) or tumor excision (Fig. 62-6C and D) is planned.

Contrast angiography is not without complications.[34] The catheter itself must be placed in a relatively large vessel, from which significant hemorrhage may occur. Likewise, the catheter may injure the vessel lumen and cause postangiographic ischemia. Injection of iodinated contrast material has been associated with refractory vasospasm, thus vasodilators often are given before contrast injection. The contrast material

itself has been implicated in postangiographic renal failure and, in some cases, anaphylactic reaction.

Newer angiographic technology has reduced the number of complications. Contrast agents that have low toxicity or are nontoxic cause fewer anaphylactic reactions. Also, less of the agent is needed when digital subtraction arteriography is performed, because this technique does not require as much contrast agent to produce an acceptable image.[35] Interventional angiography also has become popular as a therapeutic application of technology that once was used for diagnosis only. The best-known intervention is balloon angioplasty. Originally developed for coronary artery dilation, this technique has been successfully applied to the upper extremity.[36] Transcatheter infusions of thrombolytic agents for acute thrombotic and embolic disease of the upper extremity have been carried out.[37] Finally, selective embolization of feeder vessels in arteriovenous malformations has been performed as a definitive preoperative treatment for the reduction of intraoperative blood loss during planned definitive excision.

Radionuclide imaging is another traditional method of evaluating suspected vascular conditions. Injection of a small amount of contrast material, usually technetium-99m-labeled diphosphonate-1, is followed by three separate scans that provide dynamic information about perfusion of the extremity. Immediate scanning provides both arterial and venous angiograms, and delayed scanning provides information on the overall metabolic activity of the limb. Scanning is especially useful in cases in which sensitivity is required but fine resolution is not. Circumstances of this kind are encountered when determining the level of tissue viability after replantation or after an insult such as frostbite.[38] Three-phase scanning in hand surgery is particularly valuable in the assessment of CRPS. Although this condition is not an entirely vascular disorder, it may demonstrate characteristic changes on three-phase scanning.[39] Analysis of the delayed phase alone have shown sensitivities ranging from 65% to 90% and specificities from 75% to 100%. Analysis of vascular, blood pool, and delayed phase in combination have yielded sensitivity of 80.8% and specificity of 100% in acute cases of CRPS.[40] Duplex ultrasonography is a newer technique that uses traditional ultrasound technology to provide a detailed assessment of the upper extremity vasculature. It has the ability to provide images comparable in detail with those obtained in angiography. This method has several advantages. The procedure is noninvasive, inexpensive, and portable; it requires minimal setup and can be carried out quickly. However, it lacks the invasive advantages of angiography and is very operator-dependent. The procedure uses B-mode imaging, which is a more complex ultrasound technique. This application of Doppler ultrasound technology produces detailed images of the vascular tree in real time with color coding for different flow directions and velocities. The vessels can be scanned in cross section or longitudinally. The technique is applicable to both intraluminal and vessel-wall pathologic conditions. Newer contrast agents are being tested to permit the application of this technique in microvascular procedures. Currently, vessels as small as 0.5 mm can be visualized.

Magnetic resonance (MR) arteriography, a new application of MRI technology, is a noninvasive means of imaging

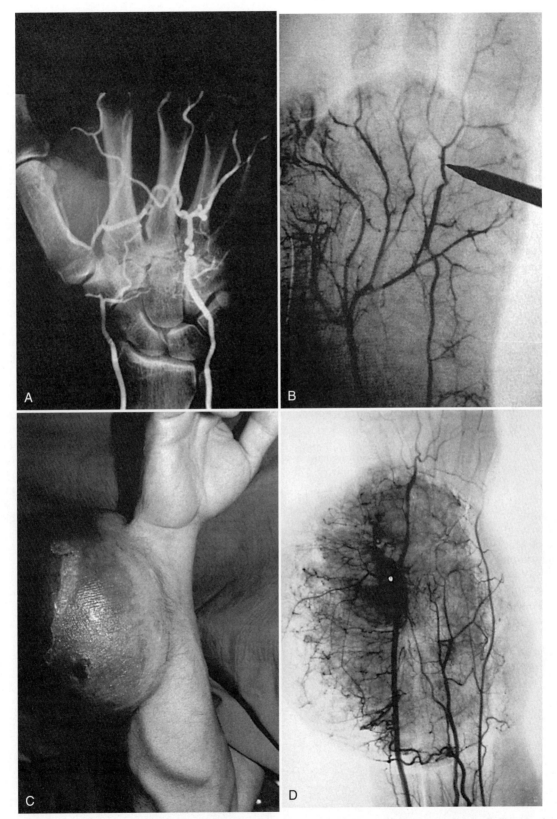

Figure 62-6 The vascular anatomy can be visualized using angiography. **A**, Normal appearance of the hand and wrist. **B**, The vascular supply to the foot is seen before toe-to-hand transfer. **C** and **D**, Gross and angiographic appearance of a large forearm mass. The latter was used to determine the surgical margin necessary for resection.

vascular disorders that was made possible by improvements in imaging sequences and in the coils used to enhance contrast. In addition, gadolinium IV contrast has been used to enhance the resolution of small vessels. One great advantage of MR arteriography is that it permits examination of the perivascular tissues for abnormalities—a capability that is especially useful when evaluating vascular masses. It is also the only modality that can view the image from any projection after it has been recorded. Its disadvantages include the amount of time required to perform the study, the claustrophobic environment of the scanner, separation of the patient from the medical team in cases of life-threatening trauma, and its expense.

Common Vascular Disorders of the Upper Extremity

Penetrating and Blunt Injuries

Critical traumatic injuries of the upper extremity that involve the arterial system are those in which distal flow is disrupted with resultant limb-threatening ischemia. In patients with such damage, treatment consists of emergent exploration and repair of the injured vessels. In contrast, noncritical injuries may remain asymptomatic or manifest subtly, presenting as upper limb claudication with prolonged exercise or overhead activity. Penetrating injury is one of the most obvious types of traumatic damage and typically is encountered as a knife or gunshot wound or a wound suffered in an industrial or motor vehicle accident. In patients with such injuries, the following seven features indicate a possible vascular injury that requires evaluation or exploration: (1) loss of distal pulses, (2) pulsatile or profuse bleeding from the wound, (3) a large hematoma at the entrance or exit wound, (4) hypotension, (5) the presence of a bruit near the wound, (6) injury to a nerve in proximity to a known vessel, and (7) proximity of the wound to vascular structures.[41] Patients with any of these seven features require evaluation with Doppler ultrasonography or angiography, or surgical exploration. Recent studies comparing ultrasonic and angiographic imaging have shown that these two methods are comparable in diagnostic sensitivity and specificity.[42] Emergent surgical exploration is indicated if distal ischemia is present.

In cases of penetrating injury to the subclavian, axillary, or brachial artery, limb-threatening ischemia usually results despite the presence of collateral vessels. Early exploration and repair is indicated (Fig. 62-7). An interposition vein graft is necessary when vessels have retracted or when a wide zone of injury precludes primary repair. Injury to the peripheral nerves may accompany the vessel damage; therefore, the surgeon should be prepared to repair these structures. Some controversy exists over the repair of "noncritical" arterial injuries in the forearm and hand. Several studies have attempted to predict the outcome based on repair of single-vessel lacerations in the forearm.[43-45] While the prognosis of these injuries varies widely depending on the mechanism and severity of injury, several studies have shown limb salvage rates from 50% up to 95% for digital, arm, and forearm vascular injuries treated acutely at trauma centers.[46,47]

Blunt trauma also may produce vascular injury. Shoulder dislocations and proximal humeral fractures may interrupt the axillary artery, and fractures of the clavicle or first rib may injure the subclavian artery. In children, supracondylar humeral fractures may compress or lacerate the brachial artery. These injuries may be avulsions of the vessels with subsequent loss of distal perfusion. Intimal injuries lacking gross vessel disruption also may result in decreased distal perfusion. In all cases of combined proximal vascular and orthopedic injury, diagnosis of the vascular injury may be overlooked because of the more obvious bony or even neurologic injury. Prompt assessment and treatment of the vascular injury may prevent limb loss, late aneurysm, or arteriovenous fistula formation. Stabilization of fractures should be performed in the same setting but before vessel repair to prevent further injury.

Compartment Syndrome

Classically, compartment syndrome of the upper extremity is not defined by injury of the vascular system. However, it

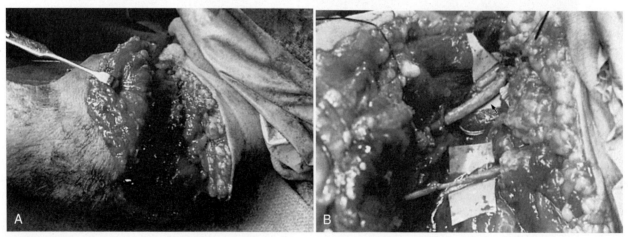

Figure 62-7 A, This limb-threatening brachial artery laceration was sustained in a machete attack. **B**, Repair was accomplished using a reversed saphenous vein graft (*arrow*).

does involve a loss of perfusion of the forearm and muscles of the hand that may have potentially devastating results. Compartment syndromes may result from a variety of traumatic insults, either blunt or penetrating. Crush injuries of the upper extremity are especially prone to develop this condition. Compartment syndrome also occurs after postischemic reperfusion of the upper extremity. Endothelial cell retraction during ischemia allows extravasation of large amounts of fluid within the enclosed fascial space, elevating interstitial pressure beyond tolerable limits.

Compartment syndrome is a clinical diagnosis that should be considered when swelling and pain in an extremity appear to exceed the amplitude of the initial injury. A well-known diagnosis mnemonic of compartment syndrome is the four P's: *Pain* with passive muscle stretch, *paresthesias*, *pallor/poikilothermia*, and *pulselessness*. Pain and paresthesias out of proportion relative to the injury are the most reliable indicators, because excellent distal pulses and tissue color may still exist with full-blown forearm compartment syndromes. The patient's hand will assume intrinsic minus posture as well.[48,49] Importantly, the presence of these symptoms may be particularly difficult to determine in children and the patient who has a head injury or is intoxicated. For this reason, several devices have been designed to measure tissue pressures. The classic construct by Whitesides et al.[50] is simple and can be made from readily available materials. A side-ported needle or slit catheter is connected to an arterial line setup and allows for clinically useful assessment of compartment pressure. Off-the-shelf compact devices with digital readouts are also available, for example the Stryker compartment pressure monitor (Stryker Medical, Kalamazoo, Mich.). Care must be taken to measure tissue pressures in all potentially involved parts of the upper extremity. There are 3 compartments in the forearm (the dorsal, volar, and mobile wad) and 10 in the hand. Any or all interosseous muscles, as well as the thenar, hypothenar, and adductor musculature, may be involved.

The tissue pressure above which compartment release should be considered is controversial. Normal tissue pressure is between 8 and 10 mm Hg. Critical pressures have been noted at levels 30 mm Hg below diastolic,[50] which translates into absolute values of 30 mm Hg[51] to 45 mm Hg.[52] Serial measurements or monitoring with indwelling wick catheters[53] have been advocated in borderline situations wherein clinical examination may be difficult. However, even though they are convenient, tissue pressure monitors should be used only in an adjunctive role. Compartment syndrome is a clinical diagnosis. Clinical suspicion, mechanism, and physical examination are the keys to expedient diagnosis. The threshold for compartment release should be low. If there is any concern for a suspected compartment syndrome, early release is reasonable.

Compartment syndrome is treated by decompression (Fig. 62-8A and B). Incisions should be extensive and provide for complete release of the involved compartments. Skin and fascia are incised along the entire length of the compartment. Often, the muscles will bulge into the open wound as a dusky mass, resuming normal color as it is allowed to escape from the restricted compartment. Release of the volar forearm—the most commonly involved compartment—should include the carpal tunnel and the proximal antebrachial fascia. Care should be taken to ensure that adequate

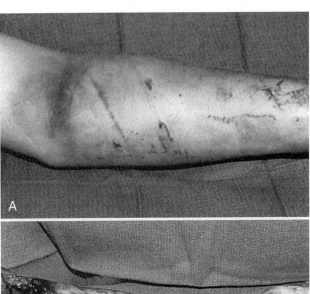

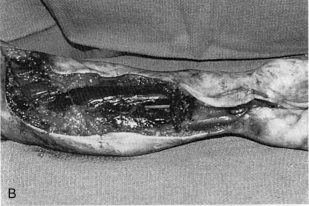

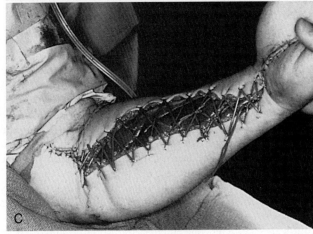

Figure 62-8 A, This young woman developed compartment syndrome after an accident in which her car rolled over and pinned her forearm. **B**, Fasciotomy was performed. **C**, After the swelling receded, the wound was approximated using vessel loops stapled to the skin edges.

release is obtained. It may be necessary to release the investing fascia of each muscle in the forearm to achieve complete release. After decompression, the wound is left open and covered with a sterile dressing or vacuum-assisted wound closure device.

The patient may require repeat operative exploration under general anesthesia to debride nonviable tissue and gain skin closure. As the swelling decreases, skin approximation may be facilitated by interweaving elastic vessel loops stapled to the skin edges and drawing the skin edges together without tension (Fig. 62-8C). As above, vacuum-assisted closure may be a helpful, though relatively expensive adjunct to aid closure. Skin grafting may be required for large defects. Return of function after decompression is excellent if surgery is performed early. However, if the condition goes unrecognized, severe neuromuscular injury can result in fibrosis and contracture. In these cases, release and advanced reconstruction of the extremity in the form of tendon transfers[54] or free-muscle transfer will be needed to restore minimal hand and forearm function.[55]

Cannulation Injuries

Cannulation of upper extremity arteries is performed for diagnostic and monitoring purposes. For example, the brachial artery is often the site of catheter introduction for coronary angiography. Passage of the cannula may injure the vessel lumen and cause the formation of a clot or internal flap that intermittently obstructs distal flow. Complications of the brachial artery cannulation occur at rates of 1.0% to 1.5%[56] and may consist of acute ischemia distal to the catheter site (Fig. 62-9), fingertip embolization and gangrene, or even vague claudicatory pain. The diagnosis can be confirmed by Doppler examination as well as by alteration in segmental arterial pressures with a significant drop at the level of the injury.

Cannulation of the distal radial artery is the most common invasive arterial procedure. Radial artery catheters are used for pressure monitoring and blood gas analysis. The complications of radial artery cannulation include thrombosis (Fig. 62-10), infection, and aneurysm formation.[14] A study of 4932 patients in the medical and surgical intensive care units showed that 1249 underwent radial artery cannulation among a total of 2119 who had arterial cannulation, just under 60%. Of these the authors found an arterial injury rate leading to loss of Doppler-audible radial artery perfusion in nearly 7% of cases. Preprocedure Allen's testing had demonstrated adequate ulnar flow, and no long-term perfusion sequelae were reported. Transient thrombosis and spasm were also reported in less than 2% of cases and resolved with supportive measures. Thrombosis may lead to distal ischemia and possible thumb loss, but it usually can be prevented by the use of small-gauge Teflon catheters. Before the insertion of any catheter, an Allen's test *must* be performed to identify digits that may be at risk for ischemia. A positive test result contraindicates catheter placement. Additionally, failed radial artery cannulation should prompt alternative means of arterial access (e.g., femoral, contralateral radial artery, subclavian). Attempts at ipsilateral arterial access in the limb may place the hand and extremity at risk.

If ischemia develops after insertion of a radial artery catheter, the catheter should be removed immediately; this alone may restore flow. However, if flow is not improved, there are two options. Arteriography may reveal a thrombosed or vasospastic artery, and salvage of the digits with intra-arterial thrombolytics or vasodilators may be achieved via the angiography catheter. Alternatively, surgical exploration of the vessel with embolectomy or resection and vein grafting may restore normal vascularity. In any case, the patient should receive anticoagulants after the procedure; heparin should be used for the first 5 to 7 days, followed by oral anticoagulants or aspirin for approximately 1 month. If the patient's condi-

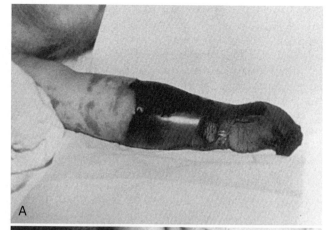

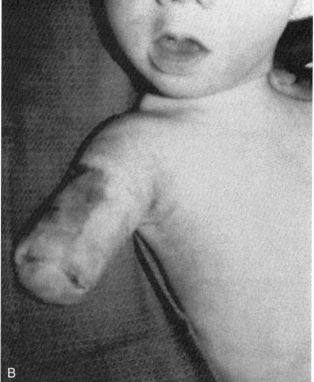

Figure 62-9 A, After cannulation of the brachial artery, this child's arm became ischemic. **B,** Amputation above the elbow was necessary.

tion does not permit anticoagulation therapy, then axillary or peripheral catheters can be inserted for infusion of vasodilating agents. Subsequent infections or aneurysms of the radial artery may be asymptomatic or be a source of distal emboli to the digits, leading to digital ischemia and necrosis. Treatment involves resection of the affected vessel with direct anastomosis or vein graft interposition.

Cannulation of peripheral veins is less subject to complications. However, peripheral IV infusions can lead to a chemical or infectious thrombophlebitis. Typically, this responds to symptomatic treatment with heat, moist wraps, and in the case of an overlying cellulitis, antibiotics. Occasionally, surgical excision is required for a painful vessel that does not respond to supportive measures. Central venous cannulation also is performed routinely for monitoring or infusion and can lead to subclavian vein thrombosis. These thromboses

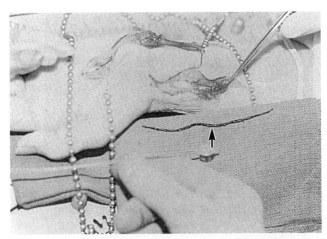

Figure 62-10 Thrombosis of the radial and ulnar arteries occurred in this patient after multiple arterial cannulations, necessitating emergent exploration, thrombectomy (*arrow*), and vein grafting of the damaged arterial segments.

may occasionally require heparin or thrombolytic agents if severe upper extremity swelling or pulmonary embolism occurs. More often, withdrawal of the catheter allows for recannulation of the central veins and resolution of symptoms. Treatment is based on acuteness of the symptoms. Systemic heparinization, thrombolysis, thrombectomy, and even resection and grafting may be required to alleviate the symptoms.

Intra-arterial Injection

Accidental arterial injection commonly occurs during attempted IV administration of recreational drugs (Fig. 62-11), and it also may occur after inadvertent cannulation of an anomalous artery in the antecubital region. The hospitalized patient who presents with acute distal ischemia after injection must be suspected of accidental intra-arterial injection.[57] After this event, a severe reaction develops whose pathophysiology is not completely understood. Three factors have been implicated. First, the particulate matter serves as an intra-arterial embolism as it travels through and blocks the smaller arteries. Second, many drugs generate a chemical arteritis, which leads to arterial thrombosis. Finally, vasospasm and inflammation are caused by material passing through the capillary bed, resulting in proximal sludging and loss of digital inflow. The differential diagnosis includes other causes of acute ischemia, trauma, embolic disease, and Raynaud's phenomenon.

Acute symptoms of intra-arterial injection may include severe burning pain, cyanosis, and tissue swelling. A concise history may be difficult to obtain because of the patient's obtundance or unwillingness to admit drug use.[58] Charney and Stern[58] recently reported on five young patients with digital ischemia and gangrene who did not have the "appearance" of the typical IV drug user. These patients initially denied attempted self-injection despite their severe symptoms. Patients admitted the injections only after repeated questioning.

The treatment of acute intra-arterial injection is somewhat controversial. Traditionally, supportive measures, including

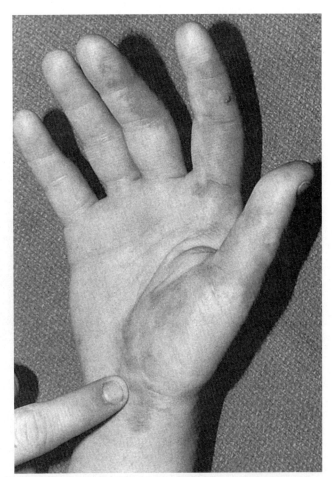

Figure 62-11 In this patient, intra-arterial injection of heroin led to digital skin loss in the region supplied by the radial artery.

sympathetic blocks, intra-arterial vasodilation, administration of thrombolytics, and anticoagulation, have been the mainstay of treatment. Arteriography and surgery are much less proven. However, during the acute period, arteriography may be used to elucidate the nature of the injury. If obstructive lesions are noted, attempts at thrombolysis or microarterial reconstruction are indicated. Diffuse injury carries a less favorable prognosis. In such cases, further supportive treatment is best and includes pain control, prevention of infection, and ultimately, amputation.

The patient who seeks treatment days to months after intra-arterial injection presents a different clinical picture. In the most severe cases the injection will result in irreversible ischemic changes, especially at the digital level. Again, supportive measures alone are indicated. Patients who have more proximal injection injuries of the brachial or forearm arterial structures and signs and symptoms of chronic ischemia, including cold intolerance, Raynaud's phenomenon, or claudication, should undergo noninvasive and arteriographic workup and microsurgical reconstruction if necessary.

Ulnar Artery Thrombosis–Hypothenar Hammer Syndrome

Entrapment neuropathy of the ulnar nerve at the wrist or elbow is the most common cause of ulnar wrist pain and

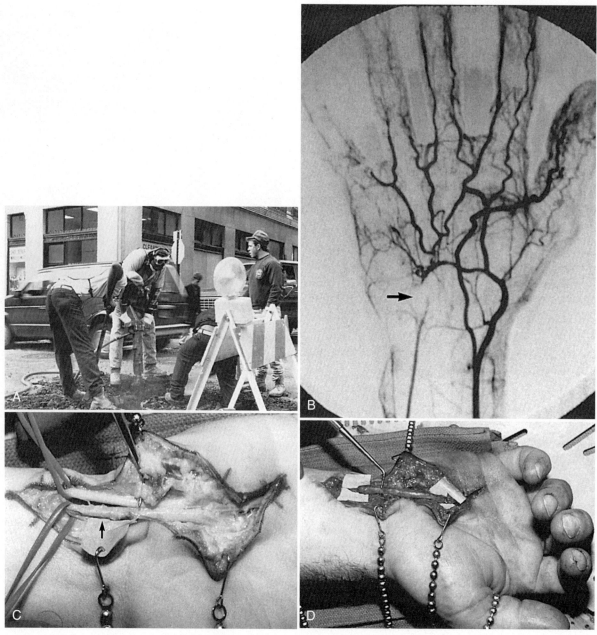

Figure 62-12 Ulnar artery thrombosis. **A**, Repetitive vibration of the palm such as that experienced during the operation of a jackhammer can cause this type of lesion. **B**, Angiogram demonstrating a blockage of flow in the ulnar artery at Guyon's canal (*arrow*). **C** and **D**, Appearance of the thrombosed artery before (*arrow*) and after resection, respectively. Note its paleness.

paresthesias. However, vascular disorders must be considered in cases wherein a palmar mass, symptoms of cold intolerance, or unilateral Raynaud's phenomenon are present. Ulnar artery thrombosis, commonly presenting as *hypothenar hammer syndrome*,[59] occurs most often in males who engage in manual labor where the palmar aspect of either hand is exposed to repetitive trauma (Fig. 62-12A). Smoking is a significant contributing factor, and reports show that 80% to 90% of patients presenting with hypothenar hammer syndrome are smokers.[60] Repetitive trauma to this area compresses the ulnar artery against the hook of the hamate with subsequent aneurysm formation or intimal injury, exposure of subendothelial collagen, and eventual thrombosis.[61] This

entity was first described by Von Rosen[62] in 1934, yet it is often overlooked in the differential diagnosis. In the absence of a history of repetitive trauma, ganglion cysts, anomalous muscular anatomy, or local arteriovenous malformation have been implicated as causes of ulnar artery thrombosis.[63,64]

The diagnosis is missed primarily because of the nonspecific presenting symptoms. Koman and Urbaniak[65] reviewed 28 patients with proven ulnar artery thrombosis and found that the correct diagnosis was made on initial examination in only half of the patients. Patients may present with pain, Raynaud's phenomenon, decreased sensation, cold intolerance, and rarely, ischemia of the ulnar hand. Symptoms may be intermittent or may progress to severe pain and ischemia at rest if the arterial thrombosis decreases digital blood flow to a significant degree. Digital ulcers or frank gangrene may develop if the thrombosis is left untreated at this stage. In Koman and Urbaniak's series,[65] 80% of patients experienced discomfort in cold weather or while holding a cold object.

The ulnar nerve may be compressed either by the expansion of the arterial wall caused by the thrombus or by a small aneurysm in the arterial wall that develops secondary to trauma. If this occurs in zone 1 of Guyon's canal, proximal to the bifurcation of the ulnar nerve, the patients will have mixed sensory and motor symptoms; this is uncommon. More distally, in zone 2, the artery is more closely associated with the motor branch of the nerve and motor symptoms will predominate or occur in isolation. However, this presentation is more commonly caused by ganglia or hook of hamate pathology. Most commonly in ulnar artery thrombosis, patients will have sensory symptoms of numbness in the ulnar digits without motor involvement. This is due to compression of the sensory branch in zone 3, distal to the bifurcation of the nerve, where the artery is closely associated with the sensory branch alone.[66]

Physical diagnostic maneuvers focus on evaluating the patency of flow to the hand as well as locating the thrombosis. Koman and Urbaniak[65] showed a positive Allen's test at the wrist with delayed or nonexistent ulnar artery inflow in every patient in their series. Doppler examination demonstrates a decreased signal in the area of Guyon's canal and obliteration of the signal at the level of the superficial arch with compression of the radial artery. Digital plethysmography is abnormal in the ulnar digits, and transcutaneous oxygen measurements are decreased. Arteriography is the gold standard for evaluation, to visualize the vascular tree, and is helpful in cases wherein distal embolism of the fingers is suspected and microvascular reconstruction is planned (Fig. 62-12B). Arteriography may eventually be supplanted by ultrasound, since excellent real-time ultrasonic evaluation is now possible.

Supportive treatment is indicated in patients with no digital ischemia, no signs of nerve compression, and those who can avoid further trauma to the ulnar side of the wrist. The majority of symptomatic patients can find relief with smoking cessation, activity modification, and oral medication. Marie et al. published an excellent review, and the largest case series, in 2007 from their experience in Rouen, France.[60] They reported 83% favorable outcome with activity modification, smoking cessation, and oral therapy with vasodilators and/or platelet aggregation inhibitors. They showed a 27.7% recurrence rate with follow-up, but successful treatment of all recurrences with modification of conservative therapies. For patients with digital ischemia or necrosis they recommended the addition of hemodilution with dextran, or heparin/low-molecular-weight heparin or a prostacyclin analogue. Vayssairat demonstrated improvement in 76.5% of these patients with this type of regimen.[67] Patients with refractory symptoms can be treated with surgical resection of thrombosis (Fig. 62-12C and D) or aneurysm, with subsequent reverse-vein grafting or primary anastomosis. Resection followed by vein grafting has shown functional recovery and graft patency of 84% at 2-year follow-up.[68] In their report, Marie et al. treated only 2 of 47 cases with surgery, since all others had been amenable to more conservative treatment.

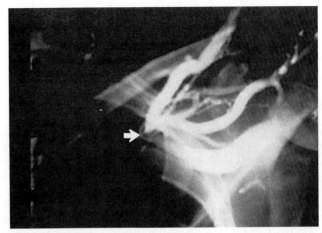

Figure 62-13 Venogram of the abducted shoulder in a patient with vascular thoracic outlet syndrome. Occlusion of the subclavian vein is evident (arrow).

Both patients treated with surgery had durable relief of their symptoms postoperatively. Finally, amputative debridement may be necessary in some cases: those that present late, when patients are unable to comply with treatment protocols (i.e., cannot stop smoking, cannot change work type), or when the extent of digit injury or infection mandate.

Vascular Thoracic Outlet Syndrome

Vascular compression at the thoracic outlet represents only 3% of all thoracic outlet problems and may be arterial (1%) or venous (2%) in origin.[69] It may have a variety of causes ranging from congenital fibromuscular bands to fracture callus. Claudication, especially with overhead activity, is the primary symptom. Distal embolization and unilateral Raynaud's phenomenon also may occur and lead to digital ischemia and gangrene. Venous obstruction may cause intermittent or persistent extremity edema. Both arterial and venous compression may be accompanied by symptoms of neurologic compression. These symptoms may be vague, so problems of the cervical spine or shoulder and peripheral nerve compression must be considered in the differential diagnosis.

Provocative testing for vascular compromise includes the elevated-arm stress test, wherein the patient holds his or her arms elevated, abducted, and externally rotated to narrow the thoracic outlet (Fig. 62-13). Overhead activity is simulated by rapidly opening and closing the hands. Vascular compression may be evidenced by muscular aching, which signifies inadequate arterial inflow. Paradoxically, venous obstruction may result in dilation of the venous vasculature with elevation of the arm. Other tests, such as the Adson's test, are less reliable because normal subjects may exhibit pulse diminution. Conversely, decreased pulse characteristics may be absent in patients with angiographic evidence of vascular occlusion. Ultrasonography and contrast angiography may be helpful to confirm the diagnosis if they show significant flow decreases when the arm is elevated from the dependent position.

The treatment of vascular compression parallels that of neurogenic thoracic outlet syndrome. Posture and stretching exercises may alleviate mild symptoms. For more severe symptoms, especially those stemming from distal embolization, operative excision of the offending structure, thrombolysis, and possible vessel grafting are indicated. The technique of thoracic-outlet decompression is well described by Whitenack et al.[70]

Vasospastic Diseases

Unlike vascular trauma or thromboembolic problems, vasospastic diseases of the upper extremity have many different etiologies linked by common symptoms, Raynaud's phenomenon. The clinical signs of classic Raynaud's phenomenon consist of a triad of cutaneous skin color changes in response to cold stimulation or stress: one or more fingers turn black or white, indicating complete lack of arterial inflow to the digit; then, the fingers gradually turn dusky blue or purple as deoxygenated blood pools in the affected digits; finally, as flow is restored, a red flush occurs that is characteristic of reactive hyperemia. Although this pattern is typical of Raynaud's phenomenon, not all patients will manifest the triphasic color changes, and any patient with complaints of "white fingers" or "cold sensitivity" should be evaluated for a vasospastic condition. Pain, especially severe pain, is not as common as are the color changes. Most patients who report pain with Raynaud's changes describe a dull aching feeling during the "attack" and/or "pins and needles" as flow is reestablished.

Interestingly, Raynaud's phenomenon is not a purely vasospastic problem. In 1862, the French physician Raynaud described this condition in 25 patients and attributed its cause to overactivity of the then recently described sympathetic nervous system.[71] In fact, most cases involve constriction of the digital arteries. Conditions in which proximal obstruction exists may reduce baseline flow to the point at which normal physiologic vasoconstrictive responses to cold produce the symptoms of Raynaud's phenomenon. Likewise, an increase in blood viscosity may decrease flow rates and result in digital pallor after a normal sympathetic response to stress. Thus, the scope of Raynaud's attacks is broadened to include not only sympathetic overdrive but also the complex interplay between local factors and general sympathetic tone.

Raynaud's phenomenon is the term used to describe the pathophysiologic cascade that presents with the classic clinical picture described above. Raynaud's disease, or idiopathic Raynaud's phenomenon, describes the situation when the phenomenon exists in isolation and not secondary to another disorder. *Raynaud's syndrome* is used to describe the occurrence of the phenomenon secondary to an underlying disease, such as in a patient with scleroderma or other collagen-vascular disease. In 1932, Allen and Brown[72,73] established minimal criteria for diagnosing Raynaud's disease: bilaterality of symptoms; absence of gangrene; absence of other primary disease, especially collagen-vascular diseases; and symptoms of at least 2 years' duration. Fingertip gangrene was later added to this list.[16]

Epidemiologic study of Raynaud's disease reveals that it most often affects women between the ages of 20 and 40 years, and it is more prevalent in colder climates. Interestingly, Raynaud's disease is more common than Raynaud's syndrome, occurring in 3% to 5% of the general population.[74]

Specific population surveys in Scandinavia and northern Europe have found that as many as 20% to 30% of healthy people complain of cold intolerance and color changes.[18] Patients who initially present with Raynaud's disease may later develop symptoms of collagen-vascular disease. Likewise, any patient with unilateral Raynaud's attacks or digital ulceration proximal to the fingertip should be suspected of having a mechanical obstruction rather than Raynaud's disease.[75]

Raynaud's phenomenon has been associated with a multitude of primary causes, including inflammatory diseases such as rheumatoid arthritis. Ingestion of drugs such as ergot, which is used to treat migraine headaches, also may cause peripheral vasospasm. More recently, vibratory occupational trauma to the digits has been associated with Raynaud's phenomenon.[76] Indeed, 50% of people in occupations such as those involving jackhammer operation will report symptoms of Raynaud's phenomenon.[77] Similarly, vibration white finger disease is associated with 125-Hz vibrations.[76] Occlusive disorders that may result in reduced digital arterial pressure (e.g., atherosclerosis, thrombosis) should be considered in the differential diagnosis.

Classically, Raynaud's syndrome is associated with collagen-vascular disease, particularly scleroderma. Of patients with scleroderma, 85% will manifest symptoms of Raynaud's phenomenon, and the attacks may be the presenting symptom in up to 50% of individuals with this diagnosis.[78] Scleroderma is associated with a constellation of problems, of which hand symptoms make up only a portion. Thorough evaluation of the patient by an internist or rheumatologist should be performed after the diagnosis has been made.

The diagnostic evaluation of the patient with Raynaud's phenomenon should begin with a thorough history and physical examination. The stimuli of the attacks, the mechanisms by which they are relieved, and whether the symptoms are unilateral or bilateral should be ascertained during questioning. Smoking, drug, and family histories may suggest an alternative primary diagnosis. Physical examination begins with observation for skin and nail changes as well as skin ulcers. All pulses should be palpated for integrity. Pulse variations may occur with positional changes of the arm. Neurologic evaluation is needed to identify signs of peripheral-nerve compression. Doppler studies and the Allen's test may reveal proximal obstruction. Provocative tests, such as placing the hands under cold running water, are rarely indicated.

Laboratory studies should include a complete blood count, erythrocyte sedimentation rate, and tests for rheumatologic abnormality, such as the presence of rheumatoid factor and antinuclear antibodies. Other tests, such as complement level determination and protein electrophoresis, also may be needed for diagnosis. Radiographic evaluation should include bilateral plain films of the hand; in addition, any other films that are prompted by clinical suspicion should be obtained. Ultrasonography is a noninvasive technique that provides excellent visualization of the arterial tree. However, arteriography is still the most commonly used means of evaluating peripheral obstruction. Noninvasive cold testing is helpful in diagnosing Raynaud's attacks and in evaluating the effectiveness of treatment. Patients with Raynaud's symptoms

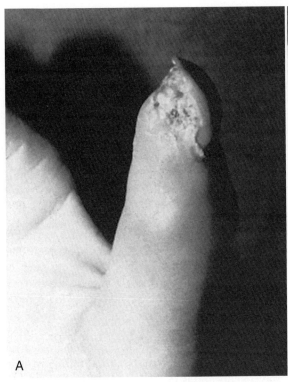

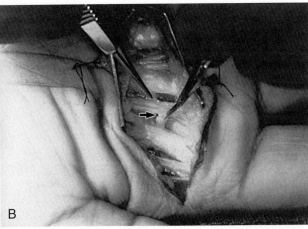

Figure 62-14 A, This digital ulcer in a patient with Raynaud's syndrome healed after the administration of oral vasodilatory medications. **B**, Peripheral sympathectomy is achieved by excising the fine network of sympathetic nerves from the digital arteries (*arrow*), thus blunting the sympathetic vasospastic constriction of the vessels.

experience an abnormal drop in digital temperature in response to cold stimulus and a prolonged recovery to baseline after the stimulus is removed.[24,79]

Treatment to alleviate symptoms and reduce frequency of attacks begins with behavioral therapy and activity modification. Keeping the fingers warm and avoiding cold stress, while obvious, must be reinforced to the patient and continually practiced. Abstaining from vasoconstrictive medications, caffeine, and cigarette smoking may be difficult for the patient but can reduce symptoms by approximately 50%. Biofeedback training also has reduced Raynaud's attacks, especially in Raynaud's disease.[80]

Medical treatment with nifedipine is used most often to prevent vasospastic events.[81] It operates by inhibiting smooth muscle contraction through blockade of calcium channels, in response to sympathetic stimulation. Nifedipine causes significant systemic side effects, the most common one being postural hypotension.

Several other medical treatments are under investigation as well. The scope of medications available to the rheumatologist to lessen frequency, severity, and duration of attack, as well as to treat and prevent ulcers and skin breakdown, is growing. Fries et al. showed statistically significant decrease in frequency of attack and duration of attacks by 33% and 45%, respectively, with use of the phosphodiesterase inhibitor sildenafil.[82] Several studies have shown the efficacy of prostacyclin antagonists such as iloprost to decrease attack frequency and severity and to improve skin condition in severe cases.[83-85] Bosentan, an endothelin receptor blocker, has been shown in two trials to significantly prevent new

ulcer formation.[86,87] This is an area of active research, and close consultation with a rheumatologist will allow these patients to benefit from these new findings.

In patients who prefer alternative therapy or do not tolerate the side effects of allopathic medical treatment, there are multiple other options. Both fish oil (omega-3 fatty acid) and evening primrose oil (omega-6 fatty acid) have been shown to raise the cold tolerance of patients and decrease frequency of attack, respectively.[88,89] Ginkgo biloba has also been shown to reduce frequency of attack in idiopathic Raynaud's disease.[90] Additionally, nonharmful alternative treatment that the patient finds beneficial should not be discouraged.

Digital ulcers are common sequelae in severe or undertreated cases. Ulcers will usually heal with conservative care (Fig. 62-14A). Such care includes whirlpool use, gentle dressing changes, and the avoidance of provocative situations. Medical therapy with topical or systemic vasodilators also may aid healing. Debridements are limited to frankly necrotic segments to preserve as much digital length as possible. Appropriate antibiotics are given for localized infection. Occasionally, recalcitrant digital ulcers require sympathectomy or microvascular reconstruction. Ultimately, pain and necrosis may result in subtotal or total amputation.

When conservative treatments fail, surgical intervention is considered. Surgical management consists of sympathectomy or microvascular reconstruction. In the past, the standard procedure consisted of sympathectomy just peripheral to the spinal cord at the level of the cervical ganglia. More recently, this paraspinal sympathectomy has been performed

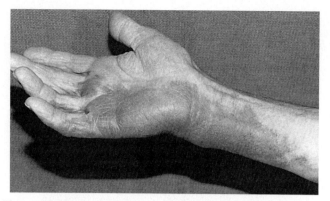

Figure 62-15 *Appearance of the capillary hemangioma, or "port wine stain."*

thoracoscopically. However, as with prior reports, the results are inconsistent, transient, and have undesirable side effects. Thune et al. in 2007 reported on their experience with thoracoscopic sympathectomy in 18 patients with severe symptoms.[91] They found an immediate effect in 83% of patients, but a recurrence of symptoms in 61%. Excessive sweating and salivation were reported by 63% and 30%, respectively. On a follow-up questionnaire, 43% of patients reported that they "regretted having the operation."

Digital sympathectomy has gained popularity since it was reported by Flatt in 1980.[25,80,94] Adventitial stripping of the common and digital vessels with separation of the connections between the nerve and artery have shown good results (Fig. 62-14B). Postoperatively, patients experience relief of pain, ulcer healing, and an increased feeling of "warmth" in their fingers.[93] Currently, sympathectomy is indicated if local sympathetic blockade improves the response to stress such as exposure to cold. Several small case series have shown that more than 80% of patients can expect improvement with sympathectomy performed by adventitial stripping of palmer and digital arteries.[94-97] With modern microvascular reconstruction techniques, elective microsurgical reconstruction has been used with benefit in patients with severe Raynaud's phenomenon with secondary ischemia and ulceration who have not had improvement with adventitial stripping sympathectomy.[13,96]

Hemangiomas and Vascular Malformations

Vascular conditions that are found predominantly in children range from the relatively benign hemangioma to the debilitating high-flow arterial venous malformation. Traditionally used terms such as *port wine stain* (Fig. 62-15) and *cavernous hemangioma* are descriptive but do not reflect the true endothelial nature of the lesions. Current reports divide congenital vascular anomalies into two categories: hemangiomas and arteriovenous malformations.[98]

In 30% of cases, hemangiomas are present as red spots at birth; however, they grow rapidly, and 90% are visible by age 4 weeks. Their growth rate is initially worrisome but usually slows with time, and they eventually involute without treatment. Seventy percent fade, many of these completely resolving by age 7. Females are affected up to five times more often than males. Historically, the lesion demonstrates a hypertro-

phic endothelium with an increased number of mast cells. A mixture of fibrous and fatty tissue with minimal vasculature remains with involution.

Symptomatic treatment is recommended. Ulcerations are uncommon and are treated with supportive wound care. The size of the lesion also may be controlled by compressive garments. Large hemangiomas that are unresponsive to local measures may lead to high-output cardiac failure. For this type of lesion, locally injected corticosteroids may hasten involution. No clear mechanism has been delineated, but lowering of circulating serum estrogens has been proposed as a trigger for resorption. Occasionally, a large hemangioma must be excised surgically in infancy[99] (Fig. 62-16).

According to Mulliken and Glowacki,[98] vascular malformations that contain normal endothelial cells also are present at birth as hemangiomas. As these normal vessels in abnormal locations grow with the child, they become more apparent and manifest in either a high- or low-flow state. Low-flow malformations consist of superficial capillary disorders; these have previously been referred to as *port wine stains*. Other low-flow malformations include the venous malformation, or cavernous hemangioma; lymphatic malformations; and mixed vascular malformations. These lesions are slow-growing and may either localize superficially in the dermis or be deep and diffuse. Both bony and soft tissue limb hypertrophy occurs and is more noticeable when the limb is in the dependent position. If the lesions are localized and small, supportive care may be sufficient. Larger, more diffuse lesions may be treated with compression, but surgical excision may be required if they are painful, and extensive debridement may be necessary. Preoperative evaluation with venography, color duplex ultrasonography, or MR angiography (Fig. 62-17A–C) may be used to define the lesion.

Arterial or high-flow malformations are rare but potentially devastating congenital vascular problems. Patients have tissue hypertrophy with palpable thrills and audible bruits. Severe pain as a result of distal ischemia from shunting or compression neuropathy occurs in most cases. Ulceration and frank gangrene may develop (Fig. 62-17D). Patients may experience high-output cardiac failure and manifest a significant decrease in pulse with compression of the feeder arteries (the Nicoladoni-Branham sign, or Branham's sign).[100]

Surgical management is the recommended treatment for large or painful lesions (Fig. 62-17E). Preoperative arteriography with possible embolization of feeder arteries is required before surgery. Surgical excision, often in multiple stages with free-tissue or skin grafts, may successfully eradicate the malformation. Simple ligation of the inflow vessels usually will not remedy the problem. Outcome varies greatly depending on the nature, extent, and complexity of the lesion. If complete excision may be performed and there is no recurrence, morbidity is only that related to surgical resection (i.e., minimal with small lesions, but possible severe morbidity in a patient with a diffuse invasive lesion requiring extensive resection). However, recurrence after an apparently successful extirpation is not infrequent. Depending on the size of the lesion, whether it is diffuse or well-circumscribed, and how amenable it is to initial complete resection anatomically, reports show recurrence in 50% to 66% of cases.[101,102] Ultimately, amputation of the extremity because of pain or severe ischemia may be necessary.[103]

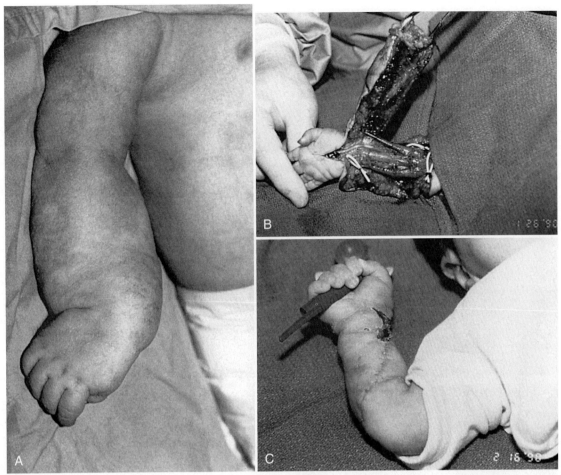

Figure 62-16 This large hemangioma of the forearm in a 6-week-old infant led to high-output cardiac failure. **A**, Preoperative appearance of the lesion. **B**, Resection and skin grafting was performed. Postoperatively, the cardiac failure resolved and the patient had normal hand function. **C**, Postoperative appearance.

Acquired Arteriovenous Fistulas

Acquired arteriovenous fistulas of the hand occur most often after a penetrating trauma. In contrast with pseudoaneurysm formation, where only arterial injury occurs, arteriovenous fistulas form after trauma to arterial and venous vessels that are in close proximity. An anomalous lumen forms between the vessels, creating a shunt proximal to the capillary bed; the result is distal ischemia or claudication and proximal venous dilation. Physical examination reveals a thrill or bruit. Ischemic pain may decrease with occlusion of either the arterial or venous feeder vessels. Diagnostic workup with color duplex ultrasonography or MR angiography will delineate the condition. Early excision allows vascular repair. Care must be taken to ligate all communicating vessels; otherwise, the fistula may recur.

Iatrogenic fistulas in the forearm and antecubital fossa used for access to renal dialysis have led to distal ischemia and tissue loss as well as compression neuropathy of the median and ulnar nerves. Early treatment, with either bending to reduce flow or revision to another site, alleviates this problem.[104,105]

Aneurysmal Disease

Aneurysms of the upper extremity are rare and have been classified according to pathologic origin (trauma, infection, or atherosclerosis), wall consistency (true or false), and location (subclavian, ulnar, or digital artery). Traumatic aneurysms (Fig. 62-18A) are the most common form of the disease; these lesions usually lack vessel wall elements and, for that reason, are called pseudoaneurysms or *false aneurysms*.[51] True aneurysms (Fig. 62-18B) have vessel walls with normal intima, media, and adventitia[106] and usually result from blunt trauma, atherosclerosis, or collagen diseases such as Marfan's syndrome.

An aneurysm presents most often as a mass. As such, all masses of the forearm must be palpated for thrills and auscultated for bruits. Doppler studies will improve the evaluation. Symptoms of distal embolization or nerve compression may be present, especially when the ulnar artery is involved.[107] The differential diagnosis of these masses includes ganglia, giant cell tumors, vascular tumors, and nerve tumors. Arteriography has been the traditional radiographic modality of choice for evaluating these masses, but noninvasive

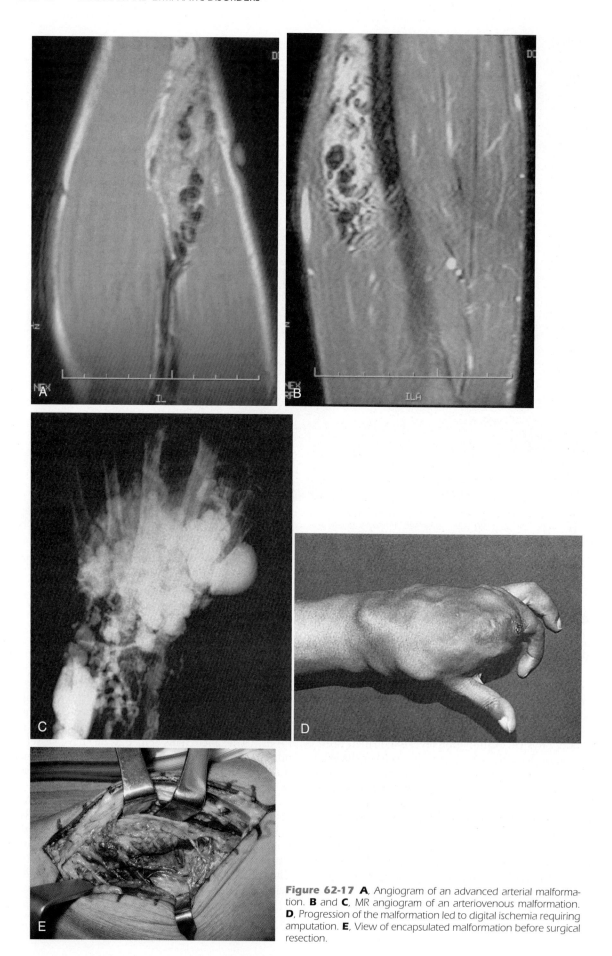

Figure 62-17 A, Angiogram of an advanced arterial malformation. **B** and **C**, MR angiogram of an arteriovenous malformation. **D**, Progression of the malformation led to digital ischemia requiring amputation. **E**, View of encapsulated malformation before surgical resection.

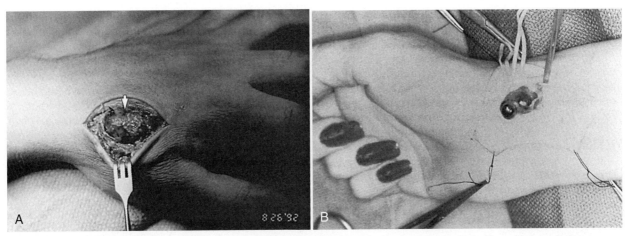

Figure 62-18 A, This traumatic aneurysm (*arrow*) developed after a stabbing that injured the radial artery in the first webspace. **B**, This true aneurysm of the radial artery developed after a blunt trauma.

assessment has been possible since the advent of duplex ultrasonography.[99]

Asymptomatic masses are simply observed, especially when they occur at the digital level. More often, however, the aneurysm will cause local pain or shower distal emboli, in which case resection and vessel ligation are performed to relieve symptoms.[108] Before ligation, the presence of adequate collateral flow must be confirmed by either preoperative Allen's testing or intraoperative plethysmography and back-flow. Microvascular reconstruction with vein grafting is necessary when adequate collateral flow is not present.

Hand Surgery in Particular Populations

Hand Surgery after Axillary Lymph Node Dissection or Radical Mastectomy

Subsequent ipsilateral hand complaints are not uncommon in patients with a history of treatment for breast cancer. Ganel et al.[109] showed that nearly 20% of patients developed carpal tunnel syndrome after axillary lymph node dissection (ALND). These problems may be related to lymphedema, which can occur in 6%-36% of patients after ALND,[110-113] but they are not confined to patients with lymphedema. More commonly, patients with a history of ALND or mastectomy present with a hand complaint, but do not have evidence of lymphedema.

Hershko et al. recently published their experience with this patient population.[114] Twenty-five patients with prior breast surgery (11 lumpectomy, 14 radical mastectomy) and ALND underwent elective hand surgery. Four of the patients had lymphedema, one of those severe. Surgery for carpal tunnel syndrome was performed in 12, and the others had surgery for a variety of hand complaints (trigger finger, de Quervain's, ganglion, etc.). No modification of technique was used; all but one operation was done with a tourniquet and local anesthesia (one patient with no lymphedema had a Bier block instead). There were no new cases of lymphedema. Two patients with preexisting lymphedema had transient

worsening that resolved in 3 months with compression stockings and physical therapy. One patient developed finger stiffness, and one had delayed wound healing in the non-lymphedema group. Dawson et al.[115] reported their experience in an ALND population of 15 women undergoing carpal tunnel release, seven of whom had lymphedema. They found no new cases of lymphedema, no worsening of preexisting lymphedema, and no infections or wound complications.

A recent survey completed by more than 600 members of the American Society for Surgery of the Hand showed that 94% of surgeons were comfortable operating on patients with prior ipsilateral ALND, and 85% were comfortable if there was preexisting lymphedema.[116] Tourniquet use was reported routinely by 94% of surgeons in patients without lymphedema and by 74% of surgeons if there was significant lymphedema. Perioperative protocol was unchanged for 50% of surgeons, whereas the other 50% added compressive postoperative therapy and or perioperative antibiotics.

Both limited case series and consensus opinion of members of the Society suggest that hand surgery may be safely performed after ipsilateral ALND. Consideration should be made for addition of compressive therapy postoperatively, especially in patients with preexisting lymphedema, and those with lymphedema should be counseled that acute exacerbation lasting several months is possible.

Hand Surgery on Patients Receiving Long-Term Oral Anticoagulants

Hand surgeons frequently encounter patients who are receiving oral anticoagulation for other medical problems. Management of these medications in the perioperative period is an important consideration. Two series have been published with regard to this patient population. Both showed that there is no need to discontinue these medications for routine outpatient hand surgery. The case series published by Smit and Hooper of 22 patients showed no bleeding complications and no other complications related to the medication.[117] A larger series by Wallace et al. showed two patients with minor bleeding problems that resolved without long-term sequelae.[118] Additionally, they found a hematoma rate consistent with published rates for Dupuytren's contracture release. Furthermore, there is also significant risk associated with discontinuing these medications needlessly.[119-121] Careful consideration to the bleeding risks of the surgery versus the patient's risk of interrupting their anticoagulation therapy must be weighed. While there are only limited data, available evidence supports continuing oral anticoagulation in patients undergoing routine outpatient hand surgery.

Summary

This chapter provides a sequential guide to the evaluation of the patient with a suspected vascular disorder. It reviews the pertinent anatomy; presents a specialized workup consisting of a guided history, physical examination, and diagnostic tests; and describes the most common vascular disorders along with their treatment protocols. Multiple specialized vascular diagnostic, perfusion, and imaging tests are also reviewed. Background, treatment, and diagnostic approach for multiple common conditions are discussed. Finally, hand surgery in particular populations is reviewed, including those receiving oral anticoagulation therapy and those with a history of axillary lymph node dissection or radical mastectomy.

REFERENCES

The complete reference list is available online at www.expertconsult.com.

Edema: Therapist's Management

JUNE P. VILLECO, MBA, OTR/L, MLDC, CHT

EDEMA DEFINED	ASSESSMENT OF EDEMA
NET CAPILLARY FILTRATION AND EFFECT ON EDEMA	TECHNIQUES FOR REDUCTION OF EDEMA
	SUMMARY
EDEMA AND STAGES OF WOUND HEALING	
PREVENTION OF EDEMA	

CRITICAL POINTS

Evaluation

Evaluation techniques should be reproducible and standardized.

Simple Lymphatic Massage

- Start and end proximally.
- Use minimal pressure needed to traction the skin.
- Pressure will vary slightly depending on skin texture.
- Strokes should be directed and open in direction of desired flow.
- Each stroke should take 2 to 3 seconds.
- Reroute edema around scar.

This chapter will cover the definition of edema, physiology, stages of wound healing, assessment of edema, and treatment techniques available to address local edema with intact (although overwhelmed) venous, arterial, and lymphatic systems.

The physiology and treatment of lymphedema is discussed separately in Chapter 64. Many of the same principles used in management of lymphedema can be applied to decrease local edema through facilitating more efficient lymphatic drainage. "Manual Edema Mobilization: Treatment for Edema in the Subacute Hand" is reviewed in Chapter 65. The reader is encouraged to refer to these additional chapters for more information on these specialized techniques.

Persistent edema presents a constant challenge to hand surgeons and hand therapists. If unresolved, it will delay healing and can result in pain and stiffness, thereby compromising functional results.

Edema Defined

Edema is the accumulation of excessive fluid in the intercellular spaces.[1,2] The process of controlling fluid accumulation involves a variety of factors that influence capillary filtration and lymph drainage. Both vascular and nonvascular processes affect fluid accumulation.

All cells are bathed in extracellular fluid. This fluid can be divided into two main components: the interstitial fluid and the blood plasma.[1,2] The interstitial fluid is outside of the closed vascular system.[3] Blood plasma is the fluid noncellular component of blood in which red blood cells, white blood cells, and platelets are suspended to collectively form total blood volume.[1,2] This circulating blood tissue permeates the vascular system and flows through the heart, arteries, capillaries, and veins.

The arterial system brings oxygen and nutrients to the cells, whereas the venous system is responsible for waste and carbon dioxide removal. The exchange of nutrients and cellular waste between the tissues and the circulating blood takes place at the level of the capillaries, primarily through diffusion and filtration. The capillary wall consists of a single layer of highly permeable endothelial cells and is surrounded by a basement membrane. The diameter of the capillary is just large enough for red blood cells and other blood cells to pass through.[1-3] Blood enters the capillaries through arterioles and metarterioles and exits through venules. It is rare that any single functional cell is more than 20 to 30 μm away from a capillary.[1,2] Oxygen and glucose are in higher

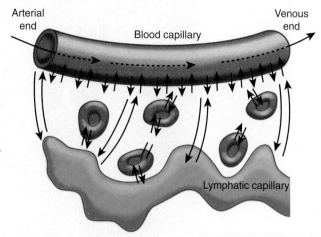

Figure 63-1 Diffusion of fluid molecules and dissolved substances between the capillary and interstitial fluid spaces. (From Guyton AC, Hall JE. *Textbook of Medical Physiology*. 9th ed. Philadelphia: WB Saunders, 1996.)

concentration in the bloodstream than in the interstitial fluid and diffuse into the interstitial fluid, whereas carbon dioxide diffuses in the opposite direction.[2,3] Proteins are too large to diffuse easily through the capillary membrane and primarily flow linearly along the capillary.[1] However, small amounts of proteins leak out of the blood capillaries into the interstitium, where they accumulate in the interstitial fluid.[1,2] The lymphatic system is responsible for returning proteins that have accumulated in the interstitial spaces back into the venous system until the system is back in balance. Lymph is fluid collected from tissues; it flows via lymphatic vessels through the lymph nodes and drains into the venous system.[1-3] Figure 63-1 illustrates the exchange process between substances in the interstitial fluid spaces with blood and lymphatic capillaries.

The spaces between cells are collectively called the *interstitium*. The fluid between cells (or interstitial fluid) is derived by filtration from the capillaries. There is a constant exchange of fluid between the intercellular tissue spaces and the blood plasma across the capillary membrane. Fluid in the interstitium is trapped by proteoglycan filaments, which cause the fluid to have the characteristics of a gel.[1,2] This "tissue gel" contains almost the same constituents as plasma, except for proteins, because proteins do not filter out of the capillaries easily. Water molecules, electrolytes, nutrients, and cellular waste *diffuse* through the interstitium rapidly, although fluid *flows* very poorly in the tissue gel.[1,2] Generally, there is only a very slight amount of fluid that is free from these proteoglycan filaments and not trapped in the tissue gel. In normal tissues, the "free" fluid is usually much less than 1%. When tissues start to develop edema, the gel can swell from 30% to 50% to accommodate the increased volume of interstitial free fluid.[1,2] After this point, the gel cannot accommodate additional fluid, and the amount of free fluid increases. The amount of the free fluid may expand to equal more than half of the interstitial fluid,[1,2] and the interstitial fluid volume can increase to several hundred percent above normal in seriously edematous tissues.[2] Pitting edema is made up of large amounts of free fluid in the tissues that can be displaced briefly by pressure, leaving a pit that slowly fills with fluid flowing back from the surrounding tissues[2] (Fig. 63-2 online). Brawny edema results when fluid in the interstitium becomes clotted with fibrinogen, preventing it from moving freely, or when tissue cells rather than the interstitium swells.[2] Brawny edema is firm to the touch.

Lymphedema refers to the specific type of edema caused by accumulation of protein-rich fluid in the extracellular space of skin and subcutaneous tissue, which results from obstruction of superficial extremity lymphatics.[4] Most edemas are caused by increased capillary filtration, which overwhelms lymph drainage (a condition called "dynamic insufficiency"). Lymphedema represents failure of the lymphatic system to drain lymph from a defined region, usually a limb, a condition called "mechanical insufficiency".[5] The lymphatic vessels are responsible for resorbing excess fluid as well as cells, proteins, lipids, microorganisms, and debris from tissues. The lymphatic system influences the volume of interstitial fluid and the interstitial fluid pressure as it compensates to balance the rate of protein and fluid leakage from the blood capillaries.

Net Capillary Filtration and Effect on Edema

Net filtration of fluid across the capillary membrane is determined by the balance between the forces that tend to force fluid outward into the interstitial spaces (filtration) and the forces that move fluid inward (resorption). Normally, the filtration pressures slightly exceed the resorption pressures, and the lymphatics balance the system by pulling excess fluid and proteins out of the interstitial spaces and returning them to the blood.[1,2]

Substances are transferred between the plasma and interstitial fluid primarily by diffusion through the capillary membrane. This diffusion provides continual mixing between the interstitial fluid and the plasma.[1,2] Lipid-soluble substances such as oxygen and carbon dioxide can diffuse directly through the cell membranes. Lipid-insoluble substances, such as chloride ions, sodium ions, and glucose, as well as water, diffuse through capillary pores or periodic intercellular clefts that connect the interior of the capillary with the exterior. These clefts or slit pores are about 20 times the diameter of a water molecule but slightly less than the diameters of plasma proteins such as an albumin molecule. The net rate of diffusion depends on the concentration difference between the two sides of the capillary membrane.

Minute vesicles are also located on the surface of the endothelial cells.[1-3] These vesicles transport plasma and extracellular fluid through the capillary wall by imbibing small amounts and then moving slowly through the endothelial cells, releasing the contents to the outer surface.[1-3] Fluid exchange depends on the properties of the capillary walls and the pressures acting across the capillary membrane. Capillary permeability is selective and is affected by pressures and relative concentrations on either side of the membrane and on the integrity of the membrane itself.[6] Capillary permeability is increased following external injury, operative trauma, and burns.[7]

The primary four pressures that influence net capillary filtration are the capillary (hydrostatic) pressure, the interstitial fluid (hydrostatic) pressure, the plasma colloid osmotic pressure, and the interstitial fluid colloid osmotic pressure. The *capillary pressure* is the blood pressure in the capillaries that tends to move fluid from the capillary outward through the membrane at any given point.[1,2,6,7] This pressure is greater at the arterial end than at the venous end of the capillary, resulting in fluid filtering out at the arterial end and being reabsorbed at the venous end of the blood capillaries.

The *interstitial fluid pressure* tends to force fluid inward through the capillary membrane when it is positive but outward when it is negative. This can be subdivided into the pressure of the fluid within the gel (integral pressure) and the free-fluid pressure. There is a slight difference between these pressures caused by the osmotic pressure of the gel. When acute edema develops, the free-fluid portion swells. Normally, in loose tissue, interstitial free-fluid pressure is slightly less than atmospheric pressure and exerts a suction force, drawing fluid out of the capillaries.[1,2] The direct cause of edema is positive pressure in the interstitial fluid spaces.[2]

Colloid osmotic or *oncotic pressures* are the pressures created by dissolved proteins, causing osmosis of fluid. The plasma colloid osmotic pressure draws fluid inward through the membrane, whereas the interstitial fluid colloid osmotic pressure draws fluid outward through the membrane. The concentration of protein in the plasma is generally two to three times that of the interstitial fluid. Approximately 75% of the plasma colloid osmotic pressure results from albumin. The plasma colloid osmotic pressure is important in preventing loss of fluid volume from the blood into the interstitial spaces.

The capillary pressure, *negative* interstitial free-fluid pressure, and interstitial fluid colloid osmotic pressure all tend to force fluid outward, whereas the plasma colloid osmotic pressure causes osmosis of fluid inward. The balance of pressure between these four forces is called the *net capillary filtration pressure*. There is usually a higher outward force (filtration pressure) at the arterial end of the capillary because of the higher capillary pressure at this end, and a higher inward force, or resorption pressure, is seen at the venous end. About nine-tenths of what is filtered out at the arterial end of the capillary is reabsorbed back in at the venous end, with the remaining fluid going through the lymph vessels.[1,2] When the net filtration pressure rises excessively, too much fluid is moved outward into the interstitial spaces for the lymphatics to manage, and *extracellular edema* results.

Abnormal leakage of fluid from the capillaries into the extracellular (interstitial) spaces can be caused by increased capillary pressure (as with arteriolar dilation, venular constriction, increased venous pressure, failure of venous pumps, or lack of active muscular activity), decreased plasma proteins (as with loss of proteins from denuded skin areas in burns and wounds), increased capillary permeability (as results from release of histamine and related substances, from kinins such as bradykinin, or from bacterial infections), or blockage of lymph return.[1-3] All of these will result in an increased volume of interstitial fluid with subsequent expansion of the extracellular fluid volume.[1,2]

Widespread edema may be caused by heart failure, loss of proteins in the urine or decreased ability to produce proteins, and excessive kidney retention of salt and water.[1-3] Trauma can cause venous obstruction or arteriolar dilation and thus result in increased capillary pressure and a higher net filtration pressure.[6] The capillary filtration pressure will also be elevated by local or general heating that causes arterial dilation. Burns not only decrease plasma proteins (as discussed earlier) but also lead to increased capillary permeability and may allow fluid to spill into the tissues as a result of damage to the integrity of the capillary endothelium or enlarged capillary pores.[6] Release of histamine, bradykinin, and substance P is part of an initial inflammatory response and will increase capillary permeability and blood flow, allowing large quantities of fluid and protein, including fibrinogen, to leak into the tissue. This in turn will cause increased interstitial fluid to accumulate.[2]

Intracellular edema can occur in conditions in which the metabolic systems of tissues are depressed or lack adequate nutrition to the cells, and it may occur in inflamed tissue areas as cell membranes increase their permeability to sodium and other ions, with subsequent osmosis of water into the cells.[1,2]

Edema and Stages of Wound Healing

The nature and treatment of edema differ for the three stages of wound healing. The stages are described here and consist of the inflammatory phase, which usually lasts the first 3 to 5 days; the fibroplastic or proliferative phase, which may last 2 to 6 weeks depending on the nature and degree of injury; and the maturation or remodeling phase, which may last from 6 months to 2 years.[8,9]

Edema is the first and most obvious reaction of the hand to injury. Most wounds have an excess of fluid content early in the healing process. Release of histamine and bradykinin increases capillary permeability and is part of a normal acute inflammatory reaction that occurs in response to tissue injury from a variety of causes, including trauma, heat, chemicals, and bacteria. Edema in the early phase of wound healing is liquid, soft, and easy to mobilize and reduce. At this stage, the excess fluid or *transudate* consists mainly of water and dissolved electrolytes.[10] This type of edema should not alarm the therapist as long as the principles of compression, elevation, use of cold, and active motion are observed to minimize pooling of blood in injured areas.[11,12] However, excessive edema can inhibit wound healing by decreasing arterial, venous, and lymphatic flow.[13]

The primary function of the inflammatory phase is to wall off the injured area, dispose of injury by-products through phagocytosis, and prepare for the fibroplastic repair phase. Chemical mediators initially cause vasoconstriction, followed by vasodilation. Increased cell permeability allows passage of fluid and white blood cells through cell walls to form plasma.[12] Leukocytes and other phagocytic cells accumulate at the site of injury to clean up the debris, and fibrinogen is converted to fibrin. Key to treatment in the inflammatory phase of wound healing is pain control and a balance between gentle active range of motion in an elevated position and rest of the involved structures. Excessive exercise in this phase can delay clot formation and increase inflammation.[12] Heat is also contraindicated in the inflammatory stage, because it will cause further vasodilation and increase membrane permeability, capillary infiltration, and arterial blood flow, which will result in additional edema.

Fibroplasia begins as early as 3 to 5 days after injury and lasts from 2 to 6 weeks, depending on the extent of the wound.[8,9] During the fibroplastic or repair stage of wound healing, repair of the injured tissue is initiated. Fibroplasia is characterized by increased capillary growth, increased fibroblasts, and new collagen synthesis. Clinically, scar production is heightened, and the wound begins to gain tensile strength.

Edema that persists into the fibroplasia phase is of particular concern to the surgeon and therapist. This edema is likely to become an ongoing problem unless early intervention is applied. The edema fluid becomes more viscous from the elevated protein content, and the excess fluid is called *exudate*.[10] The protein-rich fluid or exudate associated with edema causes fibrosis and thickening of the tissues, with subsequent shortening of structures such as ligaments and tendons. As fibrin is deposited between tissue layers, organized adhesions result between structures such as tendons and their sheaths, joint capsules, synovial membranes, and fascial layers.[6,14] Structures will continue to swell, thicken, and shorten, and eventually will be replaced by dense fibrous tissue.[11,15] The greater the edema and the longer it persists, the more extensive the scarring and the resultant pain, adhesions, disfigurement, and disability. All tissues—vessels, nerves, joints, and intrinsic muscles—become involved in a state of reduced nutrition and inelasticity. The combination of persistent edema with immobilization and poor positioning ultimately results in a stiff hand and must be circumvented.

If the lymphatic system becomes blocked or metabolites are allowed to accumulate in the interstitial spaces, colloid osmotic pressure is increased by the relative increase in concentration of proteins, again resulting in a higher capillary net filtration pressure. The coagulating effect of tissue exudates causes the interstitial and lymphatic fluid to clot, preventing the fluid from being expelled by pressure and resulting in brawny edema in the spaces surrounding the injured cells.[1] Brawny or nonpitting edema can also be caused by swelling of the tissues cells from trauma, disease, or inadequate nutrition.[1]

The final phase of healing is called the *maturation* or *remodeling phase*; it is initiated as fibroplasia subsides. In this stage, tissue remodeling and realignment are achieved by placing tensile stresses on collagen fibers. At this point, persistent, stagnant edema may have led to fibrosis with elevated protein content. Chronic edema will result in stretching of the tissue spaces, necessitating long-term use of continuous-compression garments to maintain gains made in edema reduction. If allowed to progress to the maturation phase, edema will become hard, thick, and brawny as the result of connective tissue infiltration and fibrosis. In the worst scenario, edema compromises arterial flow, causing anoxia and impaired metabolic circulation and cellular nutrition, and necrosis of tissues may ensue.

Prevention of Edema

The prevention and treatment of edema are of paramount importance during all phases of management of the injured hand.[16] Measures must be taken before edema is visible, because interstitial fluid volume will increase 30% above normal before detection.[2] According to Brand and Thompson,[17] as much as 50 mL of edematous fluid can accumulate in the hand without being noticed "by a busy therapist dealing with a succession of patients." More recently, Kelly also comments that "a 30% fluid overload may occur before swelling is visible."[18]

After surgery or trauma, the extremity should be positioned above the heart as much of the time as possible except following arterial injury/repair. In this case the hand should be slightly below the level of the heart to prevent undue pressure on the repaired artery. If the hand must be immobilized, when possible it should be positioned in the intrinsic-plus position of flexed metacarpophalangeal (MCP) joints (to 70 degrees) and extended interphalangeal (IP) joints to prevent shortening of the MCP joint collateral ligaments and IP volar plates. The wrist should be positioned in neutral or slight extension. The first webspace also must be maintained via thumb abduction and extension. This is particularly true with burn patients, whose wounds will contract as they heal. If the intrinsic-plus position is not feasible, the patient's hand should be positioned in the best approximation and the orthosis adjusted when feasible.[19] In some cases injured and repaired structures of the hand may require alternative positioning.

Active ROM and tendon gliding exercises are especially important in the fibroplasia stage of healing to prevent the development of adhesions. Orthotic positioning will help to maintain and increase ROM. All joints that are not required to be immobilized should be able to move freely in the cast or orthosis and taken through their full ROM.

Edema in its early stages is reversible. If edema can be controlled early, subsequent scar formation is minimized in comparison with the scar that forms if edema is prolonged and brawny. Postoperative efforts are directed toward minimizing edema and promoting uncomplicated wound healing. Patient education is vital. Beginning with the initial treatment in the hospital or clinic, the patient must be made aware of the factors that can exacerbate or alleviate edema.

Assessment of Edema

As discussed previously, a significant amount of edema may accumulate in a hand without visible detection.[17] For this reason, the ability to establish and measure changes in edema with standardized and reliable procedures is critical for the effective management of edema. Edema will fluctuate daily with changes in diet, activity level, water retention, temperature, and time of day. Therefore, it is important to measure both the involved and uninvolved extremities to obtain a relative comparison between the two, ideally at the same time of day and in the same position. Measures should be taken at the initial evaluation and routinely thereafter with one of the three techniques described below.

The volumeter, figure-of-eight method, and truncated circumferential method of measuring edema are all reliable techniques to measure edema. A high correlation between water displacement and geometric (truncated) formulas has been well documented.[20-26] Studies are also available that assess volumetry and truncated measures as a tool to look at change in edematous arms over a period of time. Both measures have been found to be accurate, although the methods are not interchangeable.[22,24-26] Total volumes for both of these measures are provided in units of cubic centimeters, which can be converted directly to milliliters. The figure-of-eight method provides a final measure in centimeters. A high correlation between the figure-of-eight method and volumetry has been established in three separate studies,[27-29] as well as in a study by Maihafer et al. that used slightly different landmarks.[30]

The volumeter is a standardized tool that allows the therapist to measure hand edema by measuring the amount of water the limb displaces.[31,32] Waylett-Rendall and Seibly[32] have shown that the volumeter is reliable within ± 10 mL (1%) if successive measures are performed by the same examiner. A subsequent study done by King[33] assessed the effect of water temperature on hand volume during volumetric measurement. Although there was a significant difference in volumes using extreme temperatures (41°F versus 113°F; 5°C versus 45°C), it was found that the use of "cool" (68°F; 20°C) versus "tepid" (95°F; 35°C) water does not appear to alter hand volume readings sufficiently to be of concern.[33]

The difference in volume of dominant versus nondominant hands was studied by Van Velze et al.[34] for 263 male laborers. They concluded that, on average, the left nondominant hand was 3.43% smaller (16.9 mL) than the right dominant hand for male laborers.[34]

The effect of exercise of the asymptomatic hand on volumetric and sensory status has been studied by McGough and Surwasky.[35] Their results on 20 subjects suggest that exercise influences volumetric measurements. Specifically, females in the study demonstrated a 3.6% increase in volumetrics immediately after exercise, with a decline in volume at 10 minutes after exercise to 2.4%.[35] The males in the study demonstrated a 5.2% volume increase immediately after exercise, with a decline in volume at 10 minutes after exercise to 5%. McGough and Surwasky encourage further statistical investigation on a larger scale of the role of hand dominance, gender, and age on hand volume.

It is important to follow the standardized procedure for the volumeter and to standardize alternative techniques as much as possible. The volumetric kit includes the volumeter, the 800-mL collection beaker, and a 500-mL graduated cylinder (Fig. 63-3A online). Instructions for the standardized procedure to use with the commercially available volumeters accompany each volumeter purchased from equipment companies. The volumeter should be placed on exactly the same spot on the same level surface for each use. Readings should also be taken on exactly the same spot, since most floors and tables are not completely level. The volumeter should be filled with room temperature water (68°F to 95°F) until it overflows, the overflow discarded, and the beaker placed

---

Box 63-1 Formulas for Calculating Limb Volume from Truncated Surface Measures

Formula for every 4 cm: Volume = circumference^2/π for each segment

Formula for every 10 cm: Volume = $h[(C_t \times C_t) + (C_t \times C_b) + (C_b \times C_b)]12\pi$

Where h is the height of the cone, C_t is the circumference at the top of the cone, and C_b is the circumference at the bottom of the cone, for each segment.

For example, the first cone could be the area between the MCP joints and wrist. Assuming these are 8 cm apart (height), the MCP joints (top of cone) measure 16 cm, and the wrist (bottom of cone) measures 18 cm, the formula for this segment would be:

$$8[(16 \times 16) + (16 \times 18) + (18 \times 18)]12\,\pi$$

For the next segment/cone, the wrist will now be the top of the cone, and the distal forearm at the bottom of the cone. Assuming that these landmarks are 10 cm apart and the measure at the distal forearm is 20 cm; the formula for this segment would be:

$$10[(18 \times 18) + (18 \times 20) + (20 \times 20)]12\,\pi$$

---

under the volumeter's spout. Once all jewelry has been removed from the patient's hand, the hand should be lowered into the volumeter with the thumb facing the spout and the forearm in pronation until the webspace between the middle and ring fingers firmly straddles the rod (Fig. 63-3B online). The sides of the hand should not come into contact with the sides of the volumeter. Any variations in this position should be documented. Water will overflow into the beaker. This position must be maintained until water stops spilling from the spout. The water from the beaker can than be poured into the graduated cylinder and measured. This same process is then completed with the other hand. Both hands should always be measured.[6,31,36,37]

Truncated surface measures are derived by dividing the arm into cones, determining the volume of each cone, and summing these to determine total arm volume. There are two basic formulas for this, depending on whether measures are taken every 4 cm (or less) or every 10 cm (or less) (Box 63-1). Commercial computer programs are available that automate the computations once the therapist has determined the landmarks and circumferences, or the formulas can be entered into a spreadsheet program, such as Microsoft Excel. Landmarks are recorded as the distance in centimeters measured from the third fingertip or nail bed (Fig. 63-4A) with the first landmark being at the MCP, all joints neutral as able, and the arm pronated. Additional landmarks should be taken every 4 to 10 cm. as well as anywhere that the shape of the arm changes significantly, such as the wrist and elbow. The same landmarks should be used on the uninvolved arm and in all subsequent reassessments. It is important to use

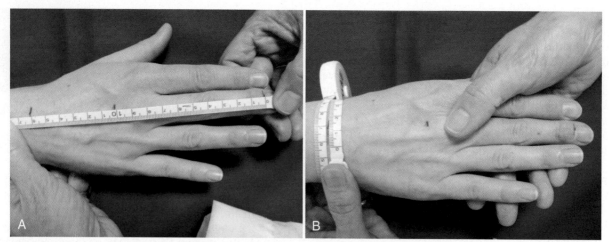

Figure 63-4 A, Landmarks are recorded in centimeters from the proximal cuticle or fingertip of the long finger, with all joints in neutral extension and the arm pronated, if able, for truncated circumferential measures. Variations in joint positioning must be noted. **B**, To enhance repeatability, circumferential measurements must be taken the same way and in the same position each time. Measurements should straddle the landmark, the tape measure should be taut without providing tension to the skin, and the portion of the extremity being measured should be parallel to the ground or table and positioned the same way as when the landmarks were determined. The tape should be placed with the higher numbers proximal to the landmark, the lower numbers distal. This therapist measures with the case of the tape measure resting just inside and below the extremity (to provide a constant and reproducible force).

the same measuring tape and to apply consistent tension. One way to accomplish this is to have the tape straddle the landmark with the larger number always proximal, and with the ball of the tape always hanging just inside and below the arm where it is being measured (Fig. 63-4B). The tape should be taut and lay flat against the skin, without being so tight as to wrinkle the skin.

Figure 63-5A to E illustrates the figure-of-eight technique as described by Pellecchia.[29] It uses four landmarks to provide one cumulative number in centimeters as a measure of edema. Measures are taken with the wrist in neutral and the fingers adducted. The tape is placed at (Fig. 63-5A) the medial wrist, distal to the ulnar styloid; crosses the ventral wrist to (Fig. 63-5B) the distal radial styloid; crosses the dorsal wrist diagonally to the (Fig. 63-5C) fifth MCP joint; and finally crosses the wrist dorsally to return to the (Fig. 63-5D) distal ulnar styloid. It is important to provide consistent tension on the tape measure.

At least one of these three measures should be appropriate for any patient with edema. All three can be used with hand edema; volumes or truncated measures can be used with edema that extends to the forearm. Truncated measures are especially useful for patients with large arms or diffuse edema that makes using the volumeter difficult, and for patients with pins, fixators, or open wounds that preclude use of the volumeter. For early-stage edema that is not observable clinically, the patient may describe heaviness or fullness in the extremity, pain, tingling, or numbness.[18] Measurements may not reflect this early-stage edema; however, the clinician should institute edema management techniques.

Techniques for Reduction of Edema

The specific techniques used to promote resolution of edema vary depending on whether the edema is in the inflammatory, fibroplastic, or maturation phase of wound healing.

The following modalities can be used in combination and are discussed in more detail below: cold, elevation, active motion, lymphatic massage, intermittent compression, continuous passive motion (CPM), compressive bandages, electrical stimulation, other electrical modalities, and hyperbaric oxygen.

Cold

Cold application may be helpful in limiting edema formation by producing vasoconstriction and reducing metabolic rate and arteriolar blood flow, reducing membrane permeability and capillary infiltration.[14,38,39] However, careful attention to vascular status is required when cold packs are used, because excessive cooling may result in tissue ischemia and damage. Cold is contraindicated in the presence of arterial compromise or repair. Cold is especially helpful during the initial inflammatory phase; it performs better than heat or contrast baths in existing studies[35,39,40] and should be used in combination with other principles of edema management, such as elevation and compression.

McMaster[38] found improved edema control with 20-minute applications of cold over 10 therapy sessions. Cote found that cold application resulted in better control of edema than heat or contrast baths.[40] Stockle[39] studied the reduction of foot or ankle edema using an intermittent impulse compression device, continuous cryotherapy, or cool packs and found reductions of 74%, 70%, and 45%, respectively. Bleakely[41] conducted a systematic review and reported that many more high-quality trials are needed to provide evidence-based guidelines in the treatment of acute soft tissue injuries. Bleakely concluded that ice was more effective than no ice after knee surgery, and more effective with exercise or electrical stimulation; moreover, Bleakely found little evidence to suggest that ice with compression was more effective than compression alone. Ice or cold packs are used with an interface lining such as a towel between the skin and the pack. The duration of use is usually for 10 to 15 minutes.

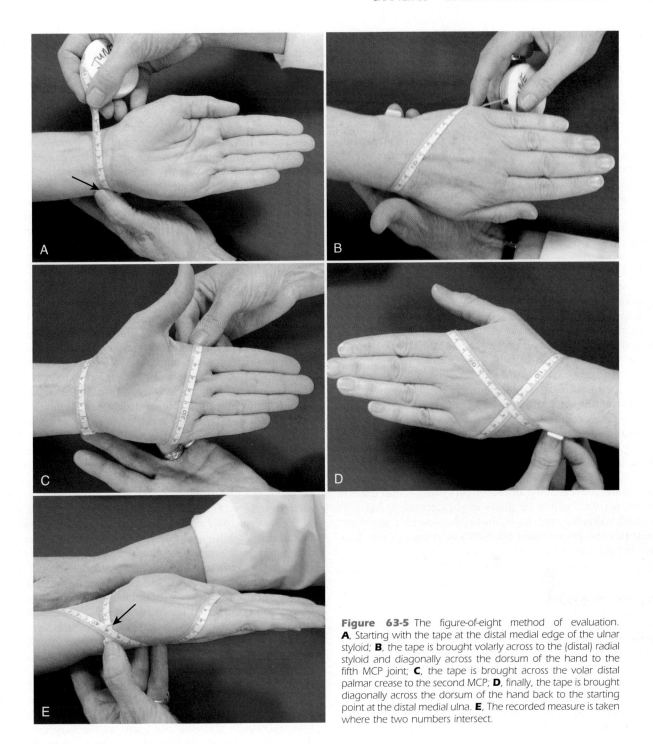

Figure 63-5 The figure-of-eight method of evaluation. **A**, Starting with the tape at the distal medial edge of the ulnar styloid; **B**, the tape is brought volarly across to the (distal) radial styloid and diagonally across the dorsum of the hand to the fifth MCP joint; **C**, the tape is brought across the volar distal palmar crease to the second MCP; **D**, finally, the tape is brought diagonally across the dorsum of the hand back to the starting point at the distal medial ulna. **E**, The recorded measure is taken where the two numbers intersect.

Elevation

Elevation uses gravity to enhance venous and lymphatic flow out of traumatized areas. Elevation is especially indicated in early-stage edema such as immediately after surgery. For elevation to be effective, a gentle decline from distal to proximal with the entire limb slightly above the level of the heart should be achieved. In other words, the hand should be slightly higher than the wrist, the wrist should be slightly higher than the elbow, and the elbow should be positioned slightly higher than the shoulder. Pillows or wedge supports can be used to position the extremity appropriately at a table or in bed. If arterial systems are compromised or if elevation causes ischemia of the extremity, the level of elevation will have to be altered. When arterial occlusion is diagnosed, the arm should be lowered below the heart. When venous occlusion is diagnosed, the extremity should be elevated.[42] While increased edema is empirically evident with dependent positioning, there are no actual studies that demonstrate decreased edema formation with elevation above the heart.[43] However, the complications of edema are much more difficult to treat than the prevention of edema, and it is prudent to utilize simple procedures such as elevation at least to the level of the heart to minimize the possibility of this development.

Precautions must be observed for the replanted arm, hand, or digit. In this case excessive elevation is to be avoided, because it can stress the arterial system. Elevation for the transplanted limb should be at the level of the heart and modified according to the patient's arterial and venous status.[44] Healthy replanted digits are warm and pink. Arterial occlusion may be indicated by a cool, pale digit, whereas venous insufficiency is associated with a dusky hue in the replanted part. The therapist should instruct the patient to make sure that the elbow is not kept in a flexed position, because this may create an obstruction to venous drainage. A sudden increase in edema or an alteration in color or temperature should be reported immediately to the surgeon.[11]

In addition to facilitating venous and lymphatic outflow from the limbs, elevation decreases the hydrostatic pressure in the blood vessels, which in turn decreases the capillary filtration pressure at the arterial end.[7] As discussed previously, hydrostatic pressure occurs in the vascular system because of the weight of blood in the vessels.[3] Peripheral venous and arterial pressures are influenced by gravity. The pressure in any vessel held below heart level is increased by gravity, and the pressure in any vessel held above the level of the heart is decreased by gravity.[3] When the hand is lower than the heart, the intravascular pressure is increased, in turn increasing the capillary filtration pressure.[7] Consequently, interstitial fluid will accumulate in the dependent hand. In contrast, keeping the limb above the level of the heart decreases the intravascular pressure and decreases the capillary filtration pressure.[3]

Active Motion

Active exercises create muscle pumping, soft tissue movement, and compression of veins and lymphatic vessels, all of which are helpful in edema control.[44-47] Strong muscular contractions assist in venous and lymphatic drainage.[47] Active motion prevents stagnation of tissue fluids that can result from lack of use.

Schuind and Burny[48] state that the postcapillary blood pressure facilitating venous return is less than 15 mm Hg, whereas the hydrostatic pressure opposing venous return from the dependent hand is approximately 35 mm Hg. Active movement is required to produce venous return.[48] There is also data supporting the benefits of exercise in enhancing lymph flow and improving resorption.[5,49] It is important to include the more proximal joints in a ROM program. These joints will become stiff if not taken through their ROM, and active pumping of the proximal muscles will help clear any proximal edema, thus allowing more efficient drainage of distal edema. An effective exercise that incorporates elevation and active motion of the digits and shoulders is to have the patient elevate both arms over the head and make firm fists at least 25 repetitions each hour.[11,50]

Light cardiopulmonary exercise will stimulate the lymphatic system and assist with fluid uptake via the thoracic duct, which penetrates the diaphragm.

Simple Lymphatic Massage

Lymphatic massage can mobilize tissue fluid and increase lymphatic flow.[7] Lymphatic massage can increase the frequency of lymphatic vessel contraction, thereby increasing the transport capacity of the lymphatic system.[19,51] Stimulation of the lymphatic system through massage has been shown to be helpful in both the lympedema population[53] and the hand therapy population.[53] Simple lymphatic drainage concepts can be applied to local edema and are discussed below.

Superficial lymphatic capillaries have anchoring filaments that attach them to the surrounding tissue. Stretch to the overlying skin causes "clefts" in the capillary walls to open and accept fluid from the surrounding tissue. Only minimal pressure is needed to stimulate this process. In fact, Eliska[54] has shown that pressure above 60 mm Hg will cause mechanical occlusion of the capillaries and be counterproductive to fluid reabsorption. The exact force required for an optimal response will vary slightly depending on skin texture but should be the minimum force required to traction the skin without sliding on the skin. In Dr. Vodder's words, "The drainage must be performed softly, harmoniously, rhythmically, and with supple hands. ... The hands should be so supple and alive that the dry skin can be massaged."[55] While the exact pressure must be adapted to the findings, it should never elicit pain.[55] A variety of types of strokes can be used, but the simplest is the stationary circle, variably referred to as a U or J or L stroke. The bottom of the stroke at the base of the J or L catches the skin distally, and then longitudinal traction is provided to the skin in a proximal direction to the limit of the skin's elasticity. Massage should never be painful, and the individual strokes should always go in the direction toward the regional lymph nodes. The palmar surface of the hand should be used when possible, or several fingers together for smaller areas so as to avoid point pressure.

Before providing simple lymphatic massage to the local area of edema, it is important to create a path for the edema. A useful analogy is a traffic jam caused by a wreck up the street. Before backed-up traffic can begin to move, the wreck has to be pulled off the highway. Once it is cleared away, the traffic farthest ahead (the most "proximal" traffic) will move first, eventually allowing the traffic at the very end (most distal) of the jam to flow again. Likewise, regional lymph nodes have to be stimulated to increase uptake proximally and provide a path for distal edema to follow. It is important to start (clear) proximally, work distally to the local edema, and then move this edema proximally by providing light, proximally directed, skin tractioning massage strokes to the skin between the edema and the regional lymph nodes. Simple lymphatic drainage should start and end proximally. Each stroke should be performed slowly and take 2 to 3 seconds, to allow for refilling and emptying of the lymphatic vessels (see video online).[51] With successive strokes, the therapist will be able to feel the underlying edematous tissue soften and flatten. It is also important to remember that edema will have to be rerouted around scars/incisions, since it cannot go through scars. Each skin area should be massaged a minimum of 5 to 10 times, with more attention to specific areas as needed.

Simple lymphatic massage is contraindicated any time stimulation of the circulatory system must be minimized or avoided. This includes, but is not limited to, co-morbidities such as deep vein thrombosis, pulmonary embolism, untreated infection, untreated cancer, chronic heart failure, or renal failure. Simple lymphatic massage is specific to local edema for the hand therapy population with an intact lymphatic system and is not appropriate for generalized edema or lymphedema. The reader is encouraged to review Chapters 64 and 65 for further information on these highly specialized techniques.

Massage techniques such as retrograde massage, tube wrapping, and string wrapping are to be avoided.

Intermittent Pneumatic Compression

Intermittent pneumatic compression may be helpful in decreasing edema during the inflammatory phase by facilitating the lymphatic system's ability to resorb proteins, cellular components, and fatty acids and by assisting in the removal of these during the fibroplasia phase.[12] Intermittent compression has been shown to be an effective adjunct to lymphatic massage to reduce lymphedema in conjunction with lymphatic massage,[52,56,57] and as an adjunct to edema with high-voltage electrical stimulation,[59] although there is variability as to the treatment protocols with regard to pressure, duration, and frequency.[13,47,49,58-60] Its efficacy with the hand therapy population has been mixed.[58,59,61] Intermittent compression increases tissue hydrostatic pressure and acceleration of the lymphatic and venous flow.[7] This in turn drives lymphatic fluid back into the venous system. However, while intermittent compression is able to displace fluid, it does not stimulate the lymphatic system directly and does not increase uptake of proteins.[60] As a result, gains made with intermittent compression pumping with protein-rich edemas may not be stable and may reverse quickly as proteins continue to pull fluid back into the interstitial spaces. To be effective, the intermittent pump pressure must be greater than the 25–mm Hg[29] mean capillary pressure and should not exceed 60 mm Hg in patients with an intact lymphatic system. One of the problems with intermittent compression pumps is that it is difficult to measure exactly how much pressure is transferred to the lymphatic vessels through the skin, which will be different for brawny edema than for pitting types of edema. Segers et al.[62] found wide discrepancies between the target pressure as set by the controls and the actual pressures delivered inside the cuff chambers, with the actual pressures being as much as 80% higher. As mentioned previously, excessive pressures may damage the lymphatic vessels and result in further increases in edema. Intermittent compression should be used cautiously and primarily with patients who are not able to master self lymphatic massage.

Treatment duration guidelines range from 30 minutes to 2 hours for the patient with acute edema. Leduc et al.[60] advise that pneumatic compression not exceed 40 mm Hg for patients with compromised lymphatic systems. The limb should be elevated during treatment with intermittent com-

pression. The compression-to-release ratio is usually 3:1 or 4:1.[13] The amount of pressure must be adjusted according to each patient's diagnosis and condition. Intermittent pneumatic compression should be used with caution with acute injuries, since premature use can result in increased bleeding.[10] Acute fractures are a relative contraindication, since the pressure could result in unwanted movement/displacement of the fracture. Stable fractures can begin with a low amount of pressure once enough healing has taken place to tolerate the pressure, but the treatment should be carefully supervised by the therapist. The presence of open wounds does not prohibit intermittent pressure as long as sterile dressings are used. Felt pads can be positioned around pins to prevent pressure on them. More chronic edema will require higher pressures and longer treatment times.

Several different models of pneumatic pumps provide compression, including single-chamber and multichamber pumps. A multichamber sequential-pressure sleeve inflates from distal to proximal and is theoretically more effective at returning fluid to the lymphatic system by preventing back-flow. One concern with the single-chamber unit is that it may merely redistribute fluid into areas of low hydrostatic pressure and spread the edema over a larger area.[63]

Intermittent compression is contraindicated in patients with infection or with any patient who has a medical condition who may not be able to safely handle the additional pressure or additional fluid load into their circulatory system. This includes patients with congestive heart failure, cardiac or renal insufficiency, pulmonary edema, deep vein thrombosis, or vascular compromise. It should be used with caution in patients with impaired sensation.

Continuous Passive Motion

CPM is another method available for the therapist to consider to reduce hand edema in postoperative patients, especially patients who have undergone surgical release procedures such as tenolysis or capsulectomy. This group of patients may be predisposed to the development of adhesions and hand stiffness. Hand CPM units include parameters that can be set by the therapist to control the specific ROM desired and velocity of movement. Many units include an MCP joint block to isolate IP joint motion. CPM is most effective during the early phases of wound healing and early scar formation. CPM in the pain-free ROM allows for improved gliding, nutrition of tissues, and scar lengthening.[64] CPM may also have a role with patients who have an impaired ability to actively use their hand, such as patients who have hemiplegia secondary to a cerebrovascular accident.[46] Passive ROM will maintain joint mobility in the specified range and can improve lymphatic flow.

Compressive Bandages

In the acute stage of wound healing, compression limits the amount of space available for swelling to accumulate.[12] Compression may decrease fibroblast synthesis of collagen by decreasing the blood flow and causing local hypoxia,[13] which is especially important in the fibroplasia phase. Pressure may mechanically force fluid out of the tissue.[13] In the later stages of wound healing, compression maintains gains made in edema reduction by reducing capillary filtration. Compressive garments help reinforce tissue hydrostatic pressure and facilitate venous and lymphatic flow. The use of compressive garments or wrapping is especially important with brawny (fibrotic) edema and should always be used following pneumatic pumping or lymphatic massage to maintain reductions in edema.

Various compressive dressings are available commercially. These include compressive stockinets, tubular elastic bandages, finger sleeves, pressure garments and gloves, short-stretch bandages, finger sleeves and wraps, self-adherent bandages, and Isotoner gloves (Isotoner, Cincinnati, Ohio), among others.[47] Short stretch bandages provide more support and controlled compression than elastic wrapping for the arm. Any type of circular elastic bandages, such as tubigrip tubular bandages, have the potential to create a tourniquet effect and should be used cautiously and monitored carefully; these types of compressive garments should be limited to alert patients during waking hours so as to allow for appropriate monitoring of circulation.

For stubborn or brawny edema, foam or chip bags made from small pieces of varied-density foam can be used under a wrap to soften these areas. Light foam over a larger area will improve tolerance to the wrap by distributing the forces, while dense foam over a problem area such as the back of the hand provides more compression. Chip bags provide significant local pressure and are especially helpful for brawny areas but may be less tolerated. As with any bandaging, the extremity should be wrapped from distal to proximal to assist with lymphatic and venous drainage, and a spiral or figure-of-eight technique (not circular) should be used.

Specialized soft finger wraps such as Elastomull (BSN Medical, Inc., Charlotte, North Carolina) can be used to facilitate lymphatic function and provide gentle compression to the hand without restricting ROM. These wraps anchor at the wrist and cross the dorsum of the hand to start at the small finger or thumb, depending on the direction of the wrap (Fig. 63-6). This type of wrap provides superior ability to provide even pressure while accommodating to changes in joint position. While originally intended as a technique to include all the digits, this same technique can be applied to a single edematous digit. These finger wraps can be worn safely in a reliable patient with normal sensation for 24 hours.

Self-adherent wrap is another alternative for small areas, such as edematous digits. Care must be taken not to apply tension while wrapping, because this can restrict circulation. Patients must be instructed to carefully monitor the finger for circulation. There are two techniques for using self-adherent wrap; 1-inch wrap can be applied in an overlapping spiral (see Fig. 63-7 online), or, for patients who have difficulty applying this technique, a larger wrap can be wrapped once around the finger and cinched (distal to proximal) to provide more gentle compression (Fig. 63-8 online). Lowell[65] reports improved results in edema control using Coban (3M, St. Paul, Minnesota) over standard dressings for a patient with bilateral hand burns.

Compressive garments are contraindicated for patients with arterial compromise, new skin grafts, or unhealed burn wounds.

All forms of external compression must be monitored by the patient to make sure that capillary flow is not restricted. The patient who is using compression wrapping at home must be instructed to look for any signs of compromised circulation, such as changes in color, coldness, or numbness in the fingertip(s).

Electrical Stimulation

High-voltage pulsed direct current (HVPC) has been hypothesized to decrease edema by reducing microvascular permeability to plasma proteins.[45,66-69] It is hypothesized that the current reduces edema by repelling negatively charged proteins in the edematous interstitial spaces.[67,69] It is suggested that when the negative polarity of HVPC repels negatively charged cells and protein, a fluid shift occurs.[67] High-voltage current includes intensities greater than 100 V. Research results are mixed.

The effect of HVPC in reducing edema has been assessed in animal experiments with frogs, rats, and hamsters.[45,60,66,68,70] Other rat studies have yielded disappointing results. Mohr,[71] Cosgrove,[72] and Cook[73] did not find significant differences using subcontraction high voltage with Sprague-Dawley rats. A recent study by Hahm[74] found that using low-frequency electrical stimulation of acupoint sites for Sprague-Dawley rats resulted in decreased edema at 6 and 12 hours postinjury, but that high-frequency (5× muscle twitch) electrical stimulation did not have an effect on edema. Thorton[75] found that different strains of rats responded differently to electrical stimulation and that Sprague-Dawley rats did not respond whereas other strains did. Chu et al.[76] studied the effect of direct current on wound edema after full-thickness burn injury in rats and found that direct electric current had a beneficial effect in reducing wound edema after burn injury but that at least 8 hours of treatment were required to achieve a sustained maximum effect.

Human studies include work by Stralka, Griffen, Faghri Cheing, and Man.[58,69,77-79] Stralka et al.[69] conducted a study on the use of HVPC in reducing chronic hand edema in conjunction with a wrist orthosis that demonstrated significant decreases for hand edema and pain following treatment. Griffin et al.[58] compared the effectiveness of a single-treatment HVPC, intermittent pneumatic compression, and placebo-HVPC. Differences between the HVPC and placebo-HVPC group approached but did not reach statistical significance ($P = 0.04$). Reduction in hand edema was significant for the intermittent pneumatic compression group compared with the placebo-HVPC group, at the $P = 0.01$ level. Faghri[77] studied the effects of neuromuscular stimulation (NMS)-induced muscle contraction and elevation and concluded that NMS was more effective for reduction of edema than elevation alone for hand edema in flaccid cerebrovascular accident patients. However, Geurts[80] found Fagri's statistics "insufficient and at specific points erroneous." Man[79] found no significant difference with NMS used with ankle sprains.

Transcutaneous electrical nerve stimulation has not been found helpful with treatment of edema.[81]

All patients who are candidates for electrical modalities must be cleared medically before initiating this type of therapy. The use of electrical modalities is contraindicated in patients who have a pacemaker, cardiac arrhythmias,

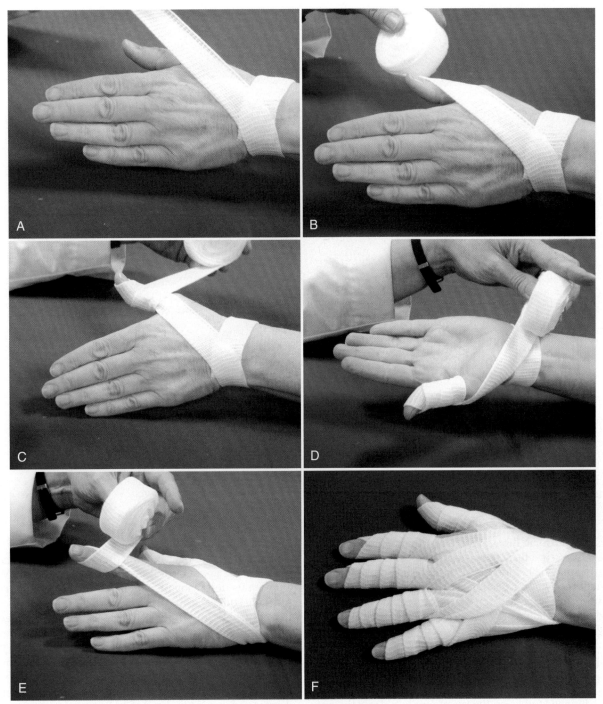

Figure 63-6 A, Elastomull is anchored at the wrist and wrapped diagonally across the back of the hand to (**B**) the outermost aspect of the distal thumb. **C**, The wrap is then spiraled around the thumb from distal to proximal with each layer overlapping the previous layer by one-half width. **D**, From the base of the thumb the wrap continues around the base of the wrist, leaving the palm free. **E**, This technique is continued for each of the digits, each time anchoring around the wrist and leaving the palm free. **F**, Dorsal view of completed wrap.

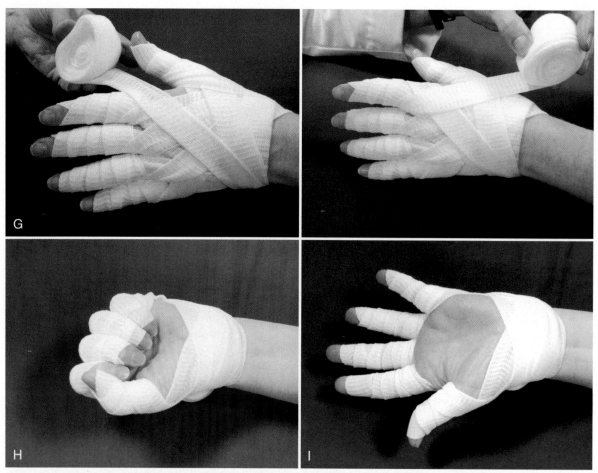

Figure 63-6, cont'd G (1 and 2), For additional support at the webspaces, additional wrap can be anchored at the wrist and wrapped once around each finger. **H**, The finger wrap provides gentle compression without limiting motion, and is well tolerated. **I**, Volar view of completed wrap with palm free.

seizures, myocardial disease, or any other condition that may be adversely affected by current. Although electrical stimulation may be helpful in decreasing edema in any of the three stages of wound healing, it has been suggested that intensities that produce muscle contractions should be avoided in the inflammatory phase because they may increase clotting time.[12]

Low-Level Laser Therapy and Ultrasound

Previous human studies on the use of low-level laser therapy for edema control primarily following ankle sprains has yielded mixed results and has not provided any conclusive support for using low-level laser therapy with musculoskeletal conditions.[10,82] More recently, positive results were obtained by Sergioulas[83] with ankle edema and Ozkan[84] with edema following injury to digital flexor tendons; these studies have used different treatment parameters and instrumentation.

The nonthermal effects of ultrasound include acoustic streaming and cavitation.[85] Nonthermal ultrasound modulates membrane properties, alters cellular proliferation, and produces increases in proteins associated with inflammation and injury repair including vasodilation of arterioles and activation of adhesion molecules.[85] Fyfe and Chahl[86] found significant but short-term reductions in the edema response using .79 Hz applied for 2 or 4 minutes with male (Wistar) albino rats following injections of silver nitrate. Human research studies using ultrasound to reduce ankle edema have utilized a variety of parameters and have yielded conflicting results.[10] Hashish[87] applied very low level ultrasound at .1 W/cm^2 following bilateral surgical extraction of molars and achieved greater edema reduction in the placebo group than the test group. Additional research is needed to determine the best parameters and efficacy of ultrasound to decrease edema in the hand therapy population.

In summary, there are a variety of modalities available to assist in edema reduction, but more research is needed to determine the appropriate treatment parameters and overall efficacy with specific approaches to upper extremity edema. The reader is referred to Chapter 117 in this text for further information on the use of physical agents in hand rehabilitation.

Hyperbaric Oxygen Therapy

Hyperbaric oxygen (HBO) therapy is a treatment wherein the entire body is treated with 100% oxygen at greater than normal atmospheric pressures. This treatment increases the concentration of oxygen in the blood plasma and cells. HBO has a potential role with any condition wherein blood flow and oxygen delivery are compromised. In a double-blind randomized, placebo-controlled study, Kiralp et al. found HBO therapy to be an effective and well-tolerated method for decreasing pain and edema in patients with chronic regional pain syndrome.[88]

Summary

The best treatment of edema is to prevent and minimize its occurrence through the use of atraumatic surgical techniques, appropriate postoperative dressings and positioning, judicious and monitored use of cold, comfortable elevation, and early motion when possible. If edema persists, the patient should be instructed in lymphatic massage and an appropriate level of continuous compression. A variety of other clinical treatment options can be considered to further enhance arterial systems, venous return, and lymphatic flow. Therapists must be judicious in selecting the most appropriate approaches for each patient given the level of supportive evidence in the literature, other treatment considerations, and clinical time constraints. Control of edema is essential to optimize the benefits of therapy and, ultimately, hand function.

REFERENCES

The complete reference list is available online at www.expertconsult.com.

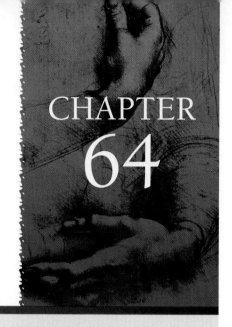

Management of Upper Extremity Lymphedema

HEATHER HETTRICK, PhD, PT, CWS, FACCWS, MLT

ETIOLOGY OF LYMPHEDEMA
EXAMINATION
INTEGUMENTARY CONSIDERATIONS
LYMPHEDEMA INTERVENTIONS

APPROACHES FOR RISK REDUCTION
COMMON FUNCTIONAL IMPAIRMENTS AND
  RECOMMENDATIONS FOR MANAGEMENT
SUMMARY

CRITICAL POINTS

- A healthy lymphatic system is generally able to prevent or decrease the amount of acute edema. Under normal conditions, the transport capacity of the lymphatic system is approximately 10 times greater than the physiologic amount of the lymphatic loads.
- The decisive difference between lymphedema and virtually all other types of edema is the high content of plasma proteins in the interstitial fluid.
- The diagnosis of lymphedema is made in most cases by patient history, systems review, inspection, palpation, and a few select noninvasive tests such as volume or girth measurement.
- Tissue lesions common in lymphedema, caused by the impaired lymph vascular system and/or other co-morbid conditions, may present as simple superficial excoriations to multifarious ulcers with complex etiologies.
- Compression is the cornerstone of lymphedema therapy.
- Complete decongestive therapy is a two-phase intervention for lymphedema that is noninvasive, highly effective, and cost-effective that can reduce and maintain limb size.
- The goal of exercise is to improve lymphatic flow without adding undue stress to the impaired lymphatic system.

Lymphedema is a chronic, incurable condition that is characterized by an abnormal collection of fluid owing to an anatomic alteration of the lymphatic system.[1] Throughout the world, it is estimated that one person in 30 is afflicted with lymphedema.[2] Lymphedema can lead to significant impairments in function, integumentary disorders, pain, and psychological issues. Appropriate identification and intervention of this disease can improve functional and aesthetic outcomes and patient quality of life. This chapter describes the function of the lymphatic system and the etiologies of lymphedema. Examination, intervention, and preventive measures are discussed, as well as impairments associated with lymphedema and other complications involving the upper extremity.

Etiology of Lymphedema

The lymphatic system has two main functions. First, it provides significant immune function by protecting the body from disease and infection via production, maintenance, and distribution of lymphocytes. The second function is the facilitation of fluid transport from the interstitial tissues back into the bloodstream. This fluid transport maintains normal blood volume and eliminates chemical imbalances in the interstitial fluid.[3] The substances transported by the lymphatic system are called lymphatic loads (LL) and consist of protein, water, cellular debris, and fat (from the digestive system). These lymphatic loads are filtered by regional and central lymph nodes before reentry into the venous blood system.

The lymphatic capillaries, the beginning of the lymphatic system, abound in the dermis at the dermal-epidermal junction, forming a flat, two-dimensional continuous network over the entire body with the exception of the central nervous system and cornea.[3] Unlike blood capillaries that consist of continuous tubules of endothelial cells, lymphatic capillaries consist of overlapping endothelial cells (Fig. 64-1). A surrounding fiber net of anchoring filaments, arranged around the lymph capillaries, enables these vessels to stay open at the junction between the overlapping cells even under high tissue pressure[4] (Fig. 64-2). The lymphatic loads are resorbed by the lymph capillaries and flow into larger lymph vessels

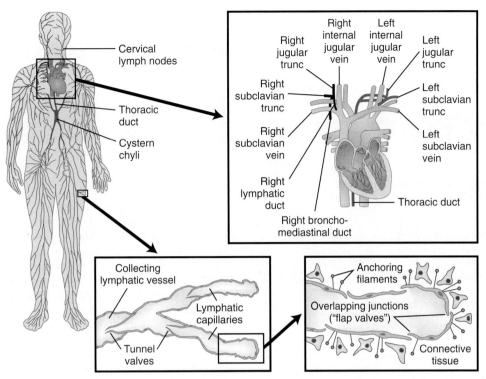

Figure 64-1 Lymph capillaries.

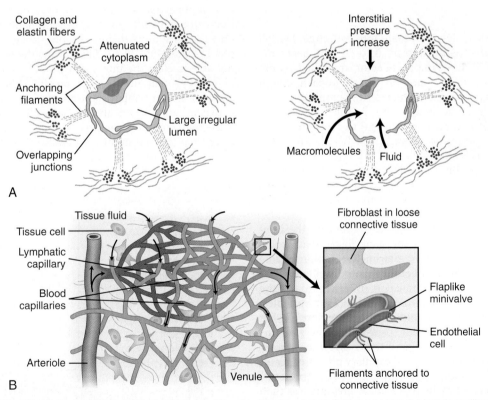

Figure 64-2 Anchoring filaments. **A,** A cross-section of lymph capillary showing how lymph fluid moves into the lymph capillary. **B,** The relationship of the lymphatic system with the circulatory system.

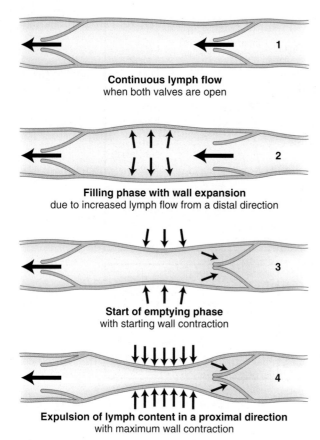

Continuous lymph flow
when both valves are open

Filling phase with wall expansion
due to increased lymph flow from a distal direction

Start of emptying phase
with starting wall contraction

Expulsion of lymph content in a proximal direction
with maximum wall contraction

Figure 64-3 Lymphangiomotoricity.

Table 64-1 Starling's Equation: $J_v = K_f [P_c - P_{if} - \sigma(\pi_p - \pi_{if})]$

Legend	Definition
$P_c - P_{if}$	Hydrostatic pressure gradient
$\pi_p - \pi_{if}$	Colloid osmotic pressure gradient
K_f	Permeability of water and small solutes
σ	Permeability of plasma proteins
J_v	Capillary filtrate
J_L	Lymphatic return
$J_v > J_L$	Edema

called precollectors, which then drain into collectors. Lymph collectors have valves, spaced every 6 to 20 mm. Segments between two valves in a lymph collector are called lymph angions. The contraction of smooth muscle in each angion (called lymphangiomotoricity) generates the propulsive force of lymph flow along the lymph vessel. The frequency of contraction of lymph angions at rest is 6 to 10 contractions per minute.[5] The propulsion directs the lymph fluid into regional and central lymph nodes to be filtered (Fig. 64-3). Ultimately, the lymph fluid empties into the venous system through the left and right venous angles, i.e., at the junctions between the subclavian and jugular veins at the level of the clavicles.

The amount of lymphatic load transported by the lymphatic system is dependent on the same forces that propel blood in the blood capillaries. Starling's equation (Table 64-1) describes the balance or equilibrium of capillary filtration and reabsorption.[4,6] The transport of fluid through the membrane of blood capillaries depends on four variables: blood capillary pressure, colloid osmotic pressure of the plasma proteins, colloid osmotic pressure of the proteins located in the interstitial tissue, and tissue pressure.

Ultrafiltration is defined as blood capillary pressure greater than the colloid osmotic pressure of plasma proteins. Reabsorption is defined by blood capillary pressure less than the colloid osmotic pressure of plasma proteins.[4]

A shift in Starling's equilibrium toward an increase in ultrafiltration (such as occurs in cases of inflammation or venous hypertension) or decreased colloid osmotic pressure (associated with hypoproteinemia) can cause an increased amount of lymphatic load, placing a higher burden on the lymphatic system. A healthy lymphatic system is generally able to prevent or decrease the amount of acute edema. Under normal conditions, the transport capacity (TC) of the lymphatic system is approximately 10 times greater than the physiologic amount of the lymphatic loads. This is known as the functional reserve (FR) of the lymphatic system[4] (Fig. 64-4). As long as the lymphatic load remains lower than the transport capacity of the lymphatic system, the lymphatic compensation is successful. If the lymphatic load exceeds the transport capacity, edema will occur. This is called dynamic insufficiency of the lymphatic system; the lymph vessels are intact but overwhelmed (Fig. 64-5). The result is edema, which can usually be successfully treated with elevation, compression, and decongestive exercises (any basic exercise to facilitate the muscle pump).[4]

Lymphedema is caused by mechanical insufficiency or low-volume insufficiency of the lymphatic system. The transport capacity drops below the physiologic level of the lymphatic loads (Fig. 64-6). This means the lymphatic system is not able to clear the interstitial tissues, and an accumulation of high protein fluid is the result. This is recognized as lymphedema or lymphostatic edema.[4] The decisive difference between lymphedema and virtually all other types of edema is the high content of plasma proteins in the interstitial fluid. Over time (several months to years), this can lead to fibrosis of all affected tissue structures and is readily evident in the

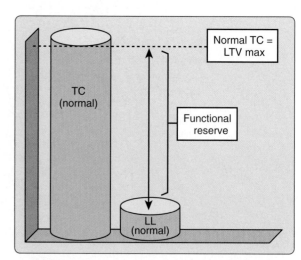

Figure 64-4 Functional reserve of the lymphatic system. LTV, lymph time volume.

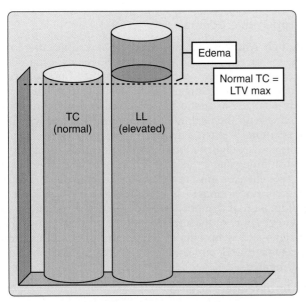

Figure 64-5 Dynamic insufficiency.

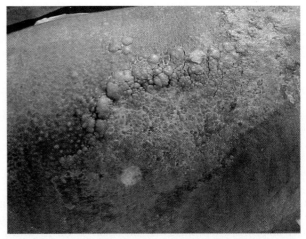

Figure 64-7 Skin changes with lymphedema. The image depicts dry skin, hyperkeratosis, fibromas, and papillomas. (The image above is a copyrighted product of Association for the Advancement of Wound Care [www.aawcone.org] and has been reproduced with permission.)

texture and consistency of the involved integument[7] (Fig. 64-7).

Sometimes the etiology of edema is uncertain, and there is no clear clinical distinction between lymphedema and other types of edema. Some swelling may be a mixture of both edema and lymphedema, as occurs when the functional reserve of the lymphatic system is exceeded and the lymph transport capacity is compromised.[8] The progression of lymphedema from the first perception of "heaviness" by the patient and nonresolving edema to irreversible fibrotic changes takes time. In an effort to standardize the associated integumentary changes, staging and classification systems have been developed. The staging system is used clinically to describe the subjective and objective integument changes.

The classification system is used for unilateral limb involvement and is based on circumferential limb measurements. Tables 64-2 and 64-3 show the stages and severity classification systems for lymphedema. Early accurate diagnosis, patient education, and appropriate treatment will decrease the amount of time needed to achieve limb reduction, skin changes, and overall improvement or restoration of function.[3]

The etiology of lymphedema is currently classified into two major categories: primary and secondary lymphedema. Primary lymphedema is caused by a condition that is either hereditary or congenital. In the United States, it is estimated that approximately 2 million people have primary lymphedema.[9] Eighty-three percent of primary lymphedema cases

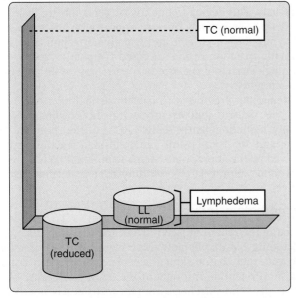

Figure 64-6 Mechanical insufficiency.

Table 64-2 Stages of Lymphedema

Stage	Description
0	Latent or subclinical condition: swelling is not evident despite impaired lymph transport.
I	Reversible lymphedema: early accumulation of protein-rich fluid, elevation reduces swelling; tissue pits on pressure.
II	Spontaneously irreversible lymphedema: proteins stimulate fibroblast formation; connective and scar tissue proliferate; minimal pitting even with moderate swelling.
III	Lymphostatic elephantiasis: hardening of dermal tissues, papillomas of the skin, tissue appearance elephant-like. (Not everyone progresses to this stage.)

Adapted from the International Society of Lymphology Consensus Document on Diagnosis and Treatment of Peripheral Lymphedema, 2003.

Table 64-3 *Severity of Lymphedema Stages*

Classification	Description
Minimal	<20% increase in limb volume
Moderate	20%–40% increase in limb volume
Severe	>40% increase in limb volume

Adapted from the International Society of Lymphology Consensus Document on Diagnosis and Treatment of Peripheral Lymphedema, 2003.

manifest before the age of 35 (lymphedema praecox)[10] and 17% manifest after the age of 35 (lymphedema tardum). The onset of primary lymphedema can occur at birth (Milroy's disease or Meige's syndrome), but most often the onset is during puberty or around the age of 17 years. Eighty-seven percent of all cases of primary lymphedema occur in females, and the lower extremities are more often involved than other body parts.[11]

Secondary lymphedema is caused by some identifiable insult to the lymphatic system.[11] Secondary lymphedema etiologies include inflammation, infection, radiation therapy, surgery, filariasis (parasitic infection), trauma, iatrogenic alterations, artificial self-induced lymphedema, benign or malignant tumor growth, and chronic venous insufficiency.[11] Approximately 2.5 to 3 million people in the United States have been diagnosed with secondary lymphedema.[9] One third of patients who undergo mastectomy (with lymph node resection) secondary to breast cancer develop secondary lymphedema of the upper extremity (the reported incidence varies depending on study parameters).[12] Radical lymph node dissection with prostate cancer causes lymphedema of one or both legs and often the genitals in more than 70% of the cases.[13] Secondary lymphedema is usually unilateral; however, it may present in both limbs. It is important to note, however, that involvement of the limbs and presentation of the edema is generally not symmetrical. One limb will appear larger, and it is this limb that should be addressed first with respect to intervention strategies.

Lymphedema can lead to numerous health-related and emotional problems. Of concern is the high risk of infection and skin changes associated with chronic lymphedema, particularly for patients who do not receive appropriate intervention. Fluid accumulation in the tissues is an ideal medium for pathogen growth, and cellulitis and venous-type ulceration (particularly of the lower extremities) can be a common occurrence for patients with lymphedema. Patients also experience embarrassment and social barriers because of the increased limb size, discomfort, diminished movement and function of the affected limb or limbs, and difficulty donning and doffing clothing, each of which may compromise a person's quality of life.[8]

Differential Diagnosis of Breast Cancer–Related Edemas

(Adapted from Linda T. Miller, *Management of Breast Cancer Related Edemas*, 5th Edition).

Postoperative Edema

Although lymphedema can occur at any time after treatment for breast cancer,[14] postoperative edema, often called acute lymphedema, occurs within the first 6 weeks after breast cancer surgery. Mild postoperative edema and subtle changes in tissue are expected and often transient, resolving with the healing of the surgical site and lymphatic regeneration.[15] Often, therapeutic interventions such as simple active range of motion (ROM) exercises and appropriate positioning may be all that is necessary to assist in resolving the edema. Any individual who undergoes axillary, breast, or chest surgery is considered to be at risk for the development of lymphedema in the trunk quadrant and upper extremity of the affected side. Patient education about the signs and symptoms of lymphedema as well as proper management and protection of the limb at risk should be implemented.

Cording-Related Edema

At approximately 2 to 3 weeks after the axillary dissection, many patients will experience pain along the anteromedial aspect of the involved upper extremity,[16] which appears to follow a neurovascular pattern. Cordlike, superficial, fibrous bands usually develop, which are often visible and palpable, especially through the anterior elbow and ventral forearm. Pain associated with cording, also known as sclerosing lymphangitis,[16,17] is often described as a "drawing" or "pulling" feeling, which extends from the axilla to the fingers. Shoulder flexion with the elbow extended becomes increasingly difficult because of tightness of the cords.

These cordlike bands usually soften and often disappear at approximately 8 to 12 weeks. However, mild moist heat applied to the outstretched arm, followed by gentle, skillful stretching of the cords and soft tissue, can provide a dramatic decrease in pain and increase in ROM in only a few therapy sessions.

Often, cording-related edema is most noticed initially in the ventral forearm and radial hand and is commonly described as "painful," fitting the pain pattern as described previously. This edema frequently presents during the first 3 months postoperatively but can appear with the same signs and symptoms years later and usually corresponds to some traumatic irritation of the sclerosed lymphatic vessels, such as a quick stretch of the arm or an attempt to lift something that is too heavy.

Edema that presents with cording as its underlying cause must be treated concurrently with the cording. Manual therapy, including gentle passive ROM of the shoulder with elbow and wrist extension and mild skin traction, can be followed by the appropriate edema techniques. When treated early and appropriately, cording-related edema usually resolves.

Chemotherapy-Induced Edema

Edema of the arm or adjacent trunk may develop in patients undergoing certain chemotherapy regimens. Corticosteroids such as dexamethasone and glucocorticoids may cause short-term fluid retention throughout the body.[18,19] Because of the axillary dissection, drainage from the ipsilateral lymph vessels may be impaired. Any increase in fluid in the compromised area can tip the balance in favor of an edematous condition.

At the first sign of edema, management techniques should be initiated. Treatment success may be hampered as long as the patient continues to receive chemotherapy. However, once chemotherapy is concluded, the edema can resolve with continued treatment.

Emphasis must be placed on early detection and treatment of these acute edemas. They often will resolve with skillful, early intervention. However, if allowed to progress, even these early edemas can go on to become chronic conditions.

Chronic Lymphedema

Lymphedema occurs between the deep fascia and the skin. In addition to a decrease in lymphatic transport capacity, there is also a decrease in macrophage activity and an increase in the action of fibroblasts.[20,21] The accumulating protein creates an environment for chronic inflammation and progressive fibrosis of the tissues. Fibrosis of the initial lymphatic vessels and collectors leads to a failure of the endothelial junctions to close and valvular dysfunction in the deeper collecting vessels. This results in the failure of the vessels to remove proteins from the interstitium.[22] As the condition progresses, protein continues to accumulate, forming a network of fibrosclerotic tissue.

Other histologic changes, such as deep fascial thickening, occur as edema progresses. Changes such as circumference and tissue texture can easily be detected and documented. However, before the development of such obvious symptoms, an increase in the infection rate (recurrent cellulitis) may indicate an impending lymphedema.[20,21]

Examination

A thorough physical examination and clinical history are essential in correctly diagnosing lymphedema and thereby choosing the appropriate interventions.[23] The diagnosis of lymphedema is made in most cases by patient history, systems review, inspection, palpation, and a few select noninvasive tests such as volume or girth measurement. Diagnosis of upper extremity lymphedema is usually evident, especially with a history of axillary, breast, or chest surgery. At present, the only clinical test that has been shown to be a reliable and valid method to diagnose lymphedema is Stemmer's sign.[24,25] This is a thickening of the skin over the proximal phalanges of the toes or fingers of the involved limb and the inability to "tent" or pick up the skin (Fig. 64-8).

If the result is positive, it is a definite indication of lymphedema; if it is negative, lymphedema might still be present, but not yet advanced enough to cause Stemmer's sign.[26] When Stemmer's sign is absent, it is appropriate to treat the edema with conventional interventions of elevation, rest, and compression. If the edema does not respond to conventional interventions, it should be monitored and regular reassessment should be conducted because the underlying pathology may be early lymphedema.

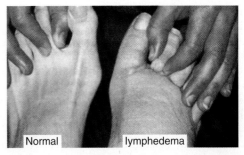

Normal | lymphedema

Figure 64-8 Stemmer's sign. (The image above is a copyrighted product of the Association for the Advancement of Wound Care [www.aawcone. org] and has been reproduced with permission.)

A thorough history is essential to correctly identify lymphedema. The history should include the following:

- Onset of the symptoms (swelling, heaviness of limb), length of time since initial onset, and the triggering event (i.e., a bee sting, sprained wrist, recent surgery or trauma) if known.
- Medical history including traumatic events and surgery. This should also include all current medications, health risk factors, and coexisting problems (i.e., cancer diagnosis, obesity, cardiac problems, venous insufficiency), and family history.
- Pain and/or associated discomfort. Significant pain may suggest additional tests and measures to determine whether a secondary problem exists such as venous or arterial compromise and an underlying orthopedic condition. Most patients with lymphedema report heaviness and associated discomfort in lieu of pain because of the large amounts of fluid in the tissues.
- Functional status and activity level. Does the patient report a loss in function or difficulty performing activities of daily living because of the swelling? How active or inactive is the patient and what type of activities does he or she enjoy and/or participate in?
- Review of social habits such as smoking, diet and nutritional habits, and physical fitness/weight management strategies. A diet does not exist for lymphedema, but a low-sodium diet in combination with good hydration and nutritional habits is recommended.[27]
- Treatment and intervention history. Some interventions may have led to an exacerbation of the symptoms, such as improper compression, sole use of a pneumatic compression pump, thermal modalities, and/or deep massage.[28]

After the history, a brief systems review should be performed. Specifically, a review of the cardiopulmonary, integumentary, musculoskeletal, and neuromuscular system will help the clinician to identify health problems that may require referral to another health professional, and it may help to identify specific tests and measures to use to complete a thorough patient assessment. In addition, it is important to review the patient's affect, cognition, language, and learning style to optimize the examination and intervention strategies.

Tests and measures that should be included for patients with lymphedema or those at risk of the development of lymphedema follow.[29] Characteristic findings common with lymphedema include the following:

- Integumentary integrity. Extensive palpation and inspection including texture (rough, orange peel–like), color (red, brown, darker than person's natural color), pitting status (slow or hard to pit), fibrosis (hardening of the skin and tissues), temperature (involved limb may feel warmer on palpation), deepening of skin folds (skin may fold over wrist joint similar to a rubber band effect), nail quality (thickened and/or discolored), Stemmer's sign, and presence of cysts/fistulae, papillomas, or ulcers (defects in the integument such as lesions and benign growths).
- Anthropometric characteristics. Volume measurements using water displacement and girth measurements comparing circumferential limb segments of the involved and noninvolved limbs are the most common noninvasive assessments of the lymphedematous limb.[30] If the involvement is bilateral, baseline measurements should be taken of both limbs for future comparison. Tonometry (measurement of fluid mobility by recording the tissue deformation) and bioelectrical impedance analysis (amount of extracellular water and total water content) are newer methods that can assist with detecting subclinical lymphedema.[31,32]
- Joint integrity and mobility, muscle performance, ROM, and posture. Patients with lymphedema can present with significant limitations on manual muscle testing and goniometry because of the heaviness of the limb from the excessive fluid burden. Biomechanical compensations and overuse of the noninvolved limb can negatively affect joints and posture.
- Pain. Pain should be differentiated from discomfort or heaviness. The location is important to determine whether the pain is related to the lymphedema or another problem. The use of a Visual Analogue Scale can objectify the patient's pain response and help to differentiate pain from discomfort. Pain may be related to other patient co-morbidities (i.e., peripheral vascular disease, orthopedic or neuromuscular pathologies), or it could be an indicator of infection (i.e., cellulitis). Further evaluation should explore the true nature of the pain so that the appropriate intervention can be implemented.
- Arousal, mentation, and cognition. These are important because patient education and compliance are paramount for successful management. Patients require extensive education and support to learn how to manage lymphedema and how to prevent exacerbations and/or associated complications. Verbal instruction, demonstration, and patient-appropriate literature will help to empower patients with lymphedema.
- Ventilation, respiration, and circulation. A pulmonary review (part of the systems review) will determine the patient's tolerance to deep breathing and resisted breathing, which are components of lymphedema intervention.
- Sensory and reflex integrity. These are particularly important with associated complications such as diabetes and circulatory disorders so as to recognize and prevent further injury.
- Motor function. Establishing the patient's functional baseline will promote individualized exercise prescription, aiding in compliance and positive outcomes. In clinical practice, it seems that the larger the lymphedematous limb is, the more common and advanced the compensations and impairments present in fine and gross motor skills.
- Orthotic, prosthetic, supportive devices, assistive and adaptive devices. Identification of need will assist with the rehabilitation and prevention components of treatment by improving safety and facilitating independence.
- Aerobic capacity and endurance. Establishing baseline will promote individualized exercise prescription, thus assisting with compliance and improved outcomes.
- Self-care and home management. It is imperative to determine the needs of the patient to effectively implement treatment interventions. The patient's ability or lack of ability to participate will directly affect the course of care, particularly self-management of lymphedema.
- Community and work/school integration or reintegration and environmental, home, and work/school barriers. Patient and family education, modification of lifestyle, and maintenance and prevention strategies should consider the patient's home and work/school life for optimal results.[28]

Integumentary Considerations

Meticulous skin and nail care is a significant part of lymphedema intervention and prevention. The goal is to prevent skin breakdown and infection. However, many patients present with skin lesions because of the destructive nature of chronic lymphedema and the excessive fluid burden on the tissues. The excess fluid commonly associated with chronic lymphedema increases the diffusion distance and the distance that oxygen, nutrients, and blood are required to travel from the capillaries to the cells and tissues of the skin. A high fluid burden on the tissues could also result in systemic infection because stagnant fluid is present for pathogen growth. Tissue lesions common with lymphedema, caused by the impaired lymph vascular system and/or other co-morbid conditions, may present from simple superficial excoriations to multifarious ulcers with complex etiologies. Vascular and inflammatory ulcers, fungating wounds, radiation burns, minor traumas, and failed surgical sites are all potential skin lesions that may present in patients with lymphedema.

If wounds are present on a lymphedematous limb, lymph drainage and compression can help to decrease the severity of the ulceration.[1] Appropriate wound management combined with specific lymph drainage around the ulcer helps to rid the wound of cellular debris and toxins.[5] Care should be taken to drain the fluid away from the ulcer to prevent wound congestion, and additional drainage techniques should be used on the proximal extremity to promote the lymphatic flow toward regional lymph nodes. (Specific drainage techniques are discussed in the section on lymphedema interventions.)

Cellulitis is the most common complication of primary and secondary lymphedema. Cellulitis is a painful inflammation of the soft tissue that is characterized by expanding local erythema, palpable local lymph nodes in 50% of the cases, and associated fever and chills.[13] Caused by an acute *Streptococcus* infection, the smallest injuries can be the portal of entry for the bacteria, leading to a local or systemic infection. Seventy percent of cellulitis cases are caused by simple injuries such as cuts, abrasions, insect bites, local burns, and interdigital mycosis.[13] Treatment requires local antibiotics and/or persistent systemic antibiotic therapy in addition to patient education about preventive measures because recurrence is frequent, thereby further limiting lymph transport capacity.[13]

Local wound infection is common because the moist/wet environment is conducive to pathogen growth. Treatment involves addressing the underlying infection, if present, with appropriate systemic and topical antibiotics. Local wound care should involve managing the oftentimes copious exudate while maintaining adequate compression. Hydrofibers, alginates, and other absorptive dressings should be considered in the presence of exudating wounds. Four-layer bandage systems (e.g., Profore, Smith & Nephew, Largo, FL; and Dyna-Flex, Johnson & Johnson, New Brunswick, NJ) are effective for absorbing excess drainage and provide the necessary and vital compression. With compression and control of lymphedema, the associated wounds will heal in the majority of cases.[1] Once the systemic and/or local infection has resolved, specific lymphedema interventions (manual lymph drainage, compression, exercise, and skin and nail care) should begin or resume.

Compression is the cornerstone of lymphedema therapy. The degree of swelling and the presence of skin breakdown, diabetes, arterial insufficiency, and chronic congestive heart failure must be considered.[1] Short-stretch bandages, long-stretch bandages, cotton padding, self-adherent crepe dressings, and combination wraps are among the various compression bandages used in the treatment of lymphedema. In applying compression, frequently reassessing the condition of the limb (i.e., limb size reduction) and matching the dressing to the patient's diagnosis and wound status is critical.[1]

With respect to compression, bandages differ in elasticity and extensibility. Bandages also have varying amounts of resting and working pressure. Resting pressure is pressure exerted on the skin by the elastic when put on stretch, whether the patient is moving or activating a muscle pump. Working pressure is pressure exerted on the skin when contracting muscles push against a compression bandage. Short-stretch bandages have a high working pressure and low resting pressure. Short-stretch bandages (e.g., Comprilan, BSN-Jobst, Inc., Charlotte, NC) stretch 20% of their original length compared with long-stretch bandages (e.g., Ace wraps) that stretch up to 190% of their original length. When the limb is at rest, short-stretch bandages supply a comfortable degree of support (without a tourniquet effect), but the total pressure increases significantly when the muscles contract against fixed resistance. This creates an effective, intermittent massage that forces interstitial fluid into functioning lymph collectors. Therefore, the compression wrap becomes a dynamic part of the wound dressing or treatment for patients with lymphedema.[1]

Lymphedema Interventions

Once the diagnosis of lymphedema has been made, it is essential that the appropriate interventions be used to address the patient's impairments. Treatment should involve specific interventions for lymphedema, integument management strategies, and rehabilitation for functional impairments. Long-term management requires prevention and maintenance strategies to decrease the risk of exacerbations, infections, and other associated impairments.

Lymphedema is a manageable disease with the appropriate treatment and intervention. The goal of lymphedema therapy is to get the patient back to a subclinical or latency stage, regardless of his or her diagnosed stage or classification. In most cases, this can be readily achieved with complete decongestive therapy (CDT). CDT is a two-phase intervention for lymphedema that is noninvasive, highly effective, and cost-effective that can reduce and maintain limb size.[33-35] The proposed benefits of CDT include opening collateral lymphatic drainage pathways, increased pumping by the deep lymphatic pathways, and a reduction and breakdown of fibrotic tissue.[23,34]

Phase I, or the intensive phase, involves meticulous skin and nail care, manual lymphatic drainage (MLD), bandaging, exercise (in bandaging), and the use of a compression garment (at the end of phase I). Phase II, or the self-management phase, involves the patient wearing a compression garment during the day, bandaging at night, exercise (in the garment or bandage), meticulous skin and nail care, and self-MLD as needed.[35]

MLD is a specialized manual technique based on the physiologic principles of lymph flow and lymph vessel emptying. MLD affects the lymph system by moving lymph fluid around blocked areas toward collateral vessels, anastomoses, and uninvolved lymph node regions; increasing lymph angiomotoricity; increasing the volume of transported lymph fluid; increasing pressure in the lymph collector vessels; improving lymph transport capacity; and potentially increasing arterial blood flow.[34,36-42]

In Europe, phase I of CDT includes twice-daily visits for an average of 4 to 6 weeks. In the United States (because of health-care constraints), CDT is limited to daily visits for 3 to 4 weeks for the upper extremity and 4 to 6 weeks for the lower extremity.[35] Phase II begins when phase I ends (a plateau in limb reduction as indicated by weekly girth measurements) and may continue for as long as 18 months after CDT initiation. The duration and intensity of treatment depend on the clinical stage of lymphedema. Stages I and II (mild and moderate lymphedema) are more easily managed than stage III (severe lymphedema). Patient compliance is paramount, and management is a lifelong process. The stages and classifications help health-care professionals to determine the intensity of the therapy as well as plan the potential duration of the interventions.

Functional limitations should be addressed according to patient needs. Often, as the limb(s) reduces in size, function is improved. However, patients often require basic exercise prescription to improve strength, flexibility, and cardiovascular health.

Several other interventions are worthy of discussion as they are often implemented for the management of edematous and lymphedematous limbs. These include intermittent compression pumps, diuretics, and physical agents.

Intermittent Pneumatic Compression

Intermittent pneumatic compression pumps can be harmful to patients with lymphedema when they are used inappropriately. These pumps successfully mobilize fluid; however, proteins may remain in the affected tissues. This can promote more fluid to accumulate because proteins are hydrophilic, causing the area to become even more fibrotic. If a pump is used without MLD, the mobilized fluid may collect in the torso from the upper extremity or in the groin area from the lower extremities. The pumps do not reroute lymph fluid, as does MLD. It is highly recommended to only use a pump at the end of phase II of CDT in combination with MLD. The pump should not be used to decongest, but to maintain the benefits of CDT.

Diuretics

A second treatment consideration is the use of diuretics. Diuretics also mobilize fluid out of the affected areas and increase the blood volume. The proteins, however, remain in the affected tissues, drawing in more water, which ultimately leads to more fibrosis. Some patients may have co-morbidities that require the use of diuretics, such as congestive heart failure, certain kidney disorders, or high blood pressure. As long as the physician is managing the patient for the specific condition that requires a diuretic, then the diuretic should be continued. If the diuretic is solely being used to manage lymphedema, it is important to discuss other treatment options such as CDT with the physician and suggest that the diuretic be discontinued.

Approaches for Risk Reduction

Patients must be educated about the risk reduction practices and risk factors as currently understood. Patients must also avoid activities that can cause a further decrease of the transport capacity of the lymph vessels or unnecessarily increase the lymphatic fluid and protein load of the lymphatic system in an affected region.[28]

Patients should be properly educated regarding exercise and activities of daily living that are safe and beneficial for them to perform. The goal of exercise is to improve lymphatic flow without adding undue stress on the impaired lymphatic system. Exercise programs should be prescribed and progressed at a pace to ensure compliance and where the effects of the exercise can be monitored and altered if required. Individual exercise programs should be adjusted to the patient's fitness level and directed by a therapist or clinician with knowledge on exercise progression, lymphedema contraindications, and risk factors.

Risk reduction strategies and adherence to maintenance programs are essential to decrease the risk of exacerbation and/or injuries that can lead to infection and subsequent lymphedema.

The National Lymphedema Network (NLN) published a Position Statement of Lymphedema Risk Reduction Practices in 2006.[43] The recommendations published in this position statement are listed below with express permission by the NLN to reprint the content.

1. Skin care: avoid trauma/injury to reduce infection risk.
   a. Keep extremity clean and dry.
   b. Apply moisturizer daily to prevent chapping/chafing of skin.
   c. Attention to nail care; do not cut cuticles.
   d. Protect exposed skin with sunscreen and insect repellant.
   e. Use care with razors to avoid nicks and skin irritation.
   f. If possible, avoid punctures such as injections and blood draws.
   g. Wear gloves while doing activities that may cause skin injury (i.e., washing dishes, gardening, working with tools, using chemicals such as detergent).
   h. If scratches/punctures to skin occur, wash with soap and water, apply antibiotics, and observe for signs of infection (i.e., redness).
   i. If a rash, itching, redness, pain, increased skin temperature, fever, or flulike symptoms occur, contact your physician immediately for early treatment of possible infection.
2. Activity/lifestyle
   a. Gradually build up the duration and intensity of any activity or exercise.
   b. Take frequent rest periods during activity to allow for limb recovery.
   c. Monitor the extremity during and after activity for any change in size, shape, tissue, texture, soreness, heaviness, or firmness.
   d. Maintain optimal weight.
3. Avoid limb constriction
   a. If possible, avoid having blood pressure taken on the at-risk extremity.
   b. Wear loose-fitting jewelry and clothing.
4. Compression garments
   a. They should be well fitting.
   b. Support the at-risk limb with a compression garment for strenuous activity (i.e., weight lifting, prolonged standing, running) except in patients with open wounds or with poor circulation in the at-risk limb.
   c. Consider wearing a well-fitting compression garment for air travel.
5. Extremes of temperature
   a. Avoid exposure to extreme cold, which can be associated with rebound swelling or chapping of skin.
   b. Avoid prolonged (longer than 15 minutes) exposure to heat, particularly hot tubs and saunas.
   c. Avoid placing limb in water temperatures above 102°F (38.9°C).
6. Additional practices specific to lower extremity lymphedema
   a. Avoid prolonged standing, sitting, and crossing legs.
   b. Wear proper, well-fitting footwear and hosiery.
   c. Support the at-risk limb with a compression garment for strenuous activity except in patients with open wounds or with poor circulation in the at-risk limb.

Note: Given that there is little evidence-based literature regarding many of these practices, the majority of the recommendations *must* at this time be based on the knowledge of pathophysiology and decades of clinical experience by experts in the field.

Common Functional Impairments and Recommendations for Management

Lymphedema can significantly affect a patient's functional status and quality of life. Because lymphedema is a progressive disease, early intervention and identification of the disease are important to improve patient outcomes. Once limb reduction has been achieved with CDT, associated functional limitations should be addressed.

Because of the significant size of some lymphedematous limbs, patients often have difficulty with activities of daily living. Involvement of the upper extremity can often affect gross and fine motor skills involving the phalanges, wrist, elbow, and shoulder, rendering basic skills difficult, if not impossible. Additionally, patients often are deconditioned and have limited cardiovascular endurance. Initiating CDT to reduce limb size will facilitate improvements in function and activities of daily living. Providing patients with appropriate assistive devices will enhance safety and reduce complications related to biomechanical compensations. Basic exercise prescription for cardiovascular endurance and strengthening will provide overall improvement in mobility tasks and enhance home and community skills.

Other impairments associated with lymphedema include limitations in ROM (because of large fluid volumes), decreased strength (related to diminished use), and difficulty with upper extremity function and activities of daily living when the lymphedema is present in the hand and/or arm. ROM should improve as limb volume decreases. Individualized exercise prescription including ROM and therapeutic exercise will improve function by restoring range and strength for both fine and gross motor activities. Compliance with exercise prescription is improved if activities are broken down into short-duration yet frequent sessions throughout the day. In addition, lifestyle modifications and adherence to compression therapy will augment functional outcomes.

Summary

Lymphedema is often referred to as a hidden epidemic; however, it is a manageable disease. Identification and intervention at any stage can improve functional and cosmetic outcomes. Recognizing and addressing the associated impairments related to lymphedema will enhance outcomes and patient satisfaction. Additionally, patient education and compliance with treatment is paramount for the successful management of this disease.

REFERENCES

The complete reference list is available online at www.expertconsult.com.

Manual Edema Mobilization: An Edema Reduction Technique for the Orthopedic Patient

CHAPTER 65

SANDRA M. ARTZBERGER, MS, OTR, CHT AND
VICTORIA W. PRIGANC, PhD, OTR, CHT, CLT

REVIEW OF THE LITERATURE
THEORETICAL FOUNDATION: ANATOMIC AND
    PHYSIOLOGIC SUPPORT
MANUAL EDEMA MOBILIZATION CONCEPTS

CASE EXAMPLES
FREQUENTLY ASKED QUESTIONS ABOUT MANUAL
    EDEMA MOBILIZATION
CONCLUSION

CRITICAL POINTS

- All edema is not the same.
- Stimulation of the lymphatic system is necessary to decrease subacute and chronic edema.
- The proteins associated with subacute and chronic edema need to disperse through the lymphatic system, as they are too large to permeate the venous system.
- The initial lymphatic system is superficial, fine, and fragile, therefore firm compression may collapse the system.
- Diaphragmatic breathing, light massage, and exercises help to stimulate the lymphatic system.

Manual edema mobilization (MEM) is a lymphatic stimulation technique used for recalcitrant subacute or chronic limb/hand edema in the orthopedic population. The phrase popularized by Watson-Jones in 1941,[1] "Oedema is glue," summarizes the importance of reducing edema in swollen hands because persistent edema can contribute to fibrosis, stiffness, and limited range of motion (ROM). Historically, many edema treatment techniques were developed with the rationale that the technique "stimulated the venous and lymphatic systems,"[2-4] giving the impression that one technique would affect both systems equally. However, current literature now describes differences between how the venous and lymphatic systems remove excess fluid,[5] thereby lending credence to the fact that not all edema reduction techniques work for all types of edema. Clinically, therapists have seen that some edemas reduce with little effort, whereas others progress into a gel-like and fibrotic state regardless of intense therapy. This phenomenon can be puzzling and frustrating for therapists. However, an understanding of the different types of edema and an understanding of the differences between the venous

system and lymphatic system with regard to edema reduction can help therapists understand why some common edema treatment techniques may not work on all types of edema (Table 65-1). The purpose of this chapter is to describe the MEM technique, which is an edema reduction technique used to stimulate the lymphatic system to decrease subacute and chronic edema in the orthopedic population.

Review of the Literature

History

MEM was first described in the late 1990s as a method of decreasing subacute and chronic edema in orthopedic patients through stimulation of the lymphatic system.[6,7] Using lymphatic treatment techniques for orthopedic patients to decrease subacute and chronic edema in people with healthy but overloaded lymphatic systems is relatively new. However, although the concept of MEM is relatively new, the history of MEM from a physiologic perspective is closely linked with historical revelations regarding the lymphatic system.

Throughout the 17th and 18th centuries, scientists, anatomists, and physicians described the role of the lymphatic system as part of the circulation system within the body,[5,8,9] with lymph flowing from tissues, through the lymphatics, and into the bloodstream.[10] Additionally, during this time frame, the connection between the lymphatic system and edema was also appearing in the literature.[11] Treatment techniques designed to capitalize on this link between the lymphatic system and edema started appearing in the literature during the 19th and 20th centuries, as several massage therapists and physicians designed different manual techniques to stimulate the lymphatic system for edema reduction purposes.[5,12] The most well-known lymphatic

Table 65-1 Types of Edemas Seen by Hand Therapists

Type	Etiology	Clinical Description and Stages
Inflammatory edema (high-plasma protein edema)	Trauma to tissue as a result of injury, infection, or surgical procedure. The result is high capillary permeability, imbalance in Starling's equilibrium, and an overload of the intact lymph nodes and lymph system because of excess plasma proteins flowing into the interstitium. There is also temporary obstruction and/or damage to the surrounding lymphatics that decreases protein uptake.[51-53]	**Acute:** Typically lasts from insult to 72 hours. Initially there is flooding of damaged tissue area with electrolytes and water. These low-protein substances readily diffuse by osmosis back into the venous system and thus respond well to elevation because elevation decreases hydrostatic pressure, thus reducing the flow of fluid into the interstitium.[54] This type of edema also responds to light retrograde massage, icing, and bulky hand dressings. Shortly after insult, low levels of plasma proteins begin to invade the area.[44]
		Subacute: Edema that lasts more than 72 hours to a week is considered subacute edema. It contains excess plasma proteins that disrupt Starling's equilibrium.[52] Lymphatic transport out of the involved area is further compromised because of damage or destruction of the lymphatics resulting from the initial trauma, scar formation, compression from a cast, excessive tissue loss, etc. Fibroblasts are activated by the proteins trapped in the interstitium and produce collagenous tissue.[12] If untreated, it can progress from a soft spongy state (slow to rebound from being pitted is characteristic of a lymphatic congested area) to a dense gel-like state. To decrease this type of edema, the lymphatics must be specifically stimulated such as through an MEM program.
		Chronic Edema: Edema lasting 3 months or longer is considered chronic. It is characterized as brawny (hard, indurated) and can become fibrotic (unable to pit). This type of edema can be reversed with MEM and adjunctive techniques to soften tissue
Lymphedema (high-plasma protein edema)	Often associated with lymphadenectomy and/or lymph node radiation, primary lymphedema, or filariasis. Foldi et al.[25,55] described it as a "low output failure of the lymph vascular system."	Classified by grades. Grade I: pitting that reduces with elevation; no fibrosis. Grade II: does not reduce with elevation, fibrosis; ranges from moderate to severe with elephantiasis as the extreme of this grade.[14] Magnetic resonance imaging and isotopic lymphoscintigraphy show that lymphedema occupies the epifascial compartment.[56] Thus, fibrosis of a joint rarely occurs.
Stroke edema (complex edema)	Initially a simple low-protein edema from accumulation of fluid in the tissue as a result of the loss of muscle pump, dependency positioning, etc. If edema is not reduced, increased tissue hydrostatic pressure compromises lymph flow capacity, and then edema can become gel-like and indurated.	A simple pitting edema that is perpetuated by the loss of motor function (muscle pump) and eventually can become gel-like and then fibrotic.
Edema from kidney or liver disease (decreased plasma proteins)	Caused by decreased plasma proteins in the interstitium (i.e., loss of proteins through the urine as in nephrotic syndrome) or failure to produce plasma proteins (as in liver disease).[21]	This is a pitting edema. MLT or MEM is not appropriate treatment.
Edema resulting from cardiac conditions	Heart failure, etc.[21]	Often seen as bilateral pitting edema around the ankles/feet. However, other conditions can also produce this bilateral swelling. MLT or MEM is not appropriate treatment.

Note: The table shows that all edemas are not alike: there are types of the edemas such as high protein and low protein; there are stages labeled acute, subacute, and chronic that reflect component changes in the edema; there are cardiac and renal edemas and lymphedema; there are comorbidities that affect the edema reduction or increase it. When a therapist understands these factors, he or she will no longer treat all edemas alike by just trying one technique after the other without a physiologic rationale. This is the new learning and challenge in treating orthopedic hand and arm edema.

massage technique, known today as manual lymphatic drainage (MLD), was developed in the 1960s through a collaboration of different German health care specialists.[12] Since then, variations of the MLD technique have been reported in the literature under terms such as decongestive lymphatic therapy, complex decongestive physiotherapy, and lymph drainage therapy.[5,13,14] Recently, the term *manual lymphatic treatment* (MLT) has been increasingly used in scientific publications[5] to describe principles common to all schools of lymphatic drainage, and, therefore, despite the numerous acronyms, all these aforementioned techniques

are designed to stimulate the lymphatic system through the application of light compression bandages, light massage, exercises, and skin care.[5,13,14]

Existing Research

Currently, there is one published quasiexperimental study on MEM.[15] This study demonstrated statistically significant reductions in edema in four of the five subjects by using a single-subject design study when MEM was entered into the standard treatment protocol.[15] Additionally, there is one published case study on MEM demonstrating how MEM can be incorporated into a treatment program for a patient with multiple traumas to the upper limb.[16] Although MEM is starting to appear in the literature as an effective treatment option for specific patient populations,[16,17] there is still a need for continued research on the use of lymphatic therapies for orthopedic patients because such research may alter how therapists initially treat orthopedic edema.

Theoretical Foundation: Anatomic and Physiologic Support

MEM is built on the same theoretical foundation as manual lymphatic therapies.[6,7,18] The anatomical and physiological support for manual lymphatic therapies is that stimulation of the lymphatic system is necessary to decrease high-protein edema.[5,19] Normally, plasma proteins, which are proteins found in the blood, are present in lower concentrations in the interstitial fluid compared with the microvessels.[20] Typically, the concentration of these larger proteins in the interstitial spaces remains low because these proteins do not diffuse easily through the microvessels.[21,22] However, after an injury, the inflammatory response changes the permeability of the microvessels, allowing these plasma proteins to leak into the interstitial spaces.[22,23]

These plasma proteins that leak into the interstitium are too large to permeate the venous system[5,24] and need to be disposed of through the lymphatic system[21,20] because a primary role of the lymphatic system is to dispose of matter that is too large for the venous system.[5,20,21,24] However, after an injury, the lymphatic system may be damaged or overloaded, which can hinder its ability to dispose of these larger plasma proteins.[5,25] If these plasma proteins remain in the interstitium, the colloid osmotic pressure, which is "the pressure to diffuse exerted by proteins and macromolecules,"[5] of the interstitial fluid increases.[21] This increase in the interstitial colloid osmotic pressure subsequently draws more fluid into the interstitial spaces.[19,22,23,26] Therefore, if these proteins remain in the interstitium, the edema will persist because of the pull of fluid into the interstitium.[25] Prolonged stagnation of plasma proteins in the interstitium leads to chronic inflammation.[27] As stated by Casley-Smith and Casley Smith,[19] "If edema lasts several weeks, this promotes chronic inflammation with its aftermath of excess fibroblasts and collagen deposition in the tissue."

The lymphatic tissue drainage system consists of three levels of structures. The lymph capillaries, called the initial lymphatics and precollectors, make up the first level.[14,28] These structures are finger-shaped, closed at one end, netlike vessels located in the interstitium that directly or indirectly drain every part of the body.[21] The vessels consist of a single layer of overlapping endothelial cells that have connector filaments anchoring them to surrounding connective tissue[14,29] (Fig. 65-1). The flaplike junctions formed by the overlapping endothelial cells open when the local interstitial pressure changes. When the junctions open, fluid flows in, changing the internal pressure of the lymphatic from low to high, thus closing the flaplike junctions.[21,29]

Lymph then enters the deeper tube-shaped collector lymphatics. The collector lymphatics have walls consisting of three layers. The inner layer is called the intima or endothe-

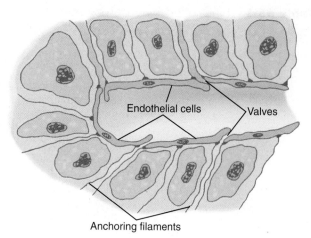

Figure 65-1 Special structure of the lymphatic capillaries that permits passage of substances of high molecular weight into the lymph. (From Guyton AC, Hall JE. *Textbook of Medical Physiology.* Philadelphia: WB Saunders; 1996.)

lium.[30] The media or middle layer consists of smooth muscle and thin strands of collagen fibers[30] that respond to the stretch reflex. The outer layer, called the adventitia, is formed by connective tissue.[21] Every 6 to 20 mm within the tube-shaped collectors are valves that prevent the backflow of lymph.[30] The space, or chamber, between the valves is called a lymphangion.[31] As fluid enters a lymphangion, it fills the segment, stimulating a stretch reflex of the medial smooth muscle layer. The ensuing contraction causes the proximal valve to open and propel the lymph to the next proximal lymphangion[30,31] (Fig. 65-2). At rest, lymphangions pump 6 to 10 times per minute.[21] However, with muscle contraction from exercise, lymphangions can pump 10 times that amount.[14,21]

The collector lymphatics propel lymph to the nodes.[29] The nodes consist of a complex of sinuses that perform immunologic functions. After leaving the nodes, lymph either enters the venous system through lymph-venous anastomoses or continues to move into deeper lymphatic trunks and eventually returns to the blood circulatory system via the left and right subclavian veins.

Anatomically, the trunk is divided into four lymphatic quadrants, or lymphotomes (drainage territories).[14] These consist of left and right upper quadrants, called thoracic lymphotomes, and left and right lower quadrants, called

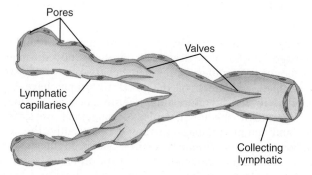

Figure 65-2 Structure of lymphatic capillaries and a collecting lymphatic, showing also the lymphatic valves. (From Guyton AC, Hall JE. *Textbook of Medical Physiology.* Philadelphia: WB Saunders; 1996.)

abdominal lymphotomes.[14] The thoracic lymphotomes extend from the anterior midline to the vertebral column on both the left and right sides of the upper trunk. Lymph drains within the lymphotomes from superficial to deeper vessels that connect to nodes. Between the lymphotomes are watershed areas (i.e., dividing areas) where normal drainage is away from the watershed, moving toward the nodes.[32,33] There are only a few superficial and deep connecting lymph vessels across watershed areas, but there are superficial collateral vessels.[14] These collateral connections across watersheds are very important because when there is lymph congestion, they provide alternative pathways to uncongested lymph vessels. The extremities also have lymphotomes. The upper extremity lymphotomes drain mainly into the axillary nodes. Detail of this information and more extensive drawings can be found in the work of Kubik.[33]

Lymph from the right thoracic lymphotome, right upper extremity, and right side of the head drains into trunks that eventually empty into the right lymphatic duct. This duct empties into the right subclavian vein and into the superior vena cava of the heart. Both lower extremities, both abdominal lymphotomes, the left thoracic lymphotome, and the left side of the head drain into the thoracic duct, which is the largest lymphatic vessel in the body and extends from L2 to T4.[30,33] The thoracic duct empties into the venous system at the juncture of the left subclavian and jugular veins. As described by Chikly,[5] "the lymphatic system is therefore a second pathway back to the heart, parallel to the blood venous system."

The lymphatic system is described as "a 'scavenger' system that removes excess fluid, debris and other materials from the tissue spaces."[21] It is an alternate path for those substances that are too large to be disposed of through the venous system.[24] There is a close link, therefore, between an adequately functioning lymphatic system and edema because "oedema can only occur if the lymphatic system has failed."[14]

Therefore, the overall theory of lymphatic therapies, including MEM, is to remove plasma proteins from edematous areas by stimulating the lymphatic system, which subsequently enables these proteins to leave the interstitial spaces and enter the lymphatic structures. By ridding the interstitial spaces of these hydrophilic proteins, subacute and chronic edema decreases.

Differences Between MLT and MEM

Despite physiologic similarities between MLT and MEM, there are differences worth noting. One difference between the MLT technique and the MEM technique is the patient population. MLT techniques were originally devised for individuals with lymphedema, which is a high plasma protein edema associated with a mechanical obstruction or insufficiency of the lymphatic system.[32] MEM was designed for orthopedic patients with subacute and chronic edema in whom the lymphatic system is intact but temporarily overloaded.

Another difference between the MLT techniques and the MEM technique is the length of the treatment. Because MLT is used on people with a permanently insufficient lymphatic system, the treatment sessions are longer and more involved because large amounts of fluid may need to be rerouted throughout the body. Conversely, because the MEM technique is used on people with intact lymphatic systems, the treatment sessions are shorter and typically involve moving less fluid. Also, unique to MEM is the use of pump point stimulation, which helps to eliminate the extensive massage time spent on an involved extremity because of the simultaneous stimulation of areas in the body with concentrated lymphatic structures. When using MEM on someone with subacute edema that has been present for 3 to 4 weeks, it is not unusual to see the edema decrease after two 20-minute sessions, especially if the patient is compliant with the home MEM program. These shorter treatment sessions are conducive to the needs of today's clinicians in the orthopedic setting.

Manual Edema Mobilization Concepts

The basic MEM technique consists of diaphragmatic breathing, light skin-traction massage, exercise, pump point stimulation, and a self-management program. Adjunctive methods such as chip bags, low-stretch bandaging, and Kinesio taping may also be used for patients with chronic edema, when lymph softening techniques are necessary. To effectively use the MEM treatment method, therapists need an understanding of the physiologic and anatomic rationale underlying the five basic treatment concepts as related to lymphatic stimulation (Table 65-2).

MEM Treatment Concept 1: Diaphragmatic Breathing

Description

All MEM sessions begin with deep, diaphragmatic breathing. This "belly" breathing involves breathing in deeply through the nose, causing the abdomen to expand, and then slowly exhaling through "pursed" lips. Feeling or seeing the rise and fall of the abdomen can help the therapist ensure that the patient is correctly performing the technique.[34,35]

Anatomic/Physiologic Support. Respiration changes tissue pressure,[33] and thus lymphatic absorption is stimulated.[29] The thoracic duct is the largest and one of the deepest lymphatic structures. It lies anterior to and parallel with the spine beginning at L2 and terminating into the left subclavian vein at approximately T4.[30] Diaphragmatic breathing, also known as the pulmonary pump,[5] changes pressure within the thoracic duct.[5,33] The thoracic duct functions on hydrodynamic principles.[33] Therefore, the pressure differential created from diaphragmatic breathing helps propel the lymph centrally toward the subclavian veins.[36] These pressure changes in the thoracic duct then create a vacuum (suction), pulling lymph from the peripheral structures centrally.[14,28,33]

MEM Treatment Concept 2: Light Skin-Traction Massage

Description

A light skin-traction massage is a massage so light that no blanching or indentation of the skin occurs yet it is firm enough to move the skin, thereby preventing the hand from sliding on the skin. The light skin-traction massage

Table 65-2 Anatomic and Physiologic Rationale for Manual Edema Mobilization Premises

	Anatomic Rationale	Physiologic Rationale
Premise 1: diaphragmatic breathing		Tissue-pressure changes open the interendothelial gaps of the initial lymphatics, allowing proteins to enter the lymphatic system
		Diaphragmatic breathing can change the interstitial pressure
		Respiration moves lymph through the largest and deepest lymphatic structures
Premise 2: light skin massage	Initial lymphatics are located within the dermoepidermal layer	Tissue-pressure changes open the interendothelial gaps of the initial lymphatics, allowing proteins to enter the lymphatic system
	Initial lymphatics can collapse with firm pressure	Light massage can change the interstitial pressure
Premise 3: exercise	Lymphangions are muscular units found in the collector lymphatics	Tissue-pressure changes open the interendothelial gaps of the initial lymphatics, allowing proteins to enter the lymphatic system
		Exercises can change the interstitial pressure
		Muscle activity stimulates the deeper lymphatic vessels
		Lymphangions have a higher rate of contraction or "pumping" during exercise
Premise 4: pump point stimulation	Refer to Table 65-3	Fluid moves from an area of higher concentration to an area of lower concentration
Premise 5: low-stretch bandaging	See Premise 2.	Changes in interstitial pressure increase initial lymphatic protein absorption. Neutral warmth softens indurated tissue increasing lymph flow

technique involves a rhythmical massage that forms U shapes on the skin, with the opening of each U in the direction of lymphatic flow proximally to an uninvolved or previously decongested area. The massage technique should remain light and should follow lymphatic pathways.

Clearing U Massage. Initially, the therapist performs the MEM massage technique (the U technique) in one segment of the body, starting proximally (or centrally) and moving distally down the segment. This proximal- (or central-) to-distal massage technique is referred to as the "clearing Us," and its purpose is to clear the lymphatic system within that segment. The clearing Us technique consists of performing five consecutive U massages in the most proximal (or central) location within that segment, then performing another five U massages just distal to the previous five, and continuing in this manner down to the distal portion of that segment. For example, if edema is in the right hand, the clearing Us would start with five Us at the left shoulder region, then five at the left clavicle, five over the sternum, five over the right clavicle, five at the right shoulder region, and so on down the arm until the therapist reached the hand.

Immediately after performing the clearing U massage technique in each section (trunk, upper arm, elbow, forearm, hand), active and/or passive exercises that move the joints and muscles associated with the recently cleared body segment are performed. In the example given, active and/or passive shoulder flexion, shoulder abduction, elbow flexion/extension, wrist flexion/extension, and fisting exercises would be performed after the clearing U massage.

Once the clearing U massages have been performed throughout the entire segment and the active and/or passive exercises have been performed, that segment is then considered cleared. The purpose of clearing a segment is to open and clear out the lymphatic pathways to allow the flow of lymph into the central structures.

Flowing U Massage. After a segment has been cleared, the therapist changes the direction of the massage technique to promote the flow of lymph through the recently cleared segment. During the flow portion, the U massage is performed distally to proximally (or centrally) within the newly cleared segment. This distal-to-proximal (or -central) massage technique is referred to as "flowing Us," and it consists of performing one U massage in a distal location within the cleared segment, then performing another U massage just proximal to the previous one, and continuing up to the most proximal portion of the segment. At this point, the sequence is repeated until five U massages have "flowed" up the cleared segment.

In the previous example, after the right arm had been cleared, the therapist would perform one U massage over the dorsum of the right hand, then over the right volar wrist, the right volar forearm, the right cubital tunnel, the right volar upper arm, the right shoulder, the right clavicle, the sternum, the left clavicle, and then finally the left axilla. This entire sequence would then be performed a total of five times to "flow" the lymph up the right arm over to the left axilla, so it drains centrally. Flowing U massage consists of sequential Us (one following another) starting in the distal part of the segment being treated and moving proximally past the nearest set of lymph nodes. The flowing can be described as "waltzing" up the arm. After the five flowing Us have been performed within a segment, active and/or passive exercises associated with the body area are performed.

Differences Between Clearing U Massage and Flowing U Massage. Although the clearing U massage and the flowing U massage are performed in the same segmental area, they differ from each other in two ways. First, the clearing U massage is performed in a proximal- (or central-) to-distal fashion, whereas the flowing U massage is performed in a distal-to-proximal (or -central) fashion. Second, the clearing U massage consists of performing five U massages in each location before moving distally, whereas the flowing U massage consists of performing only one U massage distally within a segment, and then moving sequentially up the segment until the proximal (or central) portion of that segment is reached. The flowing U massage sequence is then repeated a total of five times (Figs. 65-3 through 65-5).

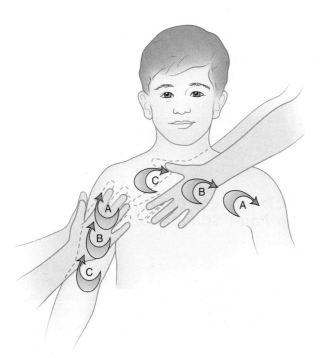

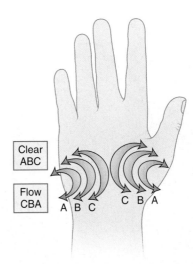

Figure 65-5 Palm: Lateral side of the therapist's thumbs are placed along the lateral sides of the patient's first and fifth metacarpals. Clear A, B, C and flow massage C, B, A sliding across the flexor retinaculum to the outside edges of the hand. Flow massage the dorsum of the hand to the mid-forearm.

Figure 65-3 Trunk: Clear A, B, C, and flow C, B, A. Upper arm: Clear A, B, C by tractioning the skin from posterior to the biceps. Flow massage C, B, A up to the sternum or to the uninvolved quadrant.

Anatomic/Physiologic Support

The light skin-traction massage influences the lymphatics on a superficial level. As mentioned earlier, the initial lymphatics are the small lymphatic channels that create a meshlike network[14,33] throughout the dermoepidermal layer of the

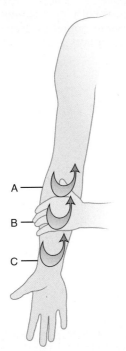

Figure 65-4 Forearm: Clear A, B, C. Flow massage C, B, A. Clear elbow node five times and continue massage to the biceps or the head of the humerus. Pronate the forearm and repeat the same sequence on the dorsum of the arm.

skin.[5] Attached to these small lymphatic channels are the anchoring filaments, which connect these cells to the surrounding tissues, and between these cells are junctures known as interendothelial gaps[5] (Fig. 65-6). As tissue pressure changes, the anchoring filaments assist in opening these interendothelial gaps,[5,33] thereby allowing fluid within the interstitial spaces to enter the lymphatic system.[37] Therefore, any mechanism that changes interstitial pressure ultimately stimulates lymphatic flow, and massage is one of those variables reported to change tissue pressure.[14,38]

Additionally, because the initial lymphatics are considered "feather fine" fragile vessels,[5] firm pressure can collapse them. Miller and Seale[39] found that a pressure of 60 mm Hg initiated lymphatic closure, with complete closure at 75 mm Hg.[39] Furthermore, it has been demonstrated that a 3- to 5-minute massage at 70 to 100 mm Hg on edematous tissue caused temporary damage to the endothelial lining of the initial and collector lymphatics.[40] Therefore, the MEM massage technique is light, just enough to move the skin without blanching it.

MEM Treatment Concept 3: Exercise

Description

Active and/or passive exercise is an integral part of MEM. The MEM exercise routine normally begins with trunk exercises immediately after the diaphragmatic breathing. The active/passive exercises then move to the periphery and correlate with the area on the body recently massaged with the clear and flow techniques. For example, if the MEM massage technique was just performed over the volar aspect of the wrist, then active and/or passive wrist flexion and extension would occur immediately after the massage.

Anatomic/Physiologic Support

Similar to light massage, muscle contractions also influence tissue pressure, allowing fluid to flow into the initial

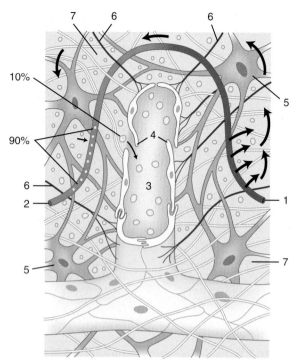

Figure 65-6 Incorporation of the lymph capillary in the interstitium. 1, Arterial section of the blood capillary; 2, venous section of the blood capillary; 3, lymph capillary; 4, open intercellular groove–swinging tip; 5, fibrocyte; 6, anchor filaments; 7, intercellular space. *Small arrows* indicate the direction of the blood flow; *large arrows* indicate the direction of the intercellular fluid flow. (From Kubic, S. Anatomy of the Lymphatic System. In: Foldi M, Foldi E, Kubik S (eds). *The Textbook of Lymphology for Physicians and Lymphedema Therapists*, 2003 Elsevier Gmbh, Munchen.)

lymphatic system by opening the interendothelial gaps.[14] Additionally, after the fluid enters the initial lymphatics, it then travels through deeper lymphatic vessels, the collector lymphatics[5,14,33] (Fig. 65-7). At the level of the collector lymphatics, the lymphatic system has muscular units known as

lymphangions. Simultaneous muscle activity has been found to stimulate the deeper layers of the lymphatic system[14] because the lymphangions have a higher rate of contraction or "pumping" during exercise,[41] and lymphatic flow can increase by 10 to 30 times through the lymphangions with exercise.[5,30] Exercise then stimulates the superficial lymphatics by altering tissue pressure and stimulates the deeper lymphatics, which aids in propelling the lymph through the deeper vessels.[14]

MEM Treatment Concept 4: Pump Point Stimulation

Description

In the extremities, there are areas of concentrated lymphatic bundles or lymphatic nodes (Table 65-3). The term *pump point stimulation* refers to simultaneously massaging two areas of concentrated lymphatic structures versus one set of lymphatic structures as in clear and flow massage. These are points of stimulation done in a U-shaped pumping motion. For instance, after the light skin-traction massage of clear and flow is done across the upper trunk, pump point stimulation is performed on the involved extremity followed by flow massage to a proximal site and exercise of the muscles in the area. The concept underlying pump points is based on the theory that massage creates a locally negative pressure gradient, thereby draining the lymphatic system distally[18,41] (Figs. 65-8 and 65-9). The MEM study,[15] which primarily included the use of pump point stimulation, showed a decrease in post orthopedic edema.

Anatomic/Physiologic Support

Although there is currently no anatomic research that supports the use of pump points to decrease edema, there is speculation by the authors that the observed decrease in

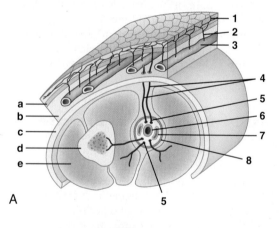

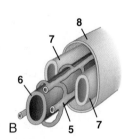

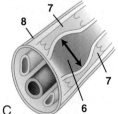

1 Capillaries of the skin ⎫
2 Precollector   ⎬ Superficial system
3 Collector   ⎭
4 Perforating vessels
5 Deep lymphatic system
6 Artery
7 Accompanying veins
8 Vascular sheath
a Cutis b Subcutis c Fascia d Bone e Muscle

Figure 65-7 Structure of the lymphatic system. Layers **(A)**, content of the vascular sheath **(B)**, lymph transport by arterial pulsation **(C)**. (From Kubic, S. Anatomy of the Lymphatic System. In: Foldi M, Foldi E, Kubik S (eds). *The Textbook of Lymphology for Physicians and Lymphedema Therapists*, 2003 Elsevier Gmbh, Munchen.)

Table 65-3   Correlation of Pump Points to Lymphatic Nodes/Bundles

Pump Point[18]	Lymphatic Nodes/Bundles[33]
Medial, anterior deltoid	Deltoideopectoral lymph nodes Axillary nodes are in this general area
Posterior deltoid	Dorsolateral upper arm bundle
Cubital node	Superficial cubital lymph nodes
Triceps insertion	Located between the proximal areas of the radial and ulnar forearm bundles The exception: Does not directly correlate with a specific set of lymphatic nodes or bundles
Volar wrist	Median forearm bundle
Dorsum of hand	Long transverse collaterals between the radial and ulnar collectors

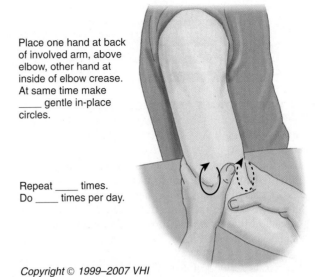

Place one hand at back of involved arm, above elbow, other hand at inside of elbow crease. At same time make ____ gentle in-place circles.

Repeat ____ times.
Do ____ times per day.

Copyright © 1999–2007 VHI

Figure 65-9 Upper extremity pump point 3 with caregiver assist.

edema after pump point stimulation may be the result of changes in pressure gradients. The circulatory system, which includes the lymphatic system, functions on pressure gradients, meaning that substances diffuse across cell membranes from areas of higher concentration to areas of lower concentration. This diffusion is known as Starling's forces or Starling's equilibrium.[5] The permeability of membranes and changes in hydrostatic and colloid osmotic pressure (either in the capillaries or the surrounding tissue) influence how fluid diffuses across capillaries.[14] It is known that the interendothelial gaps open when total tissue pressure is low and close when total pressure is high.[14] Therefore, it is plausible that creating a locally negative pressure gradient in the lymphatic system could entice fluids to flow from the tissues (the area with a higher pressure gradient) into the lymphatic system (the area with a lower pressure gradient). The authors speculate that simultaneously massaging these areas of increased lymphatic structures (referred to as pump points) creates a negative pressure gradient, although there is currently no supporting literature for this speculation.

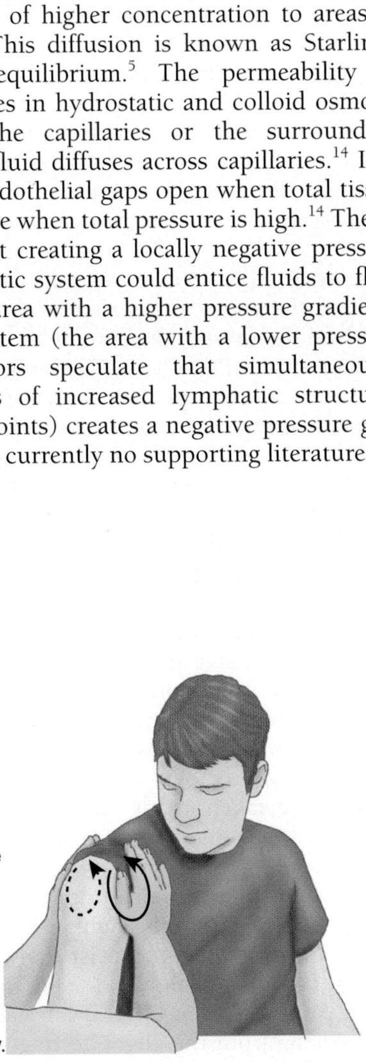

MEM Treatment Concept 5: Low-Stretch Bandaging

Description

Low-stretch arm and/or finger bandages are applied to an edematous limb if after two MEM treatment sessions, the edema has not decreased significantly, refills shortly after treatment, or induration (hardness of tissue) remains. Low-stretch bandages look like an Ace bandage in color and thickness but are 100% cotton and, because of the weave, have only a 20% stretch factor. Because these bandages have little stretch, they provide a compressive counterforce to an expanding muscle belly. This counterforce causes a change in interstitial pressure, which stimulates the lymphatics to absorb fluid and other materials from the interstitium. When the muscle belly relaxes, the bandages only contract 20% and thus do not give a strong force that could collapse the initial lymphatics. Light compression is obtained from the layering of multiple bandages, not from the applied stretch. The MEM bandaging system usually consists of three layers. The first two layers are stockinette and cast padding. The third layer consists of one or two short stretch bandages placed in a gradient pattern, thereby providing greater compression distally. For bandage use guidelines, see the "Frequently Asked Questions" section.

Anatomic/Physiologic Support

Leduc and colleagues[26,43] found that the combination of multilayered bandages on the forearm combined with exercise increased protein absorption by the lymphatic capillaries. Additionally, external pressure[39] and temperature[28] also facilitate lymph movement because it has been shown that the flow of lymph within the vessel is best between 22°C and 41°C (71.6°F and 105°F) and sharply slows down or stops below and above those temperatures.[28] Thus, bandaging can influence protein absorption by providing light compression and perhaps by providing a buildup of body heat that is within the mid-range of ideal temperature to mobilize lymph.

Place one hand on front, other hand on back of involved shoulder: palms at armpits, fingers pointing toward top of shoulder. At same time make ____ gentle in-place circles.

Repeat ____ times.
Do ____ times per day.

Copyright © 1999–2007 VHI

Figure 65-8 Upper extremity pump point 1 with caregiver assist.

CONTRAINDICATIONS AND PRECAUTIONS TO CONSIDER

Contraindications

Do not do MEM

- If an infection is present because there is the potential to spread the infection
- Over areas of inflammation because of the likelihood of increasing the inflammation and pain. In this case, do MEM proximal to the inflammation to decrease congested fluid, thus decreasing congestion and pain.
- If there is a blood clot or hematoma in the area because there is a chance of activating or moving the clot.
- If the patient currently has congestive heart failure, severe cardiac problems, renal failure, severe kidney disease, liver disease, or pulmonary problems because there is the potential to overload these already failing systems. These people usually have low protein edemas, and MEM is for high protein edemas.
- If there is active cancer; a controversial theory notes the opportunity to spread the cancer. Absolutely never do MEM if the cancer is not being medically treated and always seek a physician's advice.
- If the patient has primary lymphedema (congenital) or secondary lymphedema (i.e., post-mastectomy). To successfully treat this condition, it involves knowing how to reroute lymph to other parts of the body and how to perform specific treatment techniques that are beyond the scope of this chapter.

Precautions

Be aware that with MEM, there is the potential to:
- Increase the feeling of morning sickness during the first trisemester of pregnancy because of increased movement of fluid throughout body
- Alter blood sugar levels in someone with diabetes
- Lower blood pressure further in patient with preexisting low blood pressure

Contraindications to MEM

The precautions/contraindications related to MEM are those universal to most massage programs and specific to the impact of moving large volumes of fluid through the system (Box 65-1). A physician should always be consulted if the therapist is concerned about the patient's present or past cardiac or pulmonary status. For instance, if there is a significant volumetric difference between the two extremities, a therapist should inform the physician that there is the potential to move that much fluid through the heart and lungs. The physician should be asked whether this would compromise the patient's cardiac status.

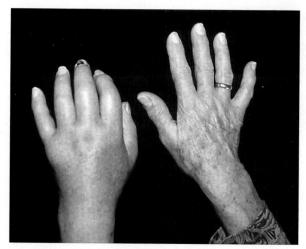

Figure 65-10 Mrs. M.G. before manual edema mobilization and therapy. (Courtesy Janine Hareau, PhD, PT, OT.)

Case Examples

The results of using MEM can be seen in the following case examples. The first case example, Mrs. M.G., shows the results of using MEM and low-stretch bandaging exclusively at the beginning of treatment, with progression to ROM and modalities once edema reduction started. The second example, Matthew, demonstrates the effect MEM can have in one session with early subacute edema.

Mrs. M.G. M.G. is a 75-year-old woman who was referred to hand therapy 8 weeks after a left (L) hand infection that involved the thumb, thenar eminence, and first dorsal interosseous space (Fig. 65-10). The infection was resolved after a series of antibiotics. The exact cause of the infection was never determined but was thought to be related to a (L) thumb nail bed infection. An evaluation revealed severe hand inflammation, severe swelling in the left hand thenar eminence and over the dorsum of the hand, a "spongy pitting" dorsal hand and digit edema, shiny taut tissue on the dorsum of the hand and digits, a visual analog scale (VAS) pain rating of 8 out of 10, active flexion ranging 0 to 20 degrees for each joint of each digit, full active extension to 0 of all digits, pain prohibiting passive flexion, no functional use of the hand, and sensory limitations ranging from decreased to loss of protective sensation throughout the entire hand. The hand pain prevented Mrs. M.G. from sleeping throughout the night for 8 weeks. Left and right comparison girth measurements were taken at the elbow, palm, wrist, and proximal phalanx of each digit. These girth measurements were totaled for each upper extremity from the elbow to the fingertips. The total girth measurement for the left was 102.5 cm compared with 89 cm on the right, a 13.5-cm girth difference.

The initial treatment consisted of performing MEM proximal to the inflammation and using low-stretch bandaging to the forearm and hand. After 2 consecutive days of treatment, total edema from the elbow to fingertips decreased 3.5 cm. Mrs. M.G. had no pain and was able to sleep throughout the night for the first time in 2 months. One month later, the total left lower arm and hand girth was only 3 cm greater

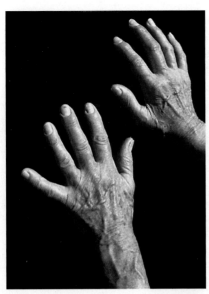

Figure 65-11 Mrs. M.G. 2 months later at discharge. (Courtesy Janine Hareau, PhD, PT, OT.)

than that of the right. In other words, Mrs. M.G. lost 10.5 cm of girth from the initial 13.5-cm girth difference between the two extremities. After the 2 days that it took to reduce the initial edema, an exercise program was initiated, which included isometric exercises and tendon gliding for 1 week. This exercise program promoted joint/tendon motion without causing tissue inflammation. Beginning the second week of treatment, a progressive exercise program was started that included electrical stimulation and the use of a continuous passive motion machine. At the end of 2 months of treatment, sensation throughout the hand had improved, ranging from normal light touch to decreased light touch, and the patient had complete active flexion and extension ROM of all digits (Fig. 65-11). At the 1-year follow-up, reevaluation revealed that the left hand girth was 1 cm less than that of the right hand.

Matthew. Matthew is a 42-year old construction worker whose right middle finger was caught in an up and down moving cylinder device. As a result of the injury, he sustained a traumatic boutonniere deformity. One and a half weeks later he sought hand therapy. The evaluation revealed a total circumference girth difference between the right and left middle fingers of 3 cm. Active and passive proximal interphalangeal (PIP) ROM was 30/90 degrees. Passive PIP extension beyond −30 degrees was too painful to pursue. Active distal interphalangeal (DIP) range with PIP blocked into extension was 0/20 degrees.

After the evaluation, a 20-minute MEM program was performed by the therapist. This program consisted of diaphragmatic breathing; massage of the supraclavicular areas (terminus); trunk exercise; bilateral axilla massage; MEM clear and flow massage to the uninvolved axilla across the chest; pump points 1, 3, 4, and 5 followed by flow massage and exercise; two specific MEM techniques to the hand/finger; MEM flow massage to the uninvolved axilla; and fisting above the head. There was a visible and measurable 50% decrease in edema in the right middle finger when mea-

surements were taken at the end of this first treatment. The same evaluation revealed that the PIP could be passively extended to 5 degrees from full extension, causing a VAS pain rating of 2 on a scale of 10, and active PIP ROM improved to 10/100. A custom simple safety pin type orthosis enabling functional use while doing construction work was fabricated for the patient. The home program consisted of two appropriate ROM exercises for the PIP and DIP plus a very brief 5-minute MEM program to do twice daily (Fig. 65-12).

The patient cancelled a follow-up appointment the next week because of his work schedule. He stated that he did not think that he needed to reschedule because swelling was "all down in his finger." Also, he informed the therapist that he could fully bend and straighten the finger at all joints. He did experience moderate finger pain at the end of a work day, but this was relieved by doing the brief MEM home program and wearing the orthosis at night. The patient was informed that he should continue wearing the orthosis 7 days per week, 24 hours per day for at least 2 more weeks.

Three weeks later, the therapist ran into the patient in the grocery store. The patient showed her that he had full ROM of the right middle finger, no pain, and only did the brief MEM program and/or wore the orthosis when the finger swelled or to reduce pain from "overstretching" at work tasks.

Frequently Asked Questions About Manual Edema Mobilization (Table 65-4)

Who are candidates for MEM? Patients who have stagnant high-protein edema are candidates for MEM. This includes patients who have edema beyond the normal acute phase that is not reducing with the usual acute-phase treatment methods (see Table 65-1). MEM can also be used to prevent edema and/or reduce the amount of edema for the trauma or post-surgical hand problems that are beyond the acute phase, meaning those whose edema is barely visible or not visible at all, but are being seen for other treatment needs such as ROM. The lymphatics have a safety valve function[5,28] and can take on considerably more than the usual 10% of excess interstitial fluid before they become overloaded and edema becomes visible. From this it can be theorized, but research is needed, that doing MEM on the trunk and upper arm and performing pump point stimulation at the beginning of one or two sessions can decongest lymphatics that are reaching maximum capacity, thereby preventing a lymphatic overload that would likely have resulted in edema. Clinically, it is commonly seen that those patients with minimal or nonvisible edema will say "my hand feels lighter" or "my fingers move easier" after a MEM treatment.

Would MEM be effective in reducing edema in the acute stage? During the acute stage (72 hours or less), fibrin plugs prevent lymphatic uptake by the initial lymphatics surrounding a wound.[44] Therefore, if the edema is acute, uptake near the wound may not occur. However, at a minimum, MEM would stimulate and clear the proximal lymphatic pathways, and this might be helpful. In a study by Hutzschenreuter and Brummer,[45] tissue on two groups of sheep was lacerated and

Breathing-2   Diaphragmatic-sitting or standing

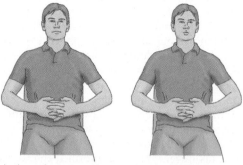

Inhale through nose making navel move out toward hands. Exhale through puckered lips, hands follow navel in.

Repeat __3__ times. Rest __3__ seconds between repeats. Do __2__ times per day.

Neck-1 Terminus

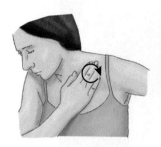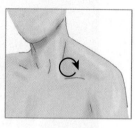

In hollow above uninvolved collarbone, using flat fingers make __10__ slow, gentle, light in-place circles. Repeat on involved side.

Repeat __2__ times. Do __2__ times per day.

Trunk-2 Side bend with towel

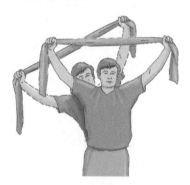

Stand or sit, arms extended above head, holding stretched towel. Bend to one side. Hold stretch for __3__ seconds. Repeat, bending to other side. Do not push head forward.

Repeat __2__ times. Do __2__ times per day.

Axillary-2 Two at a time

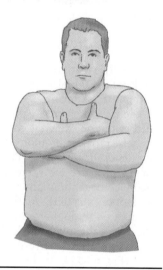

Cross arms placing weight of flat hand with flat fingers at center of both armpits making __10__ in-place circles.

Do __2__ times per day.

Arm/hand-2 elbow: cubital crease nodes

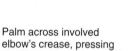

Palm across involved elbow's crease, pressing slightly harder on inside of elbow make __10__ in-place circles.

Repeat __2__ times. Do __2__ times per day.

Pump point-10 UE pump point five without caregiver assist (modified)

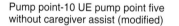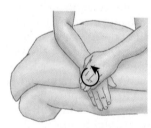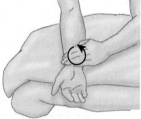

With involved hand palm side down, place other hand on top. Make __10__ in-place circles. Repeat on palm side of wrist.

Repeat __2__ times. Do __2__ times per day.

Figure 65-12 Matthew's home program. MCPs, metacarpophalangeals; UE, upper extremity.

Arm/hand-32   Hand: fingers-clear

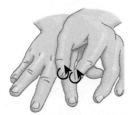

Involved palm down, hold first bone of involved finger(s) between thumb and index of other hand, lightly lift skin from under to top of involved finger and make __10__ in-place circles.

Repeat __3__ times. Do __2__ times per day.

Arm/hand-33   Hand: volar MCPs to elbow nodes-sweep

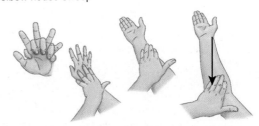

Sweep __10__ times from horizontal palm lines, through web spaces, across top of hand, turning arm palm up continue to elbow nodes.

Do __2__ times per day.

Arm/elbow-1   Upper arm: make fist overhead

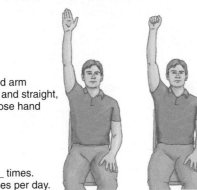

With involved arm above head and straight, open and close hand __10__ times.

Repeat __2__ times.
Do __2__ times per day.

Copyright © 1999–2007 VHI

Figure 65-12, cont'd

sutured. One group was administered MLD from day 1 postoperatively, whereas the control group received no MLD. There was no difference in edema reduction in either group until the end of the first week. Then, in the following weeks, the MLD group had a significantly greater increase in fluid movement and edema reduction than the control group. Thus lymphatic stimulation had no effect on reducing edema in the acute inflammation stage (less than 72 hours), but did affect the edema reduction within a week. This study provides further insight into the effectiveness of lymphatic massage performed in the acute stage of wound healing.

When should MEM begin? Usually 1 week after surgery/trauma as long as there is no infection, the sutures have been removed (so dehiscing of healing tissue does not occur), and there are no other contraindications. Because the lymphatic system can become congested before edema is visible, performing MEM on the trunk and stimulating pump points 1 and 3 one week after surgery/trauma might decongest the lymphatic system proximally and thus lessen or prevent future edema.

How can a therapist determine whether edema is high in protein? An edema that is "spongy" and has slow tissue rebound when indented is often a high-plasma protein edema. The best way to determine the type of edema is to look at the etiology and determine whether there are coexisting edemas (e.g., cardiac edema).

Do I always begin MEM at the trunk, even when there is just edema in the finger (e.g., from a finger fracture)? Yes, because when there is visible or barely visible edema, lymph congestion can often be palpated as proximal as the posterior deltoid. This edema needs to be moved out first so that the more distal edema can move proximally. Sometimes this has to be done only once (i.e., the first treatment session). The next session would begin with diaphragmatic breathing, proximal trunk exercises, pump point 1, and axillary and cubital node massage, and then MEM would begin at the volar forearm.

What are pump points? This is a term coined to describe a massage technique that appears, in the authors' opinion, to get a faster flow of congested lymph out of an area.[18,42,46,47] Refer to concept 4 and Tables 65-2 and 65-3 for more information related to pump points.

For a geriatric patient with multiple diagnoses, should I perform MEM on the entire extremity in one session? No, you could easily overload the cardiopulmonary system. Often this edema moves out of an area quickly because it is a complex edema. Thus, treating only one segment the first time and observing whether any complications occur are recom-

Table 65-4   Activating Lymph Uptake Review

Whys	Rationale	Clinical Application
Why keep pressure light?	Initial and precollector lymphatics must be stimulated to open and close to uptake lymph[21]; it is not a passive filtration/osmosis system	Keep compression light to avoid collapse of the dermis layer lymphatics[39,40]
Why are stimuli needed to facilitate lymphatic pumping?	Initial lymphatics have no pumping mechanism of their own and must be stimulated to open and close to uptake the large molecules and fluid from the interstitium. Collector lymphatics are capable of pumping.[30,31]	Initial lymphatic uptake and flow are increased by mild stimulation,[25] such as massage, light compression, and muscle contraction. Collector lymphatic rate of pumping is increased by surrounding muscle contraction.[30]
What start proximally?	Research by Pecking et al.[57] showed that in a postmastectomy lymphedema case, the speed of lymphatic transport from the involved hand increased immediately if the contralateral normal quadrant was treated by MLD. They also reported a 12% to 38% uptake in the involved limb when the contralateral axillary nodes were massaged.	Start light (no blanching or indenting of tissue) skin massage very proximal to the edema. Start stimulation in the noninvolved contralateral quadrant.
Why proximal exercise?	Exercise and diaphragmatic breathing cause changes in the intrathoracic pressure, which draw lymph centrally.[28]	Create a proximal suctioning effect by beginning exercises at the trunk.
Why massage nodes?	Lymph fluid passes through lymph nodes that can give 100 times the resistance to the flow of fluid as the thoracic duct.[14] Nodes can become a "bottleneck" or "kink in the hose" to the flow of lymph.	Use heavier (full weight of hand, not forceful pressure) massage at the nodes.
Why exercise?	Exercise can increase lymph transport speed 10 times.[30]	Exercise muscles in the segment just massaged to help speed movement of lymph proximally and thus clear distal congestion more rapidly.
Why low-stretch multilayer bandages?	Leduc et al.[26,43] found that the combination of multilayered bandages on the forearm and exercise increased protein absorption. Optimal temperatures to facilitate lymph movement are between 71.6° and 105.8°F or 22° and 41°C.[28]	When induration is present, consider using low-stretch bandages to increase protein absorption during exercise and for the buildup of neutral warmth and light compression with prolonged use for increasing lymph mobility.

mended. Complications to look for would be signs of congestive heart failure, decreased blood pressure, and decreased blood sugar level for the diabetic patient. If none occurs, the therapist may decide to gradually include more segments in further treatment. A MEM course is needed to teach how to safely work with this population and how to modify other aspects of MEM.

How long should I do MEM? The first session may take 20 minutes and consist of MEM in the trunk (diaphragmatic breathing, trunk exercise, bilateral axillary massage, clear and flow massage across the upper trunk axilla to axilla pathway, trunk exercise, diaphragmatic breathing) and then pump point 1 with flow back to the uninvolved axilla plus shoulder and trunk exercises. Usually hand edema will begin to reduce or soften because of this proximal work. The patient is taught a home program to do several times daily. At the next session, MEM might be performed on the entire extremity, and the patient is instructed in an expanded home therapy program. Subsequent treatments might involve the therapist doing MEM on the trunk and pump points and then beginning extensive MEM just proximal to the edema. Care must be taken not to add treatment techniques that could cause reinflammation of tissue (e.g., an overly aggressive strengthening program). A Kinesio taping program is an excellent addition to MEM to have more continuous lymphatic stimulation as the patient performs routine daily tasks.

When are low-stretch bandages used? After two or three MEM sessions, bandages might be advised if (1) tissue remains indurated, (2) edema recurs because of the presence of plasma proteins, (3) tissue has lost its elasticity from being stretched for a prolonged period and thus refills with tissue fluid, or (4) there is decreased motor function.

What are chip bags and what is their function? These are items described by Casley-Smith and Casley-Smith.[14] Chip bags can consist of pieces of 1-inch foam of various densities that are enclosed in a stockinette bag and placed on the skin over indurated areas of edema. The chip bags can be secured with a low-stretch bandage or can be worn under an elastic glove. This gives light stimulating compression and retains body heat, resulting in further tissue softening.

Can one of the various types of elastic/cotton stockinette tubes be a substitute for a low-stretch bandage? Yes, for minimal edema. The tube does not have gradient pressure. It must not be too tight, which would result in collapsing the initial lymphatics. A clinical guide regarding tightness is that the therapist should be able to get his or her whole hand under the proximal end of the elastic/cotton stockinette tube with a comfortable, not excessive, compression felt on his or her hand. The distal end of the tube might have to be tapered with stitching to accommodate the shape of the arm. Two methods have been used clinically to prevent rolling down of the tube on the extremity that could cause more edema distally. A 2-inch wide piece of foam strapping material is *lightly* placed around the proximal end of the tube 1 inch below the top of the tube. The proximal end of the tube material is then overlapped (cuffed) on to the foam strap. This helps to secure the tube from rolling proximally down the arm. The same thing is also possible using a 3- to 4-inch wide piece of Coban bandage that the therapist *completely* stretches all the elastic out of and *lightly* places around the arm at the proximal end of the tube bandage and then folds the tube end over the top of the Coban, as described previously.

If the patient previously had lymphedema from a mastectomy and then has a hand injury and/or surgery on the same side and the edema gets worse, can I effectively use MEM? No, MEM does not teach rerouting around areas of node removal or around fibrotic radiated tissue. The therapist must seek the help of a person adequately trained in MLT techniques.

How is rerouting around scar done? The goal is to reroute congested lymph around areas of tissue damage into adjacent functioning lymph capillaries (lymphatics). The therapist begins clear and flow massage proximal to the incision or congested site. Then the therapist creates a vacuum, drawing the congested lymph around the scar by having her proximal hand form Us near where the lymph is to be directed toward a node, and the other hand is just proximal the edematous area performing flowing Us toward the proximal hand.

If current edema control techniques are working, why change to MEM? The challenge is to reexamine the success of these techniques in light of what stimulates the lymphatics. Fisting above the head is often prescribed to reduce edema.[48] A closer examination of this technique reveals motion beginning proximal to the trunk and proceeding distally as the scapula rotates along with stretching of the trunk and arm muscles and ending with distal active muscle contraction from fisting as the arm is extended above the head. This technique follows the principles that stimulate lymphatic flow. Are elastic gloves effective because they are loose fitting, giving light compression and thus stimulating the lymphatics? Is use of the pneumatic pump effective because the pressure is set at 35 mm Hg or less rather than diastolic pressure, which exceeds the pressure needed to collapse the lymphatics and prevent lymph uptake? Is the retrograde massage effective because it is being used on a low-protein edema such as early stroke edema or on very early stages of subacute edema before stagnation of lymph occurs? Is the use of sponge-type finger wraps effective to soften hard edema and scars because they are providing prolonged light compression and neutral warmth? Possibly all of these techniques would make the more distal edema reduce faster if a couple of sessions included MEM on the trunk, upper arm, and pump points because of the decongesting effect on the proximal nodes and lymphatics.

What is the number 1 mistake therapists make when performing the MEM technique? Therapists forget that edema is congested significantly proximal to the visible edema and so do not start the MEM at the uninvolved axilla and clear and flow massage across the chest to the uninvolved axilla. Starting MEM at a set of nodes just proximal to the visible edema will just congest the lymph more proximally and it will return. A pathway must be created so that the more distal edema can move proximally. A useful analogy is that of a clogged sink filled with nondraining water (edema). When the clog in the pipe (proximal congestion) is eliminated, the water (edema) drains out of the sink.

Conclusion

There are four key factors related to subacute and chronic edema that validate the use of lymphatic therapies on people with orthopedic subacute and chronic edema. First, it has been shown in an animal model that if excess plasma proteins remain in the interstitium, they can cause chronic inflammation,[32] possibly leading to fibrosis.[32] Second, orthopedic subacute and chronic edemas are high-protein types of edema with increased plasma proteins in the interstitium.[14,44] Third, it is well documented that the role of the lymphatic system is to remove these excess plasma proteins and other lymph constituents from the interstitium.[5,14,21,30,33] Fourth, existing research from the lymphedema literature validates techniques that effectively stimulate lymphatic uptake for people with lymphedema, thereby diminishing the interstitial plasma proteins.[5,14,25,49,50] These four key factors provide the foundation for MEM, which is a technique that adapts lymphatic drainage principles for application to the orthopedic population. The clinical results have been very positive, and MEM opens a door to another facet of orthopedic edema reduction that needs further research and clinical publications.

REFERENCES

The complete reference list is available online at www.expertconsult.com.

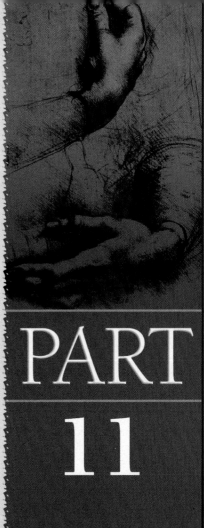

Stiffness of
the Hand

Pathophysiology and Surgical Management of the Stiff Hand

KENNETH R. MEANS, JR., MD, REBECCA J. SAUNDERS, PT, CHT, AND THOMAS J. GRAHAM, MD

PREVENTING THE STIFF HAND
GENERAL THERAPY CONSIDERATIONS
CHARACTERISTICS OF STIFFNESS OF THE SMALL
    JOINTS: PIP AND MCP JOINT STIFFNESS

THUMB STIFFNESS
STIFFNESS OF THE HAND INTRINSICS
HAND STIFFNESS IN PATIENTS WITH DIABETES
CONCLUSIONS

CRITICAL POINTS

Indications For Surgical Management

Failure to progress with further nonoperative treatment options; typically 4 months or longer from time of injury or initial surgery

Priorities

Regain passive motion first, then active motion

Pearls

High degree of patient motivation required before embarking on surgical release and postoperative therapy

Healing Timelines and Progression of Therapy

If no critical structures require protection, therapy progresses as the skin/soft tissue and degree of patient comfort allow

Pitfalls

Failing to identify the primary cause of the particular stiffness before attempting surgical correction

Precautions

Resist the temptation (and often patient pressure) to "jump in early" with regard to surgical management of stiffness; the best results will come to those who wait (again, typically 4 months and plateau in therapy/orthotic use; if either criterion is not yet met, continue nonoperative treatment if possible)

Timing for Return to Work/Activities of Daily Living

Once skin and soft tissues are healed and the patient is comfortable, activities may be increased as tolerated. We use as a general rule of thumb that once range of motion (ROM) is more than 50% to 75%, we start strengthening and once strength is more than 50% to 75%, we allow the patient to begin resuming normal work/sports activities. Of course individualized plans will be required and may necessitate functional capacity evaluations for specialized work situations.

There is not a more universally agreed-upon challenge among patients and professionals who are brought together by injuries and disorders of the hand than combating stiffness. Loosely identified by loss of motion, the type of stiffness about which we write has many dimensions: discomfort, altered tissue dynamics, potential elements of neurovascular dysfunction, and functional compromise. Short-term motion loss accompanying any form of injury or intervention to the hand is to be anticipated. Swelling, pain inhibition, and the need for protection by initial orthotic use all contribute to posttraumatic stiffness. When the tissue response and functional capabilities do not return after a reasonable time and an assiduous pursuit of an advanced rehabilitation program, then surgical solutions may have a role.

It may be at first counterintuitive to approach a problem that has swelling and fibrosis as basic components by contemplating a surgical solution. There is no avoiding the concept that "surgery is injury," but a controlled approach to release of contracted or immobile structures can be the last and most logical alternative when nonoperative care has failed to optimize outcome.

It should be remembered that releases of the joints themselves only address passive ROM. The intact function of the extensor and flexor systems is still required to actively range the joints. This means that, after a joint release, if passive motion is regained but active motion is still lacking, then extensor and/or flexor tenolysis or other reconstruction is required to regain active motion. An analogy for patient discussions is that the joints are like the wheels of a car, and the tendons are the engine. Typically we try to get the wheels (joints) able to spin as smoothly as possible first. If the wheels are locked up, no matter how hard you run the engine, they will not spin. Once the wheels are freely mobile, we rely on the engine (tendons) to maintain the advances that are made with animating the joints. If the engine is not working, we will need to "power" it with a separate procedure (tenolysis), which is covered in other chapters. In this chapter, we focus on selected concepts, challenges, and complications related to hand stiffness. A thorough description of the anatomy and biomechanics of the hand is essential to the understanding of the development, presentation, and treatment of stiffness and can be found in Chapter 1. The key facets of surgical planning, technical elements of operative care, and a balanced approach to rehabilitation are explored. This chapter also serves as an update and expansion of the excellent contributions by our colleague, Dr. Peter Innis, in the last edition of this text.

Preventing the Stiff Hand

Preventing the development of stiffness is part of the ideal management of all injuries to the hand.[1] Unfortunately, despite the best efforts of the surgeon, therapist, and patient, some degree of stiffness after any substantial hand injury is nearly inevitable. Principles of treatment include reduction of edema through elevation of the hand above heart level and the use of compressive dressings as the skin and soft tissues allow; positioning and orthotic use as needed, and institution of ROM as soon as possible.

The early reduction of hand edema is critical in the prevention of stiffness. When there is fluid about and within the metacarpophalangeal joint (MCPJ), the joint assumes a posture of extension because this is the position in which the joint can hold the largest volume of fluid. As the MCPJ assumes its extended posture, the proximal interphalangeal joint (PIPJ) and distal interphalangeal joint (DIPJ) tend toward semiflexion as the extensor tone is decreased and the flexor tone is increased at these joints. If left in these positions for an extended period of time, the surrounding capsuloligamentous structures of the joints will become contracted. This is why the edematous, posttraumatic hand will gravitate toward MCPJ extension and interphalangeal joint (IPJ) flexion contractures if left unchecked.

Elevation of the hand to reduce edema should be at or above the level of the heart, both during the day and when sleeping. A sling may be useful but can also be detrimental when used continuously by restricting the movement of the shoulder and elbow. When a sling is used, it should be cinched high so the hand is at or above heart level and the patient should be instructed to perform ROM exercises for the proximal uninvolved joints when out of the sling to prevent loss of motion.

An orthosis is placed on the hand with the finger MCPJ in flexion, the IPJs in extension, and the thumb in abduction whenever possible. This orthosis position counters the nonfunctional posture described previously.

If fractures or injuries to the bone and joint structures are intrinsically stable or adequately stabilized surgically, then an early postoperative motion program can be instituted. In some cases, the injured part and adjacent joints may need to be immobilized for a period of time to allow healing, but motion of the uninvolved and unimmobilized joints should be started as soon as possible to prevent loss of motion and to help to decrease edema.

General Therapy Considerations

The following chapter covers in detail the therapist's role in the management of the stiff hand. The following are some general therapy considerations that are important to emphasize relative to surgical management.

It is important to keep in mind functional ROM when setting goals for the significantly stiff hand. A study by Hume and colleagues[2] identified functional ROM of the hand for 11 activities of daily living (ADL) using both standard and electrogoniometric methods. They found functional flexion postures averaged 61 degrees at the MCPJ, 60 degrees at the PIPJ, and 39 degrees at the DIPJ. The amount of flexion for the thumb averaged 21 degrees at the MCPJ and 18 degrees at the IPJ. Patients who are unable to achieve these functional ranges may require built-up handles for ADL utensils and specific vocational tool use.

Evaluation of the stiff hand should include the following: active and passive ROM, edema, pain, sensibility, flexor and extensor tendon gliding and length, and intrinsic muscle function and length. Chapter 6 provides a detailed description of the clinical examination of the hand.

Prolonged edema is one of the most common causes of stiffness in the hand. Simons and colleagues[3] described three different venous pumping systems in the hand and specific exercises to activate each one. In all the subjects, an increase in the velocity of venous return occurred when individual systems were activated. The deep venous system in the palm can be activated with isometric intrinsic muscle contraction by adducting the digits against resistance. The superficial dorsal and superficial palmar systems are activated the most by external compression. The authors showed that these systems also act together and produce the greatest effect during fist formation. The effects during fist formation were found to be potentiated by abducting the digits.[3]

Kinesiotaping is another proposed method of controlling edema when wound healing permits.[4] This helps alleviate pain and is theorized to facilitate lymphatic drainage by microscopically lifting the skin during active motion. Pressure and irritation may be taken off the neural and sensory receptors, which results in decreased pain. Pressure is gradually taken off the lymphatic system, which aids in lymphatic return. Further research is needed to support the use of kinesiotaping for edema control.

Orthoses are frequently used in the management of stiffness of the hand. The following chapter covers in detail the use of orthoses in the management of hand stiffness. In general, the type of orthosis used and the schedule of use is individualized depending on a number of factors such as the

Table 66-1 Guideline for Interpretation of the Modified Weeks Test[11]

PROM Increase (degrees)	Orthotic Technique
20	No orthosis
15	Static orthosis
10	Dynamic orthosis
0–5	Static progressive orthosis

The degree of increase in passive range of motion (PROM) following a thermal modality, exercise, and sustained end range positioning is used to determine the need for or the orthotic technique to be used to further increase passive ROM of a stiff joint.

Table 66-2 Digital Functional Assessment

Result	% TAM	Finger TAM (degrees)	Thumb TAM (degrees)
Excellent	85–100	220–260	119–140
Good	70–84	180–219	98–118
Fair	50–69	130–179	70–97
Poor	<50	<130	<70

From Freeland A. *Hand Fractures: Repair, Reconstruction and Rehabilitation.* Philadelphia: Churchill Livingstone; 2000:13.
TAM, total active motion.

phase of healing after injury or surgery and whether the purpose of the orthosis is protective or corrective. Orthoses can be static, dynamic, and static progressive.[5,6] Flowers proposed an algorithm to guide therapists in their splint selection based on clinical assessment of tissue compliance using a modified Weeks test.[7] This procedure involves taking a passive ROM measurement of the stiff joint before any exercise or modality, i.e., a "cold reading." A second reading is taken after treatment including a thermal modality and exercise followed by sustained positioning of the stiff joint at the end of its available motion. The two readings are compared to determine the gain in ROM, which reflects tissue compliance and the severity of stiffness. Orthoses are chosen based on the degree of tissue compliance (Table 66-1).

Colditz[4,5] described a casting technique used to help facilitate a more normal pattern of motion as well as increased ROM for use with the significantly stiff hand. The technique, called casting motion to mobilize stiffness, is described in detail in the following chapter.

The Digit Widget is an external fixator-type device used to increase ROM typically for PIP flexion contractures. It is used after an unsuccessful trial of orthosis use or before surgical release for severe flexion contractures to facilitate the surgery. Pins are surgically inserted into the patient's bone distal to the target joint (Fig. 66-1). The frame is affixed to the pins and strapped to the hand, and rubber bands are applied. These bands exert a constant extension torque on the PIP joint.

Patients should be monitored closely after the application of any type of orthosis for signs of inflammation including erythema, heat, increased pain or edema, decreased active/passive ROM, and decreased sensation. When any of these signs or symptoms are present, the orthosis should be checked for proper fit and pressure distribution. ROM should be reassessed every 2 to 3 days to monitor progress and the effectiveness of the orthosis. Plateaus in ROM gains may indicate the need for a different orthosis design and/or change in exercise program. It is important to frequently review the patient's home program of orthosis wear and exercise to ensure compliance.

Exercises after surgery for stiffness are selected and begun based on the surgical procedure performed. For example, ROM exercises, both passive and active, are indicated after surgical release of a stiff and contracted joint(s). With tenolysis of adherent and scarred tendons, isolated and differential tendon-gliding exercises must be included as well. It is important to know the preoperative pattern of stiffness and what was achieved at surgery to appropriately set goals for therapy. Exercises are typically begun as soon as possible postoperatively. See Chapters 40 and 68 for therapy after flexor and extensor tenolysis and MCPJ and IPJ capsulectomies.

Outcomes of surgical procedures of the stiff hand can be assessed by using the End Result Committee of the American Society for Surgery of the Hand values for digital functional assessment (Table 66-2).[6]

Characteristics of Stiffness of the Small Joints: PIP and MCP Joint Stiffness

For both the MCP joints and PIP joints, it is essential to confirm that there is not significant bone and/or cartilage damage at the articular surfaces that could be limiting ROM. In these instances, soft-tissue releases alone are contraindicated because increasing ROM without addressing articular issues will lead to more pain and rapid destruction of the remaining articular cartilage. Instead, articular reconstruction in the form of osteotomies, cartilage transplants, or microfracture or other techniques must be used in concert with soft-tissue procedures. If salvage of the joint is not possible or feasible, then arthrodesis or arthroplasty are considered.

PIP Joint Stiffness

The stiff and contracted PIP joint creates significant functional impairment. Even a seemingly innocuous PIPJ injury such as a collateral ligament sprain can lead to surprisingly significant amounts of PIP joint pain, swelling, and stiffness.

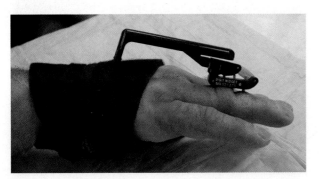

Figure 66-1 Clinical photo of the Digit Widget. (Courtesy James P. Higgins, MD.)

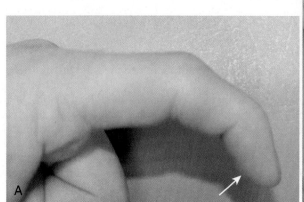
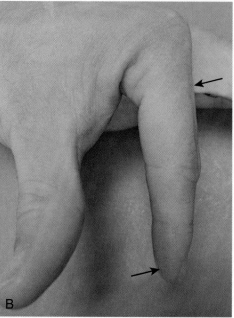

Figure 66-2 Extrinsic flexor tendon adhesion/tightness limiting PIP joint extension. **A,** With the MCP joint extended, the PIP joint assumes a posture of flexion and cannot be extended further due to flexor tendon adhesion and tightness. **B,** PIP joint extension improves with metacarpophalangeal (MCP) joint flexion.

The difficulty in overcoming a PIP joint flexion contracture is due in part to the relative weakness of the extensors compared with the flexors. For this reason, the "safety position" of the hand requires that the PIP joint be positioned in full neutral extension unless contraindicated, depending on the injury.

Surgical Considerations for the Stiff PIP Joint

If sufficient time and therapy have been given to a stiff PIP joint but a significant limitation remains, surgical intervention is considered. A minimum of 4 months of intense therapy after an injury or surgery is prudent unless there are specific reasons to accelerate the decision for surgery. If progress is able to be documented beyond 4 months, therapy is continued until a plateau in progress occurs.[8] At this point, a determination is made as to whether the residual limitations are sufficient to consider surgical release. This decision is made in concert with the patient, therapist, and surgeon. Consideration of the impact that the residual limitation has on the patient's function combined with the potential for improvement with surgical intervention weighed against the intraoperative and postoperative effort expected are all involved in the decision to proceed with surgical intervention.

A limitation that is intrinsic to a joint must be distinguished from that which is from an extrinsic factor such as tendon adhesions. In the case of limited PIP joint extension, if the finger is flexed at the MCP joint and the PIP joint can be extended passively, then the limited PIP joint extension is secondary to flexor tendon adhesions (Fig. 66-2). If the limitation is unchanged regardless of whether the MCP joint is flexed or extended, then it is considered intrinsic to the joint and releases as described in the following section are appropriate (Fig. 66-3). It is important to note that limited PIP joint extension may be caused by both intrinsic and extrinsic factors. See Chapter 6 for a detailed discussion of clinical examination of the hand.

A PIP joint extension contracture is characterized by limited PIP joint flexion. The limitation may be caused by tightness or adherence of the extensor tendons, intrinsic tendons, or joint capsuloligamentous structures. If the limitation is lessened by MCP joint extension and worsened by MCP joint flexion, extrinsic extensor tendon tightness or adhesions are suspected (Fig. 66-4). If the limitation in PIP joint flexion is worsened by MCP joint extension and improved with MCP joint flexion, intrinsic tendon tightness is suspected (Fig. 66-5). If the limited PIP joint flexion is unaffected by MCP joint flexion or extension, then it is intrinsic to the joint itself, and releases as described in the following are used (Fig. 66-6).

Surgical Management of PIP Joint Flexion Contractures

The contributors to PIP joint stiffness include all tissues volar to the axis of PIP joint rotation. Each level and type of tissue

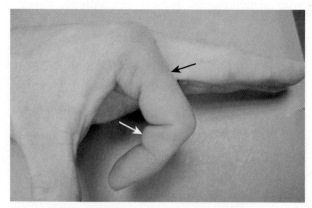

Figure 66-3 Flexion contracture of the proximal interphalangeal (PIP) joint due to capsuloligamentous contracture. The PIP flexion contracture is not improved by metacarpophalangeal joint flexion.

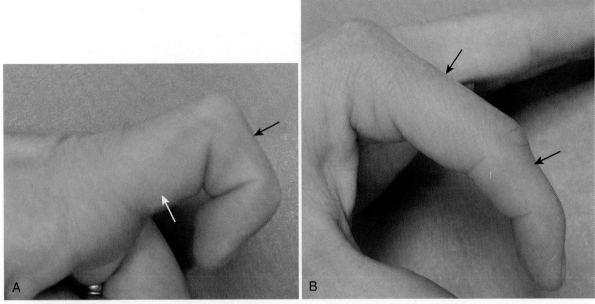

Figure 66-4 Limitation of PIP joint flexion caused by extrinsic extensor tendon tightness/adhesions. **A,** PIP joint flexion is possible with the MCP joint in extension. **B,** PIP joint flexion is limited with the MCP joint flexed due to extensor tendon adhesions or tightness.

need to be identified and a plan for its release and reconstruction devised. Although other options for surgical release exist, such as the TATA procedure (Téno-Arthrolyse Totale Antérieure or anterior tenoarthrolysis), most surgeons typically follow the technique and principles as espoused by Curtis[9] in his classic paper and expanded on by others. As each structure is sequentially released, the degree of improvement is assessed. If correction is inadequate, the releases continue in order. Specialized considerations, such as PIPJ stiffness in the setting of a boutonnière deformity, are considered in other chapters in this text.

Skin. Stiffness resulting from primary skin problems (Dupuytren's contracture or burns) or those resulting from multiple previous operations or simply long-term joint flexion may warrant special consideration, but the basic skin handling is decided more by the degree of contracture than its etiology. The following are surgical guidelines with modifications made based on individual characteristics of each case.

- Contracture of less than 30 degrees. There is probably no incision that could not be used and take care of all goals: access to joint, neurovascular protection, and coverage. Those more familiar with the standard Bruner-type incision may wish to use it, whereas those comfortable with the mid-axial incision will certainly find it extremely fitting.
- Contractures of 30 to 60 degrees. More attention needs to be paid to skin coverage when contractures reach this

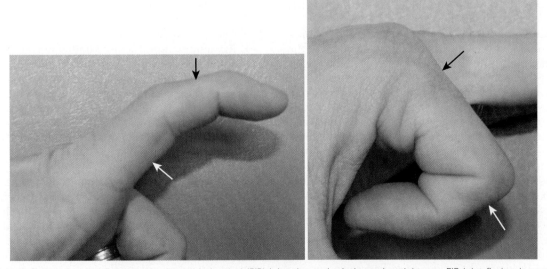

Figure 66-5 Limitation in flexion of the proximal interphalangeal (PIP) joint due to intrinsic tendon tightness. PIP joint flexion is more limited with metacarpophalangeal (MCP) joint extension **(A)** and improves with MCP joint flexion **(B)**.

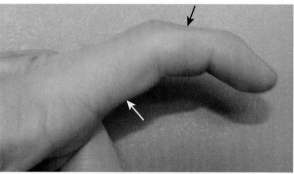
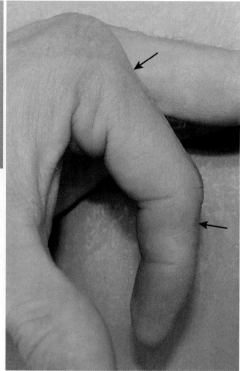

Figure 66-6 Extension contracture of the proximal interphalangeal (PIP) joint due to capsuloligamentous stiffness. The PIP joint extension contracture (limited PIP joint flexion) is unaffected by metacarpophalangeal (MCP) joint extension or flexion.

degree. The standard Bruner-type incision is technically difficult to perform and somewhat dangerous because of incisions crossing the flexor surface in the setting of typical volar displacement of the neurovascular bundles. We have used two incisions with success: (1) the mid-axial incision and (2) a modified Bruner-type incision in which the radially or ulnarly based chevron portions start and end at the digital flexion creases and the apices of the incision stop at the volar midline. This allows effective lengthening of the skin column at the terminus of the case by extending an incision from the apex transversely to the opposite mid-axis, then advancing the flap in the manner of a V-Y.

- Contractures of 60 to 90 degrees. Again, two basic incision types have been successful in our hands: (1) the mid-axial incision can still yield adequate skin coverage, but the apertures that may be open proximally and distally may be unacceptably large or in locations that are disadvantageous, and (2) the H-incision. In this latter option, bilateral mid-axial incisions are made and connected by a transverse incision (usually made over the mid-P1 or mid- P2 level). As with the appropriately performed single mid-axial approach, the neurovascular bundles are left dorsal. After the deep release work is completed, there will be a rectangular aperture requiring a skin graft.
- Contractures greater than 90 degrees. The more successful the release of these advanced contractures during the operative session, the more difficult skin coverage becomes. Again, we have had some success

with using the mid-axial incision, even for these severe cases. The H-incision could work with more extensive grafting. Even elective skeletal shortening (usually through arthrodesis) is a consideration.

- Also important to consider with the soft-tissue sleeve of the digit are the neurovascular structures. For particularly long-standing and/or severe flexion contractures, there may be considerable shortening or tethering of the digital arteries and nerves. In this case, a complete intra-operative release of the flexion contracture is usually still possible, but a static progressive extension orthosis may be required so that these structures may slowly adapt to the relative lengthening that the flexion contracture release provides.
- Ray amputation. Having photographs of successful ray amputations readily available in the clinic can be an invaluable tool to educate patients for whom this could be a logical consideration for the "parasitic" stiff finger. We consider ray amputation a reconstructive, more than a terminal or salvage, procedure. It must be in the portfolio of considerations for advanced and recalcitrant problems.

Tendon Sheath and Flexor Tendons. Once the skin sleeve has been opened, the tendon sheath is encountered. A window is made to include the A3 pulley and the contracted cruciate (C1 and C2) pulleys between the A2 and A4 pulleys. Small sections of these latter pulleys may be released to achieve adequate exposure. A Ragnell or similar smooth retractor is used to pull the flexor digitorum superficialis and profundus separately through the proximal and distal flexor sheath to release any adhesions. This step is important to eliminate another possible contributor to the flexion contracture while also allowing for as much active flexor tendon excursion postoperatively as possible.

Volar Plate/Checkrein Ligaments. Classically, the flexor tendons are now retracted so that the palmar aspect of the PIP joint is exposed. The checkrein ligaments are seen proximal to the volar plate and along the radial and ulnar aspects of the proximal phalanx. These structures are elevated off of the proximal phalanx in a proximal-to-distal direction until the proximal edge of the volar plate is reached. If there is still insufficient correction of the contracture, then the volar plate is released in a proximal-to-distal direction, maintaining its attachment to the palmar lip of the base of the middle phalanx.

Alternatively, we have favored focusing our surgical attention on the P2 insertion of the volar plate. By first incising the entire distal aspect of the plate from the middle phalanx, then carrying the longitudinal incision proximally in the interval between the volar plate and accessory collateral ligaments on the radial and ulnar side, the joint is usually both well released and adequately exposed. We believe that this affords us with two important benefits: (1) the volar plate, with its proximal anchoring, is still available to us in case we need it for PIP joint reconstruction (e.g., volar plate arthroplasty), (2) it decreases the chance of vincular injury, which almost certainly occurs with the proximal dissection of the so-called checkrein ligaments—less bleeding should translate to less scarring.

Collateral Ligaments. The collateral ligaments represent the final option for release of the PIP joint flexion contracture. The accessory collaterals are released first, followed by subtotal or complete release of the proper collaterals if necessary.

Once all structures that have required release have been addressed, the final ROM and stability of the PIP joint are determined. If radical release was needed, including sacrifice of the collaterals, there may be significant radial/ulnar instability. As long as flexion/extension stability is maintained, an aggressive postoperative motion protocol is still used with ranges purely in this plane of motion and while protecting against radial/ulnar stresses with buddy straps, dynamic orthoses, or otherwise. If extension instability is present in the form of dorsal subluxation of the middle phalanx at the PIP joint, then dorsal extension block orthotic positioning or pinning may be used with progressive extension in therapy postoperatively. In these cases, it is important to not allow the flexion contracture to recur, typically by allowing 10 to 15 more degrees of extension per week.

Surgical Management of PIP Joint Extension Contractures

Although less common than flexion contractures, an extension contracture of the PIP joint can be just as significantly limiting for a patient. A stepwise approach is still prudent. We use a mid-axial incision if both flexion and extension contractures will need to be addressed. If there is an isolated extension contracture, we perform a dorsal curvilinear incision centered on the PIP joint. With this approach, a large dorsal flap is created, allowing access to the entire dorsum of the joint. An extensor tenolysis is performed next, with special care to maintain the central slip insertion at the dorsal base of the middle phalanx. If following extensor tenolysis there is insufficient passive flexion then formal release of the joint is performed. By elevating the lateral bands centrally/dorsally, windows in the dorsal joint capsule between the central slip and the collateral ligaments can be created with a scalpel on the dorsal radial and ulnar aspects of the joint. A Freer elevator or similar tool is placed sequentially in the radial and ulnar aspects of the joint and intra-articular adhesions are released. Again, care is exercised to maintain the central slip insertion. The elevator tool is gently allowed to slide palmarly inside the PIP joint until it reaches the palmar aspect of the joint. Further volar release into the retrocondylar sulcus at the volar-proximal aspect of the proximal phalanx head may be necessary. Doing this allows the retrocondylar sulcus to receive the base of the middle phalanx as the joint flexes. If passive flexion is still limited, then release of the accessory and proper collateral ligaments is performed, typically by release of their origin off the proximal phalanx head.

MCP Joint Stiffness

Fortunately the MCP joint is not typically as challenging as the PIP joint with regard to stiffness. Also, debilitating stiffness is not as commonly encountered with this joint. Contrary to the PIP joint, loss of flexion is the issue that is usually seen with MCP joints. A dorsal incision is made centered on the MCP joint. If several MCP joints require release, a long transverse incision may be used. Full-thickness skin flaps are elevated above the radial and ulnar aspects of the extensor hood. The extensor tendon can undergo tenolysis proximally and distally to ensure that it is not contributing to loss of flexion. The ulnar sagittal band is typically incised so as to not violate the weaker radial sagittal band and avoid ulnar subluxation of the extensor tendon. Once the sagittal band is opened, the extensor is retracted radially so that the MCP joint capsule is exposed. Alternatively, the extensor tendon may be split longitudinally, revealing the MCP joint capsule. The dorsal capsule can be incised longitudinally and a Freer elevator or similar tool is used to release the capsular adhesions. A complete excision of the dorsal capsule may be performed, if needed, to allow flexion of the MCP joint. The elevating tool of choice can also be used to slide along the articular surface of the metacarpal head in a dorsal-to-volar direction to free up volar adhesions. It may even be necessary to slide the tool along the volar surface of the distal metacarpal to release the retrocondylar sulcus of the metacarpal head and allow it to accept the base of the proximal phalanx in flexion. Finally, release of the collateral ligaments from their origin at the metacarpal head may be required.

When MCP joint flexion contractures are present, they are usually due to something other than joint stiffness, i.e., something extrinsic to the joint. This is usually the case with skin contracture, such as in Dupuytren's disease, posttraumatic longitudinal scarring of the palmar skin, or flexor tendon adhesions.

Thumb Stiffness

The thumb is considered to be responsible for 40% or more of overall hand function. Fortunately, a large ROM at all thumb joints is not a requirement for function. In fact, there is significant variation in the general population, especially with thumb IP joint and thumb MCP joint flexion and extension, with some patients demonstrating minimal active or passive ROM at one or both joints while still maintaining excellent performance.

The most debilitating form of stiffness of the thumb is loss of opposition and webspan secondary to thumb webspace adduction contracture. Again, a systematic approach to thumb adduction contracture is recommended. As each surgical step is taken, passive ROM is assessed and the releases stop once adequate motion is restored. Skin is addressed first, often with a large Z-plasty, to make more skin length available to the distal webspace skinfold line between the thumb and index rays. Next, the dorsal fascia overlying the first dorsal interosseous (DI) muscle is incised. If necessary, the first DI muscle can be completely released from the thumb metacarpal. A formal release of the adductor pollicis may be required. This is accomplished by first identifying and protecting the princeps pollicis artery after the radial artery dives between the two heads of the first DI. Next, the adductor pollicis is divided. Alternatively, the adductor pollicis may be released off of the middle finger volar metacarpal. This provides an adequate release while still allowing the origin of the adductor to scar down in the palm and potentially maintain some function as opposed to complete release of its insertion on the thumb metacarpal. A capsular release of the thumb carpometacarpal (trapeziometacarpal) joint may be required. The final potential step for a first webspace release is trapeziectomy, which unlocks the thumb carpometacarpal joint. Ligament reconstruction and/or interpositional arthroplasty are according to the surgeon's choice. Sometimes advanced soft-tissue coverage options must be considered if extensive releases are required (Fig. 66-7).

Stiffness of the Hand Intrinsics

Tightness of the intrinsic musculotendinous system of the hand may be seen as a primary or secondary entity. Its primary form is often seen in athletes, musicians, or other individuals who are often overexerting the intrinsic muscles of the hand. As the overexertion continues, the muscle–tendon units may become shortened, leading to intrinsic tightness. This is often clinically manifest by vague discomfort in the hand or a sense of fatigue as activities continue for any length of time in one sitting. Secondary stiffness of the hand intrinsics typically occurs after major trauma to the hand, such as a gunshot wound and crush injury. Intrinsic muscle injury followed by edema and eventual fibrosis and even muscle necrosis is the genesis of the stiffness. Often in these cases the MCP joints or PIP joints themselves may also be stiff such that dedicated contracture release of the joints may be required at the same time as the intrinsic tendon release.

When surgical release is required, incisions are made on the dorsal aspect of the MCP joints. A single transverse inci-

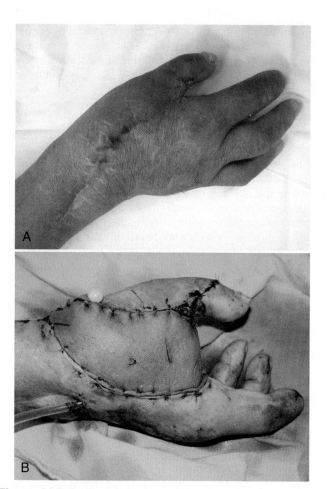

Figure 66-7 A, B, Clinical photographs of a severe first webspace contracture treated with extensive releases and a lateral arm free flap. (Courtesy of James P. Higgins, MD.)

sion may be used if multiple digits will need release. Dissection proceeds palmarly on either side of the MCP joint until the intrinsic tendons are reached. The ulnar- and radial-sided interosseous tendons are released first. For the small finger, the tendon of the abductor digiti minimi also needs to be released. If after these releases at the MCP joint, there is still inadequate passive PIP joint flexion because of intrinsic tendon tightness, then separate releases of the lateral bands just proximal to the PIP joint level may be required as well.

Hand Stiffness in Patients With Diabetes

A patient with diabetes has a proclivity for hand stiffness. This may be seen in the form of chronic trigger digits (stenosing tenosynovitis) in which pain and mechanical changes in the flexor tendon system limits ROM. It is not uncommon for patients to present with a digit locked in flexion or a digit than cannot be flexed due to the long-standing tenosynovitis. Eventually a PIP joint flexion contracture may develop in these patients. These cases can be surgically managed with A1 pulley release and postoperative therapy/orthosis wear directed at the PIP joint. If the flexion contracture is significant and likely to be recalcitrant to nonoperative treatments, then formal surgical release in the same setting may be warranted. Patients with diabetes also have a higher incidence of Dupuytren's contracture.

A generalized tendency toward limited joint ROM intrinsic to the joints themselves has also been seen in patients with all forms of diabetes mellitus.[10] This is often termed limited joint mobility (LJM) or Rosenbloom's syndrome and is thought to be unique to patients with diabetes.[11] LJM can be observed throughout the upper extremity but may be most pronounced and functionally limiting in the hand. The presence and severity of LJM have been correlated with age and male sex as well as with duration of diabetes and degree of glucose control.[12,13] LJM has also been variably linked to a higher risk of concomitant or eventual development of other diabetic complications, such as nephropathy, neuropathy, and retinopathy.[14,15] The mainstays of treatment are nonoperative, including edema control methods and orthosis wear as needed, and strict glucose control is prudent in general.[16] Use of an aldose reductase inhibitor may also be beneficial and should be at the discretion and direction of the patient's endocrinologist and/or primary care physician.[17] One should proceed with surgical intervention with significant trepidation, given the possible postoperative complications as well as likely comorbidities present that increase anesthesia and surgical risk factors. Surgery is typically reserved for those with significant functional impairments that affect ADL. In these cases, the surgical principles discussed in the previous sections should be applied as needed for particular joint stiffness. Again, the risks of surgical intervention must be carefully analyzed relative to potential benefits.

Conclusions

Treatment of the stiff hand remains a challenge for physicians, therapists, and especially patients, and prevention is the best medicine. Fortunately, we do have several "arrows in our quiver" to address the stiff hand, each being used appropriately as the severity and chronology of the stiffness dictate. The need to develop a strong working relationship among the physician, therapist, and patient cannot be overstated because these challenges will test the patience of all those involved in their care.

REFERENCES

The complete reference list is available online at www.expertconsult.com.

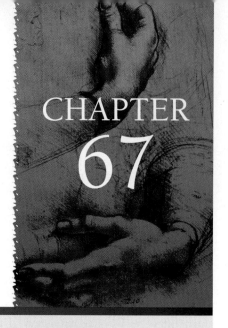

CHAPTER 67

Therapist's Management of the Stiff Hand

JUDY C. COLDITZ, OTR/L, CHT, FAOTA*

THE CHALLENGE OF THE STIFF HAND
DEFINITION OF STIFFNESS
STIFFNESS AND THE STAGES OF WOUND
    HEALING
EVALUATION AND TREATMENT OF EARLY
    STIFFNESS

EVALUATION AND TREATMENT OF THE
    CHRONICALLY STIFF HAND
SUMMARY

CRITICAL POINTS

- Effective rehabilitation of the stiff hand requires that the effects of immobilization be minimized while not overloading healing tissue.
- Interosseous muscle tightness frequently contributes to limited finger flexion. One should assume that interosseous muscle tightness contributes to the limited motion until it can be proven otherwise.
- In the chronically stiff hand, tissue adherence and stiffness, chronic edema, and maladapted cortical patterning are interdependent problems. To be successful regaining mobility of the stiff hand, all three problems must be altered simultaneously.

The Challenge of the Stiff Hand

Clinical experience confirms certain risk factors for stiffness in the hand. The more tissue traumatized, the greater the likelihood of stiffness.[1] Severe trauma injuring bone and multiple soft tissue layers usually requires longer periods of immobilization because of the need to regain skeletal stability. The decrease in tissue elasticity that accompanies increasing age creates less tolerance for the insult of trauma.[2] Infection that extends the wound beyond its mechanically created boundary creates adherence between multiple remote

tissue planes. Although we know these basic facts, many questions about stiffness in the hand remain unanswered: Why do some patients have great difficulty regaining motion long after others have returned to normal function? How can we identify what amount of motion, at what frequency, and with what duration will maximize individual patient results? We do know, as did Sir Charles Bell in 1883, that "the mechanical properties of the living frame, like the endowments of the mind, must not lie idle, or they will suffer deterioration."[3] Prolonged immobilization is the greatest enemy of hand mobility. Our challenge is to devise a treatment program that provides balanced stimuli to elicit a positive response.

Definition of Stiffness

The term *stiff* is used commonly when describing the hand lacking full mobility. The word *stiff* is usually reserved to describe the physical property of matter whose close molecular structure makes it rigid, resisting deformation when an external force is applied. Stiffness of the hand is not an increased rigidity of the tissues themselves[4] but a constraint created by crosslinking of the previously elastic configuration of the collagen fibers.[5]

Collagen provides most of the tensile strength of the tissue in the hand. Collagen fibers themselves are inelastic, but movement between the collagen fibers imparts elasticity to the tissue. Normal hand motion occurs when these strong, dense connective tissue structures glide relative to one another.[6] Stiffness is caused by the fixation of the tissue layers so that the usual elastic relational motion is restricted by crosslinks binding the collagen fibers together.[5,7-11]

*The author appreciates the thoughtful review of and revision suggestions for this chapter by Kevin Park, OTR/L, CHT; Karen R. Roeming, MA, OTR, CHT; and Ingrid Wade OTR/L, CHT.

INTRAMOLECULAR CROSSLINKS

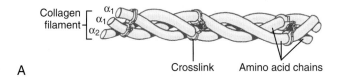

A

INTERMOLECULAR CROSSLINKS

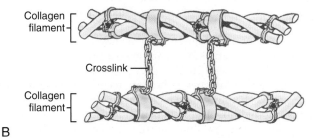

B

Figure 67-1 A, Collagen crosslinking occurs between amino acid chains within one collagen filament (weak crosslinks) and (**B**) between collagen filaments, locking them to one another (strong crosslinks). (From Hardy MA. The biology of scar formation. *Phys Ther.* 1989; 69:1020.)

Peacock and Cohen[11,12] provide an excellent analogy for the concomitant strength and elasticity of normal collagen. They compare collagen fibers to the strength of the relatively inelastic nylon thread used to make women's nylon stockings. Significant elasticity of the stocking fabric is created by the way in which the nylon threads are knitted together. Collagen crosslinking does not change the collagen fibers themselves (analogous to the nylon thread), but it restricts the movement of one fiber (thread) in relation to another (Fig. 67-1).

Stiffness and the Stages of Wound Healing

Tissue injury creates a relatively extended period of heightened collagen synthesis, degradation, and deposition within a wound as compared with the rate of this process within normal uninjured tissue.[12] Healing tissue progresses through three stages: inflammatory, fibroplasia, and remodeling (or maturation).[13] Although these are chronologic stages, they do not follow a precise timeline unless the wound has no complications.

During the inflammatory stage the wound prepares to heal, during the fibroplastic stage the tissue structure is rebuilt, and during the remodeling stage the final tissue configuration develops.[14] In the ideal circumstance a healing wound progresses through these stages in an orderly and timely manner. Wounds with massive tissue injury, infection, absence of wound closure, or delayed healing, or wounds requiring repeated surgery or lacking proper wound hygiene, have extended stages of healing far beyond the ideal time frame. Therapists treating complex injuries cannot follow the chronology of a wound and assume a certain stage;

instead they must be able to evaluate the characteristics of the wound or healing scar and determine the appropriate stage to devise appropriate therapy.

In the uncomplicated wound, the initial inflammatory phase of wound healing is completed within a few days. Randomly oriented, matted collagen fibrils unite the injured structures during this early phase of healing, although fibers cannot be visualized through the light microscope until the fourth or fifth day after injury. Because the intercellular forces are weak, wounds may be disrupted with ease during this stage.[6] Most surgical wounds are protected with immobilization until the wound healing has begun.

In the uncomplicated wound the fibroplasia stage begins at the end of the first week of healing, when the fibroblast begins replacing the macrophage as the most common cell type. About 2 days later fibroblasts begin the process of collagen synthesis and outnumber the granulocytes and macrophages in the wound. The fibroblasts evolve into myofibroblasts and are responsible for collagen fiber synthesis and concurrent contraction of the wound edges. Capillaries reestablish within the wound, forming a dense network. Collagen fibers are laid down between the capillaries, forming the scar needed to keep the wound closed. By the end of the second week, the wound is filled with newly synthesized but disorganized collagen fibers invading all areas of the wound.[6,15,16] Although the strength of the wound remains diminished (at 3 weeks an incised and sutured wound has less than 15% of its ultimate tensile strength),[6] the random orientation of the collagen fibers limits their movement relative to one another. At this stage the scar is not strong and cannot tolerate excessive stress. If wound circumstances are ideal, the fibroplastic stage (also called the proliferative stage) occurs within the first week after the wound is created. However, in complex wounds or wounds with complications, this period is greatly extended.

Joint stiffness and tissue adherence palpated during this stage can be described by a soft end-feel at the limitation of passive motion. This tissue responsiveness occurs because the crosslinking of the collagen fibers is weak and stress causes the collagen fibers to align themselves with the direction of stress. The fluctuant end-feel of the passive joint limitation results primarily from edema filling the interstitial spaces and thus limiting full passive mobility. Because of the diminished strength of the healing tissue, excessive force can tear the fibrils, causing more injury and reviving the inflammatory process. Any force must be applied slowly and gently, and be sustained for a brief period of time. During fibroplasia, intermittent active motion is the ideal means of applying stress to the disorganized collagen to encourage realignment. More resistive motions can be coaxed by the application of a gentle sustained force applied using orthotic mobilization. Young scars can be altered morphologically by conditions of stress that are ineffective in older scars.[17]

In the uncomplicated wound the maturation stage usually begins between 3 and 6 weeks after surgery or injury. In the hand with delayed healing, infection, multiple tissue trauma, or multiple surgeries, the beginning of the maturation phase may be prolonged many weeks or months. As the cell population decreases, the number of scar collagen fibers increases.[6] The total collagen accumulation then stabilizes and remains constant. At this stage collagen deposition is accompanied by collagen degradation, creating equilibrium. Alteration in the architecture of scar collagen fibers occurs as the scar matures. The tissue continues to respond to applied stress, but the response is greatly diminished as compared with the earlier stages. Physical changes are caused by changes in the number of covalent bonds between collagen molecules (see Fig. 67-1). Scars remain metabolically active for years, slowly changing in size, shape, color, texture, and strength,[6] and ultimately begin to resemble normal tissue.

Wounds that are well into the maturation stage exhibit a hard end-feel when passive joint motion is applied. The joint motion does not yield to gentle force and stops abruptly. This response to palpation requires more consistent application of force to effect change. In the early part of the maturation stage, intermittent serial static or static progressive use of an orthosis can effectively mobilize the stiff hand. More complex injuries and more resistive chronically stiff hands require a more consistent application of gentle force, requiring a different approach. A nonremovable cast is recommended to consistently direct active force across stiff joints. This technique, casting motion to mobilize stiffness (CMMS), is discussed later (see "Evaluation and Treatment of the Chronically Stiff Hand").

Evaluation and Treatment of Early Stiffness

The demarcation line between the early stiff hand and the chronically stiff hand is difficult to pinpoint. In the following sections the early stiff hand is discussed separately from the chronically stiff hand, because the treatment approaches suggested differ greatly. Regardless of the stage of stiffness, manual examination is required to determine exactly which anatomic structures are limiting motion. The early stiff hand that is past the acute stage of healing but continues with edema, joint stiffness, and/or tissue adherence remains relatively immobile. This immobility may result from lack of functional use, pain, fear, or continued protection of healing tissue. A cycle is established in which inactivity leads to stiffness and adherence. This leads to continuing edema, which leads to continued inactivity (Fig. 67-2). In most postsurgical hand patients, changing one of these three factors readily breaks this cycle. For example, reducing edema allows greater potential for movement, which decreases inactivity and in turn decreases stiffness and tissue adherence. As the therapist

and patient work together on each of the three factors, the other factors are directly influenced and the mobility of the hand returns.

Edema

Treatment of the stiff hand cannot begin without a thorough understanding of the causes of edema and the factors that influence it. Because its presence is a primary cause for immobility of the injured hand, edema reduction to create potential for motion is always a primary component of treating the stiff hand.

The reader is encouraged to review the other chapters about the lymphatic system and treatment for edema in this text (see Chapters 63 and 65). Key points are briefly reviewed here to support edema reduction recommendations made later in this chapter. These recommendations may differ from some long-held treatment beliefs.

Edema is excess fluid in the interstitium (the spaces between cells).[18-21] Because one-sixth of the body consists of spaces between cells,[20] there is significant room for expansion when the spaces are filled with edema. The injured hand normally develops edema as a result of increased capillary permeability, which allows leakage of fluid and protein into the tissue spaces.[20] The presence of mild postoperative edema actually facilitates wound healing by causing a moderate increase in the strength of the healing wound and an increase in macrophages and fibroblasts.[18,22] Greater amounts of edema destroy the continuity of the wound, breaking the fibrin seal and the integrity of the sutures.[18]

The lymphatic system is an intricate network of lymphatic conduits that drain excess fluid and other substances, including cells, proteins, lipids, microorganisms, and debris from the tissues to maintain homeostasis.[20,21]

Following an injury, the lymphatic system is often overwhelmed by the rate of capillary filtration and cannot carry the volume of fluid as fast as it is produced. This results in the development of edema. This normal edema production in response to injury is to be clearly differentiated from lymphedema, caused by lymphatic obstruction that causes protein to accumulate in the tissue spaces, which gives rise to osmosis of the fluid out of the capillaries.

Movement of lymph fluid through the lymphatic system is aided greatly by external forces—adjacent muscle contraction, tissue compression (e.g., gentle massage, bandaging), and general stimulation (e.g., arterial pulsations, body movement)—because the lymphatic system itself has no active pump. If wound healing progresses without complication, edema begins to subside and motion is regained. However, injured hands that develop significant stiffness do not follow this path, and inflammation and edema persist.

Pitting versus Nonpitting Edema

Before the development of externally visible pitting edema, the interstitial spaces must first become filled with fluid. This filling of the interstitium with lymphatic fluid increases the internal pressure, eliminating the ease of movement before edema is visible externally. Although this interstitial edema cannot be visually appreciated or measured as easily as pitting edema, it plays a significant role in preventing full motion of the hand.

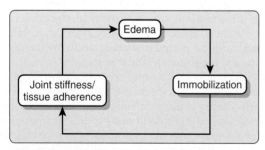

Figure 67-2 In the early stiff hand, three factors interplay to create stiffness: edema, immobilization, and joint stiffness–tissue adherence. Changing any one factor alters the cycle of stiffness.

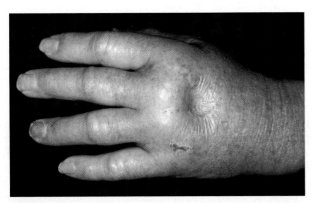

Figure 67-3 Pitting edema is best observed on the dorsum of the hand after sustained pressure with the thumb.

Most of the interstitial fluid is trapped within the interstitial tissue gel. When edema exists in pockets of free fluid outside the interstitial spaces, it "pits" with pressure. These pockets of free fluid can hold more than half of the volume of the interstitial fluid.[20] One common location of pitting edema is on the dorsum of the hand, where the loose dorsal skin pocket provides ample space for pockets of free fluid to accumulate. Manual pressure placed on the dorsal pocket causes the fluid to move, leaving an indentation (or pit)—thus the term *pitting edema* (Fig. 67-3).

Evaluation of Edema

External pitting edema can be measured accurately via water displacement.[23,24] Measurement of pressure created by interstitial edema is impossible to accurately measure. A precise observational examination is far more useful in appreciating the level of interstitial edema.

Careful inspection of both hands (Fig. 67-4), comparing the general appearance, gives an insightful view of the presence of interstitial edema. Loss or diminution of normal small skin wrinkles, tautness or obliteration of the dorsal finger joint creases, and obscurity of metacarpal head definition and of the dorsal finger extensor tendons are recordable observations of the presence of interstitial edema.

The presence of interstitial edema can be felt if the examiner palpates both hands simultaneously with eyes closed.

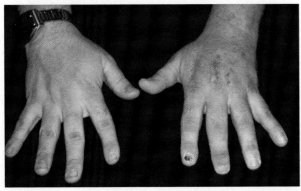

Figure 67-4 Visual comparison of the injured and uninjured hands shows differences in skin wrinkles and creases, metacarpal head definition, and prominence of dorsal extensor tendons.

Comparable fullness of the tissues is palpable, creating diminished tissue mobility in the injured hand. (In contrast, pitting edema is felt as fluctuant.) Active and passive joint motion is limited by a tangible fullness of the space, creating a soft feel to the end-range of joint motion. An experienced clinician can discern by palpation whether edema is the primary cause for limited passive joint motion.

Unfortunately, such palpation does not allow objective, quantifiable measurement, so that accurate comparison examinations and documentation of edema reduction are impossible. Some therapists use circumferential measurements of a digit, palm, or wrist, but the lack of reliability makes such measurements useful only as an approximate indicator of progress. If such measurements are used, the anatomic location of the measuring tape must be recorded and a repeatable amount of force applied to the measuring tape at each examination.

Edema Control Techniques

Minimizing the negative effects of immobilization caused by edema is the most useful initial treatment for the injured hand. Elevation, active muscle contraction, external pressure from various sources, and stimulation via gentle light massage can prevent the accumulation of excessive edema. Understanding which edema reduction technique to use when and the optimal type of force or pressure to use throughout the stages of healing is key to successful prevention of the stiff hand. Readers are urged to review the chapters on edema in this book (Chapters 63 and 65).

Elevation. Immediately following injury and/or surgery, immobilization of the tissues is usually necessary to allow completion of the inflammatory phase of healing without disrupting the healing wound.

Interstitial fluids tend to accumulate in dependent parts because the increased intravascular pressure increases capillary filtration.[19,25] Even a normal hand can develop edema if it is immobile and dependent.[26] Thus, elevation of the immobilized hand minimizes edema. The postcapillary blood pressure that facilitates venous return is less than 15 mm Hg of hydrostatic pressure. If the hand is in a dependent position, the pressure opposing the venous return is approximately 35 mm Hg of hydrostatic pressure.[20]

Elevation of the extremity, i.e., hand above the elbow, elbow above the heart, is the single most useful postoperative instruction to decrease the hydrostatic pressure in the vessels.[25] Patients must be instructed carefully on the precise definition of elevation. The concept of a drop of water being able to run downhill to the heart without ever encountering an uphill run helps patients visualize adequate elevation.

Maintaining the arm in a sling is not adequate elevation and encourages the extremity to become quiescent. It is far more productive to instruct the patient to maintain elevation during the day by using pillows or books and reserve the use of a sling for brief periods of ambulation. During this time, intermittent active motion of the proximal joints should be encouraged to ensure that joint motion is maintained and large proximal muscle groups are recruited to assist venous and lymphatic flow.

When the surgical dressing is removed and intermittent active motion of the injured part is begun, intermittent elevation is still necessary to assist edema reduction. There is often a practical quandary. The hand is edematous and active motion is encouraged, but the patient is also instructed to elevate the hand, which is in an inactive position for the extremity. A balance can be achieved by instructing the patient to do active pumping exercises intermittently with the hand and arm elevated and to elevate the hand when not using it actively. Prolonged periods of using the hand in a dependent position with minimal active motion are to be avoided at this stage because of the difficulty maintaining the pumping balance.

Active Motion: Pumping versus Gliding Motion. Active muscle pumping near the site of edema is the single most important stimulus for increasing lymphatic flow. However, active motion across the site of injury immediately after surgery may disrupt healing and often cannot be immediately employed. Because there are no muscles within the digits, skin movement and tissue compression from active flexion is the stimulus required for increased lymphatic flow in the digits. When digital motion must be limited to protect healing structures, gentle pressure to the digit, elevation, and active muscle contraction in adjacent uninjured areas must substitute for active motion of the digit itself. With many digital injuries, the metacarpophalangeal (MCP) joint may safely be allowed full motion. This permits the patient to perform pumping exercises of digital adduction and abduction, and MCP joint flexion and extension, which contracts the adjacent proximal intrinsic muscles. Conversely, blocking the MCP joints in extension assures active flexion forces are directed to the interphalangeal (IP) joints to effectively mobilize the digital edema. If a well-conformed orthosis is applied to stabilize the MCP joints in extension, the molded volar orthosis surface provides appropriate pressure to the dense lymphatic network in the palm. This palmar pressure further assists in the reduction of digital edema.

In a randomized study of patients who started shoulder range of motion (ROM) immediately versus 7 days after axillary dissection for cancer, those waiting 7 days had less wound drainage, fewer days of drainage, and earlier postoperative discharge than patients who started immediately following surgery. There was no difference in the outcome of ROM in the two groups.[27] This study suggests that active motion should appropriately be delayed when tissue injury or surgical dissection is extensive.

The muscles proximal to the wrist are larger than the intrinsic muscles of the hand and thus more effective stimulators of the lymphatic system. As long as the vascular status of the hand is stable, intermittent active motion of proximal muscles is begun as early as possible following surgery. Waste products that are evacuated from the injured hand are more effectively moved through the lymphatic system with this intermittent active motion. Passive ROM does not stimulate muscle contraction and, for that reason, cannot be substituted for active motion to reduce edema.[28]

When active motion of the injured part is allowed, elevation and proximal pumping must be continued until enough motion is present at the injury site to allow local pumping sufficient for adequate lymphatic flow. Patients who exercise the injured part of the hand while elevated see a dramatic edema reduction as they gain motion at the site of injury.

Compression. In addition to active muscle contraction providing intermittent internal compression to the lymphatic conduits, gentle external pressure also aids in lymphatic flow. Excessive pressure restricts lymphatic flow. For this reason, large compressive bandages are applied postoperatively to maintain gentle pressure to the hand. As one would expect, the use of external pressure alone, in the absence of active pumping, provides little long-term change. However, the use of external pressure as an adjunct to active motion often can interrupt the edema cycle, allowing potential for full active motion.

External wraps or elastic garments, external orthoses or bandages, or gentle external massage provide external pressure treatment. In the past, recommendations have been made for firm retrograde pressure to "push" the edema out of the hand. This concept should be abandoned and a concept of gentle external pressure should be adopted to facilitate lymphatic flow. See Chapters 63 and 65 on edema treatment for additional treatment suggestions.

Compressive Bandage. Surgical dressings and other forms of immobilization are used to provide necessary rest so newly injured tissues are protected from external forces and can begin the healing process. When a wound has delayed healing, some form of bandaging that continues to supply gentle compression is advisable. When a patient presents with significant pitting edema (regardless of the stage of healing), the quantity of edema present in the tissues is so great that mobilization of the joints is futile until the edema is reduced. Although the foremost goal is mobilization of the hand, a brief period of partial immobilization in a bulky compressive dressing that distributes pressure to all tissues

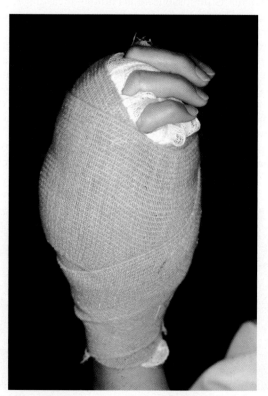

Figure 67-5 A bulky dressing may be used overnight or for a few days to provide prolonged but gentle compression for effective edema reduction.

is a wise initial treatment (Fig. 67-5). The fingers are gently wrapped with a self-adherent elastic bandage before multiple layers of fluffed gauze squares are placed between the digits and also applied dorsally and volarly. A gauze wrap around the hand and wrist compresses the fluffed gauze squares. The fingers are left free to flex and extend at the IP joints, but the motion of the MCP joints is limited temporarily by the bandage. Elastic bandages and/or plaster of Paris slabs may be added to the exterior of the dressing for more specific support and compression. In significant pitting edema, the consistency of pressure provided by such a nonremovable overnight dressing can assist in dramatic edema reduction.

If edema is a result of excessive manipulation of the hand causing a prolonged inflammatory response, a short period of rest and immobilization in a compressive bandage reduces both edema and inflammation. This approach allows a better starting point for upgrading motion and the use of other gentle edema reduction techniques. It may seem contradictory to immobilize a stiff swollen hand. The immobilization is necessary, because it is the most effective way to provide conformed pressure that will reduce the edema to a level at which productive active motion is possible.

Orthoses. Immobilization decreases initial edema, reduces pain, and permits tissue repair without the stress of external forces. The use of immobilization orthoses during the acute stages of wound healing can provide effective rest and compression in addition to accurate positioning to protect healing structures or to maintain a balanced position. If orthoses are applied with straps, the lymphatic vessels can be occluded by the pressure of the strap.[29] Pitting edema distal or proximal to a strap is a sign that strap pressure is impeding lymphatic flow. A safer alternative is the use of a wide elastic wrap or a molded thermoplastic piece that covers both dorsally and volarly. This distributes pressure rather than localizing it to a strap. When applying a hand-resting orthosis to an edematous hand, it is best to hold it in place by wrapping a wide elastic bandage at an angle along the full length of the orthosis. Later, when the edema has subsided, straps may be applied. This application technique is also effective for orthotic fabrications on the edematous elbow.

A removable immobilization orthosis made from dorsal and volar plaster of Paris slabs provides the most precise positioning, intimate fit, and even distribution of pressure possible[30] (Fig. 67-6). As edema subsides, this plaster of Paris splint is serially changed to safely gain new joint positions. Either a plaster of Paris or thermoplastic immobilization

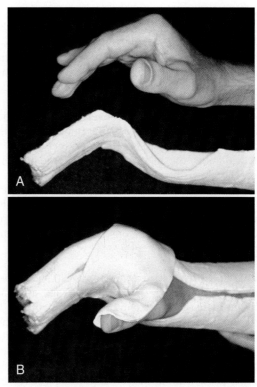

Figure 67-6 A, Volar plaster slab positions the hand. **B,** The hand is held precisely in position by the addition of a dorsal slab and an (optional) smaller slab to position the thumb.

orthosis can assist in optimal positioning and provide gentle distributed pressure while still protecting healing tissues from stress.

External Wraps. Self-adherent elastic wraps are commonly used to control edema in the hand and especially in the digits. Any self-adherent elastic wrap must be applied lightly with particular caution so that it does not constrict blood flow or restrict active motion. It is the consistency of light pressure, not the intensity of pressure that is important. It is particularly important to explain this concept to patients and have them demonstrate independent light application of the self-adherent elastic wrap before leaving the clinic.

A single layer of the self-adherent elastic wrap can be applied by wrapping either a 3- or 4-inch width around the digit and gently pinching it together on the dorsum of the

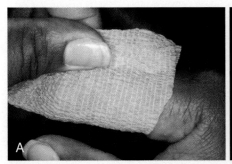 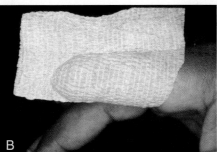 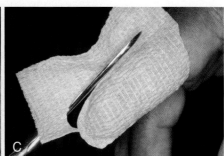

Figure 67-7 A and **B,** Self-adherent elastic wrap is applied to the injured digit by pinching the material together on the dorsum of the finger. **C,** The material is trimmed to make a small unobtrusive seam.

finger and trimming to a narrow seam (Fig. 67-7). This application allows easier adjustment of the tension with the one hand the patient has available than does the wrapping of multiple overlapping layers. One or two layers of tubular stockinette sized to fit the finger and applied underneath the self-adherent elastic wrap will offer a more gentle contact with the skin during movement of the digit.

Gloves. Elastic gloves are a convenient and inexpensive means of providing external pressure. Since one glove does not fit all patients and there is a lack of direct contact of the glove in the palm, the fit of the glove should be carefully assessed. The glove should fit like a loose second skin, providing a very gentle traction to the skin when the hand is moved within it. U.S. suppliers now market various brands of inexpensive edema gloves that are appropriate for use with the edematous hand. Tight constrictive gloves should be avoided.

Gentle External Massage.

All hand therapists should become thoroughly familiar with the gentle-massage approach of manual lymphatic therapy techniques (see Chapters 63–65). Originally developed as a means of facilitating lymphatic flow in patients with chronic lymphedema, this gentle facilitatory massage can be helpful with many hand trauma patients, most of whom have normal lymphatic anatomy.

After the acute healing phase has subsided, patients with isolated injuries may require only a short period of gentle massage. Patients with extensive crush injuries or large wound areas where the lymphatic anatomy is altered are ideal candidates for longer-term manual edema mobilization techniques (see Chapters 63–65) to facilitate lymphatic flow around injury areas to reestablish lymphatic flow. Above all else, vigorous, forceful massage as recommended by many in the past should be abandoned. Superficial lymphatic vessels are thin, fragile structures that may be further destroyed by vigorous therapy.[31]

Mobilizing the Early Stiff Hand

Although many treatment techniques have been developed to mobilize the stiff hand, no basic research supports any particular exercise treatment regimen to regain mobility.[9,10] Two basic principles for postoperative rehabilitation are imperative: The effects of immobilization must be minimized, and healing tissue must not be overloaded.[32]

Benefits of Early Motion

After injury, limited early movement reestablishes tissue homeostasis, increases venous and lymphatic flow, increases tensile strength of the wound, and directs the alignment and orientation of collagen fibers.[7,15,20,33-35]

In the early postoperative period, the beneficial effects of motion can be provided either by active or continuous passive motion (CPM), but active motion must quickly assume the dominant role if the patient is to resume functional use. The challenge is to allow enough motion to nullify the negative effects of immobilization but prevent excessive motion that will impede normal healing.

Beginning with Arem and Madden,[17] many studies have validated the concept of controlled stress to promote favorable collagen orientation and to increase tensile strength of the healing tissue. Unknown, however, is how much, how many repetitions, how often, how long, and to what extent motion should be carried out for optimal stress application to influence tissue. If we knew how to precisely apply stress, postoperative therapy would be more efficient and productive.[6] At this time, the guideline for the parameters of stress application must be the observation of a positive influence on the tissue and the absence of a renewed inflammatory response.

Early active motion should be precise, preventing substitution motions of the uninjured looser joints. For active motion to be productive in the stiff hand, it is usually necessary to block the looser joints. Active motion should be to the easy maximum end-range and should be repeated intermittently throughout the day. Frequent repetitions during each exercise period or extremely frequent exercise periods are not indicated early in rehabilitation. As a general guideline, the more acute the injury and the more inflamed the tissues, the more intermittent the active motion should be. As edema subsides and active motion is tolerated without an increasing inflammatory response, more frequent motion is indicated. The schedule for the balance between rest and motion depends on the tolerance of the tissue for increased frequency of motion, which can be determined only by a gentle trial-and-error method.

Importance of Preventing or Resolving Interosseous Muscle Tightness

A discussion of the stiff hand is incomplete without a focus on the most frequent cause of finger stiffness: Interosseous muscle tightness (commonly, but incorrectly, called "intrinsic tightness"). The interosseous muscles reside within a tight fascial compartment between the metacarpal bones. These small interosseous muscles have limited excursion, making them relatively intolerant to the adaptive shortening that occurs as a result of immobilization. Direct trauma to the metacarpal area may also create injury or ischemia to these muscles, causing potential for an even greater severity of interosseous muscle tightness.

Full finger flexion demands elongation of the interosseous muscles. If the interosseous muscles are tight, full finger flexion is limited by the tightness. Since the line of pull of the interosseous muscles is volar to the MCP joint and dorsal to the IP joints, interosseous muscle tightness is determined by defining the amount of passive proximal interphalangeal (PIP) joint flexion when the MCP joint is flexed and then determining if this amount of PIP joint flexion is less when the MCP joint is simultaneously brought into passive hyperextension. This is the position of maximum elongation of the interosseous muscles.

Lack of full finger flexion is often assumed to be caused only by joint stiffness and/or lack of full glide of the extrinsic flexor tendons, and testing for interosseous muscle tightness is overlooked. Since interosseous muscle tightness from either direct injury or adaptive shortening frequently contributes to limited finger flexion, one should always assume this is contributing to the limited motion until it can be proven otherwise.

Instead of working on active and passive end-range composite finger flexion, the most appropriate approach to resolving stiffness of the fingers may be to block the MCP

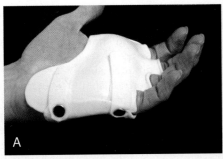
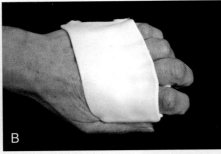
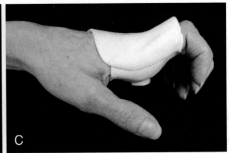

Figure 67-8 A, Ulnar-volar view of an orthosis to allow active elongation of both the interosseous and lumbrical muscles. Note overlapping ulnar-sided closure, intimate contour of orthotic material in palm, and block over proximal phalanx allowing full PIP joint flexion. **B**, Dorsal view of orthosis shows intimate contour and well-distributed pressure over all MCP joints. **C**, Radial-lateral view shows position of MCP joint hyperextension. In the stiff hand, MCP joint hyperextension may have to be serially regained. (Copyright Judy C. Colditz, 2008.)

joints in extension while allowing full IP joint flexion. An exercise orthosis that blocks the MCP joints in extension is appropriate for the newly injured hand. For more severe and long standing interosseous muscle tightness a nonremovable cast may be required. (See "Dominant Interosseous Flexion Pattern".)

The complex subject of interosseous muscle tightness versus lumbrical muscle tightness, and methods for testing, quantifying, and resolving interosseous muscle tightness are beyond the scope of this chapter, and the reader is referred to other sources.[36]

Blocking Motions

Unlike most of the large joints in the body, the small joints of the hand are moved by muscles crossing multiple joints. Because muscle pull results in the movement of the joints with the least resistance, muscle excursion will affect proximal mobile joints before affecting stiffer distal joints. Manual blocking transfers the muscle force to the targeted stiff joint, enabling the patient to experience glide at the site of restriction. For example, when the MCP joint is blocked during finger flexion, extrinsic flexor glide is directed across the IP joints rather than allowing MCP flexion directed by the interosseous muscles (Fig. 67-8). If blocking is an early part of treatment, many patients require only intermittent manual blocking exercises to regain balanced motion. If joint stiffness and/or tissue adherence is persistent, a blocking orthosis offers a longer period of sustained redirected active motion across the stiff joints to regain balanced motion (see Fig. 67-8).

Balance of Exercise and Rest

The primary guideline for exercise progression should be the status of the hand after exercise. If edema, pain, and stiffness increase after exercise (or any treatment), the hand is not yet ready for that level of stress. Conversely, if the patient experiences sustained increased comfort and mobility, the amount of exercise is appropriate for the stage of recovery and may be slowly upgraded. Most patients can sense a positive tissue response versus a negative one and modify their exercise regimen accordingly to maintain the positive response.

Proprioceptive Feedback

When working to regain finger flexion, proprioceptive feedback is essential. Providing resistance to finger flexion to increase the patient's proprioceptive sense of digital motion is beneficial. This is particularly critical in the presence of diminished sensibility. This type of feedback can be accomplished by the patient holding an object slightly smaller than the available range of finger flexion. Use of a padded handle that demands some effort to be held firmly will allow use of the hand for eating and self-care activities while demanding slightly more finger flexion than is readily available. The size of the handle is decreased as the patient gains flexion range.

Muscle Isolation and Pattern of Motion

Patients who experience stiffness of the hand following injury invariably feel that a strong muscle pull is required to overcome the stiffness. Unfortunately, this excessive effort recruits the strongest muscles and overpowers the weaker muscles (Fig. 67-9). Co-contraction of muscles is a common result of excessive effort. The patient must first be taught that a gentle pull isolates the desired muscle and that exercise for strengthening comes later in therapy. The patient learns a clear difference between a strong global pull that is ineffectual and a gentle but sustained precise pull that reestablishes muscle balance. Understanding this difference between the "right" and the "wrong" way to exercise ensures that the patient repeats the exercise correctly at home. It may be helpful to have the patient pull intensely and let the stronger muscles overpower to appreciate the contrast with the gentler isolation exercises.

Patients whose limbs have been immobilized in a cast following a distal radius fracture provide a practical example. The weakened wrist extensor muscles cannot adequately stabilize the wrist in extension to allow the finger flexor muscles to flex the digits. When the patient is asked to extend the wrist, the finger extensor muscles substitute for the wrist extensor muscles because they have been unrestrained in the cast and are stronger (see Fig. 67-9). If edema and finger stiffness are accompanying complications, little progress can be made with finger motion until the patient can stabilize the wrist with the wrist extensor muscles.

Low-Load, Prolonged Stress

It is often stated that therapy should apply a low-load, prolonged stress to accomplish plastic deformation of the tissues.[37-39] Early in the fibroplasia stage of healing, before collagen crosslinking is well established, intermittent active motion is usually enough stress to favorably alter the

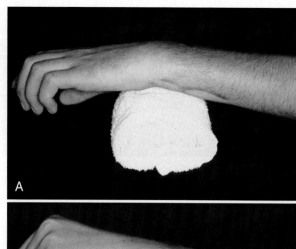

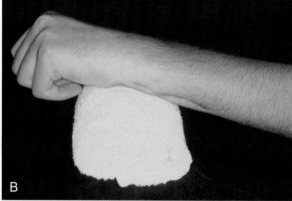

Figure 67-9 A, After Colles' fracture, a patient attempts wrist extension but uses extrinsic finger extensors instead of wrist extensor muscles. **B**, When the patient maintains full finger flexion, he or she can isolate the wrist extensor muscles.

crosslinking. Later in healing, when excess collagen crosslinking limits motion, low-load, prolonged stress favorably modifies the crosslinks and the collagen fibrils slip over each other.[40] This slippage is accomplished by active exercises that provide a concentrated force application to achieve maximum joint motion and soft tissue glide, which allows slippage of the crosslinks. This may be gained in a number of ways. If the tissues do not mobilize in response to blocked active exercise, orthotic mobilization that provides a gentle force for a longer period may be indicated. If the stiffness is persistent, a nonremovable cast promotes cyclic motion directed to the stiffer joints. This concentration of active force across stiff joints can mobilize even the most resistant of joints. (See "Evaluation and Treatment of the Chronically Stiff Hand" section.)

Passive Range of Motion

Although joint motion can be maintained by either active or passive motion,[41] passive motion provides limited glide of the tissue planes other than the periarticular structures. Increasing passive motion does not necessarily increase active motion.

As with other therapeutic techniques, there are no research data to dictate the ideal force, speed, and duration of passive motion.[5] Although passive joint motion often is prescribed to overcome post-traumatic joint stiffness, no research supports the efficacy of either intermittent passive motion or

CPM to reduce joint stiffness.[9] Aggressive passive motion of the hand is detrimental and should be avoided.[8,28]

Passive motion in the injured hand should be defined as the gentle encouragement of tissues to reach a maximum available length. The amount of force should respect the resistance of the tissues, and the position should be increased only when the tissues relax and decreased resistance is felt. When edema is diminished, any gentle passive joint motion should be done with accompanying gentle traction to the joint to allow room for one joint surface to glide over the other without compression. One gentle, prolonged hold will allow the motion to be repeated actively more effectively than many repeated quick sudden passive stretches. Quick, forceful stretches result in tissue damage and should be avoided at all times.

In the hand with more mature stiffness caused by increased collagen crosslinking, the brief intermittent nature of passive motion is ineffective and should be avoided. This seems contradictory, because one assumes that the stiffer the joint the more force is required to mobilize it. Rather than increased force, it is the increased duration of a low-level force that best creates change. When patients with significantly stiff hand joints undergo passive ROM during a therapy session, there is an immediate response of tissue mobilization. However, when the patient returns, the progress gained in the previous session has not been retained. A study of stiffness in rabbits after tibia fracture compared ankle stiffness between joints undergoing CPM and joints that remained immobile in a cast. The ankles receiving CPM demonstrated immediate reduced stiffness, but over time the stiffness in the CPM group was progressively and significantly greater than the group immobilized.[9] This study suggests that further investigation is warranted regarding the long-term effects of passive ROM on stiff joints.

Active Range of Motion

Active ROM has multiple advantages over passive ROM. Active motion stimulates the lymphatic system, diminishing edema, and more quickly returns the hand to a state of homeostasis. Active motion also requires normal reciprocal glide of soft tissue structures such as tendons and ligaments. Another advantage of active motion is the continued association of the motor cortex to the active muscle contraction. Patients sustaining injury who are unable to use normal muscle recruitment patterns move in maladapted patterns. If maladapted movement continues, the motor cortex learns the maladapted motion and defines it as normal. A period of only 9 weeks will alter the motor cortex patterning.[42] The earlier the patient is able to recruit the appropriate muscle pattern, the greater the patient's potential to recapture full mobility.

Joint Mobilization

Although manual joint mobilization is advocated by many for the treatment of stiff joints of the hand, manual mobilization of the small joints of the hand is best reserved for specific capsular tightness with no accompanying inflammation. When motion is limited as a result of edema, manual joint mobilization may be ineffective and can lead to an increased inflammatory response. Joint mobilization without accompanying edema reduction does not increase the available room for movement. There are no published data on the effectiveness of joint mobilization in reducing joint stiffness. Nor are there any data that suggest harm.

Benefits of CPM

Because joint motion is needed to preserve joint lubrication,[7,40] CPM often is used postoperatively to treat joint pathology. Neither laboratory nor clinical studies have shown that CPM is useful for treating joint stiffness once it has occurred.[10,43] Therefore, CPM is appropriately reserved for the immediate postoperative period to prevent complications rather than to resolve stiffness. Readers are referred to the archives on the companion Website for the chapter *Continuous Passive Motion for the Upper Extremity: Why, When, and How* by LaStayo and Cass from the 5th edition.

Pathologic Patterns of Motion in the Early Stiff Hand

Loss of Wrist Tenodesis Pattern

The exquisite balance of muscle forces crossing the wrist and fingers creates a reciprocal motion called *tenodesis*. Finger extension occurs with wrist flexion as a result of the increased tension on the extrinsic extensor muscles when the wrist flexes. Conversely, when the wrist extends, tension is increased in the extrinsic flexor muscles that flex the fingers. This reciprocal action establishes the normal grasp and release pattern of the hand.

With stiffness, the tenodesis balance in the hand is frequently affected. In a minor injury, tenodesis is regained as motion at the injury site improves. In more severe injuries requiring long periods of immobilization, many joints may become stiff and the muscles crossing them become weak, altering the reciprocal balanced motion.

The wrist is the key joint to reestablishing the tenodesis balance in the hand. Without the ability to stabilize the wrist in extension, the finger flexor muscles cannot transfer enough power to regain finger flexion. Usually the primary goal is to regain digital flexion for grasp and manipulation of objects. However, when the fingers and the wrist all have limited motion, active finger flexion is not possible without first gaining some wrist extension (Fig. 67-10).

Intrinsic-Plus Pattern

During normal finger flexion, IP joint flexion dominates before significant MCP joint flexion begins.[41] If the hand is edematous and extrinsic flexor glide is limited (commonly seen after immobilization of wrist fractures or flexor tendon repair), the patient will initiate finger flexion with MCP joint flexion, and little IP joint flexion occurs. In this pattern of motion the interosseous and lumbrical muscles are never elongated to their maximum length, and they adaptively shorten, making the mobilization of the IP joints even more difficult.

Early treatment—consisting of activities, exercises, and/or orthoses that block MCP joint flexion and require IP joint flexion (unless contraindicated by surgical repairs)—can convert global finger flexion into specific glide across the IP joints (see Fig. 67-8). In the chronically stiff hand, longer

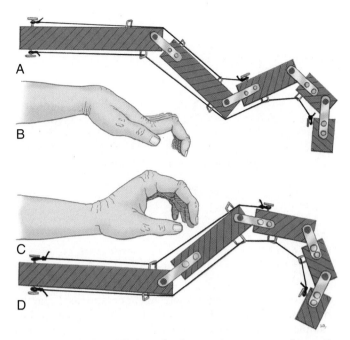

Figure 67-10 A and **B**, Loss of wrist extension creates tension on the extrinsic extensor muscles, and finger flexion is lost. **C** and **D**, With the wrist in extension, the tension on the finger flexors facilitates digital flexion. (From Bunnell S. *Surgery of the Hand*, 2nd ed. Philadelphia: JB Lippincott, 1948: p. 84)

periods of intervention may be necessary to change the pattern of motion. (See section on "Evaluation and Treatment of the Chronically Stiff Hand.")

Intrinsic-Minus Pattern

When the intrinsic muscles are not actively participating in digital flexion, isolated MCP joint flexion is absent. Flexion occurs first at the IP joints, and only after full IP joint flexion do the extrinsic flexors pull the MCP joint into flexion. This may result from denervation of the intrinsic muscles, but in the stiff hand it is more commonly a result of isolated capsular tightness of the MCP joints or the restraint created by adherence of the extensor tendons on the dorsum of the hand. Blocking the wrist so that flexion forces from the extrinsic flexors can be directed to the MCP joints is required to actively mobilize the MCP joints. Without MCP joint flexion the intrinsic hand muscles cannot participate in the digital flexion.

Evaluation and Treatment of Joint Stiffness and Decreased Tissue Glide

Joint Tightness

Joint tightness is identified by manually examining the passive ROM of a joint to determine whether the passive ROM changes as proximal and distal joint positions are altered. If the joint ROM does not change, isolated joint tightness is present (Fig. 67-11).

Clinical reality usually provides a combination of joint tightness and other external constraints, such as muscle–tendon unit tightness or tendon adherence. An experienced therapist can determine the balance and mix of the many

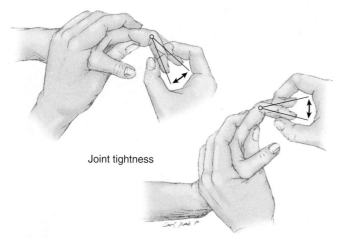

Joint tightness

Figure 67-11 *Joint capsular tightness is defined when the range of passive joint motion is the same regardless of the position of proximal and distal joints.*

tissues that are limiting motion. Accurate appraisal may be limited until certain joint motions have been regained. For example, PIP joint flexion must be gained before the full extent of interosseous muscle tightness can be determined.

Accurate, repeated ROM measurements must be the means of monitoring improvement.[44] If there is a large discrepancy between the active and passive ROM, the emphasis should lie on active pull-through. If the active and passive ROM are equal, it may be appropriate to gain passive motion via mobilization orthotic positioning. Increased passive motion can also be achieved by blocking the more flexible joints, allowing active motion to reduce joint stiffness, which in turn increases passive ROM.

Manual Treatment. The degree of trauma to the joint capsule and the stage of healing determine whether the palpated resistance to full-joint motion is the expected amount of joint stiffness. When joint tightness is evaluated, a distinction should be made between a joint with a soft end-feel and one

with a hard end-feel. A *soft* end-feel refers to a joint whose stiffness is characterized by a soft and springy end to the passive joint motion. This soft end-feel joint tightness results from edema within the joint capsule and the early stages of collagen crosslinking. With active motion and an intermittent low-load stress, the capsular joint structures can regain independent glide. *Hard* end-feel joint tightness has less edema present and is primarily a result of more mature collagen crosslinking. When moved to its maximum ROM, there is an abrupt and well-defined end point to the passive test. The hard end-feel joint requires more prolonged periods of mobilization in an orthosis to gain motion or more sustained periods of cyclical active motion. (See the section on "Evaluation and Treatment of the Chronically Stiff Hand.")

It is appropriate to apply manual gentle passive ROM to joints with a soft end-feel. If the joint edema is minimal, gentle prolonged passive stretching to soft end-feel joints can allow more active motion to be transmitted across the stiff joint. In many cases this is enough influence to resolve joint stiffness. In the joint sustaining minor trauma, early intermittent gentle passive motion may produce full active motion without further intervention.

Joint Mobilization via Use of an Orthosis. If active and passive mobilization techniques are not successful or if the joint resistance is significant when initially evaluated, mobilization orthotic positioning to regain capsular length in one direction may be essential to regain joint motion. The motion with the greatest resistance is the least likely motion to be regained with only active and intermittent passive stretching, and this motion should be the target of mobilization via use of an orthosis. Wrist joint extension, MCP joint flexion, and IP joint extension are often the most resistant joint motions, and must be given orthotic priority to balance the strength of the more powerful opposing muscles.

Mobilizing orthoses directed toward isolated joint tightness requires that only the involved joint be included in the orthosis (Fig. 67-12A). Orthoses may be applied that provide

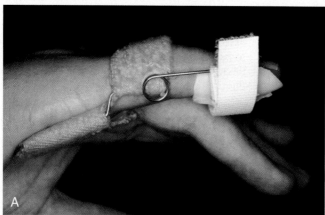
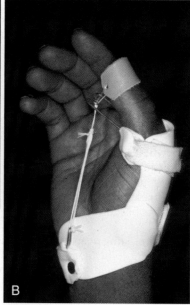

Figure 67-12 A, A dynamic PIP extension-mobilization orthosis effectively gains PIP joint extension without including other joints. **B**, An orthosis stabilizes the MCP joint of the thumb while dynamically mobilizing the IP joint into flexion.

a dynamic, serial static, or static progressive force. Dynamic force applied by rubber band or spring traction is a soft application of force appropriate for joints with a soft end-feel. If joint edema is present, serial static orthoses can gain joint motion concurrent to providing edema reduction via gentle joint compression. Joints with greater resistance respond favorably to prolonged application of serial static orthoses, or may respond to static progressive orthoses. Serial static or static progressive orthoses should be reserved for extension mobilization positioning, since compression of the joint in the maximally flexed position is poorly tolerated. A dynamic force may be more comfortable for the patient at the end-range of joint flexion than an unyielding static progressive force, because flexion dramatically increases intra-articular pressure[45] (Fig. 67-12B). (See Chapters 123 through 125 for further discussion regarding use of orthoses for mobilization of joints.)

Muscle–Tendon Unit Tightness

Muscle–tendon unit tightness is shortening of the muscle–tendon unit from origin to insertion, limiting full simultaneous motion of all joints crossed by the muscle–tendon unit. The muscle is the elastic part of this unit, which shortens with disuse. This tightness commonly occurs as a result of immobilization or restricted motion following injury or surgery. If a muscle–tendon unit is left in a short position in the presence of tissue inflammation, the tendon will also become adherent along its entire path, even if there is no direct trauma to the tendon or tendon bed. Specific trauma to the tendon or tendon bed, however, creates distinct adherence at the site of injury. Tendon adherence thus may be isolated to the point of trauma or extend over a larger area of more extensive trauma or immobilization in the presence of inflammation. Tendon adherence affects movement only of the joint(s) distal to the point of adherence. Although both muscle–tendon unit tightness and tendon adherence may have similar clinical presentations, careful examination identifies the exact location of the problem.

Evaluation. Both tendon adherence and muscle–tendon unit tightness are demonstrated by a distinct difference between the passive distal joint motion when the proximal joints are positioned in flexion versus extension (Fig. 67-13).

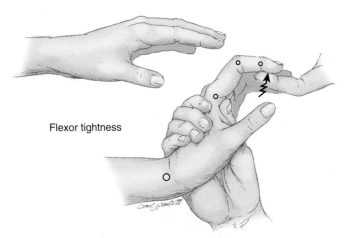

Flexor tightness

Figure 67-13 Tightness of the extrinsic flexor muscles is seen when finger extension is limited when the wrist is extended but unimpeded when the wrist is in a neutral position or in flexion.

The most proximal joint crossed by the muscle–tendon unit is the key to appraising tightness. For example, with tightness of the extrinsic extensor muscles, the fingers will be unable to flex as far with the wrist in flexion as when the wrist is in extension. The opposite is true for extrinsic flexor muscle tightness; with wrist extension, finger extension is limited by the shortness of the extrinsic flexor muscle–tendon unit(s). But when the wrist is flexed, the fingers can extend. To achieve an effective stretch of the extrinsic flexor muscles, the wrist must be held in extension while the fingers are also gently but firmly held in maximum extension (Fig. 67-14A).

The same principle holds for the interosseous muscles in the hand, with the MCP joint key to evaluating interosseous muscle tightness. Because the interosseous muscle–tendon units run volar to the axis of the MCP joint and dorsal to the axis of the PIP joints, the maximum stretch of this muscle–tendon unit occurs when the MCP joint is held in maximum extension (e.g., hyperextension) and the PIP joint is passively flexed. If the range of passive PIP joint flexion is less when the MCP joint is held in full extension, the interosseous muscles are tight (Fig. 67-15). Examining the patient's contralateral uninjured finger for interosseous muscle provides a baseline for that individual's normal interosseous muscle–

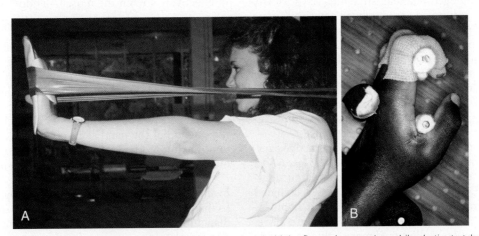

Figure 67-14 A, Stretching long-flexor tightness may combine an orthosis to hold the fingers in extension while elastic stretches the wrist into extension. **B**, A pegboard stabilizes various joints to allow the patient to apply prolonged active stretch for IP joint tightness and intrinsic muscle tightness.

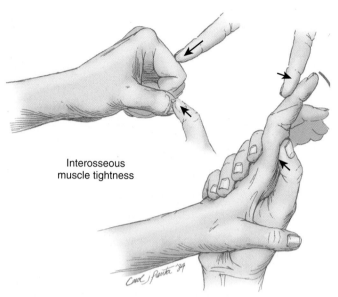

Interosseous
muscle tightness

Figure 67-15 *Interosseous muscle tightness is noted when PIP joint passive flexion is less when the MCP joint is extended (or hyperextended) than when it is flexed.*

tendon unit length.[36] This varies considerably among normal individuals.

Treatment.

Tightness. Because muscle–tendon unit tightness usually results from immobility of the hand, intermittent passive stretching following by active blocked motion often alleviates mild muscle–tendon unit tightness. This is true especially when stretching is started early after the injury or surgery. The stretch must be prolonged[46] and followed by active use of the muscle through the stretched range.

Tendon adherence seen early usually can be eliminated by a prolonged stretch to glide the tendon through its maximum range. Such stretching must be delayed if the tendon has been repaired. If, when stretching tendon adherence, the therapist feels a palpable release of the adherence, the stretched position should be maintained and then slowly incrementally positioned until the response subsides. This sudden slipping of the tissue layers can be felt as the gentle force is sustained through the increasing range. It should be strongly emphasized that this prolonged manual stretching is a slowly applied force and is continued based only on a positive tissue response. The therapist can palpate the diminished resistance in the tissues. The patient should be comfortable throughout this procedure, feeling pulling and perhaps slight discomfort, but never pain. Patients with early tendon adherence may experience a dramatic improvement in motion after such a prolonged stretch. More commonly, one does not see this sudden dramatic response but instead sees slow improvement over a longer time with repeated stretching.

Both passive mobilization via an orthosis and active exercise can elongate muscle–tendon tightness (see Figs. 67-12 and 67-14). Orthoses to diminish muscle–tendon unit tightness require that all joints crossed by the tightness be included in the orthosis. Orthoses for muscle–tendon unit tightness should be easily adjustable or replaceable as gains are made. Mobilization via orthoses is discussed more fully later in this chapter.

Adherence. A tendon may be adherent anywhere along its path. Motion to decrease the adherence is accomplished only by joint motion distal to the adherence. This can be active motion of the joints distal to the adherence that actively pulls on the adherent tendon, or it can be passive motion of the joints distal to the adherence, which are moved in the direction opposite to the active motion (i.e., passive extension if a flexor tendon is adherent). This insight allows correct positioning for exercise and determines the joint(s) to be included in any orthosis. Mobilization via orthoses to decrease tendon adherence is effective only in regaining distal glide of an adherent flexor or extensor tendon. To gain proximal glide, the patient must isolate and strengthen the correct muscle to regain full excursion of the adherent muscle–tendon unit.

Adherence after flexor tendon repair provides an example of the type of active motion necessary to gain proximal glide of an adherent tendon. Commonly, after flexor tendon repair the patient flexes strongly with the unimpeded interosseous muscles, and minimally glides the extrinsic flexor tendons, especially if the injury has been within the flexor sheath (zone II). Commonly the MCP joint fully flexes before the IP joints reach full flexion. When tendon healing permits, blocking the MCP joint in extension to demand flexor tendon excursion across the distal joints is mandatory (see Fig. 67-8A and Fig. 67-14B). Tendon-gliding exercises[47,48] that require independent glide of the profundus and superficialis tendons relative to one another and of the profundus tendon relative to the underlying bone must be included. Early gentle resistance provides helpful feedback to ensure correct motion and begins to strengthen the weakest muscle unit. When tendon healing is complete, neuromuscular electrical stimulation may be used if a feedback effect is desired and muscle fiber recruitment is inadequate.

Mobilization via an Orthosis. Use of an orthosis to decrease tendon adherence need include only the joints distal to the site of adherence. An example would be dorsal adherence of an extensor tendon over a healed metacarpal fracture. Orthotic positioning of all finger joints in flexion to glide the tendon distally would not require inclusion of the wrist, because the adherence is distal to the wrist. In contrast, if the problem is tightness of the extrinsic extensor muscles, the wrist must be positioned in some flexion within the orthosis to effectively stretch the muscle–tendon unit.

Skin and Scar Tightness and Adherence

All wounds heal with internal and external scar. Depending on the size, location, and extent of scar, external scars (especially linear scars) may limit joint motion. Even if the scar is not adherent to the underlying joint(s), the length of the scar may not allow multiple joints to move in the same direction simultaneously. For example, a split-thickness skin graft on the dorsum of the hand can tether the skin so that either IP joint flexion or MCP joint flexion is possible, but simultaneous MCP and IP joint flexion is not possible.

Evaluation. Skin tightness is assessed by positioning joints so that the limiting scar must elongate to a maximum length. Blanching, palpable tightness, or immobility of the scar or skin displays the extent of tightness (Fig. 67-16). If skin tightness is limiting joint motion, placing the skin in its

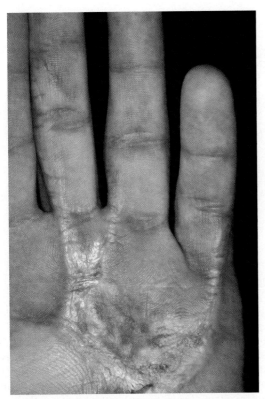

Figure 67-16 Blanching of the skin at the MCP joint demonstrates scar adherence and tightness.

shortest position allows increased joint motion proximally or distally. This motion is diminished as either joint is positioned to elongate the involved skin. This limitation may be difficult to determine in a severe injury that creates both skin tightness and joint tightness.

Manual Treatment. External scars are visually evident but must be palpated to determine their mobility and character. All new external scars will be adherent to the underlying bed and will have decreased oil and sweat production. In large scars, the lack of lubrication and adherence causes the scar to be dry and intolerant to frictional forces. As the scar reaches maturity and can tolerate friction, gentle direct massage with an appropriate lubricant is the treatment of choice.

Orthotic Mobilization for Skin Tightness. Unlike other tightness often alleviated by intermittent stretch, skin tightness usually requires prolonged holding of the skin at its maximum length. Use of an orthosis is mandatory to accomplish this. Prolonged serial static orthotic positioning with a positive-pressure interface mold provides the best force to realign the collagen fibers. Any orthosis to elongate skin and scar tightness must also position the joints at the proximal and distal ends of the tightness to allow full elongation of the tissue.

In the hand such prolonged positioning with the skin in the longest position is difficult to achieve. The need for increased mobility and strengthening of the hand must be balanced with the need for prolonged scar elongation. At a minimum, such mobilization positioning orthoses should be worn during sleep. In the initial stages of wound contraction the orthosis may be required 23 of 24 hours if the graft or scar covers a large area and/or multiple joints. As tissue matures, the duration of orthosis wear may be slowly decreased to nighttime only. The rigid effect of an orthosis counteracts myofibroblast pull[49] and decreases scar proliferation and contraction.

General Principles of Passive Orthotic Mobilization of the Early Stiff Hand

Therapists must have a wide spectrum of treatment skills to mobilize stiffness in the hand. If the patient is seen early after a simple injury, often no passive mobilization with an orthosis is required. However, patients with greater tissue damage commonly require orthotic positioning to optimize functional motion. It must be emphasized that use of an orthosis alone is not adequate treatment but must always be in conjunction with an individualized exercise program. Because scar can be modified by stress application,[17] passive orthotic mobilization may be an important part of regaining mobility of the severely injured hand. Unfortunately, all orthoses, even those applying passive mobilization, impose immobilization and constriction, and the good of the orthosis must outweigh the negative effects of restriction and immobilization.[8] Orthotic mobilization applied early postinjury that repositions joints with serial application is the safest early means of mobilizing healing tissue.

Each orthosis applied to the injured hand must be designed based on the mobilization goals for that hand.[50] Therapists must possess analytic skills, manual construction skills, and biomechanical knowledge to apply well-fitting and well-designed orthoses. Adequate discussion of orthotic fabrication far exceeds the scope of this chapter, but important points are discussed in the following sections.

Tissue Response to Orthotic Mobilization

Human tissue responds to the application of mechanical force. Because collagen tissue is elastic by virtue of the weave configuration of the larger subunits,[11] short-duration force applied to collagen fibers elongates the tissue but provides no alteration of the collagen fiber construct. This is the elastic response.[37,51] If the force is applied over a prolonged period, the plastic response occurs. The tissue retains all or part of the elongated position. The amount of temporary versus long-term change of tissues depends on the intensity and duration of the applied load.[33,38]

Optimal deformation is with the application of an intermittent low-load stress for defined periods of time.[33,37,46,52] One can understand this principle by thinking how a rubber band, when quickly stretched, returns to its original length; a rubber band held stretched does not return to its original length as quickly or as completely.

The dilemma is that prolonged positioning imposes immobilization. The challenge is to balance periods of passive orthotic mobilization with periods of active movement to ensure the maintenance of passive gains. Passive orthotic mobilization must apply a low magnitude of force to avoid stimulation of the inflammatory response that increases edema and fibrosis.

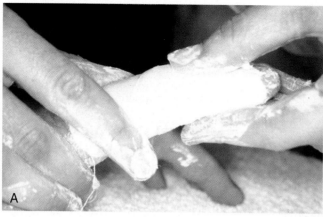
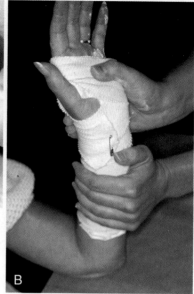

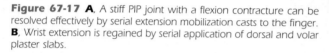

Figure 67-17 A, A stiff PIP joint with a flexion contracture can be resolved effectively by serial extension mobilization casts to the finger. **B**, Wrist extension is regained by serial application of dorsal and volar plaster slabs.

Force Application in Orthotic Mobilization

Although it is possible to measure the amount of force being applied with an orthosis, there is currently no way of measuring either the optimal amount of stress needed or the optimal application time of the stress to bring about the most rapid agreeable scar modification. The critical question is not the amount of force we are applying but the pressure exerted on the skin where the force is applied.[8] This point-of-force application becomes the limiting factor. Although one can measure how much pressure can be tolerated before skin necrosis occurs, this is of indirect value because mobilization orthoses are applied intermittently. Pressure becomes relatively unimportant in the presence of intermittent application.[8,53] Fess has demonstrated that experienced therapists consistently choose greater amounts of force for application to more mature scar.[54] Flowers and LaStayo have introduced the idea of total end-range time (the amount of time a restricted joint is held at maximum length), suggesting that future orthosis prescriptions will specify both the amount and duration of force application.[38] Glasgow et al. demonstrated a statistically significant greater effect of longer versus shorter applications of total end-range time in resolving joint contractures in a prospective randomized trial.[55] Until we have a means of measuring the amount of resistance in the tissues and developing a rationale for the maximum desirable force, the patient's tissue response to the force application remains the primary guideline to force application.

The patient must understand that the goal is not to tolerate increasing amounts of tension but rather to tolerate low tension for longer periods. After an initial adjustment period, a patient's tissues should comfortably increase tolerance to the prolonged passive-mobilization force. The patient should be aware of the sensation of stretching while wearing the orthosis but should not experience pain. A motivated patient will eagerly wear an effective, well-fitting orthosis.

Types of Mobilization Orthoses

A therapist can choose from three types of passive mobilization orthoses (serial static, dynamic, and static progressive)

or can choose a splint that provides active redirection. In the early stiff hand, active redirection can be accomplished by a removable exercise orthosis (see Fig. 67-8), and more chronic stiffness requires a nonremovable cast. Understanding the mechanical effect of each type of orthosis allows the therapist to choose the most effective means of regaining motion while facilitating healing.

Serial Static Mobilization Orthoses. A serial static orthosis immobilizes joints in a stationary position. The orthosis is applied with the tissue at its maximum length and is worn for long periods of time to allow the tissue to adapt[8,56] (Fig. 67-17). After a period of tissue accommodation, either a new orthosis is applied or the old orthosis is remolded to hold the tissue at a new maximum length. Although the orthosis is stationary, the repeated repositioning of the joint(s) increases the length of the tissues.

Dynamic Mobilization Orthoses. A dynamic orthosis applies force to a specific joint or joints. A stretched rubber band, spring, or wire coil generates the continuous force (see Fig. 67-12). As joint motion changes, the force of the orthosis continues. Although the force is constantly pulling while the orthosis is applied, the application of force is intermittent because the orthosis is periodically removed.[57] In the early stiff hand where collagen crosslinking is immature, intermittent dynamic force application effectively restores tissue mobility. In the hand with more mature stiffness, the intermittent nature of the force application is often inadequate to effect desired change.

For dynamic force application to mobilize the tightest structures, the hand must at times be positioned awkwardly in the orthosis. The intermittent nature of dynamic force application allows such awkward positions to be tolerated, because active therapy combines with the orthotic positioning program to regain balanced motion. Use of a dynamic orthosis is the technique of choice when passive motion of the joints is responsive to manual stretch and inflammation has subsided.[51,58]

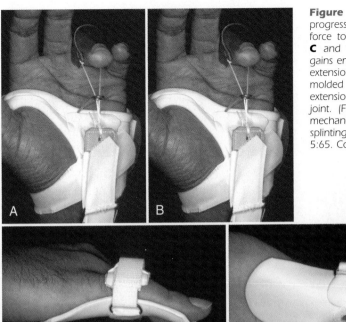

Figure 67-18 A and **B**, Static progressive orthosis applies flexion force to gain MCP joint flexion. **C** and **D**, Serial static orthosis gains end-range proximal IP joint extension, because volar piece is molded in a position of greater extension than is available to the joint. (From Colditz JC. Efficient mechanics of PIP mobilisation splinting. *Br J Hand Ther.* 2000; 5:65. Copyright 2000.)

A period of therapy to regain active tendon pull-through and edema reduction while increasing the tolerance to stress readies the hand for dynamic mobilization in an orthosis. If the dynamic orthosis is applied too early or with too much force, it can escalate the inflammatory response.

Static Progressive Mobilization Orthoses. Static progressive mobilization orthoses may appear identical to dynamic mobilization orthoses, but the applied force is not dynamic (Fig. 67-18). Instead of the constant pull of a rubber band or spring, the tension on the joint is an adjustable static force. The force may be applied via hook-and-loop fastener or with commercially available components that adjust in small increments. When tension is applied, the joint is positioned at its maximum end-range. The force is adjusted when the tissue response allows repositioning to a new length.

Static progressive orthoses are effective for joints with limited motion when there is significant resistance at the end of the passive stretch. Static progressive orthoses are especially recommended when positioning to regain end-range joint extension of the small joints of the hand (see Fig. 67-18C and D). As with other passive mobilization orthoses, the patient removes the orthosis and works on active glide or may use another orthosis to gain another direction of motion. Prolonged stretch at the end of the ROM is what gives the joint its full easy motion in both directions. The earlier the hand is ready for static progressive positioning, the shorter the time required to regain motion. The longer after injury that positioning is initiated, the longer the orthosis will have to be worn to regain the motion.

Choosing Mobilization Orthoses Based on the Stage of Healing

The stress appropriate to mobilize tissues differs in each clinical stage of healing. Static immobilization splints rest inflamed tissues during initial healing to provide protection and to allow inflammation to subside. If the desired position of immobilization cannot be obtained initially, serial static mobilization orthoses can safely reposition joints of the hand without providing undue stress to healing tissues. When injury is extensive and inflammation is prolonged, the rest provided by the orthosis is of continuing value. The process of tissue healing and maturation proceeds at variable rates in individuals, and many patients may have a prolonged inflammatory response.[58] After the initial inflammation subsides, the injured tissues begin the proliferative stage of healing. Cells are multiplying at a rate higher than normal. During this stage, correctly applied stress has its optimal benefit in determining the length, orientation, and relationship of the collagen fibers. If patients do not respond sufficiently to gentle manual passive stretching and active exercise, the gentle force of a dynamic orthosis is usually all that is required. If there is any indication of a continuing inflammatory response (e.g., fluctuant edema, reddened joints, pain with joint motion), a serial static orthosis should be chosen to provide a balance of rest while also repositioning joints.

As the tissue matures and joint motion has significant resistance with a hard end-feel, the prolonged force of serial static or static progressive orthotic positioning is necessary. A truly resistive joint is best treated with a serial static ortho-

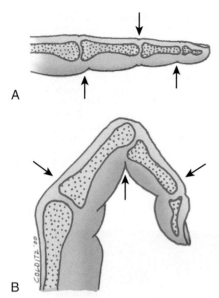

Figure 67-19 A, The three points of force for PIP joint extension orthotic positioning places the middle point of force directly on the extensor surface of the joint and the two opposite forces palmarly—as far from the joint as possible. **B**, The three points of force for PIP joint flexion orthotic positioning are in the same location, but on opposite surfaces to those for extension. (From Colditz JC. Efficient mechanics of PIP mobilisation splinting. *Br J Hand Ther*. 2000;5:65-71. Copyright 2000.)

sis that is not removed by the patient. Although the static progressive orthosis also provides prolonged positioning at the maximum passive length, its periodic removal allows the tissue to resume the original resting length. These recommendations are based on clinical experience and not on empirical research results. A recent study comparing dynamic to static progressive elbow mobilization via orthotic positioning demonstrated no difference between these two methods.[59]

A new technique of mobilizing stiffness, casting motion to mobilize stiffness (CMMS), is appropriate for the chronically stiff hand unresponsive to traditional therapy techniques. This is discussed in a subsequent section.

Basic Principles of Orthotic Mobilization

Because passive orthotic mobilization is often an integral part of effective therapy for the stiff hand, the basic principles of mobilization by orthosis are discussed in this section. The reader is directed to more in-depth information on this topic available from numerous sources.[57,60-71]

The effectiveness of any mobilization orthosis is limited by the accuracy of the design, fit, and force application. Every orthosis that immobilizes or mobilizes a joint must use three points of pressure for each joint.[62] The middle force is applied directly at the axis of the joint. Without crossing another joint, the two opposite forces are placed as far away from the middle force as possible for maximum efficiency (Fig. 67-19).

Orthotic fabrication for extension mobilization or immobilization places the middle force over the dorsum of the joint axis, and the opposing forces are placed on the volar surface as far away as possible without crossing over another mobile joint (see Fig. 67-19A). Because there is little natural padding on the dorsum of the hand, pressure over the joint must be carefully placed and be well molded to be comfortable.

The three points of pressure for flexion mobilization orthotic fabrication are the reverse of those used for extension: Volarly over the axis of the joint with the two opposing forces applying pressure dorsally as far away from the joint as practical (see Fig. 67-19B). The difficulty in flexion mobilization orthotic fabrication is the impossibility of applying force directly over the volar aspect of a joint while also allowing room for the joint to fully flex.

Unlike extension mobilization orthoses, where the forces are almost in direct opposition, the forces may be almost at right angles in flexion mobilization orthoses. This is especially true when flexing the joints of the hand (Fig. 67-20). If the forces are at a right angle, the orthosis base shifts distally before the stiff joint moves unless the orthosis base is adequately secured.

Distributing Pressure Evenly. The palmar surface of the hand, with its thicker and more adherent skin and with the presence of the thenar and hypothenar muscles, can tolerate pressure more easily than the dorsum of the hand. The skin on the dorsum of the hand is thin and highly mobile. The dorsum of the hand also has multiple bony prominences that tolerate pressure poorly. For example, in low-profile dynamic or static progressive PIP joint extension mobilization designs, the orthosis is molded contiguously over the MCP joints to distribute pressure over as much of the dorsal surface as possible. The leading edge of the block ends exactly at the joint axis so that all the force is specifically directed to the precise anatomic location.[62] Well-distributed pressure over the dorsal hand tissues is better tolerated than the concentrated pressure of a strap. Pressure on the neurovascular bundles of fingers can be minimized by constructing finger loops of a firm material and attaching string to both sides.[64]

Another example of effective pressure distribution is the use of dorsal and volar plaster slabs for serial repositioning of the wrist (or wrist and fingers). The molded volar and dorsal pieces distribute pressure over both surfaces. The three points of pressure needed to immobilize the wrist (two volarly that are proximal and distal to the wrist and one dorsally over the wrist) are widely distributed by the molded

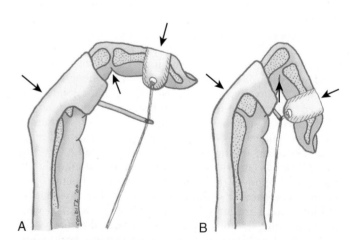

Figure 67-20 A and **B**, The line of force application for PIP joint flexion mobilization changes based on the angle of maximum passive flexion of the joint. (From Colditz JC. Efficient mechanics of PIP mobilisation splinting. *Br J Hand Ther*. 2000;5:65-71. Copyright 2000.)

contours (see Fig. 67-17B). This is in contrast to the use of a volar slab with a strap concentrating the force over the dorsal wrist area.

Providing Constant Tension. Even distribution of pressure is the primary factor to ensure comfort with force application. Avoiding sharp edges or ill-fitting molded shapes will enhance comfortable prolonged wear. Attention to construction detail coupled with listening to the patient and modifying the orthosis readily in response to the patient's comments will ensure maximum wear and comfort.

The tolerance to the force of dynamic or static progressive mobilization orthoses usually relates to the amount of force application. Using the minimum force the patient can tolerate for increasing amounts of time is preferable to using increasing amounts of force. The patient's goal should be increased wearing time before force is increased. Conversely, if the patient cannot comfortably wear the orthosis beyond a few minutes and the orthosis fits well, the force should be decreased.

Ease of Adjustment. Any passive mobilization orthosis must be easy to remold, inexpensive to replace, and quick to adjust. Because the goal is increased motion, the orthosis must be adaptable to the anticipated change. Low-temperature thermoplastic materials with memory allow quick remolding and adjustments to adapt to new positions, decreased edema, or to relieve unwanted pressure. Unfortunately, thermoplastic materials with memory also limit the intimate conformity of the material to the small shapes of the hand. The use of plaster of Paris for specific clinical applications allows quick construction of a new orthosis with minimal materials cost and provides the ultimate shape conformity.[72]

Brass rods used as outriggers for dynamic or static progressive mobilization orthoses allow quick adjustments by bending the wire (Fig. 67-21). For example, as finger joint flexion increases, the line of pull of the finger loop must be directed closer toward the palm. Alternatively, as finger extension improves, the dorsal outrigger must be shortened and placed more proximally.

Providing a Force Perpendicular to the Long-Bone Axis. The construction of a dynamic or static progressive mobilization orthosis requires attention to a few additional mechanical principles. To mobilize a joint, one must provide a pull at a 90-degree angle to the axis of the long bone that is the distal articulation of the joint in question[64] (Fig. 67-22). The outrigger is positioned as close to the point of force application as possible. The outrigger redirects the line of pull and keeps the line close to, and parallel with, the orthosis base. This system is of value only if a secure orthosis base has been applied that is intimately conformed, has well-distributed pressure, and accurately stabilizes the proximal joints.

The outrigger will deform before the tissue elongates if either the outrigger or its attachment to the orthosis base is unstable. Outrigger stability is directly correlated to length of the outrigger and the manner of attachment to the base. Attaching the outrigger over a large area of the orthosis base and to the distal edge of the orthosis contributes to maximum outrigger attachment stability.

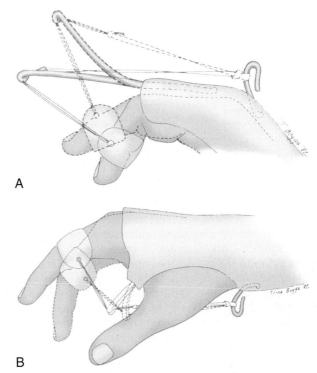

A

B

Figure 67-21 Ease of adjustment of low-profile wire outrigger system is accomplished by bending the wire outrigger. This allows maintenance of a 90-degree line of pull when either extension (**A**) or flexion (**B**) is gained. (From Colditz JC. The biomechanics of a thumb carpometacarpal immobilization splint: design and fitting. *Am J Occup Ther.* 1983;37:182-188. Reprinted with the permission of the American Occupational Therapy Association, Inc. Copyright 1983.)

Wearing Tolerance. When applying a passive mobilization orthosis, one must observe two areas of progress. First, the patient must be able to tolerate the orthosis comfortably for increasing periods of time. If this does not occur, the orthosis either needs adjustment or is the wrong type. Intolerance also may suggest that the orthosis has been applied at the wrong time in the healing process. Second, precise goniometric

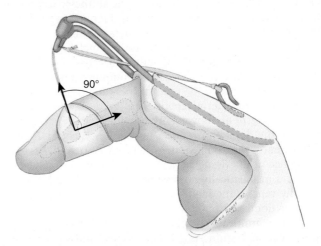

Figure 67-22 To extend the PIP joint, a low-profile dynamic (or static progressive) orthosis provides a line of pull at a 90-degree angle to the distal end of the middle phalanx. (From Colditz JC. The biomechanics of a thumb carpometacarpal immobilization splint: design and fitting. *Am J Occup Ther.* 1983;37:182-188. Reprinted with the permission of the American Occupational Therapy Association, Inc. Copyright 1983.)

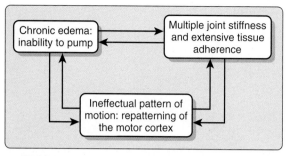

Figure 67-23 In the chronically stiff hand, three factors are interdependent, and effective mobilization requires that all factors are addressed simultaneously.

measurements must be taken before application of the orthosis. If there are no measurable gains for a few weeks after application, the orthosis is not effective. Reevaluation of the type of orthosis, the fit, and the patient's tolerance is merited.

Many patients are encouraged by the rapid gains of motion in response to orthosis application. They become discouraged when they remove the force of the orthosis and the deformity recurs. Patients should be instructed that to maintain gains of motion made while wearing the orthosis, its prolonged use as well as concomitant active exercises will be required. (See Chapters 123 through 125 for further discussion regarding use of orthoses for mobilization of joints.)

Evaluation and Treatment of the Chronically Stiff Hand

Clinical experience and review of the literature suggests three factors that interplay to perpetuate stiffness in the chronically stiff hand (Fig. 67-23). First, there is stiffness limiting movement in multiple joints, often including uninjured joints. Adherence of multiple soft tissue layers is palpable, adding constraints to limited passive joint motion. Intermittent manual mobilization or use of a mobilization orthosis provides only a temporary reduction of the stiffness. Second, the lack of active motion has diminished the pumping ability of the lymphatic system, and chronic edema permeates all tissue planes, even sites remote from the original injury. Edema reduction efforts prove temporary, because the stiffness limits active motion and lymphatic pumping cannot be maintained. Third, because the joint stiffness and tissue adherence have caused long-term repetition of an awkward and ineffectual pattern of movement, the ineffectual pattern has become the dominant motion in the motor cortex. Even if the patient wants to move in a balanced, normal pattern, the resistance from tissue adherence and the chronic edema makes it mechanically impossible to do so. The patient continually repeats the ineffectual pattern of movement, and it remains dominant.

In the chronically stiff hand, these three factors of tissue adherence and stiffness, chronic edema, and motor cortex patterning are interdependent. Changing one factor alone does not change the other factors. If mobility of the stiff hand is to be regained, all three factors must be altered simultaneously (see Fig. 67-23). Such chronic stiffness can be dramatically reduced using a technique called CMMS, developed by

the author.[72,73] The CMMS technique is appropriate for the chronically stiff hand unresponsive to traditional therapy techniques.

Casting Motion to Mobilize Stiffness

CMMS is the use of plaster of Paris casting to selectively immobilize proximal joints in a desired position while constraining distal joints so that they move within a productive direction and range.[72,73] Unlike more traditional treatment methods, the CMMS technique simultaneously mobilizes stiff joints, reduces edema, and generates a new pattern of motion to revive the cortical representation of normal motion. Traditional manual mobilization techniques and mobilization orthoses are less effective in the chronically stiff hand than in the newly stiff hand, because these techniques are intermittent and address only one problem at a time.

The CMMS technique contradicts traditional treatment theory in several ways. First and most dramatically, active motion regains both active and passive joint motion. No passive motion, modality, or manual treatment is applied. Because the cast immobilizes proximal joints and allows only the stiff joints to move in the range and direction needed, motion is isolated and part of the hand is immobilized. Typically, therapists believe that immobilization of any joint is to be avoided and motion in all directions should be gained concurrently. CMMS focuses on gaining the motion that is needed most, which may temporarily cause loss of motion in the other direction or loss of motion in the immobilized joints. This approach also contradicts the common assumption that one should never allow gains in one direction of motion at the expense of the other direction. In the chronically stiff hand, the balance of motion is overwhelmingly in favor of the stiff pattern. The constrained motion within the cast allows the opposite pattern of motion to become dominant, while simultaneously mobilizing adherent tissues and evacuating the stagnant edema. Reeducation of a more normal pattern of motion is facilitated by the restraints imposed by the cast and, when the patient is weaned from it, the motions temporarily lost while in the cast return (unless there is some specific anatomic injury preventing such return). In cases of altered anatomy following injury the therapist must be convinced that the reconstructed anatomy has the potential to return to the balanced motion before applying the CMMS technique. The same concern is not applicable to stiffness of uninjured joints resulting from immobilization.

CMMS can successfully mobilize severe stiffness that is unresponsive to traditional treatment.[74] Because the patient is mobilizing only with active motion, treatment is not painful. Therapy sessions consist of reevaluation, cast changes, and home instructions, creating a cost-effective treatment approach that is overwhelming for neither the therapist nor the patient. As functional motion is regained, a very slow weaning from the cast wear is begun and the functional use of the hand continues the progression of mobilization.

To accurately convey the appropriate application of the CMMS technique, the rationale of the technique is discussed, followed by discussion of the clinical application of the technique.

Joint Stiffness and Tissue Adherence

Unlike other therapy approaches to reduce joint stiffness, CMMS uses only active motion to mobilize stiff joints. Therapists do not expect active motion alone to have the ability to mobilize a stiff joint that has an abrupt hard end to passive motion. Perhaps this disbelief arises from the assumption that, if active motion could resolve joint tightness and tissue adherence, it would have already done so. However, without the constraint of the cast directing movement to the stiffest joints, the patient will unavoidably move the more mobile joint(s) first, leaving the stiff joint with the least power and excursion during active motion. The fact that frequent cyclic active movement alone mobilizes significant joint stiffness is the most persuasive aspect of the CMMS technique.

The relative immobility of the chronically stiff hand allows development of the well-known negative effects of immobilization (see Fig. 67-23). In particular, the lack of normal stress to the tissues allows excessive crosslink formation within the collagen matrix, creating increased mechanical resistance to motion. When the hand is positioned within the cast, cyclic active motion across the stiff joints applies positive stress to the tissues, altering the crosslinking, and tissue resistance diminishes.[16,35,75] Because the only motion occurring at the joint is motion within the range needed, all active movement reinforces gains in ROM. In the acutely injured hand, intermittent blocking exercises are enough to accomplish this, but in the chronically stiff hand the nonremovable cast provides the consistency needed for active motion to successfully mobilize stiff joints.

Mobilization orthoses applied to the chronically stiff hand apply an intermittent force at the end of the joint motion in one direction only. Unfortunately, the mobilization orthosis also imposes immobilization during this time, because no active tissue gliding is occurring. When the orthosis is removed, the patient reverts to the ineffectual pattern of motion, nullifying the gains of passive motion made while wearing the orthosis. The negative aspects of orthotic mobilization in the chronically stiff hand are compared with the positive aspects of the CMMS technique in Table 67-1.

As discussed previously, CPM has proven the effectiveness of long-term cyclic loading applied acutely after injury to prevent joint stiffness,[43,45,76] but its usefulness for reducing stiffness has not been demonstrated.[10,43] Undoubtedly, this is because the patient with a stiff hand reverts to the nonfunctional pattern of movement upon discontinuation of the CPM, providing no reinforcement to improved joint mobility. Intermittent blocked motion has long been used by therapists to achieve precise tendon glide across joints. The CMMS technique simply provides a sustained blocking exercise rather than an intermittent one. The CMMS technique combines stiffness reduction with simultaneous cortical repatterning of the active motion.

Because of its intermittent nature, manual passive ROM is ineffective in changing joint stiffness in the chronically stiff hand. Although there may be an immediate positive response to manual application of passive ROM in patients with chronic stiffness, they do not maintain passive gains made in a previous therapy session. Although the effects of stress deprivation on connective tissues can be prevented by both passive and active joint motion,[5] there is no proven correla-

Table 67-1 A Comparison of the Disadvantages of Mobilization Orthotic Positioning with the Advantages of the CMMS Technique in the Chronically Stiff Hand

Disadvantages of Mobilization Orthotic Positioning	Advantages of CMMS
Mobilization of Stiff Joints	
1. Immobilizes stiff joint(s) at end range.	1. Active motion mobilizes joint at end of range.
2. Applies force in one direction only.	2. Active motion is possible in two opposite directions.
3. Prevents active excursion of the soft tissues and tendon(s) across the joint.	3. Active motion allows repeated excursion.
Reduction of Chronic Edema	
1. Applies localized constrictive force.	1. Applies well-distributed, light, sustained pressure and provides pseudo-massage.
2. Can apply excessive passive force.	2. Cannot apply excessive force.
3. Active lymphatic pumping is lacking.	3. Active motion facilitates lymphatic pumping.
4. Inflammatory response may be prolonged.	4. Diminished tissue inflammation is observable.
Repatterning of Motor Cortex	
1. Allows no active motion.	1. Desired active motion occurs.
2. Intermittent use allows pathologic motion to recur when orthosis is removed.	2. Nonremovable cast allows adequate time and repetitions for cortical repatterning.
3. No effort is directed toward regaining normal tenodesis motion.	3. Weaning proceeds only as patient can maintain normal tenodesis motion.

CMMS, Casting motion to mobilize stiffness.

tion between the application of passive motion and increased active motion in the chronically stiff hand. In the chronically stiff hand, because of the lack of differential reciprocal tissue glide during passive motion, passive ROM does not result in increased active ROM. If applied repeatedly and forcefully, passive ROM prolongs the inflammatory response in the chronically stiff hand.

To regain passive motion, it has been assumed that stiff joints must be held at length by applying a low-load, prolonged stress with a mobilization orthosis.[8] A positive relationship between the total time a joint is held at end-range and decreased tissue resistance to passive motion has been demonstrated.[38,55] However, a positive relationship between active motion and increased total end-range time has not been proven. End-range active cyclic loading[77] across stiff joints provided by the CMMS technique provides an effective low-load and more prolonged force, though cyclic in nature. Not only does motion occur in the range needed, but the constraint of the cast restricts the joints from returning to the position of adaptive shortening.

The principle of using a cast to limit motion in one direction to increase active motion in the other direction has been used only in the larger joints of patients with spastic muscles. King[78] reports the use of a drop-out elbow cast for spastic elbow contracture of 90 degrees of flexion. In 12 days the

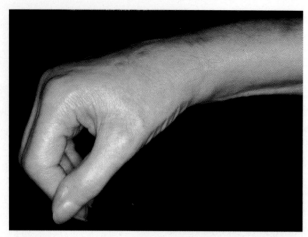

Figure 67-24 *A chronically stiff hand shows an absence of a normal tenodesis pattern and the resulting ineffectual pattern of motion when finger flexion is attempted.*

contracture was reduced to 12 degrees of flexion. Others report similar improvement in motion and also report a calming effect on the spasticity as a result of cast application.[79-81]

Edema

The chronically stiff hand is characterized by atrophic, shiny skin with diminished or absent joint creases, mild pitting (or nonpitting) edema, and firmness to palpation of the tissues throughout the hand as compared with the contralateral uninjured hand (Fig. 67-24). Edema within the joint capsule limits joint motion. When inflammation persists, pain with motion encourages patients to hold joints immobile in the most comfortable position.[14,18,82,83]

Prolonged edema continues because limited active motion restricts the pumping ability of the lymphatic system. Additionally, severe hand trauma may include direct injury to the lymphatic system. With prolonged edema, excess fibrosis from the lingering presence of high-protein edema further impedes the flow of fluid and proteins through the tissue channels to the initial lymphatics,[18,21,84] resulting in a low-grade chronic inflammation.[20] Although patients who have sustained trauma to the hand may have injury to the local lymphatic system, the proximal lymphatic system is normal. Lack of motion in the hand reduces the distal-to-proximal pumping that moves the lymphatic fluid to the more proximal lymphatic vessels. The CMMS technique resembles the effects of bandaging and gentle superficial massage used in manual lymphatic therapy techniques to evacuate the lymphatic fluid to more proximal areas.[85]

Active motion is the single most effective stimulator of the lymphatic system.[20,28] The CMMS technique reduces edema by redirecting active motion to the stiffest area, which is usually the more distal joints. The absence of muscles in the digits requires that skin motion and tissue compression produced by digital flexion provide physical stimulation of the superficial lymphatics. The concurrent contraction of the intrinsic hand muscles helps move the lymphatic fluid proximally. Active movement of unconstrained proximal joints that are not in the cast continues the distal-to-proximal lymphatic pumping.

In addition to active motion of the distal joints, consistent light compression of the tissues by the cast and movement of the skin relative to the cast padding stimulates lymphatic flow.[31,86] The intimately molded contour of the plaster of Paris cast provides constant light tissue pressure to facilitate lymphatic fluid movement in the delicate initial lymphatics of the skin. Gilbert[87] describes the lymphatic network of the palm and fingers as much more abundant than its dorsal counterpart. The firmness of the plaster of Paris in the palm during active finger flexion may provide a more effective means of lymphatic stimulation to the hand than other treatment approaches.

Movement of the hand within the cast provides a pseudo-massage of the skin as the hand moves against the soft padded, but unyielding, contour of the cast. Because the initial lymphatics are thin, fragile structures, they are collapsed easily by vigorous massage,[18,31] and such gentle but frequent facilitatory movement provides the appropriate amount of stimulation while eliminating the possibility of overly vigorous and destructive edema reduction techniques. The fact that the cast is nonremovable provides constant stimulation during cyclic active motion.

Additionally, the insulating quality of the cast provides neutral warmth, retaining body heat.[78,81] Because a direct relationship exists between ambient temperature and the permeability of the initial lymphatics,[88,89] this factor may also assist in increasing lymphatic flow. In addition, neutral warmth may assist in general tissue relaxation and/or facilitate tissue elongation.[78,81,90] During the weaning phase, patients usually elect to wear the bivalved cast, stating that the warmth, comfort, and ability to move correctly within the cast is a comforting experience.

Because the accumulation of plasma proteins is a cause of chronic inflammation,[91] stimulation of the lymphatic system by the movement within the cast reduces the observable redness and the pain associated with joint motion. The reduced pain encourages active joint motion, which in turn becomes more comfortable.

Change in the Pattern of Motion

Perhaps the most significant but least appreciated difference between the recently injured hand and the chronically stiff hand is the change in the pattern of active motion of the hand (Fig. 67-25). Local tissue adherence and/or joint tightness prevent normal synergistic motion. In chronic stiffness this maladapted pattern has been repeated long enough that the definition of movement in the cerebral motor cortex has been altered. In the chronically stiff hand this altered pattern of motion restricts both motor and sensory feedback input. Limited use of the hand creates feedback deprivation similar to rigid immobilization.[92,93]

Neuroscience literature has proven that animals and humans trained in movement combinations magnify the cortical representations of the motor areas predominantly used, and that lack of use decreases the cortical area.[94-97] For example, squirrel monkeys given a repetitive fine motor task increase cortical representation of the small muscles of the hand while simultaneously decreasing the representation of the larger proximal muscles.[98] The first dorsal interosseous muscle in the reading hand of Braille readers has a larger

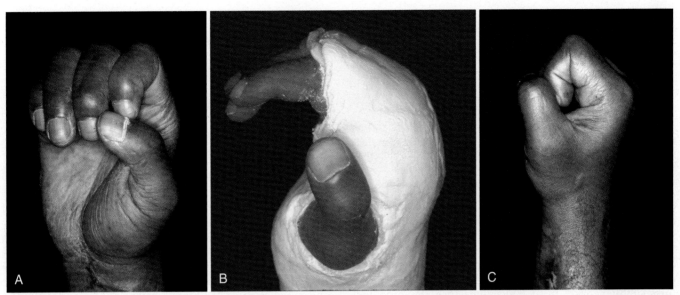

Figure 67-25 A, Chronically stiff hand 7 months after flexor tendon and nerve injury at the volar wrist shows limited passive motion and poor ability to stabilize wrist in extension. **B**, Cast provides optimal position for active mobilization of fingers into flexion. **C**, Resulting range and pattern of flexion (note tenodesis is present) after a few weeks of cast wear.

cortical representation than in the nondominant hand of the same person or in the hands of control subjects who do not read Braille or are not blind.[99]

It is therefore logical that the altered pattern of motion created by tissue adherence in the chronically stiff hand provides the opportunity for diminished cortical representation of the previous normal pattern of active motion. At the same time, the cortical area controlling the newly dominant muscle(s) enlarges. The constrained motion within the CMMS cast demands repetition of correct muscle activation, providing prolonged active movement necessary to repattern the somatosensory cortex. Although cortical representation changes rapidly based on use, for repatterning to become an ingrained automatic dominant motion, the motion must be repeated for long periods during the day and over many days or weeks.[98,100-104] Repatterning is enhanced by conscious, close attention to the desired active motion.[105] Unattended repetitive motion and passive motion result in little or no significant plasticity changes in the cortex,[106,107] explaining why passive motion may be ineffectual in the chronically stiff hand. In the absence of permanent peripheral injury (i.e., amputation or denervation), the altered pattern can be quickly retrained to the original "normal" because the original cortical connection patterns persist and can easily be reactivated.[103]

Because of the long standing feedback deprivation that has caused abnormal movement pattern changes in the somatosensory cortex, regaining motion is both a complex mechanical and a cerebral issue. All too often hand therapists assume that the problem is only mechanical or related to the peripheral tissues, and are frustrated when traditional mobilization techniques are not successful.

The same dysfunctional patterns of motion are seen in the chronically stiff hand as in the newly injured hand. A wrist tenodesis pattern often is absent or altered. Wrist flexion is commonly observed when finger flexion is attempted. The key to directing normal digital movement with the CMMS

cast is stabilization of the wrist in slight (20–30 degrees) extension. Even when the stiffness is localized to a single PIP joint, the wrist must be included in the cast to direct the force and tendon excursion to the stiff joint. Because the wrist is the largest joint crossed by the extrinsic muscles, its position is critical to directing excursion to the smaller joints. Positioning the wrist in slight extension takes stretch off the weakened wrist extensors[56] and positions them so that they can fire synergistically with the finger flexors. If passive wrist extension is limited, a period of serial casting to bring the wrist into slight extension is required before application of the CMMS cast.

The mechanical problems of joint stiffness and tissue adherence are well described in the previous section on evaluation and treatment of early stiffness, and are described here only in relation to the desired design of the CMMS cast.

Dominant Interosseous Flexion Pattern

Normal finger flexion is initiated by the extrinsic flexor muscles, specifically the flexor digitorum profundus (FDP). The IP joints flex considerably far before significant MCP joint flexion is included.[41,108] One of the most common pathologic patterns of motion typically observed in the stiff hand is digital flexion dominated by the interosseous muscles where finger flexion is initiated at the MCP joint(s) instead of at the distal interphalangeal (DIP) joint(s). If the patient has difficulty gliding the FDP tendons across the stiff IP joints, this reinforces the interosseous muscle dominance. Because the normal arc of finger flexion exhibits significant IP joint flexion before MCP joint flexion, patients demonstrating a pathologic pattern of dominant MCP joint flexion have their casts applied with the MCP joints blocked in extension.

A position of MCP joint extension reinforces extrinsic flexor tendon glide and provides maximum active tension on the flexor tendons.[109] Blocking the MCP joints in extension recreates the correct initial phase of digital flexion by isolat-

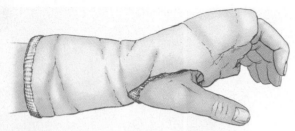

Figure 67-26 Initial cast to facilitate long-flexor glide and to mobilize IP joints includes the MCP joints, maintaining them in extension. (Copyright Judy C. Colditz, 2008.)

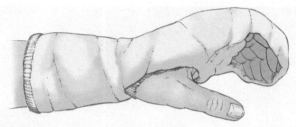

Figure 67-28 A dorsal hood made of plaster of Paris is positioned over the fingers so the DIP joints are in a starting position of relatively greater flexion than the PIP joints. This positioning facilitates initiation of finger flexion at the DIP joint(s). (Copyright Judy C. Colditz, 2008.)

ing the FDP muscle, facilitating profundus glide within the digit for IP joint motion, and preventing dominant interosseous muscle (MCP joint flexion) pattern (Fig. 67-26).

In the severely stiff hand with limited passive joint motion, diminished flexor tendon glide, and severe interosseous muscle tightness, it is difficult to mobilize all of these structures simultaneously. In such a circumstance, the initial cast should block the MCP joints in slight flexion (Fig. 67-27). If initially the MCP joints are positioned in full hyperextension, it is more difficult for the patient to pull against the interosseous muscle and joint tightness, and initiate motion with the extrinsic flexor muscles. Blocking the MCP joint in slight flexion allows the FDP tendon to increase its glide and mobilize the stiff IP joints before also being required to pull against the interosseous muscle–tendon unit tightness. It is simply mechanically overwhelming in the severely stiff hand to start with the MCP joints in hyperextension.

Some patients cannot actively initiate IP flexion with the profundus muscles when the MCP joints are stabilized in extension. Although these patients are few, they have the most severe stiffness. To help the patient isolate and gain glide of the FDP tendon(s), a dorsal hood is placed over the IP joints (Fig. 67-28). This hood simply positions the DIP joints in relatively greater flexion than the PIP joints, so when the patient pulls away from the dorsal hood, the motion is initiated first with the FDP muscle(s). The patient is instructed to flex the IP joints by first moving the fingernails away from the hood.

The purpose of the dorsal hood is not to serially push the joints into more flexion but instead to capture the normal relative starting position of active IP joint motion. The hood positions the IP joints in the ideal relationship to one another to assure that finger flexion is instigated by the FDP muscles.

Once IP joint motion is partially regained and excursion of the extrinsic flexors is reestablished within the finger, positioning the MCP joints in full extension (hyperextension) in the cast is necessary to elongate the interosseous and lumbrical muscles (Fig. 67-29). A stepwise treatment approach is the most effective; allow the FDP tendon to increase its glide and mobilize the stiff IP joints before also being required to pull against the interosseous muscle–tendon unit tightness.

When full IP flexion is possible while the MCP joints are held hyperextended, the MCP joint immobilization may be slowly discontinued (see later comments on weaning) and full composite finger flexion allowed. This should be considered only when the patient is able to spontaneously initiate flexion with the FDP muscles.

Some patients may however present initially with reasonable IP joint ROM and FDP tendon glide. These patients do not need to wear a cast with the MCP joints blocked in slight flexion but can immediately begin using the "intrinsic muscle stretch" cast in Figure 67-29.

In the severely stiff hand the range of finger flexion may dramatically improve when the MCP joints are blocked in the initial cast. This dramatic mechanical mobilization may tempt the therapist to begin early weaning and to think that a cast with the MCP joints held in hyperextension is unnecessary. This treatment route will be a disservice to the patient, as it is impossible to have severe chronic limited finger flexion without developing secondary interosseous muscle tightness.

Limited digital motion present in all chronically stiff hands will cause the interosseous muscles to adaptively shorten. After the patient has regained digital flexion using the profundus muscle(s), or if finger flexion is present

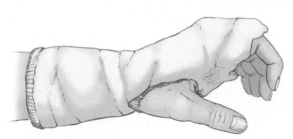

Figure 67-27 A cast positioning the MCP joints in slight flexion is desirable as a starting position if interosseous muscles are extremely tight and/or IP joint tightness is severe. This same cast position with slight MCP flexion is desirable when wanting to gain both flexion and extension of a stiff proximal IP joint. (Copyright Judy C. Colditz, 2008.)

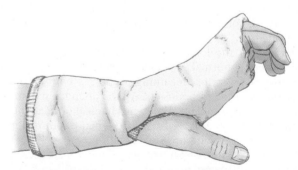

Figure 67-29 After FDP tendon glide and IP joint mobility are regained, the hand is positioned in the cast with the MCP joints in full extension (hyperextension) to allow cyclic active motion to reduce tightness of both the interosseous and lumbrical muscles. (Copyright Judy C. Colditz, 2008.)

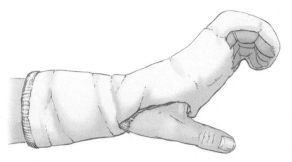

Figure 67-30 If the patient has had great difficulty isolating the extrinsic flexor muscles and regaining active IP joint flexion, it may be desirable to continue the hood as part of the cast used to elongate the intrinsic muscles. (Copyright Judy C. Colditz, 2008.)

but not full, a cast to position the MCP joints in maximum extension (hyperextension) but to allow full IP joint flexion is applied so cyclic active digital flexion elongates both the interosseus and lumbrical muscles (see Fig. 67-29). The lumbrical muscle is in its longest position when the profundus muscle is actively contracting (as a result of the proximal movement of the origin of the lumbrical muscle on the profundus tendon) while the MCP joints are in extension and the IP joints are flexed. Thus, the active hook position elongates both of these intrinsic hand muscles. If the intrinsic finger muscles are extremely tight or the patient had great difficulty in regaining profundus glide, a dorsal hood may also be attached to this cast design (Fig. 67-30). The hood is infrequently needed at this stage. Although this cast position of MCP joint hyperextension does not support functional use of the hand, its use is mandatory to reach the ultimate goal of normal ROM and functional use of the hand.

Almost all surgical and therapy texts stress the importance of positioning the MCP joints in flexion to maintain the maximum length of the collateral ligaments. Inclusion of the extended MCP joints in the cast is contradictory to this traditional teaching. It is the increased IP active motion resulting from this position that reduces edema and demands glide of the tendons of the intrinsic muscles across the MCP joint, two factors that outweigh the temporary immobilization of these joints. Much of the cause of limited MP joint flexion is probably edema within the joint capsule, which is loose in extension but compressed in flexion. By blocking the MCP joint in full extension with the cast providing a contoured palmar pressure, edema within the MCP joints is reduced while the intrinsic muscle tendons are gliding past the MCP joint. Active IP joint flexion with the MCP joints blocked in extension demands elongation of the interosseous and lumbrical muscles. Active IP extension with the MCP joint in full extension also demands maximum muscle contraction of the interosseous muscles. Blocking the MP joints in full extension while allowing active IP joint flexion and extension thus elongates and tones the interosseous muscles. Since the interosseous muscles are the prime MCP joint flexor muscle(s), when casting is discontinued, MCP joint flexion can be regained without further specific intervention toward mobilizing the MCP joints into flexion. The only exception is if there is the presence of specific dorsal adherence resulting from dorsal trauma.

The inability to initiate finger flexion with the profundus muscles is commonly seen in the stiff hand following immobilization for a distal radius fracture or other trauma. In the initial CMMS cast, the desired relational position of DIP and PIP joint flexion may not be attainable because of joint stiffness, especially the DIP joint. After a few days in the cast the patient will gain digital flexion, but it is usually with the flexor digitorum superficialis (FDS) muscles rather than with the FDP muscles. If this occurs, the addition of a small piece of plaster of Paris or thermoplastic material over the distal edge of the dorsal hood (just over the distal phalanx) will aid in greater DIP joint flexion as the patient moves cyclically. It is important that each time the patient actively flexes, the fingernails move away from the dorsal hood before the PIP joint moves. The patient must look at and think about initiating this active motion to regain glide of the FDP tendon(s).

The complex decision-making process of applying the CMMS technique for the most common problem of regaining digital flexion in the chronically stiff hand is illustrated in Figure 67-31. This illustration only applies to stiff hands lacking full finger flexion.

Dominant Extrinsic Flexion Pattern (or Intrinsic Minus)

Although the dominant intrinsic flexion pattern discussed above is the most common pattern of stiffness seen in the hand, other patterns of stiffness present that require other cast designs to effect change.

When MCP joint flexion is limited either by capsular tightness or by adherence of the extrinsic extensor system, the intrinsic muscle power to the IP joints is eliminated, explaining the term "*intrinsic*-minus pattern." The intrinsic muscles cannot get into position to provide force for digital control, and the extrinsic muscles dominate the pattern of motion.

To regain MCP joint flexion, the wrist cast is applied in slight extension and a dorsal hood is placed only over the proximal phalanges, positioning them at their easy available maximum passive flexion range (Fig. 67-32). Care must be taken to assure the cast does not extend too far distally on the palmar surface, thus blocking MCP joint flexion. The patient works to actively pull the proximal phalanx away from the dorsal hood while flexing only the PIP joint with the superficialis muscle. The patient is instructed to place the fingertips on the cast and to "slide" the fingertips proximally. This exercise isolates the interosseous muscles, and cyclic loading increases the range of MCP joint flexion.

As MCP joint flexion increases, the cast may be changed to create a starting position of somewhat greater MCP joint flexion (Fig. 67-33). A small pad can also be inserted between the proximal phalanx and the dorsal block to position the MCP joints in slightly more flexion. The purpose is not to serially position the MCP joints in maximum flexion and hold them there, but instead to position the MCP joints in slightly greater flexion so active MCP joint flexion is within the end-range. The cast never holds the MCP joint immobile, because there is always room for the movement into and away from end-range flexion.

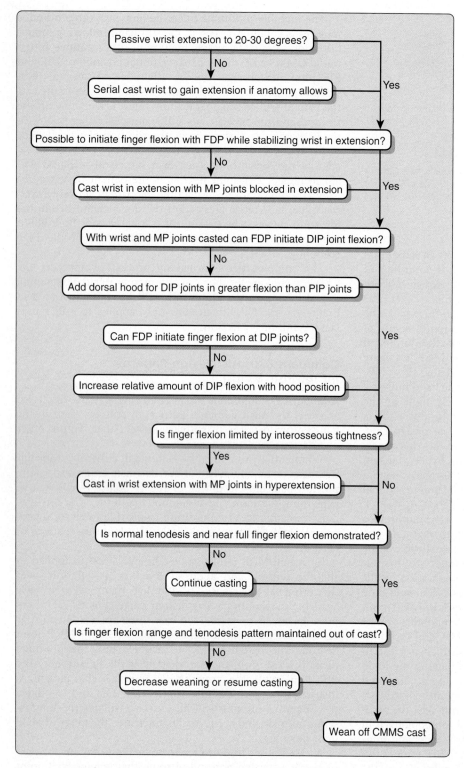

Figure 67-31 Algorithm outlining the decision-making process for the application of the CMMS technique to regain finger flexion in the chronically stiff hand. (Copyright: Judy C. Colditz, 2008.)

Dominant Isolated Interphalangeal Joint Tightness

When injury is at or near a joint, isolated capsular tightness can prevent or restrict joint movement. The muscle–tendon units that normally move the joint shift their power to the adjacent unrestricted joints, diminishing the force available to mobilize the stiff joint(s). In such a circumstance the CMMS cast is applied to block all proximal joint movement (see Fig. 67-27). The wrist and all digits are included, so the overflow from the adjacent digital movement helps the patient initiate the joint motion needed. In extreme cases (seen primarily in children), the distal joints may also have to be constrained. If the patient has difficulty initiating active motion because of the severity of the joint stiffness, a dorsal

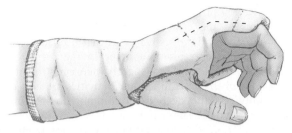

Figure 67-32 MCP joint flexion is regained by allowing cyclic active MCP joint flexion away from a dorsal block. (Copyright Judy C. Colditz, 2008.)

hood may be needed to direct the desired range and direction of motion (see Fig. 67-28). This is only rarely required.

Traditional treatment for capsular tightness usually focuses on gaining one direction of motion at a time. Gains in one direction often create a loss of motion in the opposite direction. Energy is then directed toward resolving the lost motion, which in turn cancels out the initial gains, making the entire process minimally successful. The greatest advantage of the CMMS approach is the ability to simultaneously gain both flexion and extension in a stiff distal joint. This gain of reciprocal motion reestablishes the two-way differential glide of the tissues, and both active and passive joint motion is reestablished.

Clinical Application of CMMS

General Principles

Because the extrinsic flexors and the extrinsic extensor muscles strongly influence digital motion, the wrist must always be included in the cast and positioned in slight extension so the extrinsic muscle power is directed toward the digits. It is this position that facilitates the most effective transmission of force to the joints of the hand to mobilize them into flexion. Even if the stiffness is limited to only one digit, the other digits should be included in the cast to allow the cortical representation of the uninjured digits to assist with accurate motion.[103] The only exception to this may be to allow slightly greater freedom of motion in the index finger if the stiffness is isolated to the ulnar digits.

It is important to use plaster of Paris for the CMMS technique because of its inherent intimate molding ability.[72] Other synthetic casting materials are more rigid and have

sharp edges. Thermoplastic splinting materials should not be substituted for the plaster of Paris, because they are readily removed and allow for poor skin tolerance to prolonged wear. Only in cases in which the stiffness is not yet chronic and shorter periods of exercise are effective can the principles of the CMMS technique be applied with thermoplastic materials.

To regain joint mobility, significant time is required. In Noyes' study of immobilization of monkey knees, it took one year to fully resolve the flexion contracture.[35] The most challenging principle for hand therapists is the amount of time in a cast required to result in permanent change in active motion for the chronically stiff hand. Although the mechanical change is usually relatively rapid, the cortical change needed for the motion to be permanently retained requires a prolonged period of repeated constrained motion. Patients with chronic stiffness may wear the cast for many weeks or a few months with few or no cast changes. When more acute injuries are being treated, tissue responds rapidly to intervention. In the chronically stiff hand, effective change takes much longer.

Treatment Guidelines

It is difficult to relay detailed treatment protocols for the CMMS technique, but general guidelines are given in the following sections. Each treatment sequence is based on the patient's individual diagnosis, specific causes of tightness and/or lack of glide, pathologic pattern of motion, and response to the CMMS treatment. The therapist must be able to critically evaluate the stiff hand and determine the exact anatomic structures limiting motion. This knowledge determines the specific position needed to harness productive active motion within a cast. The algorithm flow chart (see Fig. 67-31) is an example of the thought process applicable to a stiff hand with limited finger flexion and interosseous muscles tightness.

Cast Design. The design of the CMMS cast is determined by the pattern of motion and locus of tightness (see Figs. 67-26 through 67-30, 67-32, and 67-33). The position for immobilizing proximal joints is not arbitrary. For example, if the PIP joint of the little finger is primarily lacking extension, one might choose to immobilize the MCP joint in significant flexion to facilitate proximal excursion of the dorsal apparatus across the joint and invite greater participation of the extensor digitorum communis. If the PIP joint of the little finger primarily lacks flexion, placing the MCP joint in full extension (or even hyperextension) drives more extrinsic flexor force across the joint toward flexion. If both flexion and extension are equally limited in the little finger PIP joint, a position of about 45 degrees of MCP joint flexion would give the best mechanical advantage for mobility of the PIP joint in both directions.

An arbitrary time period for cast wear is initially chosen. The cast is then removed to reevaluate the active pattern of motion. Observation of the new, altered, active pattern of motion determines the desired position of the proximal joints and the position of any dorsal blocks in the next cast. When the next cast is applied, usually only the position of the MCP and IP joints is changed, and the new wrist cast is applied in the same slightly extended position. The exception

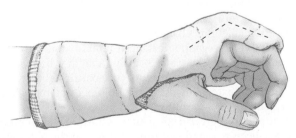

Figure 67-33 When the initial range of MCP joint flexion is regained, the MCP joints are positioned in somewhat greater flexion so they can be exercised in the available end-range of flexion. (Copyright Judy C. Colditz, 2008.)

to this would be if there is an element of extrinsic flexor or extensor muscle tightness that requires a change of wrist position.

Time in the Cast. The most challenging aspect of the CMMS treatment for therapists is the amount of time required in the cast to repattern the motor cortex. Initial mechanical gains will be rapid, and the therapist will be tempted to immediately begin the weaning process. Experience has proven that this approach is fruitless, because the patient immediately reverts to the old maladapted pattern of motion that has remained dominant in the motor cortex. Stiffness returns.

It is important to take into account the duration of time the hand has moved in the stiff altered pattern. The longer this nonproductive pattern has been present, the longer the time required in the cast for the cortical change to be enduring. Most patients require a minimum of 2 to 4 weeks of full-time casting, although the design of the cast may be changed during this time. Patients with prolonged chronic stiffness may require 6, 8, or more weeks of full-time casting. Although this seems like a protracted period for the therapist, one must keep in mind that it is really a short period relative to the time the stiffness has been present.

Weaning Process. After a prolonged period of full-time cast wear, a period of slow weaning must occur to ensure that the patient can retain the active motion gained. Because of weakness from the chronic stiffness and from partial immobilization in the cast, the patient will quickly fatigue and revert to the previous maladaptive pattern of movement. Initially, time out of the cast should be short. The frequency of short time periods out of the cast should be increased before each time period is increased.

When the patient can display the desired ROM out of the cast while also demonstrating a spontaneous tenodesis pattern, slow weaning can begin. The cast is sawn on the radial and ulnar aspects, but the underneath padding and stockinette are cut only on the radial side. The edges of the sawn cast are covered with adhesive tape to secure the padding and stockinette and to cover the raw edges of the plaster of Paris. Circumferential hook-and-loop straps are then applied. The cast can then be removed and reapplied to allow weaning to slowly begin (Fig. 67-34).

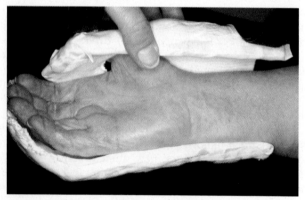

Figure 67-34 When the patient is ready to begin weaning from the CMMS cast, the cast can be made removable by bivalving it and applying hook-and-loop straps to secure it when reapplied.

The weaning process starts with brief (about 15-minute) periods out of the cast a few times a day. The patient works actively on nonresistive tasks that use the tenodesis pattern and concentrates on moving in the correct active pattern. After 1 or 2 weeks of slightly increasing the number of times out of the cast, functional activities are added that purposefully use the desired motion but do not provide excessive resistance. The patient learns to identify when the pattern of motion is disintegrating, and returns to the cast. Awareness of how the hand should be used ensures that all motions out of the cast reinforce the gains made while in the cast.

Therapists are cautioned at this time to avoid focusing on regaining motion in the opposite direction. Contractures of the PIP or other joints will probably be present as a result of the time in the cast. If efforts are immediately directed toward eliminating the joint contractures as the weaning begins, that effort will cancel the effectiveness of the time in the cast. Only when the desired motion has been regained and the patient can maintain the motion out of the cast is any effort directed toward regaining motion in the opposite direction. In most cases the motion will slowly return with normal hand use. Therapists also should be cautioned that it is futile during the weaning period to revert to manual treatment techniques. The focus should remain on functional active motion.

Invariably, patients who are weaned too quickly will require a period of repeat casting. The treatment principles of the CMMS technique are so contradictory to traditional teaching that it will require a dramatic change in thinking to become comfortable with this treatment technique.

Contraindications

The CMMS technique should not be used unless the therapist has skill in the application of a safe and comfortable plaster of Paris cast and its safe removal. The cast must be applied perfectly, with well-distributed pressure affording perfect comfort. Precision is required to adequately block the small joints of the hand while allowing full motion of the adjacent joints. Excessive exothermic reaction of the hardening plaster of Paris must be avoided.[110-113] Claustrophobic patients may not be able to tolerate the confines of the cast, and the technique should be applied judiciously to this population. The circumferential cast should never be applied to acute injuries, especially if vascular instability is present. It may be used in select postsurgical cases such as flexor tenolysis to facilitate correct tendon glide, but only after a few days in the postoperative compressive dressing.

This technique should not be indiscriminately applied to all patients with chronic stiffness. In the cases of severe trauma, the anatomic changes from an injury may eliminate the potential for regaining balanced motion, and the loss of motion created by the CMMS casting may not be regained. Elderly patients with significant osteoarthritis may have some residual extension loss of the IP joints, and they should be treated with more caution.

Historically, a great deal of time, effort, and pain endurance has been required to restore motion to the chronically stiff hand.[8] In the era of increasing cost-benefit analysis, the amount of motion regained relative to the time and energy expended on treatment must be an efficient return. The

CMMS treatment method simplifies the treatment approach, and even a severely stiff hand can be mobilized with only a few therapy visits and cast changes extended over a number of months. It is important to note that the CMMS treatment method was developed by the author and although there is sound theoretical basis and the author's clinical experience supporting this technique, its use warrants prospective clinical research studies to demonstrate its effectiveness.

Summary

Understanding the causes of stiffness in the hand and choosing the type and timing of intervention is fundamental to successful mobilization of the stiff hand. A gentle approach to the tissues of the hand aimed at reducing edema and avoiding stimulation of the inflammatory response is required. The ability to influence and improve motion of the hand is the result of appropriate responses to the processes occurring in the hand. Gentle manual stretching, active motion, and use of the hand in conjunction with timely mobilizing orthoses can effectively transform the newly stiff hand into a mobile one. When the stiffness is prolonged and chronic joint tightness and tissue adherence limit motion, when chronic edema prolongs the inflammatory effect, and when the stiffness allows only a nonfunctional pattern of motion, these complex interrelated problems can be addressed with the newer technique of CMMS.

The delicate balance between tissue glide and freedom of motion can be restored, even after severe hand injuries, if the therapist provides a program of treatment based on a sound understanding of, and respect for, tissue response and the healing continuum.

REFERENCES

The complete reference list is available online at www.expertconsult.com.

Postoperative Management of Metacarpophalangeal Joint and Proximal Interphalangeal Joint Capsulectomies

NANCY CANNON, OTR, CHT

Critical Points

- Patients should identify functional goals for the elective procedure and the therapist must ensure the goals are foremost in the therapy treatment program.
- A comprehensive, custom-designed rehabilitation program is essential for an excellent, functional outcome.
- Effective edema control serves as the chief priority the initial three weeks following surgery to effectively limit pain, allow greater range-of-motion, and limit the formation of scar tissue.
- Custom-fabricated orthoses, both for immobilization and mobilization purposes, play an integral role in a successful outcome.
- Specific tendon gliding exercises are essential for maximizing tendon excursion and limiting tendon adherence when tenolyses are performed in conjunction with the capsulectomy.

Historical Overview

A review of the literature shows that some of the earliest metacarpophalangeal (MCP) joint capsulectomy procedures were performed by Shaw[1] in 1920 and Fowler[2] and Pratt[3] in the 1940s. This reconstructive procedure was often performed secondary to severe hand trauma from war injuries. Since then, other authors have written on the subject.[1,2,4-15] Most of the publications have a limited review of the surgical procedure and the outcomes.

Some of the early articles cited in the literature for proximal interphalangeal (PIP) joint capsulectomies were by Curtis[16] in 1966, Rhode and Jennings[17] in 1971, Sprague[18] in 1976, and Young and colleagues[19] in 1978. The elective procedure was offered to patients to enhance functional performance of the hand.

There are limited written works on the rehabilitation for MCP joint and PIP joint capsulectomies. Laseter,[20,21] Gorman,[22] and Saunders[23] published the most thorough reviews of therapy after these procedures. Laseter contributed comprehensive chapters on the subject in the second and third editions of this textbook. Other authors have briefly addressed the postoperative therapy.[3-6,8,9,14,18,19,24-30]

Dorsal MCP Joint Capsulectomy

This procedure is recommended primarily for stiff joints in which the surfaces of the head of the metacarpal and base of the proximal phalanx of the MCP joint are relatively normal and the anatomic relationship of the bones has been preserved.[2,3,14,30,31] However, other authors[7,16,24,32] believe that the procedure can be performed even when radiographs reflect considerable joint damage.

Dorsal MCP joint capsulectomies are indicated when the MCP joint has an extension contracture with significant functional limitation in MCP joint flexion secondary to thickening and contracture of the dorsal capsule, adhesions of the extensor tendons over the dorsum of the hand or the MCP joint, contracture of the collateral ligaments (primarily the cord portion), and skin contracture or scarring over the dorsum of the hand as seen with burns.[7,22,24,32]

Some of the more common diagnoses requiring dorsal capsulectomy are metacarpal fractures, proximal phalanx fractures (primarily at the base), soft tissue or bony crush injuries of the hand, nerve palsies, zone V and VI extensor tendon repairs, Volkmann's contracture, burns, skin contractures, and distal radius fractures with secondary pain and residual stiffness of the hand.

A number of authors believe that it is unlikely that the procedure will add valuable function to the hand when 60 to 75 degrees of active and/or passive range of motion (ROM) already has been achieved before capsulectomy.[7,24,30-32] Through the years, I have observed a large number of patients with 50 to 60 degrees of passive MCP joint flexion before surgery who ultimately obtained significant improvement in functional use of the hand after the procedure. This has been particularly true when limitation with the MCP joint involves the ring and small fingers. Restoring flexion of the ring and small fingers is invaluable for maximizing hand function.

Contraindications

The chief medical contraindication to this procedure is arthritis. The procedure is not indicated to improve ROM in a digit limited by arthritis. In addition, patients who are not highly motivated and do not have specific functional goals for the procedure would not be favorable candidates for this elective procedure. This contraindication would be true of all elective surgical procedures for which intensive postoperative rehabilitation is necessary after the surgery.

Anatomy of the MCP Joint

A thorough understanding of the bony and soft tissue anatomy at the MCP joint level is essential for appreciating the surgical procedure and establishing an effective postoperative treatment regimen (Fig. 68-1).

The MCP joint is a diarthrodial joint with two freedoms of motion in flexion and extension and abduction and adduc-

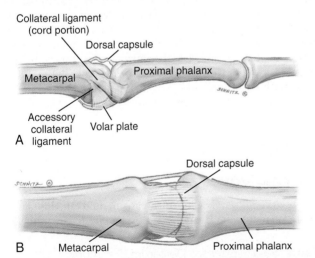

Figure 68-1 A, Lateral view illustrates the relationship of the collateral ligaments, dorsal capsule, and volar plate at the metacarpophalangeal (MCP) joint with the MCP joint in a neutral position of 0 degrees of extension. **B**, Dorsal view illustrates the bony configuration and relationship of the metacarpal and proximal phalanx. The bony relationship between the metacarpal head and the base of the proximal phalanx differs slightly at each digit.

tion.[33] Unlike the PIP and distal interphalangeal (DIP) joints, which have a consistent degree of stability throughout the arc of motion, the MCP joint has a relatively significant amount of lateral and rotational mobility, which is at its greatest in extension and is relatively eliminated in full flexion. This is because of its bony anatomy and surrounding soft tissue structures.[34]

Bony Anatomy

The bony anatomy of the metacarpal head is configured slightly differently in each of the metacarpals.[35] The metacarpal heads have a smooth and asymmetrical shape. In the index finger, the metacarpal joint surface rotates in a slightly ulnar direction, whereas the ring and small finger metacarpal heads are rotated slightly radially, which allows the fingers to converge toward the middle finger with a common resting point for grasping. This is an important anatomic relationship to be observed with fabrication of dynamic flexion orthoses for the MCP joints. Within the joint itself, the spherical convex contour of the metacarpal head articulates with the concave articular surface of the proximal phalanx. As flexion occurs at the MCP joint, the potential for direct contact between the two bones increases. In part, this is because the surface of the metacarpal head is twice as wide on the volar surface compared with the dorsal portion.

Soft Tissue

Ligaments

The ligamentous support of the MCP joint is composed of a main collateral ligament and an accessory collateral ligament arising eccentrically off the metacarpal head on the radial and ulnar sides of the joint. The main collateral ligament (cord portion) originates on the metacarpal head and inserts on the volar and lateral base of the proximal phalanx.[34] The accessory collateral ligament originates on the metacarpal head and inserts primarily into the volar (palmar) plate. The main collateral ligaments are redundant in MCP extension and taut in MCP flexion. As the MCP joint flexes, these ligaments must stretch over the wide tubercles and volar base of the metacarpal head. The main collateral ligament in particular becomes increasingly taut as the MCP joint reaches 45 degrees of flexion (Fig. 68-2).

Volar Plate

The volar plate, or palmar plate, is a fibrocartilaginous structure on the volar surface of the MCP joint. Distally, the structure is firmly secured to the proximal phalanx and is reinforced by fibers from the accessory collateral ligaments. Proximally, its attachment with the metacarpal head is loosely secured. This permits the laxity necessary for MCP joint hyperextension. The deep transverse metacarpal ligament acts as an added soft tissue support structure for the volar plate and MCP joint.[34]

Dorsal Capsule

The dorsal capsule consists of dense connective tissue. The structure is relatively redundant in extension and becomes taut in flexion. The capsule serves as a support structure for the MCP joint.

MCP JOINT EXTENSION

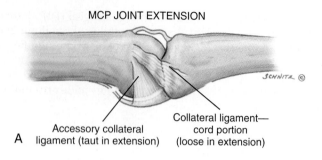

A

Accessory collateral ligament (taut in extension)

Collateral ligament— cord portion (loose in extension)

MCP JOINT FLEXION

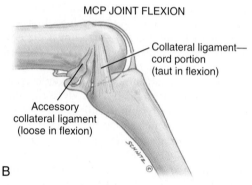

B

Collateral ligament— cord portion (taut in flexion)

Accessory collateral ligament (loose in flexion)

Figure 68-2 A and **B**, The laxity and redundancy of the collateral ligaments in metacarpophalangeal (MCP) joint extension and tautness in full flexion. The cord portion of the collateral ligament is loose in extension and becomes increasingly taut as 45 degrees of flexion is achieved. The accessory collateral ligament actually has its greatest tension through the initial 45 degrees of flexion and thereafter has slightly less tension.

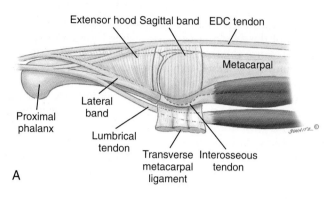

Extensor hood   Sagittal band   EDC tendon

Metacarpal

Proximal phalanx

Lateral band

Lumbrical tendon

Transverse metacarpal ligament

Interosseous tendon

A

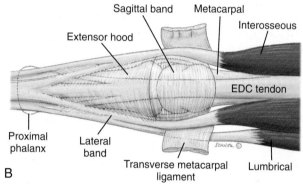

Sagittal band   Metacarpal

Interosseous

Extensor hood

EDC tendon

Proximal phalanx

Lateral band

Transverse metacarpal ligament

Lumbrical

B

Figure 68-3 A, The lateral view reflects the soft tissue structures that surround and support the metacarpophalangeal (MCP) joint dorsally, volarly, and laterally. **B**, The dorsal view shows the intricate relationship of the extensor mechanism to the dorsal capsule and MCP joint. EDC, extensor digitorum communis.

Muscles/Tendons

In extension, the MCP joint inherently maintains stability through the intrinsic muscles. To a lesser degree, added stability is provided through the extrinsic flexors and extensors crossing the MCP joint. Both the extrinsic and intrinsic muscles assist with active flexion and extension at the MCP joint level (Fig. 68-3).

Tendon excursion of the extensor digitorum communis (EDC) is important to keep in mind, particularly when an extensor tenolysis accompanies the MCP joint capsulectomy[36,37] (Table 68-1). With the proper exercises, maximum excursion of the EDC can be obtained, thereby preventing adherence of the EDC to adjacent soft tissue and/or bony structures.

Beyond the EDC, it is valuable to recognize the added contribution of the extensor indicis proprius (EIP) and extensor digiti quinti (EDQ). Both of these muscles are innervated by the radial nerve.

Preoperative Assessment

Hand surgeons should consider including an assessment by the hand therapist as part of the initial evaluation process for patients referred with hand stiffness. The therapist can evaluate the patient's past therapy regimen and determine whether additional therapy can positively influence the stiff MCP joints and potentially eliminate the need for surgery. Conversely, the therapist can reinforce the need for the elective procedure through the objective evaluation and assessment of the patient's therapy program.

The preoperative assessment should include (1) the patient's pertinent medical history; (2) active and passive ROM of all digits and the wrist; (3) evaluation for possible intrinsic tightness and extrinsic extensor tightness; (4) manual muscle testing of the extrinsic flexors, extensors, and intrinsic muscles; (5) the patient's current pain level and history of pain; (6) integrity of the skin; (7) notation of any previous infection and risk of recurrence; (8) functional performance level of the hand in activities of daily living (ADL), along with vocational and avocational activities; and (9) the patient's desired functional goals of surgery.

Surgery

Terminology

A *capsulectomy* is excision of a capsule and, in this case, a joint capsule.[38] The Latin derivation is *capsule*, meaning "the

Table 68-1   Extensor Digitorum Communis Tendon Excursion: Metacarpophalangeal Joint

	Index	Long	Ring	Small
Bunnell et al., 1956[57]	15 mm	16 mm	11 mm	12 mm

joint capsule," and *ectomy*, meaning "cutting, excision." Thus, with a capsulectomy, there is surgical excision of a portion of the joint capsule along with the soft tissue structures intricately associated with the joint. *Capsulotomy*, on the other hand, is an incision, but not excision or removal, of soft tissue structures. It is not uncommon, however, for these terms to be used interchangeably.

Procedure

A thorough understanding of the operative procedure is essential to effectively manage the postoperative therapy. A number of authors have described their surgical approach for MCP joint dorsal capsulectomies.[5,14,28,32,39,40] The reader is referred to Chapter 66 for a complete description of the surgical management for MCP joint contractures. The following is an overview of one surgical approach for dorsal MCP joint capsulectomies.[8,9]

- A longitudinal incision is made along the dorsal aspect of the affected joint or joints (Fig. 68-4A, online).
- The extensor hood is incised, and the extensor tendon is either retracted laterally to the joint or split longitudinally to gain visual exposure of the joint (Fig. 68-4B, online).
- The synovium and the dorsal capsule are exposed and excised (Fig. 68-4C, online).
- The collateral ligaments are excised in a balanced fashion along the cord portion just beneath and on both sides of the tubercle of the metacarpal head. The distal portion of the cord is left attached to the accessory portion of the collateral ligament (Fig. 68-4D, online).
- As passive flexion is attempted, if the MCP joint opens like a book instead of the proximal phalanx gliding along the head of the metacarpal (as seen with normal joint biomechanics), then a periosteal elevator or curved dissector is passed around the volar aspect of the metacarpal head to free the adhesions between the metacarpal head and the volar plate (Fig. 68-4E, online). This will correct the problem.
- The wound is closed. If the extensor tendon has been split longitudinally, it is reapproximated and sutured before skin closure.
- In cases of extensive dissection, consideration may be given to placing drains along the surgical area to enhance drainage and secondarily reduce postoperative edema, risk of hematoma, and ultimate scar-tissue formation.
- In severe cases in which a certain degree of rebound or tendency to resist passive flexion occurs, consideration may be given to percutaneous pinning of the joint in flexion for a limited time before initiating therapy.[19,25,41]
- A bulky compressive dressing is evenly applied, positioning the MCP joints in 45 to 75 degrees of flexion.
- If postoperative pain is a concern (based primarily on the patient's history of pain after the initial injury or surgery), consideration may be given to postoperative transcutaneous electrical nerve stimulation (TENS) along the appropriate peripheral nerve distribution.

If an extensor tenolysis is needed, the tenolysis would be performed before the capsulectomy. In some cases, extensor tendon adhesions may be the primary restriction to passive flexion, and an extensor tenolysis alone may prevent the need for capsulectomy.

Hand Therapy

Postoperative Therapy

To establish an effective postoperative course of rehabilitation, the therapist and surgeon should thoroughly discuss the patient's surgery. The therapist must have a complete understanding of the extent of surgery performed, any residual limitations to full passive flexion, potential concerns related to joint stability, and any additional surgical procedures (e.g., tenolysis, intrinsic releases). Based on this information, the initial postoperative therapy program can be established.

Examination

An objective examination should be performed during each treatment session after surgery. It is critical to monitor active and passive ROM, edema with circumferential measurements along the distal palmar flexion crease or along the MCP joints, pain with a visual analog scale or by rating the pain on a scale of 0 to 10, and the wound (size and appearance). The objective examination is essential to monitor the patient's progress and the effectiveness of each treatment method.

As part of the initial examination, the therapist should have a full understanding of the patient's goals and objectives for the surgery. With this information, the therapist can effectively design the rehabilitation program prioritizing these goals.

Edema Management

Control of postoperative edema during the initial 10 to 14 days after surgery is of great importance (Fig. 68-5). Effective edema management is key to a successful outcome. During the initial inflammatory phase and, more important, during

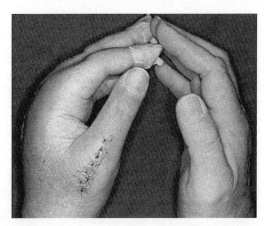

Figure 68-5 *Moderate edema is noted in the left hand, which underwent dorsal capsulectomies to the index through small finger metacarpophalangeal (MCP) joints along with the thumb MCP joint, compared with the right hand. Dorsal edema is common after MCP joint capsulectomies for the initial 10 to 14 days after surgery.*

the fibroplasia phase of wound healing, the fibroblasts and fibrin lay down collagen, affecting the suppleness of the soft tissue structures and forming restrictive adhesions. Effective edema management minimizes the formation of adhesions, decreases the pressure and resistance to passive joint motion, and favorably influences the orientation of collagen fibers as active and passive ROM exercises are incorporated in the therapy program.

When excessive edema is present, there is heightened pain and increased risk of wound separation and subsequent infection. It is critical to effectively manage the edema so that it will not interfere with the course of rehabilitation.

One particularly effective method for controlling postoperative edema in the hand and forearm is a carefully and evenly applied light compressive dressing (Fig. 68-6, online). The dressing is changed at each therapy visit and is worn for the initial 10 to 14 days after surgery. Once the light compressive dressing is discontinued, elastic stockinettes may be worn on the hand and forearm along with an edema glove to assist with managing persistent edema.

In addition to the light compressive dressings and elastic stockinettes, elevation and interdigital massage (between the metacarpals and along the length of the volar and dorsal aspects of the hand) are effective for managing the boggy edema often noted after surgery. With the massage, it is important to avoid direct contact with the sutures and to avoid skin separation along the suture line.

To manage digital edema, finger socks or Coban are applied and worn between exercise sessions (Fig. 68-7, online). The edema at this level will generally subside within 2 to 3 weeks.

Wound Care

In most instances, wound care can be accomplished through the use of postoperative light compressive dressings. The dressings serve as the sterile barrier between the wound and contaminants in the environment. When possible, the Xeroform, which is often placed over the sutures before the bulky dressing is applied, is left in place to provide added wound protection (Fig. 68-8, online).

Occasionally, when extensive surgery is required, significant dorsal edema may create a limited degree of wound separation. These wounds generally have an uneventful course and heal readily by secondary intention.

On occasion, a hematoma will occur. In these instances, it is important to express the hematoma to prevent an environment for infection. With the use of sterile technique, hematomas may be manually expressed by slightly separating the sutured skin edges and gently rolling a 4 × 4-inch sterile gauze pad with light pressure along the skin to express the hematoma or the hematoma may be aspirated by the physician with a needle and syringe. After expression of the hematoma, the wound must be monitored carefully for signs of infection. A course of prophylactic antibiotics is not uncommon.

In traumatic injuries in which extensive surgical dissection is necessary (i.e., combined capsulectomies and tenolyses in multiple digits), a Hemovac drain may be placed in the surgical area for 1 to 3 days to allow drainage and evacuation of the residual bleeding. This is valuable in reducing the risk of the development of a hematoma and excessively dense scar tissue postoperatively.

Pain Management

Effective edema management is one means for controlling the postoperative pain associated with MCP joint capsulectomies. In addition, TENS has proven to be beneficial in reducing postoperative pain (Fig. 68-9, online). High-rate, conventional TENS settings, with electrode placement along the peripheral nerve distribution of the surgical area, has repeatedly proven effective in the authors experience.[42]

The surgeon may choose to use an in-dwelling pain catheter to control the postoperative pain along with a regimen of oral narcotics for the initial days after surgery.

Exercises

The bulky compressive dressing should be removed within the initial 24 to 48 hours after surgery to initiate ROM exercises. It is important to begin the exercises before the close of the inflammatory phase of wound healing and before active participation of the fibroblasts in laying the framework for the formation of new collagen. Initiating early controlled motion will aid in the alignment and orientation of the newly forming collagen and will ultimately affect the final arc of motion.

Important to include in the postoperative exercise regimen are the following active, active-assisted, and passive ROM exercises (Fig. 68-10):
• Composite flexion and extension of the digits
• MCP joint flexion/extension with the interphalangeal (IP) joints extended
• MCP joint flexion/extension with the IP joints flexed
• Abduction/adduction of the digits

The exercises should be performed slowly, maintaining the end ROM between 5 and 10 seconds.

When capsulectomies have been performed to the index and small fingers, it is important to isolate the EIP and EDQ through independent extension of the index and small fingers. In addition, ROM exercises for the wrist should be performed. Wrist exercises should include isolated active and passive ROM along with simultaneous wrist and finger flexion, followed by wrist and finger extension. These exercises will provide for independent and maximum excursion of the extrinsic extensors and are especially necessary to include when extensor tenolysis accompanies the capsulectomy.

Exercising for 10 to 15 minutes every 2 hours has proven effective on a clinical basis. The rest period between exercise sessions allows the wound to "quiet down" and the inflammation to somewhat subside before the initiation of the next exercise session. In addition, the muscles have more than an adequate recovery period before the next exercise session.

Patients need to understand that the ROM achieved in the first 10 to 14 days after surgery becomes more difficult to maintain 3 to 4 weeks postoperatively as the soft tissues heal. This is related to the wound-healing process and proliferative nature of the new collagen after the initial 2 weeks after surgery. Patients will be more understanding and less likely to be discouraged if this has been explained in advance.

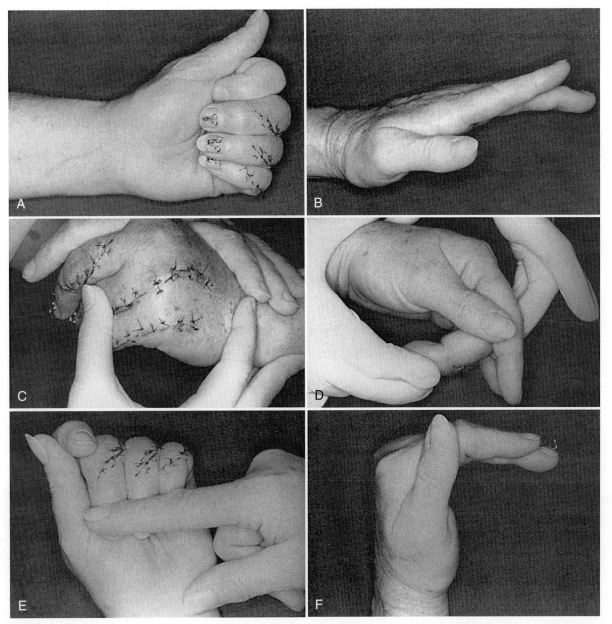

Figure 68-10 Active and passive range-of-motion exercises are initiated within the inflammatory phase of wound healing with occasional exception. Exercises valuable to include in therapy are demonstrated. **A,** Active flexion. **B,** Active extension. **C,** Passive metacarpophalangeal (MCP) joint flexion. **D,** Composite passive flexion. **E,** Composite passive flexion. **F,** MCP joint flexion with the interphalangeal (IP) joints extended.

Occasionally, patients will have a sluggish start with the postoperative therapy program. Factors such as nausea secondary to anesthesia or the pain medications, postoperative pain, and edema may inhibit progress. In these cases, the initial therapy program may need to include an exercise session at some point during the night, in complement to the daily exercise schedule. This may be necessary to ensure that the patient continues to makes gains in motion each day.

Functional activities should be stressed along with the ROM exercises early in the postoperative therapy program. Unlike many other surgical procedures in which protection of anatomic structures is essential, this procedure can permit relatively normal use of the hand without risk of damage to soft tissue or bony structures. Therefore, the earlier that the

hand begins performing functional activities, the sooner the hand will have restored functional use in normal ADL. In the clinic, functional exercises that emphasize MCP joint flexion with IP joint extension should be encouraged.

Strengthening exercises for the long flexors, extensors, and intrinsics may be initiated after the edema and pain have subsided. To minimize ongoing edema and/or pain, strengthening is delayed until 6 to 8 weeks after surgery. Putty, hand exercisers, and hand weights are effective for enhancing the overall strength of the hand and forearm. As for initiating a work-conditioning program, it tends to be more valuable when initiated no earlier than 6 to 8 weeks after surgery. The delay allows residual inflammation and edema to resolve before commencing repetitive lifting and heavy use of the hand.

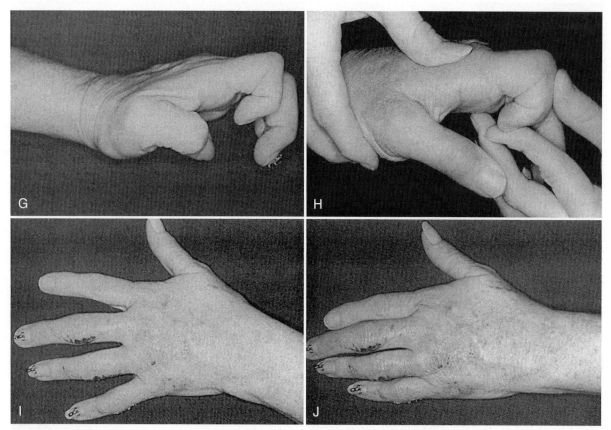

Figure 68-10, cont'd G and **H**, MCP joint extension with IP flexion (active/passive). **I**, Abduction of the digits. **J**, Adduction of the digits.

Orthotic Devices

With dorsal MCP joint capsulectomies, the use of orthoses serves three basic and important purposes: (1) immobilization to reduce inflammation and thus decrease pain and edema, (2) immobilization of the surgical area in a position that maximizes the passive flexion achieved in surgery and maintains lengthening of the soft tissue structures, and (3) dynamic mobilization to passively enhance joint ROM.

Clinically, I have found it effective to position the hand in a safe-position orthosis between exercise sessions and at night during the initial 3 to 4 weeks after surgery (Fig. 68-11, online). This places the MCP joint collateral ligaments on optimal stretch. Occasionally, the MCP joints can be positioned in as much as 90 degrees of flexion, but, more commonly, the hand is positioned in approximately 75 degrees at the MCP joint level.

Immediately after surgery, the MCP joints may not achieve the desired level of flexion because of the postoperative dressing, edema, and/or discomfort. It is important to serially adjust the orthosis in increased flexion at each treatment session until maximum flexion is achieved.

When it is difficult to achieve full flexion of the MCP joints, a dynamic flexion orthosis may be added to the therapy program (Fig. 68-12). The orthosis may be added as early as the first postoperative day, if necessary. The degree of limitation in passive flexion determines the daily time requirements for wearing the orthosis. In severe cases in which the hand is resistant to full passive flexion, the dynamic orthosis may be worn between exercise sessions during the day. Rarely is it worn at night because of potential discomfort, bulkiness of the orthosis, and risk of heightened edema or circulatory problems.

Because immobilization can quickly lead to heightened joint stiffness, orthosis wear should be gradually eliminated at the earliest reasonable time. This should be done as each orthosis has fulfilled its intended purpose. The time frame will vary, but usually within the initial 3 weeks, the orthosis-wearing time may be decreased each day until the orthosis is no longer needed. The safe-position orthosis is usually continued at night for 8 to 10 weeks.

Another form of passive stretching that has proven effective and that may negate the need for dynamic orthosis wear is a simple procedure referred to as *taping* (Fig. 68-13, online). Either dorsal taping or composite taping may be performed. Both are effective for limbering up the hand before an exercise session.

Scar Management

A valuable method of scar management after MCP joint capsulectomies is scar massage and scar retraction with lotion. Scar massage includes deep massage along the length of the scar, horizontally across the scar, and in circular clockwise and counterclockwise motion. Scar retraction also may be performed to mobilize the soft tissues (Fig. 68-14, online). With scar retraction, the patient performs active ROM while the therapist (or the patient after being taught) mobilizes the

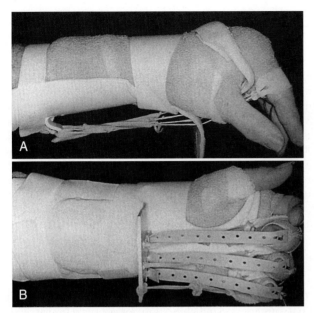

Figure 68-12 Dynamic flexion orthosis positioning may focus on the metacarpophalangeal (MCP) joints alone (**A**) or may be applied in a composite fashion (**B**) when extrinsic extensor tightness is present or when dorsal capsule tightness is present at both the MCP and proximal interphalangeal joint levels.

skin in the direction opposite the active motion. The goal is to mobilize the skin and free subcutaneous adhesions. In addition, Dycem may be used with scar retraction to better stabilize the skin.

Silicone products such as Otoform and 50/50 may be applied under orthoses or dressings to remodel the dorsal scar and aid in remodeling the collagen fibers. Scar remodeling products such as these are worn at night for approximately 8 weeks after suture removal and wound closure.

Modalities

Neuromuscular Electrical Stimulation

Neuromuscular electrical stimulation (NMES) may be used to assist with active ROM at the MCP joint level in both flexion and extension (Fig. 68-15, online). With MCP joint capsulectomies, it is more frequently used to maximize the proximal excursion of the EDC and the long flexors with the goal of maximizing MCP joint ROM. Muscle stimulation also may be used for the intrinsics to facilitate isolated MCP joint flexion.

Effective treatment parameters that I have used include the following: waveform, asymmetrical biphasic; pulse rate, 35 to 40 pulses per second; rise time, 2 seconds; on time, 15 seconds; off time, 20 seconds; intensity, set at a level that creates a strong motor response yet is well within the patient's comfort level; and time, 15-minute session. It is common for the NMES to be used three to four times daily as a part of the home exercise program.

Ultrasound

Occasionally, when patients heal quickly and form dense scar after surgery, it becomes difficult to maintain supple joints and tendon gliding. In these instances, ultrasound has been especially beneficial.

Ultrasound serves as a deep heating agent, elevating the temperature of the soft tissue structures.[43] The deep heat allows for greater passive suppleness and elasticity of the soft tissues. Clinically, the following parameters for using ultrasound have met with positive success: frequency, 3.0 MHz; intensity, 0.7 to 1.0 W/cm^2; continuous mode; and treatment time, 8 minutes.

Continuous Passive Motion

Continuous passive motion (CPM) units have proven to be clinically effective in reducing postoperative pain and edema and ultimately may increase joint ROM. Recognizing that there are a variety of hand CPM units on the market, it is important to determine which unit will effectively produce the desired motion. In the case of MCP joint capsulectomies, the goal is to decrease pain and edema and maximize ROM at the MCP joint level.

It is important to realize that few CPM units, if any, create a full arc of motion with composite flexion to the distal palmar flexion crease and full extension. This is because of the anatomic length differences in the digits. That the CPM unit may not achieve a complete arc of motion need not preclude its use. CPM units have repeatedly proven effective in reducing pain and edema. Therefore, it is one treatment method to be considered for the patient who has significant edema and pain during the initial week to 10 days after surgery. After this time, the therapy program should be reevaluated. The CPM unit may have accomplished its intended purpose. This allows the therapy program to place greater emphasis on specific ROM exercises, orthosis wear, and alternative edema management and pain management methods.

Interestingly, Schwartz and Chafetz[44] in 2008 reported no statistically significant ROM benefit with CPM after tenolysis with capsulectomy or capsulectomy alone. Their research focused on changes in ROM, duration of therapy, and number of therapy visits.[44]

Motivation

To maximize the success of the procedure, the patient must be self-motivated and have specific goals in mind for the procedure (i.e., improvement in performing specific functional tasks). These goals should be charted and the patient advised as to whether the goals are realistic and achievable.

In addition to the patient's self-motivation, the therapist must play an active role in motivating the patient to achieve the desired goals. The patient's overall success may depend on the therapist's ability to keep him or her actively involved in the early postoperative therapy regimen and to maintain that active participation 6 to 8 weeks later.

Results after MCP Joint Capsulectomy

A limited number of articles can be found in the literature relating to the results after MCP joint capsulectomy. In 1979, Gould and Nicholson[25] reported a series of 100 patients with dorsal MCP capsulectomies. In their series, the MCP joints were pinned in flexion for 10 to 14 days. With all diagnostic categories, the authors achieved a mean gain of 21 degrees of active and 29 degrees of passive MCP joint motion after the procedure. The greatest gains were seen in those 11 to 20 years of age. From a diagnostic perspective, greater gains were seen with the one stroke patient in their series (51.5 degrees passively) and with the five burn patients (36 degrees and 42 degrees passively). The least gains were seen with reflex sympathetic dystrophy (3 degrees actively and 28 degrees passively) and with fractures and crush injuries (18 degrees actively and 20 degrees passively). The authors stated that most patients could be flexed to 90 degrees intraoperatively, but this was rarely maintained postoperatively.

Young and colleagues[19] reported in 1978 on 10 patients with 24 dorsal MCP joint capsulectomies. After the procedure, the MCP joints were placed in flexion and pinned for 14 days before ROM exercise was begun at this level. The overall increase in passive ROM at the MCP joint level was 48 degrees. The greatest gain was seen in the lacerations and "other" category (71 degrees in each category and closed fractures 60 degrees passively). The least gain was seen in the open fracture category (a gain of 37 degrees passively).

Buch,[45] in his series, reported a minimum average increase of 30 degrees passively in MCP joint ROM. Results were significantly less notable when skin grafting was performed in association with the capsulectomy.

In 1947, Fowler[2] described his results as "excellent with 80% to 90% of motion confidently expected if local tissues are good and the mechanics of the hand satisfactory." Fowler did not include compiled clinical results with the article. Postoperative management consisted of rigid orthosis wear or traction with the MCP joints in flexion for 3 weeks before ROM exercise was begun at the MCP joint level.

I have found dorsal MCP joint capsulectomies to be a reliable and effective procedure for enhancing overall functional performance of the hand in the majority of cases. The superior results are seen in young patients (up to 25 years old), in patients requiring exclusively capsulectomy in a single or multiple digits, and where the articular surfaces of the MCP joint are relatively normal. Maintaining the results achieved in surgery is certainly a challenge, however, and becomes increasingly difficult with crush injuries to the dorsum of the hand that require extensive extensor tenolyses along with the MCP joint capsulectomies. PIP joint capsulectomies may even be necessary concurrently with the MCP joint capsulectomies. In such cases, the ring and small fingers tend to be the greater challenge in maintaining the MCP joint flexion, and yet functionally they are the most critical.

The goal need not be to achieve a complete arc of motion from 0 to 90 degrees. The goal may be to simply make the arc of motion more functional for the patient. Crush injuries are a good example of this point. In these cases, there may be a certain degree of destruction to the articular surface of the MCP joint, and it may be unrealistic to anticipate restoring full motion. What can be accomplished, however, is for the arc of motion to be altered in increased flexion and thus be of greater functional value to the patient.

Functional ROM

It is helpful to remember what is considered functional ROM for the joints of the hand. Functional flexion averages 61 degrees at the MCP joint level, 60 degrees at the PIP joint level, and 39 degrees at the DIP joint level.[46] In the thumb, functional flexion is 21 degrees at the MCP joint level and 18 degrees at the IP joint level. These arcs of motion are based on common ADL. Although they do not specifically address individual vocational and avocational pursuits, they do provide a basic guideline for functional performance measures of the hand. One should assess the individual and special needs of each patient in considering the surgery, and in cases in which the surgery is performed, the goal must be to strive for the highest functional performance levels.

Case Report

A 63-year-old man presented to the office 3 months after his initial surgery and rehabilitation for a crush injury, which included a fourth metacarpal fracture. There were significant limitations in ROM restricting the patient in daily activities and avocational interests. In particular, he had the most difficulty carrying objects in his hand and was unable to play golf because he could not grip the club. Preoperative active and (passive) ROM revealed the following (in degrees) in the MCP joints: 0/45 (55) in the index finger, 15/50 (60) in the long finger, 20/35 (45) in the ring finger, and 10/30 (40) in the small finger.

Surgery consisted of extensor tenolyses and dorsal MCP joint capsulectomies of the index through small fingers. A bulky compressive dressing was placed postoperatively, and the patient was referred to therapy the following day.

Once the bulky dressing was removed, an initial evaluation was performed, consisting of ROM measurements, wound and pain assessment, edema measurements, and obtaining his medical history. Based on the physician's orders, surgery performed, and initial evaluation, the following treatment program was established:

- Edema control for the forearm and hand with a light compressive dressing and digit-level edema control with finger socks
- Active and passive ROM exercises emphasizing isolated MCP joint motion; composite passive flexion and extension; isolated tendon excursion of the EDC, EIP, and EDQ; and intrinsic stretches
- Dynamic flexion orthosis for the MCP joints to be worn four times daily for 45 minutes (Fig. 68-16D)
- Safe-position forearm-based orthosis positioning the MCP joints in maximum flexion to be worn between exercise sessions and dynamic orthosis wear

On the third postoperative day, the patient presented with significant edema, notably on the dorsum of the hand (see Fig. 68-16A). A hematoma was present and manually expressed using sterile technique (see Fig. 68-16B, C). Draining of hematomas is critical to minimizing the risk of infection and excessive scar formation.

By the third postoperative week, the patient's wound had healed uneventfully. There were dense adhesions along the dorsum of the hand. Scar mobilization techniques, including

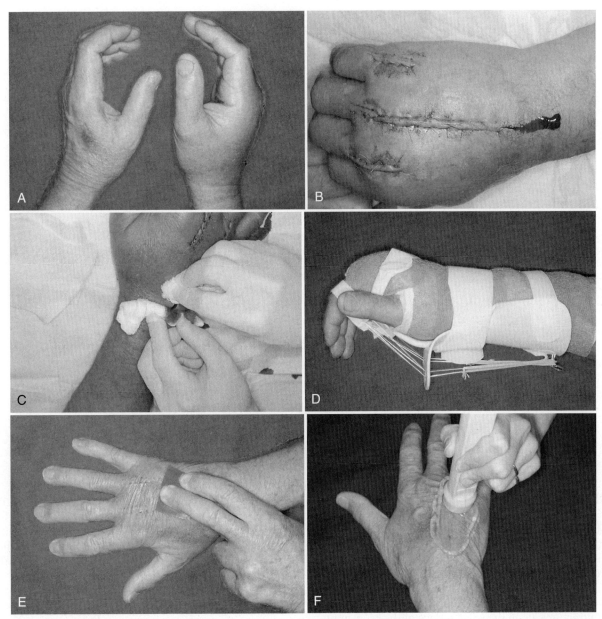

Figure 68-16 *Case example. A 63-year-old man underwent dorsal metacarpophalangeal (MCP) joint capsulectomies and extensor tenolyses of the index through small fingers.* **A**, *On the first postoperative day, moderate edema was noted and typical for the extent of surgery.* **B**, *A hematoma was present on the dorsum of the hand on the third postoperative day.* **C**, *The hematoma was manually expressed using a sterile technique.* **D**, *Wrist immobilization orthosis with dynamic MCP joint flexion was added to the therapy program within the first week to enhance passive flexion of the MCP joints.* **E**, *Dycem was used to assist with scar mobilization in the area where the skin was densely adherent to the underlying scar tissue.* **F**, *Ultrasound was used as a deep heat to enhance the elasticity of the adhesions and secondarily increase motion with the hand in extension as well as in flexion.*

scar massage with lotion, scar retraction using Dycem to mobilize the skin opposite the direction of the tendon gliding (see Fig. 68-16E), and ultrasound for deep heat to enhance the elasticity of the underlying soft tissue structures (see Fig. 68-16F), were added to the therapy program.

Interval therapy visits continued for 10 weeks. The patient had a successful final outcome (see Fig. 68-16G–I). He was able to use his hand successfully in functional activities, including golf. A reassessment at 5 months revealed the following active and (passive) ROM (in degrees) of the MCP joints: 0/75 (75) in the index finger, 30/80 (85) in the long

finger, 20/80 (85) in the ring finger, and 15/80 (80) in the small finger.

With elective surgeries such as this, it is important to keep in mind the functional goals that the patient desires from surgery. Therapy should focus on continually upgrading and modifying the treatment program to meet these objectives.

Equally important, the orthosis used during the course of therapy to maximize and maintain MCP joint flexion must be *gradually* eliminated over a span of time (30–45 days), or the patient may lose key motion achieved in therapy.

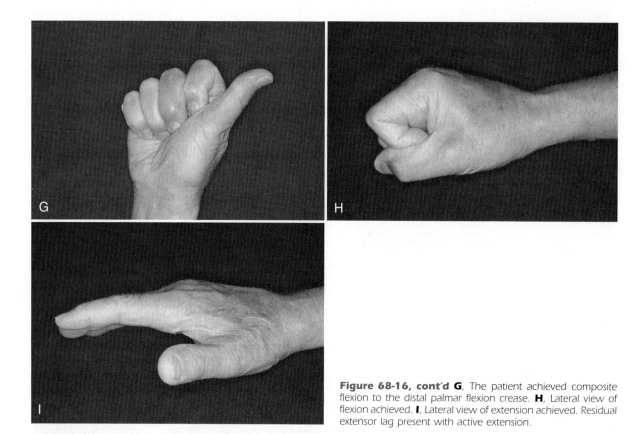

Figure 68-16, cont'd G, The patient achieved composite flexion to the distal palmar flexion crease. **H**, Lateral view of flexion achieved. **I**, Lateral view of extension achieved. Residual extensor lag present with active extension.

Volar MCP Joint Capsulectomy

Volar MCP joint capsulectomies are performed far less frequently. Some of the more common diagnoses or conditions requiring volar capsulectomy are longstanding intrinsic contractures with secondary contracture of the volar plate, burns, Volkmann's contracture, Dupuytren's contracture, crush injuries, spasticity, prolonged immobilization, soft tissue contractures along the volar surface of the MCP joints, and burst injuries to the palm.[36,47,48] Descriptions of the surgical approach to MCP joint volar capsulectomies have been reported in the literature.[4,15,41]

In most cases, postoperative therapy may be initiated within 24 hours after surgery. Edema and pain control measures, as previously described, may be used throughout the course of therapy. The orthotic position of choice will be in extension. For night wear, an orthosis positioning the MCP and IP joints in full extension is recommended. During the day, between exercise sessions, a dynamic extension orthosis positioning the MCP joints in extension should prove effective. Exercises should consist of unrestricted active and passive ROM, including emphasis on intrinsic stretches both actively and passively. The intrinsic stretches are particularly critical because intrinsic releases are generally needed along with the volar capsule release. Within 4 to 6 weeks, the extension orthosis may gradually be eliminated, with the goal of completely discontinuing the extension orthoses by 10 to 12 weeks after surgery.

The overall prognosis is good for restoring MCP joint extension without risking loss of MCP joint flexion. The greatest difficulty is in patients with longstanding, chronic intrinsic contracture and poor soft tissue on the volar surface that may require grafting and delayed therapy intervention.

Summary: MCP Joint Capsulectomy

Excellent ROM at the MCP joint level affords patients enhanced functional use of the hand. By carefully assessing the patient's preoperative status, one can determine the added functional value that surgery offers the patient. After a decision is made to perform the procedure, the motivated patient most likely will have an outcome that meets his or her functional needs. This assumes that the postoperative treatment plan is carefully orchestrated and monitored by the physician and therapist in conjunction with the patient.

PIP Joint Capsulectomy

Injuries to the PIP joint are quite common in the hand. In most instances, after medical management and the intervention of therapy, the patient has restored ROM and function of the hand. In the instances in which there is a residual passive limitation in PIP joint ROM, consideration may be given to performing a capsulectomy.

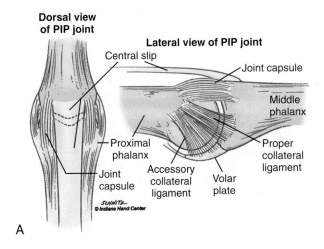

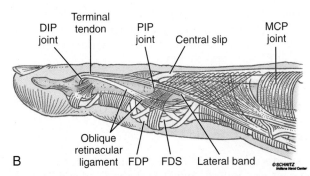

Figure 68-17 A, Illustration depicting anatomic structures surrounding proximal interphalangeal (PIP) joint of the digit. **B**, Lateral view of the anatomic structures at the PIP joint level and along the proximal and middle phalanx. DIP, distal interphalangeal; FDP, flexor digitorum profundus; FDS, flexor digitorum superficialis; MCP, metacarpophalangeal.

Diagnoses that are more vulnerable to residual joint stiffness requiring a secondary procedure include proximal and middle phalanx fractures (particularly intra-articular fractures), fracture dislocations of the PIP joint, avulsion of the central slip, zone II flexor tendon injuries with lacerations into the volar plate, Dupuytren's disease with involvement of the PIP joint, longstanding ulnar nerve palsy or combined ulnar and median nerve palsy, and skin contractures secondary to burns or soft tissue injuries.

Capsulectomies at the PIP joint level are performed both dorsally and volarly. A dorsal capsulectomy is performed to achieve increased passive flexion with a volar capsulectomy to increase passive extension. The goal of each procedure is to considerably improve function of the hand.

PIP Joint Anatomy

It is important to understand the anatomy of the PIP joint and corresponding structures. The illustration depicts the anatomic structures intimate to the PIP joint (Fig. 68-17). The extensor mechanism, dorsal capsule, collateral ligaments, volar plate, flexor digitorum superficialis, and flexor digitorum profundus are all clearly illustrated. It is critical to

recognize the relationship of these anatomic structures when considering the rehabilitation program.

Dorsal PIP Joint Capsulectomy

Surgery

Numerous articles have been written on dorsal PIP joint capsulectomies.[5,8,9,28,35,48,49] The reader is referred to Chapter 66 for a complete description of the surgical management for PIP joint contractures. The following summarizes one surgical approach as described by Idler.[8,9]

To perform a dorsal PIP joint capsulectomy, an incision is made over the dorsal aspect of the PIP joint. Dissection is made through the skin and subcutaneous tissue to the extensor mechanism. Once visualized, the transverse retinacular fibers are released along the volar margin of the lateral bands both radially and laterally. The lateral bands are elevated to visualize the joint capsule. The joint capsule is incised along the distal portion of the dorsal head of the proximal phalanx. If necessary, the joint capsule is excised. If this procedure does not achieve satisfactory passive flexion of the PIP joint, the collateral ligaments are gradually released dorsally to palmarly off the proximal phalanx. In addition, the extensor mechanism may require tenolysis to achieve full passive flexion without "rebound." It is not uncommon to perform a tenolysis in conjunction with the capsulectomy (Fig. 68-18).

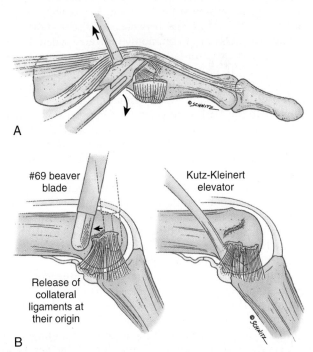

Figure 68-18 A, Surgical approach for performing a dorsal proximal interphalangeal joint capsulectomy. With the extensor mechanism elevated, the blade is inserted into the joint space, releasing the dorsal capsule from its attachments to the head of the proximal phalanx. **B**, The collateral ligaments are released from its attachment to the head of the proximal phalanx. Two instruments are illustrated.

Therapy

Therapy commences 24 to 36 hours after surgery. The bulky compressive dressing is replaced with a light compressive dressing to the hand and forearm, along with a digital dressing. The digital dressing often consists of sterile 1-inch gauze and 1-inch Coban or finger socks. It is important to apply a dressing that does not restrict ROM.

The initial exercises consist of active, active-assisted, and passive ROM to the entire hand for 10 to 15 minutes every 2 hours. Beyond composite flexion and extension, the patient is instructed to exercise with the MCP joints passively positioned in approximately 60 to 75 degrees of flexion while actively extending the PIP joints into maximum extension. It is emphasized to be equally forceful with active extension as with flexion. There should be a balanced effort with both arcs of motion. With the extensors having appreciably less power than the flexors, it is important to emphasize equal active effort in both directions.

When an extensor tenolysis is performed in conjunction with the dorsal capsulectomy, *isolated* passive flexion of the PIP joint is emphasized as opposed to *composite* passive flexion initially to minimize or avoid increasing the preoperative limitation in active extension. Within 7 to 10 days, composite passive flexion is added. For extension, an ideal outcome is maintaining active extension within 5 degrees of the preoperative active extension.[6]

An extension orthosis is custom fabricated and fitted to wear between exercise sessions and at night. Typically, this is a hand-based orthosis crossing the MCP joint and extending to the distal phalanx. On occasion, a dynamic orthosis is fabricated with light tension on the rubber band to assist with achieving full extension at the PIP joint. The dynamic orthosis may be worn during and between exercise sessions. The dynamic orthosis is most commonly indicated when there is concern that an extensor lag may increase and become problematic at the PIP joint level.

Additional orthosis wear is often necessary to increase passive PIP joint flexion. Most commonly, a forearm-based orthosis with the MCP joint positioned in extension is fabricated. Dynamic traction is added to mobilize the PIP joint into flexion and, as necessary, the DIP joint. The orthosis is worn for intervals of time during the day. The frequency and duration for wearing the orthosis are based on the passive limitation and joint "end feel." Wearing the dynamic orthosis three to four times daily for 30 to 45 minutes is a common starting point for the orthosis. An alternative wearing schedule would include wearing the dynamic orthosis for 10 to 15 minutes before each exercise session to enhance passive mobility before commencing specific exercises.

Within the initial 6 weeks after surgery, the goal is to begin weaning the patient out of the orthosis. To discontinue all orthosis use by 10 to 12 weeks is the goal in therapy.

Figure 68-19 reviews the case report of a patient who was hit by a bus and incurred multiple injuries, including a soft tissue crush degloving injury to the dorsum of her hand. Initially managed elsewhere, she presented 5 months post-injury. Significant joint stiffness with arthrofibrosis of the PIP joints had developed. At 6 months post-injury, she underwent extensor tenolyses, dorsal PIP joint capsulectomies, and

ulnar intrinsic releases of the index, long, ring, and small fingers.

Results

Clinically, dorsal PIP joint capsulectomies, with or without extensor tenolysis, are quite effective for enhancing functional use of the hand and restoring ROM. Reports in the literature reflect favorable results with the procedure as well.[26,50,51] Mansat and Delprat[52] reported their findings after dorsal PIP joint capsulectomies. The average ROM gain with flexion was 28 degrees. Preoperatively, the average extension was 19 degrees, with the flexion at 34 degrees. Postoperatively, the extension was 8 degrees and flexion 62 degrees. The motion improved to a more functional arc of motion. Gould and Nicholson[25] reported their outcomes after dorsal capsulectomies at the PIP joint. In 47 digits, they had a 21-degree gain passively and 14-degree gain actively. Creighton and Steichen[6] reported an average improvement of 34 degrees in flexion 6 months after extensor tenolysis and dorsal PIP joint capsulectomy.

Volar PIP Joint Capsulectomy

Surgery

As described by Idler,[8,9] either Brunner's incision or a midlateral incision is used along the proximal and middle phalanx of the digit to perform a volar PIP joint capsulectomy. Dissection is carried down through the subcutaneous tissue to the flexor sheath. A portion of the flexor sheath is excised along the area of the PIP joint. As needed at this point, a flexor tenolysis of the flexor digitorum superficialis and profundus may be performed, if necessary. This is followed with dividing the check-rein ligament. If the PIP joint does not passively extend after this procedure, the volar plate is released from the accessory collateral ligaments. Should passive PIP joint extension remain limited, the collateral ligaments are gradually released along the lateral aspect of the proximal phalanx (Fig. 68-20).

A number of other surgeons have described in the literature their surgical approach to volar PIP joint capsulectomies.[5,27,28,52-54]

Therapy

Therapy commences within 24 to 36 hours after surgery. The bulky compressive dressing is removed. A light compressive dressing along the forearm and hand is applied to moderate the postsurgical edema. A digital-level dressing is applied consisting of sterile gauze and either 1-inch Coban or finger socks. Emphasis is placed on edema control and pain management in the initial days after surgery. Effective control of pain and edema can rather predictably ensure a successful outcome of this procedure when the patient actively follows the custom-designed rehabilitation program.

Exercises are initiated that consist of active, active-assisted, and passive ROM to the digits and wrist every 2 hours for

Text Continues on p. 937.

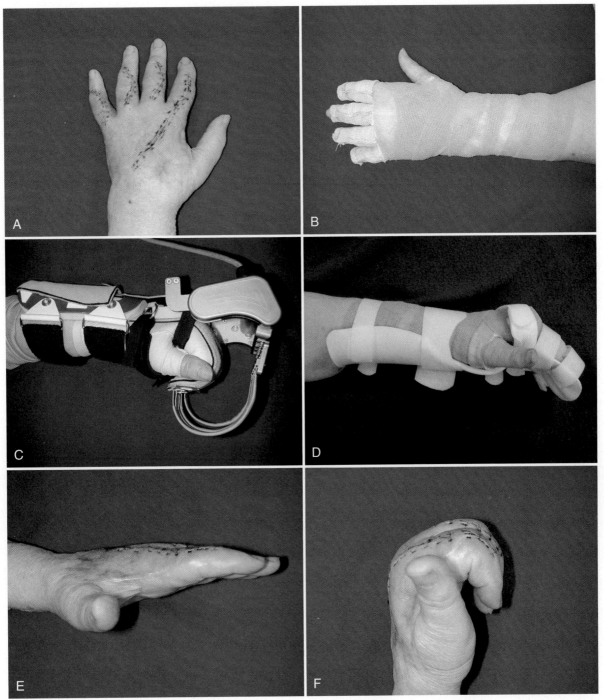

Figure 68-19 Case example. A 75-year-old woman with a workers' compensation injury of a nondominant hand crushed by a bus with a resultant degloving injury to the dorsum of her hand. She developed secondary joint stiffness and arthrofibrosis, particularly at the proximal interphalangeal (PIP) joint level and reported limited functional ability to securely grasp objects due to limited flexion. **A**, Surgery 6 months post-injury; extensor tenolyses, dorsal PIP joint capsulectomies, and ulnar intrinsic releases index–small fingers. **B**, Light compressive dressing to the forearm and hand for the initial 10 days postoperatively; sterile digital dressing and finger socks for edema control. **C**, Postoperative continuous passive motion (CPM) between exercise sessions the initial week after surgery. **D**, Forearm-based, safe-position orthosis worn at night. **E** and **F**, Active digital extension and flexion 6 days postoperatively.

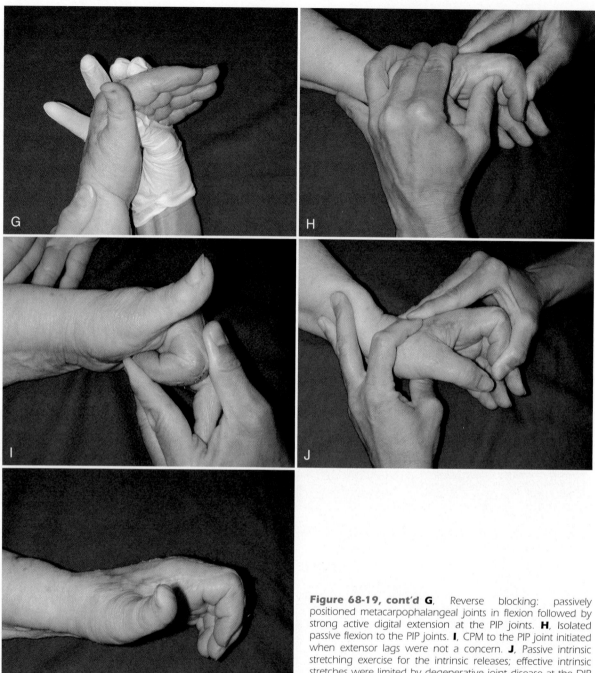

Figure 68-19, cont'd G, Reverse blocking: passively positioned metacarpophalangeal joints in flexion followed by strong active digital extension at the PIP joints. **H**, Isolated passive flexion to the PIP joints. **I**, CPM to the PIP joint initiated when extensor lags were not a concern. **J**, Passive intrinsic stretching exercise for the intrinsic releases; effective intrinsic stretches were limited by degenerative joint disease at the DIP joints. **K**, Patient attempts to perform active intrinsic exercises for the intrinsic releases.

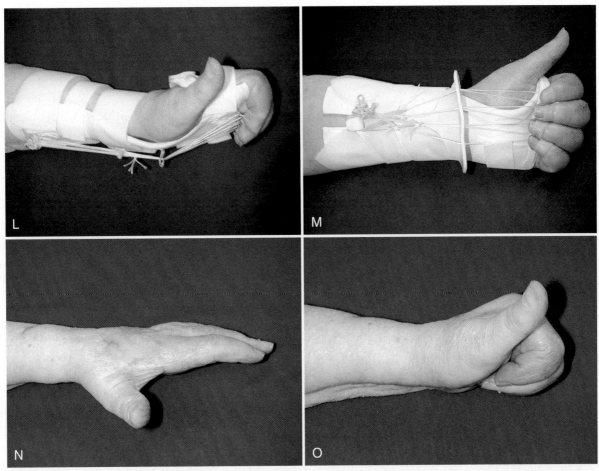

Figure 68-19, cont'd L and **M,** Dynamic interphalangeal flexion and composite dynamic flexion initiated once the CPM unit was discontinued at 1 week postoperatively. **N,** Active digital extension at 3 weeks postoperatively with an extension deficit in the index finger PIP joint. **O,** Active composite flexion at 3 weeks postoperatively remained slightly limited. Patient reported notable improvement with grasping hand-held objects at this early stage of her recovery.

10- to 15-minute sessions. Emphasis is placed on passive PIP joint extension to maximize the intended purpose of the surgery. With all exercises, it is emphasized to actively and passively hold the end range of motion a minimum of 5 seconds actively and 10 seconds passively. When a flexor tenolysis is performed in conjunction with the capsulectomy, which is common, it is equally important to emphasize active tendon-gliding exercises. Exercises include composite active flexion followed by full active extension, blocking exercises to the PIP and DIP joints for the superficialis and profundus (assuming the tendons are known to be of good quality), isolated flexor digitorum superficialis exercise, active IP joint flexion with the MCP joints extended followed by full digital extension and flexion, and composite wrist and digital flexion followed by wrist and digital extension. Exercises proximal to the wrist are encouraged at least once daily.

Wearing an orthosis between exercise sessions and at night for the initial 3 to 4 weeks after surgery is effective in minimizing the postsurgical edema, risk of wound separation, and pain. In addition, the orthosis is effective in positioning the digit(s) to maximize the intended benefit of the surgical procedure. A full extension orthosis is custom fabricated and fitted to the hand and digit(s). When multiple digits have undergone the procedure, and particularly when a tenolysis has been performed, a forearm-based orthosis that positions the digits in full extension is preferred.

Should it become apparent with ROM measurements that the PIP joint extension is not reaching the ROM achieved intraoperatively, a secondary orthosis with dynamic traction may be introduced. Initiating use of a dynamic orthosis by the third postoperative week is common. This is particularly true with releases of the small finger PIP joint and previous injuries with notable intra-articular involvement of the PIP joint. Based on the patient evaluation and the end-feel of passive extension, the therapist can determine the frequency and duration of orthosis wear. When a dynamic orthosis is indicated, wearing it between exercise sessions during the day and wearing the custom static orthosis at night are effective.

Modalities can play a role in the successful outcome after volar PIP joint capsulectomy, much like any secondary procedure in which ROM is initiated within a day or two after surgery and recovering motion fairly quickly is critical. Postoperative TENS may be helpful for pain management. NMES can be effective for enhancing active ROM. In addition, ultrasound is commonly included in therapy 2 to 3

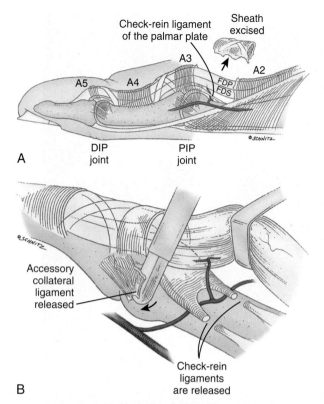

Figure 68-20 A, Illustration depicting the initial steps of a volar proximal interphalangeal (PIP) joint capsulectomy with limited resection of the flexor sheath between the A2 and A3 pulleys to expose the flexor tendons and underlying joint. **B**, The check-rein ligaments. Volar plates are released. If the PIP joint does not fully extend, the collateral ligaments are carefully released on both sides of the joint. DIP, distal interphalangeal; FDP, flexor digitorum profundus; FDS, flexor digitorum superficialis.

weeks after surgery. Patients will routinely report that the heating effect makes the soft tissues feel softer and the joints easier to move.

Results

Clinically, the more dramatic results occur when the preoperative flexion contractures are greater than 45 degrees. At this level, the digit has become a functional problem for the patient. Performing tasks with an outstretched hand are not possible, and performing simple tasks such as reaching into pants pockets may not be possible or awkward at best. Even if the joint release does not achieve full extension, if the residual joint contracture is 15 degrees or less, the patient's functional limitations are basically resolved.

The most challenging finger in which to regain full active and passive PIP joint extension is the small finger. This is particularly true when there has been a longstanding joint

contracture where the extensor mechanism has become relatively lengthened or redundant such that once the joint is released, full active extension of the PIP joint to neutral extension just cannot be achieved. Because of this, the joint cannot maintain the full extension that was achieved with surgery and the postoperative therapy.

Brüser and colleagues[53] reported their findings for volar PIP joint capsulectomy. In part, their results identified the variance in outcomes with mid-lateral and palmar incisions. Between the two approaches, the ROM gain after capsulectomy was 30 degrees in the palmar incision group and 50 degrees in the midlateral incision group.

Beyerman and colleagues[55] and Weinzweig and colleagues[56] reported their findings comparing capsulotomy and no capsulotomy with subtotal palmar fasciectomy for Dupuytren's disease. Beyerman and colleagues found that there were no statistical differences between the capsulotomy group and the noncapsulotomy group with respect to residual PIP joint contracture at the last follow-up visit. Weinzweig and colleagues reported similar findings. They showed no statistically significant difference in the percentage of contracture correction between groups.

Gould and Nicholson[25] reported on 41 patients with volar PIP joint capsulectomies. The average gain in active PIP joint extension was 13 degrees. The passive extension improved 24 degrees.

Mansat and Delprat[52] reported a multicenter study carried out at 10 hand services in France. For PIP joint flexion contractures, the mean improvement in extension at the PIP joint was 18 degrees.

Summary

Rehabilitation plays a vital role in the recovery from MCP joint and PIP joint capsulectomies. The key to a successful outcome is understanding the initial injury, the level of recovery from the initial injury, the pertinent medical history, the preoperative ROM, the patient's goals and functional expectations of the elective surgery, the surgical procedure itself, and the intraoperative ROM. This information provides the framework for establishing the optimal rehabilitation program. In addition, this information, along with how the patient progresses through the course of rehabilitation, allows the therapist to modify and upgrade the program effectively to maximize the patient's recovery. The goal is to provide a well-orchestrated rehabilitation program that is time limited and cost-effective and achieves the functional goals of the patient.

REFERENCES

The complete reference list is available online at www.expertconsult.com.

INDEX